UNIVERSITY OF SHEFFIELD
LIBRARY
WITHDRAWN FROM STOCK

Oxford Textbook of

Musculoskeletal Medicine

Free personal online access for 12 months

Individual purchasers of this book are also entitled to free personal access to the online edition for 12 months on *Oxford Medicine Online* (www.oxfordmedicine.com). Please refer to the access token card for instructions on token redemption and access.

Online ancillary materials, where available, are noted at the end of the respective chapters in this book. Additionally, *Oxford Medicine Online* allows you to print, save, cite, email, and share content; download high-resolution figures as Microsoft PowerPoint slides; save often-used books, chapters, or searches; annotate; and quickly jump to other chapters or related material on a mobile-optimised platform.

We encourage you to take advantage of these features. If you are interested in ongoing access after the 12-month gift period, please consider an individual subscription or consult with your librarian.

Oxford Textbook of Musculoskeletal Medicine

SECOND EDITION

Edited by

Michael Hutson

Specialist emeritus in Musculoskeletal Medicine,
Royal London Hospital for Integrated Medicine,
London, UK

and

Adam Ward

Consultant emeritus in Musculoskeletal Medicine,
Royal London Hospital for Integrated Medicine,
London, UK

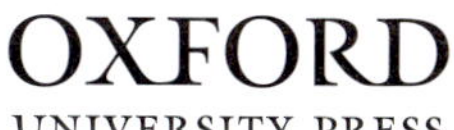

OXFORD
UNIVERSITY PRESS

Great Clarendon Street, Oxford, OX2 6DP,
United Kingdom

Oxford University Press is a department of the University of Oxford.
It furthers the University's objective of excellence in research, scholarship,
and education by publishing worldwide. Oxford is a registered trade mark of
Oxford University Press in the UK and in certain other countries

© Oxford University Press 2016

The moral rights of the authors have been asserted

First Edition published in 2005
Second Edition published in 2016

Impression: 1

All rights reserved. No part of this publication may be reproduced, stored in a retrieval system, or transmitted, in any form or by any means, without the prior permission in writing of Oxford University Press, or as expressly permitted by law, by licence or under terms agreed with the appropriate reprographics rights organization. Enquiries concerning reproduction outside the scope of the above should be sent to the Rights Department, Oxford University Press, at the address above

You must not circulate this work in any other form
and you must impose this same condition on any acquirer

Published in the United States of America by Oxford University Press
198 Madison Avenue, New York, NY 10016, United States of America

British Library Cataloguing in Publication Data

Data available

Library of Congress Control Number: 2015934703

ISBN 978–0–19–967410–7

Printed and bound in the UK by Bell & Bain Ltd.

Oxford University Press makes no representation, express or implied, that the drug dosages in this book are correct. Readers must therefore always check the product information and clinical procedures with the most up-to-date published product information and data sheets provided by the manufacturers and the most recent codes of conduct and safety regulations. The authors and the publishers do not accept responsibility or legal liability for any errors in the text or for the misuse or misapplication of material in this work. Except where otherwise stated, drug dosages and recommendations are for the non-pregnant adult who is not breast-feeding

Links to third party websites are provided by Oxford in good faith and for information only. Oxford disclaims any responsibility for the materials contained in any third party website referenced in this work.

UNIVERSITY
OF SHEFFIELD
LIBRARY

Foreword to second edition

What is your first approach when it comes to musculoskeletal conditions? Is a back strain almost always attributable to one or two dysfunctional lumbar spine segments, and is an elbow pain almost certainly correctable by injection? Or is your attitude to the back sufferer that his or her life situation, family, or employer is likely to be a problem, and the elbow pain a sign that work or domestic duties need to be changed?

This attitude of yours will probably lead you to certain chapters in this book. Thus, those who favour the anatomical, structural approach will head straight for those chapters with masterly descriptions of presentations of regional disorders, be they the shoulder or ankle or others. Or your preference may lead you to those chapters which discuss biomechanical and occupational factors, or those which discuss the psychological and social background to so many of your patients' problems. There are many jewels to be found.

The true benefit of this book will come to you, I suspect, when you finally turn to what you thought of as 'the other chapters'. Many advances have arrived in recent years, since this book's first edition, both in the understanding and best management of physical disorders, anatomical injuries, and dysfunctions—and also in the understanding of the interplay of our body's function with our life's activities, occupations, and preoccupations.

Your reading will reassure you that musculoskeletal medicine is a fascinating and rewarding specialism which amply repays study, research, and practice. This book will not always serve up easy answers, but it will entice you into thinking more deeply about what you are doing with your musculoskeletal cases. In this respect, you will see how very experienced authors admit openly that not everything is straightforward, and they show you their way of navigating the minefields—just look at Blomberg's map for the back, for example. I am glad too that, again and again, it comes through that while technical excellence is a help, it is the doctor or therapist who communicates well, who 'understands', and who takes trouble to be kind to his or her patient, who will get the best results.

Richard Ellis, London, 2015

Preface to second edition

For this second edition of the *Oxford Textbook of Musculoskeletal Medicine*, I have chosen to provide an accompanying preface, which I hope will be read as a logical sequence to the preface to the first edition. By that means, the reader will be aware of the more advanced position of musculoskeletal (MSK) medicine in 2015 compared to the situation in 2005.

At the time of writing this second preface, the general practitioner with a special interest (GPwSI) in MSK conditions has become well established in NHS service provision in the UK. The General Medical Council has engaged the Council of BIMM (British Institute of Musculoskeletal Medicine) in the development of a 'credentialling' process for practitioners with competence in MSK medicine. Additionally, discussions have led to a Master's degree and a faculty or a 'standing committee' in MSK medicine in order to provide an appropriate infrastructure to secure its future. Less encouragingly, my co-editor, Adam Ward, to whom I am indebted with respect to this second edition, has not been replaced as a consultant at the Royal London Hospital for Integrated Medicine (formerly the Royal London Homeopathic Hospital) following his retirement, a situation seen by many as a considerable disappointment in the progression of MSK medicine to specialty status.

Although it could therefore be argued that *plus ca change plus c'est la meme chose* prevails, I am more than satisfied that the contents of this second textbook, nearly 10 years after the first, are ample demonstration of the considerable advance of the body of understanding and practice of MSK practice at the present time.

In 2015, the terms 'musculoskeletal medicine' and 'manual medicine' are in common usage internationally, supported medico-politically by the International Federation for Manual/Musculoskeletal Medicine (FIMM) and, with regard to the demonstration of and advancement of the scientific content of our discipline, by the International Academy of Manual/Musculoskeletal Medicine. Clinical evaluation of musculoskeletal disorders demands specific expertise that is developed by 'hands-on' experience. Accordingly, it is recognized that there is no substitute for continued honing of haptic evaluative and therapeutic skills by repeated practice. It is worth emphasizing that the detection of relatively subtle soft tissue signs, such as loss of joint play, oedema, myofascial disturbance, and abnormal muscular and neural tension, which requires patience and much practice, brings its own rewards.

The contributors to this book have understood that the editors have encouraged an eclectic approach to this second edition, which inevitably creates an overlap between authors' contributions and, not infrequently, a base for further debate. However, a common theme has been maintained throughout, as stated in my first preface—the absolute requirement for the predication of a clinical diagnosis based upon manual examining skills.

Michael Hutson, 2015

Preface to first edition

Multi-author textbooks take some years to come to fruition. Hopefully, the wait will have been worthwhile, both for those readers who have been aware of the impending completion of the text and for the authors themselves. When 'penning' this first paragraph of the draft preface, I wrote: 'Musculoskeletal medicine is a relatively new term, encompassing much if not all of orthopaedic medicine, manual medicine, and osteopathic medicine'. Several years on, in 2005, the terms 'musculoskeletal medicine' and 'neuromusculoskeletal medicine' are in common usage. Service provision is well advanced in the UK for instance, where a new category of intermediate care provider has been established at the initiative of the Department of Health and the Royal College of General Practitioners—the general practitioner with a special interest (GPwSI) in musculoskeletal conditions. The International Federation for Manual/Musculoskeletal Medicine (FIMM) incorporated 'musculoskeletal medicine' into its title in 1995, and numerous national societies do the same: the British Institute of Musculoskeletal Medicine (BIMM) was established in 1991 when the British Association of Manipulative Medicine (BAMM) merged with the Institute of Orthopaedic Medicine (IOM).

(Neuro)musculoskeletal medicine comprises the theoretical basis, diagnosis, and treatment of disorders of the musculoskeletal system, incorporating manual diagnostics, a variety of therapeutic techniques such as manipulation and injections, and preventive and rehabilitative procedures. The intrinsic components of disorders of the musculoskeletal system are twofold: structural (pathomorphological) and functional (pathophysiological). Within the text, a comprehensive account is provided of both structural and functional disorders of the spine and of the extremities.

Early pathomorphological changes reflect adaptive processes to biomechanical stresses. *Advanced structural pathology* such as intervertebral disc prolapse, meniscus derangements, and tendinopathies are the consequences of the failure of adaptation of the soft tissues to postural and dynamic stresses. They are described in some detail in the text. When appropriate, the relevant stressors, particularly but not exclusively biomechanical, are identified and discussed.

Pathophysiological (neuromuscular) disturbances are classified using the accepted international term 'somatic (or 'segmental' when applied to the spine) dysfunction'. The recognition, diagnosis, and management of these reversible dysfunctional states, manifesting clinically as reduced joint mobility, tight muscles, disturbances of the autonomic nervous system, and abnormal neurodynamics, differentiate the discipline of musculoskeletal medicine from rheumatology. The non-surgical management of these disorders, both structural and functional, differentiates the discipline from orthopaedic surgery.

Clinical evaluation of musculoskeletal disorders demands specific expertise that is developed by 'hands-on' experience. Accordingly, it is recognized that there is no substitute for continued honing of these evaluative skills by repeated practice. For those clinicians who are new to the discipline, welcome—interesting insights await those with a receptive mental attitude (Mooney 1995).

Inexperienced physicians may experience initial difficulty accepting dysfunction as a 'disease' model. It does not have 'hard' physical signs, such as those associated with gross trauma seen in orthopaedic surgical practice, as a predominant feature (Gargan 1995). However, the detection of relatively subtle soft tissue signs, such as loss of joint play, (troph)oedema, myofascial disturbance, and abnormal neural tension, which requires patience and much practice, brings its own rewards.

The contributors to this book have international reputations in musculoskeletal medicine, particularly in those topics with which they are identified in the text. Inevitably, there is some overlap between the individual contributions, but a common theme has been maintained throughout—the absolute requirement for the predication of a clinical diagnosis based upon manual examining skills.

The concept of 'syndromes' is eschewed, although some would argue that many diagnoses, especially spinal dysfunction, are inherently syndromic. Whenever possible, the specific soft tissues associated with the dysfunctional process, their anatomical location, and aetiological factors are identified. The interaction between a decompensated musculoskeletal system and the human environment is explored with particular reference to behavioural responses to chronic pain.

A major development in recent years has been our increased knowledge of the mechanisms involved in the perception of pain, particularly pathological pain. The neurophysiological and neurodynamic abnormalities associated with (chronic) regional pain syndromes are correlated with their clinical expression in the text.

Management strategies are explored in considerable detail. The association between specific diagnoses and patients' responses to pain and dysfunction is developed. Inappropriate advice from inadequate training in musculoskeletal medicine (Hutson 1993) causes iatrogenic disease. Conversely, an active approach to management predicated upon expertise and experience, reaps its own rewards and reduces the likelihood of progression from acute musculoskeletal dysfunction to chronic pain, distress, and disability.

Although patient education is recognized as a priority, and given appropriate exposure in the text, a change in attitudes of doctors, particularly to back pain, is seen as essential (Ellis 1995). Emphasis is placed on keeping patients at work whenever possible. Specific therapeutic options, including spinal and peripheral joint manipulation and injection techniques, are described in detail, and their role identified in the wider strategem of resolution of dysfunction, pain relief, and rehabilitation.

Finally, the inclusion in the text of the best available documented research in this field provides the reader with an opportunity to integrate clinical expertise and scientific evidence, and thereby to pursue evidence-based musculoskeletal medicine as far as this is possible.

Michael Hutson, 2005

References

Ellis, R. M. (1995) Back pain. *British Medical Journal*, **310**, 1220.

Gargan, M. F. (1995) What is the evidence for an organic lesion in whiplash injury? *Journal of Psychosomatic Medicine*, **39**(6), 777–81.

Hutson, M. A. (1993) *Back pain: recognition and management*. Butterworth Heinemann, Oxford, p. vii.

Mooney, V. (1995) Prolotherapy in the spine and pelvis: an introduction. *Spine*, **9**(2), 309–11.

Contents

List of contributors

Fazal Ali
Chesterfield Royal Hospital
Chesterfield, UK

Tom Baster
Newnham Road Medical Centre
Queensland, Australia

Mark Batt
Queens Medical Centre
Nottingham University Hospitals
Nottingham, UK

Gurjit Bhogal
The Royal Orthopaedic Hospital
Birmingham, UK

Derek Bickerstaff
The One Health Group
Sheffield, UK

Heiner Biedermann
Surgeon, Private practice for Manual Medicine
Köln, Germany

Stefan Blomberg
Stockholm Clinic–Stay Active
Stockholm, Sweden

Grahame Brown
Institute of Occupational Health and School of Sport and Exercise Science
University of Birmingham
Birmingham, UK

Keith Bush
The London Clinic
London, UK

Anthony Campbell
Formerly Royal London Hospital for Integrated Medicine
London, UK

Angela E. Clough
Hull & East Yorkshire NHS Trust
UK

Peter J. Clough
Manchester Metropolitan University
Manchester, UK

Milton Cohen
St Vincent's Clinical School, UNSW Australia
Darlinghurst, New South Wales, Australia

Mark Comerford
Movement Performance Solutions
Chichester, West Sussex, UK

Thomas Crisp
BUPA Centre
London, UK

Thomas Dorman †
Formerly Internal Medicine
Paracelsus Clinic
WA, USA

Richard Ellis
Emeritus rheumatologist at University of Southampton and Salisbury District Hospital, UK

Hany Elmadbouh
The Fitzwilliam Hospital
Peterborough, UK

Raoul Engelbert
University of Amsterdam
Amsterdam, The Netherlands

Bryan English
Chief Medical Officer
Derby County Football Club
Derby, England

Thomas Findley
University of Medicine and Dentistry of New Jersey
Newark, New Jersey, USA

Jens Foell
Imperial College
London, UK

Lennard Funk
Bridgewater Hospital
Manchester, UK

Jo Gibson
Royal Liverpool and Broadgreen University Hospital Trust
Liverpool, UK

C. Chan Gunn
Division of Sports Medicine
University of British Columbia
Vancouver, B.C. Canada

Toby Hall
School of Physiotherapy and Exercise Science
Curtin University
The University of Western Australia
Australia

Richard Higgins
Claremont Private Hospital
Sheffield, UK

Michael Hutson
Specialist emeritus in Musculoskeletal Medicine
Royal London Hospital for Integrative Medicine
London, UK

Anju Jaggi
Shoulder and Elbow Service
Royal National Orthopaedic Hospital Trust
Middlesex, UK

Vladimir Janda †
Formerly Department of Rehabilitation Medicine
Charles University, Prague

Birgit Juul-Kristensen
Research Unit of Musculoskeletal Function and Physiotherapy
Institute of Sports Science and Clinical Biomechanics
University of Southern Denmark
Odense, Denmark

Jennifer Klaber Moffett (Retired)
Institute of Rehabilitation
University of Hull
Hull, UK

Martin T. N. Knight
The Spinal Foundation
Tenterden, Kent, UK

David Knott
Society of Orthopaedic Medicine
Orthopaedic Physician and Clinical Lead
Dorset Musculoskeletal Services
Dorset, England

Alena Kobesova
The Prague School of Rehabilitation
Department of Rehabilitation and Sports Medicine
2nd faculty of Medicine, Charles University
Prague, Czech Republic

Pavel Kolar
The Prague School of Rehabilitation
Department of Rehabilitation and Sports Medicine
2nd faculty of Medicine, Charles University
Prague, Czech Republic

Michael L. Kuchera
Marian University
Indianapolis, USA

Stephen M. Levin
Ezekiel Biomechanics Group
McLean, Virginia, USA.

Roderic MacDonald
London College of Osteopathic Medicine
London, UK

Chris J. Main
Keele University
Staffordshire, UK

Steve McNally
Manchester United Football Club
Manchester, UK

Puneet Monga
Wrightington Hospital
Wigan, UK

Nat Padhiar
London SportsCare, BMI The London Independent Hospital
Stepney Green, London, UK

Jacob Patijn
University Pain Centre Maastricht, UPCM
Department of Anesthesiology/Pain Management
Maastricht University Medical Centre
The Netherlands

Simon Petrides
Blackberry Orthopaedic Clinic
Milton Keynes, UK

Nicholas Peirce
Queens Medical Centre
Nottingham University Hospitals
Nottingham, UK

John Quintner
Wyllie Arthritis Centre
Western Australia

David Rabago
University of Wisconsin
Department of Medicine
Madison, Wisconsin, USA

Lars Remvig
Department of Rheumatology
University Hospital of Copenhagen
Copenhagen, Denmark

Margherita Ricci
Isokinetic Medical Group
FIFA Medical Centre of Excellence
Bologna, Italy

Diego Rizzo
Isokinetic Medical Group
FIFA Medical Centre of Excellence
Bologna, Italy

Kim Robinson
School of Physiotherapy and Exercise Science,
Curtin University
The University of Western Australia
Australia

Sjef Rutte
University Pain Centre Maastricht, UPCM
Department of Anesthesiology/Pain Management
Maastricht University Medical Centre
Maastricht, The Netherlands

Marcela Safarova
The Prague School of Rehabilitation
Department of Rehabilitation and Sports Medicine
2nd faculty of Medicine, Charles University
Prague, Czech Republic

John Tanner
The Oving Clinic
Oving, West Sussex, UK

Stefano Della Villa
Isokinetic Medical Group
FIFA Medical Centre of Excellence
Bologna, Italy

Julia Walton
Wrightington Hospital
Wigan, UK

Michael Walton
Wrightington Hospital
Wigan, UK

Adam Ward
Consultant emeritus in Musculoskeletal Medicine
Royal London Hospital for Integrative Medicine
London, UK

Paul J. Watson
Department of Health Science
Leicester General Hospital
Leicester, UK

Nefyn Williams
Bangor University
Gwynedd, UK

Michael Yelland
Griffith University
Nathan, Queensland, Australia

PART 1

Introduction to musculoskeletal medicine

Chapter 1

Fundamentals of musculoskeletal medicine

Michael Hutson

Eclecticism: deriving ideas, tastes, style, etc. from various sources; not didactic in the sense of being tediously pedantic.

(The Concise Oxford Dictionary)

So is the word 'eclectic' defined. This (second) edition of the *Oxford Textbook of Musculoskeletal Medicine* is based on the same principles as the first. It is an eclectic mix of concepts, diagnostics, and treatment of musculoskeletal disorders, written by leading proponents of their specific interests within this medical specialty and associated specialties.

Concepts of musculoskeletal medicine

'There are more things in heaven and earth, Horatio,
Than are dreamt of in your philosophy.'

Hamlet

Readers with limited knowledge of the history of the development of the diverse 'schools' of manual medicine, the core components of which are manual diagnosis and treatment of neuromusculoskeletal disorders, may be somewhat confused by the plethora of terminology used to describe the medical discipline embraced by these schools and the conceptual variants themselves. This diversity is the beauty and perhaps the frustration of musculoskeletal medicine. It epitomizes its eclecticism and reflects its philosophical challenges.

The distinctiveness of musculoskeletal medicine is undoubted and perhaps unparalleled in the medical sciences. At its heart is the recognition and management of dysfunctional states of the neuromusculoskeletal system, now formally defined as *somatic dysfunction*. The historical background of the emergence of the underlying concepts of somatic dysfunction is provided by MacDonald in Chapter 2, and the characteristics of somatic dysfunction are further identified by Kuchera in Chapter 10. In this introductory chapter, I review the development and principles of musculoskeletal medicine; in Chapter 65, I review integrated medicine, with my co-editor Adam Ward.

I wish to address the characteristics of orthopaedic medicine, osteopathic medicine, manual medicine, and musculoskeletal medicine. By this means it will become apparent that there are a number of important conceptual models common to and underpinning these disciplines: structural (pathomorphological), pathophysiological ('functional'), biomechanical, and biopsychosocial.

Orthopaedic medicine

Orthopaedic medicine was founded upon the structural (anatomic or morphological) disturbances of the neuromusculoskeletal system as defined by James Cyriax. Orthopaedic medicine may be seen as the natural consequence of the application of the disease–illness model (which has provided the framework for most medical disciplines for several centuries) to orthopaedic derangements that come under the province of the physician. It is archetypically 'allopathic' (for those readers who wish to distinguish between allopathic and osteopathic medicine).

Cyriax (1969) envisaged derangements of the intervertebral disc as the primary spinal pathology to account for the vast majority of 'simple' back pain and nerve root pain. He described the capsular and non-capsular patterns of articular disturbances at peripheral joints, and devised selective tissue tension tests to differentiate between articular, ligamentous, contractile, and neural lesions. Based on reductionist principles, his views represented a seminal breakthrough in the evaluation of lesions of the soft tissues. Conceptually (in the 1940s), this was the first time since the work of Sir William Gowers, at the end of the nineteenth century, that allopathic medicine was able to throw off the mantle of soft tissue rheumatism and the somewhat nebulous conditions it embraced such as fibrositis.

Although distinct by definition (with respect to management of musculoskeletal problems) from orthopaedic surgery, a further breakthrough made by orthopaedic medicine was in nosology. Orthopaedic medicine became recognized as the application of a unique systematized clinical evaluation (including inspection, active movements, passive movements, resisted muscle contraction, and palpation) of the soft tissues of the locomotor system. Predicated primarily on pathomorphology (such as degenerative, histopathologic, inflammatory, neoplastic, or infective lesions) with a relatively simple view of loss of function (pain, weakness, loss of movement), terminology accorded to the disease–illness model of scientific modernism. Specific diagnoses such as tendinitis, bursitis, ligament sprains, and peripheral nerve entrapment replaced fibrositis and associated syndromes.

According to Cyriax, the principal challenges to osteopathy were the basic morphological concepts of annular disc tear, nuclear disc prolapse, and dural tension as the pathologies underlying the vast majority of spinal derangements. Although Cyriax soon discarded the theory of sacroiliac derangement (for which a mobilization technique was illustrated in his first textbook only), he allowed Barbor to describe the development of sclerotherapy (prolotherapy) for ligamentous disturbances of the spine, including sacroiliac ligamentous insufficiency, in the subsequent editions of his textbook. As will be seen later, the adoption by osteopathic physicians of the concept of fibroproliferative treatment techniques for ligamentous disturbances is an example of the increasingly 'broad church' attitudes adopted by both allopathic and osteopathic medicine and demonstrated with increasing maturity by musculoskeletal medicine over recent years.

Osteopathic medicine

Osteopathic medicine, founded on the work of Andrew Taylor Still who 'threw the banner (of osteopathy) to the breeze' in 1874, represented a seminal breakthrough in conceptual thinking. It provided a radical model for ill health and disease. Although revised and redefined, Still's basic concepts continue to underpin osteopathic principles and practice. Interestingly, there has been a resurgence of interest at Kirksville Osteopathic Medical School, Missouri, USA, (founded by Still) in his original manual techniques. Stated simplistically, the rationale was that health and ill health are related to spinal function and dysfunction. However, somatic dysfunction should never be considered in isolation. Viscerosomatic reflex patterns are the very essence of osteopathic medicine.

Originally described as the 'osteopathic lesion', somatic dysfunction is now the accepted international term for the dysfunctional lesion. It is more formally defined by the Clinical Guideline subcommittee on Low Back Pain (American Osteopathic Association, 2010) as 'impaired or altered function of related components of the somatic (body framework) system: skeletal, arthrodial, and myofascial structures, and related vascular, lymphatic, and neural elements'.

Somatic dysfunction is essentially a pathophysiological phenomenon. Anatomic derangements should always be considered as contributory factors, as should adverse posture and abnormal biomechanics. Of interest is that, at the height of James Cyriax's influence in the UK in the middle and later decades of the twentieth century, there could not be two more diametrically opposed schools than osteopathic manipulative (sometimes referred to as neuromusculoskeletal) training (the branch of osteopathic medicine that focuses particularly on neuromuscular problems) on the one hand and the structuralism of orthopaedic medicine on the other. However, during and since the last two decades of the twentieth century, there has been a gradual convergence of these schools; for instance, the acceptance by allopathic medicine of dysfunctional neuromusculoskeletal states characterized by somatic dysfunction, and the incorporation of prolotherapy into advanced osteopathic training.

Manual medicine

In Europe, manual medicine was substantively influenced by osteopathic medicine. Chiropractic also played a role (Neumann 1989). An emphasis on articular dysfunction, using 'blockage' as old terminology, is a distinguishing characteristic. In this regard, there is much in common with the theories and practice advanced by John Mennell (Zohn and Mennell 1976) who, having trained in London, based his work (in the USA) on the concepts of his father (James Mennell) and the elder (Edgar) Cyriax. However, muscle hypertonus/contraction and the associated features of somatic dysfunction are consistent features in European manual medicine. The Czech school of manual medicine, led by Karel Lewit and Vladimir Janda, places a particular emphasis on muscle dysfunction. Contributions by Vladimir Janda and Alena Kobesova are included in this book (Chapters 8, 12, and 61).

In general terms, 'manual medicine' has come to be regarded as the relatively pure core model of manual diagnostics and manual therapeutics. To practitioners of manual medicine in some European countries, 'musculoskeletal medicine' is a somewhat wider subject, incorporating other management strategies such as injections.

Musculoskeletal medicine

Musculoskeletal medicine has emerged from a background of orthopaedic medicine (as previously described, developed by James Cyriax at St Thomas' Hospital, London), manual medicine, and osteopathic manipulative medicine. Musculoskeletal medicine may easily be distinguished from allied specialties such as rheumatology and orthopaedic surgery. The distinctive and underlying concepts of musculoskeletal medicine are:

- the scientific basis of function of the neuromusculoskeletal system;
- the pathophysiological and structural basis of dysfunction of the neuromusculoskeletal system.

With respect to management strategies, there is an overlap with other disciplines such as pain management and rehabilitation. There is a close working relationship with allied non-medical professions, particularly physiotherapy. Knowledge of functional anatomy, ergonomics, biomechanics, podiatry, exercise physiology, and general medicine is essential. Clinical application of this knowledge is reflected in distinctive manual diagnostic techniques. Management skills include spinal mobilization and manipulation (both allopathic and osteopathic), injections, and a wide range of other manual techniques. Complementary, mind–body, and holistic approaches to health are particularly relevant to chronic musculoskeletal disorders and are nowadays often described as 'integrated medicine' (see Hutson and Ward, Chapter 65).

In short, musculoskeletal medicine has accepted the concept of neuromusculoskeletal dysfunction, as developed by osteopathic medicine and manual medicine, but retains many of the allopathic characteristics of orthopaedic medicine. It has an established evidence base (upon which this textbook has been constructed), yet it retains the art and compassion of the healthcare professional who is well versed in the biopsychosocial as well as the biomechanical, pathophysiological, and pathomorphological models of care.

It incorporates holism and eclecticism and is an archetypal post-modern medical discipline.

Biosocial model of Engel (and other healthcare constructs)

George Engel, Professor of Psychiatry and Medicine at University of Rochester School of Medicine, Rochester, New York, threw down a challenge by identifying the need for a new medical model. In a seminal article (Engel 1977), he stated that the adherence to a model of disease was no longer adequate for the scientific tasks and social responsibilities of either medicine or psychiatry. The existing biomedical model, with molecular biology as its basic scientific discipline, embraced reductionism and mind–body dualism. It developed as medicine became 'scientific', particularly as taxonomy and other analytical scientific methods were applied to disease and suffering.

Engel proposed a biosocial model that 'takes account of the patient', the social context in which he lives, and the complementary system devised by society to deal with the disruptive effects of illness—that is, the physician role and the healthcare system. Clearly, it embraces psychosocial factors, including the status of the patient and the sick role, and addresses the apparent paradox that illness and wellness may not be related closely to 'positive' laboratory findings. It explains the variations of response by patients to health issues—from 'illness' or 'injury' to 'problems of living'. Not only has this model stood the test of time over recent decades, it is even more important now in an era of technological development and (often) dependency, in which there appears to be increasing reliance by clinicians generally, and particularly those who do not have the benefit of musculoskeletal medical training, on imaging for both diagnosis and invasive (usually injection) techniques.

Henrik Wulff developed a somewhat different view when he described the two cultures of medicine: objective facts versus subjectivity and values (1999). In clinical practice, there are scientific components (reasoning from theoretical knowledge, and reasoning from past experience—evidence-based medicine, for instance) and humanistic components based on wisdom and personal interpretation of findings from patient psychology and ethical reasoning.

McDonald (1996) went further when he suggested that physicians often make clinical decisions based on insufficient evidence-based medicine from randomized trials or epidemiological studies, and by the use of rules of thumb (or 'medical heuristics'), derived from personal theories, assumptions, experience, traditions, and lore.

My own views are similar to those of Suarez-Almazor and Russell (1998) who wrote that 'the art of medicine' is not about applying anecdotal experiences to the solution of clinical problems; it is about critically appraising the evidence in front of us and linking it to our focus of interest, the individual patient.

The biopsychosocial model of Waddell is discussed in the section 'Models of care in neuromusculoskeletal medicine' in this chapter.

Distinctiveness of musculoskeletal medicine

Numerous references are made in this textbook to the distinctiveness of musculoskeletal medicine. This is associated with improved and more widespread understanding of neural plasticity and neuromusculoskeletal dysfunction, and the application of appropriate diagnostic manual techniques to problems that more often than not present as pain syndromes.

The clinician who acquires knowledge of neuromusculoskeletal dysfunction gains insight into conditions, such as whiplash and upper limb pain, that may manifest in diverse ways, defy the established disease–illness model, and present a substantive diagnostic challenge to the 'uninitiated'.

By way of illustration, some of those dysfunctional problems that commonly cause epistemological errors in conceptual thinking, diagnosis, and management, in the absence of insight into neural plasticity, are discussed here.

Whiplash

Traumatic injuries to the musculoskeletal system caused by vehicular collisions are universal, apparently becoming more prevalent (or at the very least more frequently complained of), and subjected to insurance claims. However, they are by no means a modern phenomenon. 'Railway spine' was just as much a suitable topic for the honing and application of polemical skills in the second half of the nineteenth century as whiplash and whiplash-associated disorders are today. In the nineteenth century, opinion was divided between those physicians who were aligned to neurobiological explanations for traumatic backache and associated symptoms and those who identified psychosomatic fundamentalism as more congruent with their own beliefs (Cohen and Quintner 1996). In many respects, the debate has not moved on to any substantive degree other than for the increasing recognition of the neurophysiological basis for many symptoms that were previously unexplained. Even so, 'spinal concussion' was not too far off the mark as an expression of a disturbed spinal cord when contrasted with the modern views regarding neuronal activity in the dorsal horns.

A recognition of the concept and features of somatic dysfunction facilitates an understanding of the myriad complaints in whiplash-associated disorders ranging from dizziness, visual disturbances, and headaches; pain and dysaesthesiae in the upper limbs; discomfort in the lower back, sacroiliac regions, and buttocks—to name but a few. Temporomandibular joint dysfunction (jawlash) occurs in a significant subgroup of patients. The symptoms of vertigo, dizziness, visual disturbances, etc. are sometimes grouped together as the Barré–Lieou syndrome (Barré 1926). Proximal thoracic spinal dysfunctions are common, as are sacroiliac disturbances.

The Lithuanian experience of the low incidence of symptomatic whiplash, one year after the index event (Schrader et al. 1996), is not surprising given the intrinsic modulating effect on pain pathways of the descending cerebrospinal tracts operating outside a medicolegal context. By contrast, it is hypothesized that the inhibitory function of these tracts is often compromised by perpetuating factors that are associated with the 'advanced' culture of the Western world.

The lack of 'hard physical signs' (Gargan 1995) inhibits most orthopaedic surgeons from making a meaningful evaluation within a biopsychosocial model of 'injury' in those who continue to complain one year after the index event. Over-reliance on delta forces and other mechanistic concepts associated with the application of the laws of physics to the cervical spine (in particular) in whiplash leads to the denial of the possibility of soft tissue whiplash strains in low-velocity collisions. (I reject this argument on the basis of biological implausibility.) Without appropriate manual diagnostics, the absence of identifiable 'organic' pathology invites a suspicion (in the clinician's mind) of wilful exaggeration by the patient or frank malingering, thereby contributing (should the scepticism of the examiner be obvious to the patient), in some, to distress, chronicity of symptoms, and disability.

Upper limb pain

The concept of neuropathic arm pain is explored by Hutson in Chapter 33. Regional pain syndromes are relatively incomprehensible without an understanding of neural function, soft tissue dysfunction, and spinal dysfunction. The application of neurodynamics to a functional assessment of the neck, upper back, and upper limb is a fruitful exercise without which diagnoses are presumptive and based on exclusion. The medical profession is indebted to the work of Australian physiotherapists such as David Butler (see Chapters 15 and 56 by Hall and Robinson) who have improved our understanding of the application of basic anatomy and physiology to neuronal circuitry between the neck and the hand. Musculoskeletal physicians should at the very least become acquainted with and hopefully skilled at evaluative diagnostic manual tests for soft tissue and neural dysfunction.

Although 'adverse neural tension' has become somewhat dated as medical shorthand and medical jargon (and replaced by AND—adverse neural dynamics—in deference to improving knowledge of neural plasticity), it should meanwhile become as familiar a concept for the expression of neural sensitivity or irritability as 'dural tension' in the lower limbs (as assessed by the straight leg raise and femoral stretch test).

Back pain

That appropriate diagnostic skills are prerequisites for meaningful and effective management strategies is a theme throughout this textbook. Nowhere is this more relevant than in the diagnosis and management of back pain, particularly lower back pain (LBP). Over the last decade, the term 'non-specific' back pain has (regrettably) become established in medical practice. In this condition, clinical examination undertaken by practitioners with limited or no specific musculoskeletal medicine training or understanding of dysfunction yields no abnormalities, a situation 'confirmed' by negative serology and/or imaging. Although 'non-specific' LBP (or its companion term 'mechanical back pain') appears fixed in the current medical lexicon, it ignores the possibility of a wealth of clinical signs diagnostic of dysfunction, which when treated, for instance by mobilization, manipulation, or other means of release of soft tissue tension, produces relief of pain (Lewit 2011).

A time-consuming but potentially rewarding part of my own clinical work is to disabuse many patients of misconceptions regarding the nature of their back pain and to reverse the effects of its past mismanagement, instilled by 'conventional wisdom' of the medical profession over recent decades. These misconceptions so often arise from the discussion of 'crumbling spine', 'worn out discs', and 'arthritis' arising from X-ray appearances, paying no heed to the clinical findings in a competent musculoskeletal examination. Old habits die hard. The inculcation of healthy attitudes, appropriate rehabilitation programmes, and early return to premorbid levels of daily activities is predicated on evaluation strategies that differentiate nociceptive and neuropathic pain, and recognize the role of red flags (for serious disease), yellow flags (for psychosocial factors with particular relevance to chronicity), and illness behaviour. Rehabilitation for musculoskeletal conditions is well served by a number of authors in this textbook.

Tender points

The concept of tender points and trigger points is explored throughout this textbook. Proponents of myofascial pain syndromes (MPS) as an important diagnostic group propose a primary dysfunctional state within the muscle as the explanation for tenderness, muscle hypertonus, the jump sign, and referred pain phenomena. The proposition of primary muscle dysfunction is contested by many clinicians, and the reader is referred to Quintner and Cohen (Chapter 14) for a comprehensive review of the MPS debate and a deconstruction of untenable hypotheses.

A hypothesis with which I personally am comfortable is that tender/trigger points are, for the most part, a manifestation of tension within the musculoskeletal system, possibly in the form of secondary hyperalgesia. As such, they reflect the process of neurosensitization, whether locally, regionally, or centrally.

Fibromyalgia, which is explored in considerable detail, particularly by Jens Foell (Chapter 13), may be considered to be an expression of a widespread pain syndrome in vulnerable individuals. Regional pain syndromes also abound; for instance, neuropathic arm pain (type II work-related upper limb disorder). At a more local level, neurosensitization may well be an expression of recent neural trauma but may also arise as a consequence of local dysfunction, infection, or inflammation.

Allodynia indicates a reduced threshold to potentially nociceptive stimuli; hyperalgesia indicates reduced tolerance of nociceptive stimuli; and hyperpathia indicates a prolonged nociceptive response to provocative stimuli.

Practitioners of musculoskeletal medicine will be familiar with the ubiquitous tenderness and muscle hypertonus in the proximal scapular fixator muscles, and also in the glutei, which are common accompaniments (or responses) to gravitational or postural cervicodorsal spinal stresses and lower back stresses respectively.

Red flags and yellow flags

The terms 'red flags' and 'yellow flags' refer to the relevant factors that emerge at interview or examination of a patient that act as 'markers' for serious spinal pathology (red flags) or psychosocial factors and coping mechanisms associated with chronicity (yellow flags). Red flags include onset of back pain in the elderly, thoracic spinal pain, a history of malignancy, general ill health, weight loss, etc. Psychosocial yellow flags include social deprivation, poor job satisfaction, incorrect beliefs, a history of inappropriate or ineffective coping strategies, abnormal behaviour, and fear/pain avoidance. 'Blue flags' and 'black flags' refer to the work environment, and may be viewed as subdivisions of the yellow flag psychosocial group. Blue flags are defined as an individual's perceptions about work conditions and their impact. Black flags refer to objectively established work conditions, contracts, sickness policy, entitlements, and legislation that impact on the employee.

Illness behaviour

Behavioural responses to illness and injury are manifold. Accordingly, it is not unusual for emotional responses to be manifest by patients during contact with others, including examining clinicians. As a consequence, it is somewhat arbitrary as to when behavioural reactions identified by the examiner at interview or on clinical examination are 'abnormal'. The more common findings of established illness behaviour are hesitancy on movement (particular in response to instructions during examination), pain gesturing and vocalization, dizziness, and other somewhat inappropriate reactions.

Abnormal illness behaviour (first described by Pilowsky in 1969) is 'an inappropriate or maladaptive mode of experiencing, perceiving, evaluating or responding to one's own state of health'. It is sometimes, mistakenly, assumed to have a conscious aspect. However, a more appropriate interpretation is that abnormal illness behaviour, with its accompanying concept 'the sick role', is the overt expression of distress, misattribution, and maladaptation, often reflecting poor or exhausted coping mechanisms.

Inappropriate signs

'Inappropriate' signs in assessment of low back pain were described by Waddell et al. in 1980, but have been open to abuse. Waddell was instrumental in distinguishing 'non-organic' or 'inappropriate' symptoms and signs of abnormal illness behaviour from the symptoms and signs of 'organic pathology' or 'physical impairment' (see Box 1.1). The signs in particular have been used extensively by orthopaedists.

Unfortunately, the detection of inappropriate features, particularly inappropriate clinical signs, sometimes leads to inappropriate interpretation of the underlying clinical problem. 'Non-organic' does not necessarily equate to deliberate exaggeration or fabrication of symptoms. It should mean what it sets out to state: that there is probably no significant or relevant abnormality of tissue morphology—which, in the context of the underlying concept of neuromusculoskeletal dysfunction in this textbook, should come as no great surprise in many disorders. Additionally, in the light of our present understanding of neurosensitization, the sensory signs, and possibly most of the other 'inappropriate' signs, are capable of interpretation as abnormal neural processing.

Disability

Disability is the adverse effect on activities of daily living, particularly work, caused by illness or injury. It has a large subjective component, which is difficult, if not impossible, for the examining clinician to forecast or quantify in an individual. Reliance on demonstrable pathology (for instance by radiography or magnetic resonance imaging—MRI) is epistemologically unsound because it ignores the behavioural responses to life's problems, illnesses, and injuries. A constant theme throughout this text is 'treat the patient, not the MRI'.

Disability should be contrasted with impairment of function. Loss of function may be relatively easy to quantify (for instance, the loss of movement at a peripheral joint in a compliant patient), and sometimes more difficult (such as the evaluation of loss of movement at the lumbar spine). Nevertheless, the range of passive movements represents an objective assessment made by the examiner. Naturally, impairment of function is often a major contributor to disability but it may not be the most important factor. As previously stated, psychosocial factors are often paramount in the development and chronicity of disability.

In addition to societal factors, the role of the medical profession is often contributory. It is a truism to state that patients sometimes recover despite the 'best' attentions of the medical profession. In patients with neck and back pain, iatrogenesis is often a major aetiological, perpetuating, or aggravating factor (see 'Evidence-based medicine' in this chapter). Disability is commonly the product of dysfunction, fear avoidance, distress, and iatrogenesis.

Iatrogenesis

The following factors are often relevant to the role of the medical profession:

- failure to understand somatic dysfunction
- failure to distinguish between neuropathic and nociceptive pain
- failure to recognize illness behaviour and psychosocial factors
- failure to differentiate impairment from disability
- inappropriate labelling, misattribution, and medical jargon
- catastrophizing (by the doctor)
- unjustified restriction of activity
- buck passing (for instance, delaying therapy by use of tests or secondary referral)
- readiness or willingness to provide sickness certification.

The non-medical professions are not exempt: the domination of spinal manipulation at the expense of the inculcation of positive self-help and self-stabilization strategies in some osteopathic and chiropractic regimes leads to patient dependency. (An example of the biopsychosocial model cast aside in favour of the biomedical model.) The lack of mobilizing or manipulating techniques in some physiotherapists' armamentarium is a contrasting deficiency.

In some countries, the ill-defined status of musculoskeletal medicine and the uncertain role of the musculoskeletal physician within the medical community are factors that affect the credibility of the examining doctor, and as a consequence, the effectiveness of his or her management strategy.

Box 1.1 Symptoms of 'inappropriate' illness behaviour

- Non-dermatomal numbness and pain
- Non-myotomal ('global') weakness in the leg
- Constant symptoms
- Refractoriness to and often intolerance of treatments

Signs relating to low back pain complaints

- Lumbar pain on axial loading
- Lumbar pain on simulated rotation
- Improvement of straight leg raise on distraction
- Regional sensory changes
- Superficial widespread non-anatomical tenderness
- Regional jerky resisted muscle contraction
- Over-reaction generally

Evidence-based medicine

Evidence-based medicine (EBM) has been defined by Sackett as the conscientious, explicit, and judicious use of the current best evidence in making decisions about the care of individual patients (Sackett 1998). Universally accepted as concordant with best and most cost-effective practice at the turn of the millennium, it is equally applicable to musculoskeletal medicine. By definition, EBM is reliant upon the best available evidence being brought to bear on a patient's problems. Physicians are expected to use diagnostic techniques that are both reliable and valid, and therapies that have proven efficacy. Sackett softened his approach to EBM by stating that inherent in its practice is integration of the best available external clinical evidence from systematic research with individual clinical expertise. In view of the acceptance within musculoskeletal medicine of tacit knowledge and acquired wisdom from experience (Aristotelian 'episteme') by practitioners, it is probably more appropriate to combine expertise, experience, and evidence into the concept of evidence-informed practice (EIP).

The use of mathematics in musculoskeletal medicine has been refined by Bogduk (1999). Interobserver reliability for diagnostic examining techniques is crucial if sense is to be made of dysfunctional neuromusculoskeletal conditions. Unlike other branches of medicine, there are few gold standards for dysfunctional states. Serological, radiological, neurophysiological, and histopathological investigations may be normal in somatic dysfunction. As a consequence, validation of diagnostic techniques is dependent upon agreement on the basic characteristics of dysfunction. Despite the difficulties, critical appraisal of the evidence for its validity and usefulness is possible (see Patijn, Chapter 3).

The development and testing of hypotheses, allowing them to stand unless proven false (Popper 1959), combined with clinical observations, has provided the empiric basis of advancement of knowledge in musculoskeletal medicine in the past (Dorman 1995). Knowledge is based on evidence, which in its broadest sense includes everything that is used to determine or demonstrate the truth of an assertion, and is also context-dependent. On a deeper philosophical basis, there are problems with truth, which is contemporary and different in different cultures (cultural relativism). To quote Dawkins (1998): 'Is a truth just a so-far-unfalsified hypothesis? What status does truth have in the strange, uncertain world of quantum theory? Is anything ultimately true?' (Dawkins, R. (1998) *Unweaving the Rainbow*. Penguin Books, London.)

Regrettably, independence, objectivity, and neutrality in research are not always obvious or achievable. Emerging facts have to be 'interpreted' (given meaning and value), placed in context, and disseminated. An additional problem is that successful dissemination of knowledge is a potentially complex process: the availability of evidence and its transmission may be limited; service-level agreements may not encourage the use of evidence or guidelines; incentives (moral, ethical, or financial, for instance) may disproportionately influence decision making; credibility of opinion leaders may be variable, at best; and political support may be lacking, though it is to be hoped that hypothesis, innovation, and implementation of evidence will not be stultified unduly by political considerations.

Sometimes, in the frequent absence of 'gold standard' diagnoses in functional disorders, it is only when a putative syndromic diagnosis (that is 'recognized' by a specific test) responds to a specific therapeutic procedure that the test may be considered to be valid. This is essentially a pragmatic approach to diagnosis and management (see Blomberg, Chapter 60). For example, some clinicians (including myself) are satisfied that the three features—tenderness of the posterior superior iliac spine, reduced mobility of the sacroiliac joint, and gluteal hyperalgesia—constitute, in combination, an appropriate diagnostic test for sacroiliac joint dysfunction; but, in the absence of a gold standard diagnostic test for this condition, the subjective (patient's) approval of the results of appropriate therapy and the objective (observer's) assessment of improved sacroiliac mobility immediately after the procedure provide second-best validity for the diagnostic test.

Models of care in neuromusculoskeletal medicine

Four conceptual models are described: biomechanical, pathomorphological, pathophysiological, and biopsychosocial.

Biomechanical model

The biomechanical model of dynamic stability in which the components of the musculoskeletal system (bones, joints, ligaments, muscles, fascia, and other soft tissues) contribute to efficient load transference and, as a consequence, to movement of the body with least energy expenditure and injury risk, underpins the text of this book. However, the emphasis is on the clinical aspects of somatic disorders that arise when the body's adaptive processes to physical stresses (for instance, gravitational, environmental, work- and sports-related) are overwhelmed—rather than biomechanics. For a greater understanding of basic biomechanics of the musculoskeletal system, the reader is referred to other texts. The more advanced biomechanical concepts and their clinical application to the pelvis, developed in recent decades by Levin and Dorman (see Chapters 16 and 17) and by researchers in the Netherlands, prompts me to make reference to sacroiliac dysfunction, and to provide a short summary of recent 'trends' by way of illustration.

The concepts of *form closure* and *force closure* at the sacroiliac joint were introduced by Vleeming et al. (1990). Form closure is due to the close apposition of the joint surfaces, their 'irregular' but complementary pits, ridges, and grooves, and the wedge shape of the sacrum. Force closure is the biomechanical contribution to stability (maximal in nutation—forward movement of the base, or 'promontory', of the sacrum) made by the muscles, ligaments, and fascial systems. When shear forces at the sacroiliac joint are adequately controlled by the stabilizing effects of form closure and force closure, loads can be transmitted between the lower limbs and the trunk in a cost-effective manner. When pelvic functional stability is not achieved, and shear is uncontrolled, the 'cost' to the body is the state of functional and biomechanical decompensation, manifest as painful syndromes, particularly (but not exclusively) low back pain and somatic pelvic pain. The reader is also directed to Chapter 63 in which Mottram and Comerford address the motor control of the lower back and pelvis, the relationship between muscular balance and pain syndromes, and rehabilitation strategies for a return to dynamic stability.

The editors are excited by the introduction of new neuromuscular concepts in this second edition of the textbook. In Chapter 61, Kobesova introduces, from the Czech Republic, the concept of dynamic neuromuscular stabilization. Biederman writes on functional disorders of the spine in small children in Chapter 22. In Chapter 11, Rutte provides a stimulating insight into the practical application of biomechanics in musculoskeletal medicine, with particular reference to the Preferential Mass Mechanics Method (PMMM) used in the Netherlands.

The 'pathobiomechanics' of disorders in the upper and lower limbs is often of primary importance. This applies particularly to sports-related problems in the pelvis and lower limbs (dealt with comprehensively by Hutson and English, Chapter 34; Peirce, Chapter 37; English, Chapters 41, 43, 44, and 46; and Higgins, Chapter 42) and to both sports- and work-related problems in the shoulder and upper limbs (covered by Tanner, Chapters 28 to 30; Funk and colleagues (shoulder), Chapters 31 and 32; and Hutson et al. (upper limb), Chapter 33). Ergonomics is an associated healthcare model worthy of study in patients with shoulder and arm pain due to repetitive or stereotyped movements. Knowledge of sports technique is essential for the diagnosis, rehabilitation, and prevention of further injury in overuse conditions of the lower limb.

Pathomorphological ('structural') model

One cannot consider the nature of musculoskeletal disorders without reference to structural abnormalities. After all, 'organic pathology' has always been, and indeed continues to be, the primary focus for orthopaedists (and surgeons in general, from which corporate body orthopaedic surgeons have emerged during the last hundred years). Disorders of bone, other than stress fractures, receive scant attention in this textbook; they are dealt with very adequately in numerous orthopaedic texts. However, physicians with expertise in neuromusculoskeletal disciplines should always consider bone pathology in the differential diagnosis of axial and peripheral pain, both traumatic (or 'acute') and overuse (or 'chronic'). Examples are to be found in the text: avulsion fractures, osteochondral injuries, epiphyseal fractures, and metastatic carcinoma, for instance.

Traumatic injuries to the soft tissues, particularly in the limbs, may arise primarily as a consequence of external factors. A trip or stumble leading to a fall may cause a ligament sprain, joint dislocation, or muscle tear in members of the community of varying degrees of fitness; of course, constitutional factors may increase vulnerability to injury and reduce the rate of recovery. When repetitive stresses cause failure of the adaptive processes inherent in collagenized tissues, the degree of decompensation may be assessed functionally by clinical examination, assisted when necessary by a variety of investigative tools. Experience is required in decision making as to whether or when further investigations (with the inevitable financial cost) are desirable or necessary. Experience is essential with regard to the interpretation and relevance of pathomorphological findings (for instance, disc degeneration, disc bulge, or even frank disc prolapse in back pain, or increased uptake in bone scans of the lower limbs in runners).

Terminology changes over time to keep abreast of improved understanding of pathomorphology. An example is the current use of the term 'tendinopathy' (replacing 'tendinitis') as the consequence of overuse and/or degeneration. Disruption of collagen with histological features of degeneration, rather than an invasion of inflammatory cells, is seen in Achilles tendinopathy, patellar tendinopathy, and rotator cuff tendinopathy. Evidence has accumulated over more than a decade (see Khan et al. 1999, 2002) that rehabilitation for tendinopathy affecting the weightbearing tendons (Achilles, patellar) should comprise eccentric contraction regimes. At the shoulder, assessment and rehabilitation of rotator cuff lesions (see Gibson et al., Chapter 32) demand an evaluation of the provocative factors (associated with shoulder girdle biomechanics, ergonomics, posture, sports dynamics) involved in subacromial impingement. Ligamentous laxity at the glenohumeral joint, often acquired by sportspeople as a consequence of repeated or forceful stretching at the shoulder, is often a confounding factor in sports that demand substantive upper limb activity (Hutson 2001).

Meniscus derangements, particularly at the knee, require careful evaluation. The 'classical' presentation of a twisting sprain, joint effusion, and locking of the knee is an indication for the attention of the traumatologist or orthopaedic surgeon. Recurrent, self-resolving bouts of knee pain in the young may be assessed most effectively by arthroscopy, but in middle life and beyond, critical appraisal of the patient by the application of clinical examination techniques of the type devised by Cyriax, augmented by stress tests for cruciate insufficiency (see Bickerstaff and Ali, Chapter 36), will serve the musculoskeletal physician best. When degenerative tears of the menisci, as evident on MRI, become symptomatic, the clinician becomes increasingly reliant on a sound knowledge of functional rehabilitation. As degenerative changes in the soft tissues advance, tissue preservation and maximization of functional capacity become paramount.

Pathophysiological model

The pathophysiological model provides the framework for the construct of *somatic dysfunction*, sometimes referred to as 'functional pathology' (Lewit 2011). As neurobiology and pathoneurobiological processes are further elucidated and defined, it becomes conceptually easier (even for allopathically trained physicians) to take a leaf out of the manual therapist's book in appreciating the limitations of chasing the nociceptive source of the pain, and to think in terms of evaluating the reasons behind the overt manifestations of dysfunction. Kuchera eloquently provides both an overview and an in-depth analysis of the factors associated with somatic dysfunction in Chapters 10, 27, and 50.

The analgesic response to manual therapy is very probably associated with significant neurophysiological effects in addition to the effects on joint mechanics and the chemical environment of injured tissue. Although unproven as yet, it is postulated that for treatment of spinal dysfunction to be successful, activation of descending pain inhibitory systems may be as important as local responses at (spinal) segmental and peripheral levels. Neurodynamics is also an important consideration in disorders of the upper and lower limbs. Neural dysfunction may be the primary or a contributory cause of shoulder and/or elbow pain or of buttock and/or posterior thigh pain. No musculoskeletal examination is complete, whether for axial or peripheral pain, without a neural assessment.

Butler (2000) refers to 'an emerging new construct in neurodynamics' by advising that the neurophysiological aspects of mechanosensitivity should be considered when undertaking neural tension tests. The changing concepts, over recent decades, with respect to the upper limb neural tension tests provide the reader with an insight into how increasing recognition of neural plasticity affects our thinking. The Australian manual therapist Robert Elvey revived the concept of neural tension in the upper limb at an international manual therapy conference (Elvey 1979). 'Revival' perhaps does not do Elvey justice, but it is a fact that the London neurologist Vivian Poore wrote of arm pain in the 1870s and 1880s (a hundred years before Elvey's introduction of the term 'brachial plexus tension test'). Poore (1887) included details of tension tests for the median, ulnar, and radial nerves. The upper limb tension test was introduced by Kenneally et al. in 1988 and used by Butler in his textbook *Mobilisation of the Nervous System* in 1991. (Kenneally described the upper limb tension test as the 'straight leg raise of the arm'.) Currently, the neural tissue provocation test is used as a means of assessing mechanosensitivity of the neural tissue, though Butler demurs on the basis that neurosensitization may play a role and on the recognition that other soft tissues, besides the neural tissues, are challenged on the upper limb tests. As a consequence, Butler prefers the term 'upper limb neurodynamics testing'. The subject is reviewed and brought up to date by Hall and Robinson in Chapters 15 and 56.

The concept of secondary hyperalgesia as the pathophysiological explanation for referred tenderness (palpatory hyperalgesia) and discomfort on active and passive movements (articular hyperalgesia) has gained much ground. It reflects the increasing awareness of abnormal sensory processing. Cohen et al. (1992) can take much credit for their projection of neural dysfunction as the cause of some cases of previously undiagnosed upper limb pain.

Biopsychosocial model

The demand for an alternative to the disease–illness (biomedical) model, which had supported medical practice for centuries and was reinforced by the pathomorphological concepts of Virchow (1858), gathered pace through the 1980s. The following points became recognized:

- Contrary to the Cartesian theory of pain (subsequently—though somewhat unfairly with respect to René Descartes—described as the 'duality of pain'), pain perception and pain behaviour vary enormously from person to person.
- Pain does not equate to tissue 'injury' in most cases of back pain.
- Chronicity of back pain, also neck pain arising from whiplash, and some upper limb pain syndromes, correlates poorly with tissue injury or structural disorder.
- Psychosocial factors are better predictors of recovery or chronicity than pathomorphological considerations.
- Disability is distinct from somatic dysfunction. Although impairment of function is a component in the development of disability, there are often significant psychological, social, and iatrogenic factors.

The biopsychosocial model of pain, healthcare, and disability, for which much credit should go to Waddell and colleagues (1984, 1987), addresses these and other issues. In effect, this model is an extension of Waddell's views on the distinction between distress, disability, and dysfunction (with which I entirely concur). The psychosocial factors are explored further, elsewhere in this text. A useful synopsis is the recognition that:

- Acute pain is a complex sensory and emotional experience, often associated with distress. Although pain is distinct from disability, both are subjective phenomena.
- The chronicity and severity of pain, particularly (but not exclusively) spinal pain, correlate well with psychosocial factors that include premorbid psychological profile, environmental stresses, misattributions and beliefs, iatrogenesis, and litigation.

Pragmatism and complexity in musculoskeletal medicine

Patients' expectations in the twenty-first century are increasing. Across the spectrum of health issues, patients are very likely to have and to declare values and preferences. They expect to be involved in decision making, seeking quality of treatment that is predicated upon their individual circumstances. In parallel with patients' 'New Age' views (a phrase that ushered in the twenty-first century), there have been significant societal anxieties and cultural changes in more recent years. The widespread use of the internet by patients, to support their understanding of their medical conditions, has added another dimension to the clinician's management of musculoskeletal problems. Accordingly, clinicians need to be increasingly flexible to address the complexity of health-related problems. Herein lies an enigma. Evidence-based medicine is virtually *de rigueur* in the current decade, demanded by commissioning groups and viewed as an essential component of 'governance' (the medical profession's all-encompassing self-regulating mechanism). However, individual tailor-made treatment programmes providing value, and independent of meta-analytical medical judgements, are demanded by patients. A multidisciplinary approach is often required. Can we square the circle? To do so, we must understand the application to science of modernism, post-modernism, and complex adaptive systems ('post-normal science').

Based on the science of Galileo and Newton *inter alia*, and the philosophy of thinkers such as René Descartes and Hume in the Age of the Enlightenment, the fundamental principles of modernism were (and remain) logic, reason, rationalism, and reductionism. Theories about disease and illness are based on measurements, thereby explaining reality. If theories have no measurable components, they are essentially invalid. Much of medical practice since the eighteenth century, and continuing to this day, adopts modernist principles based on a biomedical model. Orthopaedic surgery is a prime example.

Post-modernism, on the other hand, is essentially anarchic and eclectic. It rejects dogma, rejects the concept of universal truth, and rejects modernism. Friedrich Nietzsche developed some of these principles, but there have been many subsequent advocates, in particular Lyotard and Fourcault. Specifically, post-modernism rejects the (modernist) mantra that objectivity is possible in scientific work. Objectivity is often compromised by the quest for, or the achievement of, power. Post-modernism espouses non-conformity and diversity. Such principles are congruent with complementary and alternative medicine, and to some extent with manual therapy (in its broadest sense).

Post-normal science has adopted some post-modern ideas (Laugharne 2002). However, its essential principle is that uncertainty and unpredictability are inevitable in complex systems. This often applies for instance to healthcare. The search for absolute truth is viewed with grave suspicion. In post-normal science, science itself is not rejected. However, its boundaries should be expanded to allow discourse regarding socio-cultural implications with all interested parties (of which there are many). There are numerous applications of post-normal science. In the so-called 'civilized' countries, issues such as genetically modified foods, stem cell research, and cloning have implications for society in general, engaging many stakeholders.

The introduction of complexity (in the form of uncertainty, unpredictability, and an expanded peer community)—a feature of post-normal science referred to as non-linearity— demands adaptability and flexibility on the part of the physician (Wilson and Holt 2001). This type of healthcare paradigm is known as a *complex adaptive system*, in which patients' problems vary from the simple (with a high degree of agreement between clinicians and a high degree of certainty of diagnosis) to—at the opposite extreme—'chaotic' in which there is very low agreement and a very low degree of certainty. Most cases are situated between these two extremes, demanding the need (in many cases) for multiple approaches, creativity, and (above all) pragmatism.

An appropriate problem for the study of the often complex relationships between pathomorphology and pathophysiology, and the pertinence of the complexity theory, is posterior thigh pain, or 'hamstring dysfunction'. A 'tear' or 'pull' of the hamstrings is a common problem in sport. Posterior thigh pain has a high prevalence in the general population. Why is hamstring dysfunction so often a 'pain in the butt' and/or thigh, and how do we explain its frequently recurring nature? The answer perhaps lies in the fact that whichever model or paradigm (pathomorphological, biomechanical, biopsychosocial, or pathophyisological) is chosen, there is underlying neuromusculoskeletal weakness, decompensation, or 'vulnerability'.

In the pathomorphological model, hamstring dysfunction is the consequence of intrinsic muscle deficiency, commonly a tear of the biceps femoris muscle. The severity may be based on the clinician's experience, but tissue injury is more accurately graded by MRI: Grade 1, anatomy preserved, oedema; Grade 2, muscle fibre disruption; Grade 3, haematoma. Inevitably, rehabilitation demands attention to restoration of muscle function.

In the biomechanical model, factors such as muscle fatigue, flexibility, strength, and imbalance are considered. Additionally, ageing and muscle function with respect to dynamic stability and range of movements of the hip, spine, and knee are valid issues. Gait analysis is often required in investigation. Other factors involved in aetiology are incomplete rehabilitation, inappropriate warm-up before sport, training errors, and associated issues including those enumerated in the pathophysiological model.

The biopsychosocial model, incorporating the psychological aspects of pain, is explored by a number of authors in this textbook.

In many patients, adherence to the pathophysiological model is maximally productive. This model is predicated upon neural dysfunction arising in the lower back or pelvis, and adversely affecting hamstring contraction. A likely cause of hamstring inhibition is 'false' or 'disturbed' proprioceptive input from the lower back and pelvis, particularly the spinal facet (apophyseal) joints and sacroiliac joints, and possibly from the periphery such as ankle or knee following lower limb trauma. Characteristic clinical features are spinal dysfunction, sacroiliac dysfunction, myofascial trigger points, neural dysfunction, and muscle weakness patterns, primarily of the S1 myotome. These patterns of lower limb discomfort in young adults, often sportspeople, are mostly 'pseudoradicular' insofar as there is usually no evidence of nerve root compression, merely disturbed neurodynamics, though intervertebral foraminal neural irritation (as a consequence of recess stenosis) is increasingly the cause of thigh pain in the ageing population.

Management strategies are essentially pragmatic. Treatment is directed towards the identifiable dysfunctions, commonly at the spine and pelvis. Rehabilitation should continue until restoration of full functional capacity is achieved. Treatment options include spinal and paravertebral injections in the form of epidural injections, foraminal blocks, and facet blocks. Other injections and needling techniques, particularly for trigger points, are usually helpful. Controversial treatments that are not yet validated but are gaining popularity include injections of enzymes to 'enhance reabsorption of haematomas', injections that include a homeopathic remedy 'to modulate factor P and oxygen radicals', and injections of protein-free ultrafiltrate of calf's blood 'to increase oxygen uptake, to accelerate the processes of granulation and vascularization, and to improve microcirculation'. Additionally, prolotherapy may be required for refractory or recurrent cases (see Dorman, Chapter 54; Petrides, Chapter 55; and Blomberg, Chapter 60).

Management of sclerotomal or 'pseudoradicular' syndromes is a good example of a complex adaptive system paradigm. Mobilization/manipulation, soft tissue treatment, paravertebral blocks, epidural injections, and sclerosant injections (prolotherapy) may all have a place, followed by a comprehensive rehabilitation protocol. Diverse treatments may of course be given sequentially, but many clinicians, including myself, prefer combined therapy on the basis that individual treatment modalities may have a 'synergistic' rather than additive effect. The pragmatic approach, based on an antidysfunctional management strategy, is discussed more fully by Blomberg (Chapter 60).

Hutson and Ward discuss an integrated approach to healthcare in Chapter 65. The essential characteristics of musculoskeletal medicine, as practiced by the editors of this textbook when engaged by their patients who are suffering from somatic symptoms and distress, are summarized by Foell in Chapter 5: 'the haptic exploration of the body that experiences this hurt, paired with the capacity to listen to the patient's story, and knowledge about the healthcare system itself, provides at least the basis for a good working relationship in order to bring things forth.'

References

Barré, J. A. (1926) Sur un syndrome sympathique cervical posterieure et sa cause frequente: l'arthrite cervicale. *Rev. Neurol.*, 33, 1246.

Bogduk, N. (1999) Truth in musculoskeletal medicine; truth in diagnosis—validity. *Australasian Musculoskel. Med.*, 4 (1), 32–9.

Butler, D. S. (1991) *Mobilisation of the nervous system*. Churchill Livingstone, Melbourne.

Butler, D. S. (2000) *The sensitive nervous system*. Noigroup Publications, Australia.

Clinical Guideline subcommitte on Low Back Pain, AOA, (2010).J. Am. Osteopath. Assoc. Nov;110/11: 653–66.

Cohen, M. L., Arroyo, J. F., Champion, G. D., Browne, C. D. (1992) In search of the pathogenesis of refractory cervicobrachial pain syndrome. *Med. J. Aust.*, 156, 432–6.

Cohen, M. L., Quintner, J. L (1996) The derailment of railway spine: a timely lesson for post-traumatic fibromyalgia. *Pain Rev.*, 3, 181–202.

Cyriax, J. (1969) *Textbook of orthopaedic medicine*. Williams and Wilkins, Baltimore.

Dawkins, R. (1998) *Unweaving the rainbow*. Penguin Books, London.

Dorman, T. A. (1995) Concepts in orthopaedic medicine. *Spine*, 9(2), 323–31.

Elvey, R. L. (1979) Brachial plexus tension tests and the pathoanatomical origin of arm pain. In: Idezak, R. (ed.) *Aspects of manipulative therapy*. Manipulative Physiotherapists Association of Australia, Melbourne.

Engel, G. E. (1977) The need for a new medical model: a challenge for biomedicine. *Science*, 196(4286), 129–36.

Gargan, M. F. (1995) What is the evidence for an organic lesion in whiplash injury? *J. Psychosomat. Res.*, 39(6), 777–81.

Hutson, M. A. (2001) *Sports injuries: recognition and management*, 3rd ed. Oxford University Press, Oxford.

Kenneally, M., Rubenach, H., Elvey, R. L. (1988) The upper limb tension test: the SLR of the arm. In: Grant, R. (ed.) *Physical therapy of the cervical and thoracic spine*. Churchill Livingstone, New York.

Khan, K. M., Cook, J. L., Bonar, F. et al. (1999) Histopathology of common tendinopathies. Update and implications for clinical management. *Sports Med.*, 27, 393–408.

Khan, K. M., Cook, J., Kannus, P. et al. (2002) Time to abandon the 'tendinitis' myth. *BMJ*, 329, 626–7.

Laugharne, R. (2002) Psychiatry, postmodernism and postnormal science *J. Roy. Soc. Med.*, 95, 207–10.

Lewit, K. (2011) Implementation of guidelines. *Int. Musc. Med.*, 33(3), 126–7.

McDonald, C. J. (1996) Medical heuristics: the silent adjudicators of clinical practice. *Ann. Intern. Med.*, 124, 1, 56–62.

Neumann, H.-D. (1989) *Introduction to manual medicine*. Springer-Verlag, Berlin.

Pilowsky, I. (1969) Abnormal illness behaviour. *Br. J. Med. Psychol.*, 42, 347–51.

Poore, G. V. (1887) Clinical lecture on certain conditions of the hand and arm which interfere with performance of professional arts, especially piano playing. *BMJ*, 1, 441–4.

Popper, K. R. (1959) *The logic of scientific discovery*. Harper and Rowe, New York.

Sackett, D. L. (1998) Editorial: evidence-based medicine. *Spine*, 23(10), 1085–6.

Schrader, H. et al. (1996) Natural evolution of late whiplash syndrome outside the medicolegal context. *Lancet*, 347, 1207–11.

Suarez-Almazor, M. E., Russell, A. S. (1998) The art versus the science of medicine. Are clinical guidelines the answer? *Ann. Rheum. Dis.*, 57, 67–9.

Virchow, R. (1858) *Die cellular pathologie in ihrer begrundurg auf physiologische und pathologische*. A Hirshwald, Berlin.

Vleeming, A., Volkers, A. C. W., Snijders, C. J., Stoeckart, R. (1990) Relation between form and function in the sacroiliac joint. 2: Biomechanical aspects. *Spine*, 15(2), 133–6.

Waddell, G. et al. (1984) Chronic low back pain, psychologic distress and illness behaviour. *Spine*, 9, 209–13.

Waddell, G. (1987) A new clinical model for the treatment of low back pain. *Spine*, 12, 632–44.

Waddell, G., McCulloch, J. A., Kummell, E. et al. (1980) Non-organic physical signs in low back pain. *Spine*, 5, 117–25.

Wilson, T., Holt, T. (2001) Complexity and clinical care. *BMJ*, 323, 685–8.

Wulff, H. (1999) The two cultures of medicine: objective facts versus subjectivity and values. *J. Roy. Soc. Med.*, 92, 11, 549–52.

Zohn, D. A., Mennell, J. McM. (1976) *Musculoskeletal pain: diagnosis and physical treatment*. Little, Brown, Boston.

Chapter 2

Somatic dysfunction: the life of a concept

Roderic MacDonald

N.B. In this usage, somatic does not mean pertaining to the soma (body), rather than the psyche (mind), but to structures innervated by the somatic nervous system rather than the autonomic. Embryologically, the adjective chosen might more pedantically have been 'somitic', to distinguish involvement of structures derived from primitive mesodermal somites (from which skeleton and voluntary muscle derive) rather than viscera.

Approach to writing this chapter

This chapter attempts to chart the history of an idea over a century and a half and involves judging the thoughts of people by viewing a selection of their writings and inferring the reasons for their actions. The author is resigned to the fact that sampling the mass of available sources has been an arbitrary process, so that what is presented is not claiming perfect objectivity or accuracy. However, it is hoped that the narrative will indicate that the most effective way to progress in healthcare may not be just to use the output of data from established science to formulate reviews and guidelines but also to be aware of the processes, intellectually and practically, that are necessary for the institutions of science to keep steering an optimal path, without their momentum taking them down blind alleys. Such awareness starts with the realization that theory guides science, whether it leads to a change in a manual technique or to building a multi-billion dollar particle collider. What may hinder identifying and developing the theories needed to bring about necessary changes in direction? We will try to trace the progress of ideas from conception, through dissemination, investigation, and acceptance to implementation—the competitive struggle and obstacles.

Method of writing this chapter

This chapter uses Thomas Kuhn's analysis of the development of science as a descriptive framework. Since its publication in 1962, his *Structure of Scientific Revolutions* (Kuhn 1970) has achieved wide acceptance and is particularly relevant as it relates development of knowledge to factors in societies generally, as well as in clinics and laboratories. His thesis gives a specific meaning to some terms. (Hoping to aid understanding, these terms will be briefly presented and, when used in the text, may be italicized to indicate that their *Kuhnian* meaning is being used.)

Kuhn proposed that much activity involved in accumulating scientific knowledge is guided by explanatory concepts or *paradigms* that provide a framework of expectations and methods, accepted by those using them as most relevant to the area of study. The *paradigm* provides the theoretical basis from which questions for experimenters derive, and their work will tend to use skills and equipment specifically designed to answer these questions. A paradigm that has become so accepted in an area of science that most work investigates its implications is termed a *ruling paradigm* and such focused activity, *normal science*. Research committees will usually prefer to allot scarce funds to projects that investigate plausible hypotheses and plausibility often requires concordance with the *ruling paradigm*. The concentration of training, funding, and data generation in *normal science* ensures that situations explicable by the paradigm will be unravelled efficiently. A paradigm ruling over a wide area of science may persist for centuries and determine the nature of university departments and the content of textbooks. However, there will always arise, within *normal science*, situations in which strenuous attempts to explain an observation fail. Kuhn dubbed these instances *anomalies* and said that usually, they would be explained at a future date by some modification of technique, but still within the paradigm—activity he termed *puzzle-solving*.

Considerable build-up of *anomalies* can be tolerated by scientists without threatening the *paradigm rule*,but at times, there may be some loss of confidence in it and investigations begin to waver from strictly *normal science*. The scientific community enters a state that Kuhn refers to as *crisis* when those involved may feel insecure, especially if there is societal pressure to deliver answers and resourcing is at risk. At a variable time after *crisis* onset, or occasionally a factor initiating it, some workers may become aware of another, *rival paradigm* that offers the possibility of explaining all that the *ruling paradigm* can and some of the *anomalies*. Increasing awareness of this rival may deepen *crisis* and lead to investigations seeking to confirm whether its promise can be confirmed. This often necessitates studies using other methods than *normal science*. When this happens, a phase of *extraordinary science* has begun. The scientific community remains in *crisis* until investigation ***either*** confirms the *rival paradigm*, in which case it comes to *rule* and a new era of *normal science* ensues, ***or*** *extraordinary science* fails to confirm the rival and the *ruling paradigm* lives to fight another day and *normal science* resumes under its influence. The replacing of a *ruling paradigm* ushering in a new period of *normal science*, he described as a *scientific revolution*. A *revolution* may affect a small area of science or have a wider effect of which non-scientific society becomes aware.

Kuhn's major contention was that paradigms, especially if absorbed during education, are so fundamental to how observations are understood that it may be very difficult to see any other explanation. So, the proponents of competing paradigms may find it difficult to resolve their differences rationally—to see the others' points of view—especially when evidence is not conclusive: Kuhn referred to the *incommensurability* of their explanations of observed reality.

Introduction

At first thought, the success of healthcare professional groups should depend on how much they benefit sick people. However, it is often not easy to be sure how great such benefits are or whether in fact there are harms inflicted. In reality, a treatment may be used because its benefit is plausibly predicted by science and then assumed, or there are pressures on healthcare providers to respond to a person's need even when they have no proven response available. Also, those with a professional or financial commitment to a treatment may be biased towards providing it. Among these complexities, the choice between various treatments depends on both the needs of society and also the acceptance of the concepts different professions use both to make sense of the illnesses they encounter and also to justify the therapies they use. That acceptance may be just by the professional group involved, healthcare generally, or by society at large.

We will consider in this chapter, the progress of treatments given for musculoskeletal pain and impairment in the UK over 150 years, related to their underlying concepts and the groups in which they originated. These are intertwined journeys of ideas, people, and methods: stories of discoveries, rivalries, waste of resources, and avoidable suffering which may stimulate aspiration to develop better ways for scientific medicine to progress.

Origins

In the UK, physicians, apothecaries and surgeons provided the strands of theory and practice that were joined and sanctioned as the registered medical profession by the Medical Act of 1858. Apart from this process, traditional healers and bone-setters continued to practice unofficially.

Concurrently what we would now consider to be medical science was making a major leap forward. To those who consider the advance of scientific knowledge to be due to a steady accumulation of observations revealing the truth, the state of mind of those involved may seem irrelevant but, as Kuhn has influentially described, there is always a conceptual framework or *paradigm*, a pre-conception, which guides the specific enquiry undertaken and into which each new observation is fitted. Histological and bacteriological advances of the nineteenth century generated a concept of disease as an effect of changes to the structure of the body at tissue level, often induced by infection. Consequently further investigation was focused on histological and bacteriological correlates of illness which generated an avalanche of success, inevitably distracting thought and investigation from other possible ways that health may be impaired. However this progress of medical science was slow to be translated into practice; the taxonomy of diseases progressed well ahead of the means to treat them.

Meanwhile in the United States, Andrew Still, whose medical education had been conventional for the day, launched osteopathy, a system of diagnosis and therapeutics that he developed and founded in 1874. This innovation was separate from conventional medical development and was proposed as a rejection of the therapeutics then used which Still deemed ineffective and often harmful. A basic concept integral to the discipline from its inception was the osteopathic spinal lesion, later re-named and defined as segmental somatic dysfunction (SD). This concept entails considering abnormal function of the musculoskeletal system—and its entailed neurological and circulatory elements—to be a primary factor in producing impairment of health rather than merely a secondary response to traumatic or pathological processes in the involved tissues. So, for example, a situation of pain, limitation of movement, and muscle spasm would not be assumed to be a reaction to underlying inflamed or disrupted tissue (structural pathology) but would also be considered capable of being caused by a primary change in function of the structures involved: a disturbance of physiology rather than an abnormality of histology. Further, by so-called somato-visceral effects on nerves and especially arterial supply, the spinal dysfunction was deemed to be able to affect the function of visceral organs. This view persisted, being reiterated fifty years later by Wilfred Streeter (1929), a vigorous champion of osteopathy in the UK:

> The bone-setter, unlike the osteopath, deals only with localised injury . . . The osteopathic treatment is of a broader and more comprehensive character. Its whole object is to secure the free and completely unobstructed circulation of the vital fluids within the body, not alone for the minor purpose of healing local injuries, but for the inclusive maintenance of the whole organism in health. It recognises that any derangement of the body framework or impairment of its structural integrity, by irritation or pressure upon the nerves and blood vessels, interferes with the natural flow of the vital fluids, and its technique is designed to correct such structural or mechanical maladjustments, particularly maladjustments of the spine, and thus to liberate the body's remedial forces. Osteopathic manipulations . . . effect a fundamental concord and harmony of the entire mechanism of the body, a concord not merely of the bony framework but of the secretions, ferments, chemical processes and blood and nerve supplies by which life is continued and the balance of health is maintained.
>
> (*The New Healing*, Streeter W, Methuen & Co., London, 1929, p. 147)

This chapter will look at the changing relationship of SD and those basing their treatment on it, with the concepts and practitioners of conventional medicine. It will also consider the relationship of Streeter's wide visceral application of his work to what he termed 'the minor purpose of healing local injuries' to which this textbook is devoted.

Battle commenced

The rivalry between the concept of SD and what we shall call, the structural pathology concept, was acted out in many communities. As both movements developed in the Western World, it is the USA and Europe that were most involved; the situation in the UK, between the two World Wars, was one stage set for confrontation. Doctors of Osteopathy, trained in the USA, had come to the UK and enjoyed success, so much so that there were sixty in their professional association, the British Osteopathic Association (BOA) when the Osteopathic Association Clinic was set up in 1927. Located in Westminster, London, in the former residence of the Prime Minister, Lloyd George, the Clinic was opened by George Bernard Shaw, playwright and commentator on society. His address was extensively reported in the national press (Shaw 1927a,b). He asserted that:

> Osteopathy should be part of the equipment of every doctor in the country . . . A doctor should have no right to be registered unless he has osteopathic technique at his fingers' ends.
>
> (George Bernard Shaw, *Evening Standard*, 12th February 1927)

Speaking against the restrictive practices of professions and about the medical school curriculum *vis-à-vis* osteopathic technique, Shaw stated:

> I am here to make the strongest protest against the omission of this technique to make room for a great quantity of obsolete stuff, which is there for no other purpose than to make it as difficult as possible for people to get into the profession . . . this technique should be added to the qualifications of every man allowed to practise medicine or surgery in this country.
>
> (George Bernard Shaw, *Manchester Guardian*, 12th February 1927. Reproduced with permission of Guardian News & Media Ltd.)

At this time, it was the influence of SD on visceral function, by so-called somato-visceral influences, that Still had proposed, that was the main area of contention between osteopathy and orthodox medicine. With the limited diagnostic methods of the time, many referred pain patterns from musculoskeletal sources would have inevitably been misdiagnosed as visceral conditions. Their resolution following osteopathic manipulation of symptoms that medical diagnosis had named angina, pleurisy, or problems with gall bladder or stomach, would have been hailed as a success for osteopathy against these maladies, to the chagrin of the medical doctors involved. (This observation is not denying the possibility of osteopathic methods affecting visceral maladies, but that is a separate issue from the subject of this chapter.)

Circulating anecdotes of recoveries after treatment were influential even before the internet so that, in Britain, in the years between the two World Wars, demand for osteopathic treatment soon led to those trained in the American osteopathic schools becoming outnumbered, many-fold, by people with less or no training, who could use the unprotected name of osteopathy to attract custom. To address this unsatisfactory situation, osteopaths in the UK campaigned (with influential support) for statutory regulation to give protection to both themselves and their patients. A House of Lords Select Committee (1935) considered the proposed Regulation and Registration of Osteopaths Bill, hearing twenty witnesses in the process. Evidence from the British Medical Association (BMA), by a former chairman of its council, Sir Henry Brackenbury, held that they accepted the usefulness of manipulation for some musculoskeletal conditions and they considered it should be part of the medical curriculum. However, they dismissed, as an unscientific creed, the osteopathic assertion that the spinal lesion was the single most important factor in producing visceral disease through its effects on blood circulation and neural function, and the BMA objected to osteopathic education because of its compulsory bias. Asked if medical education was not also biased, Sir Henry replied:

> It is unbiased in so far as it takes and teaches all the facts of the basic sciences and anatomy and physiology without any preconceived notions as to certain theories.

Questioned as to whether there was bias in medical science and treatment, he replied:

> No; except in the sense that if a fact seems to be accepted by the whole or almost the whole scientific world I should not feel that my scientific attainments warranted me in disagreeing with it, but I should hold it the right of a medical man to take any other view.

The Select Committee reported in July 1935: although the standard of British osteopathic training was ostensibly the main reason why the Bill failed to proceed, some conclusions on contemporaneous osteopathy were reported:

> Osteopathy is not—as is popularly supposed—a craft or art limited to the treatment of maladies or defects of the bones, joints, muscles or ligaments, etc., by manipulation; in this sphere the committee has no doubt that qualified osteopaths perform valuable services. They may even possibly be regarded as having at one time developed a technique in advance of medical science, which has been to some extent accepted by members of the medical profession who practise what is called 'manipulative surgery'. Osteopathy, however, claims to be a method of healing which is suitable for treatment of *all diseases of any description*. As the law stands, anyone is entitled to practise the art of healing, but only registered medical practitioners are entitled to hold themselves out as duly qualified to treat all diseases . . . two alternative, and to a great extent conflicting theories of healing . . . it would not be safe or proper for Parliament to recognize osteopathic practitioners as qualified, on a similar footing to registered medical practitioners, to diagnose and treat all human complaints.

So the report accepted the 'valuable service' of osteopaths in musculoskeletal conditions, but the theoretical basis of a more general application was clearly rejected when it was seen as opposing that of orthodox medicine—a victory for the structural pathology *ruling paradigm* of officially recognized medical practice.

Conventional medicine ascendant

For the next forty years, the interlinked fortunes of the SD concept and its followers were eclipsed by the great strides that conventional medical practice began to make, at last matching the advances of medical science. From being almost totally therapeutically ineffectual in 1935, by 1975, for example, the scourges of syphilis, tuberculosis, and many other infectious diseases had been conquered; diabetes, pernicious anaemia, and hypothyroidism had effective remedies; and intravenous fluid replacement and blood transfusion allowed recovery from many previously irreversible situations. Apart from cancer, the prospect of 'a magic bullet', 'a pill for every ill' seemed realistic and consequently, the credibility of those offering other forms of treatment declined to the extent that Stephen Ward, the American-trained osteopath at the centre of a major national security scandal in the 1960s, was frequently referred to in the national press as a 'quack'. As he had never purported to be a registered medical practitioner, this description implies that in the UK, the whole of osteopathy was then popularly held to be quackery: most people were unaware of the existence of an official osteopathic profession in the USA.

The influence of modifying neural function on visceral disease was given some support by the work of Speransky (1944) during the Russo-Finnish war. He had demonstrated lobar consolidation in the lungs in laboratory animals as a response to experimental lesions in the brain, and had derived a treatment whereby local anaesthesia of areas of skin in upper thoracic dermatomes had appeared to hasten recovery in lobar pneumonia faster than the early sulphonamides available. However, the effectiveness of penicillin, when it became available, put into shadow, questions of why the presence of the pneumococcus bacterium did not seem to be the critical determinant of the illness in apparently healthy people and what other factors might influence the occurrence and progress of the disease.

In conventional war, it has been said that the victor writes the history: in applications of science, only those whose methods are recognized by society to be most effective get an audience for their theories and a secure place in the standard textbooks. So we have seen, in visceral disease, when confronted with the arrival of effective medical treatment, osteopathy lost credibility and its theoretical rationale was of no general interest. Similarly, in musculoskeletal maladies, some orthodox developments seemed to favour a structural pathology paradigm, namely:

i) the recognition of intervertebral disc displacements as a significant structural pathology,

ii) the histological demonstration of inflammatory arthritis,

iii) the radiological demonstration of osteoarthritic change in joints local to pain or impairment.

Progress by *normal science* methods was apparently secure.

The corollary of the acceptance of the structural pathology paradigm was that manipulation was not a rational treatment: how could manipulation affect the cellular processes mentioned above? Manipulation of a painful osteoarthritic neck, for example, was deemed irrational and potentially harmful: how could a degenerative and inflammatory condition be improved by imposing physical force and movement on it? The medical response to a patient's report of a successful treatment was likely to consider them a gullible recipient of a placebo effect who was lucky not to sustain harm.

The osteopathic concept of SD allowed for the possibility of manipulation changing function: that dysfunction is reversible is a credo of the discipline. Andrew Still likened the manipulative effect to a master millwright remedying a faulty windmill by adjusting and aligning components, each of which is structurally sound. This mechanical analogy was useful to explain treatment to patients and also for practitioners to visualize what they did. For many years, it was popular to describe abnormal function by the departure from the usual neutral position of a joint at rest (although within the normal anatomical range, i.e. it was not a subluxation). Treatment was often seen as 'correcting' such an abnormal position. These mechanical explanations were useful enough to persist despite the failure to demonstrate any plausible mechanism for these positional aberrations. Patients were still prepared to believe that the 'bone out of place' was re-placed by the manipulation they received; this being confirmed by the accompanying click which was elevated to the status of a surrogate of successful treatment. While such simplistic analogies may be useful and persist, careful clinical observation and considerations of basic science had led to more complex theoretical models incorporating developments in neurophysiology, but these did not enter into medical discourse while the structural pathological concept was still expected, eventually, to solve the mysteries of all diseases (save for those of a psychological origin).

Accommodation with orthodoxy

In response to medical advances in visceral disease, there was a strong debate in osteopathic circles in the USA concerning the teaching of materia medica in osteopathic schools, with the curricular differences between these schools and medical schools being steadily eroded. As progressively, state by state, the graduating osteopaths became eligible for medical licensing, the training and practice of osteopathy and medicine overlapped increasingly; the quantity of pharmaceutical advertising in the osteopathic journals approached that in those of orthodox medicine, and the selling point of osteopathic medicine became that it had all the elements of orthodox medicine but with the addition of an extra osteopathic factor.

A Kuhnian analysis of these developments would suggest that, in practice, the American osteopathic profession had largely abandoned the paradigm of SD being a significant factor in illness. Whether this was so would depend on what comprised the extension to medical care—the extra osteopathic factor offered by osteopathic doctors to the American population. However, when asked to elaborate on what that factor was, it was often described in terms of the holistic medicine principles increasingly fashionable throughout western medicine from the 1960s—the self-righting properties of body systems and their inter-relatedness, especially extending to functions of the mind. This was in accordance with Still's original proposals that the interconnectedness of body systems required that it be treated as a unit with a self-healing potential. However, his further tenet, that recovery should be aided by removing aberrations of function not with drugs but with manipulation, was progressively reduced in emphasis so that the teaching and use of manipulation declined to a level that its enthusiasts within osteopathy would describe a generation of osteopaths lost to the distinctive practice that Still had formulated.

A concept may be said to exist if it has been proposed and published, but that existence is of scant importance if it is not being discussed and developed into both treatments that are taught and practiced, and testable hypotheses that go on to be evaluated by controlled trials that meet the strict criteria of the day. Education and research have costs that must be met from expected benefits. Significant research into SD was undertaken in the post-war USA when Irvin Korr, a non-osteopathic physiologist, was funded by the osteopathic profession to investigate the spinal segmental abnormalities that osteopathy had termed lesions. He did indeed demonstrate (Korr 1947) objective changes in the responses to stimuli of segmental spinal muscles that correlated with an osteopath's independent palpation diagnosis. He and his osteopathic colleague, Denslow, deserved considerable credit for their development of apparatus to monitor muscle function and to also map skin conductivity. As comparable equipment would not be available 'off the shelf' for nearly fifty years, this was truly *extraordinary science*. However, once some justification for osteopathic contentions had been produced, this activity appears to have dwindled and Korr's stance of investigating osteopathy from the viewpoint of a dispassionate scientist must have been somewhat devalued as he became an enthusiastic advocate for osteopathy. The more orthodox scientific medical community must have thought he had 'gone native'.

In the UK, the General Council and Register of Osteopaths (GCRO), as it worked for acceptance of the osteopathic profession, often took criticism from its members for choosing to emphasize the musculoskeletal aspects of osteopathic practice and for not seeking a war of words with orthodoxy over the management of visceral disease. The GCRO was a voluntary register that had been set up following the House of Lords Select Committee Report (1935) as a necessary stage in the progress towards statutory recognition. In its work to raise the profile and standards of osteopathy, the GCRO stressed its usefulness in musculoskeletal problems, to the chagrin of those osteopaths still holding to Still's original compass. However, the politically astute leadership chose not to position themselves as an easy target of medical opposition to osteopathy which continued to attack any assertion of effectiveness in treating visceral conditions. This was re-iterated in the BMA *Handbook of Medical Ethics* of 1980:

> The practice of manipulation does not involve acceptance of any particular theory of the causation of disease; osteopathy does. Because such theories are incompatible with scientific medicine, it is clearly impossible for a doctor to collaborate with an osteopath, or to use such services for his patient while maintaining effective control of the treatment.

However, the edition of 1981 had changed this entry to one provided by the author which stressed the musculoskeletal nature of most osteopathic work but left open the range of problems that might be influenced by dysfunction of musculoskeletal structures:

> Modern osteopathy maintains that it augments more conventional medicine with a number of diagnostic and therapeutic techniques based on the premise that much symptomatology of musculoskeletal origin is caused by potentially reversible dysfunction which may be more effectively treated by physical measures such as manipulation, rather than pharmacological or surgical remedies appropriate to pathological processes.

This small personal dent in the ramparts of conventional medicine was dwarfed in 1982 when Charles, Prince of Wales, was invited to be President of the BMA. Although ostensibly a ceremonial role, he used the opportunity to urge the BMA to look critically at modern medicine (1982):

> Today's unorthodoxy is probably going to be tomorrow's convention . . . by concentrating on smaller and smaller fragments of the body, modern medicine perhaps loses sight of the patient as a whole being . . .

The potential influence, on an 150-year-old association of a learned profession, of a 34-year-old with no scientific background, heir to a constitutional monarchy, might be thought tenuous, but in fact the social imperatives of the situation prevailed: the BMA would not risk appearing discourteous to an invited guest or of being caricatured as arrogant and resistant to change. So the BMA's Board of Science and Education set up a working party to assess the value of alternative therapies which reported in 1986. Concerning osteopathy it said (BMA 1986):

> Osteopathic teaching was foremost in demonstrating the value of palpation and pressure in the local examination of the spine, methods that are still not routinely taught in all medical schools, yet this simple exercise at once uncovers the possibility of local signs of abnormal function and identifies the spinal area to which a diagnosis and treatment may be directed. A comprehensive codification of techniques, all directed to obtaining the object of the relief of pain with the minimum of force is also the debt owed to osteopathy.

This apparent belief in the value of identifying abnormal function in order to use manipulative techniques to relieve pain, seems to come without any explicit acceptance of the existence or mechanisms of such abnormal function or trial evidence of effectiveness. The report's approach had perhaps to do with the BMA not wanting to challenge osteopathy in the musculoskeletal arena, as it was aware of a governmental attitude to complementary medical practices: services available in the market that should only be regulated to protect the public from false claims or harm. Also, to challenge the theoretical background of osteopathy in the largest area of its perceived effectiveness, spinal pain, it would have to propose a better theoretical basis and/or a more successful treatment. This it could not do.

Failure of the structural pathological paradigm to account for non-specific back pain

In the UK in July 1976, Members of Parliament questioned the Health Minister, David Owen, asking what measures were being taken to reduce the incidence of back pain. In reply, he announced the formation of the Working Group on Back Pain, to be chaired by Professor A.L. Cochrane. This multidisciplinary group, including a medically qualified osteopath, was convened that same year and reported in 1979. They concluded:

> 8:3 The most fundamental problem is uncertainty about the nature of back pain, of how the complaint arises, and of the significance of various attributes that may be associated with it . . . There is no satisfactory evidence that any treatment, let alone early treatment, is sufficiently effective in influencing the natural history of the condition in most acute back pain sufferers as to justify diverting resources to the establishment of crisis clinics . . . Knowledge in these areas will be improved only as a result of sustained investment in clinical and basic research studies directed at unravelling these problems . . . This gives rise to conflicts over what constitutes a scientific approach to the problem. Many painful conditions arise from well-defined pathological entities and in these circumstances it is acceptable to concentrate on the morbid state, in the hope that the pain will be controlled secondarily as the underlying pathology is modified.

However, they go on to say:

> 8:4 Pain is a subjective complaint, an emotional response to afferent input, in which evidence of pathology or other objective signs may be difficult to detect.

The influence of aetiological uncertainty on research is mentioned:

> 8:8 In developed fields of enquiry a successful application for support is required to include a testable hypothesis and a method appropriate for this purpose. However at margins of the islands of knowledge the problem is usually ill-defined and a testable hypothesis cannot usually be formulated without further observation to describe the natural phenomenon. Furthermore, until the problem has been adequately circumscribed it is not possible to assess what methods may be appropriate, even less to develop what techniques the situation may demand.
>
> (Working Group on Back Pain, Department of Health and Social Security, HMSO, London 1979, p. 18)

However, the major research initiative, both basic and clinical, that the Cochrane report had called for, did not take place. So, the structural pathological model was struggling for evidential support. Martin Roland, then a researcher in back pain (and one author of the Roland-Morris Disability Scale for the problem), summed up the situation when he said that it was progress when the medical profession admitted that in the overwhelming majority of instances of back pain, the cause was unknown.

Waiting for crisis

When such a *ruling paradigm* fails to account for observed reality and meet the needs of society, (in this case, for effective diagnosis and treatment of back pain), then Kuhn's analysis of the progress of knowledge suggests that a science-based community will not abandon it, even though the instances of *paradigm failure*, termed *anomalies*, build up. However, this build-up may begin to shake confidence in the paradigm and sow the seeds of *crisis*, especially if the arena in which it is observed is more public than just the scientific community. He suggests though that the *ruling paradigm* will only be seriously threatened when enough investigators become aware of a rival concept with sufficiently greater explanatory scope that it has potential to be the new *ruling paradigm*.

While a re-interpretation of existing data may be enough to allow such a *scientific revolution*, there is more often a period when the *rival paradigm* needs some investigation to confirm its superior fit with reality. This investigation may require a departure from *normal science* by having to focus on new aspects of the problem requiring different methods—Kuhn's *extraordinary science*. For example, to explore an SD hypothesis for back pain will need observations, not of structure, but of function (motion, force, and electromyography) to be collected, with implications for staffing, training, and equipment. Of importance to understanding these processes are factors such as the cost of entering a period of *extraordinary science*, not just to funders but also to those whose careers and reputations may be affected. These factors may suppress the onset of *crisis* or prolong it for long periods if resources cannot fund necessary investigation. On the other hand, societal pressure may hasten the process when there is an evident requirement to move towards more effective science-based answers to community needs.

While the SD hypothesis was accepted within osteopathy, there was little recognition in the medical or public domains—all osteopathic theories were thought to be addressing the causation of visceral diseases, where the structural pathological paradigm was more successful and its rival could be dismissed as implausible. Until a *rival paradigm* is seen to be at least as plausible by the leaders of an area of science, then confirmatory research is unlikely to take place and any anomalous observations will continue to be investigated using the methods dictated by the *ruling paradigm*. This *normal science* would attempt to explain musculoskeletal impairments by ever more detailed examination of structure-seeking pathological changes. With the development of computed tomography (CT) in the 1970s, closely followed by magnetic resonance imaging (MRI), structural abnormalities could be sought with a finer and finer sieve, by static images, while histology, down to electron microscopy, could refine the search further. A period of time would elapse before experience with these new technologies would fail to show that the abnormalities revealed predicted the majority of back pain experienced—who would have back pain and who would not. Further episodes of pain could come and go while, year on year, images would change little. However, if there were to be a period of *extraordinary science* investigating SD, then it would have to wait on instrumental developments. Most of the reliable methods of capturing data about function would not become generally available until the late 1990s—systems for monitoring three-dimensional motion; surface electromyography (EMG) made usable by pre-amplification; and the computer software to manage the deluge of data from these systems (data for which the painstaking work of establishing norms had hardly started). Until these phenomena ceased to be considered secondary effects of the state of the structure, they would not be seen as an important area for funding of projects.

In 1989, the Society for Back Pain Research's (SBPR) meeting in Birmingham was entitled 'Back pain—classification of syndromes'. This forum was notable for the wide range of disciplines attending including basic scientists, psychologists, osteopaths, and chiropractors, as well as medical specialists from orthopaedics and rheumatology. After presentation of a hierarchical tree representing all potential causes of back pain (divided into trauma, inflammatory, degenerative, malignant, and metabolic) by Dr Paul Pynsent (PP), Director of Research, Royal Orthopaedic Hospital, Birmingham, and Jeremy Fairbank (JT), Orthopaedic Surgeon, Oxford, open discussion followed (Fairbank and Pynsent 1990):

> Audience member (Aud.) 'You do not have any classification for functional pathology or dysfunction.'
> PP 'I do not understand what functional pathology means.'
> Aud. 'It means . . . abnormal function in the absence of morbid anatomical change.'
> PP 'If someone comes to your clinic with pain then presumably they have something wrong somewhere. It is either of psychogenic origin, or there is some inflammation of a muscle or whatever else you might like to attribute to the term "strain".'
> Aud. '. . . there are people who do not fit neatly into either trauma or degenerative, and everybody sees that.'
> PP 'If you pick up something and your back suddenly hurts, then presumably this is trauma.'
> Aud. 'Bending over to wash one's teeth is not exactly trauma, but I have had a number of people who have had back pain who simply bent over the wash basin.'
> JT 'I think most of the rest of this meeting is to do with degenerative and traumatic cause, but the two comments we have had, I have to say, are in the area of the art of medicine rather than its science. As long as people are using these terms, I do not really understand what they are talking about. It is important that we explore the scientific basis of these clinical observations.'
>
> (*Back Pain: Classification of Syndromes*. Edit. Fairbank J, Pynsent P. Manchester University Press, Manchester, UK, 1990, p. 21–2.)

So, consideration of abnormal function as a cause of back pain was not seen as scientific—the *ruling paradigm* for discourse of this subject was causation by structural pathology. The discussion just described may suggest some of the *incommensurability* between rival paradigms that Kuhn suggested could prevent rational debate among proponents.

So, the community of investigators within UK conventional medicine, while failing to find structural pathology correlates of back pain experience, were largely unaware of a contemporaneous *rival paradigm* shared by thousands of health practitioners practicing in their community in unorthodox or alternative medicine. The exclusion of such practitioners was aided by differing terminologies, few shared academic contacts, and rivalry in the claims of efficacy made to the community: it owed more to the anthropology of tribalism than an image of science as the dispassionate search for evidence and meaning.

At the London College of Osteopathic Medicine (LCOM), licensed (registered) medical practitioners of orthodox medicine had been taught osteopathic theory and practice since 1946, and so had the individual opportunities to experience discourse informed by both traditions—their orthodox background and the osteopathic tradition brought to the UK by American Doctors of Osteopathy from the beginning of the century. For many, this opportunity to see the spectrum of musculoskeletal maladies from a different viewpoint was transformative: departures from normal comfortable function were not automatically assumed to be the effect of underlying pathological processes. With the osteopathic concept that much abnormal function could be a primary condition that was reversible, they undertook treatment by manual methods and by looking at the whole body for obstacles to recovery. Many thought that by becoming familiar with the thinking and concepts of both traditions—osteopathic and conventional—they could become a useful conduit between them. However, the realities of tribalism, paralleled by the Cold War still going on around them, meant that someone not clearly in either camp was trusted by neither.

The negotiations that would lead to establishing the statutory General Osteopathic Council (GOsC), in 1993, did not involve any LCOM members. However, formation of the GOsC, although probably impossible without the profession playing down the visceral application of their work, did not imply any acceptance of osteopathic concepts concerning musculoskeletal maladies. The public required protection, osteopaths wanted recognition, and the BMA did not object: the ruling paradigms of each profession remained distinct.

While scientists may tolerate such schisms for long periods, maintaining boundaries by non-communication, the wider community, on which they depend for support, may become intolerant of theoretical argument when a clear direction for practical progress is needed. Governmental tolerance was tested when, at the beginning of the 1990s, the number of days of back-related sickness compensation in the UK had doubled over the previous five years. Paradigm failure was now compounded by societal pressure for an explanation.

A paradigm shift

For *crisis* to develop within conventional medical science, all that was required was awareness of a plausible explanation, that might lead to more effective treatment for the increase in back pain. For a decade, an alternative explanation for the persistence of non-specific back pain had been developing, a paradigm of chronicity in back pain disability as a behavioural response to psychosocial distress rather than a physical impairment. The leading proponent of this development, Gordon Waddell, an orthopaedic surgeon, summarized his explanatory paper thus (1987):

> Because there is increasing concern about low-back disability and its current medical management, this analysis attempts to construct a new theoretic framework for treatment. Observations of natural history and epidemiology suggest that low-back pain should be a benign, self-limiting condition, that low back-disability as opposed to pain is a relatively recent Western epidemic, and that the role of medicine in that epidemic must be critically examined. The traditional medical model of disease is contrasted with a biopsychosocial model of illness to analyse success and failure in low-back disorders. Studies of the mathematical relationship between the elements of illness in chronic low-back pain suggest that the biopsychosocial concept can be used as an operational model that explains many clinical observations. This model is used to compare rest and active rehabilitation for low-back pain. Rest is the commonest treatment prescribed after analgesics but is based on a doubtful rationale, and there is little evidence of any lasting benefit. There is, however, little doubt about the harmful effects—especially of prolonged bed rest. Conversely, there is no evidence that activity is harmful and, contrary to common belief, it does not necessarily make the pain worse. Experimental studies clearly show that controlled exercises not only restore function, reduce distress and illness behaviour, and promote return to work, but actually reduce pain. Clinical studies confirm the value of active rehabilitation in practice. To achieve the goal of treating patients rather than spines, we must approach low-back disability as an illness rather than low-back pain as a purely physical disease. We must distinguish the symptoms and signs of distress and illness behaviour from those of physical disease, and nominal from substantive diagnoses. Management must change from a negative philosophy of rest for pain to more active restoration of function. Only a new model and understanding of illness by physicians and patients alike makes real change possible.
>
> (G Waddell. A new clinical model for the treatment of low back pain. *Spine* 1987; 12(7):632–44)

With the perceived explosion in back-related incapacity giving impetus to the search for explanation, this paradigm was taken up by a medical/political consensus, and rapidly the emphasis in management swung towards a modification of behaviour rather than the previous policy that was either to attempt cure of the presumed structural pathology by some form of treatment (albeit usually ineffective) or to allow resolution to occur spontaneously (if it would). (In practice, many people sought treatment outside conventional medicine, from various manipulative professions, without any concern over the theoretical basis of the treatment.)

The rapidity of change in official advice showed that *paradigm change* can take place with the stage of *crisis* compressed to a minimum when those who can resource research and implementation feel impelled to drive the process. Dissemination of information within the community and confirmatory research can be resourced and fast-tracked, and the education of professionals influenced. This paradigm-led change occurred fast enough to justify Waddell's text being entitled *The Back Pain Revolution* (2004). Briefly, the principles of avoiding rest, maintaining activity, and early return to work were reinforced by a positive message that pain did not signify harm and recovery was to be expected. This policy was disseminated by an officially published booklet, 'The Back Book' (HMSO 1996). When such a policy to change the behaviour of the population and healthcare practitioners is centrally organized, the arguments in favour of it necessarily seek clarity and simplicity, so that detail in the original author's thesis may be lost; details that may seem unimportant when judging the effect of a national campaign but may be important to many individuals.

Waddell had always held that the abnormal illness behaviour of some back pain sufferers, that he proposed should be recognized and assessed, could be a normal response to undiagnosed, unimproved back pain that threatened mobility and livelihood. And yet the message cascading down to many frontline healthcare workers had often become blurred, so that persistence of so-called 'simple back pain' was judged likely to be due to psychosocial factors. Increasing distress would then reinforce that judgement rather than addressing the possibility of unrelieved peripheral pain generation. Even when you are its author, and are surfing the wave of rapid paradigm change driven by a tide of societal pressure, that does not mean you can control it. In the second edition of *The Back Pain Revolution* of 2004, Waddell has added an introduction to the chapter on the physical basis of back pain which could be seen as providing a correction to the emphasis and direction of practices that he sees resulting from his analysis of the problem (Waddell 2004, p.153):

> So there is no doubt, let me state very clearly: back pain is a physical problem. Over the past 25 years, we have focused a lot (perhaps too much at times) on psychosocial issues. Psychosocial factors influence how patients respond to back pain and they are important in low back disability, but they do not cause the pain. Back pain is not a psychological problem. Back pain starts with a physical problem in the back.
>
> (G Waddell. A new clinical model for the treatment of low-back pain. *Spine* 1987; 12(7):632–44)

He then goes on to give a clear exposition of the features of SD in the spine, concluding the chapter (Waddell 2004, p. 175):

> I believe the traditional search for anatomic sites and structural causes for pain is simply inappropriate for non-specific low back pain. That is why it has failed. More physiologic concepts of dysfunction hold much greater promise.

So, while interpretations of the biopsychosocial model still dominate the orthodox approach to back pain, especially in general practice, its main architect attempts to realign its sphere of influence to allow consideration of the concept that he acknowledges arises from alternative medicine's 'more than a century of astute clinical observation of the musculoskeletal system'. In many ways, Waddell's personal position is a counter-instance to Kuhn's suggestion that *incommensurability* is often an obstacle to a rational resolution of paradigm differences. However, it is perhaps the followers of paradigm-driven practice who, as a group, are most susceptible to that conceptual inflexibility.

Evaluating manipulation

Before the question 'why does this work?' is seriously asked, there usually needs to be an acceptance that 'this does work'. So a major factor that could enhance the plausibility of the SD paradigm and attract resources to its investigation would be convincing evidence of a substantial benefit from manipulation. It is unlikely that such an effect could have a credible explanation within the structural pathological paradigm or be mistaken for a placebo effect if control treatments were suitably designed. Research as a search for knowledge is not nearly as likely to happen as research to bring direct advantage to whoever can fund it. So, when there is a product to be licensed or promoted, industry usually funds research.

While manipulation is a commodity, it is mainly provided by individuals who felt, in the 1980s, that funding promotion of their own practices would benefit them more than contributing to a research initiative by their profession. After all they reasoned, the expectation of benefit among those already purchasing osteopathic care was probably higher than would be demonstrated by any randomized controlled trial (RCT). In 1975 (Doran and Newell) and 1985 (Gibson et al.), individual osteopaths in the UK had been involved in small published trials, administered by orthodox medical institutions, without significant benefits being demonstrated. So, it is not surprising that the GCRO was not enthusiastic about involvement in trials and, when the author addressed its council, the stated attitude to treatment trials was that osteopaths knew what they did was effective and so did their patients, so why would they allow themselves to be assessed by the hostile and ignorant conventional medical establishment that was embedded in most healthcare research facilities.

The then unique fusion of osteopathic and medical awareness at the LCOM led to a decision to fund research directly. They accepted that a lack of proven benefit from manipulation was an obstruction to acceptance of osteopathy and so supported an RCT of manipulation for non-specific back pain from which a modest temporary benefit was shown and the report of which was published in 1990 (MacDonald and Bell).

Then finally in the UK, evaluation of manipulation for back pain attracted official support. How did this happen? The actions of communities and their scientists in situations of Kuhnian *chaos* are unpredictable, and the various independent and governmental organizations and individuals who may have contributed to this happening are legion. Had it occurred due to an added positive influence or the reduction of opposition? Did those involved know how much they each had influenced the outcome? In understanding such situations, the author offers the metaphor of the Ouija board: many agencies are overtly in play but the influence of each on the outcome may not be accurately known by any. One factor was that with negotiations going on for the statutory regulation of osteopathy and chiropractic, it was undesirable for such official recognition to occur with no evidence of benefit to the community. So, the Medical Research Council (MRC) funded an RCT, published in 1990, evaluating chiropractic manipulation in non-specific low back pain (Meade et al.) and the United Kingdom back pain exercise and manipulation (**UK BEAM**) trial in 2003 (UK BEAM Trial Team 2004) which had a manipulation arm staffed by trained manipulators whether osteopaths, chiropractors, or physiotherapists. To those applying the Ouija metaphor, it will be unclear, *not only* in which direction and how hard the glass had been pushed by each agent as they contribute to the eventual summation effect, *but also* what was the motivation of those who favoured trials. Did they want manipulation demonstrated as effective or did they expect an outcome that would justify rejecting what they saw as an expensive, irrational placebo? Probably few were consciously seeking justification of any underlying concept. The results of the two MRC-funded trials showed a statistically significant benefit for manipulation but not at a level of much clinical importance, so that the plausibility of any underlying concept was hardly affected (if considered at all).

However, the large professions of chiropractic and osteopathy in the USA have finally organized research programmes and, most importantly, the OSTEOPATHIC trial from the Osteopathic Research Center, University of North Texas, was reported in 2013 (Licciardone et al.). This large RCT showed that manipulation was capable of substantial benefits at twelve weeks to some non-specific back pain subjects, with response rates approaching 2:1 for the greatest effects (> 40-mm reduction of a 100-mm pain VAS). However, analysis of treatment responses compared with those having sham treatments show that 15% of subjects were the main recipients of such benefits, approximating to a number needed to treat (NNT) of eight. Analysis identifying predictors of this response could help unravel the major problem referred to in the Cochrane Report (HMSO 1979, p. 48) of the heterogeneity of back pain causation:

factors found to predict response to manipulation may give insights into the mechanisms of the dysfunction that has been affected, and aid more cost-effective targeting of the treatment. Interestingly, most response had occurred after three treatments.

The use of responder analysis, rather than means of the outcomes of treatment groups, has been increasingly recognized as appropriate when there is significant heterogeneity: distinct aetiological groups cannot be identified by the available entry criteria and therefore normal distributions of response are not likely. Hence, the UK BEAM trial data has been re-analysed (Froud et al. 2009) and shown NNTs at least as favourable as the OSTEOPATHIC trial.

Another effect of manipulation has been discovered in the treatment of restless legs syndrome (RLS) where, at least in the short term, the osteopathic method of counterstrain has outperformed the standard drug treatments (Peters et al. 2012). This has stimulated interest in the possible modes of action of this distinctive method and led to a proposition of a mechanism of somatic dysfunction based on proprioceptive calibration errors reversible by manipulation (MacDonald 2013).

Synthesis

Contemporary practitioners of musculoskeletal medicine accept both the possible contribution of structural pathology to pain generation and also varying amplification of the ensuing disability by adverse psychosocial factors. In addition though, those who have accepted the SD paradigm into their thinking find assessing disturbance of function a necessary tool to complete the analysis of situations of musculoskeletal pain—to consider the variable contributions of disease, distress, and dysfunction to each individual's situation. There is little personal awareness of *incommensurability* of the three underlying *paradigms* until trying to communicate with someone who cannot conceive of pain arising other than in tissue damaged by trauma or inflammation. It has to be accepted, as an obstacle to that conception, that basic science has yet to demonstrate conclusively a mechanism for such pain generation that could be inserted into the medical curriculum. On the other hand, it is 35 years since the Cochrane Report pointed out that a nationally directed research effort was required to gain understanding of back pain mechanisms. Such activity as has occurred has been mainly research into analgesic and anti-inflammatory agents, and management of psychosocial factors. The inadequate response to that recommendation is in stark contrast to Professor Cochrane's worldwide influence on the emergence of evidence-based medicine.

Future

The views expressed in this chapter are perhaps too personal, based on four decades of contemporaneous observation and involvement. The vignettes of significant statements and attitudes are necessarily opportunistic, and much of that time, the author's adoption of a Kuhnian perspective may have kept his thinking (about paradigms) within that paradigm. If the resulting insights have any value, it must be that they aid progress.

The tendency of groups in applied science to use their own conceptual frameworks and languages, sometimes as a badge signifying identity and loyalty, can prevent the development and refining of ideas that comes from free discourse. This would not matter as much as it does if the groups currently accepted by society did not inevitably hold the keys to the resources of scientific education and research so that, even if they were not consciously closing down examination of new approaches, they just would not see the possibilities of a new direction for the focus of those resources.

Slavish acceptance of Kuhn's idea of *incommensurability* of the views of those adhering to rival paradigms might lead to a pessimism concerning the usefulness of scientific discourse other than the presentation of data. However, there is value in recognition that such discourse is not the dispassionate and rational examination of observations down to first principles, but that everyone carries their preconceptions into the forum. Who would not fear ridicule if they take seriously something not currently accepted and are subsequently deemed gullible, but also who does not fear being seen as an outmoded, inflexible reactionary when a new fashionable way of thinking takes over? Also, once a group has the power over resources, why would they risk ceding it to rivals in the battle to mould research towards the methods they have faith in and gain public acceptance? So is there a lack of communication leading to inward-looking groups among whom, those with power jealously guard it and those without it, relish the status of the outcast band guarding their secrets? Is there a double-bind whereby without evidence of efficacy, no group will be accepted by the scientific community, but without the compliance of that community, no valid evidence of efficacy may be forthcoming?

Recognition of these issues can lead to them being addressed by:

(a) contact between groups, with each trying to develop terms that are understood by all sides rather than using the jargon that identifies members of a group to each other;

(b) advocating spread of responsibility so that control of publicly funded research facilities is not delegated solely to mainstream;

(c) those within non-conventional groups recognizing that acceptance must to some extent be on the terms of the majority;

(d) recognizing that a concentration on treatment outcomes research exclusively, without respect for the development of underlying concepts by basic science, will hinder progress.

Finally, the recognition that disturbances of neuromusculoskeletal function can have an independent effect leads to the need to assess that function which, while slowly yielding to instrumental objectivity, in clinical practice is almost totally dependent on skills of hand and eye. To acquire those needs time and teaching which, without recognition of the primary importance of this competence, is difficult to justify in medical training. For obvious reasons, airline pilots and neurosurgeons have the necessary time devoted to their training: it is not yet so obvious what skills a doctor working in musculoskeletal pain and impairment should have. Increasing recognition of somatic dysfunction as a real and relevant entity would help to secure the survival of skills without which much of this book would be the poorer.

References

(1996) *The back book*. The Stationery Office Ltd., London.

British Medical Association. (1980) *Handbook of medical ethics*. BMA, London, p. 41.

British Medical Association. (1981) *Handbook of medical ethics*. BMA, London, p. 45.

British Medical Association. (1986) *Alternative therapy: report of the Board of Science and Education*. BMA, London, p. 55.

Doran, D. M. L., Newell, D. J. (1975) Manipulation in treatment of low-back pain: a multi-centre study. *BMJ*, 2, 161–4.

Fairbank, J., Pynsent, P. (eds) (1990) *Back pain: classification of syndromes*. Manchester University Press, Manchester, UK, p. 21–2.

Froud, R., Eldridge, S., Lall, R., Underwood, M. (2009) Estimating the number needed to treat from continuous outcomes in randomised controlled trials: methodological challenges and worked example using data from the UK Back Pain Exercise and Manipulation (BEAM) trial. *BMC Med. Res. Method.*, **9**, 35, doi:10.1186/1471-2288-9-35.

Gibson, T., Grahame, R., Harkness, J., Woo, P., Blagrave, P., Hills, R. (1985) Controlled comparison of short-wave diathermy treatment with osteopathic treatment in non-specific low back pain. *Lancet*, 1, 1258–61.

HRH The Prince of Wales. (1982)'Complementary medicine': a speech by HRH The Prince of Wales. BMA, London.

Korr, I. M. (1947) The neural basis of the osteopathic lesion. In: Korr, M., Peterson, B. (ed.) *The collected papers of Irvin*. American Academy of Osteopathy, Colorado.

Kuhn, T. S. (1970) *The structure of scientific revolutions* (2nd ed.). University of Chicago Press, Chicago.

Licciardone, J. C., Minotti, D. E., Gatchel, R. J., Kearns, C. M., Singh, K.P. (2013) Osteopathic manual treatment and ultra-sound therapy for chronic low back pain: a randomized controlled trial. *Ann. Fam. Med.*, 11, 122–9, doi:10.1370/afm.1468.

MacDonald, R. S.(2013) The positional release phenomenon and the effects of counterstrain manipulation: reflections and implications. Int. Muscul. Med., 35(3), 95–8.

MacDonald, R. S., Bell, C. M.(1990)An open controlled assessment of osteopathic manipulation in nonspecific low-back pain. *Spine*, 15(5), 364–70.

Meade, T. W., Dyer, S., Browne, W., Townsend, J., Frank, A. O. (1990) Low back pain of mechanical origin: randomised comparison of chiropractic and hospital outpatient treatment. *BMJ*, 300, 1431–7.

Peters, T., MacDonald, R., Leach, C. M. J. (2012) Counterstrain manipulation in the treatment of restless legs syndrome: a pilot single-blind randomized controlled trial; the CARL Trial. *Int. Muscul. Med.*, 34(4), 136–40.

British Medical Association, London (1935) The Osteopaths Bill. A report of the proceedings before a select committee of the House of Lords 1935. British Medical Association, London. (Reprinted from reports in the *BMJ* 9th March–20th April and 27th July 1935.)

Shaw, G. B. (1927a) Address to the British Osteopathic Association. *Evening Standard*, 12th February 1927.

Shaw, G. B. (1927b) Address to the British Osteopathic Association. *Manchester Guardian*, 12th February 1927.

Speransky, A. D. (1944) Experimental and clinical lobar pneumonia. *Am. Rev. Soviet Med.*, 2(Oct), 22–7.

Streeter, W. (1929) *The new healing*. Methuen & Co., London, p. 147.

UK BEAM Trial Team. (2004) United Kingdom back pain exercise and manipulation (UK BEAM) randomised trial: effectiveness of physical treatments for back pain in primary care. *BMJ*, 329, 1377.

Waddell, G. (1987) A new clinical model for the treatment of low-back pain. *Spine*, 12(7), 632–44.

Waddell, G. (2004) *The back pain revolution* (2nd ed.). Churchill Livingstone, London.

Working Group on Back Pain, Dept. of Health and Social Security. (1979) *The Cochrane Report*. HMSO, London, p. 18.

Chapter 3

Evidence-based medicine in Manual/Musculoskeletal Medicine: a blessing or a curse?

Jacob Patijn

Introduction to evidence-based medicine

Over the past four decades, the philosophy of so-called 'evidence-based medicine' has taken the healthcare world by storm; a prominent development that is also being gradually integrated into Manual/Musculoskeletal Medicine. Evidence-based medicine (EBM) is defined as the conscientious, explicit, and judicious use of the best evidence currently available in making decisions regarding the care of individual patients and, therefore, the practice of EBM implies combining individual clinical expertise with the best available external clinical evidence from systematic research (Sackett et al. 1996). When using the term individual clinical expertise, we mean the proficiency and judgement that individual clinicians acquire through clinical experience and practice (Sackett et al. 1996).

EBM was initially defined as contrary to clinical experience. Already by 1972, a foundation for what would later be called EBM had been created by Cochrane, who stated that too much medical care was based on interventions of dubious or unknown safety and efficacy, thus causing harm at both individual and population levels through iatrogenic injury, waste of resources, and failure to use more effective treatments (Cochrane 1972). This statement suggested that, at that time, medicine consisted of 'badly performing physicians' who provided their patients with inadequate treatment. However, some authors simply see EBM as old wine in new bottles (Grahame-Smith 1995).

EBM has been around for as long as there have been clinicians, and we have to be convinced that these clinicians used the best evidence available in the treatment of their patients. EBM as such started in the late 1980s at McMaster University in Canada and at Oxford University in the United Kingdom, in response to results of studies which showed a huge difference in medical practice for the same problem. Based on their individual experience, a later established working group at McMaster University condemned clinical decision making by doctors as hopelessly old-fashioned, and stated that the only solution was their EBM (Evidence-Based Medicine Working Group 1992). Subsequently, clinical experience was reintroduced into the philosophy of EBM by the same working group (Sackett et al. 1996). In the case of pre-EBM medical doctors, their clinical experience was, in reality, the best evidence for treating patients. In those days, this clinical experience was the most complete, easiest, and accessible source of evidence (Karthikeyan and Pais 2010).

Many types of therapeutic and diagnostic approach taught in universities were based on historical traditions rather than on solid scientific research. If a medical hypothesis survived long enough, it was eventually integrated into medical textbooks and, by the time second editions were published, it had become fact for medical students and professionals. However, over the past four decades, the nature of evidence has changed fundamentally. Due to the huge increase in medical research and rapidly developing medical and computer technology, resulting in an ever-increasing stream of scientific publications, a much improved volume of evidence has been created. At the same time, we must realize that this new evidence is not the easiest or most accessible. The problem for today's clinician is that it is almost impossible to stay medically up to date by reading all the medical advances reported in primary journals (Hooker 1997). In general medicine, for example, it would be necessary to read and examine 17 articles a day, 365 days a year (Davidoff et al. 1995). In practice, this becomes even more difficult, and an epidemiological and biostatistical way of thinking is needed in order to judge the content of publications. The consequence and reality is that, more and more often, we have to rely on the evaluation of medical research results and the conclusions of non-medical epidemiologists.

Three parallel developments have probably had a significant effect on the introduction of EBM. Since the 1960s, medicine has seen a sharp rise in new technical developments, and the consequent explosive demand for medical interventions. In addition, life expectancy has increased, resulting in a higher population over 65 years of age, and therefore a greater volume of sick people. At the same time, we are faced with the post-war baby boom generations. The end result is that health costs have risen dramatically. These developments, and the consequences of them, intentionally or unintentionally resulted in a marriage between EBM and healthcare policy makers together with health insurance companies. This can have a negative effect from the point of view that doctors fear that EBM will be adopted by healthcare managers and policy makers in order to justify healthcare costs. Even convinced proponents of EBM judge this to be a misuse of EBM, and state that the number of doctors practicing EBM in order to improve the quality and quantity of life of individual patients may increase rather than lower the cost of their care (Sackett et al. 1996). Further discussion of healthcare management falls beyond the scope of this chapter.

Let us return to the definition of EBM and consider its various constituent parts: EBM is defined as the conscientious, explicit, and judicious use of the best evidence currently available in making decisions regarding the care of individual patients and, therefore, the practice of EBM implies combining individual clinical expertise with the best available external clinical evidence from systematic research (Sackett et al. 1996).

What is (best) evidence?

At first glance, the inclusion of the word 'evidence' in the definition of EBM automatically gives the impression that we are dealing with a sense of scientific authority or truth. The scientific aspect of evidence is the collection and analysis of patient-centred published clinical research, resulting in a final conclusion that can be implemented in daily practice. Most EBM concentrates on the efficacy of all kinds of treatments. These treatments have been evaluated using randomized controlled trials (RCT) as the gold standard. Most well-known RCTs involve the evaluation of the therapeutic effects of a new kind of medication on a particular disease or clinical symptom. Therefore, the pharmaceutical industry ostensibly makes an important contribution to EBM, since it has another aim than just EBM. Before pharmaceutical companies can obtain marketing authorization for a particular product, they must provide regulatory authorities with structured evidence demonstrating safety, quality, and efficacy of the product, and be able to justify the indications and appropriate dosages and to state any contraindications (Ashby and Smith 2000). Nevertheless, most evidence about EBM is derived from such RCTs.

Despite being considered the gold standard in evidence-based practice, RCTs have their limitations, in particular when trying to prove a 'cause and effect' relationship between symptom relief and treatment (Cahana 2005). Firstly, many RCTs are carried out in heterogeneous study populations, with the consequence that both positive and negative efficacies seen in RCTs may be due to unknown subpopulations within the study population. On the other hand, in the case of too strict RCT inclusion and exclusion criteria, the final results only apply to a very small studied population. Factors such as drop out, non-compliance, and a decrease in the patient population can influence treatment outcome analysis. One limitation is that RCTs are usually carried out in a very limited proportion of the population—excluding heterogenous symptoms (which constitute the normal patient population)—and therefore do not provide an answer for problems seen by doctors in their consulting rooms.

Another aspect of RCTs is that, even in high-quality trials with clearly positive efficacy results (for example, cognitive behavioural treatment in low back pain), there may be too little effect to justify implementation into daily practice, let alone for advising individual patients. One of the most uncertain factors in RCTs is the outcome measures, and whether therapeutic intervention and outcome measure(s) are located in the same biological system. For example, how do we evaluate interventional pain treatment when we know that pain is a multidimensional biopsychosocial subjective phenomenon?

In conclusion, RCTs frequently do not reflect daily reality. This means that they usually provide answers to parts of a problem, but not to the whole problem itself. RCTs do not take account of patients' individual psychological and social problems and beliefs and other habits which will be seen in daily practice. Many other aspects of the statistical methodology of RCTs are extensively reviewed elsewhere (Goodman and Greenland 2007; Ioannidis 2005, 2007).

Nowadays, evidence-based guidelines for treatment policies have been developed for all kinds of interventions, including for lower back pain (e.g. manipulation) (Airaksinen et al. 2006). The sources of these guidelines are meta-analyses of previously performed RCTs for a particular treatment. These RCTs form the foundation for the final recommendations in the guidelines. Based on various levels of evidence (Grondon and Schieman 2010), specific recommendations are formulated for treatments of, for example, lower back pain (Airaksinen et al. 2006; Rubinstein et al. 2011). However, it should be understood that these meta-analysis-based recommendations are based on RCTs with all their aforementioned limitations and flaws. Even in the case of a positive recommendation for a particular treatment, we will never achieve a 100% cure rate, or come even close to this (Mullen and Streiner 2004): RCT results apply to 'average patients' (Feinstein and Horwitz 1997).

At the present time, when evaluating treatment efficacy, 'numbers needed to treat' (NNT) are used (Cook and Sackett 1995; Dowie 1998). NNT is the number of patients that must be treated for a particular disease with a particular therapy. NNT illustrates more clearly the relationship between statistical and clinical significance.

Our daily observations of patients raise many questions about 'best evidence', such as why do some patients improve and others do not after having received the same recommended treatment? Since we are dealing with individual patients, we should perhaps change the phrase 'use of current best evidence' in the EBM definition into 'evaluating current best evidence in decision making in the care of individual patients'. Has EBM lost the connection with the reality of daily practice, during which clinicians deal with individual patients? Among other things, our individual patients vary with regard to physiology, mental capacity, emotional stamina, time constraints, family and cultural considerations, financial status, drug and food allergies, willingness to comply, ethnic background, ability to travel, relationship resources, and side-effects to medication (Brase 2008).

More important is the question: has EBM forgotten that practitioners, when diagnosing and treating diseases, face many medical uncertainties, since the precise aetiology and/or pathophysiology of many diseases is only partly known or even lacking? In their daily practice, clinicians frequently use diagnostic procedures that are extracted from hypothetical aetiologies and/or pathophysiologies of diseases which often lack the badly needed gold standards. The same diagnostic procedures are used as inclusion criteria for study populations in RCTs. It can be questioned whether enough attention has been paid to the presence of sufficient reproducibility and/or validity of the diagnostic tests as inclusion criteria. For example, in RCTs evaluating treatment of the lower back, magnetic resonance imaging (MRI) lumbar findings are used as inclusion criteria (Canbulat et al. 2011). However, the reproducibility of MRI lumbar findings with respect to degenerative intervertebral discs is low, with kappa values of around 0.34 as a measure of inter-observer agreement (Madan et al. 2003). The same is true when using lumbar discography images as inclusion criterion (Pneumaticos et al. 2006).

In conclusion, we cannot solely rely on the findings of RCTs as the 'best available evidence', in view of all their shortcomings. Moreover, we also have to realize that what purports to be evidence can only be seen as such until other studies prove it differently, reflecting the 'limited storage life' of the 'best available evidence'.

The contribution of individual clinical expertise

Despite the general enthusiasm for EBM, it also has its share of critics. The major criticism of EBM is that it is perceived as de-emphasizing the patient's values, perspectives, and choices, as well as failing to account for individual social and biological variation (Kohatsu et al. 2004). Therefore, proponents of EBM stress that our individual clinical expertise (or knowledge) must be combined with best available evidence in making decisions about the care of individual patients (Sackett et al. 1996). The additional phrase 'individual clinical expertise' in the EBM definition is completely contradictory to those advocates of EBM who state that its goal is the standardization and not individualization of patient care (Hasnain-Wynia 2006).

Individual clinical expertise can be considered to be the sum total of all the cognitive processes involved in clinical decision making. It involves the appropriate application of knowledge and individual expertise to the problem in hand. Individual knowledge and expertise is more or less the same as that performed by physicians in the pre-EBM era, and is open to all manner of interpretation. Individual knowledge is not a static thing and is dependent on many factors, such as the experience of the physician (seniority), willingness to utilize continuous postgraduate education, and the position of the physician in the healthcare system (peripheral versus university-based). Another problem regarding the addition of 'individual clinical expertise' in the EBM definition is how to judge the quality of the clinical expertise of a particular physician. This has certainly resulted in a lively discussion on how to use the EBM definition in the treatment of individual patients. Young and newly graduated physicians, with an evidence-oriented university medical education but little practical experience, are probably more prone to use EBM as a 'medical cookery book'. This seems to be an undesirable way to simplify medical conditions. In contrast, those who have extensive experience in diagnosing and treating patients, during long careers, rely more heavily on previously acquired medical 'knowledge'. In these cases, empirically based medicine informs them of the best options, but does not carry out the decision making (Marwick 2000).

Individual clinical expertise mainly refers to the diagnostic processes in which a medical history is the most important diagnostic tool in making a correct diagnosis or differential diagnosis. Other psychosocial factors are also included in the medical history in order to provide a complete clinical picture of the patient. The physical examination will then clarify whether the supposed diagnosis can be confirmed or rejected. Complementary diagnostics, such as MRI, can clarify the differential diagnosis. However, we must realize that all diagnostic procedures, including medical history, should be evidence based. This means that they should at least be reproducible in the sense that two physicians using the same diagnostic procedure in the same patient can agree on their final judgement of the diagnostic test. This also applies to all types of imaging techniques (MRI, computed tomography (CT) scan) that frequently are used as the only diagnostic tool. Preferably, the diagnostic test should also be validated with a gold standard. Since the precise aetiology and/or pathophysiology of a disease are frequently unknown, validation of medical diagnostic procedures is generally problematic.

The consequences for healthcare systems constitute a topic that is beyond the scope of this chapter, but certainly reflect the reality of EBM. in the use of all kinds of evidence-based practical guidelines as management tools, and places a mechanism originally intended for internal use into the hands of such 'outsiders' as utilization reviewers, government, and healthcare insurers (Eddy 1990). In particular, governmental departments 'use' evidence-based practical guidelines as medical cost-reducing tools in healthcare systems that leads to computer-embedded guidelines, regulatory stimuli, and financial incentives (Brase 2008). In this way, EBM becomes synonymous with using the 'best cost-reducing' evidence in decision making in the care of individual patients. If, at the present time, EBM were to be rigorously used as the standard criterion for the cost effectiveness of the entire medical profession, many hospital departments would probably have to be closed. EBM was never intended primarily to be associated with the regulation of health costs. Introducing the cost aspect into EBM guidelines creates confusion in decision making for individual patients and diverts attention from the main aim of EBM, which is primarily content-related.

Despite the aforementioned negative aspects of EBM, the apparent shortcomings of RCTs as the gold standard for efficacy, and the (sometimes) contradictory results of systematic reviews, EBM still shows that physicians need to change their attitude towards a more critical approach within their own profession, in the sense that they need to admit to the possibilities and, more importantly, to the difficulties of diagnosing and treating their individual patients.

The principles of evidence-based Manual/ Musculoskeletal Medicine

If we apply the concept of EBM, including its features of using 'best evidence' and 'individual clinical expertise', to Manual/ Musculoskeletal (M/M) Medicine, we must realize that M/M medicine is not as clearly defined as some medical disciplines such as, for example, neurology. Nowadays, M/M medicine is characterized by a conglomerate of different schools, each with their own philosophy, their own diagnostic procedures, and their own therapeutic approaches. These approaches within M/M medicine are frequently named after the pioneers who developed the philosophy of the method, such as Lewit (2010), Janda (1979), Stoddard (1993), Maitland (Hengeveld et al. 2005; Maitland et al. 2005), Mennell (1960), Maigne (2001), Greenman (2003), Still (osteopathy) (Chila 2010; King et al. 2010), and Marsman (Rutte 2002). Moreover, in many countries, M/M medicine comprises a rather eclectic system derived from the different approaches towards it. In the United

States, for example, the osteopathic approach is a philosophy with a comprehensive and holistic form of healthcare, but which also integrates various European-based M/M medicine aspects.

Without going into the details of all the various approaches, the only aspects they apparently have in common are their manually performed diagnostics and treatments. In these diverse schools, therapeutic modalities are not restricted to a single treatment, such as manipulation/mobilization. Other therapies, such as various exercise programmes, local injections, interventional pain treatments, myofascial releasing techniques, trigger-point therapy, neural therapy, balneotherapy, and rehabilitation programmes are frequently integrated into their treatment arsenal in M/M medicine.

Having noted the inexact, diverse descriptions of M/M medicine, we must conclude that 'evidence-based manual/musculoskeletal medicine' is not a concept in which to find definite answers. In the medical literature, despite the other therapeutic modalities that exist, the best therapeutic evidence in M/M medicine is mainly associated with manipulation and/or mobilization (Airaksinen et al. 2006; Assendelft et al. 2013; Bronfort et al. 2004; Rubinstein et al. 2013). Therefore, the systematic analysis of published therapeutic trials in M/M medicine is mainly limited to manipulation/mobilization, using different levels of evidence (see Table 3.1).

For example, with respect to manipulation/mobilization of patients with chronic lower back pain (CLBP), there is some evidence (Level B) that manipulation is superior to sham manipulation for improving short-term pain and function. Moreover, there is some evidence that spinal manipulation, in addition to general practitioner (GP) care, is more effective than GP care alone in the treatment of CLBP (Level B), and it is recommended that a short course of spinal manipulation/mobilization as a treatment option for CLBP be considered (Airaksinen et al. 2006). However, for patients with acute lower back pain, spinal manipulation is no more effective than inert interventions, sham manipulation, or when used together with another intervention (Rubinstein et al. 2013).

Levels of evidence relating to the efficacy of manipulation in CLBP are subsequently integrated into all kinds of national and international healthcare guidelines, comprising various recommendations for its use in the treatment of CLBP. Depending on the country concerned, recommendations can differ markedly with regard to daily practice. This suggests that other factors beyond the scientific analysis of therapeutic results in systematic reviews are decisive in the final recommendations. One of the problems with these defined 'levels of evidence' is that different formats regarding the levels have been published by the same research institute, suggesting an arbitrary application (Vet et al. 2003). An additional problem is the reproducibility of the procedure of assessment of the level of evidence. The inter-observer agreement regarding different levels of evidence is low, with a kappa value of 0.33, resulting in the fact that different formats of levels of evidence can result in completely contradictory conclusions regarding the efficacy of the same treatment (Ferreira et al. 2002). Another problem facing the groups producing these national or international guidelines is how they understand the problem and therapy they are analysing. Moreover, their personal attitude may influence the solution when heterogeneous research data are concluded. For daily practitioners in M/M medicine, these kinds of observations do not make it any easier to interpret and integrate the recommendations of national guidelines on manipulation in CLBP, the more so because they are not familiar with the various types of epidemiological and statistical analysis methods used in their development.

Apart from all the aforementioned critical comments on integrating the best evidence of efficacy, it should be taken into account that every treatment in M/M medicine needs a correct indication. This treatment indication should be based on diagnostic procedures, regardless of the school of M/M medicine from which they originate. An important condition with respect to these diagnostic procedures in different schools of M/M medicine is their proven reproducibility. The same is true of the reproducibility of the anatomical location or segmental level of the spine at which the treatment is applied. For example, RCTs in manipulation and/or mobilization frequently do not use the reproducible diagnostic procedures common in M/M medicine to define their study populations, and do not provide data on how they standardize the anatomical location at which the manipulation is to be applied. In a recent RCT evaluating manipulation in patients with cervicogenic headache, only the general criteria of the International Headache Society were used to define the study population. No data on specific (M/M medicine) diagnostic findings were provided when defining the cervicogenic headache population, and no information was available in the 'Material and method' section of the paper on standardization of the treatment (Haas et al. 2010). The absence of this diagnostic reproducibility in RCTs probably explains both the positive and negative efficacy outcomes of manipulation and/or mobilization in spinal pain disorders.

If we want M/M medicine to be more evidence based, we first have to focus our attention on diagnostic procedures, regardless of training in M/M medicine.

Table 3.1 Levels of evidence for therapy (see Higgins and Green 2011)

Level A	Generally consistent findings provided by (a systematic review of) multiple high-quality randomized controlled trials (RCTs).
Level B	Generally consistent findings provided by (a systematic review of) multiple low-quality RCTs or non-randomized controlled clinical trials (CCTs).
Level C	One RCT (of either high or low quality) or inconsistent findings from (a systematic review of) multiple RCTs or CCTs.
Level D	No RCTs or CCTs.

(Higgins, J. P. T. and Green, S. (2011) *Cochrane Handbook for Systematic Reviews of Interventions*, Wiley.)

Evidence-based diagnostic procedures in Manual/Musculoskeletal Medicine

Numerous textbooks have been written on M/M medicine, and will be used to form the basis of the numerous courses provided by educational systems in this field. The problem is that, after a number of editions have been published, the hypotheses, with their derived diagnostic tests and therapeutic interventions, become the benchmark for students and professionals in M/M medicine, despite the lack of such scientific evidence as the reproducibility and validity of the diagnostic tests.

Nowadays, the blessing of EBM in M/M medicine is that it urges us to develop a more critical attitude towards the content, possibilities, and impossibilities of our profession. The present reality in M/M medicine is that different schools have developed different

Table 3.2 Diagnostic tests for sacroiliac (SI) joint dysfunction taught at different schools of manual/musculoskeletal medicine

SI Tests in Prone Position	SI Tests in Supine Position	SI Test in Neutral Sitting Position
Midline Sacral Thrust Test	Patrick Test	Sitting Flexion Test
SI Joint Play Test	Hip Flexion Adduction Test	PSIS Inequality Test
Prone Knee Flexion Test	SI Translation Test	SI Test in Dynamic Upright Position
Cranial Shear Test	Gaelen's Test	Standing Flexion Test
SI Compression Test	SI Thigh Thrust Test	Spine Test
Ischial Tuberosity Level Test	Supine Long Sitting Test	Retroflexion/Lateral Flexion Test
Four Point Sacral Motion Test	Iliac Crest Height Test	Gillet Test
	Supine Leg Length Test	Pelvic Distortion/Cervical Rotation Test
	Hip Rotation	

diagnostic tests for the same joint. This is clearly illustrated in the case of sacroiliac (SI) joint tests, for example (Table 3.2). Most of these SI tests purport to diagnose the hypomobility of the SI joint and/or the joint as the primary source of pain (Lewit 2010).

Table 3.2 illustrates a fundamental problem in M/M medicine, as defined in the following statement:

> There are many different schools of manual/musculoskeletal medicine in many different countries of the world, with too many different diagnostic procedures and many different therapeutic approaches.

The consequence of this statement is five-fold:

1. Many schools of M/M medicine teach their characteristic diagnostic procedures within their educational systems (including instructional courses). Most of these diagnostic tests have not been proven to be reproducible. The question therefore arises of whether potentially non-reproducible tests are transferable to students. In reproducibility studies, it is often seen that no sufficient overall agreement regarding a test (the percentage of observers agreeing to the test results) can be reached in order to obtain as good a kappa value as possible as a measure for inter-observer agreement. Educational systems should remove these kinds of tests from their instructional course materials. If teaching potentially non-reproducible tests, instructional courses provide M/M medicine practitioners with inadequate diagnostic tools for treating their patients. This can lead to situations where, based on non-reproducibly performed tests, one practitioner can decide to treat a patient with M/M medicine while another does not. Therefore, in M/M medicine, it is essential that educational systems become evidence based.

2. Due to the lack of good reproducibility, validity, sensitivity, and specificity studies, the mutual comparison of diagnostic procedures between schools is completely impossible. Scientific exchange and fundamental discussions between these various schools, based on solid scientific methods, are practically impossible at the present time. Such a situation seriously hampers the development of a definitive specialty of M/M medicine.

3. The absence of validated diagnostic procedures in M/M medicine leads to heterogeneously defined study populations in efficacy trials. Therefore, the comparison of efficacy trials, using the same therapeutic approach (for example, manipulation), is completely impossible.

4. The lack of validated diagnostic procedures from the various schools of M/M medicine, ill-defined therapeutic approaches, and low-quality RCT study designs are the main causes of weak 'best evidence' in the proven efficacy of different treatments used in M/M medicine.

5. If the present situation in M/M medicine should continue, this will lead to a slowing down of the badly needed process of professionalization, and M/M medicine could become obsolete. National and international guidelines will give a negative recommendation with regard to the use of M/M medicine in spinal-related pain syndromes and other diseases and, whether or not it is justified, this will have financial consequences for the daily practitioner in M/M medicine, since healthcare organizations and companies will remove M/M medicine from their protocol. Government and medical service providers may use EBM to the disadvantage of patients when they agree only to fund what has been proven by EBM, which usually means information from RCTs (Kruger 2010). If EBM is used for 'evidence-based purchasing', it will create tension between the best interests of the individual versus the population (Saarni and Gylling 2004).

It should be clear that EBM in medicine in general, and M/M medicine in particular, should focus more on diagnostic procedures with respect to *reproducibility and validity*.

Many diagnostic procedures in the various schools of M/M medicine are based on a particular hypothesis and/or philosophy. For example, various SI tests were developed to test the mobility of the SI joint. Reduced mobility of this joint is thought to be one of the aetiologies of CLBP (Goode et al. 2008). However, it is questionable whether all these tests (see Table 3.2) take account of SI hypomobility (Tullberg et al. 1998). Indeed, cadaver studies have shown the existence of mobility of the SI joint (Smidt et al. 1997). Even in older subjects, there was still a significant amount of sacroiliac motion. However, this motion was too insignificant for the manual detection of sacroiliac asymmetries, even for clinicians with good palpatory and observational skills. In M/M medicine, it can be questioned whether it really tests what it is supposed to test, as suggested by a hypothesis, which in its turn is derived from the prevailing philosophy of a school of M/M medicine. This is called the validity of a test. Validity is determined by measuring how well a test performs against the gold or criterion standard. For a particular clinical test, the criterion standard could be a radiological or surgical finding. The absence of gold standards also constitutes a problem in M/M medicine. Gold standards are essential for both general medicine and M/M medicine in order to provide a scientific basis for hypotheses and their derived diagnostic procedures and treatments. However, before evaluating the validity of a test, it first has to be proven to be reproducible.

In the past decade, an increasing number of reproducibility studies have been published using the kappa value as a measure for inter-observer agreement (Cohen 1960). However, the reality for M/M medicine is that, based on the evaluation of systematic reviews, European guidelines do not, for example, recommend spinal palpatory tests in the diagnosis of lower back pain (Airaksinen et al. 2006). Most of the studies use kappa statistics to assess the reproducibility of a diagnostic procedure (Cohen 1960). In many of these reproducibility studies, evaluating the same diagnostic procedure, a large range of kappa values is found, varying from −0.09 to +1.00 (Patijn and Ellis 2001). In a reproducibility study, if a kappa value of less than 0.60 is found (Landis 1977), the authors conclude that the test has no clinical value. One of the major problems in reproducibility is the dependency of the kappa value on the prevalence of the index condition (P_{index}), which is unknown in advance.

In order to illustrate this problem in more detail, the background of some reproducibility studies is discussed. Figure 3.1 shows the results of a theoretical reproducibility study. Two observers, A and B, carry out the same test in 40 subjects. Observers can agree (Yes/Yes and No/No) or disagree (Yes/No and No/Yes) about the test carried out in the same patient. The levels of agreement and disagreement are shown in a 2×2 contingency table (see Figure 3.1). The P_{index} is calculated using a special formula, as shown in Figure 3.1. This formula includes the positive tests (Yes/Yes, Yes/No, and No/Yes) of the 2×2 contingency table. The relationship between the kappa value and the P_{index} is illustrated in the curve in Figure 3.2.

As already stated, all kappa values found in reproducibility studies to be below the level of 0.60 (see dotted line in Figure 3.2) are thought to have no clinical value. However, if the P_{index} is too low (too few positive tests found) or too high (too many positive tests found) (see blue dots in Figure 3.2), the kappa value will always be below the cut-off level of 0.60 and can even become negative (Patijn and Remvig 2011). This means that, in the majority of the reproducibility studies included in systematic reviews, conclusions have been made based on inappropriate data taken from these studies. Therefore, the European recommendations not to use spinal palpatory tests in the diagnosis of lower back should be reconsidered (Airaksinen et al. 2006).

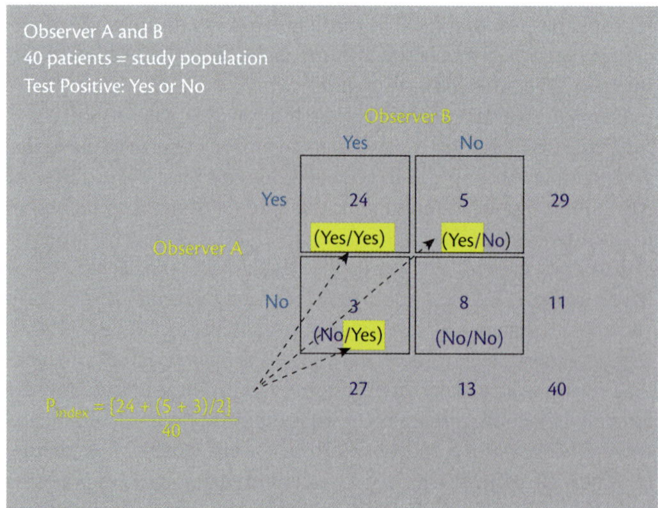

Figure 3.1 The results of a reproducibility study with 40 patients, one test, and two observers (A and B), presented in a 2×2 contingency table to calculate the P_{index}.

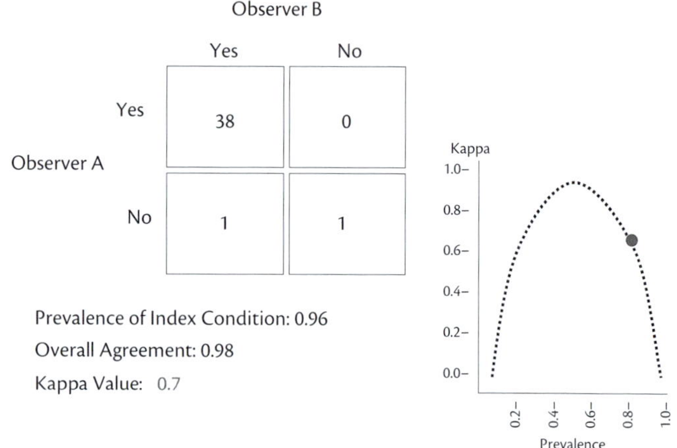

Figure 3.2 Relation between kappa value and prevalence index of the index condition P_{index}. The dotted line is the cut-off level of 0.60. The blue dots indicate low kappa values (arrows) in case of a low (left blue dot) or high (right blue dot) P_{index}.

The International Academy for Manual/Musculoskeletal Medicine has developed a standardized protocol for reproducibility studies in which a solution is provided for tackling the problem of the prevalence of the index condition in these kinds of studies (IAMMM 2011; Patijn et al. 2005). The feasibility of this standardized protocol has been proven in several reproducibility studies (Bakhtadze et al. 2011; Patijn et al. 2005; Vind et al. 2011). For practitioners of M/M medicine, reproducibility studies only showing low kappa values, with no mention of the prevalence of the index condition P_{index}, have no value for their daily practice.

When discussing evidence-based M/M medicine, reproducibility studies of its diagnostic procedures are essential. In particular, reproducible diagnostic procedures are important for defining clinical syndromes. These well-defined clinical syndromes can be used in RCTs to evaluate the efficacy of a treatment. In addition, reproducible diagnostic procedures can be used for validity studies. For example, reproducible global passive cervical rotation tests can be validated with devices that quantify the range of cervical motion. Clinical syndromes defined by medical history and reproducible diagnostic procedures will provide a way to research the philosophy of schools of M/M medicine, and result in the badly needed gold standards in M/M medicine. Until then, estimation of the specificity and sensitivity of diagnostic procedures is possible. At this time, individual clinical experience in M/M medicine meets external clinical evidence. The ability of the practitioner to recognize clinical syndromes based on reproducible diagnostics provides him/her with the tools needed to obtain the best evidence for treatment modalities.

The future of evidence-based medicine in Manual/Musculoskeletal Medicine

The inclusion of a chapter on EBM in a textbook on M/M medicine does not mean that the contents of the other chapters are invalid due to their lack of scientific evidence. The present trend in EBM should stimulate the practitioner in M/M medicine to become more critical about his daily practice. By integrating external evidence into his personal experience, he can acquire more in-depth information on the aetiology of his patients' complaints. By defining clinical syndromes based on reproducible diagnostic procedures, he can apply explicit treatment and, consequently, obtain some prediction of the outcome of his therapy.

On the other hand, it is the task of the scientists at the various schools of M/M medicine to perform reproducibility, validity, specificity, and sensitivity studies. They transfer this information to their students by integrating it into their educational systems.

EBM must never evolve into a 'cost-cutting-based medicine'. Quite rightly, there is fear that EBM will be misused by health insurance companies and healthcare managers in order to cut the costs of healthcare, particularly with respect to an alternative discipline such as M/M medicine. This is not only a misuse of EBM but also a fundamental misunderstanding of its aims. Applying EBM to all disciplines of regular medicine, with the idea of cutting costs, will very likely lead to disastrous problems in healthcare. In this way, EBM becomes a curse to the daily practitioner of M/M medicine.

Using EBM in M/M medicine in the correct way will lead to the further development of our profession. Validated diagnostic procedures become interchangeable between the different schools of M/M medicine. Efficacy trials, based on homogeneous populations, will become mutually comparable. Good practitioners of M/M medicine will use both their indispensable expertise and the best scientific evidence available at that time to provide their patients with the best care possible.

Integrating 'evidence-based medicine' as a tool for developing a more critical attitude towards the possibilities and impossibilities of diagnostic and therapeutic daily care by a practitioner of M/M medicine should be regarded as a blessing.

References

Airaksinen, O., Brox, J. I., Cedraschi, C., et al. (2006) Chapter 4. European guidelines for the management of chronic nonspecific low back pain. *Eur Spine J*

Ashby, D., Smith, A. F. (2000) Evidence-based medicine as Bayesian decision-making. *Stat Med* 19, 3291–305.

Assendelft, W. J., Morton, S. C., Yu, E. I., Suttorp, M. J., Shekelle, P. G. (2013) WITHDRAWN: Spinal manipulative therapy for low-back pain. *Cochrane Database Syst Rev* 1, CD000447.

Bakhtadze, M. A., Patijn, J., Galaguza, V. N. (2011) Inter-examiner reproducibility of the segmental motion palpation springing test for side bending at level C2–C3. *International*

Brase, (2008) 'Evidence-based medicine': rationing care, hurting patients. 1–16.

Bronfort, G., Nilsson, N., Haas, M., et al. (2004) Non-invasive physical treatments for chronic/recurrent headache. *Cochrane Database Syst Rev* CD001878.

Cahana, A. (2005) Ethical and epistemological problems when applying evidence-based medicine to pain management. *Pain Pract* 5, 298–302.

Canbulat, N., Sasani, M., Ataker, Y., et al. (2011) A rehabilitation protocol for patients with lumbar degenerative disk disease treated with lumbar total disk replacement. *Arch Phys Med Rehabil* 92, 670–6.

Chila, A. G. (ed.), American Osteopathic Association. (2010) *Foundations of osteopathic medicine* (3rd ed). Lippincott Williams & Wilkins.

Cochrane, A. L. (1972) *Effectiveness and efficiency: random reflections on health services*. London: Nuffield Provincial Hospitals Trust.

Cohen, J. (1960) A coefficient of agreement for nominal scales. *Educ Psychol Measure* 20, 37–46.

Cook, R. J., Sackett, D. L. (1995) The number needed to treat: a clinically useful measure of treatment effect. *BMJ* 310, 452–4.

Davidoff, F., Haynes, B., Sackett, D., Smith, R. (1995) Evidence based medicine. *BMJ* 310, 1085.

Dowie, J. (1998) The 'number needed to treat' and the 'adjusted NNT' in health care decision-making. *J Health Serv Res Policy* 3, 44–9.

Eddy, D. M. (1990) Practice policies: where do they come from? *JAMA* 263, 1265–72 *passim*.

Evidence-Based Medicine Working Group. (1992) Evidence-based medicine. A new approach to teaching the practice of medicine. *JAMA* 268, 2420–5.

Feinstein, A. R., Horwitz, R. I. (1997) Problems in the 'evidence' of 'evidence-based medicine'. *Am J Med* 103, 529–35.

Ferreira, P. H., Ferreira, M. L., Maher, C. G., Refshauge, K., Herbert, R. D., Latimer, J. (2002) Effect of applying different 'levels of evidence' criteria on conclusions of Cochrane reviews of interventions for low back pain. *J Clin Epidemiol* 55, 1126–9.

Goode, A., Hegedus, E. J., Sizer, P., Jr. (2008) Three-dimensional movements of the sacroiliac joint: a systematic review of the literature and assessment of clinical utility. *The Journal of Manual & Manipulative Therapy*, Vol. 16 No. 1 (2008), 25–38.

Goodman, S., Greenland, S. (2007) Why most published research findings are false: problems in the analysis. *PLoS Med* 4, e168.

Grahame-Smith, D. (1995) Evidence based medicine: Socratic dissent. *BMJ* 310, 1126–7.

Greenman, P. E. (2003) *Principles of manual medicine. Publisher Williams & Wilkins, Baltimore, USA*.

Grondin, S. C., Schieman, C. (2010) Evidence-based medicine: levels of evidence and evaluation systems. In: *Difficult decisions in thoracic surgery*. M.K. Ferguson (ed.) Springer-Verlag London, pp. 13–22.

Haas, M., Spegman, A., Peterson, D., Aickin, M., Vavrek, D. (2010) Dose response and efficacy of spinal manipulation for chronic cervicogenic headache: a pilot randomized controlled trial. *Spine J* 10, 117–28.

Hasnain-Wynia, R. (2006) Is evidence-based medicine patient-centered and is patient-centered care evidence-based? *Health Serv Res* 41, 1–8.

Hengeveld, E., Banks, K., Maitland, G. D. (2005) *Maitland's peripheral manipulation*. Butterworth-Heinemann, London-Boston.

Higgins, J. P. T., Green, S. (2011) *Cochrane handbook for systematic reviews of interventions*. John Wiley.

Hooker, R. C. (1997) The rise and rise of evidence-based medicine. *Lancet* 349, 1329–30.

International Academy of Manual Musculoskeletal Medicine (IAMMM) (2011) *1.Reproducibility and validity: protocol formats for diagnostic procedures in manual musculoskeletal medicine*. Available at: <http://iammm.net>.

Ioannidis, J. P. A. (2005) Why most published research findings are false. *PLoS Med* 2, e124.

Ioannidis, J. P. A. (2007) Why most published research findings are false: author's reply to Goodman and Greenland. *PLoS Med* 4, e215.

Janda, V. (1979) Muskelfunktionsdiagnostik. Acco, Leuven, Belgium

Karthikeyan, G., Pais, P. (2010) Clinical judgement and evidence-based medicine: time for reconciliation. *Indian J Med Res* 132, 623–6.

King, H. H., Jänig, W., Patterson, M. M. (2010) *The science and clinical application of manual therapy*. Elsevier Amsterdam.

Kohatsu, N. D., Robinson, J. G., Torner, J. C. (2004) Evidence-based public health. *Am J Prev Med* 27, 417–21.

Kruger, M. (2010) The ethical approach to evidence-based medicine. *S Afr J Clin Nutr*, 23(1): 1–2.

Landis, J. (1977) The measurement of observer agreement for categorical data. *Biometric*, Vol. 33, No. 1 (Mar., 1977), pp. 159–174.

Lewit, K. (2010) *Manipulative therapy: musculoskeletal medicine*. Churchill Livingstone/Elsevier, Amsterdam.

Madan, S. S., Rai, A., Harley, J. M. (2003) Interobserver error in interpretation of the radiographs for degeneration of the lumbar spine. *Iowa Orthop J* 23, 51–6.

Maigne, J.-Y. (2001) Soulager le mal de dos, Masson, Paris.

Maitland, G. D., Hengeveld, E., Banks, K., English, K. (2005) *Maitland's vertebral manipulation*. Butterworth-Heinemann, Boston.

Marwick, C. (2000) Will evidence-based practice help span gulf between medicine and law? *JAMA, 2000 vol. 283 (21) pp. 2775–2776.*

Mennell, J. M. (1960) *Back pain*. Little, Brown and Company, Boston Toronto.

Mullen, E. J., Streiner, D. L. (2004) The evidence for and against evidence-based practice. *Brief Treat Crisis Interven* 4, 111–21.

Patijn, J., Ellis, R. F. (2001) Low back pain: reproducibility of diagnostic procedures in manual/musculoskeletal medicine. *J Orthop Med* 23, 36–42.

Patijn, J., Remvig, L. (2011) *Reproducibility and validity: protocol formats for diagnostic procedures in manual/musculoskeletal medicine*, Available at: <http://iammm.net>.

Patijn, J., Pragt, E., Ruud, B. (2005) Reproducibility studies in manual/musculoskeletal medicine: a new method for kappa independence from prevalence. *J Orthop Med* 27, 11–16.

Pneumaticos, S. G., Reitman, C. A., Lindsey, R. W. (2006) Diskography in the evaluation of low back pain. *J Am Acad Orthop Surg* 14, 46–55.

Rubinstein, S. M., Terwee, C. B., Assendelft, W. J. J., de Boer, M. R., van Tulder, M. W. (2013) Spinal manipulative therapy for acute low back pain: an update of the Cochrane review. *Spine* 38, E158–77.

Rubinstein, S. M., van Middelkoop, M., Assendelft, W. J. J., de Boer, M. R., van Tulder, M. W. (2011) Spinal manipulative therapy for chronic low back pain: an update of the Cochrane review. *Spine* 36, E825–46.

Rutte, S. (2002) Een visie op de Marsman-methode.

Saarni, S. I., Gylling, H. A. (2004) Evidence based medicine guidelines: a solution to rationing or politics disguised as science? *J Med Ethics, 2004 vol. 30 (2) pp. 171–175.*

Sackett, D. L., Rosenberg, W. M., Gray, J. A., Haynes, R. B., Richardson, W. S. (1996) Evidence based medicine: what it is and what it isn't. *BMJ* 312, 71–2.

Smidt, G. L., Wei, S. H., McQuade, K., Barakatt, E., Sun, T. (1997) Sacroiliac motion for extreme hip positions: a fresh cadaver study. *Spine, 1997 vol. 22 (18) p. 2073.*

Stoddard, A. (1993) Manual of osteopathic practice, Hutchinson, LOndo, Melbourne, Sydney, Auckland, Johannesburg.

Tullberg, T., Blomberg, S., Branth, B., Johnsson, R. (1998) Manipulation does not alter the position of the sacroiliac joint: a roentgen stereophotogrammetric analysis. *Spine, 1998 vol. 23 (10) p. 1124.*

Vet, H., Tulder, M. W., Bouter, L. M. (2003) Levels of evidence—intellectual aid or absolute judgement?, Journal of Clinical Epidemiology, 56(9), 917–918.

Vind, M., Bogh, S. B., Larsen, C. M., Knudsen, H. K., Sogaard, K., Juul-Kristensen, B. (2011) Inter-examiner reproducibility of clinical tests and criteria used to identify subacromial impingement syndrome. *BMJ Open* 1, e000042.

Chapter 4

Musculoskeletal primary care

Nefyn Williams

Introduction to musculoskeletal primary care

Many musculoskeletal specialists only consider primary care to be a source of patient referral. However, musculoskeletal disorders comprise 15–20% of all consultations with a general practitioner (GP) (Jordan et al. 2007; Royal College of General Practitioners 2007) and it has been estimated that 50% of these patients are managed by GPs without referral. GPs are also well placed to carry out triage, gatekeeping, and signposting to other services. They manage patients with multiple morbidities and coordinate complex pathways of care. Together with primary care nurses, the core treatments they provide for musculoskeletal problems include: prescriptions for analgesia, non-steroidal anti-inflammatory drugs, pain-modifying agents, disease-modifying drugs for inflammatory disorders; advice and education about healthy behaviours such as the promotion of weight loss and exercise; cardiovascular risk assessment and osteoporosis screening for patients with inflammatory arthritis; regular monitoring of blood tests for patients on disease-modifying drugs.

The assessment and management of musculoskeletal problems in primary care can be considered in terms of the Royal College of General Practitioners' core competencies (RCGP 2013), which are:

- Primary care management
- Person-centred care
- Specific problem-solving skills
- Comprehensive approach
- Community orientation
- Holistic approach

Musculoskeletal primary care management

Definition

In contrast to specialist musculoskeletal practice, primary care provides general medical care which lacks specificity for any particular organ system. A widely used definition of primary care is that it is 'first-contact, continuous, comprehensive, and co-ordinated care provided by populations undifferentiated by gender, disease, or organ systems' (Starfield 1994).

Primary care as gatekeeper

Primary care is the first tier of a health system, based in the community, provided by general medical practitioners, practice nurses, and other members of the multidisciplinary primary healthcare team. Healthcare systems in which primary care has a central role achieve better health outcomes, higher satisfaction with service users, and lower costs. These benefits are in large part due to the gatekeeping role whereby patients only consult a secondary care specialist after being referred by their primary care practitioner. As specialists order more investigations and perform more procedures, and as these have a monetary cost and the risk of iatrogenic harm, so the gatekeeper role reduces overall costs and adverse events. The downside of this gatekeeper role is the risk of under-treatment by failing to refer on those who would benefit.

Manage primary contact with patients and deal with unselected problems

GPs are often presented with musculoskeletal symptoms which are difficult to differentiate into distinct diagnostic categories. This may be because these symptoms are self-limiting, distorted by early treatment or changed circumstance, intermediate between existing diagnostic labels, a mild or atypical variant of known pathology, not yet understood, or some combination of these (Hungin 2004; Kroenke and Mangelsdorff 1989). Diary studies reveal that individuals tend to develop a new physical symptom on average every five to seven days, the vast majority of which do not result in a consultation. Those individuals who consult doctors are more likely to have had a recent stressful life event (Pennebaker 1983). Individuals with high levels of psychological distress are more likely to notice and complain about internal bodily sensations (Barsky 1999; Pennebaker 1983). The degree of psychological distress is linked to both the number and severity of symptoms (Katon et al. 2001) and healthcare use (Frostholm et al. 2005).

Cover the full range of musculoskeletal conditions

A broad range of musculoskeletal problems can present to primary care. Occasionally, serious pathologies present and it is important that GPs can distinguish these from the majority of less serious non-specific conditions. Examples of serious pathologies include: infection such as septic arthritis, discitis, or osteomyelitis; cancer such as bony metastases; and neurological compromise such as the cauda equine syndrome. These are usually suspected by the presence of 'red flag' symptoms, whose use has spread from their original use in low back pain triage (NICE 2009) to other regions. The next group are specific pathological diagnoses such as lumbar nerve root pain or sciatica, osteoarthritis of the hand, hip, or knee and also inflammatory arthritis such as rheumatoid disease and ankylosing spondylitis. Prompt recognition of inflammatory arthropathy is important because prompt treatment improves long-term prognosis. Similarly, conditions such as internal derangement of the knee and ruptured Achilles tendon should be referred early to an orthopaedic surgeon. Some acute systemic inflammatory conditions can be appropriately treated in primary care, such as polymyalgia rheumatic and gout. Common regional soft-tissue problems such as tennis elbow and trigger finger can also be managed in primary care. Rare connective tissue disease such as lupus may present with non-specific symptoms and affect other organs such as skin, kidneys, and blood vessels. Several musculoskeletal conditions in children present at typical ages, and need to be differentiated from variants of normal.

However, it is often difficult to give patients discrete pathological diagnoses when they present to primary care with musculoskeletal symptoms, and it is often more convenient to give a regional pain syndrome label. The back is the commonest reason for consultation, followed by the knee, chest, and neck (Jordan et al. 2010). In children, the main regional problem is the foot. Widespread pain is common, with 5% of the population consulting with pain from several regions, which is more prevalent in older age groups, females, and in those with chronic pain (Carnes et al. 2007). Epidemiological studies of the general population have demonstrated that most people with a chronic regional pain syndrome also have pain in another region (Kamaleri 2008; Macfarlane 1999). In the case of back pain, patients presenting with back pain plus pain elsewhere are six times more likely to have a poor outcome than patients with back pain alone (Thomas et al. 1999). Patients with such 'chronic widespread pain' are also more likely to have typical associated features of fibromyalgia, such as multiple tender points, fatigue, poor sleep, low mood, and irritable bowel.

Coordinate care with other professionals in primary care and with other specialists

Other musculoskeletal clinicians working in the community include physiotherapists, osteopaths, chiropractors, and acupuncturists, some of whom may be based in primary care or indeed be primary care clinicians. As well as referral to secondary care musculoskeletal services, there are also intermediate care services which are often based in community facilities (Goodwin and Smith 2011).

Person-centred musculoskeletal primary care

Adopt a person-centred approach with patients, in the context of their circumstances

According to McWhinney, person-centred care is at the heart of family medicine (McWhinney and Freeman 2009). This stresses the uniqueness of each patient and that their illness can only be understood in terms of their individual context, taking into account their personal preferences and expectations. Person-centred care emphasizes a long-term, continuous relationship between doctor and patient. Unlike episodic care, it takes a longitudinal approach which can span a whole lifetime. At its best, it allows a long-term therapeutic relationship to develop which makes full use of familiarity and time as diagnostic and therapeutic tools. This relationship should be based on participation rather than paternalism, respecting a patient's autonomy. Consultation skills should emphasis communication; setting priorities in partnership. Satisfaction with care is strongly linked with this focus on patient centredness.

Challenge unhealthy beliefs and behaviours

Health information should be delivered effectively to promote better outcomes. Patients' unhelpful beliefs should be challenged; for example, that their spine is crumbling. Fear is often more disabling than the pain itself in musculoskeletal disorders and fear avoidance beliefs should be identified and challenged. Unhealthy behaviours such as activity avoidance should also be recognized, and more helpful strategies promoted to improve function and maintain physical activity, for example. A treatment plan should be agreed with goals that facilitate self-management.

Specific problem-solving skills in musculoskeletal primary care

Relate decision-making processes to the prevalence of illness in the community

Knowledge of the prevalence and incidence of common musculoskeletal disorders within the community population (see Table 4.1) should be combined with knowledge of the common findings obtained from taking a clinical history and examination of the musculoskeletal system. Time is limited in primary care consultations, so the history and physical examination should be focused on the affected region. The primary care clinician should be familiar with the examination routines described in the later sections of this book for each musculoskeletal region. In addition, there is a rapid screening examination for all of the musculoskeletal system which can be performed within the time constraints of the primary care consultation called the GALS screen (gait, arms, legs, and spine) (Arthritis Research UK).

In contrast to hospital specialists, when solving problems, GPs have to tolerate uncertainty, explore probability, and marginalize danger; hospital specialists have to reduce uncertainty, explore possibility, and marginalize error.

Intervene urgently when necessary

The concept of 'red flags' was first used in the management of low back pain to highlight worrying clinical features suggestive of serious spinal pathology that warrant further investigation (NICE 2009). Their use need not be restricted to back pain and they can be adapted for other regions of the musculoskeletal system.

Manage conditions that may present early and in an undifferentiated way

As can be seen from Table 4.1 and as discussed earlier, much musculoskeletal illness presents to primary care in the form of undifferentiated symptoms. The long-term doctor–patient relationship in primary care is invaluable in the diagnostic process. It provides knowledge of the type, frequency, and manner of previous

Table 4.1 Prevalence of musculoskeletal disorders per 100,000 person years at risk

Condition	Prevalence in population >16 years old	95% confidence intervals
All musculoskeletal disorders	13,275	13,215–13,336
Soft-tissue rheumatism and chronic widespread pain	4068	4034–4104
Back pain	3747	3715–3779
Osteoarthritis	1724	1702–1746
Rheumatoid disease	215	207–223
Polymyalgia rheumatic	165	159–172
Osteoporosis	135	129–141
Ankylosing spondylitis	37	34–40
Systemic lupus erythematosus	13	12–15
Scleroderma	6	5–7
Gout	6	4–7

Data sourced from Jordan KP, Clarke AM, Symmons DP, Fleming D, Porcheret M, Kadam UT, Croft P. Measuring disease prevalence: a comparison of musculoskeletal disease using four general practice consultation databases. *Br J Gen Prac* 2007; 57: pp. 7–14.

presentations by the patient, and also allows the use of time as a diagnostic tool. Owing to the vague undifferentiated nature of much musculoskeletal illness, the primary care clinician must be tolerant of a degree of diagnostic uncertainty (Flocke et al. 2002).

Make effective and efficient use of diagnostic and therapeutic interventions

Investigations have a limited role in the diagnosis and management of musculoskeletal problems in primary care. Plain radiographs are usually not indicated for patients with low back pain in the absence of 'red flag' symptoms. Similarly, there is a poor correlation between the radiographic features of osteoarthritis of the knee on the one hand and pain and functional loss on the other. Decision-making tools are available in some circumstances; for example, the 'Ottawa Rules' are guidelines for deciding whether a patient with a foot, ankle, or knee injury should be offered a plain X-ray to diagnose a possible fracture (Ottawa Hospital Research Unit). Also, blood tests have only a limited role in the diagnosis and management of inflammatory disorders such as rheumatoid disease and polymyalgia rheumatic. Indeed, negative blood tests should not delay the early referral of a suspected inflammatory polyarthropathy.

Comprehensive approach to musculoskeletal primary care

Manage multiple complaints and pathologies simultaneously

Primary care clinicians do not just concentrate on the musculoskeletal system, but address multiple complaints and comorbidities and coordinate care across different sectors and between specialists. This means that GPs should consider musculoskeletal comorbidity such as osteoarthritis when treating other chronic illness. Treatment of musculoskeletal disorders using non-steroidal anti-inflammatory drugs (NSAIDs) can cause problems in terms of gastrointestinal ulceration and bleeding, increased cardiovascular risk, renal impairment, and drug interaction. Mental health problems that influence and exacerbate musculoskeletal health should be identified, such as depression, health anxiety, and fear avoidance. Patients with rheumatoid disease should be safely prescribed disease-modifying agents with careful monitoring for adverse effects; GPs should be aware of the increased cardiovascular and fracture risk for these patients. They must minimize the impact of patients' symptoms on their well-being by taking into account personality, family, daily life, economic circumstances, and physical and social surroundings. A useful model for primary care consulting is that the GP deals with the presenting complaint, the manner in which the patient uses the health service, other relevant chronic illnesses, and then health promotion and disease prevention (Stott and Davis 1979).

Apply health promotion and disease prevention strategies appropriately

In the case of musculoskeletal care, the promotion of health and well-being involves avoiding excessive weight gain, maintaining a healthy diet (including exposure to sufficient sources of calcium and vitamin D), and promoting physical activity. This should include empowering patients and the promotion of self-care including educational information from charities such as Arthritis Research UK (Arthritis Research) and patient support organizations such as Arthritis Care (Arthritis Care).

Manage and coordinate health promotion, prevention, cure, care, and rehabilitation

Coordination of care means that GPs must not just manage disease and prevention, but also coordinate rehabilitation by other therapists and agencies. GPs need to work with patients in their rehabilitation and safe return to work using occupational support services.

Community orientation in musculoskeletal primary care

General medical practices are based in localities with a defined practice population, so GPs should reconcile the health needs of individual patients with the health needs of the community in which they live; balancing these with available resources. GPs are aware of the physical environment where their patients live and need to understand the relationship between health and social circumstances of the practice population. They should also be aware of the main employers in their locality and the effect of work on musculoskeletal conditions; for example, osteoarthritis of the hip in farm workers, osteoarthritis of the knee in miners, vibration white finger from the use of hand-held percussive or powered tools. They should be knowledgeable about the local availability of services and the potential health effects where these services are deficient. In addition, they should understand the effect of musculoskeletal problems leading to work incapacity and its impact on patients' health, their families, and the local community. GPs need to encourage patients to remain at work whenever possible, and to facilitate a patient's return to work by providing consistent advice and the prompt use of occupational health services and other local interventions that minimize work loss. The recently introduced 'fit notes' have replaced illness certification, and these encourage the use of altered working environments and staged return to work to facilitate this (Department for Work and Pensions 2010). Community orientation is also about the tensions that may exist between individual wants and needs and the needs of the wider community.

Holistic approach to musculoskeletal primary care

Biopsychosocial models

Psychological factors such as stress are known to affect the neuroendocrine and immune systems (Haleem et al. 2000) and appear to enhance inflammatory processes in autoimmune disease such as rheumatoid arthritis (Zautra et al. 1998). Psychosocial risk factors such as distress, low mood, and the tendency to communicate bodily distress in response to psychosocial stress (so-called somatization) are important in the development of persistent musculoskeletal pain and disability. When patients consult with musculoskeletal problems, the GP should always consider the physical, psychological, social, occupational, and financial effects on individuals, their carers, and families. They should also be aware of cultural differences in the expression of emotional distress and the presentation of pain and loss of function. Some authors also believe that the biopsychosocial model should also have a spiritual or existential dimension, which is about helping people whose sense of meaning and purpose is challenged by illness (Murray et al. 2003).

Tools for identifying psychosocial factors

To aid identification, these psychosocial factors have been described in terms of different coloured flags (Kendall et al. 2009) to complement the concept of 'red flags' described earlier for clinical features suggestive of serious spinal pathology:

- Yellow flags (personal factors)
  - Thoughts—such as catastrophizing; dysfunctional beliefs and expectations concerning pain, work, and healthcare; negative expectation of recovery; preoccupation with health
  - Feelings—such as worry, distress, low mood, fear of movement, uncertainty about the future
  - Behaviours—such as reporting extreme symptoms, passive coping strategies, serial ineffective therapy
- Blue flags (occupational factors)
  - Employee—such as fear of re-injury, high physical job demand, low expectation of resuming work, low job satisfaction, low social support or social dysfunction in the workplace, perception of high job-related 'stress'
  - Workplace—lack of job accommodation or modified work or employer communication with employee
- Black flags (contextual factors)
  - Misunderstandings and disagreements between key players (including healthcare)
  - Financial and compensation problems
  - Process delays
  - Over-reactions to sensationalist media reports
  - Spouse or family member with negative expectations, fears, or beliefs
  - Social isolation or dysfunction
  - Unhelpful policies or procedures used by the employer

A simple screening tool (STaRT Back (Hill et al. 2008)) has been developed to screen patients with low back pain for prognostic indicators, categorizing them into three categories:

1. low risk of chronicity requiring primary care advice, reassurance, and medication only;
2. medium risk, with physical obstacles to recovery requiring referral for physiotherapy;
3. high risk, with psychological obstacles to recovery which require a psychological component to their treatment.

Difficulties using the biopsychosocial model

In routine clinical care, the biological, psychological, and social components of illness may be interpreted and managed separately, rather than in an integrated manner. Significant symptoms of anxiety or depression are present in 25–52% of primary care patients (Kessler 1999) but many go unrecognized because over half present with physical rather than psychological symptoms. This is partly due to time constraints, but also because the biomedical model in which disease can be viewed independently from the person who is suffering from it, and from his or her social context, remains deeply entrenched in contemporary medical practice and teaching (McWhinney and Freeman 2009). Over-reliance on the biomedical model may result in over-investigation and referral for unnecessary opinions and procedures, which may have adverse effects, as well as waste resources. Inappropriate pathological labelling can also increase psychological morbidity and the likelihood of somatic fixation. One method to tackle this, particularly in the area of medically unexplained symptoms, is in re-attribution, where patients are made aware of the psychosocial contribution to their symptoms (Fink 2002), and also by explaining the concept of somatic dysfunction, which is based on the idea that symptoms can arise from abnormal functioning of the musculoskeletal system that are not dependent upon structural pathological processes (Greenman 1996).

Primary care physiotherapy

Despite the large musculoskeletal burden in primary care, undergraduate training in this area is limited, fragmented, and from a secondary care perspective (Goh et al. 2004). There is often insufficient time, and many GPs lack the skills to diagnose and manage these conditions. In addition, musculoskeletal conditions have not been prioritized in the performance-related component of GPs' remuneration—the Quality Outcomes Framework (QOF). Other professions based in the community, such as physiotherapy, also consider themselves to be primary care professionals. Their advantage is that they provide musculoskeletal knowledge, expertise, and treatment skills. They bring a different philosophy of management which is less embedded in a traditional medical, disease-centred model of care, such as the International Classification of Diseases, and deals more with patients' degree of functional ability, using the International Classification of Functioning (ICF)(World Health Organisation). Increasingly, physiotherapists are accepting self-referrals from patients in the community, bypassing the GP's gate-keeper role. The disadvantages are that these community physiotherapists are not generalists, in that they focus on the musculoskeletal system or a particular patient group such as the frail elderly. Also, there is a danger that GPs will become further deskilled in the management of this patient group.

Vision for the future of musculoskeletal primary care

If primary care is to meet the challenge of managing musculoskeletal patients using the RCGP core competencies, then all GPs need to be competent in musculoskeletal diagnosis and biopsychosocial management. Musculoskeletal skills can be developed through postgraduate education, and courses are available from the Primary Care Rheumatology Society and the British Institute of Musculoskeletal Medicine. In addition, many GPs work in intermediate care and secondary care clinics, and then use the specialist skills they have acquired in their own practices, acting as a practice resource, accepting in-house musculoskeletal referrals. Community physiotherapists and intermediate care clinics should be used not only for referrals but also as an educational resource. Musculoskeletal problems could be managed more proactively in primary care if included in the QOF. Much musculoskeletal care could be shifted to more of a rehabilitation model using the ICF.

References

Arthritis Care (www.arthritiscare.org.uk)

Arthritis Research UK (www.arthritisresearchuk.org/)

Barsky AJMD, Borus JFMD. Functional somatic syndromes. *Ann Intern Med* 1999; 130:910–21.

Carnes D, Parsons S, Ashby D, et al. Chronic musculoskeletal pain rarely presents in a single body site: results from a UK population study. *Rheumatology (Oxford)* 2007; 46:1168–70.

Department for Work and Pensions (DWP). *Statement of fitness for work*. London: DWP, 2010. Available at: <http://www.dwp.gov.uk/docs/fitnote-gp-guide.pdf>.

Fink P. Assessment and treatment of functional disorders in general practice: the extended reattribution and management model—an advanced educational program for nonpsychiatric doctors. *Psychosomatics* 2002; 43:93–131.

Flocke SA, Miller WL, Crabtree BF. Relationship between physician practice style, patient satisfaction and attributes of primary care. *J Family Practice* 2002; 51:10.

Frostholm L, Fink P, Christensen KS, et al. The patients' illness perceptions and the use of primary health care. *Psychosom Med* 2005; 67: 997–1005.

GALS. Arthritis Research UK. The musculoskeletal examination: GALS http://www.arthritisresearchuk.org/health-professionals-and-students/student-handbook/the-msk-examination-gals.aspx#sthash.NpFKR9E9.dpuf

Goh L, Samanta A, Cavendish S, Heney D. Rheumatology curriculum: passport to the future successful handling of the musculoskeletal burden? *Rheumatology* 2004; 43:1468–72.

Goodwin N, Smith J. Developing a national strategy for the promotion of integrated care. The evidence base for integrated care. London: The King's Fund and the Nuffield Trust; 2011. Available at: <http://www.nuffieldtrust.org.uk/sites/files/nuffield/evidence-base-for-integrated-care-251011.pdf>.

Greenman PE. *Principles of manual medicine* (2nd ed). Baltimore MA: Williams and Wilkins, 1996.

Haleem S, Kaplan H, Pollack M. Moderating effects of gender and vulnerability on the relationships between financial hardship, low education and the immune response. *Stress Med* 2000; 16:167–77.

Hill JC, Dunn KM, Lewis M, et al. A primary care back pain screening tool: identifying patient subgroups for initial treatment. *Arthritis Rheum* 2008; 59:632–41.

Hungin P. The therapeutic illusion: self-limiting illness. In: Jones R, Britten N, Culpepper L, et al. (eds) *Oxford textbook of primary medical care* (1st ed). Oxford: Oxford University Press; 2004, pp. 210–4.

ICF. World Health Organization. Towards a common language for functioning, disability and health (ICF). Geneva: WHO, 2002.

Jordan KP, Clarke AM, Symmons DP, et al. Measuring disease prevalence: a comparison of musculoskeletal disease using four general practice consultation databases. *Br J Gen Prac* 2007; 57:7–14.

Jordan KP, Kadam UT, Hayward R, Porcheret M, Young C, Croft P. Annual consultation prevalence of regional musculoskeletal problems in primary care: an observational study. *BMC Musculoskel Disord* 2010; 11: 144

Kamaleri Y, Natvig B, Ihlebaek CM, Bruusgaard D. Localised or widespread musculoskeletal pain: does it matter? *Pain* 2008; 138:41–6.

Katon W, Sullivan M, Walker E. Medical symptoms without identified pathology: relationship to psychiatric disorders, childhood and adult trauma, and personality traits. *Ann Intern Med* 2001; 134:917–25.

Kendall NAS, Burton AK, Main CJ, et al. (on behalf of the Flags Think Tank). *Tackling musculoskeletal problems: a guide for the clinic and workplace*. London: The Stationery Office, 2009.

Kessler D. Cross sectional study of symptom attribution and recognition of depression and anxiety in primary care. *BMJ* 1999; 318:436–9.

Kroenke K, Mangelsdorff D. Common symptoms in ambulatory care: incidence, evaluation, therapy and outcome. *Am J Med* 1989; 86:262–6.

Macfarlane GJ. Generalised pain, fibromyalgia and regional pain: an epidemiological view. *Bailliere's Best Pract Res Clin Rheumatol* 1999; 13:403–14.

McWhinney IR, Freeman T. *A textbook of family medicine* (3rd ed). Oxford: Oxford University Press, 2009.

Murray SA, Kendall M, Boyd K, Worth A, Benton TF. General practitioners and their possible role in providing spiritual care: a qualitative study. *Brit J Gen Prac* 2003; 53:957–9.

Ottawa rules. Ottawa Hospital Research Institute. Ottawa ankle rules. www.ohri.ca/emerg/cdr/docs/cdr_ankle_poster.pdf

Pennebaker JW. *The psychology of physical symptoms*. New York: Springer-Verlag, 1983.

Red flags for back pain. National Institute for Health and Care Excellence (NICE) Clinical Knowledge Summaries. Back pain – low (without radiculopathy) 2009 Assessing for serious risks. http://cks.nice.org.uk/back-pain-low-without-radiculopathy#!diagnosissub:2

Royal College of General Practitioners (RCGP). *RCGP curriculum 2010* (revised 14 August 2013). London: RCGP, 2013. Available at: <http://www.rcgp-curriculum.org.uk/PDF> (accessed January 2014).

Royal College of General Practitioners (RCGP). *Birmingham Research Unit weekly returns service annual prevalence report 2007*. Birmingham: RCGP, 2007.

Starfield B. Is primary care essential? *Lancet* 1994; 344(8930):1129–33.

Stott NCH, Davis RH. The exceptional potential in each primary care consultation. *J Roy Coll Gen Prac* 1979; 29:201–5.

Thomas E, Silman AJ, Croft PR, Papageorgiou AC, Jayson MI, Macfarlane GJ. Predicting who develops chronic low back pain in primary care: a perspective study. *BMJ* 1999; 318:1662–7.

Zautra AJ, Hoffman JM, Matt KS, et al. An examination of individual differences in the relationship between interpersonal stress and disease activity among women with rheumatoid arthritis. *Arthritis Care Res* 1998; 11:271–9.

Chapter 5

The social determinants of pain: from body work to social work

Jens Foell

Introduction and overview to the social determinants of pain

An old medical adage states 'the sick, the poor, and the old will always be with us'. Add 'female' to this list and the scene is set for the social determinants of pain, which broadly reflect categories of social disadvantage.

This chapter explores musculoskeletal pain in the community and will consider questions such as: How common is musculoskeletal pain (and how sure are we of this)? What are its consequences? Whose problem is it? How can it be prevented? How and to what extent does its distribution relate to the distribution of work within the healthcare professions and between medical and social care? How do different health and welfare systems address the problem?

It should already be clear that this is not a biomedical account of musculoskeletal pain. The focus in this chapter is on the 'social', on what is widely known as the 'biopsychosocial' model of pain (Engel 1977). It explores the social determinants of chronic pain and presents a case that these 'social' factors deserve much greater attention in the therapeutic encounter than is usually assumed. Sociosomatic medicine—that is the relationship between the body and the society in which the body is living—is the topic of this chapter; this is distinct from psychosomatic medicine (Schaefer 1966).

Using musculoskeletal pain as an index condition, I explore the modifiable and non-modifiable factors contributing to the emergence of chronic problematic pain (van Hecke et al. 2013; Barker et al. 2014). Pain which is widespread in individual bodies is also widespread in the population; estimates range between 10% and 35% (Ospina and Hartstall 2002). Players in the health industry may see this as an opportunity to market their drugs, interventions, and educational programmes. The high prevalence of chronic pain, coupled with its 'chronicity', makes it an attractive target for pharmaceutical companies; an estimated 530 million pounds per year is spent on non-cancer analgesics in the UK alone (BBC 2013). However, the medicalization of the pain experience is fraught with difficulty, especially since most interventions for chronic pain have very limited evidence of effectiveness (Borsook and Kalso 2013; Williams et al. 2011). This chapter will go some way towards addressing why the medicalization of musculoskeletal pain is so problematic. In particular, it will outline why this approach, however seductive its appeal, serves neither patients nor doctors well.

Social aspects of musculoskeletal pain

How common is (widespread) musculoskeletal pain in the general population?

Musculoskeletal disorders play a significant role as part of the rising burden of non-communicable diseases alongside cardiovascular, metabolic, and mental health conditions (Murray et al. 2012). The overarching term 'musculoskeletal disorders' includes categories of heterogeneous aetiology, such as inflammatory arthritides (including seropositive and seronegative arthropathies), tendinopathies, fractures, osteoarthritis, low back pain, and regional pain syndromes of all sorts. The focus of this chapter is on chronic musculoskeletal pain associated with polysymptomatic distress.

Low back pain and knee pain are the commonest causes of pain in the locomotor system (Brooks 2006). The prevalence of osteoarthritis of the knee has been estimated as 13% for women and 10% for men (Zhang and Jordan 2010). As expected, the figures vary depending on sample selection, definition, and methodology. Risk factors for the onset of symptomatic osteoarthritis include obesity, age, previous trauma, and female gender (Blagojevic et al. 2010). A recent systematic review investigating the global prevalence of low back pain suggested caution regarding the interpretation of the results (Hoy et al. 2012). The variations in anatomical definition of low back pain and the duration of pain prevent a simple answer; the range of figures oscillates between 11.9 ± 2.0% as point prevalence and 23.2 ± 2.9% for one-month prevalence (Hoy et al. 2012). Prevalence estimates are further complicated by issues relating to the robustness of original data sources (the accuracy of clinical coding, for example), and variations related to method of data collection. Postal surveys may yield very different results from data extraction from clinical systems. Depending on definition, sampling frame, and survey methodology, the range of estimates varies between 10% and 35% of the adult population (Ospina and Hartstall 2002). The heterogeneity of the definitions and methodologies makes the interpretation of these findings difficult. A recent systematic review and meta-analysis of chronic widespread pain in the general population analysed these aspects in great detail and estimated chronic widespread pain at 10% point prevalence. It is well recognized that self-reporting via questionnaires leads to higher levels of reported pain than face-to-face-interviews, which in turn lead to higher levels of reported pain than morbidity coding in medical databases (Mansfield 2013).

Does musculoskeletal pain occur in isolation?

Musculoskeletal pain rarely occurs at only one site in the body (Carnes et al. 2007; Raftery et al. 2011). However, the structure of short medical interactions which are typical of general practice (including a recent trend towards 'one consultation, one problem') tends to encourage patients to report single-site pain (Rohrbeck et al. 2007). Unless there is a deliberate invitation by the doctor to uncover pain at different sites of the body, the issue of widespread pain is easily missed, as is the opportunity to explore the potentially important relationship between pain at one site and pain at another. If the conceptual lens of the practitioner is widened to incorporate problems in other body regions and organ systems, the potential is opened for a wider range of diagnoses on one hand, and opportunities to co-create meaning on the other hand. Furthermore, enquiry into the intensity of pain, its duration, and the distribution across different body sites can have important implications for the patient's prognosis (Mallen et al. 2007). In the context of stratified care (i.e. different care packages for subgroups of patients), this is an important conversation to have (Muller et al. 2013). If for example, psychological factors like 'catastrophizing' form a significant part of the pain experience, it is wise to offer these patients therapies with psychological components (Bair et al. 2013; Foster et al. 2014).

Many patients suffering from chronic pain, especially those who are older or poorer, have more than one coexisting pathology (multimorbidity) or more than one manifestation of a single pathology (comorbidity) (Valderas et al. 2009). These patients present a difficult problem for service providers. The structure of health services in most industrialized societies, where services are organized around specialisms and distributed over a range of care providers, adds an institutional layer of complexity to the problem and contributes (harmfully and somewhat artificially) to the framing of these patients as 'difficult', 'undesirable', or 'heartsink' (Koekkoek et al. 2011). To add to an already complicated picture, each medical specialism has its own repertoire of taxonomies and discourses to make sense of soft-tissue complaints. The wide variation in terminology and explanatory models may increase the confusion which people affected by persistent pain often report (Toye et al. 2013).

Poverty and pain

The association between pain experience and socioeconomic status is well documented (Assumpcao et al. 2009; Macfarlane et al. 2009; Poleschuck and Green 2008). The severity of chronic pain and markers of poverty are correlated (Bridges 2012). Which modus operandi is in place? Is it related to the area one is living in? (Eachus et al. 1999; Urwin et al. 1998) Is it mediated by educational status? (Brekke et al. 2002; Roth and Geisser 2002) To what extent is status within the social hierarchy and personal control over workload predictive of the experience of pain? (De Vogli et al. 2007) Is the association between low socioeconomic status mediated by material factors like transport, access to services, exposure to adverse environmental circumstances? (Jordan et al. 2008) Or are emotions the key players in the emergence of problematic pain in association with low socioeconomic status? (Keefe et al. 2001)

The literature suggests a variety of processes mediating between social rank and pain characteristics (Schurer et al. 2014). All of the aforementioned factors—area, educational status, and control over workload—have been shown to have an effect on the prevalence and intensity of pain in a population. This also holds true for relative poverty (the difference in material status within a population), even in populations that are affluent overall. Indeed, the sharpness of the social gradient or the width between the richest and poorest within a society has been shown to affect health outcomes of the society as a whole, including the better off! (Wilkinson and Pickett 2007)

Cultural diversity

Increasing cultural diversity of the population adds another dimension to interactions about musculoskeletal pain, and is worthy of special attention (Meeuwesen et al. 2007; Priebe et al. 2011; Rechel et al. 2013). This, it turns out, is not just an issue of ethnic diversity or different cultural scripts about how pain is experienced or presented, since the picture is complicated by the overrepresentation of patients from ethnic minorities in populations of low socioeconomic status. The challenges presented by the combination of social disadvantage, cultural barriers, and language barriers in healthcare consultations have been reported extensively (Kai et al. 2007). Musculoskeletal pain in combination with mental health problems adds to the complexity. 'Idioms of distress'—the multiple ways in which bodies display distress—often include somatic pain (Nichter 2010). The process of making sense of this situation in interactions between clinician and patient, in order to arrive at what Clark has called 'fusion of horizons', is often a long process and one which is facilitated by continuity of care (Clark 2008). Continuity of care remains primarily within the realm of general practice (Uijen et al. 2012).

Musculoskeletal pain is often the presenting complaint for complex traumatic experiences, even torture (de C Williams 2013). Disclosure of such sensitive issues as past or present exposure to physical and psychological violence needs a safe environment to facilitate managing the consequences (Crosby 2013). Musculoskeletal pain in combination with other symptoms such as headaches, visceral pain, and genitourinary pain is relatively common, and should guide the curiosity of the practitioner towards enquiring about traumatic situations in the background. Whether the polysymptomatic presentation is considered as an indicator for the presence of central sensitization or as an 'idiom of distress', it needs thorough assessment and careful negotiation of management strategies (Aggarwal et al. 2006; Hinton and Lewis-Fernandez 2010). Stress-related physical and mental symptoms have a high prevalence amongst refugees (9% for post-traumatic stress disorder (PTSD), 5% for major depression) (Fazel et al.).

Social suffering and musculoskeletal pain

Spectrum bias: the social dimension

The degree to which clinicians have to engage with social disadvantage varies widely given that practices serve local communities which tend to be characterized by particular (and often rather narrowly defined) socioeconomic characteristics (Carr-Hill et al. 1996). The gap is even wider when one compares musculoskeletal services in a public-funded setting with those delivered in the private sector. Whereas hands-on therapies such as manual medicine or acupuncture are easily accessible and frequently sought and delivered in the latter, they are rarely funded or commissioned in the public sector (Bishop et al. 2012). Inequities are reported regarding access to various components of musculoskeletal services, ranging from joint replacement surgery to access to self-management programmes (Ackerman and Busija 2012).

It is well recognized that chronic widespread pain can be a manifestation of a spectrum of stress-related disorders (de Kloet et al. 2005; McFarlane 2007). The ability to cope with adversity, to maintain stability through change, is closely related to the resources available to the sufferer and issues of social and financial capital (McEwen 2010). Factors such as adverse childhood experiences or exposure to domestic violence or intimate partner violence shape the illness trajectory over a lifetime, and this extends to the life of children involved (Bardes et al. 2001; Coker et al. 2005; Davis et al. 2005; Ellsberg et al. 2008; Jones et al. 2009; Kirkengen 2008; McBeth et al. 1999; Von Korff et al. 2009). The experience of being excluded is known to intensify the pain experience, and this has been shown to be true even in experimental conditions with healthy volunteers (Eisenberger et al. 2003). Migrants from war-torn countries frequently experience both types of disadvantage—the sequelae of past trauma and the experience of present disenfranchisement in the host society (Bhui et al. 2003; Cook and England 2004; Kirmayer 2002, 2007; Löfvander and Furhoff 2002).

The severity of the pain experience and the ability to live the life one wants to live despite adversity, is associated with socioeconomic status. The scope of practice in socially deprived areas or in services intended for marginalized people (e.g. outreach services for people affected by homelessness or for refugees) needs to reflect this reality; a 'one size fits all' approach is unlikely to address the particular complexities of life at the margins of society (Feldman 2006; Fiscella and Epstein 2008). A group of general practitioners (GPs) looking after disadvantaged communities in Scotland recently formed an association, under the banner of the 'deep end', with the aim of addressing the social determinants of health in the populations they serve (Mercer et al. 2007; Watt 2004, 2011, 2012). This includes a variety of linked approaches, ranging from allowing more time in medical appointments in order to address complexity within continuity of care, to a multifaceted approach to support vulnerable families who frequently experience 'multiple jeopardy' and close organizational alignment with social services (Marcenko et al. 2012). Legislative approaches, such as welfare policy, try to address similar problems on a macropolitical level (Deep End Steering Group 2013).

Epistemologies of pain and suffering

Although commonly juxtaposed, 'pain' and 'suffering' are usually regarded as different categories of experience. The term 'pain'—at least in medical circles—tends to be associated with neurophysiological processes, explained in terms of scientific phenomena such as central sensitization. By contrast, suffering conveys a more existential meaning, lending itself less readily to this kind of scientific reasoning (Porter 1993; Wall 1999). From a sociological viewpoint, suffering is seen as 'the cultural struggle to reconstitute a positive sense of meaning and purpose for self and society against the brute force of events in which these are violated and destroyed' (Wilkinson 2005). Suffering is often (but clearly not always) the result of what a person has physically and emotionally endured, and in a way is 'testimonial to what has happened' (Candib 2002). The damage inscribes itself into the bodies in various ways—some reversible and amenable to biomedical technologies, some irreversible, and here to stay (Kleinman 1995). This situation, in which social hurt cannot be removed with medical means from the body or from the life of the patient, invites an alternative framework for interactions: this alternative framework draws on anthropological concepts of suffering (Delvecchio Good et al. 1992). Clifford Geertz summarized it in his quote 'man is an animal suspended in webs of significance that he himself has spun' (Geertz 1994). The existential issues, in contrast, are situated either in the realm of psychological approaches or in the under-researched area of pastoral care and holding work (Cocksedge et al. 2011).

The biopsychosocial model has been criticized for lumping conflicting approaches together in a medicalizing concept (Armstrong 1987). The term 'biopsychosocial' embraces all these aspects. The sequence of the components seems to indicate a hierarchy, and also different accountabilities. 'Bio' is the domain of biomedical interventions, 'psycho' shifts the accountability to the engaging patient, whereas 'social' stands for the overwhelming but unmodifiable forces of environment and society. What can be done then about the 'S' in the biopsychosocial (BPS) model? At least one way to address these factors is the active and dedicated engagement in processes of social administration. This includes an awareness of the 'politics of diagnosis' in matters relating to housing, work, and access to health, as much as dedicated work to influence these social determinants of health.

Competition and consensus: healthcare services for musculoskeletal pain

The range and purpose of musculoskeletal services

Services addressing musculoskeletal matters are delivered in the medical sector, the fitness industry, and in the realm of complementary and alternative medicine. The organizing principal, broadly speaking, may be wellness or illness. The agenda may be performance enhancement or injury prevention, help with maintaining a balance in body–mind–environment interactions, or treatment which follows a biomedical diagnosis. The boundaries between these sectors are at times blurred; for example, some purpose-built medical centres include a gym for patients, and the 'entrepreneurial' practice may employ a range of complimentary practitioners. Each different professional grouping brings with it a particular 'professional vision' that is an interpretation of the phenomenon under scrutiny (e.g. musculoskeletal pain) that is shaped by a range of socially constructed discursive practices particular to that professional group—in other words, 'practices for seeing' (Goodwin 1994). There is physiotherapy as a profession, which grew alongside the medical profession and has gained independent status in some countries. There are independent practitioners like chiropractors and osteopaths, whose core skills consist of the handling of soft tissues. There are also fitness instructors, massage therapists, independent acupuncturists, complementary therapists, and healers who treat muscular aches and pains. Primary care provides access to medical services on a community level. Specialist medical services and physiotherapy are available under various access criteria via third-party funding, but also as independently accessed services (which still may require a referral from primary care). Osteopaths and chiropractors operate predominantly in the private sector. Massage therapists, healers, and fitness instructors commonly rely on 'out of pocket' treatments to generate their income. These service configurations have an effect on the provider–client interaction.

The historical roots of musculoskeletal knowledge systems

Many hands-on therapist-delivered musculoskeletal practices have their ideological roots in systems which have an uneasy relationship with the reductionist approach of Western biomedicine. Therapies like massage, acupuncture, osteopathy, and chiropractic are commonly accessed by people who are bothered by musculoskeletal ailments. These interaction-rich, hands-on, therapist-delivered therapies are based on models which differ in their fundamental assumptions from orthodox biomedical practice. It must be said at this point, that what constitutes 'orthodox' or 'heterodox' practice is not stable across time and place. The hallmark of biomedicine is the foundation on Western scientific practice. Anatomy and physiology are the core disciplines in scientific Western medicine. All scholarly medical systems before 1800 were based on the assumption of a balance of vital forces. Medical practice consisted of manipulating these forces, which went by a range of names such as 'humours', 'vapors', 'pneuma', or 'qi'. The significant paradigm change occurred after the French revolution, when the attention shifted away from an enquiry based on symptoms to the examination of the body, or from the lived (subjective) experience to the (apparently) 'objective' physical signs. The physician's question shifted from 'What's the matter with you?' to 'Where does it hurt?'. A medical diagnosis could now be made by subordinating the subjectivity of the patient, since 'truth' was to be discovered in the patho-anatomical correlation. The post-mortem examination instructed the gaze of the medical practitioner (Foucault 1986). Ultimate truth was seated in the dead body, and hospitals were the institutions in which this knowledge was generated. Diseases were localized alterations from the norm. The diseased organ, extracted from the dissected cadaver and displayed in a jar in a pathology collection, epitomizes this approach.

This new agenda of establishing an objective account of the state of the tissues diminished the assumed authority of the patient over his bodily knowledge. It also affected the physician's experience in interpreting these accounts, which were enriched by the clinical examination. History taking and examination are still today the basic building block of medical encounters, but this process is often further objectified by laboratory investigations. For a huge proportion of musculoskeletal complaints, it is not possible to validate the experienced distress by technological investigations; there is no jar in a pathology museum labelled 'fibromyalgia'. This invalidation of the lived experience, or rather its 'subordination' beneath the superior account of the physician and his technological artefacts, is particularly problematic, since it places constraints on what it is possible to accomplish or explain and may, in turn, be potentially harmful to patients (Colloca 2007; Williams 2009).

Musculoskeletal therapies include a heterogeneous set of health-care practices with roots in traditional medicine in various medical cultures, such as bone setting and mechanotherapy in the West, or acupuncture in the East. The genealogical lineage of physiotherapy as a discipline leads to continental Europe after the Napoleonic wars. Incorporating the educational ideas of Jean-Jacques Rousseau into a system of physical and moral development was the core agenda in the pedagogic systems of philanthropic reformers like J.C.F. GutsMuths in Germany and Per Ling in Sweden (Brodin 2008; Terlouw 2007). These educational systems were used in the institutions to form young bodies, school and military, and also as therapeutic tools to deal with orthopaedic conditions such as curvatures of the spine or malformations of the feet. The ideological components of nature therapy included the therapeutic use of air and water alongside massage. 'Physiotherapy' as a term to describe these practices was coined in 1851 by the German military physician Lorenz Gleich (Juette 1996). It sits conceptually close to naturopathy as an eclectic medical discipline, which is characterized by using stimulation therapies. The discipline of physical medicine and rehabilitation has its ideological roots in this historical formation.

Spinal irritation conceptualized the spine as a source of irritation for nerves, the body structure with the highest status in nineteenth-century medical thinking (Allan and Waddell 1989). Two messianic Midwesterners developed holistic therapeutic systems in contrast to the reductionist agenda of European laboratory medicine. Osteopathy and chiropractic originated in the medical climate of nineteenth-century Northern America. A.T. Still founded osteopathy as a method to achieve equilibrium of form and function of the musculoskeletal system. D.D. Palmer developed chiropractic as a reactive and preventative system to address obstructions of nerves, which have consequences for the physiological functioning of the body (Howell 1999). These systems originated in the United States in the context of a pluralistic medical market place with fierce competition within orthodox medicine and between professions.

Acupuncture and moxibustion (the therapeutic application of mugwort incense as heat treatment on specific body sites) came to the attention of Western medical elites as a by-product of the colonization of Eastern markets. Wilhelm ten Rhyne was a physician attached to the Dutch East India Trade Company, and he published *De acupunctura* in 1683 (Schullian 1979). Western medicine in those times combined high status for the scholarly medical elite with dangerous and ineffective treatments. Doctors were therefore all too often the subject of satire. Ten Rhyne described, with the eyes of an academic insider, the practices of an alternative knowledge system. The medicine he saw in Japan involved piercing the skin with needles at defined points according to a belief system he did not understand. Skin piercing was common practice in Western medicine: cupping and phlebotomy by lancets or leeches belonged to standard medical interventions. The Eastern worldview, however, was very different and could not easily be mapped onto Western conventions. This is well illustrated by the use of a familiar example—taking the pulse. This common practice for both Eastern and Western practitioners involves placing a finger on the wrist to feel the patient's pulse. However, the knowledge system to interpret the differences in soft-tissue movement diverges substantially. One system draws conclusions on mechanical actions of the heart, blood pressure, and stiffness of the arterial walls. The other system infers changes of the inner workings of the relationships between organ systems, which include morphological non-existing organs like the triple burner. These differences in interpretive paradigms between Eastern and Western traditions have existed since antiquity

(Kuriyama 2002). Losses in translation from Chinese or Japanese into Latin, and from Latin into English, were unavoidable. Western medical acupuncture—the translation of an Eastern medical practice into a Western scientific model—was on the cards more than 300 years ago (Bivins 2001).

Professional regulation, governance, and scientific method

It should be clear by now that musculoskeletal pain is a contested field, and that in a pluralistic healthcare arena, this breeds competition between healthcare providers for patients (or 'clients' depending on the nature of the service contract). The competition may be for lucrative segments, such as working with elite athletes or delivering 'bespoke' wellness services for the well off. There is also competition for the masses of people that are covered by basic insurance. However, this is not just a competition driven by financial interests; there is also competition for the authority to interpret bodily experience.

Evidence-based medicine has firmly established the place of probabilistic statistics as a means to evaluate the efficacy and effectiveness of treatments, and this has become a crucial tool in healthcare politics (Harrison et al. 2002). The randomized controlled trial (RCT) is at the centre of this endeavour. Evidence-based medicine poses a particular challenge to complex interventions formed by multidimensional therapy (and the therapist). Their multidimensional character makes them less readily amenable to blinding, standardization, and randomization (Fregni et al. 2010). Access to a research infrastructure also becomes a prerequisite to keep therapies and methods on the market. Physiotherapy is one musculoskeletal profession which has been successful in establishing its academic credentials. Research institutions and governmental bodies are not exclusive for one or the other profession. Current developments see a blurring of professional boundaries in the delivery, research, and administration of healthcare. What happened first in the realm of orthodox medicine—the closely interrelated combination of research and its interpretation and application in guidelines and pathways—is now gradually happening in the sector of complementary and alternative medicine. Acupuncture and spinal manipulation for the treatment of low back pain, for example, have been widely investigated and informed the development of evidence-based treatment guidelines (Furlan et al. 2005; Rubinstein et al. 2011).

The stakeholders in the field of musculoskeletal care

Unlike specialisms such as ophthalmology or urology, the field of musculoskeletal medicine is not (yet) generally regarded as a specialism in its own right, and neither is it a coherent community of practice (Lave and Wenger 1991). This is at least, in part, because the field does not consider a single-organ or a single-treatment approach but crosses numerous disciplinary traditions, each with their own emphasis, their own set of approaches to treatment, and, crucially, different understandings of the meaning and nature of 'sickness' and 'health'. Orthopaedic surgeons are specialized in surgical interventions; rehabilitation specialists, in coordinating strategies for regaining function, dealing with multisystemic disability. Physiotherapists are experts in assessing movement and function, and favour exercise-based therapies. Pain specialists focus on injection therapies and advanced pharmacotherapy and work in hospital-based multidisciplinary teams. Sports and exercise specialists predominantly focus on exercising as a means to address problems of the body that is already engaging in purposeful loading strategies. Occupational health specialists deal with the problems of work, be it from an ergonomic or a psychological perspective. Psychologists have their expertise in the psychological dimensions of human relationships. Osteopaths, chiropractors, some physiotherapists, and also doctors trained in manipulative techniques apply hands-on procedures to the tissues in order to restore or optimize function. General practitioners see musculoskeletal pain in the context of the person as a whole (including significant others), manage prescribing and referrals, and add their knowledge as expert generalists. This list is not exhaustive but demonstrates that no specialism can claim authority over the field of musculoskeletal medicine. It is therefore of paramount importance to establish a discourse, which allows the separate and disparate skills and knowledge bases to synergistically interact with each other for the sake of the benefit of the patient.

At present, what these separate specialisms have in common is that they are exposed to similar dilemmas—for example, how to interact effectively with the person as a whole, taking the complexity of musculoskeletal pain into account. They also share the commonality of not being entitled, trained, or paid to address all facets of these painful, multifaceted conditions. What may be regarded as a 'holistic' practice is inevitably a small, relatively tightly defined area of expertise, and care is still fragmented as a result. The absence of definite authority over the knowledge field of musculoskeletal medicine places every actor in a position of limited influence. This in itself is not a bad thing, if the actors in the field can agree on core competencies and safe approaches, which facilitate transition of care and reduce semantic confusion for patients.

Complexity and continuity of care—relationships and information

Chronic pain often coexists with depression and anxiety (Arnow et al. 2006; Bair et al. 2008; Dominick et al. 2012; Gerrits et al. 2014). Unfortunately, this combination challenges the way healthcare is organized. Healthcare practitioners looking after the body may touch the person; helpers concerned with the mental state will mainly talk. Access to specialist services, embodied by the presence of a coordinated multidisciplinary team including psychology and physiotherapy services, is the standard to achieve for these situations. Cross-sectional surveys and clinical audits have revealed that this is the exception, not the norm (Price et al. 2012).

> Complexity is the rule in the co-morbid pain patient, not only for diagnosis, but also for management needs to be integrated across disciplines. In an era of super-specialisation, where there is a risk of treating diseases specifically and separately, we must acknowledge the essential role of a unifying clinician, who can sum up and coordinate all the specialist interventions for a pain patient. (Giamberardino and Jensen 2012)

The work of unifying, coordinating, making sense, negotiating, and listening is highly skilled labour (Cocksedge 2005). It needs psychological flexibility, health-systems literacy, high information-processing skills, and last, but not least, kudos and status. Haggerty describes the role of the main coordinator to be

> . . . the provider with the most comprehensive knowledge, typically the general practitioner or the family doctor . . . What matters for continuity is that the designation and the role of the coordinating person should be visible to the patient and to others in the system. (Haggerty 2012)

UNIVERSITY OF SHEFFIELD LIBRARY

Vulnerable patients and those with complex multimorbidities are most affected if continuity of care is hampered. Good communication and sharing of information are needed (Freeman 2011). Good care needs trust between clinician and patient. Trust between clinicians is needed to make care transitions useful (Calman and Rowe 2008). However, sensitive biographical information (for example, the disclosure of intimate partner violence) or, in other words, the patient's narrative, is not a value-free dataset, to cut and paste from one organization to another, from one relationship to another (Brody 1994). Care coordination is therefore much more than time spent with the patient. It is also time spent for the patient and on behalf of the patient, which often involves the skilful work of dealing with the dynamics of incompatible information systems.

The social determinants of pain: why is the personal political?

How does the social get under the skin? And into the muscles? The association between low socioeconomic status and mortality (alongside other health outcomes, such as birthweight) is well established; there are numerous examples demonstrating the stark contrasts in life expectancy between wealthy or poor parts of the same city (such as between Newton Mearns and Dalmarnock in Glasgow, or even the drop in life expectancy along the Jubilee Line in London, moving in an eastward direction) (Hanlon et al. 2006; Office for National Statistics 2008).

The World Health Organization (WHO) defines the social determinants of health as

> . . . the circumstances, in which people are born, grow up, live, work and age, and the systems put in place to prevent and treat illness. These circumstances are in turn shaped by a wider set of forces: economics, social policies, and politics. (Commission on Social Determinants of Health 2008)

How these forces interact in detail is unknown. One epidemiological study concludes that psychological factors mediate between socioeconomic status and chronic widespread pain (Davies et al. 2009). This supports a model featuring predominantly psychosocial factors. However, the hypothesized link between the perception of stress, physiological stress systems, and polysymptomatic distress has not been demonstrated by measuring biomarkers (Aggarwal et al. 2013). Materialist or neo-materialist frameworks, in contrast, look at material factors (housing, transport, access to public services, nutrition) as main variables in this interplay of body, mind, and environment (Lynch et al. 2000). Nancy Krieger includes a life-course dimension in her ecological model of health inequalities (Llosa et al. 2013). 'Embodiment' is the term she uses to describe the relationship between individual bodies and the environment which shapes people's lives (Krieger 2005).

Social justice continues to have a pivotal role in the social determinants of health, regardless of the weighting of individual factors and the hierarchy of their connections. It affects both equity (fair and equal access to common goods) and inequality (the asymmetrical distribution of means). The lack of social justice is the fuel in the fire of persistent distress of humans as social animals. Alcohol use and violence, for example, are more predominant in societies with stark contrast between rich and poor (Wolf et al. 2014). Wilkinson and Pickett point to the association between income inequality and public health outcomes (2006). The social gradient, they argue, does not only affect the lower strata of society, it has an effect on society as a whole.

The ascent of the civil rights movements and feminism, in particular, directed the interest of justice into what had previously been described as private matters. The way in which power relationships influence seemingly private matters, such as sexuality and reproductive work, became a publicly debated topic. Sexual abuse and domestic violence, matters which have been attributed to private relationships, outside the public domain, became public matters. This is mirrored in the drive to include domestic/interpersonal violence into the catalogue of matters which need to get addressed in medical frameworks (Duxbury 2011; Feder et al. 2011; Garcia-Moreno et al. 2006; Kendall-Tackett et al. 2003; Malpass et al. 2014; Shefet et al. 2007; Taft et al. 2013). Screening for domestic violence is now advocated in current public health guidance of the National Institute of Health and Social Care Excellence (NICE) (2014).

Wilkinson and Pickett demonstrate, in comparisons between and within countries, how inequality and unfairness is associated with health outcomes such as obesity, teenage pregnancies, literacy, and mental health. This is a product of relative poverty (the difference between social ranks) in contrast to absolute poverty (access to basic life commodities such as shelter and nutrition). Pain is not explicitly mentioned as a category, but the association between chronic pain and variables linked to relative poverty (obesity, low educational attainment, isolation, exclusion) has already been mentioned extensively. It means that the consequences of discrepancies in wealth distribution affect also the wealthy; that social relationships permeate the boundaries between the classes. Although Wilkinson and Pickett did not consider patients with chronic pain explicitly, I hope I have made clear that there is a strong association between the prevalence of chronic pain and several of the variables which feature in this epidemiological work. The logical conclusion would be that chronic musculoskeletal pain is less an issue in more equal societies. However, does this hold true?

The welfare state paradox

At this point, it is useful to step back and compare and contrast the various ways in which health and social care are laid out in different economies. It pays attention to the roles of the state, the family, and the market in welfare provision (Esping-Andersen 1990). Welfare state typologies commonly distinguish between Scandinavian (social democratic), Anglo-Saxon (liberal), Bismarckian (conservative), and Southern countries (Ferrera 1996). The Scandinavian model features a strong interventional role for the state in promoting social equality through a redistributive social security system. Continental European conservative models (Germany, Austria, France) aim to maintain existing social patterns; unemployment allowance, for example, is delivered as a percentage of preceding earnings. In liberal welfare models, this is not the case. Here, unemployment allowance is delivered at a flat rate and not related to previous earnings.

These different approaches reflect different underpinning ideologies regarding the contribution of family, kinship, state, and market economy to the welfare system. A survey of 65,000 people across 218 regions in 21 countries, exploring the perception of their global health, concluded that 90% of the perceived health is related to individual factors, 10% to system factors (Eikemo et al. 2008). What is the role of health systems in particular within the fabric of the welfare state? Wide variations exist regarding public/private ownership, remuneration policies (fee for service vs. capitation), state involvement, coverage, and governance (Thomson et al. 2012).

Primary care has been identified as the key mechanism of effective healthcare delivery (Starfield et al. 2005). It features equal access to healthcare, affordability, and continuity of care as essential components (Kringos et al. 2010). Comparative transnational health systems' research on European primary care systems concluded that these systems are associated with high healthcare expenditure, reduced growth rates in healthcare spending, reductions in unnecessary hospitalizations, and reduced socioeconomic inequality in self-rated health (Kringos et al. 2013). However, 'self-rated health' is a subjective variable. Hard facts, such as the discrepancy of mortality rates between the social strata, support the notion that despite advances in other areas such as housing and access to culture, health inequalities persist in developed welfare regimes. (Beckfield and Krieger 2009). A variety of hypotheses try to explain these findings and include health selection as a consequence of increased social mobility (adoption of healthy lifestyles by the ones who move up in social rank), mathematical artefacts, psychosocial and neo-materialist explanations, a life-course perspective, and also the material consequences of immaterial factors, such as cultural capital (Bambra 2011; Mackenbach et al. 2008). How does the social get under the skin? This question arises again, and it becomes linked with the old feminist slogan, 'the personal is political' (Mackenbach 2010).

Summarizing the social determinants of pain

In this chapter, I have dealt with what I have called the sociosomatic aspects of illness—the complex relationship between the body and the society in which the body is living. Using musculoskeletal pain as an index condition, I have explored the modifiable and non-modifiable factors contributing to the emergence of chronic problematic pain (van Hecke et al. 2013). I have applied an eclectic range of conceptual and disciplinary lenses to make sense of suffering, guided primarily by a curiosity to understand how the social gets under the skin, or what Kirkengen refers to as the 'biology of poverty' (Kirkengen 2008).

By juxtaposing descriptions of different strategies which aim to alleviate the effects of chronic pain, ranging from hands-on therapies (with the individual) to welfare state provision (for the collective), I have moved from body work to social action, and in doing so, have exposed the extent to which efforts underpinned primarily by a commitment to the biomedical model fall short of being able to explain—let alone provide a solution for—the patient with chronic musculoskeletal pain. It seems that social hurt cannot be removed from the body by medical means. It is not the patient who is the 'difficult' problem. These patients *become* problematic *because* they do not neatly 'fit' existing compartmentalized organizational structures. Chronic pain is not necessarily 'unexplainable', as so often concluded in the medical context (Dowrick 2011; de C Williams and Johnson 2011). Rather, it may only *become explainable* (and therefore remediable) by explicit reference to a multilayered, multiperspectival, multidisciplinary approach. The issues that need attention lie deeply hidden in the thicket of workforce organization and in processes of social administration. A greater focus on the 'S' in the biopsychosocial model of illness invites a concept of pain which encompasses much more than the identification of maladaptive processes.

The poor, the old, and the sick will always be with us. So what might be done to improve the lot of patients who endure chronic and unremitting musculoskeletal pain? Perhaps one approach would be to widen the range of expertise on offer at the chronic pain clinic, to ensure that attention is paid to those aspects of patients' lives which often remain partially or, at worst, wholly unexplored in current service models. If a robust effort was made to include all the relevant professional perspectives, then I suggest it is highly likely that the 'chronic pain clinic' would look rather less like a 'clinic' than it typically does at present.

However—and here comes more than a consolation—we always do all that is possible to improve matters: the haptic exploration of the body that experiences this hurt, paired with the capacity to listen to the patient's story, and knowledge about the healthcare system itself, provides at least the basis for a good working relationship in order to bring things forth.

References

Ackerman IN, Busija L. Access to self-management education, conservative treatment and surgery for arthritis according to socioeconomic status. *Best Practice & Research Clinical Rheumatology* 2012; 26(5):561–83; doi: 10.1016/j.berh.2012.08.002.

Aggarwal VR, Macfarlane GJ, Tajar A, et al. Functioning of the hypothalamic–pituitary–adrenal and growth hormone axes in frequently unexplained disorders: results of a population study. *European Journal of Pain* 2013; doi: 10.1002/j.1532-2149.2013.00413.x.

Aggarwal VR, McBeth J, Zakrzewska JM, et al. The epidemiology of chronic syndromes that are frequently unexplained: do they have common associated factors? *International Journal of Epidemiology* 2006; 35(2):468–76; doi: 10.1093/ije/dyi265.

Allan DB, Waddell G. An historical perspective on low back pain and disability. *Acta Orthopaedica Scandinavica Supplementum* 1989; 234:1–23.

Armstrong D. Theoretical tensions in biopsychosocial medicine. *Social Science & Medicine* 1987; 25(11):1213–8.

Arnow BA, Hunkeler EM, Blasey CM, et al. Comorbid depression, chronic pain, and disability in primary care. *Psychosomatic Medicine* 2006; 68(2):262–8; doi: 10.1097/01.psy.0000204851.15499.fc.

Assumpcao A, Cavalcante A, Capela C, et al. Prevalence of fibromyalgia in a low socioeconomic status population. *BMC Musculoskeletal Disorders* 2009; 10(1):64.

Bair MJ, Poleshuck EL, Wu J, et al. Anxiety but not social stressors predict 12-month depression and pain severity. *Clinical Journal of Pain* 2013; 29(2):95–101.

Bair MJ, Wu J, Damush TM, et al. Association of depression and anxiety alone and in combination with chronic musculoskeletal pain in primary care patients. *Psychosomatic Medicine* 2008; **70**(8):890–7; doi: 10.1097/PSY.0b013e318185c510.

Bambra C. Health inequalities and welfare state regimes: theoretical insights on a public health 'puzzle'. *Journal of Epidemiology and Community Health* 2011; 65(9):740–5; doi: 10.1136/jech.2011.136333.

Bardes CL, Gillers D, Herman AE. Learning to look: developing clinical observational skills at an art museum. *Medical Education* 2001; 35(12):1157–61; doi: 10.1046/j.1365-2923.2001.01088.x.

Barker C, Taylor A, Johnson M. Problematic pain—redefining how we view pain? *British Journal of Pain* 2014; 8(1):9–15; doi: 10.1177/2049463713512618.

Beckfield J, Krieger N. Epi + demos + cracy: linking political systems and priorities to the magnitude of health inequities—evidence, gaps, and a research agenda. *Epidemiologic Reviews* 2009; 31(1):152–77; doi: 10.1093/epirev/mxp002.

Bhui K, Abdi A, Abdi M, et al. Traumatic events, migration characteristics and psychiatric symptoms among Somali refugees. *Social Psychiatry and Psychiatric Epidemiology* 2003; 38(1):35–43; doi: 10.1007/s00127-003-0596-5.

Bishop FL, Amos N, Yu H, et al. Health-care sector and complementary medicine: practitioners' experiences of delivering acupuncture in the public and private sectors. *Primary Health Care Research & Development* 2012; FirstView:1–10; doi: 10.1017/S1463423612000035.

Bivins R. The needle and the lancet: acupuncture in Britain, 1683–2000. *Acupuncture in Medicine* 2001; 19(1):2–14.

Blagojevic M, Jinks C, Jeffery A, et al. Risk factors for onset of osteoarthritis of the knee in older adults: a systematic review and meta-analysis. *Osteoarthritis and Cartilage* 2010; 18(1):24–33; doi: 10.1016/j.joca.2009.08.010.

Borsook D, Kalso E. Transforming pain medicine: adapting to science and society. *European Journal of Pain* 2013; 17(8):1109–25; doi: 10.1002/j.1532-2149.2013.00297.x.

Brekke M, Hjortdahl P, Kvien T. Severity of musculoskeletal pain: relations to socioeconomic inequality. *Social Science Medicine* 2002; 54(2):221–8.

Bridges S. Chapter 9: Chronic pain. In: *Health survey for England—2011; health, social care and lifestyles*. London: Health and Social Care Information Centre, 2012.

Brodin H. Per Henrik Ling and his impact on gymnastics. *Svensk Medicinhistorisk Tidskrift* 2008; 12(1):61–8.

Brody H. 'My story is broken; can you help me fix it?': medical ethics and the joint construction of narrative. *Literature and Medicine* 1994; 13(1):79–92.

Brooks P. The burden of musculoskeletal disease—a global perspective. *Clinical Rheumatology* 2006; 25(6):778–81; doi: 10.1007/s10067-06-0240-3.

Calnan M, Rowe R. Trust relations in a changing health service. *Journal of Health Services Research & Policy* 2008; 13(suppl 3):97–103; doi: 10.1258/jhsrp.2008.008010.

Candib LM. Working with suffering. *Patient Education and Counseling* 2002; 48(1):43–50; doi: 10.1016/s0738-3991(02)00098-8.

Carnes D, Parsons S, Ashby D, et al. Chronic musculoskeletal pain rarely presents in a single body site: results from a UK population study. *Rheumatology* 2007; 46(7):1168–70.

Carr-Hill R, Rice N, Roland M. Socioeconomic determinants of rates of consultation in general practice based on fourth national morbidity survey of general practices. *British Medical Journal* 1996; 312:1008–12.

Clark J. Essay: Philosophy, understanding and the consultation: a fusion of horizons. *British Journal of General Practice* 2008; 58:58–60.

Cocksedge S, Greenfield R, Nugent GK, et al. Holding relationships in primary care: a qualitative exploration of doctors' and patients' perceptions. *British Journal of General Practice* 2011; 61(589):e484–e91; doi: 10.3399/bjgp11X588457.

Cocksedge S. *Listening as work in primary care*: Oxford: Radcliffe Press, 2005.

Coker AL, Smith PH, Fadden MK. Intimate partner violence and disabilities among women attending family practice clinics. *Journal of Women's Health* 2005; 14(9):829–38; doi: 10.1089/jwh.2005.14.829.

Colloca L. Nocebo hyperalgesia: how anxiety is turned into pain. 2007.

Commission on Social Determinants of Health. Closing the gap in a generation—health equity through action on the social determinants of health. Geneva: WHO, 2008.

Cook A, England R. Pain in the heart: primary care consultations with frequently attending refugees. *Primary Care Mental Health* 2004; 2(2):107–13.

Crosby SS. Primary care management of non-English-speaking refugees who have experienced trauma: a clinical review. *Journal of the American Medical Association* 2013; 310(5):519–28; doi: 10.1001/jama.2013.8788.

Davies KA, Silman AJ, Macfarlane GJ, et al. The association between neighbourhood socio-economic status and the onset of chronic widespread pain: results from the EPIFUND study. *European Journal of Pain* 2009; 13(6):635–40.

Davis DA, Luecken LJ, Zautra AJ. Are reports of childhood abuse related to the experience of chronic pain in adulthood? A meta-analytic review of the literature. *The Clinical Journal of Pain* 2005; 21(5):398–405.

De Vogli R, Ferrie JE, Chandola T, et al. Unfairness and health: evidence from the Whitehall II Study. *Journal of Epidemiology and Community Health* 2007; 61(6):513–8; doi: 10.1136/jech.2006.052563.

Deep End Steering Group. Deep End Report 21: GP experience of welfare reform in very deprived areas In: Watt G, Orr R, (eds.) *Deep End Report*. Glasgow: University of Glasgow, 2013, p. 15.

Delvecchio Good M-J, Brodwin PE, Good BJ, et al. *Pain as a human experience: an anthropological perspective*. Berkeley: University of California Press, 1992.

Dominick CH, Blyth FM, Nicholas MK. Unpacking the burden: understanding the relationships between chronic pain and comorbidity in the general population. PAIN 2012; 153(2):293–304; doi: 10.1016/j.pain.2011.09.018.

Dorner TE, Muckenhuber J, Stronegger WJ, et al. The impact of socio-economic status on pain and the perception of disability due to pain. *European Journal of Pain* 2011; 15(1):103–9; doi: 10.1016/j.ejpain.2010.05.013.

Dowrick C. Persistent pain: the need for a cooperative approach. *British Journal of General Practice* 2011; 61(591):639–40; doi: 10.3399/bjgp11X601488.

Duxbury F. Domestic violence, PTSD, and diagnostic enquiry. *British Journal of General Practice* 2011; 61(589):496–7; doi: 10.3399/bjgp11X588385.

Eachus J, Chan P, Pearson N, et al. An additional dimension to health inequalities: disease severity and socioeconomic position. *Journal of Epidemiology and Community Health* 1999; 53(10):603–11; doi: 10.1136/jech.53.10.603.

Eikemo TA, Bambra C, Judge K, et al. Welfare state regimes and differences in self-perceived health in Europe: a multilevel analysis. *Social Science & Medicine* 2008; 66(11):2281–95.

Eisenberger NI, Lieberman MD, Williams KD. Does rejection hurt? An fMRI study of social exclusion. *Science* 2003; 302(5643):290–2.

Ellsberg M, Jansen HAFM, Heise L, et al. Intimate partner violence and women's physical and mental health in the WHO multi-country study on women's health and domestic violence: an observational study. *The Lancet*; 371(9619):1165–72; doi: 10.1016/S0140-6736(08)60522-X.

Engel G. The need for a new medical model: a challenge for biomedicine. *Science* 1977; 196(4286):129–36; doi: 10.1126/science.847460.

Esping-Andersen G. *The three worlds of welfare capitalism*. Princeton: Princeton University Press, 1990.

Fazel M, Wheeler J, Danesh J. Prevalence of serious mental disorder in 7000 refugees resettled in western countries: a systematic review. *The Lancet*; 365(9467):1309–14; doi: 10.1016/S0140-6736(05)61027-6.

Feder G, Davies RA, Baird K, et al. Identification and Referral to Improve Safety (IRIS) of women experiencing domestic violence with a primary care training and support programme: a cluster randomised controlled trial. *The Lancet* 2011; 378(9805):1788–95.

Feldman R. Primary health care for refugees and asylum seekers: a review of the literature and a framework for services. *Public Health* 2006; 120(9):809–16; doi: 10.1016/j.puhe.2006.05.014.

Ferrera M. The 'Southern model' of welfare in social Europe. *Journal of European Social Policy* 1996; 6(1):17–37; doi: 10.1177/095892879600600102.

Fiscella K, Epstein RM. So much to do, so little time: care for the socially disadvantaged and the 15-minute visit. *Archives of Internal Medicine* 2008; 168(17):1843–52; doi: 10.1001/archinte.168.17.1843.

Foster NE, Mullis R, Hill JC, et al. Effect of stratified care for low back pain in family practice (IMPaCT Back): a prospective population-based sequential comparison. *The Annals of Family Medicine* 2014; 12(2):102–11; doi: 10.1370/afm.1625.

Foucault M. *The birth of the clinic*. London, 1986.

Freeman GK. Holding relationships in general practice: What are they? How do they work? Are they worth having? *British Journal of General Practice* 2011; 61(589):487–8; doi: 10.3399/bjgp11X588240.

Fregni F, Imamura M, Chien HF, et al. Challenges and recommendations for placebo controls in randomized trials in physical and rehabilitation medicine: a report of the international placebo symposium working group. American Journal of Physical Medicine and Rehabilitation 2010; 89(2):160–72; doi: 10.1097/PHM.0b013e3181bc0bbd.

Furlan AD, van Tulder MW, Cherkin DC, et al. Acupuncture and dry-needling for low back pain. *Cochrane Database of Systematic Reviews* 2005(1):Cd001351; doi: 10.1002/14651858.CD001351.pub2.

Garcia-Moreno C, Jansen HAFM, Ellsberg M, et al. Prevalence of intimate partner violence: findings from the WHO multi-country study on women's health and domestic violence. *The Lancet* 2006; 368(9543):1260–9; doi: 10.1016/s0140-6736(06)69523-8.

Geertz C. Thick description: toward an interpretive theory of culture. *Readings in the Philosophy of Social Science* 1994:213–31.

Gerrits MMJG, van Oppen P, van Marwijk HWJ, et al. Pain and the onset of depressive and anxiety disorders. *Pain* 2014; 155(1):53–9; doi: 10.1016/j.pain.2013.09.005.

Giamberardino MA, Jensen TS. *Pain comorbidities—understanding and treating the complex patient*. Seattle: IASP Press, 2012.

Goodwin C. Professional vision. *American Anthropologist* 1994; 96(3):606–33; doi: 10.1525/aa.1994.96.3.02a00100.

Haggerty JL. Ordering the chaos for patients with multimorbidity. *British Medical Journal* 2012; 345; doi: 10.1136/bmj.e5915.

Hanlon P, Walsh D, Whyte B. Let Glasgow flourish—a comprehensive report on health and its determinants in Glasgow and West Central Scotland. Glasgow: Glasgow Centre for Population Health, 2006, p. 360.

Harrison S, Moran M, Wood B. Policy emergence and policy convergence: the case of 'scientific-bureaucratic medicine' in the United States and United Kingdom. *The British Journal of Politics & International Relations* 2002; 4(1):1–24; doi: 10.1111/1467-856x.41068.

van Hecke O, Torrance N, Smith BH. Chronic pain epidemiology—where do lifestyle factors fit in? *British Journal of Pain* 2013; doi: 10.1177/2049463713493264.

Hinton D, Lewis-Fernández R. Idioms of distress among trauma survivors: subtypes and clinical utility. *Culture, Medicine and Psychiatry* 2010; 34(2):209–18; doi: 10.1007/s11013-0-9175-x.

Howell JD. The paradox of osteopathy. *New England Journal of Medicine* 1999; 341(19):1465–8; doi:10.1056/NEJM199911043411910.

Hoy D, Bain C, Williams G, et al. A systematic review of the global prevalence of low back pain. *Arthritis & Rheumatism* 2012; 64(6):2028–37; doi: 10.1002/art.34347.

Jones GT, Power C, Macfarlane GJ. Adverse events in childhood and chronic widespread pain in adult life: results from the 1958 British Birth Cohort Study. *Pain* 2009; 143(1–2):92–6

Jordan KP, Thomas E, Peat G, et al. Social risks for disabling pain in older people: A prospective study of individual and area characteristics. *Pain* 2008; 137(3):652–61; doi: 10.1016/j.pain.2008.02.030.

Juette R. *Geschichte der alternativen medizin—von der volksmedizin zu den unkonventionellen therapien von heute*. Muenchen: C.H.Beck, 1996.

Kai J, Beavan J, Faull C, et al. Professional uncertainty and disempowerment responding to ethnic diversity in health care: a qualitative study. *PLoS Med* 2007; 4(11):e323; doi: 10.1371/journal.pmed.0040323.

Keefe FJ, Lumley M, Anderson T, et al. Pain and emotion: new research directions. *Journal of Clinical Psychology* 2001; 57(4):587–607; doi: 10.1002/jclp.1030.

Kendall-Tackett K, Marshall R, Ness K. Chronic pain syndromes and violence against women. *Women & Therapy* 2003; 3(1–2):45–56; doi: 10.1300/J015v26n01_03.

Kirkengen A. Inscriptions of violence: societal and medical neglect of child abuse—impact on life and health. *Medicine, Health Care and Philosophy* 2008; 11(1):99–110; doi: 10.1007/s11019-07-9076-0.

Kirmayer LJ. Editorial: Refugees and forced migration: hardening of the arteries in the global reign of insecurity. *Transcultural Psychiatry* 2007; 44(3):307–10.

Kirmayer LJ. The refugee's predicament. *L'Evolution Psychiatrique* 2002; 67(4):724–42.

Kleinman A. *Pain and resistance—the delegitimation and relegitimation of local worlds. Writing at the margin—discourse between anthropology and medicine*. Berkeley: University of California Press, 1995, pp. 120–46.

de Kloet ER, Joels M, Holsboer F. Stress and the brain: from adaptation to disease. *Nature Reviews Neuroscience* 2005; 6(6):463–75.

Koekkoek B, Hutschemaekers G, van Meijel B, et al. How do patients come to be seen as 'difficult'?: a mixed-methods study in community mental health care. *Social Science & Medicine* 2011; 72(4):504–12; doi: 10.1016/j.socscimed.2010.11.036.

Krieger N. Embodiment: a conceptual glossary for epidemiology. *Journal of Epidemiology and Community Health* 2005; 59(5):350–5; doi: 10.1136/jech.2004.024562.

Kringos D, Boerma W, Hutchinson A, et al. The breadth of primary care: a systematic literature review of its core dimensions. *BMC Health Services Research* 2010; 10(1):65.

Kringos DS, Boerma W, van der Zee J, et al. Europe's strong primary care systems are linked to better population health but also to higher health spending. *Health Affairs* 2013; 32(4):686–94; doi: 10.1377/hlthaff.2012.1242.

Kuriyama S. *The expressiveness of the body and the divergence of Greek and Chinese medicine*. New York: Zone Books, 2002.

Lave J, Wenger E. *Situated learning: legitimate peripheral participation*. Cambridge University Press, 1991.

Llosa AE, Ghantous Z, Souza R, et al. Mental disorders, disability and treatment gap in a protracted refugee setting. *The British Journal of Psychiatry* 2014; 204(3):208–13; doi: 10.1192/bjp.bp.112.120535.

Löfvander MB, Furhoff A-K. Pain behaviour in young immigrants having chronic pain: an exploratory study in primary care. *European Journal of Pain* 2002; 6(2):123–32; doi: 10.1053/eujp.2001.0309.

Lynch JW, Smith GD, Kaplan GA, et al. Income inequality and mortality: importance to health of individual income, psychosocial environment, or material conditions. *British Medical Journal* 2000; 320(7243):1200–4; doi: 10.1136/bmj.320.7243.1200.

Macfarlane GJ, Norrie G, Atherton K, et al. The influence of socioeconomic status on the reporting of regional and widespread musculoskeletal pain: results from the 1958 British Birth Cohort Study. *Annals of the Rheumatic Diseases* 2009; 68(10):1591–5; doi: 10.1136/ard.2008.093088.

Mackenbach JP, Stirbu I, Roskam A-JR, et al. Socioeconomic inequalities in health in 22 European countries. *New England Journal of Medicine* 2008; 358(23):2468–81; doi: 10.1056/NEJMsa0707519.

Mackenbach JP. New trends in health inequalities research: now it's personal. *The Lancet* 2010; 376(9744):854–5; doi: 10.1016/S0140-6736(10)60313-3.

Mallen CD, Peat G, Thomas E, et al. Prognostic factors for musculoskeletal pain in primary care: a systematic review. *British Journal of General Practice* 2007; 57(541):655–61.

Malpass A, Sales K, Johnson M, et al. Women's experiences of referral to a domestic violence advocate in UK primary care settings: a service-user collaborative study. *British Journal of General Practice* 2014; 3(620):e151–e158; doi: 10.3399/bjgp14X677527.

Mansfield K. Identifying chronic widespread pain in primary care—a medical record database study [Doctor of Philosophy]. Keele University, 2013.

Marcenko MO, Hook JL, Romich JL, et al. Multiple jeopardy: poor, economically disconnected, and child welfare involved. *Child Maltreatment* 2012; 17(3):195–206; doi: 10.1177/1077559512456737.

McBeth J, Macfarlane GJ, Benjamin S, et al. The association between tender points, psychological distress, and adverse childhood experiences—a community-based study. *Arthritis and Rheumatism* 1999; 42(7):1397–404.

McEwen BS. *Neurobiology of interpreting and responding to stressful events: paradigmatic role of the hippocampus*. John Wiley & Sons, Inc., 2010.

McFarlane AC. Stress-related musculoskeletal pain. *Best Practice & Research: Clinical Rheumatology* 2007; 21(3):549–65; doi: 10.1016/j.berh.2007.03.008.

Meeuwesen L, Tromp F, Schouten BC, et al. Cultural differences in managing information during medical interaction: how does the physician get a clue? *Patient Education and Counseling* 2007; 67(1–2):183–90; doi: 10.1016/j.pec.2007.03.013.

Mercer SW, Fitzpatrick B, Gourlay G, et al. More time for complex consultations in a high-deprivation practice is associated with increased patient enablement. *British Journal of General Practice* 2007; 57:960–6.

Morgan CL, Conway P, Currie CJ. The relationship between self-reported severe pain and measures of socio-economic disadvantage. *European Journal of Pain* 2011; 15(10):1107–11; doi: 10.1016/j.ejpain.2011.04.010.

Muller S, Thomas E, Dunn KM, et al. A prognostic approach to defining chronic pain across a range of musculoskeletal pain sites. *Clinical Journal of Pain* 2013; 29(5):411–6.

Murray CJL, Vos T, Lozano R, et al. Disability-adjusted life years (DALYs) for 291 diseases and injuries in 21 regions, 1990–2010: a systematic analysis for the Global Burden of Disease Study 2010. *The Lancet* 2012; 380(9859):2197–223.

NICE. Domestic violence and abuse—how services can respond effectively (PH50). In: *Excellence* NIoHaC, (ed.) Manchester, 2014.

Nichter M. Idioms of distress revisited. *Culture, Medicine and Psychiatry* 2010; 34(2):401–16; doi: 10.1007/s11013-0-9179-6.

Office for National Statistics, Public Health England. *Taking the Jubilee Line route to health inequalities*. 2008. Available at: <http://www.lho.org.uk/LHO_Topics/National_Lead_Areas/HealthInequalitiesOverview.aspx>.

Ospina M, Harstall C. Prevalence of chronic pain: an overview. HTA Edmonton: Alberta Heritage Foundation for Medical Research, 2002.

Poleshuck EL, Green CR. Socioeconomic disadvantage and pain. *Pain* 2008; 136(3):235–8; doi: 10.1016/j.pain.2008.04.003.

Porter R. Pain and suffering. In: Bynum W, Porter R, (eds.) *Companion encyclopedia of the history of medicine*. London: Routledge, 1993, pp. 1574–91.

Price CH, Olukoga B, Williams O, Bottle A. *A national pain audit final report 2010–2*. London, 2012, p. 66.

Priebe S, Sandhu S, Dias S, et al. Good practice in health care for migrants: views and experiences of care professionals in 16 European countries. *BMC Public Health* 2011; 11:187.

Raftery MN, Sarma K, Murphy AW, et al. Chronic pain in the Republic of Ireland—community prevalence, psychosocial profile and predictors of pain-related disability: results from the Prevalence, Impact and Cost of Chronic Pain (PRIME) Study, Part 1. *Pain* 2011; 152(5):1096–103; doi: 10.1016/j.pain.2011.01.019.

Rechel B, Mladovsky P, Ingleby D, et al. Migration and health in an increasingly diverse Europe. *The Lancet* 2013; 381(9873):1235–45; doi: 10.1016/S0140-6736(12)62086-8.

Rohrbeck J, Jordan K, Croft P. The frequency and characteristics of chronic widespread pain in general practice: a case control study. *British Journal of General Practice* 2007; 57(535):109–15.

Roth RS, Geisser ME. Educational achievement and chronic pain disability: mediating role of pain-related cognitions. *Clinical Journal of Pain* 2002; 18(5):286–96.

Rubinstein SM, van Middelkoop M, Assendelft Willem JJ, et al. Spinal manipulative therapy for chronic low-back pain. *Cochrane Database of Systematic Reviews* 2011; (2);doi: 104/10.1002/14651858.CD008112.pub2. Available at: <http://onlinelibrary.wiley.com/doi/10.1002/14651858.CD008112.pub2/abstract>.

Schaefer H. Grundsätzliches zum problem der soziosomatik. In: Thauer R, Albers C, (eds.) *Soziosomatik der kreislaufkrankheiten*. Steinkopff, 1966, pp. 1–11.

Schullian DM. Wilhelm Ten Rhyne's 'De acupunctura': an 1826 translation. *Journal of the History of Medicine and Allied Sciences* 1979; XXXIV(1):81–92; doi: 10.1093/jhmas/XXXIV.1.81.

Schurer S, Shields MA, Jones AM. Socio-economic inequalities in bodily pain over the life cycle: longitudinal evidence from Australia, Britain and Germany. *Journal of the Royal Statistical Society: Series A (Statistics in Society)* 2014; doi: 10.1111/rssa.12058.

Shefet D, Dascal-Weichhendler H, Rubin O, et al. Domestic violence: a national simulation-based educational program to improve physicians' knowledge, skills and detection rates. *Medical Teacher* 2007; 29(5):e133–e138; doi: 10.1080/01421590701452780.

Starfield B, Shi L, Macinko J. Contribution of primary care to health systems and health. *Milbank Quarterly* 2005; 83(3):457–502; doi: 10.1111/j.1468-0009.2005.00409.x.

Taft A, O'Doherty L, Hegarty K, et al. Screening women for intimate partner violence in healthcare settings. *Cochrane Database of Systematic Reviews* 2013; (4); doi: 10.1002/14651858.CD007007.pub2. Available at: <http://onlinelibrary.wiley.com/doi/10.1002/14651858.CD007007.pub2/abstract>.

Terlouw TA. Roots of physical medicine, physical therapy, and mechanotherapy in the Netherlands in the 19th century: a disputed area within the healthcare domain. *Journal of Manual & Manipulative Therapy* 2007; 15(2):23–41.

Thomson S, Osborn R, Squires D, et al. *International profiles of health care systems*. New York: The Commonwealth Fund, 2012.

Toye F, Seers K, Allcock N, et al. Patients' experiences of chronic non-malignant musculoskeletal pain: a qualitative systematic review. *British Journal of General Practice* 2013; 63(617):e829–e841; doi: 10.3399/bjgp13X675412.

Uijen AA, Schers HJ, Schellevis FG, et al. How unique is continuity of care? A review of continuity and related concepts. *Family Practice* 2012; 29(3):264–71; doi: 10.1093/fampra/cmr104.

Urwin M, Symmons D, Allison T, et al. Estimating the burden of musculoskeletal disorders in the community: the comparative prevalence of symptoms at different anatomical sites, and the relation to social deprivation. *Annals of the Rheumatic Diseases* 1998; 57(11):649–55; doi: 10.1136/ard.57.11.649.

Valderas JM, Starfield B, Sibbald B, et al. Defining comorbidity: implications for understanding health and health services. *The Annals of Family Medicine* 2009; 7(4):357–63; doi: 10.1370/afm.983.

Von Korff M, Alonso J, Ormel J, et al. Childhood psychosocial stressors and adult onset arthritis: broad spectrum risk factors and allostatic load. *Pain* 2009; 143(1–2):76–83; doi: 10.1016/j.pain.2009.01.034.

Wall P. *Pain: the science of suffering*. London: Weidenfeld and Nicolson, 1999.

Watt G. General practice and the epidemiology of health and disease in families. *British Journal of General Practice* 2004; 54:939–44.

Watt G. Alcohol problems in very deprived areas. *British Journal of General Practice* 2011; 61:407–7; doi: 10.3399/bjgp11X578089.

Watt G. Reflections at the deep end. *British Journal of General Practice* 2012; 62(594):6–7; doi: 10.3399/bjgp12X616210.

British Broadcasting Corporation. *What is the price of your pain relief?* BBC One 'Watchdog', 2013.

Wilkinson I. *Suffering—a sociological introduction*. Cambridge: Polity, 2005.

Wilkinson RG, Pickett KE. Income inequality and population health: a review and explanation of the evidence. *Social Science & Medicine* 2006; 62(7):1768–84; doi: 10.1016/j.socscimed.2005.08.036.

Wilkinson RG, Pickett KE. The problems of relative deprivation: why some societies do better than others. *Social Science & Medicine* 2007; 65(9):1965–78; doi: 10.1016/j.socscimed.2007.05.041.

de C Williams AC, Johnson M. Persistent pain: not a medically unexplained symptom. *British Journal of General Practice* 2011; 61(591):638–9; doi: 10.3399/bjgp11X601479.

de C Williams AC, van der Merwe J. The psychological impact of torture. *British Journal of Pain* 2013; 7(2):101–6; doi: 10.1177/2049463713483596.

Williams NH. Words that harm: words that heal. *International Musculoskeletal Medicine* 2009; 31(3):99–100; doi: 10.1179/175361409x12472218840366.

Williams SJ, Martin P, Gabe J. The pharmaceuticalisation of society? A framework for analysis. *Sociology of Health & Illness* 2011; 33(5):710–25; doi: 10.1111/j.1467-9566.2011.01320.x.

Wolf A, Gray R, Fazel S. Violence as a public health problem: an ecological study of 169 countries. *Social Science & Medicine* 2014; 104:220–7.

Zhang Y, Jordan JM. Epidemiology of osteoarthritis. *Clinics in Geriatric Medicine* 2010; 26(3):355–69; doi: 10.1016/j.cger.2010.03.001.

Chapter 6

A patho-anatomical approach to chronic lumbar spinal pain—an Australian perspective

Tom Baster

Introduction to chronic lumbar spinal pain

Australian musculoskeletal statistics

Acute and chronic musculoskeletal conditions are one of the most prevalent health issues in many societies, comprising a large component of the workload of health professionals and a large component of health expenditure. In the most recent Australian Bureau of Statistics national health survey (2004), musculoskeletal conditions were more prevalent than any other condition of the national health priority areas. About 31% of Australians reported suffering from one or more of 'arthritis', 'chronic back conditions', and 'osteoporosis', and these were the main disabling condition in more than one in three Australians with a disability. They are a major area of health expenditure ($A4.6 billion 2004–05).

Of those prevalence figures, there was a slight female predominance (33%) compared to males (29%), and about 50% was reported as 'arthritis' (both osteoarthritis and rheumatoid arthritis), while the other 50% was reported as 'chronic back problems'. Prevalence was higher in older Australians and there was a modest increase in osteoarthritis with age. Indigenous Australians had a slightly higher rate of chronic musculoskeletal conditions compared to the non-indigenous population, and there was a higher rate in economically disadvantaged areas versus those less disadvantaged.

In terms of disability, 6.8% of the Australian population reported disability from chronic musculoskeletal conditions; this being higher than for any other medical condition, including diabetes and heart disease. About one third of people reporting a chronic musculoskeletal conditions felt they had a profound or severe limitation in mobility and self-care.

Specifically with regards to lower back pain (LBP), an electoral roll survey of 3000 Australians in 2001 revealed a point prevalence of 25.6%, a 12-month prevalence of 67.6%, and a life-time prevalence of about 80%. Of those surveyed with back pain, about 10% reported having a high level of disability (Walker et al. 2004).

Provision of health services

Care of this large number of patients in the Australian population is fragmented, and patients have direct access to a variety of health and allied health services that attempt to treat such conditions. In general terms, physiotherapists, chiropractics, osteopathists, myotherapists, acupuncturists, and general practitioners all diagnose and treat both acute and chronic musculoskeletal conditions, with each using a slightly different model and understanding of the underlying condition. The Australian taxpayer-funded Medicare health payment system currently restricts reimbursement of costs for any treatments to those incurred by the medical profession. However, under certain circumstances, patient costs will be reimbursed if the general practitioner (GP) has referred the patient to physiotherapy or similar via a 'chronic diseases care plan'. Private health insurance schemes also provide reimbursement for allied health costs. Prescription of potent analgesics and injection of therapeutic agents is restricted to registered medical practitioners. Medicare funding for investigations such as radiology is also restricted to the latter.

For an Australian GP, about 3.3% of consultations (3.9 million encounters in 2009–10) are related to the management of back problems (Britt 2009). Some Australian GPs have undertaken postgraduate training in musculoskeletal conditions and some practice full-time treatment of such disorders.

The approach detailed in this chapter does not necessarily reflect that taken by many GPs practicing in Australia. It is based on the use of an understanding of the underlying anatomical pathology, the prevalence figures for the structures causing LBP, combined with sensitivity and specificity figures. This information is used to help provide a clinical diagnosis and guide treatment choices.

A patho-anatomical approach to chronic lumbar spinal pain

Acute low back pain

The primary role of the GP in the assessment and management of the patient with acute low back pain is to exclude red flag conditions (see Box 6.1). The majority of cases (>95%) will present with non-specific pain and the current guidelines for management are to avoid investigations such as radiology, prescribe simple analgesics, and encourage normal activities as much as possible (see Box 6.2). It is not reasonable or useful to pursue a patho-anatomical source in such cases.

Chronic low back pain

In the GP assessment of chronic low back pain (cLBP), the presence of red flags (see Box 6.1) should again be assessed and investigated. Symptoms suggestive of spinal stenosis (leg and back pain associated with walking and relieved by stopping or forward flexion), radicular pain, and radiculopathy should be sought. However, the usual presentation of cLBP has no such features, and in developing a systematic approach to these cases, three basic questions need to be addressed clinically. These include considering exactly what, in terms of the anatomical causes of cLBP, is actually presenting; how a diagnosis can be made; and then, the treatment options available.

Prevalence

Virtually every structure in the lumbar spine has been implicated over the years as a possible cause of cLBP. This includes such structures as the thoracolumbar fascia, various ligaments, muscle strains and tears, muscle 'imbalance', kissing spinous processes, and more. However, detailed studies using precision diagnostic blocks has shown that most cases can be attributed to discs, facet joints, and the sacroiliac joints. Various studies have reported the prevalence figures from these anatomical structures and some of these (from Schwarzer, Manchikanti, and others) are shown in Table 6.1.

Box 6.1 Red flags for possible serious spinal pathology

- age <20 years or >55 years
- trauma—falls/vehicle accidents
- increasing level of pain
- previous cancer, weight loss, steroid or intravenous drug use
- systemically unwell
- cauda equina symptoms—loss of sphincter control, saddle anaesthesia, progressive motor weakness
- inflammatory disorders—especially ankylosing spondylitis, psoriasis

Box 6.2 Management of acute low back pain

- assess for red flags
- reassure—expectation of recovery over a few weeks
- avoid 'loaded' labels (e.g. 'slipped disc', 'disc prolapse', 'sciatica')
- prescribe simple analgesics—paracetamol (second-line NSAIDS, Cox2, opioids)
- encourage normal activities—avoid encouraging bed rest
- review after 1–2 weeks
- do not order imaging

Considering the figures in Table 6.1 (e.g. discogenic 39%, 26%, and 42% = average 35%; facet 32%, 40%, 31%, and 27% = average 32%) and for an older clinical population, fan easily remembered approximate ratio of 40:40:20 can be used. Thus, of ten patients seen clinically with cLBP, on average four will have discogenic pain, another four will have facet pain, and the remaining two cases

Table 6.1 Prevalence figures of anatomical structures implicated in chronic low back pain

Author	% Discogenic	% Facet	% SIJ/other	Refs
Schwarzer	39	32	21	(Schwarzer et al. 1994a,b, 1995)
Manchikanti	26	40	2	(Manchikanti et al. 1999)
Depalma	42	31	18	(Depalma et al. 2011)
Manchukonda		27		(Manchukonda et al. 2007)
Maigne			18.5	(Maigne et al. 1996)
Simopoulos			25	(Simopoulos et al. 2012)

Data sourced from: Depalma MJ, Ketchum JM, Saullo T. What is the source of chronic low back pain and does age play a role? *Pain Med* 2011; 12(2):224–33. Available at: <http://www.ncbi.nlm.nih.gov/pubmed/21266006>.

Maigne JY, Aivaliklis A, Pfefer F. Results of sacroiliac joint double block and value of sacroiliac pain provocation tests in 54 patients with low back pain. *Spine* 1996 Aug 15; 21(16):1889–92.

Manchikanti L, Pampati V, Fellows B, Bakhit CE. Prevalence of lumbar facet joint pain in chronic low back pain. *Pain Physician* 1999;2(3):59–64.

Manchukonda R, Manchikanti KN, Cash KA, Pampati V, Manchikanti L. Facet joint pain in chronic spinal pain: an evaluation of prevalence and false-positive rate of diagnostic blocks. *J Spinal Disord Tech* 2007 Oct; 20(7):539–45.

Schwarzer AC, Aprill CN, Derby R, Fortin J, Kine G, Bogduk N. Clinical features of patients with pain stemming from the lumbar zygapophysial joints. Is the lumbar facet syndrome a clinical entity? *Spine* 1994a; 19(10):1132–7.

Schwarzer AC, Aprill CN, Derby R, Fortin J, Kine G, Bogduk N. The relative contributions of the disc and zygapophyseal joint in chronic low back pain. *Spine* 1994b; 19(7):801–6.

Schwarzer AC, Aprill CN, Bogduk N. The sacroiliac joint in chronic low back pain. *Spine* 1995; 20(1):31–7.

Simopoulos TT, Manchikanti L, Singh V, et al. A systematic evaluation of prevalence and diagnostic accuracy of sacroiliac joint interventions. *Pain Physician* 2012 May; 15(3):E305–344.

will be most likely sacroiliac-related. In a younger patient population, there will be a higher ratio of discogenic cases and less facet-related cases, and these ratios will need to be adjusted accordingly. Importantly, it seems that, in the large majority of patients, there will be only one underlying anatomical cause for pain (Schwarzer et al. 1994a,b).This simplifies the clinical assessment considerably.

Prevalence figures are important in assessing the utility or otherwise of a clinical test or investigation in the diagnosis of cLBP, and indeed for other medical conditions. Of equal importance are the published sensitivity and specificity figures. Both prevalence and the sensitivity and specificity results are used to calculate the post-test probability of the condition being present in an individual patient. This can then be used as a guide in clinical decision making. For example:

Prevalence of disc pain = 40% (i.e. probability 0.4 or odds = 0.4/1–0.4 or 0.667)

MRI with findings of moderate loss of nuclear signal and disc bulge

Sensitivity = 79.8% (the number found by magnetic resonance imaging (MRI) divided by total number with discogenic pain found by provocative discography)

Specificity = 79.3% (the number rejected by MRI divided by total number rejected by provocative discography) (O'Neill et al. 2008)

Bayes theorem enables the calculation of the post-test probability (see Box 6.3).

Using the figures already given for an MRI investigation (odds 0.667, sensitivity 0.798, and specificity 0.793):

post-test odds = 0.667*0.798/(1–0.793) = 2.57

or the post-test probability = 2.57/(1 + 2.57) = 72%

By ordering an MRI investigation and receiving a report of reduced nuclear signal and a disc bulge, the diagnostic probability increases from an initial 40% to about 72%. While this is an improvement in the diagnostic process, such a figure might give pause as to the appropriate use of this investigation in a particular clinical case.

Diagnosis

The literature indicates that history and examination are of dubious value in the determination of the possible underlying pathology. Facet arthrosis is present in 100% of patients after the age of 60 and present in almost 60% beyond about the mid twenties (Eubanks et al. 2007). Similarly, degenerative lumbar discs are ubiquitous in the older population, regardless of patient symptoms (Hicks et al. 2009).

A few useful clinical clues might however be provided by the presence and absence of various signs and symptoms. For example, the probability of facet pain is increased by the presence of age >65 years, pain not increased by straining, not worsened by forward flexion, and relieved by rest (Revel et al. 1998). Classically, discogenic LBP is band-like in distribution, worse in the morning, worse with straining, and aggravated by standing in flexion (Kosharskyy and Rozen 2007). Younger age group is also predictive of discogenic aetiology. Sacroiliac (SI) joint pain is considered to be sited below the belt line and localized by the patient to around the posterior superior iliac spine area (Dreyfuss et al. 2004). Overall however, no clinical signs or symptoms can be used to definitively diagnose a patho-anatomic cause in an individual case.

Box 6.3 Bayes theorem for calculating post-test probability

Post-test odds = pre-test odds* likelihood ratio

Likelihood ratio +ve = sensitivity/1-specificity

Likelihood ratio –ve = 1-sensitivity/specificity

Facet pain—diagnosis and treatment

Diagnosis

As this is currently the most readily treated condition, it is worthwhile to consider this in the initial assessment of a patient with cLBP, especially if the patient is in the older age bracket. Based on clinical suspicion and initial odds of about 40%, the available investigations will be determined by the answers to two questions:

- Is facet pain present?
- Which joint or joints are involved?

The gold standard for diagnosis of two or three local anaesthetic blocks/facet joint is not practical in the clinical setting due to the number of procedures required; neither is it cost- or time-effective. Simple maths indicates that to screen the lower three facets properly requires up to 12 computer tomography (CT)/fluoroscopic or ultrasound-guided injections. A single block can be used instead but the significant number of false positives that can occur, about 38%, need to be recognized (Schwarzer et al. 1994c). Similarly, plain X-ray and CT are also of little diagnostic utility with the universal prevalence of facet arthrosis in the general population.

Single-photon emission computer tomography

A type of bone scan known as single-photon emission computer tomography (SPECT) is available in many centres and can be utilized for the purpose of detecting facet joints with increased radioisotope uptake as an indication of a probable active arthritic, and thus painful, process. SPECT uses a dual-head gamma camera to create a 3D image and this can provide anatomical localization to the different components of the vertebral bony structures. It can also be useful to detect active discogenic disease. The effective radiation from this procedure is about 6.4 mSv. Australian background radiation is around 1.5 mSv/year and a lumbar CT exposes the patient to considerably more (of between 9–45mSv) than a SPECT investigation (Australian Nuclear Science and Technology Organisation).

In an older study, that does not fulfil 'gold standard' diagnostic methods, SPECT sensitivity was reported to be 100%, with a specificity of 71% (Holder et al. 1995). Using such figures and the initial prevalence of 40% in the cLBP population gives a post-test probability of a facet diagnosis of about 70%. This figure can be calculated in the same way as the example given previously in this chapter (see 'Prevalence' in the 'Chronic low back pain' section). Other studies using SPECT as a basis for diagnosis and treatment indicate that this investigation provides improved clinical outcomes in terms of reduction in injections given and better pain relief (see Table 6.2).

Magnetic resonance imaging

There have been a few reports that MRI findings can be of assistance in diagnosing facet pain. A finding of a mottled appearance of a facet joint on MRI has a 0.9 specificity but only a 0.59 sensitivity

Table 6.2 Using SPECT as a basis for diagnosis and treatment

SPECT +ve significant pain relief	SPECT −ve significant pain relief	No SPECT significant pain relief	Refs
95%	47%		(Dolan et al. 1996)
86%	12.5%	41%	(Pneumaticos et al. 2006)

compared with SPECT (Kim and Wang 2006). There seems to be no association with facet hypertrophy and SPECT activity. Calculation of the post-test probability of 80% indicates that an MRI report of a mottled appearance of a facet joint is clinically useful.

TreatmentIntra-articular facet injection of local anaesthetic and steroid

As an initial treatment, this option has been shown to be effective in providing pain relief for several months following a positive SPECT result (Ackerman and Ahmad 2008). There are similar levels of pain relief to radio-frequency neurotomy in the short to medium term (Civelek et al. 2012). Intra-articular steroid and local anaesthetic can be useful as a trial of therapy, where access to radio-frequency neurotomy is limited or where patient out-of-pocket costs are a consideration. The procedure can be performed under fluoroscopy, CT guidance, or even ultrasound (Yun et al. 2012). Technically, it can be difficult to access the intra-articular space in the presence of osteophytes or other degenerative changes, and undoubtedly in many cases, there is a spill of anaesthetic on to other nearby structures which confounds the clinical assessment.

Medial branch block and radio-frequency neurotomy

This is the mainstay of the effective treatment for facet pain (see Figure 6.1) and is performed by interventional radiologists in major radiology practices in Australia and also by some anaesthetists. It involves the appropriate block of the two medial branches of the dorsal rami that supplies each facet joint. For example, to block the L4–5 facet joint requires that the medial branch from both the L3 and L4 nerve roots be addressed. It is important to check that the correct medial branches have been anaesthetized in an individual case in assessing the clinical effect.

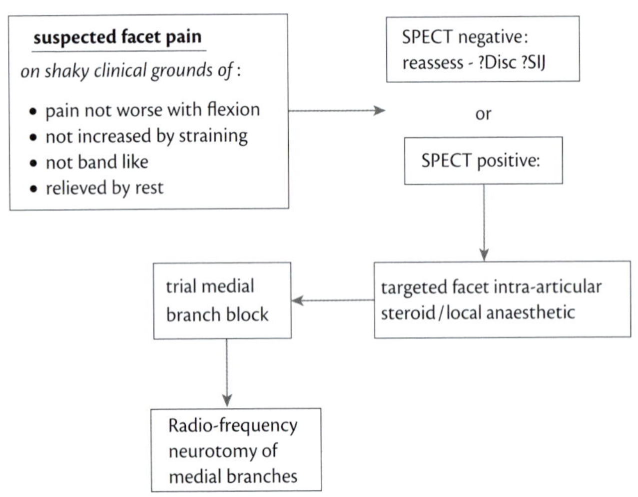

Figure 6.1 Algorithm for facet pain.

Discogenic pain—diagnosis and treatment

Diagnosis

The next group of patients to consider will present with discogenic pain, about 40% on initial prevalence figures, but probably considerably higher than this in the presence of a negative SPECT result.

Clinical examination is once again of minimal value but mention is made of two possibilities.McKenzie method

This technique is especially of use in the assessment of acute LBP with radicular symptoms, but can also be utilized in cLBP if a discogenic cause is suspected. It involves considering the change in the patient's pain in response to repetitive end-range movements. These are typically unidirectional. If the pain improves, in the sense that it becomes centralized, then this is considered to be an indication that conservative therapy will be successful. Conversely, symptom aggravation in all directions of testing and no significant centralization is considered to be negative for a response to non-surgical treatments. In patients with limited or no peripheral symptoms, this method however is of limited application (Wetzel and Donelson 2003).

Correlation of the McKenzie method with discography indicates that of about 50% of patients who centralize pain, 74% will have positive discography; another 25% who exhibit peripheralization (i.e. pain increased in the lower limb or foot) have a 69% positive discogram result; and of the final 25% who exhibit no change when tested by the McKenzie method, only 12.5% are found to have a positive discogram. The latter finding is considered by the McKenzie school to indicate there is a non-discogenic basis to the patient's pain (Donelson et al. 1997).

Bony vibration

This technique involves application of a vibrating instrument (the original instrument used was an electric toothbrush with a blunt end) to the tip of the spinous process and determining patient report of concordant pain. Sensitivity and specificity figures from two studies from the same research group were reported, with sensitivity of 0.96 and specificity of 0.72 in the first study, and sensitivity of 0.88 and specificity of 0.75 in the second (Yrjämä and Vanharanta 1994; Yrjämä et al. 1997). Using the figures from the second study provides a post-test probability of discogenic back pain when utilizing this method of bony vibration testing of 70%. This is an improvement on the initial probability and is of some use clinically, especially as this procedure can be readily applied as part of the patient physical examination.

If clinically relevant, two other investigations can be used.

Discography

The gold standard for diagnosis for a discogenic cause of cLBP is provocative discography, where the suspected disc is injected with contrast and is slightly pressurized. If the patient reports concordant pain from the procedure and when adjacent discs are similarly tested, no pain is reproduced, the diagnosis of discogenic pain is considered to be confirmed (Ivie et al. 2011).

However, clinically, it is inappropriate to undertake such an investigation in most patients, unless the patient is being considered for surgery, as there are several risks attached. These include the fairly low risk of a discitis and acute disc protrusion, but a more real concern is long-term disc deterioration from the injury inflicted to the disc by the insertion of the procedural needle. As the method requires needle insertion into adjacent discs that are asymptomatic, this could result in an iatrogenic-caused long-term deterioration (Carragee et al. 2009; Poynton et al. 2005). Further deterioration of the symptomatic disc is probably of lesser concern.

Magnetic resonance imaging

While MRI is considered to be the most useful non-invasive investigation, asymptomatic discs can appear abnormal, and a disc shown to be painful by discography can appear normal on MRI (Brightbill et al. 1994). In the presence of moderate to severe loss of nuclear signal, there is reasonable correlation with the gold standard provocative discography, as the earlier example illustrated. There is also good correlation with high-intensity zones (hiz) and modic changes (Chen et al. 2011).

MRI is readily accessible to most medical practitioners in Australia. Whilst Medicare currently restricts reimbursement of patient costs to those referred for this investigation by specialists, the out-of-pocket cost has decreased considerably over recent years and many patients are directly referred by their GP for an MRI of the lumbar spine, regardless of the cost.

Treatment

Apart from referral of severe persistent cases to specialists for consideration for fusion or disc replacement, there are currently fairly limited options for the treatment of discogenic pain in primary practice. The technique known as Intradiscal Electrotherapy, while seemingly effective, is only available currently in research facilities. Other treatment options are mentioned here.

McKenzie exercises

There is some evidence for short-term benefit from McKenzie-specific exercises, especially in patients who have shown centralization (Long et al. 2004). However, over the longer term, such exercises do not seem to continue to be effective in providing pain relief.

Caudal and interlaminar epidurals

These well-established treatment techniques continue to provide useful pain relief for discogenic pain. In two recent (2012) randomized double-blind trials of 120 patients/trial who were confirmed to not have facet and sacroiliac pain and also who did not have disc herniation or radiculitis, results indicate significant pain relief and improvement in function over a two-year period. The average number of procedures was about six per year for the caudal epidurals and four per year for the interlaminar epidurals. There seems to be no advantage in using steroid with the anaesthetic agent selected (Manchikanti et al. 2012a,b). Caudal and interlaminar epidurals can be performed readily under fluoroscopy, and caudal epidurals, with adequate aseptic technique, can be performed in a consulting room, especially in those patients who have a readily palpated sacral hiatus.

Sympathetic blocks

The innervation of the lumbar disc is both segmental via the sinuvertebral nerve, especially to the posterior aspect, and with a significant sympathetic supply of the lateral and anterior parts. Several Japanese studies have shown some possible clinical benefit of blocking the sympathetic supply at L2 level by the ablation of the rami communicans (see Figure 6.2). A UK study, however, seems to refute any benefit of this treatment. A summary of results from Simopoulos et al. (2005), Nakamura et al. (1996), Oh and Shim (2004), and Richardson et al. (2009) is provided in Table 6.3.

The negative study by Richardson, which failed to find any clinical effect from the procedure, used a combination of lignocaine, steroid, and clonidine. Clonidine, while traditionally considered to have a synergistic effect with lignocaine, has been shown to be antagonistic at the dorsal root ganglion level (Hiruma et al. 2008). This possibly explains the outcome, whereas the Japanese studies have indicated a benefit.

If this procedure is being considered, a trial block at L2 with local anaesthesia, to assess a response prior to any ablation, would be prudent. A recent review has given this treatment a positive recommendation for clinical use (Kallewaard et al. 2010).

Sacroiliac pain—diagnosis and treatment

Diagnosis

The International Association for the Study of Pain proposes the following criteria for the clinical diagnosis of SI joint pain:

- pain in the region of the SI joint
- pain reproduced by clinical tests that selectively stress the joint
- the patient reports pain relief after selective delivery of local anaesthetic

Table 6.3 Clinical effect of sympathetic blockadeat L2 level by the ablation of the rami communicans

Trial	Number of patients	Diagnosis method	Results	Note	Refs
Simopoulos	5	+ve provocative discography	50% decrease in pain for 4/12 months		(Simopoulos et al. 2005)
Nakamura	33	MRI	Decrease in pain for 1 month		(Nakamura et al. 1996)
Oh and Shim	49	Failed IDET	50% decrease in pain	Blocked L4 and L5 levels	(Oh and Shim 2004)
Richardson	12	+ve provocative discography	No effect		(Richardson et al. 2009)

Data sourced from: Dolan AL, Ryan PJ, Arden NK, et al. The value of SPECT scans in identifying back pain likely to benefit from facet joint injection. *Br J Rheumatol* 1996 Dec; 35(12):1269–73.

Pneumaticos SG, Chatziioannou SN, Hipp JA, Moore WH, Esses SI. Low back pain: prediction of short-term outcome of facet joint injection with bone scintigraphy. *Radiology* 2006 Feb; 238(2):693–8.

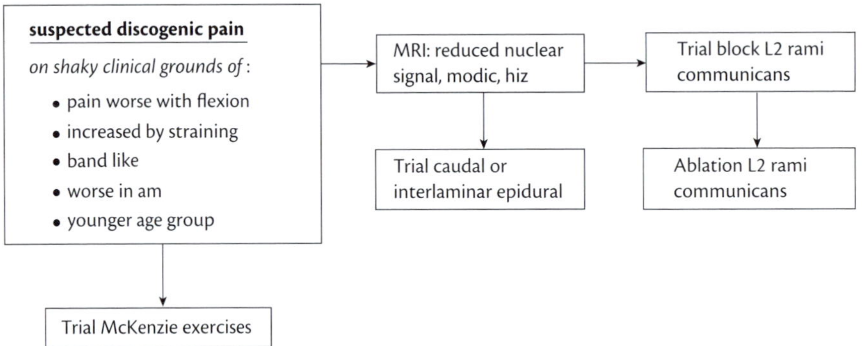

Figure 6.2 Algorithm for discogenic pain.

The clinical tests that, in combination, improve the probability of a SI joint diagnosis are as follows:

- **Distraction test**—patient supine—push down and out on both anterior superior iliac spines.
- **Posterior pelvic pain provocation test**—patient supine—flex hip and knee to 90° and apply a posterior shearing stress to the SI joint through the femur. Avoid excessive adduction of the hip as combined flexion and adduction is normally painful.
- **Gaenslen's sign**—patient supine—the hip is maximally flexed on one side and the opposite hip is extended over the side of the examination couch. This stresses both SI joint and both hips and stretches the femoral nerve on the side of the hip extension. Hip joints and femoral nerve can then be excluded using other tests.
- **Compression test**—patient lying on side—downward pressure is applied to the uppermost iliac crest, directed to the opposite iliac crest.
- **Sacral thrust**—patient prone—anteriorly directed thrust over the sacrum.

Positive tests are reproduction of the patient pain. If three of the five tests are positive, this gives a 91% sensitivity, a 78% specificity, and post-test odds of about 60% (assuming a pre-test prevalence of about 20%) (Laslett 2008).

Intra-articular local anaesthetic

This is considered to be the gold standard investigation but, as with facet joint investigations, there can be a high incidence of false positives with the use of a single trial block, and this needs to be recognized clinically. However, Mitchell et al, report that a positive first block will predict 85% of a positive second block, and there is a similar figure for a negative first block predicting a negative second (Mitchell et al. 2010). Thus practically, a single block investigation can be used.

Treatment

Treatment of SI joint pain follows the same general outline as for facet pain cases—intra-articular injections of anaesthetic and steroid agents. It provides pain relief in about 67% of cases for only a few months however (Liliang et al. 2009).

Trial of intra-articular anaesthesia can also be followed by radio-frequency neurotomy of the innervation of the joint (see Figure 6.3). This involves the dorsal branches of L4 and L5 and lateral branches of S1–3 (Cheng et al. 2012; Karaman et al. 2011). Pain relief of about 50% for 3–6 months can be achieved (50).

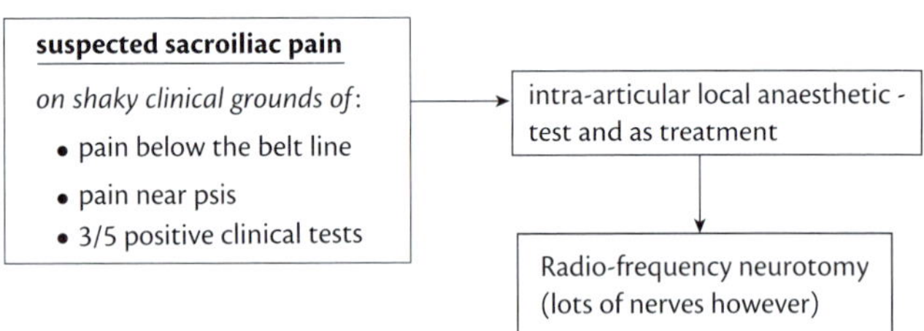

Figure 6.3 Algorithm for sacroiliac pain.

Conclusions about the patho-anatomical approach to chronic lumbar spinal pain

Chronic lumbar spinal pain is a common presentation in Australian general practice and a systematic approach is needed to identify the different types and provide effective treatment. The approach presented in this chapter is based on an understanding of the underlying pathology, with the use of published sensitivity and specificity figures possibly leading to improved clinical choices and better outcomes for patients. However, two of the three main causes of chronic back pain are still difficult to treat effectively.

References

Ackerman WE, Ahmad M. Pain relief with intraarticular or medial branch nerve blocks in patients with positive lumbar facet joint SPECT imaging: a 12-week outcome study. *South Med J* 2008; 101(9):931–4.

Australian Bureau of Statistics. *National Health Survey 2004–5*. Available at: <http://www.abs.gov.au/ausstats/abs@.nsf/Latestproducts/4823.0.55.001Main%20Features12004–5?opendocument&tabname=Summary&prodno=4823.0.55.001&issue=2004–5&num=&view=> Australian Nuclear Science and Technology Organisation (ANSTO). <http://www.ansto.gov.au/nuclear_information/about_nuclear_science/measuring_radiation>.

Brightbill TC, Pile N, Eichelberger RP, Whitman M Jr. Normal magnetic resonance imaging and abnormal discography in lumbar disc disruption. *Spine* 1994; 19(9):1075–7.

Britt H, Australian Institute of Health and Welfare, University of Sydney, BEACH (Program), Australian GP Statistics and Classification Centre. *General practice activity in Australia 2009–10*. Canberra, ACT: Australian Institute of Health and Welfare and University of Sydney; 2009.

Carragee EJ, Don AS, Hurwitz EL, et al. 2009 ISSLS prize winner: does discography cause accelerated progression of degeneration changes in the lumbar disc: a ten-year matched cohort study. *Spine* 2009; 34(21):2338–45.

Chen J, Ding Y, Lv R, et al. Correlation between MR imaging and discography with provocative concordant pain in patients with low back pain. *Clin J Pain* 2011; 27(2):125–30.

Cheng J, Pope JE, Dalton JE, Cheng O, Bensitel A. Comparative outcomes of cooled versus traditional radiofrequency ablation of the lateral branches for sacroiliac joint pain. Clin J Pain. 2013 Feb;29(2):132-7

Civelek E, Cansever T, Kabatas S, et al. Comparison of effectiveness of facet joint injection and radiofrequency denervation in chronic low back pain. *Turk Neurosurg* 2012; 22(2):200–6.

Depalma MJ, Ketchum JM, Saullo T. What is the source of chronic low back pain and does age play a role? *Pain Med* 2011; 12(2):224–33; doi: 10.1111/j.1526-4637.2010.01045.x. Available at: <http://www.ncbi.nlm.nih.gov/pubmed/21266006>.

Dolan AL, Ryan PJ, Arden NK, et al. The value of SPECT scans in identifying back pain likely to benefit from facet joint injection. *Br J Rheumatol* 1996; 35(12):1269–73.

Donelson R, Aprill C, Medcalf R, Grant W. A prospective study of centralization of lumbar and referred pain. A predictor of symptomatic discs and anular competence. *Spine* 1997; 22(10):1115–22.

Dreyfuss P, Dreyer SJ, Cole A, Mayo K. Sacroiliac joint pain. *J Am Acad Orthop Surg* 2004; 12(4):255–65.

Eubanks JD, Lee MJ, Cassinelli E, Ahn NU. Prevalence of lumbar facet arthrosis and its relationship to age, sex, and race: an anatomic study of cadaveric specimens. *Spine* 2007; 32(19):2058–62.

Hicks GE, Morone N, Weiner DK. Degenerative lumbar disc and facet disease in older adults. *Spine* 2009; 34(12):1301–6.

Hiruma H, Shimizu K, Takenami T, Sugie H, Kawakami T. Effects of clonidine on lidocaine-induced inhibition of axonal transport in cultured mouse dorsal root ganglion neurones. *Br J Anaesth* 2008; 101(5):659–65.

Holder LE, Machin JL, Asdourian PL, Links JM, Sexton CC. Planar and high-resolution SPECT bone imaging in the diagnosis of facet syndrome. *J Nucl Med* 1995; 36(1):37–44.

Ivie CS, Gianoli D, Pino CA. Provocative discography as predictor of discogenic pain and therapeutic outcome. *Tech Reg Anesthesia Pain Man* 2011; 15(1):12–9.

Kallewaard JW, Terheggen MAMB, Groen GJ, et al. 15. Discogenic Low Back Pain. *Pain Practice* 2010; 10(6): 560–79.

Karaman H, Kavak GO, Tüfek A, et al. Cooled radiofrequency application for treatment of sacroiliac joint pain. *Acta Neurochir (Wien)* 2011; 153(7):1461–8; doi: 10.1007/s00701-011-1003-8. Available at: <http://www.ncbi.nlm.nih.gov/pubmed/21479801>.

Kim KA, Wang MY. Magnetic resonance image-based morphological predictors of single photon emission computed tomography-positive facet arthropathy in patients with axial back pain. *Neurosurgery* 2006; 59(1):147–56.

Kosharskyy B, Rozen D. Lumbar discogenic pain. Disk degeneration and minimally invasive interventional therapies. *Anasthesiol Intensivmed Notfallmed Schmerzther* 2007; 42(4):262–7.

Laslett M. Evidence-based diagnosis and treatment of the painful sacroiliac joint. *J Man Manip Ther* 2008;16(3):142–52.

Liliang P-C, Lu K, Weng H-C, Liang C-L, Tsai Y-D, Chen H-J. The therapeutic efficacy of sacroiliac joint blocks with triamcinolone acetonide in the treatment of sacroiliac joint dysfunction without spondyloarthropathy. *Spine* 2009; 34(9):896–900.

Long A, Donelson R, Fung T. Does it matter which exercise? A randomized control trial of exercise for low back pain. *Spine* 2004; 29(23):2593–602.

Maigne JY, Aivaliklis A, Pfefer F. Results of sacroiliac joint double block and value of sacroiliac pain provocation tests in 54 patients with low back pain. *Spine* 1996; 21(16):1889–92.

Manchikanti L, Cash KA, McManus CD, Pampati V, Benyamin R. Fluoroscopic lumbar interlaminar epidural injections in managing chronic lumbar axial or discogenic pain. *J Pain Res* 2012a; 5:301–11.

Manchikanti L, Cash KA, McManus CD, Pampati V. Fluoroscopic caudal epidural injections in managing chronic axial low back pain without disc herniation, radiculitis, or facet joint pain. *J Pain Res* 2012b; 5:381–90.

Manchikanti L, Pampati V, Fellows B, Bakhit CE. Prevalence of lumbar facet joint pain in chronic low back pain. *Pain Physician* 1999; 2(3): 59–64.

Manchukonda R, Manchikanti KN, Cash KA, Pampati V, Manchikanti L. Facet joint pain in chronic spinal pain: an evaluation of prevalence and false-positive rate of diagnostic blocks. *J Spinal Disord Tech* 2007; 20(7):539–45.

Mitchell B, McPhall T, Verrills P. Radiofrequency neurotomy for sacroiliac pain: a prospective study. *J Sci Med Sport* 2010;12 :6–7.

Nakamura SI, Takahashi K, Takahashi Y, Yamagata M, Moriya H. The afferent pathways of discogenic low-back pain. Evaluation of L2 spinal nerve infiltration. *Br J Bone Joint Surg* 1996; 78(4): 606–12.

O'Neill C, Kurgansky M, Kaiser J, Lau W. Accuracy of MRI for diagnosis of discogenic pain. *Pain Physician* 2008; 11(3):311–26.

Oh WS, Shim JC. A randomized controlled trial of radiofrequency denervation of the ramus communicans nerve for chronic discogenic low back pain. *Clin J Pain* 2004; 20(1):55–60.

Pneumaticos SG, Chatziioannou SN, Hipp JA, Moore WH, Esses SI. Low back pain: prediction of short-term outcome of facet joint injection with bone scintigraphy. *Radiology* 2006; 238(2):693–8.

Poynton AR, Hinman A, Lutz G, Farmer JC. Discography-induced acute lumbar disc herniation: a report of five cases. *J Spinal Disord Tech* 2005; 18(2):188–92.

Rathmell JP. The promise of an effective treatment for sacroiliac-related low back pain. *Anesthesiology* 2008; 109(2):167–8.

Revel M, Poiraudeau S, Auleley GR, et al. Capacity of the clinical picture to characterize low back pain relieved by facet joint anesthesia. Proposed criteria to identify patients with painful facet joints. *Spine* 1998; 23(18):1972–6; discussion 1977.

Richardson J, Collinghan N, Scally AJ, Gupta S. Bilateral L1 and L2 dorsal root ganglion blocks for discogenic low-back pain. *Br J Anaesth* 2009; 103(3):416–9.

Schwarzer AC, Aprill CN, Bogduk N. The sacroiliac joint in chronic low back pain. *Spine* 1995; 20(1):31–7.

Schwarzer AC, Aprill CN, Derby R, Fortin J, Kine G, Bogduk N. Clinical features of patients with pain stemming from the lumbar zygapophysial joints. Is the lumbar facet syndrome a clinical entity? *Spine* 1994a; 19(10):1132–7.

Schwarzer AC, Aprill CN, Derby R, Fortin J, Kine G, Bogduk N. The relative contributions of the disc and zygapophysial joint in chronic low back pain. *Spine* 1994b; 19(7):801–6.

Schwarzer AC, Aprill CN, Derby R, Fortin J, Kine G, Bogduk N. The false-positive rate of uncontrolled diagnostic blocks of the lumbar zygapophysial joints. *Pain* 1994c; 58(2):195–200.

Simopoulos TT, Malik AB, Sial KA, Elkersh M, Bajwa ZH. Radiofrequency lesioning of the L2 ramus communicans in managing discogenic low back pain. *Pain Physician* 2005; 8(1):61–5.

Simopoulos TT, Manchikanti L, Singh V, et al. A systematic evaluation of prevalence and diagnostic accuracy of sacroiliac joint interventions. *Pain Physician* 2012; 15(3):E305–44.

Walker BF, Muller R, Grant WD. Low back pain in Australian adults: prevalence and associated disability. *J Manip Physiol Ther* 2004; 27(4): 238–44.

Wetzel FT, Donelson R. The role of repeated end-range/pain response assessment in the management of symptomatic lumbar discs. *Spine* 2003; 3(2):146–54.

Yrjämä M, Tervonen O, Kurunlahti M, Vanharanta H. Bony vibration stimulation test combined with magnetic resonance imaging. Can discography be replaced? *Spine* 1997; 22(7):808–13.

Yrjämä M, Vanharanta H. Bony vibration stimulation: a new, non-invasive method for examining intradiscal pain. *Eur Spine J* 1994; 3(4):233–5.

Yun DH, Kim H-S, Yoo SD, et al. Efficacy of ultrasonography-guided injections in patients with facet syndrome of the low lumbar spine. *Ann Rehabil Med* 2012; 36(1):66–71.

PART 2

Structural pathology; dysfunction; pain

Chapter 7

Introduction to structural pathology

David Knott

Changes in body mechanics

Alterations to the normal anatomy, such as spinal curvatures or inequality of leg length, will potentially change the mechanical stresses acting upon related soft tissue structures including joints, muscles, tendons, ligaments, and nerves. The degree of additional stress will usually be related to the degree of anatomical alteration—the body will be able to adjust and compensate for relatively minor changes. Biomechanical problems occur more commonly, though not exclusively, in the lower limbs and spine. So for example, a shortened leg may lead to the initiation of, or aggravation of, low back pain or to premature osteoarthritis of the hip joint (Friberg 1983). The management of this type of problem should involve an expert assessment of the biomechanical changes and then, where possible, correction—using a variety of methods including physiotherapy, occupational therapy, orthotics, and occasionally surgery. In addition, practical modifications to the patient's home or work environment may be necessary in some cases.

We will now consider how individual tissues can be affected by structural abnormalities.

Arthritis

The term *arthritis* implies an inflammatory process occurring within a joint and will typically present with pain, and possibly with swelling, stiffness, and reduced range of movement. Arthritis can have numerous causes with different mechanisms by which the joint becomes inflamed but with very similar clinical presentations. The term *arthrosis* describes a degenerative joint which may or may not present with pain and reduced range of movement but which is not inflamed and will not usually be swollen. Arthrosis is a very common, though not inevitable, feature of the ageing process.

The presentation of arthritis may be acute, sub-acute, or chronic and may be mild or severe in terms of pain and swelling (see Table 7.1). As arthritis (and arthrosis) progresses, usually the range of movement of the joint reduces in a pattern that is both predictable and reproducible for that particular joint—the so-called *capsular pattern* as described by James Cyriax (1982).

In the management of arthritis, some treatments can be considered as generic modalities (e.g. rest, ice, heat, analgesia, anti-inflammatory medication and/or injections) and can be applied to many different types of arthritis since they treat symptoms and/or generic pathological processes. Other treatments are condition-specific, as in rheumatoid arthritis or septic arthritis, targeting the underlying specific pathological process.

Let us now consider the more common types of arthritis (see Table 7.1).

Osteoarthritis

Osteoarthritis (OA) is a common condition and is frequently encountered in most musculoskeletal practice. OA is more common in women than men and becomes more common with advancing age. The Framingham Osteoarthritis Study in 1990 showed that the prevalence of radiographic OA increases with age from 27% in people younger than 60 years to 44% in those older than 70 years. In addition, this study showed that 2% of women with a mean age of 71 develop radiographic knee OA every year, compared with 1.4% of men, and 1% of women develop symptomatic knee OA every year, compared with 0.7% of men. In a general practice UK study, the prevalence of currently recorded diagnosis of knee OA in patients >45 years old was 1.1%, and the estimated prevalence of all those currently registered with the practice who had had knee OA diagnosed at some point was 5.5%.

Osteoarthritis has traditionally been considered to be a 'wear and tear' type problem and patients find this concept easy to understand. In reality, it can be more complex. The primary underlying abnormality seems to be an age-related change in the water and protein make-up of articular cartilage (chondrocytes and matrix) and synovial fluid linked to a deterioration in the ability of the cartilage cells to repair themselves. In addition to this, other factors can either predispose an individual to develop OA or to accelerate its progress. These include:

- Congenital abnormalities of joints/bones
- Increased mechanical stress upon a joint from deformity or obesity

Table 7.1 Differential diagnosis* of a monoarthritis

Acute/rapid onset	Septic arthritis	
	Gout	
	Pseudogout	
	Haemarthrosis	As in trauma, anticoaguants, blood dyscrasia, etc.
Chronic/slow onset	Chronic infective (e.g. TB)	
	Chronic inflammatory	Especially seronegative types
	Osteoarthritis	
	Internal mechanical	e.g. meniscal pathology at knee

* To achieve the correct diagnosis, a combination of history, examination, and relevant investigations (FBC, ESR/CRP, aspiration, imaging) will give the answer.

- Increased mechanical stress from heavy and/or repetitive work or sport
- Damage to the joint from trauma or surgery
- Damage to the joint from other diseases such as rheumatoid arthritis
- Maybe genetic factors in some patients—with some types of OA more than others (e.g. hands, hip)
- Rarer causes such as bleeding into the joints in haemophilia or deposition of iron in haemochromatosis.

Histologically, the cartilage covering the articular surfaces becomes gradually thinned and, in severe cases, will be completely worn away exposing bone underneath. Changes occur in the subchondral bone including the development of cysts, sclerosis, and microfractures. Small pieces of bone and/or cartilage may separate from the joint surface leading to loose bodies within the joint. (See Figure 7.1.) Synovium may become inflamed and hypertrophied and the amount of synovial fluid produced may increase, leading to a clinically detectable effusion. Normally however, both the quantity and quality of synovial fluid is reduced. Bony growth around the joint margins (osteophytes) commonly occurs, leading to joint enlargement and deformity and clinically recognizable features such as Heberden's nodes at the finger distal interphalangeal (DIP) joints.

Chondrocyte damage or degeneration causes release of digestive enzymes which damage collagen and degrade proteoglycan molecules such as hyaluronic acid in the matrix fluid. Attempts at repair with chondrocyte proliferation and increase in matrix component synthesis occur but this repair process fails to keep pace with the degenerative process and increasing joint damage ensues. There may be an inflammatory element to the degenerative process, although this is not as prominent as in an inflammatory arthritis such as rheumatoid. Certainly one can detect increases in the levels of pro-inflammatory chemicals such as cytokines and prostaglandin E2 (PGE2). A normally quiescent osteoarthritic joint may, however, become inflamed if subject to trauma or overuse.

Any synovial joint may develop OA, but weight-bearing joints such as the hips and knees and those given a lot of use such as the small joints of the hand, are most commonly affected. Clinical symptoms will typically be pain, swelling, and stiffness after periods of immobility. Visual changes may include swelling and there may be resultant deformity (see Figure 7.2). It must be remembered, however, that significant numbers of people with radiological joint damage do not have any pain—why is this? Although the principal histological changes in OA are within the cartilage, this tissue does not have any significant blood or nerve supply. Other tissues, such as synovium and bone, are more likely sources of pain. Current thinking is that pain in OA is complex and is influenced both by local factors and activation of central pain-processing pathways (Sofat 2011).

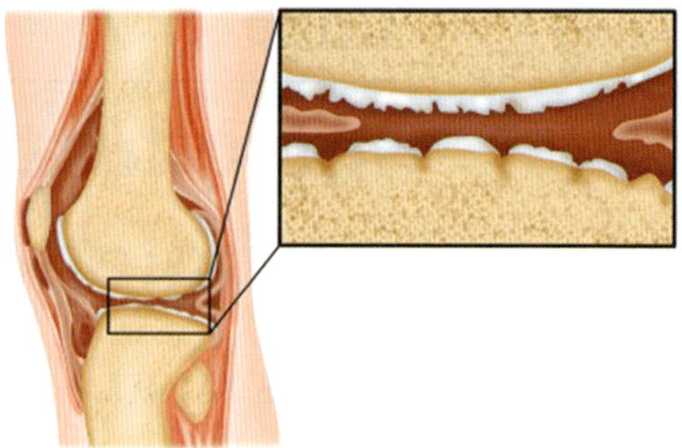

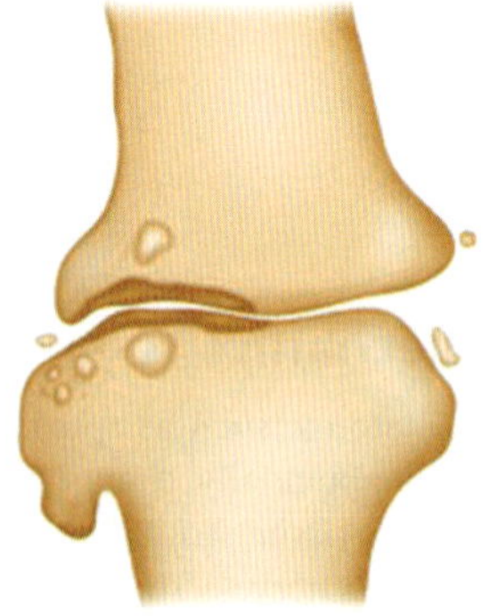

Figure 7.1 Diagrammatic representation of OA changes in knee joint.

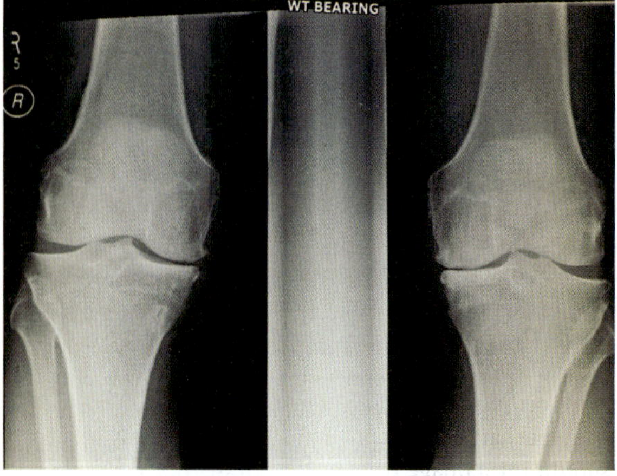

Figure 7.2 X-ray showing bilateral knee OA, more severe in the left knee. The osteophytes and joint space narrowing are clearly seen.

Treatment principles for OA are:

- Relief of pain with simple analgesics such as paracetamol and/or non-steroidal anti-inflammatory drugs (NSAIDs); physical modalities such as heat or cold may also be helpful.
- Reduced joint loading which may be best achieved by lifestyle changes including weight reduction where appropriate, muscle strengthening, and use of appliances and splints in some cases.
- Corticosteroid injections can be helpful, especially where an inflammatory element is seen to be present, but also sometimes in 'cold', apparently non-inflamed joints—the reasons for this latter efficacy is not entirely clear.
- Other pain-relieving measures such as acupuncture or transcutaneous electrical nerve stimulation (TENS) may be helpful to some.
- Hyaluronic acid injections (HA). Theoretically, these reverse the diminution and degradation of naturally occurring HA with symptom relief and (perhaps) slowing down of the degenerative process. However, the evidence for efficacy is mixed and concerns as to cost effectiveness limits use in NHS practice.
- Orthopaedic surgery, commonly in the form of joint replacement, for more severe cases not responding to conservative measures and causing significant pain and/or disability.

Treatment needs to be holistic with any associated medical conditions (e.g. depression, obesity) or social factors (e.g. housing needs) taken into account. An overview of recommendations is given in the National Institute for Health and Clinical Excellence guidelines of 2008 (NICE 2008).

Rheumatoid arthritis

Rheumatoid arthritis (RA) is the second most common form of arthritis in the UK, behind OA, affecting perhaps 2–3% of the population. The overall incidence of RA using 2010 criteria (American College of Rheumatology (ACR)/European League Against Rheumatism) was 40 in 100 000; (54 in 100 000 for women and 25 in 100 000 for men). In women, the peak age of incidence was younger than in men, with highest rates between ages 45–74. In men, incidence appeared to increase with age, with highest rates in men over 65 years old (Humphrey 2012).

RA is a chronic, autoimmune, and complex inflammatory disease leading to bone and cartilage destruction. The precise cause is unknown but it seems to be a combination of genetic susceptibility, environmental factors, and abnormal immune response to a presumed bacterial or viral trigger. Multiple genes are associated with disease susceptibility, with the human leukocyte antigen (HLA) locus accounting for 30–50% of the overall genetic risk. Inflamed joints are infiltrated by a heterogeneous population of cellular and chemical mediators of the immune system, such as T cells, B cells, macrophages, cytokines, and prostaglandins. Inflammation of the synovium is marked and proteolytic enzymes are produced. This process will potentially lead to joint damage and destruction with subsequent deformity. Painful swollen joints and marked morning stiffness are common features. To avoid this, it is important that RA is diagnosed and treated at an early stage before significant damage occurs. Fortunately, referral systems and more effective treatments mean patients with suspected RA are now seen early by rheumatologists and treatment commenced. As a result, the classical deformities of RA are much less common than in the past.

The mainstay of management in RA is, therefore, early recognition followed by the use of specific disease-modifying anti-rheumatic drugs (DMARDs) such as methotrexate. In recent years, the use of more powerful biological agents has significantly improved the outlook for RA patients with more difficult or resistant disease. Analgesics, NSAIDs, and sometimes corticosteroid injections can also have a role, as can physiotherapy and appliances, where appropriate. Management of RA is usually in secondary care—both for the initial diagnosis and commencement of treatment, and also for subsequent monitoring. The role of the general practitioner is more one of recognition of suspected RA, prompt referral, and then holistic support, as necessary, of the patient and their family.

Other inflammatory arthritis and spondyloarthropathy

There is a range of inflammatory arthropathies and also spondyloarthropathies (where the spine is involved) that share some similarities with RA but are *seronegative* (absent rheumatoid factor). Pain, morning stiffness, and the likelihood of progressive joint damage are shared to varying degrees. The better known ones include psoriatic arthritis (see Figure 7.3) and anklylosing spondylitis. The joint/spine disease may be associated with other medical conditions including iritis, urethritis, and inflammatory bowel disease. Suspicion of these conditions should lead to a referral to a rheumatologist.

Traumatic arthritis

The term 'traumatic arthritis' can cover a wide spectrum of clinical presentations and histological changes. Severe trauma can result in

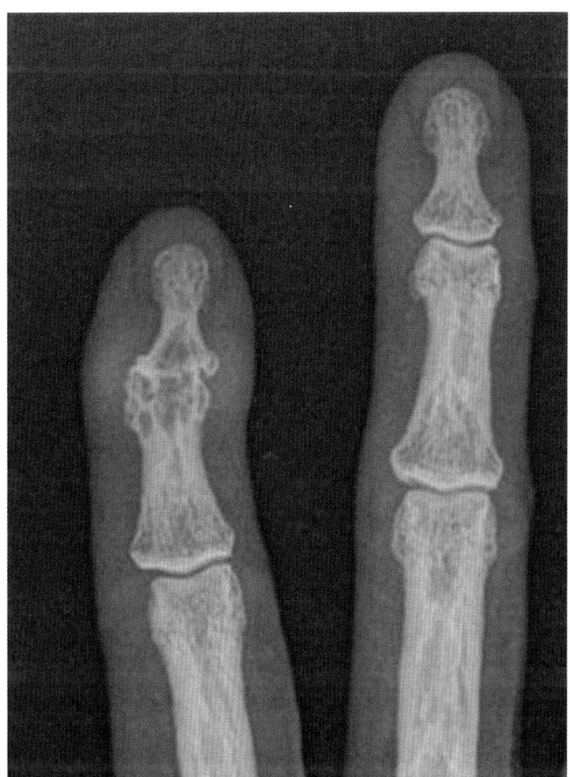

Figure 7.3 Distal interphalangeal joint arthritis associated with psoriasis.

fractures involving the articular surface, disruption of the articular cartilage, rupture of internal ligaments, and haemarthrosis. Injuries of this nature are serious and will usually require the attention of an orthopaedic surgeon. Treated or not, they will potentially predispose the joint to the development of OA.

However, in musculoskeletal practice, this term is also used to describe an acute or sub-acute presentation of a painful and often swollen joint following less severe trauma such as a sprain. The trauma has usually involved damage to the joint capsule and/or capsular ligaments with resultant inflammation and effusion. These changes will usually settle with time, rest, ice, and anti-inflammatory drugs. If not, injection of corticosteroids can be very effective in hastening recovery. There is also a school of thought, especially within sports medicine, that injecting hyaluronic acid, either into the joint or peri-articular, can be helpful at this stage, and there is some evidence to support this (Petrella 2007). The clinician must not overlook the possibility of intra-articular damage to important structures such as cruciate ligament rupture at the knee, or fracture involving a joint surface. Very rapid swelling after the injury (especially at the knee), with resultant haemarthrosis, may lead one to suspect this. If the trauma has been severe, there may be ligament laxity and joint instability.

Other forms of arthritis

Gout

Gout affects approximately 1% of the UK population and, in men, has an incidence of 1–3 per 1000 people. It is more common in men than in women and increases in incidence with age (1 in 14 older men and 1 in 35 older women). The underlying abnormality is a raised level of uric acid in the blood with deposition of crystals of sodium urate in the synovial lining of joints, leading to inflammation (see Figure 7.4). The raised uric acid levels are either due to increased production or to reduced elimination. Potential causes include:

- obesity
- hypertension, especially if treated with thiazide diuretics
- diabetes
- hyperlipidaemia
- genetic factors—gout may be familial
- impaired renal function
- a diet rich in purines
- excess alcohol intake

Diagnosis may be suspected clinically in a typical case—sudden onset of a very painful, swollen, and exquisitely tender first metatarso-phalangeal (MTP) joint—but if other joints are affected, it is often less clear-cut. Full blood count and serum urate should be checked (though this may be normal during an attack), but the only pathonomonic diagnostic feature would be the finding of uric acid crystals in joint fluid. However, aspirating an acutely inflamed first MTP joint would be very uncomfortable for the patient and in practice is rarely done.

Treatment is to modify any underlying factors, if possible, and to treat pain and inflammation during attacks using analgesia, (high-dose) NSAIDs, or possibly an intra-articular steroid injection. Colchicine is an old-fashioned, but still potentially useful treatment for patients who cannot tolerate NSAIDs. If attacks are frequent, then lowering the serum uric acid with a drug such as allopurinol can be considered.

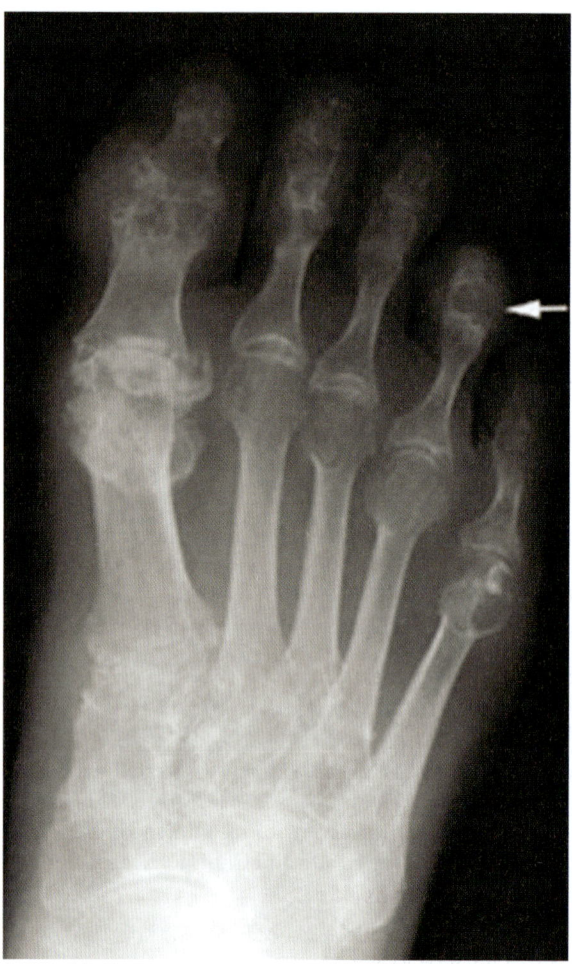

Figure 7.4 Degenerative change, para-articular erosion (arrowed), and soft tissue swelling in a case of gout.

Pseudogout

Pseudogout is similar to gout but with deposition of crystals of calcium pyrophosphate. It is also known as calcium pyrophosphate deposition disease (CPPD). Again, age and genetics are involved and also possibly other factors such as:

- excess iron storage as in haemochromatosis
- low magnesium levels in the blood
- hyperparathyroidism
- hypercalcaemia
- hypothyroidism

Unlike gout, larger joints such as the knee, hip, or shoulder are more commonly affected than the smaller ones. Diagnosis is often suggested by calcification of articular cartilage on X-ray, but again definitive diagnosis would have to be by examination of synovial fluid for the characteristic crystals. Calcification of the cartilage in the knee is a not infrequent chance finding on X-ray in an otherwise asymptomatic patient. Treatment is of the pain/inflammation with NSAIDs or cortisone injections, as needed.

Septic arthritis

Septic arthritis is a rare but serious condition, with an incidence of 2–10 per 100,000 in the UK. It will usually follow either surgery or joint injection and is more likely in patients with any cause of immune suppression or dysfunction, including common conditions such as diabetes, old age, and alcohol abuse (2003, 2006). Septic arthritis has a considerable morbidity (mainly long-term joint damage) and some mortality associated with it—figures of 31.6% and 11.5% respectively in one UK study (Weston et al. 1999). Treatment of septic arthritis is a hospital procedure involving drainage and lavage of the joint with intravenous antibiotic therapy.

Tendon pathology

Tendinopathy

This term refers to disease affecting the tendons. There are two main types to be considered:

- tendonitis—an inflammation of the tendon
- tendonosis—a degeneration of the tendon

The majority of tendon conditions seen in everyday musculoskeletal practice in the UK, especially with an increasingly elderly population, tend to be tendonosis rather than tendonitis, with little evidence of inflammation (Khan and Cook 2000). Sometimes there is a mixture of the two pathologies in the same patient.

Tendonitis and tenosynovitis

This inflammatory condition of the tendon and/or its sheath is usually caused by overuse and tends to present acutely or sub-acutely. True tendonitis is clinically uncommon, most cases being more chronic and more appropriately termed tendonosis. Symptoms include pain, worse on use, and stiffness after resting. There may well be visible swelling and redness, and palpable crepitus.

Histologically, tendonitis and tendon-sheath synovitis are characterized by acute oedema and hyperaemia of the paratenon with infiltration of inflammatory cells. After hours to a few days, fibrinous exudate fills the tendon sheath.

Treatment initially is with analgesia and oral or topical NSAIDs, combined with rest and maybe application of ice. If the condition is slow to settle, a steroid injection could be considered, especially if there is also a tenosynovitis as in De Quervain's tenosynovitis at the wrist. The condition will normally resolve within days or at most, a few weeks. If it continues much longer, then it is likely that there is also an element of tendinosis.

Tendonosis

This is much more common than tendonitis. Tendonosis becomes increasingly common with age and is often multifactorial in its aetiology. Commonly, there is a combination of relative overuse of the tendon, combined with extrinsic factors such as injury or friction, and/or intrinsic factors such as relatively poor blood supply and poor biomechanics causing increased tensile stresses. It is thought that repetitive micro tearing combined with an inadequate or chaotic healing response is involved. Increased tendon cell death with a higher apoptotic index has been found in some cases of tendinopathy (Lian et al. 2007). Genetic factors probably play a role in predisposing some people to tendon injury and tendinopathy (September et al. 2007). Common clinical sites are the rotator cuff at the shoulder, common flexor and extensor tendons at the elbow, and the Achilles tendon.

Tendonosis is tendon degeneration without clinical or histological signs of an inflammatory response. Tendonosis can also be associated with paratenonitis (e.g. in the Achilles tendon). To the naked eye, tendons may appear normal, or may be thickened and swollen. There are not usually any outward signs of inflammation such as redness or warmth. At operation, such tendons can appear duller and more yellow or brown than usual. Histologically, various changes are seen:

- The total amount of collagen is decreased (breakdown exceeds repair) and the ratio of Type III to Type I collagen is abnormally high.
- The amounts of proteoglycans and glycosaminoglycans are increased, leading to a higher than usual water content.
- The normal parallel fibre structure is disorganized with evidence of both collagen repair and collagen degeneration. Microtears and collagen fibre separations are seen—many of the collagen fibres are thin, fragile, and separated from each other.
- The number of fibroblast cells is increased; the tenocytes have a different appearance as the cells are actively trying to repair the tissue.
- There is increased vascularity.

Figure 7.5 shows a normal Achilles tendon, whereas Figure 7.6 shows a considerably thickened tendon with altered pattern of collagen, and Figure 7.7 shows a similar tendon in cross-section.

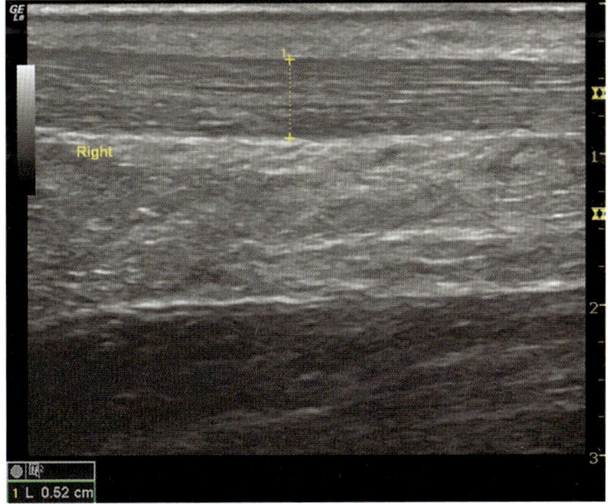

Figure 7.5 Normal Achilles tendon.
(Reproduced courtesy of Martyn Speight.)

The degenerative changes result in the tendon having reduced tensile strength and is more prone to injury, tearing, and even rupture. The tendon may or may not be painful—if so, the pain may come from nociceptor stimulation as a consequence of the disordered collagen or maybe as a result of release of irritant non-inflammatory chemicals.

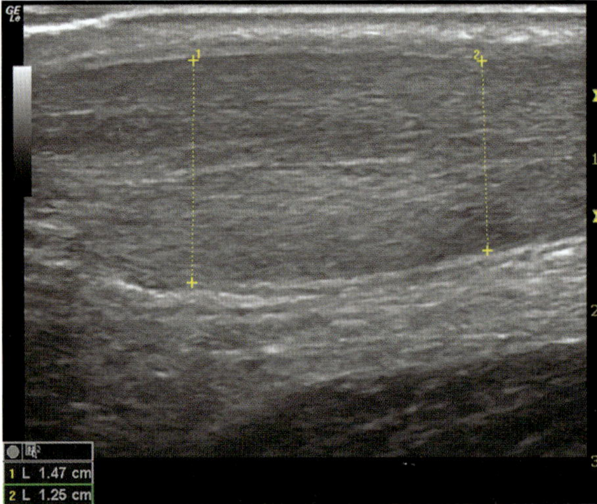

Figure 7.6 Achilles tendonosis.
(Reproduced courtesy of Martyn Speight.)

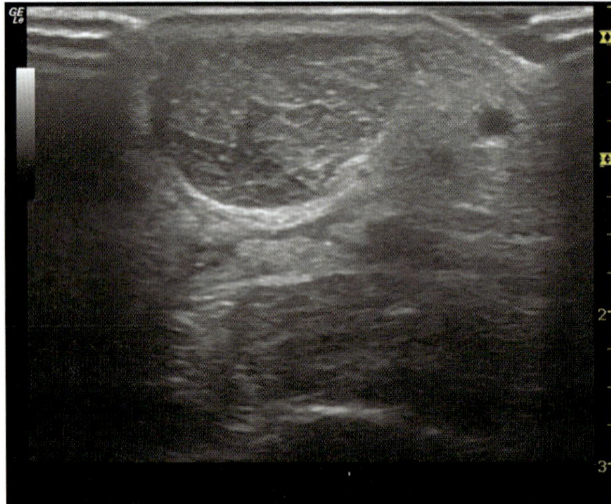

Figure 7.7 Achilles tendonosis.
(Reproduced courtesy of Martyn Speight.)

Many treatments are used for tendinopathy; when many treatments are available, it tends to mean that none are perfect! The following are commonly used:

- Physiotherapy, especially in the form of eccentric exercises, is perhaps the most successful (Mafulli and Longo 2008). Success is proportional however to physiotherapist expertise and patient compliance.
- Steroid injections are widely used and are generally held to be helpful in the short term (approximately 4–6 weeks); however, their long-term effectiveness is not known, and quality of evidence for their use remains poor and controversial. Clinically, they commonly give a period of pain relief that may be seen as a 'window of opportunity' in which to commence other, usually physical, therapies aimed at longer-term management. Injection treatment used alone will result in a high incidence of symptom recurrence.
- Other conservative treatment options available for the management and treatment of tendinopathy include:
  - rest (especially if coexistent inflammation)
  - ice
  - massage therapy (deep transverse frictions)
  - NSAIDs
  - ultrasound therapy or other electrotherapy
  - taping (to reduce loading)
  - prolotherapy (Rabago et al. 2009)
  - blood injection (Rabago et al. 2009)—autologous blood or platelet- rich plasma
  - topical glyceryl trinitrate
  - extracorporeal shockwave therapy (Chung and Wiley 2002).
- Surgical treatment—tends to be used as a last resort when conservative methods have failed (e.g. tennis elbow release or Achilles tendon debridement).

Evidence for all these treatments tends to be mixed and clinical preference will often be based on personal and colleague experience of success. Fortunately, many cases of tendonosis are self-limiting clinically and will improve with time.

Muscle pathology

Muscle strain

Muscle injuries are relatively common, with the calf and hamstrings perhaps being the most often affected and sporting activity of some kind the most common cause. Muscle strains may be graded from 1 to 3 depending upon the degree of damage to muscle fibres—1 being mild and 3 being complete rupture.

Treatment is with initial rest, maybe with ice if there is considerable swelling and bruising, followed by controlled mobilization and rehabilitation, ideally under the management of a physiotherapist. In the much less common case of complete rupture, surgical intervention could be needed. Deep transverse frictions can have a useful role in preventing adverse scar tissue formation in the acute–subacute phase, or breaking up any such scar in the chronic case.

Myopathy

This term covers a wide range of conditions including neuromuscular problems such as muscular dystrophies and mitochondrial abnormalities, and also more inflammatory conditions such as polymyositis and dermatomyositis. These conditions are more normally managed by neurologists and rheumatologists rather than musculoskeletal physicians, although physiotherapy often plays an important part. Patients taking statins to lower their blood lipids are at increased risk of myopathy—although the risk is small—estimated at 32 extra cases of myopathy per 10,000 users (Hippisley-Cox 2010).

Ligaments

Patients with ligament problems normally present in musculoskeletal medicine as a consequence of injury. They may be seen acutely following a sprain, or more chronically with continuing pains or instability following previous injuries. They can also present as a result of chronic biomechanical stress from deformity. The anterior talo-fibular ligament at the ankle and the medial collateral at the knee present most commonly.

Ligaments maintain stability at joints and, by nature of their elastic properties, also allow functional movement. If however, the ligament is placed under an intolerable stretch, as in an injury (sprain), then it may be damaged. Ligament sprains can be graded as:

- Grade 1—a relatively minor injury with damage to a few fibres producing fairly localized inflammation and pain.
- Grade 2—more extensive damage to more fibres with resultant partial tear of the ligament. Clinically, there is more swelling and bruising.
- Grade 3—Severe damage with complete rupture of the ligament. Clinically, there is pain, swelling, bruising, and joint instability.

Following an acute ligament injury, the body's repair process starts almost immediately, with an initial inflammatory response lasting for about 3 days. It is then followed by a proliferative/repair phase lasting a few weeks and then, finally, by a remodelling phase as the repaired ligament adapts to the function required of it. This latter phase can take many months. Analgesia and 'RICE' (rest/ice/compression/elevation), followed by early controlled mobilization with physiotherapy supervision, where appropriate, is the best management. Steroid injection is contraindicated in the acute situation, as it will potentially suppress the early parts of the repair process. Usually, normal function and integrity are restored, but problems can potentially arise if either:

- The ligament is badly damaged and is either completely ruptured or significantly lax following repair. Joint instability is then likely to result with maybe recurrent injury, pain, and swelling. Chronic joint instability will predispose the joint to premature development of OA. Management is to restore stability, perhaps conservatively with strengthening exercises, restoration of proprioception (where appropriate), and maybe provision of splints. Prolotherapy (where the oseoligamentous junctions are injected with an irritant pro-inflammatory substance with resultant strong and dense scar tissue) can also be used to treat and tighten/strengthen weak, lax ligaments. In severe cases, surgical repair may be necessary.
- The ligament apparently heals with a stable joint, but pain is experienced in a chronic fashion, especially after exercise. In this instance, it is likely that adverse scar tissue has formed, limiting the normal function of the joint. The preferred management is physiotherapy (deep transverse frictions of the ligament, followed by manipulation to rupture the adverse scan tissue, followed by mobilization), although steroid injection could be used in some cases of chronic ligament strain.

Bursitis

There are approximately 160 bursae located at points of potential soft tissue friction around the body, usually where tendons or muscles cross bone. Some bursae are more prone than others to become painful—common examples being the subacromial bursa at the shoulder, or the trochanteric and gluteal bursae at the hip. Bursae are lined with synovial cells and if subjected to physical trauma or friction can show inflammation and increased synovial fluid production. However, as with tendons, evidence of actual inflammation is not always seen and sometimes pathology in adjacent tissue, particularly tendonosis, may be the real cause of the pain—not the bursa at all. Reflecting this, for many clinicians, the preferred term at the hip, for example, is 'greater trochanteric pain syndrome' rather than 'trochanteric bursitis'.

The bursitis may present as an acute condition, usually through overuse or occasionally as a response to trauma, but is more commonly seen as a chronic condition associated with degenerative change and/or poor biomechanics as at the subacromial bursa in the shoulder.

Treatment can be with rest combined with either NSAIDs or steroid injections in the short term, then followed by physical therapy to address underlying faulty biomechanical issues and/or activity modification. There is conflicting evidence as to whether ultrasound-guided steroid injections are more effective than unguided (or perhaps more accurately, anatomical-landmark-guided) injections (Chen et al. 2006). Often, there is convincing evidence of better placement with ultrasound, but much less convincing evidence of better outcome. Sometimes bursitis is a chronic or recurrent problem and a surgical solution is ultimately needed, especially if there is coexistent tendon pathology (for example, subacromial decompression at the shoulder).

Intervertebral discs

James Cyriax considered the intervertebral disc to be the source of low back pain in 90% of cases (Cyriax 1982). This idea became less popular when many low back pain patients were found to have relatively normal myelograms—especially as it was thought, at the time, that the disc was not innervated (although this had been suggested by Inman and Saunders as long ago as 1947) and could, therefore, only cause pain if it prolapsed and pressed on adjacent structures. With the advent of magnetic resonance imaging (MRI) scanning, and also the realization that at least the outer portion of the disc is innervated, it is apparent that the disc itself may be a source of pain. Maybe Cyriax had a point, although the exact proportion of cases of back pain originating in the intervertebral disc cannot be known with any certainty.

The intervertebral disc consists of an outer annulus that is composed of alternating oblique sheets of collagen fibres, and also contains elastic fibres—about 10% by weight (see Figure 7.8). The nucleus pulposus is composed of a few cartilage cells and collagen fibres dispersed in a semi-fluid ground substance (Bogduk 1997). In children and young adults, the nucleus has a relatively high water content (70–90%) but with increasing age—as early as the third decade—the water content decreases and the nucleus becomes less fluid. In addition, the annulus becomes more 'fragile' and prone to develop cracks or 'fissures' in response to tortional stress. Increased tortional strain may prompt disruption of the annulus with resultant pain and maybe bulging into the spinal canal. The nucleus may prolapse into the fissure of the annulus, which then bulges out into the canal, or the nucleus can form a true herniation through the fissure into the spinal canal. There is evidence that release of nuclear material into the spinal canal will cause an inflammatory response resulting in local spinal and radicular pain.

If the disc bulges directly backwards, it will first stretch the posterior longitudinal ligament and, subsequently, the anterior dura mater. Both of these structures are innervated and pain-sensitive and can cause localized low back pain—'lumbago'. Owing to the way in which these central structures are supplied by anastamosing

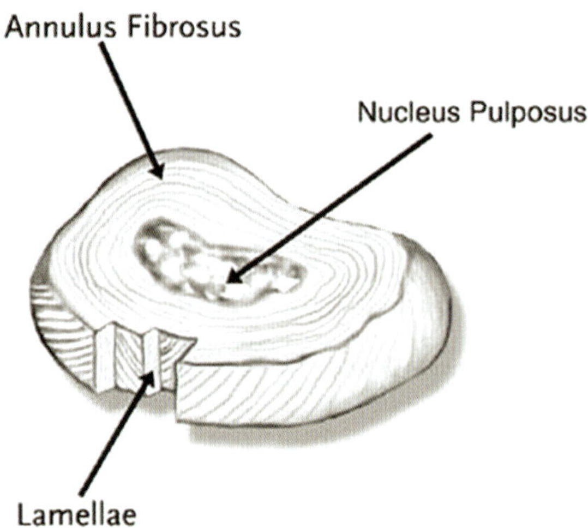

Figure 7.8 Composition of the intervertebral disc.

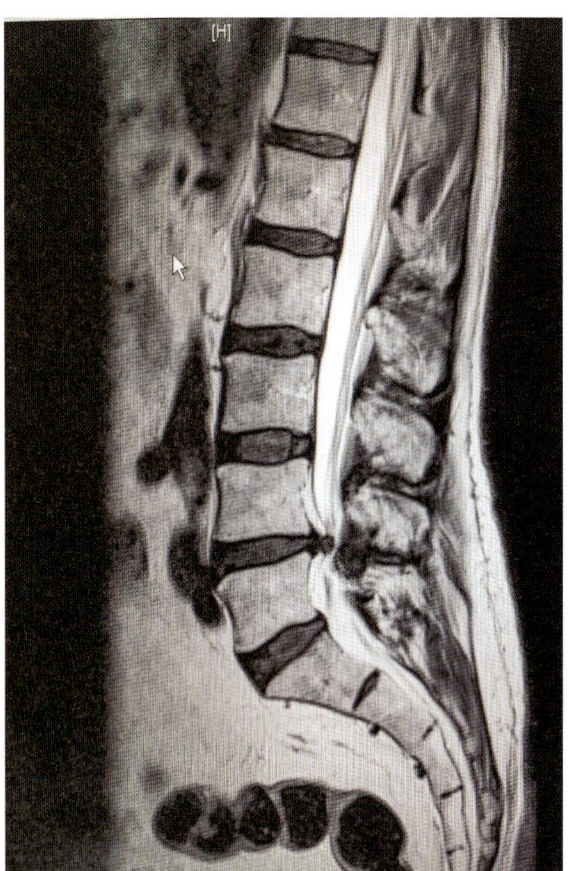

Figure 7.9 Saggital MRI showing prolapsed L4/5 disc.

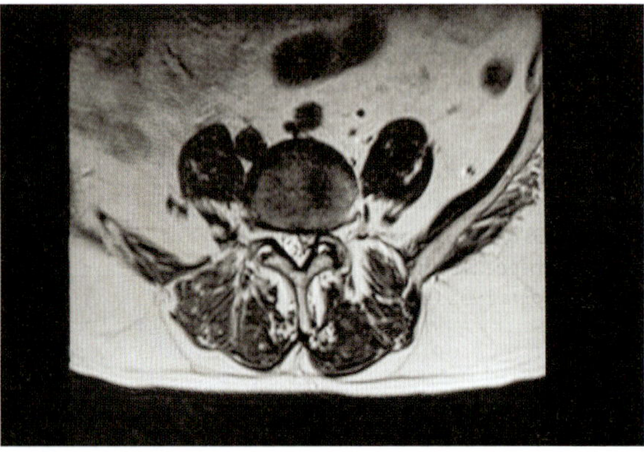

Figure 7.10 Axial view showing (the same) left L4/5 paracentral disc prolapse as in Figure 7.9.

sinuvertebral nerves, this pain tends to be poorly localized and can be central or bilateral, and is likely to be multisegmental. If the disc bulge is larger or moves laterally (because it is constrained by the relatively strong posterior longitudinal ligament), pressure may then be placed upon the nerve root dural sleeve causing segmentally referred pain in the appropriate limb. This is the explanation for the classic pattern of intervertebral disc prolapse with initial back pain followed by leg pain, with the back pain often diminishing. If the disc bulge presses more firmly, then the nerve root itself can be affected with resultant segmental radicular pain, numbness, pins and needles, and/or weakness. If the ligament is weak or ruptures, then a large central prolapse can occur into the spinal canal (see Figures 7.9 and 7.10) with the possibility of cord or cauda equina compression. Occasionally, the disc bulge or prolapse occurs first in a posterolateral, not a posterior, direction; in this case, leg pain will be the initial presentation, and there may be little if any back pain. This scenario is more common in the cervical than in the lumbar spine.

Disc injuries show a considerable propensity to recover. A small study by Saal in 1990 showed that the majority of disc herniations reduced in size over a period of 1–2 years (Saal et al. 1990). A larger study by Bush in 1992 showed similar findings, with 76% of disc herniations and 26% of disc bulges showing partial or complete resolution over 12 months (Bush et al. 1992). A review by Jacobs in 2011 concluded that whilst early surgery for disc herniations may speed recovery, there is no statistical difference between operated and non-operated patients at 1–2 years (Jacobs et al. 2011). The only indication for urgent surgery is cauda equina compression. It remains to be clarified which other patients benefit from surgery rather than conservative care, but it is probably those with definite stenosis of the central spinal canal or lateral recess.

Nerves

Nerve tissue is generally considered not to be pain-sensitive unless it has been sensitized by previous pathology such as inflammation or ischaemia. Otherwise, pressure on a nerve will tend to produce parasthesiae, numbness, and, if marked, weakness in the muscles supplied. The nature and distribution of any symptoms so produced will depend upon which portion of a nerve pathway is compressed:

- If the spinal cord is compressed, then there is usually no pain. Parasthesiae are produced in a multisegmental and usually bilateral distribution. These will be hard for the patient to localize—they will usually be in the limbs but without any clear aspect or edge to them. There may be an associated upper motor neurone (spastic) weakness with physical signs such as increased reflexes and tone, extensor plantar response, and clonus at the ankle.

- If a nerve root it compressed, then there will be unilateral and segmental referral of parasthesiae and numbness. Beyond being segmental, the symptoms are not well localized due to dermatome overlapping (they are likely to have aspect), e.g. anterior or posterior, but no well-defined edge. Weakness, if present, will be of reduced tone (flaccid) type and reflexes will be reduced or absent. Pain (from the dural nerve root sleeve) will also be segmental. If the nerve root itself is sensitized, then lancinating segmental pain may result.
- If a nerve trunk is compressed, then mild discomfort/numbness will result but paraesthesiae are the main symptom, often being worse when the pressure is subsequently released. Then, a shower of painful paraesthesiae will be experienced in the appropriate dermatome. The affected area will be localized to some extent—said to have 'aspect but no edge'. The severity and duration of the symptoms will be related to the degree and duration of compression to which the nerve trunk was subjected.
- If a peripheral nerve is compressed, then there will be parasthesiae and numbness in the distribution of that nerve (as in carpal tunnel syndrome, for example) and it will be possible to 'map' this much more accurately than with nerve root or trunk symptoms. The affected area of skin will have both 'aspect and edge'. The severity and frequency of such symptoms is related to the degree of pressure on the nerve, as is any muscle weakness. Discomfort may also be experienced as in carpal tunnel syndrome.

Persistent pressure upon a nerve can, if untreated, lead to permanent damage within the nerve. Animal models have shown that pressure on a peripheral nerve will initially produce endoneurial oedema, followed by eventual demyelination and fibrosis if left unrelieved for long periods (Rempel and Diao 2004). Relief of pressure, once these chronic changes have developed, will then not result in restoration of normal nerve function.

References

Bogduk N. (1997) *Clinical anatomy of the lumbar spine and sacrum,* Churchill Livingstone, New York.

Bush K, et al. (1992) The natural history of sciatica associated with disc pathology. A prospective study with clinical and independent radiological follow up. *Spine* 1992 Oct; 17(10):1205–12.

Chen, et al. (2006) Ultrasound-guided injections in the treatment of subacromial bursitis. *Am J Physic Med Rehab* 85(1):31–5.

Chung P, Wiley JP. (2002) Extracorporeal shockwave therapy: a review. *Sports Med* 32(13):851–65.

Coombes BK, et al. (2010) Efficacy and safety of corticosteroid injections and other injections for management of tendinopathy: a systematic review of randomised controlled trials. *The Lancet* 2010 Nov; 376(9754):1751–67.

Cyriax J. (1982) *Textbook of orthopaedic medicine, Vol. 1.* Baillière Tindall, London.

Friberg. (1983) Clinical symptoms and biomechanics of the lumbar spine and hip joint in leg length inequality. *Spine* 8:643–5.

Hippisley-Cox J. (2010) Unintended effects of statins in men and women in England and Wales. *BMJ* 340:c2197.

Humphreys JH, et al. (2012) The incidence of rheumatoid arthritis in the UK: comparisons using the 2010 ACR/EULA classification criteria and the 1987 ACR classification criteris. Results from the Norfolk Arthritis Register. *Ann Rheum Dis* 2013; 72:1315–1320.

Jacobs, et al. (2011) Surgery versus conservative management of sciatica due to a lumbar herniated disc: a systematic review. *Eur Spine J* 20(4):513–22.

Khan KM, Cook J. (2000) Overuse tendon injuries: where does the pain come from? *Sports Med Arthroscop Rev* 8:17–31.

Lian, et al. (2007) Excessive apoptosis in patellar tendinopathy in athletes. *Am J Sports Med* 35(4);605–11.

Mafulli N, Longo UG. (2008) How do eccentric exercises work in tendinopathy? *Rheumatology* 47:1444–5.

National Institute for Health and Clinical Excellence (NICE). (2008) *NICE clinical guideline 59—osteoarthritis.*

Petrella. (2007) Periarticular hyaluronic acid in acute ankle sprain. *Clin J Sports Med* 17(4):251–7.

Rabago, et al. (2009) A systematic review of four injection therapies for lateral epicondylosis: prolotherapy, polidocanol, whole blood and platelet-rich plasma. *Br J Sports Med* 43:471–81.

Rempel D, Diao E. (2004) Entrapment neuropathies: pathophysiology and pathogenesis. *J Electromyo Kinesiol* 14:71–5.

Saal JA, et al. (1990) The natural history of lumbar intervertebral disc extrusions treated nonoperatively. *Spine* 1990 Jul; 15(7):683–6.

September, et al. (2007) Tendon and ligament injuries: the genetic component. *Br J Sports Med* 41:241–6.

Sofat N, et al. (2011) What makes osteoarthritis painful? The evidence for local and central pain processing. *Rheumatology* 2011 Dec; 50(12):2157–65.

Weston VC, Jones AC, Bradbury N, Fawthrop F, Doherty M. (1999) *Ann Rheum Dis* 58:214–9.

(2003) The management of septic arthritis. *Drug Ther Bull* 41(9): 65–8.

(2006) Guideline for the management of the hot swollen joint in adults with a particular focus on septic arthritis. *J Antimicrob Chemother* 58(3):492–3.

Chapter 8

Dynamic neuromuscular stabilization and the role of central nervous system control in the pathogenesis of musculoskeletal disorders

Marcela Safarova, Alena Kobesova, and Pavel Kolar

Introduction to dynamic neuromuscular stabilization

Three levels of sensorimotor control within the central nervous system (CNS) can be distinguished. The spinal and brainstem levels control general movements and primitive reflexes during the neonatal stage. The analysis of newborn's spontaneous general movements and the assessment of primitive reflexes are crucial for screening and early recognition of risk for an abnormal development. Recognizing the very early signs of abnormal development and introducing early functional treatment may help avoid or minimize serious structural and functional consequences.

The subcortical level of CNS motor control plays an important role after the newborn stage and matures mainly during the first year of life. This allows for basic trunk stabilization, a prerequisite for any phasic movement, and for locomotion function of the extremities. Analyzing the quality of postural-locomotion patterns allows for recognizing individuals who are developing central coordination disturbance (CCD). If left untreated, CCD often results in structural abnormalities and fixation of abnormal postural-locomotion patterns which are rather difficult to change later. Treatment administered during the first year of life may prevent such undesirable consequences. On the subcortical level, orofacial muscles and afferent information are automatically integrated within postural-locomotion patterns.

Finally, the cortical, or the highest level of motor control, increasingly becomes activated. Cortical control (including the cerebellum, mainly the neocerebellum) is important for the individual qualities and characteristics of movement. It also allows for isolated segmental movement as well as relaxation. A child with impaired cortical motor control may be diagnosed with developmental dyspraxia or developmental coordination disorder.

Dynamic neuromuscular stabilization (DNS) is a neurophysiological approach that utilizes human ontogenetic models (for example, developmental motor patterns) for both the diagnosis and treatment of dysfunction in the locomotor system in newborns, infants, and adult patients.

Spinal and brainstem levels of motor control

Approximately 70% of children develop normally after birth (Banaszek 2010; Bouwstra et al. 2009; Imamura et al. 1983; Vojta 2008). Early diagnosis based on Vojta serves as a diagnostic tool to assess the quality of development in early childhood. This assessment consists of:

1) assessment of the child's spontaneous motor skills,
2) assessment of positional reactions, and
3) assessment of the dynamics of primitive reflexes.

Currently, the diagnostics based on Vojta are used for an early recognition of atypical motor development. The screening also allows for early administration of appropriate therapy (during the first six months of life), which can prevent fixation of atypical movement patterns (Vojta 2008) and decrease the risk for abnormal motor as well as structural development.

Postural activity (spontaneous motor behaviour of a newborn)

Development of motor skills usually dates to the onset of postnatal development. Movement, however, develops already in the prenatal period. A rich repertoire of movement patterns is formed in the prenatal period. The postnatal development is merely a direct and logical continuation of this development (Prechtl and Hopkins 1986). Although the newborn also uses the higher levels of motor control, the spinal and brainstem levels are utilized especially in the first four weeks (Kobesova and Kolar 2013). This is demonstrated by a presence of innate automatisms in the infant's spontaneous motor skills, which consist of newborn, simple, global movement patterns that Prechtl referred to as general movements (GMs) and primitive reflexes.

Prechtl, in his studies, substantiates that intact and normally developing CNS is a necessary prerequisite for good quality of movement patterns or GMs (Bos et al. 1998). A developing nervous system spontaneously generates a volume of motor activity, even in the absence of external sensory information. The assessment of quality and intensity of GMs is one of the most effective functional examinations of nervous system's integrity in the first months of life (Bos et al. 1998; Bouwstra et al. 2010; Nakajima et al. 2006; Prechtl et al. 1993). It is a non-invasive and inexpensive examination, by 4-D ultrasonography, that allows for assessment of the quality and level of maturation of the developing brain already present in the prenatal period (Abo-Yaqoub et al. 2012). Clinically, the assessment of GMs' quality is usable mainly in the early infant period in children with normal development, as well as in children with severe involvement. The assessment of the quantity, quality, frequency, amplitude, and other characteristics of GMs serves as a specific and sensitive indicator for normal further development, development of minimal brain dysfunction, or central paresis (Prechtl and Einspieler 1997). Prechtl described, in detail, the features of GMs that are characteristic in individual developmental stages, including the prenatal period, the initial eight postnatal weeks, and later stages up to the twentieth postnatal week. Prechtl unambiguously defined normal as well as atypical GMs that suggest pathological neuromotor development.

GMs in the prenatal period and the time around due date are characterized by movement of the entire body which may last from several seconds to minutes. There is a varied sequence of movements of the lower and upper extremities, neck, and the trunk. Their onset is gradual, and the strength, intensity, and speed begin and end gradually. The movements are smooth, appear elegant, and give an impression of complexity and variability. Writhing movements dominate from the time of due date to 8 weeks after birth and are characterized by small to medium amplitude and slow to medium speed. Usually, they have an elliptical character, which gives the impression of a twisting motion. Fidgety movements appear at 6–20 weeks (most often at 9–15 weeks) and are described as circular movements of the head, trunk, and the extremities of small amplitude, medium speed, and varied movement acceleration in all directions. They continue to be present when the infant is awake and does not focus on something that caught their attention (Prechtl 2001).

The newborn (first 4 weeks of life) in supine and in prone position demonstrates asymmetrical posture, is unsteady, nearly in constant motion, and is able to change head position. In prone position (Figure 8.1A), the slope of the shoulder and pelvic girdle axes changes as does the convex trunk curvature during contralateral head rotation. The head is rotated towards one side, the cervical spine is bent backwards, thus in lateroflexion. The trunk rests on the mat, the xiphoid process is weightbearing, the spine lacks kypholordotic curvatures. The hands are in contact with the mat. The hand forms a fist with the thumb in the palm of the hand and the wrist in ulnar deviation and palmar flexion. The elbow (in maximal flexion) points above the mat, the forearm rests in pronation. Shoulders are elevated and protracted. The shoulder joint is in internal rotation and extension. The pelvis is in ventral flexion and it is positioned higher than the cervical spine due to the arrangement of the lower extremities. The hips and knees are in flexion, the femoral bones form an abduction angle slightly less than 90°, and the hip is in internal rotation. The ankle is in dorsiflexion and pronation.

A newborn in supine position (Figure 8.1B) demonstrates a global movement and emergence of primitive kicking. This mobility has no specific aim or purpose. The head is bent back and always rotated to one side. The side towards which the head is rotated usually demonstrates convex trunk curvature. The shoulders are in protraction, internal rotation, and elevation. Upper extremities are in elbow flexion; the elbow can push into the mat. The hand is in a fist with the thumb in the palm of the hand and the wrist is in ulnar deviation and palmar flexion. The newborn cannot lay the entire surface of the trunk on the mat as the spine is positioned in extension. The pelvis is tilted forwards and sloped. The lower extremities are actively held in hip and knee flexion. The abduction angle between the femurs is slightly below 90° (45° on each side). The foot is in dorsiflexion if the movement is into hip flexion. If the newborn demonstrates primitive kicking (alternating lower extremity movement in a sagittal plane) and the hip is moving into extension, the foot is in plantar flexion. Foot pronation and supination positioning also change depending on

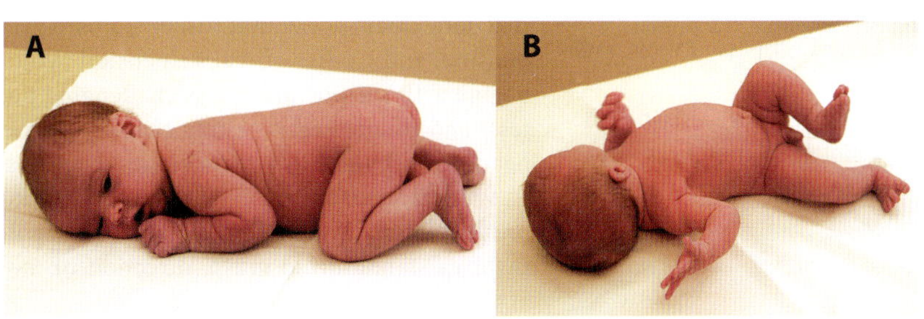

Figure 8.1 (**A**) Physiological newborn, typical prone position; (**B**) Physiological newborn, typical supine position.

the newborn's movement; a newborn cannot maintain a neutral position.

In the 1950s, Arsavskij and Krjuckova published an article about the newborn's ability to gradually turn towards a light. A newborn can track a light without global movement of the entire body. This is not only a movement of the eyes or the head or a learned movement, but rather, an innate programmed and highly coordinated process. As Vojta writes: '. . . without their knowledge, Arsavskij and Krjuckova showed that a newborn has the ability of coordinated control of body positioning' (Vojta 2008; Vojta and Peters 2007). Recent studies describe the character of visual stimulus without other contexts, with posture and its control (Kremenitzer et al. 1979). It has been shown that a newborn maintains visual contact only for a few seconds, depending also on their postural situation. The newborn visually fixates if a more advantageous postural position is provided manually. Postural body positioning is a vital foundation for all motor skills (Vojta and Peters 2007).

Primitive reflexes

Primitive reflexes are reflex movement patterns that develop as a motor reaction to a specific afferent stimulus. Primitive reflexes are usually typical for early childhood and are mostly represented in the first 4–6 weeks after birth. Some reflexes are present from birth. We know that some are also present in the prenatal period. Some reflexes cease as the CNS matures, others remain the entire life, and yet others are present only under pathological conditions. The persistence of certain reflexes beyond their expected time of physiological presence, or their absence during such time, often suggests pathological CNS development. The development of a certain characteristic picture or a type of central paresis (CP) can be predicted based on the assessment of primitive reflexes. There are three basic groups of primitive reflexes:

- Orofacial reflexes: Babkin reflex, rooting reflex, searching reflex, and sucking reflex.
- Tonic reflexes: suprapubic reflex, crossed extension reflex, stepping automatism, primitive upright reaction (lower extremity), Galant reflex.
- Grasping reflexes: palmar grasp reflex and plantar reflex.

Other primitive reflexes include Moro reflex lift reaction, heel reflex, doll's eyes reflex, acoustic-facial reflex, and visual-facial reflex.

The development of orofacial automatisms is closely linked to postural development. The lack of orofacial reflexes during the neonatal stage should be unambiguously considered as a clear sign of disrupted CNS function. Their persistence through to the beginning of the third trimester is also a clear sign of pathological development. Problems with breathing, swallowing, and chewing can be the first indicators of cerebral palsy (Vojta and Schweizer 2009).

Table 8.1 summarizes individual primitive reflexes, describes the way they are elicited, illustrates their physiological motor response, and gives the timeline for their physiological duration (Schulz 2013; Vojta 2008; Vojta & Schweizer 2009).

Similarly to the spontaneous motor patterns in the neonatal stage, a number of primitive reflexes are organized at the spinal and brainstem levels. Later, as the CNS matures, higher subcortical and cortical CNS structures and functions inhibit these primitive motor patterns, leading to a gradual cessation of primitive reflexes or, more precisely, their integration into the patterns controlled by the higher CNS centres. Some of these reflexes can once again manifest themselves as a result of regression to the spinal and brainstem levels of control during a cranial trauma, cerebrovascular accident, or degenerative or other extensive brain injury. The presence of primitive reflexes beyond their physiological timeline of occurrence and, on the other hand, their absence during early development are also signs of atypical CNS development.

The assessment of primitive reflexes is non-invasive, simple, efficient, and important, mainly in the neonatal stage. The greater the presence of pathological characteristics in primitive reflexes, the greater the risk of atypical CNS development and stronger the indication for early rehabilitation intervention. Primitive reflexes can become fixated as part of the infant's spontaneous motor skills if therapy is not indicated in time. Motor patterns of primitive reflexes do not allow for purposeful support, stepping forward, and grasping functions and pose a crucial obstacle in the normal development of postural-locomotion functions.

In the first months of development, the assessment of primitive reflexes is considered more valuable than the assessment of tendon reflexes, which may not be particularly significant for the assessment of the quality of CNS development during this period (Leonard and Hirschfeld 1995). Especially the first month of life is characterized by a spectrum of primitive reflexes. Zafeiriou et al. (1995) recommend the following eight reflexes as the most reliable during this time period: the palmar grasp reflex, plantar reflex, Galant response, asymmetric tonic neck reflex, suprapubic extensor reflex, crossed extensor reflex, Rossolimo reflex, and the heel reflex.

Postural reactions

Postural reactions represent an infant's automatic motor response to a passive change in body position. In a clinical picture, they completely correlate with the level of spontaneous motor skills and elicitation of primitive reflexes. It can be said that the assessments of spontaneous motor skills, postural reactions, and primitive reflexes represent only different ways of evaluating the CNS function.

During the assessment of postural reactions, the infant is lifted from either prone, side-lying, or supine positions above the therapeutic table. To ensure validity of the evaluation, all seven postural tests (PT) are routinely administered. These tests were compiled and modified by Vojta. They include the following: the traction test, Landau reaction, axillary suspension, Vojta's side tilt reaction, Collis horizontal suspension, Peiper-Isbert vertical suspension, and Collis vertical suspension (Vojta 2008). The testing begins with the posturally less challenging postural test (traction test) and progresses to testing that involves the infant tilting its head down by a quick manoeuvre (Peiper-Isbert reaction, Collis vertical suspension). The infant is then immediately put back on the table. Through a predictable, clearly defined method that involves standardized grasp, direction of movement, and speed

Table 8.1 Primitive reflexes

Physiological reflexes	Stimulation	Motor response	Physiological time frame / Pathological time frame	Positive response: Illustration
Orofacial Reflexes				
Babkin reflex	Light pressure into the palm; head is in neutral position	Mouth opening without additional facial expressions; ipsilateral head rotation toward stimulated side with unilateral stimulationition	0-4 weeks / Persistence beyond 6 weeks	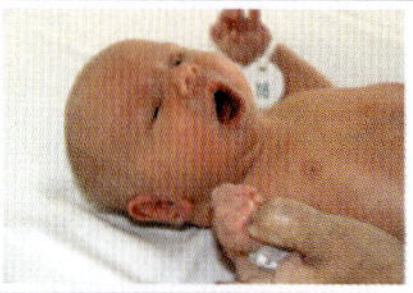
Rooting reflex	Stimulating areas of upper and lower lip with a moist finger; stimulation of right and left corner of mouth	Tongue moves in the direction of stimulation; tongue must be unwound	0-3 months / Absence of reflex or persistence beyond 6 months	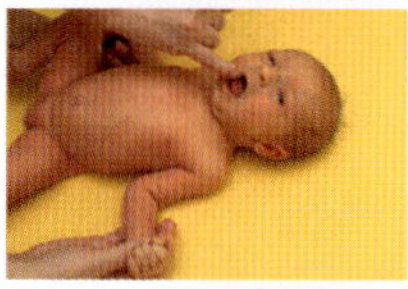
Searching reflex	Tactile stimulus on the face in the proximity of mouth	Child turns toward direction of stimulation, expressionless reaction	0-4 weeks / Absence of reflex	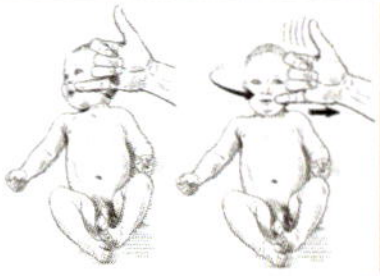 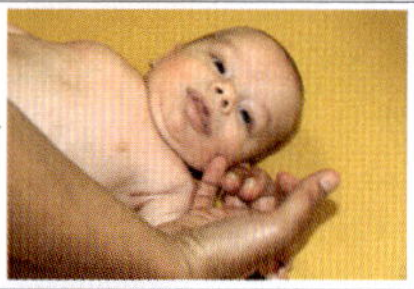
Sucking reflex	Oral stimulation with a moist finger	Child sucks the finger (6-8 swallowing contractions is the norm)	0-3 months / Absence of reflex or persistence beyond 6 months	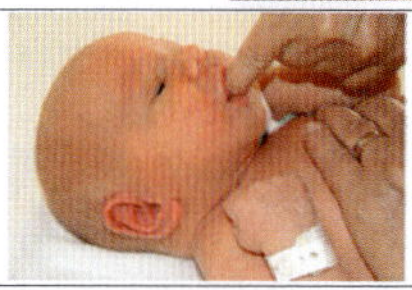
Tonic Reflexes				
Suprapubic reflex	Child is in supine. Light pressure is exerted on the cranial aspect of symphysis pubis	Lower extremities move into hip adduction, extension and internal rotation, knee extension, ankle plantar flexion and fanning of toes.	0-4 weeks / Persistence beyond 3 months	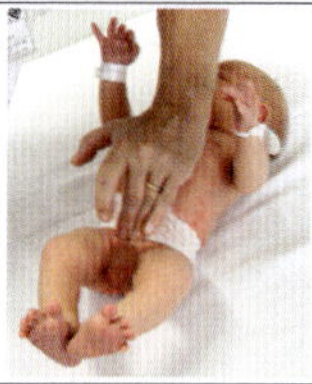
Crossed extension reflex	Child is in supine. Lower extremity is held in flexion,adduction and some internal rotation. The therapist applies pressure through the femur into the acetabulum.	Extension of contralateral lower extremity, internal rotation, adduction, tendency toward plantar flexion, big toe extension and toe abduction.	0-6 weeks / Persistence beyond 3 months	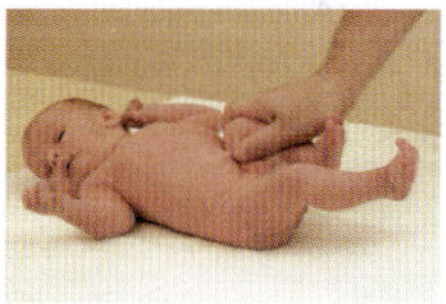
Stepping Automatism	Weight bearing through the forefoot of one lower extremity and trunk swaying over the weight bearing extremity	Contralateral extremity moves into triple flexion	0-4 weeks / Persistence beyond 3 months	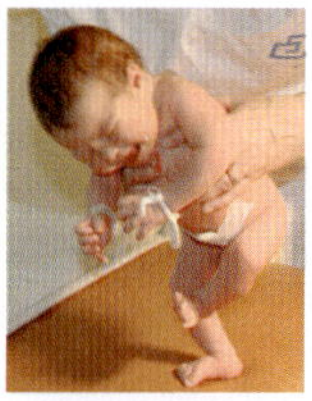
Primitive support of the lower extremities	Stand the child on the heels, weight bear through the soles of the feet.	Homologous extension of lower extremities	0-4 weeks / Persistence beyond 3 months	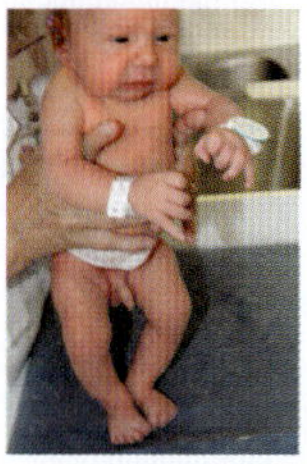

Table 8.1 (Continued) Primitive reflexes

Physiological reflexes	Stimulation	Motor response	Physiological time frame / Pathological time frame	Positive response: Illustration
Galant reflex	Child is positioned prone over the therapist's forearm, the therapist stimulates the skin along the vertebrae from the inferior angle of the scapula to the thoracolumbar junction	Lateral flexion of the trunk toward the side of stimulation; trunk movement is accompanied by movement of all extremities in neonatal stage	0-4 m during 4th month, the reflex weakens; it should be absent starting in the 6th month. / Persistence beyond 6 months	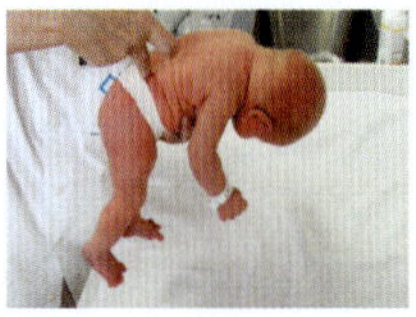
Grasping Reflexes				
Plantar reflex	Slight pressure on the plantar aspect of the foot in the area of the 3rd metatarsal head	Flexion of the MT and IP joints of the foot	0.-8. to 9. Months Until the time of support function of lower extremities	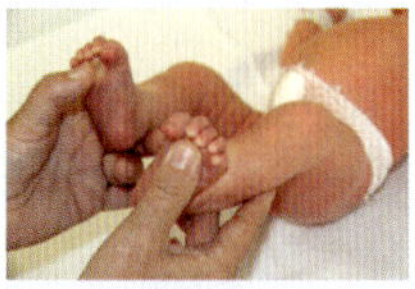
Palmar grasp	Slight pressure into the palm of the hand. Dorsum of the hand should not be stimulated.	Flexion of the MC and IP joints of the hand, grasp.	0-3months; At the time, when the child begins actively grasp the reflex weakens; it should be negative at 6 months; / Persistence beyond 6 months	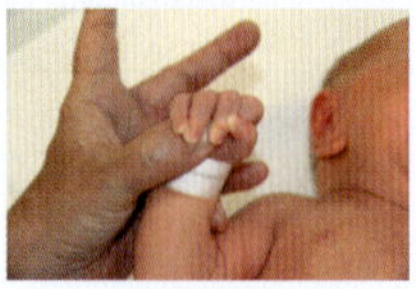
Other Reflexes				
Moro reflex	Above-threshold stimulus (light, noise, sudden movement of a diaper from underneath the infant, sudden drop of the head in a backward direction, etc.)	A-First phase consists of abduction and external rotation of the upper extremities; the head is positioned in midline and shows movement into flexion, lower extremities move into triple flexion. B-Next phase is the so called „hugging"phase with upper extremities moving into adduction. Spine is erect. Then, the body moves into its original position.	0-6 weeks / Persistence beyond 3 months	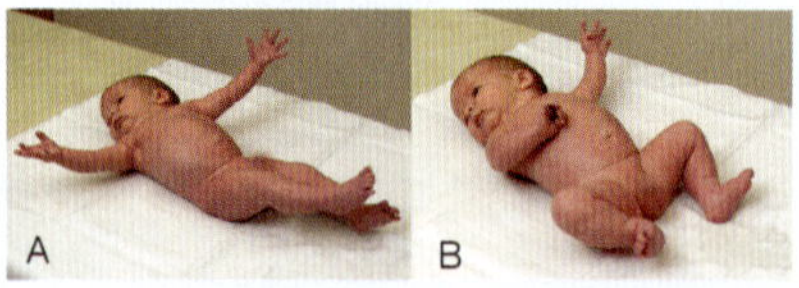 A B
Lift reaction	Child is lifted above the table while holding the sides of the trunk without contact of paravertebral muscles	With trunk movement upward, lower extremities move into flexion. With trunk movement in a downward direction, lower extremities move into extension.	0-4 months / Persistence beyond 6 months	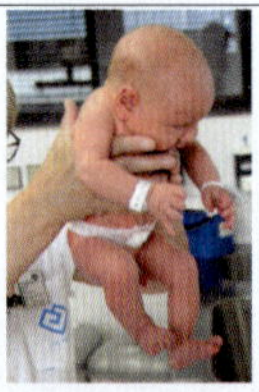
Heel reflex	Lower extremity joints are in neutral alignment. The therapist taps the heel in the direction of the long axis of the tibia (in supine).	Extremity moves into extension.	0-6 weeks / Persistence beyond 3 months	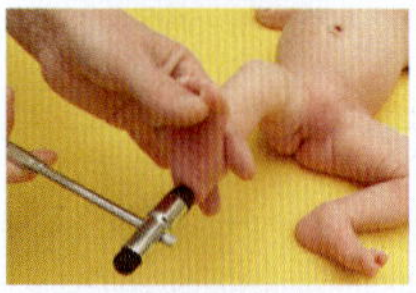
Doll's eyes phenomenon	Slow, passive head rotation	Eyes lag behind the movement; eyes look in the direction opposite to the head rotation)	0-4 weeks, reflex fades with onset of visual fixation / Persistence beyond 6 weeks	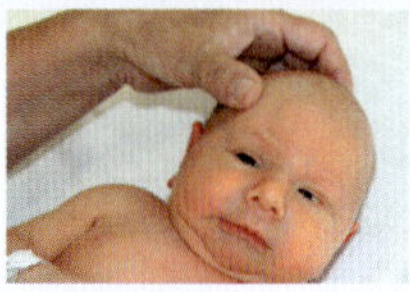

(*Continued*)

Table 8.1 (Continued) Primitive reflexes

Physiological reflexes	Stimulation	Motor response	Physiological time frame / Pathological time frame	Positive response: Illustration
Acoustic-facial reflex	Clapping next to the child's ear	Symmetrical blinking of the eyes	Since day 10; persists entire life / If it is negative after 4 months	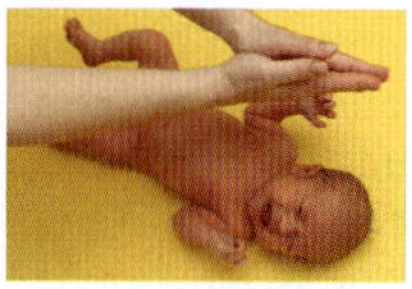
Visual-facial reflex	Quick movement of the therapist's open hand (30 cm distance) in front of the child's face. This cannot include reaction to air movement.	Symmetrical blinking of the eyes	Since month 3; persists entire life. Must be present at the onset of second trimester. Should be strongly positive at the end of second trimester. / If it is negative after 6 months	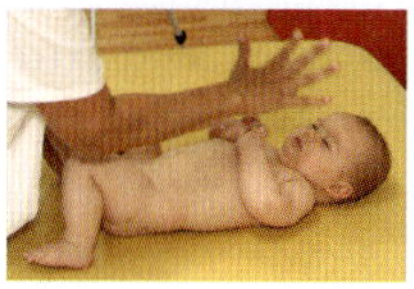
Always Pathological If Present In A Full-Term Infant.				**Reflex Testing** **Positive Reflex**
Palm reflex	Tap on the open palm; forearm is perpendicular to the frontal plane	Quick, phasic extension of the upper extremity with flexion reaction of the fingers	Can be physiologically present in infants born between 32-40 weeks of gestation. It is always negative at due date.	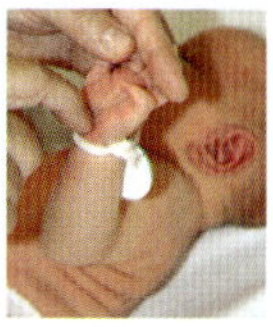 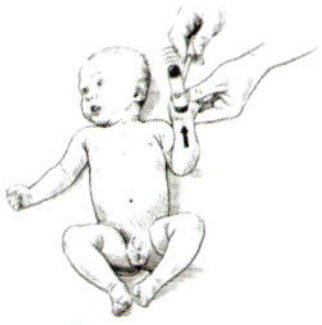
ATNR	Passive head rotation while the trunk is stabilized.	Facial-side extremities are in internal rotation and adduction in key joints, extension in mid-joints, ankle plantar flexion and inversion and toe extension. Hand is in ulnar deviation, fingers form a fist and thumb is in adduction. Occipital-side extremities are in the same position with the exception of mid-joints (elbow and knee), which are in flexion.	Not part of physiological development.	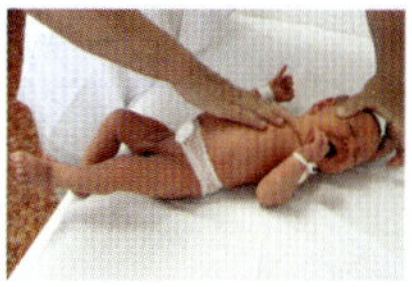 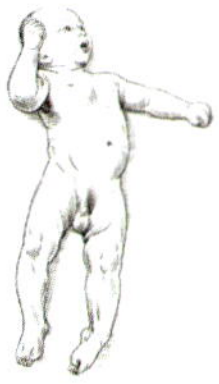
STNR	Passive head flexion with the thorax stabilized.	Upper extremities: shoulders are protracted, internally rotated and extended, elbow flexed, wrist in flexion, hand forms a fist with thumb adduction. Lower extremities: hips are extended, internally rotated and adducted, knee extended, ankle plantarflexed and inverted and toes extended.	Not part of physiological development.	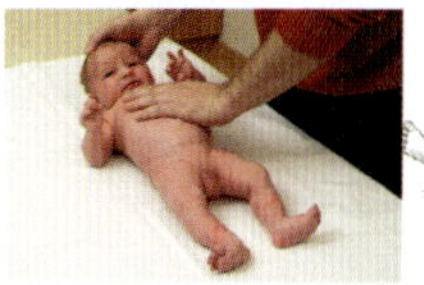 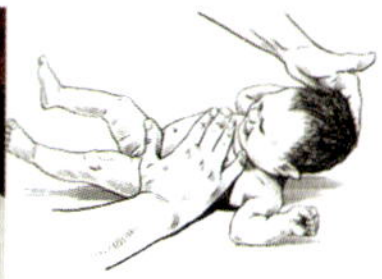
Rossolimo	Light strumming across the tips of toes on the plantar aspect.	MTP flexion and IP joint extension	Not part of physiological development.	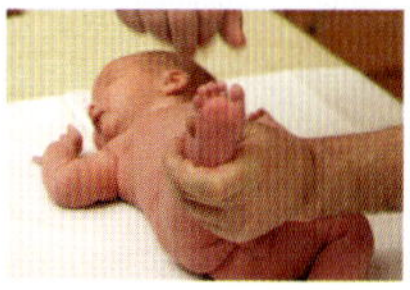 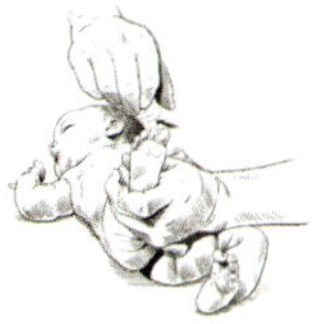
Primitive upright reaction of upper extremities	In supine, the child's arms are flexed, elbow supported in extension and wrist in extension. Pressure is exerted into the palm.	Counter pressure is felt into extension of all upper extremity joints	Not part of physiological development.	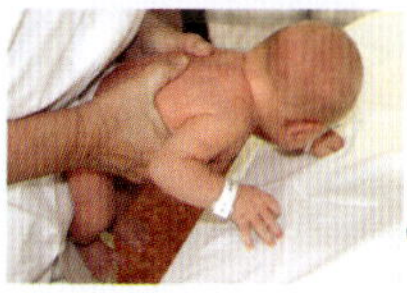 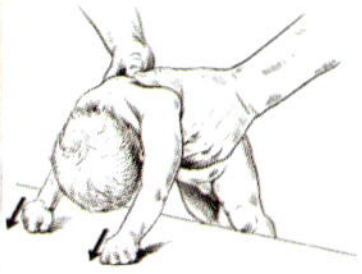

Abbreviations: (ATNR) asymmetrical tonic neck reflex; (IP) interaphalangeal; (MT) metatarsal; (MTP) metatarso-phalangeal; (STNR) symmetrical tonic neck reflex.

of movement, the infant suddenly gets into a different, extreme postural situation. The infant's first movement reaction, as well as their reaction to the sudden change in position, is observed. An experienced therapist can administer the test within 90 seconds with minimal stress to the infant. Same age, healthy infants always demonstrate a uniform response. The reaction is replicable. Certain uniformity can also be seen in infants with similar type of involvement (infants with spastic form of CP react similarly; a group of infants with hypotonic syndrome react alike), but the variability of atypical responses is wider than when compared to the norms attributed to a healthy infant's development. Reactions (head, trunk, and extremities) of infants of certain age are described precisely and in detail (Vojta 2008). A certain 'map' of postural reactions is formed based on the same stimulus. A deviation from a described norm is assessed as an atypical postural reaction.

The assessment of postural reactions pertains not only to a neonatal stage but is a part of evaluation of motor skills during the entire first year of life (Banaszek 2010). For illustration, Table 8.2 outlines the different reactions of infants with different levels of CNS maturity: a newborn and a 6-month-old infant. Note the difference in quality of postural stabilization (trunk muscle coordination), spinal uprighting, positions of head and upper and lower extremities, and integration of the orofacial system in the global reaction. A complete chart of postural reactions depicting physiological responses typical for 0–12 months of developmental age and pathological responses typical for certain types of CP can be found at <http://www.vojta.com>.

Table 8.2 Differences in postural reactions in a physiological newborn and a 6-month-old baby

Positional reactions	**Newborn**	**6-month-old baby**
Traction Test		
Landau Reaction		
Axillary Suspension		
Vojta s Tilt Reaction		

(Continued)

Table 8.2 (Continued) Differences in postural reactions in a physiological newborn and a 6-month-old baby

Positional reactions	Newborn	6-month-old baby
Collis Horizontal Suspension	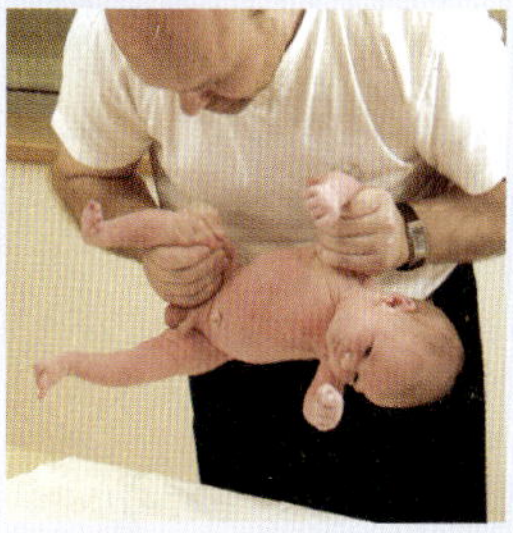	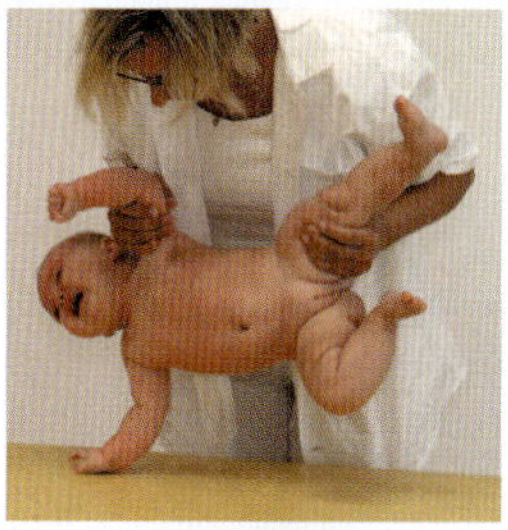
Peiper- Isbert Vertical Suspension	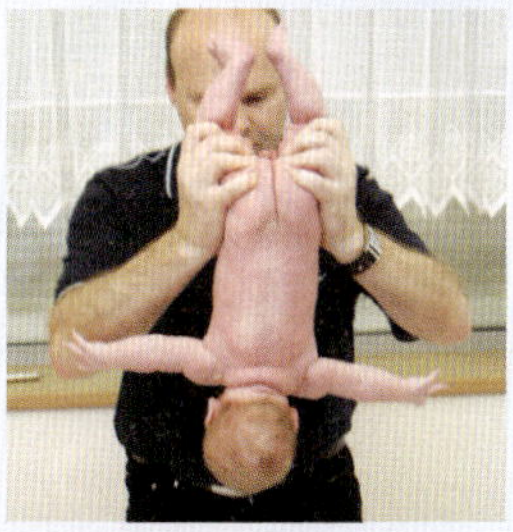	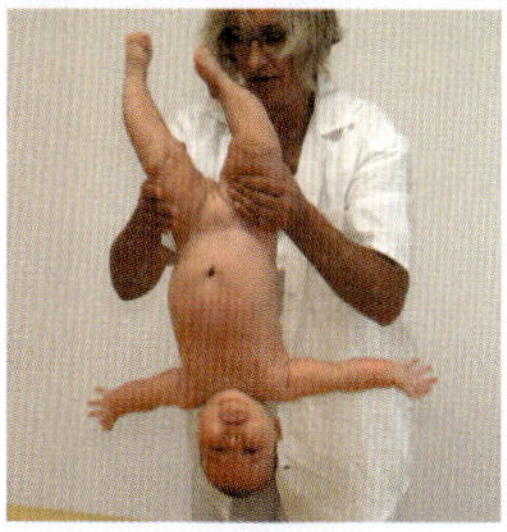
Collis Vertical Suspension	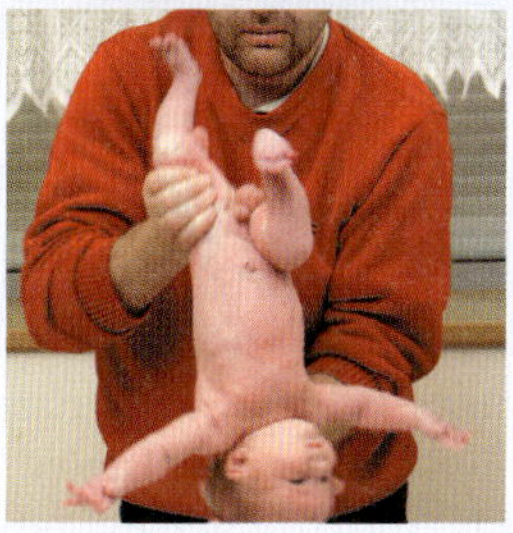	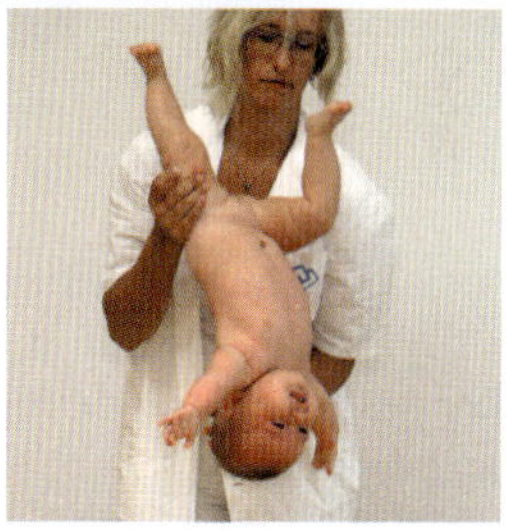

In a newborn, trunk stabilization has not yet matured and, therefore, the head and extremities do not oppose gravity in a coordinated and controlled way; Moro (and other) primitive reflexes are often expressed as part of the global pattern. In a 6-month-old infant, the more matured CNS allows for balanced muscular co-contraction (trunk stabilization) resulting in a better position of extremities and head control against gravity.

Zafeiriou et al. (1998) confirmed, in their study Vojta's observation, that the development of infants with more than five atypical postural tests in the first month of life significantly correlates with development of a spastic or hyperkinetic form of CP. Infants with less than three abnormal postural tests statistically correlate with a group of normally developing infants. This trend persisted with subsequent evaluations during the first year of life (Zafeiriou et al. 1998). Further, Vojta states that central paresis does not develop if the postural tests occur normally. Even the most minimal CNS damage has to manifest itself within the first weeks of life in order to possibly lead to development of CP. The damage would manifest itself by a disruption in postural reactivity and reflects in atypical models of postural tests (Vojta 2008).

The evaluation of postural reactions needs to be perceived as a complex CNS statement. This is why the quality of postural reactions, dynamics of primitive reflexes, and the quality and level of spontaneous mobility of the infant always correspond. A scenario, in which all postural tests are atypical and, at the same time, the infant's mobility is within normal limits, cannot occur. The interdependence of these evaluations can be described in examples. A positive tonic palmar grasp is present from birth to approximately 4.5 months of age. In humans, this reflex serves as a foundation for phylogenetic function but does not serve any purposeful function (Futagi et al. 2012). At the time, when the palmar grasp reflex is positive, the infant is unable to purposefully grasp and manipulate an object or even use the hand for support function. The reflex begins to weaken around 4 months of age and ceases completely by 6 months of age.

During the sixth month of age, an infant can spontaneously support him or herself on the palm of their hand, and grasp an object using the entire hand and purposefully manipulate it (Vojta and Schweizer 2009). A purposeful grasp starts developing from the fourth month of age. The infant reaches to the side; purposeful motor skills and hand sensitivity develop from the ulnar to the radial aspect of the hand. At this time, during Collis horizontal suspension test, the bottom arm is in abduction and the hand approximates and turns towards the mat as if the infant would like to support him or herself on the open hand (Figure 8.2). However, this reaction is very fast (as a response to a sudden change in body position) and it is not a conscious reaction by the infant. This contact of the bottom hand with the mat is not observed in an infant with a persistent tonic grasp reflex. Further, neither purposeful support function of the hand nor a grasp can be observed in the infant's spontaneous movement (Vojta 2008).

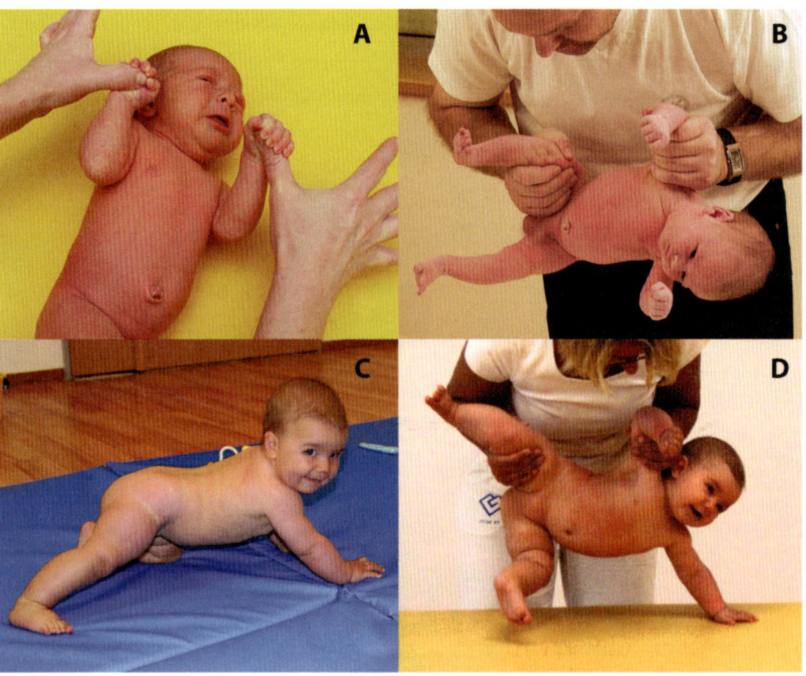

Figure 8.2 Integrity between primitive reflex and postural reaction: (**A**) Positive grasping hand reflex in a newborn; (**B**) Horizontal Collis postural reaction in a newborn—grasping reflex of the bottom arm is part of postural reaction; (**C**) Posturing of a 6-month-old infant whose palms serve for active support and primitive grasping hand reflex is fully inhibited (i.e. negative); (**D**) Horizontal Collis postural reaction in a physiological 6-month-old infant—bottom hand serves for support, primitive grasping reflex is inhibited (compare bottom hand position with the newborn in Figure 8.2A).

Postural reactions, primitive reflexes, and spontaneous motor skills illustrate the level and quality of CNS maturity. Similarly, the contexts of other postural tests, primitive reflexes, and spontaneous motor skills can be described.

Any infant demonstrating deviations from the norm during clinical assessment of postural reactions, primitive reflexes, and spontaneous motor skills is, in general, classified as an infant with CCD. CCD can be classified into four categories (see Table 8.3) based on the number of atypical reactions during postural tests and the number of atypical primitive reflexes. Even the mildest form of CCD can include rare cases that develop into CP. The number of pathological cases in individual groups steeply climbs based on involvement (Vojta 2008). Imamura reported that in untreated children with the mildest involvement (CCD1), CP develops in 2.8%; in CCD2, 4.5%; in CCD3, 30.7%; and in the severe group (CCD4) in 37.5% of children (Imamura et al. 1983). Vojta also mentions the study by Tomi, who evaluated 5485 children in 1979. Children classified in CCD3 and CCD4 (79 total) underwent therapy using Vojta method which was initiated no later than at 5 months of age. Therapy was administered to 64 children and 4 developed central paresis (0.073 percentile) (Vojta 2008).

Infants demonstrating CCD, especially CCD3 and 4, should begin treatment as soon as the signs of abnormal development are recognized. Bobath's neurodevelopmental treatment or Vojta concepts, for example, can be utilized in order to normalize postural-locomotion function as soon as possible to prevent further abnormal functional development as well as consequent structural deformities. It is important to educate the parents on daily handling and a home programme for the infant. The younger the infant, the greater the potential for neuroplasticity. Therefore, it is important to start rehabilitation early to take advantage of neuroplasticity before poor postural-locomotion patterns become fixed and structural consequences follow.

Table 8.3 Central co-ordination disturbance categories

CDD	CDD1–very mild	CDD2–mild	CDD3–moderate	CDD4–severe
Postural tests	1–3 abnormal PT; partial preservation of normal models	4–5 abnormal PT; partial preservation of normal models	6–7 abnormal PT; partial preservation of normal models	7 abnormal PT; no partial preservation of normal models
Dynamics of primitive reflexology	Intact	25% disturbed	60% disturbed	All primitive reflexes are disturbed
Indication for therapy	None; monitor development and perform regular check-ups	None; monitor development and perform regular check-ups	Indicated immediately	Indicated immediately

CCD—central co-ordination disturbance; PT—postural tests

Subcortical level of motor control

The newborn stage ends 28 days after birth. According to Vojta, to assess the spontaneous motor skills of an infant, the emphasis is placed on the quality of upright body posture within the gravitational field and to it is linked quality of support and phasic movement of the grasping or stepping-forward extremity. This foundational postural-locomotion function, allowing for purposeful movement, is linked to the subcortical and later cortical level of CNS control. Depending on the level of CNS maturity, a certain age corresponds to characteristic global postural-locomotion models that the infant spontaneously uses. Therefore, these are not learned movement skills, but rather a manifestation of CNS maturity, which is a genetically determined process.

Gradually, as the CNS matures, other muscle synergies automatically begin to function. This process is gradual and continuous. For example, an infant gradually abandons the primitive, neonatal flexed position of the pelvis and the scapula gradually descends caudally. During the third month, a muscle synergy matures that allows for pelvic, spine, and trunk positioning into a neutral position, especially in a sagittal plane. This involves a muscle synergy between the diaphragm, abdominal musculature, pelvic floor, deep neck flexors, and the spinal extensors (see Figure 61.1, Chapter 61, in this book). This muscle synergy, especially the significance of the diaphragm in this context, is scrutinized by many authors (Hodges 2003; Kolber and Beekhuizen 2007).

While in the neonatal stage, the diaphragm is solely a respiratory muscle; at the end of three months, it already fulfils simultaneous respiratory, postural, and sphincter roles. Later, the postural activity of the diaphragm begins to also be used independently of breathing (Kolar et al. 2011). This combined function is very challenging and often disrupted. A certain preference of vital, respiratory function can occur at the expense of the postural and sphincter functions. Postural weakness of the diaphragm can lead to an atypical postural development and, at the same time, a number of such children present with gastroesophageal reflux (spitting up). The diaphragm does not get involved homogenously in trunk bracing. Significant differences exist even in healthy individuals in the extent of respiratory and non-respiratory movement of the diaphragm. Individuals with insufficient ability to contract the diaphragm during trunk bracing pose a greater predisposition for onset of low back pain (Kolar et al. 2011).

The time around three months of development is considered to be very important from the aspect of postural functions. At this time, the infant's ability to maintain the lower extremities in a supine position, or the head while in a prone position above the mat, matures. The way in which the infant stabilizes their trunk, spine, and pelvis is critical. At this stage, if the diaphragm already fails in its postural function, this is compensated for by other muscles, usually the paravertebral muscles. This stereotype can easily become fixed if it is not identified early and corrected by therapy. In the end, it can lead to a chronic overloading of the spine as a result of unbalanced internal forces acting on the spine during postural activity.

Physiologically, the diaphragm descends caudally during postural activity. It flattens and acts as a piston as a result of a concentric contraction. The pelvic floor concentrically works against the diaphragm. This simultaneous activity is continued by an eccentric contraction of the abdominal muscles that act as a flexible but firm band and conform to the compression of the intra-abdominal content from both the cranial and caudal aspects. Increased intra-abdominal pressure, as a result of this postural muscle activation, ensures stabilization of the lumbar and lower thoracic spine during movement and an active body posture within gravitational field. The upper thoracic and cervical spines are stabilized by a balanced, simultaneous activity of cervical flexors and extensors, especially their deep layers (see Figure 61.1, Chapter 61, in this book). Thus, it is important whether a person adopts the correct synergy of postural muscles to provide quality and effective trunk stabilization during all movements or, an imbalanced, pathological synergy that will, in the end, lead to low back pain and undesirable structural (degenerative) changes.

Trunk stabilization in a sagittal plane precedes any conscious movement. This is a prerequisite for efficient movement. This muscle synergy is triggered automatically without our consciousness. Characteristic global ontogenetic models of the essential stabilization function of the trunk, spine, and the pelvis with continuous locomotion function of the extremities include the following: medial epicondyle support in prone position at 3 moths (Figure 8.3A), lateral grasp at 4.5 months (Figure 8.3B), transition from prone to supine position at 5–6 months (Figure 8.3C), support on extended upper extremity with palms open at 6 months (Figure 8.3D), side sitting at 7.5 months (Figure 8.3E), tripod at 8 months (Figure 8.3F), crawling at 8–10 months (Figure 8.3G), cruising (side-stepping) at 10 months (Figure 8.3H), and independent locomotion between 12–14 months (Figure 8.3I). Based on empirical evidence, these global models are demonstrated at the above mentioned ages in 50% of normally developing children. At two weeks later, it is 75% of children (Vojta 2008).

The evaluation based on the DNS concept assesses the presence of the global model, its symmetry, and quality. A non-ideal model suggests a non-ideal quality of CNS maturation (in such a case, the child is classified in CCD). The aforementioned postural-locomotion patterns are important not only to assess the child's development, but also to serve as models of an ideal postural-locomotion pattern for an adult within the DNS system. Developmental positions corresponding to 3–12 months of age are used in DNS for diagnosis as well as therapy of children and adult patients (see Chapter 61).

A less than ideal muscle synergy in sagittal stabilization, corresponding to three months of age, has consequences for all subsequent global models, as well as adulthood. An adult patient then uses their muscles without correct coordination during any phasic movement with a risk of microtrauma during young age. Later, they develop a risk of chronic overload or even degeneration, especially in the lower lumbar segments. Ultimately, this leads to chronic low back pain, which is economically considered a crucial disorder given the number of patients and the level of chronicity (Ekstrom 2008). This is the reason why the quality of sagittal stabilization in all children during their first year of life should be monitored and any pathology should be promptly corrected through physical therapy, prior to the pathological patterns becoming fixated.

The movement model of sagittal stabilization is continued by the development of postural locomotion function. All our movements are carried out in two ways: a contralateral (Figure 8.4A) or an ipsilateral (Figure 8.4B) pattern. These patterns develop separately until the seventh month. The contralateral pattern develops in a prone position and the support

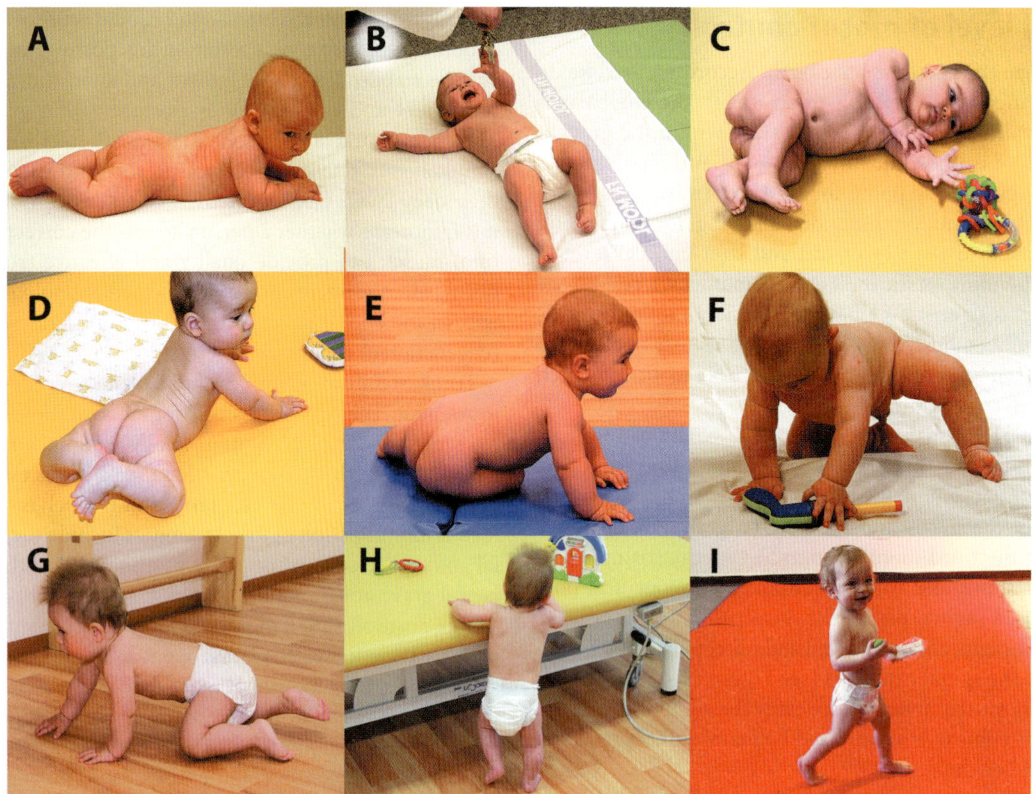

Figure 8.3 Typical postural patterns corresponding to a particular developmental age: (**A**) Prone position, support on humeral epicondyles and symphysis (3 months); (**B**) Supine position, infant grasping from the side and midline (4.5 months); (**C**) Side-lying, infant grasping across the midline (5 months); (**D**) Prone position, support on open palms and medial femoral condyles (6 months); (**E**)Side-sitting (7.5 months); (**F**) Tripod (8 months); (**G**) Crawling (8–10 months); (**H**)Side-walking (10 months); (**I**) Independent gait (12–14 months).

extremities are always opposite of each other, meaning contralateral (i.e. right upper and left lower extremity) and similarly phasic (left upper and right lower extremity). The step-forward extremities work in an open kinetic chain, while the support extremities work in a closed kinetic chain. The ipsilateral pattern develops from a supine position, in which all extremities work in an open kinetic chain initially (Figure 8.3B). Gradually, as the body moves to a side-lying position (Figure 8.3C) and the bottom upper and lower extremities are weighted, these extremities become support, while the top extremities fulfil a phasic (reaching, stepping) function (Figure 8.4B). In side-lying, the support or step-forward extremities are always on the same side of the body. It should be noted here that this ideally occurs in conjunction with a quality muscle synergy ensuring sagittal stabilization of the trunk, spine, and pelvis.

After the seventh month of age, the ipsilateral and contralateral patterns interconnect in a spontaneous movement; for example, when the child transitions from side-sitting (Figure 8.3E) (ipsilateral pattern in the middle of the eighth month) to tripod (Figure 8.3F) or to quadruped (contralateral pattern) and begins creeping (Figure 8.3G).

During the support and phasic movements of extremities, the CNS automatically uses a muscle synergy that sets the segments into a neutral position. This not only involves positioning the individual joints in relation to one another, but also the global mutual relations, such as the position of the trunk, spine, and pelvis. Therefore, in a non-ideal development, even as early as the first months of life, an atypical model of stabilization can be formed, such as the open scissors syndrome (see Figure 61.3, Chapter 61, in this book). This syndrome is typically found in patients with chronic low back pain (see Chapter 61). Similarly, anterior positioning of the thorax or shifting the thorax posteriorly in relation to the pelvis is also inefficient.

From a more localized perspective, in case of a non-ideal development, typical deviations in anatomical shapes can be found as a result of formative influences of muscles on the skeleton, such as increased anteversion angle of the femoral neck, tilted tibial plateau, or a shallow hollowing on the scapula. From a more regional perspective, for example, when assessing the position of the pelvis in relation to the femur, an abnormal sacral angle or pelvic incidence can develop. Poor posture, flat feet, or pelvic anteversion in late childhood or even in adulthood are then not a random and isolated finding, but rather a logical consequence of incorrect muscle activity controlled by the CNS.

Here again, the importance of early adequate treatment must be emphasized. In very young infants who cannot yet cooperate, Bobath's neurodevelopmental treatment approach or Vojta reflex locomotion concept can be utilized, as well as handling based on DNS developmental principles (see Chapter 61). Later, once the child matures and becomes an active participant, various concepts

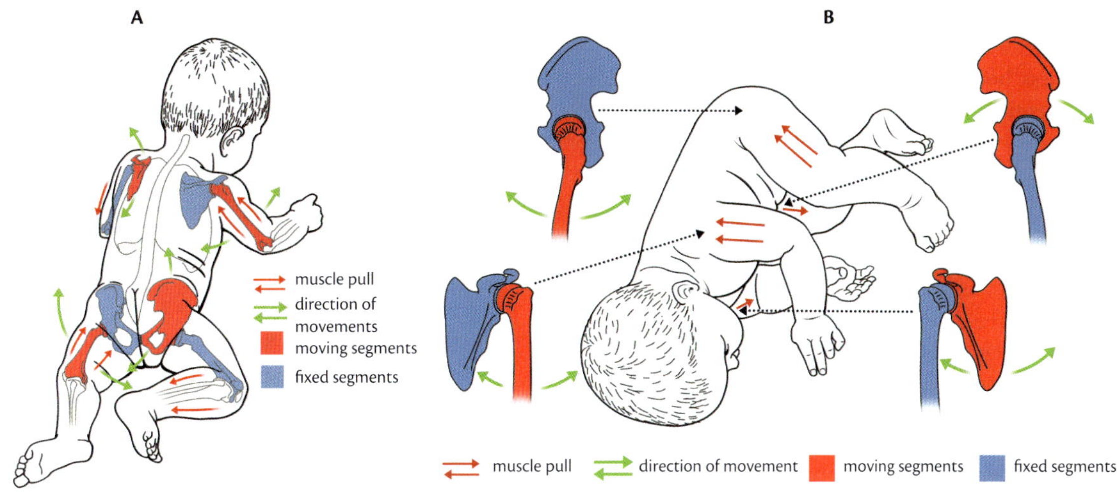

Figure 8.4 (**A**) Contralateral postural-locomotion pattern; (**B**) Ipsilateral postural-locomotion pattern.

based on developmental kinesiology emphasizing proper quality of stabilization, respiratory, and locomotion patterns can be utilized.

Cortical level of motor control

The cortical level of motor integration presents the highest level of CNS control. It begins to play a leading role in motor control after one year of age (Müller et al. 1991). It incorporates gnostic function, such as multisensory integration, allowing for body image, self-location, and first-person perspective to form (Ionta et al. 2011) as well as for decisiveness in the performance of deliberate motor function. The cortex is strongly involved in the cognitive phase of motor sequence learning (Wander et al. 2013). If the subcortical level of motor control allows mainly subconscious automatic stabilization (postural) function combined with respiratory and sphincter diaphragmatic and pelvic floor functions, the cortical function allows for individual variability of movement. The cortex allows for purposeful and deliberate modification of postural, respiratory, and phasic functions. The quality of body perception that is organized mainly on a cortical level determines the quality of phasic movement, the ability to perform isolated movement in only one segment, and the ability to relax. In rehabilitation, the quality of cortical motor control is crucial as it determines the patient's capacity to follow the clinician's instructions and to comply with the therapeutic protocol. This level of motor control is also critical in sports performance and training. Flexible adaptation of motor behaviour is highly required in most sports. In particular, stimulus discrimination, motor response selection, and inhibition processes are crucial where inhibition activity in the prefrontal cortex may play an especially important role (Di Russo et al. 2006).

Sensory (gnostic) function

Even with the eyes closed, we can 'read' our body (Mon-Williams et al. 1999). We can quite accurately describe our posture; we are exactly aware of our zones of support or body contact with the surroundings; we can detect every minor movement of any part of our body; we can differentiate a slight change in direction or speed of motion; and we can differentiate weight, position, and motion of an object. This ability is called somatognosis or body awareness, and it greatly depends on quality of proprioception and mechanoception. With our eyes closed, we can demonstrate the size of our body proportions. For example, we should be able to quite precisely draw the size of our foot, hand, mouth, or any other body part. We can 'read' a joint position (Mon-Williams et al. 1999) and repeatedly perform the same movement without visual control. These principles are critical in both sport performance and rehabilitation. Quality of somatognosis is very individual. The better the body image, the more precise and efficient the movement. Clumsiness and poor coordination may be related to abnormal proprioceptive control (Adib et al. 2005). Skin perception also influences our motion (Edin and Johansson 1995). Skin input contributes to both dynamic position and velocity sense (Cordo et al. 2001).

Derangement of body representation as a result of abnormal cortical organization has been reported in complex regional pain syndrome (Bultitude and Rafal 2010) and in phantom limb pain (Moseley and Wiech 2009), but may be an important factor in other, more frequent pain syndromes. Body awareness is related to a patient's ability to cope with chronic pain. Patients who have difficulty following therapeutic instructions or who need a longer time to learn how to perform exercises correctly (and still may not master them despite individual training sessions) may have poorer prognosis for total recovery. Therefore, in the DNS approach, we allow for self-treatment procedures only if the patient understands the exercise well and can perform it with good quality. Repetition does not make perfect, it makes permanent. Poor self-treatment may promote pathology instead of leading to recovery. It is recommended to check the quality of body perception in patients with 'non-specific pain', since the distortion in the perception of their body awareness may be an important aetiological factor and must then be addressed by therapy (Lauche et al. 2012). Moseley demonstrated that patients with phantom limb pain or complex regional pain syndrome (CRPS) showed increases in tactile acuity, normalization of cortical reorganization and decreased pain after sensory discrimination training (Moseley and Wiech 2009). When treating patients with back pain, very often the perception at a specific segment is restored after manipulation or mobilization, which, in turn, allows for a longer-lasting effect of the manual technique applied.

To clinically assess body awareness, we suggest several quick tests. For proprioception, position the patient's body (or just a painful body part—e.g. arm) in a certain position. Trace this position (Figure 8.5) and then move this body part out of this primary position. Then, ask the patient to attain the starting position again as accurately as possible. Measure any deviations. For body image estimation, you may use a dowel, asking the patient to demonstrate different body diameters with their eyes closed. For example, by sliding the top hand up the dowel, the patient can be asked to demonstrate the same distance as the width of his/her hips or shoulders, foot size, or trunk width or length (Figure 8.6). Or simply ask the patient to show the distance, lengthwise, of the widest part of their mouth, from one corner to the other. Then compare it to the actual size of the patient's body. When a discrepancy is noted, the particular body part should be trained. For example, practice repeated slow movements in different ranges and in different directions, paying full attention to this body part and its movement.

To check tactile perception, assess graphesthesia. Ask your patient to identify a number or a letter written on the skin with your fingertip. Graphesthesia may be compromised only in certain (e.g. painful) body areas and can be trained using various tactile stimulations of different amounts and quality.

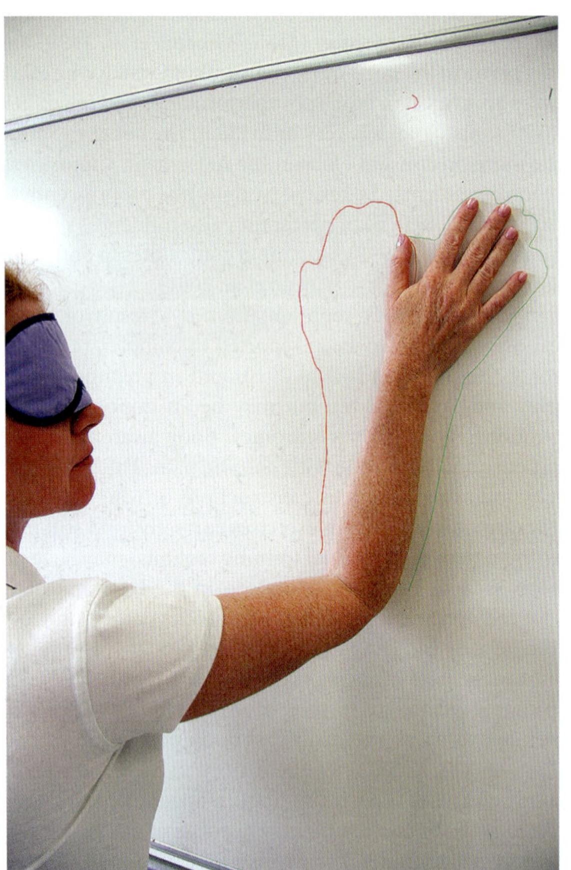

Figure 8.5 Proprioception (sense of position) test. Position a patient's body part in a certain position and trace this position (red line). The patient is then instructed to relax and attain their resting position. Then, with their eyes closed, the patient is asked to move their tested body part into the same position as previously placed by the therapist (green line). Ideally, the red and green lines are identical.

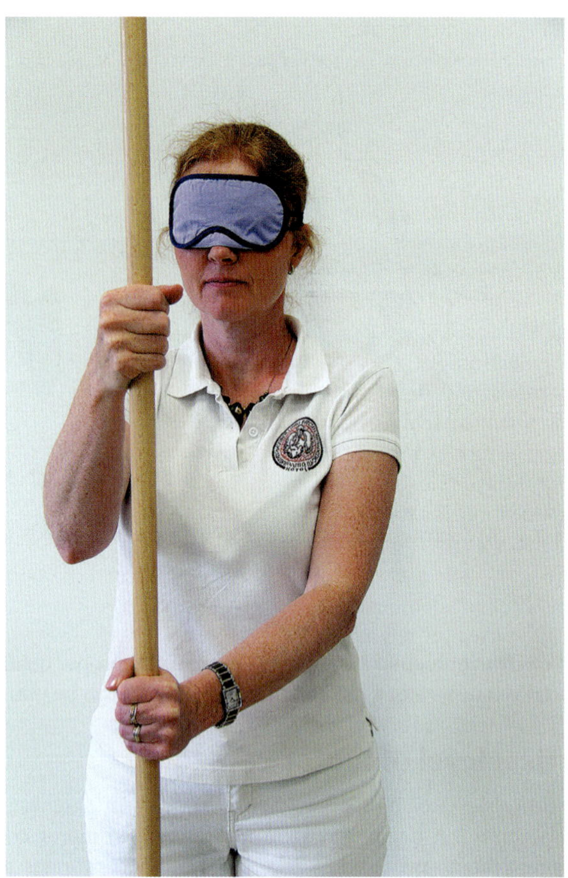

Figure 8.6 Body awareness test. The patient is instructed to demonstrate different body diameters on a dowel, with their eyes closed. Compare with the patient's true size.

Visual perception is also essential for purposeful movement (Mon-Williams et al. 1999). It allows for estimation of distance and speed as well as facilitation of an adequate and coordinated motor response within our surroundings. For example, the earlier a goalkeeper sees an approaching ball, the quicker the estimate of the angle, direction, and speed of the ball, the better the chance of catching it. This ability, however, may be quite non-homogenous. While some parts of the visual field can be perceived very well (e.g. when the ball is coming from the sides), others may be restricted (e.g. from above). In such a scenario, the goalkeeper will be more likely to let in goals when the ball is arriving from above. Training the quality of visual perception from above would then be a key aspect to success. Experienced athletes in sports involving moving objects have shown greater skill when using visual information to anticipate the direction of a moving object than non-experienced athletes of such sports (Ghasemi et al. 2011; Moreno et al. 2005). Visual perception and integration at the cortical level enables us to mimic body positions, movements, or gestures of another person, which is a critical aspect in sport and rehabilitation.

To clinically assess a patient's visual perception, you may demonstrate a certain (slightly complicated) postural situation and ask the patient to mimic it immediately and precisely. Some patients may have a great difficulty imitating posture and movement. In such a case, the rehabilitation treatment should focus on the patient's initial positioning and movement course. Patients with poor body awareness and/or with insufficient visual perception should not receive complicated self-treatment protocols. Rather, they benefit from a more individual approach and need to be instructed carefully, by a clinician, on how to exercise correct movement, starting from a proper position. Education in home programme progression needs to be rather slow.

Vestibular perception is important not only for postural balance (Angelaki and Cullen 2008) but also for vertical line perception. The perception of the visual vertical is altered in individuals with idiopathic scoliosis (Cakrt et al. 2011) and may play a role in the development of scoliosis. Whether an individual with idiopathic scoliosis perceives the vertical line differently because of the scoliosis, or if the scoliosis is in fact a consequence of abnormal vertical line perception, is a topic open to discussion. Verticality misperception related to poor balance can be an important factor in neurological patients (e.g. after stroke) (Bonan et al. 2006). Patients after whiplash injury demonstrate abnormal execution of postural synergies because they rely excessively on visual input due to the deficit in vestibular and proprioceptive activity (Madeleine et al. 2004). Even acoustic perception influences our posture and movement. Deafness may affect balance (Selz et al. 1996). Deaf individuals primarily use visual and somatosensory information to maintain their postural control (Suarez et al. 2007). Many rehabilitation approaches, including computer programs with feedback, are available to train balance strategies.

Scientific research papers (Angelaki and Cullen 2008; Cakrt et al. 2011; Cordo et al. 2001; Ghasemi et al. 2011; Mon-Williams et al. 1999; Moreno et al. 2005; Suarez et al. 2007) demonstrate how greatly the quality of somatosensory information and processing influences the quality of motion. We find it important to perform at least a brief clinical screening of sensory perception in patients with chronic musculoskeletal pain. We suggest to quickly assess each modality and treat if necessary. Not only movement but also sensory perception, integration, and interpretation can be trained, which in turn may help to normalize quality of postural-locomotion function.

Motor (executive function)

The sensory system constantly scans the environment to inform the CNS about an actual body position in order to select and carry out proper and precise movements and to provide ongoing feedback during movement. Altered multisensory CNS integration may result in poor motor planning, poor motor re-education (Polatajko and Cantin 2005), or difficulty performing motor tasks. Harris suggests that discrepancy between the awareness of motor intention, muscle and joint proprioception, and vision may itself result in pain (Cornwall et al. 2006; Harris 1999). Such individuals cannot adjust their muscle strength to the actual demand and usually activate too many unnecessary muscles for stabilization, making the movements inefficient. They demonstrate poor diadochokinesis as well as poor fluency and speed modification. A person with altered sensory integration can barely perform selective movements in only one joint or segment (Figure 8.7). They usually present with great difficulty relaxing certain muscles which may, in the end, lead to painful syndromes, though it remains unclear how stiffness and pain are related (Cacciatore et al. 2011).

While McGill states that increased axial stiffness can reduce low back pain by stabilizing the spine (McGill 1998), other authors suggest that pain results from increased loading of axial tissues due to excessive axial stiffness (Marras et al. 2004; van Dieen et al. 2003a,b).

It seems to be important to not only have sufficient initial muscle tone to stabilize the spine and to avoid injury but also display

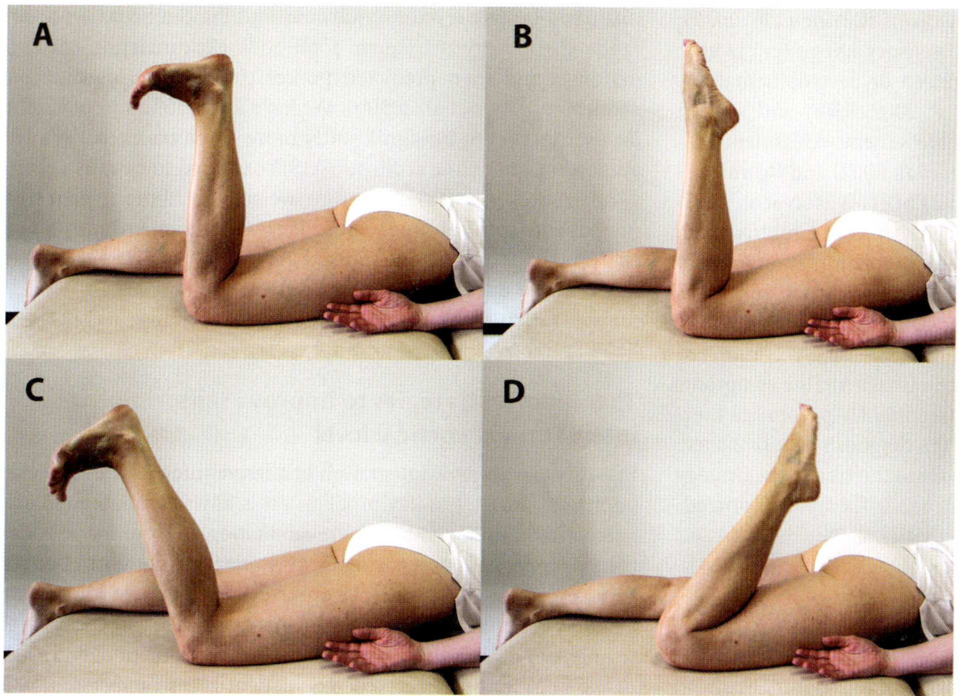

Figure 8.7 Example of a selective movement test in the ankle: (**A,B**) Physiological situation—the individual can perform selective movement in the ankle without synkinesis in other joints; (**C,D**) Abnormal situation—ankle movement and knee motion occur at the same time. Sometimes, the effort to perform selective movement may involve the contralateral extremity or the trunk (in this case, e.g. anterior and/or posterior pelvic tilt may occur when the individual aims to move only the ankle).

sufficient dynamic modulation to prevent excessive loading during movement (Cacciatore et al. 2011). Janda introduced a system of tonic and phasic muscles with tonic muscles having a tendency to develop trigger points and hyperactivation (Page et al. 2010a). Tonic muscles are mainly large, superficial postural muscles that in dynamic tests (see Chapter 61) often demonstrate hyperactivity. Patients with chronic pain often show inability to relax those muscles even in posturally simple positions (e.g. supine). In such cases, in addition to treating the trigger points, treatment should include teaching the patient how to purposefully, consciously relax those muscles that tend to be overactivated prior to introducing stabilization and exercises modifying movement patterns. Therapeutic relaxation on the basis of the CNS may allow for significant pain relief (Kettenmann et al. 2007).

Research shows that insufficient uni- or multisensory integration at the cortical level may lead to painful syndromes within the locomotor system (Flor et al. 1997; Imamura et al. 2009). Injuries, degenerative joint disorders, enthesopathies, orthopaedic problems resulting from chronic overload and repetitive stress injuries, including focal dystonia, are the typical consequences (Byl et al. 1996; Harrris 1999; Topp and Byl 1999). These disorders are usually considered to be primary diagnoses rather than a consequence of an altered sensorimotor integration and CNS control, which is more likely to be the real aetiology. The therapy then only targets 'the diagnosis' rather than the primary aetiology. Consequently, the chosen therapy usually ends up being unsuccessful in the long run. We are in agreement with Harris (Harris 1999) who suggests that in the presence of pain without relevant structural pathology, instead of treating the painful body part with analgesics and anti-inflammatories, therapy might be directed towards restoring the integrity of cortical information processing.

Developmental dyspraxia or developmental coordination disorder

According to Levine et al., deprivation of the sensory cues during development perturbs topographically organized connections between sensory fibres and spinal interneurons (Levine et al. 2012). In childhood, insufficient uni- or multisensory integration is usually diagnosed as developmental dyspraxia or developmental coordination disorder (DCD) (Gibbs et al. 2007; Kirby and Sugden 2007; Polatajko and Cantin 2005). The Movement Assessment Battery for Children (MABC) (Henderson et al. 2007) and Bruininks-Oseretsky Test of Motor Proficiency (BOTMP) (Wilson et al. 1995) can be used to diagnose developmental dyspraxia. Children with DCD who are involved in sports often complain of non-specific symptoms such as exhaustion, acute headache, vertigo, and nausea, especially during increased athletic activity (Gibbs et al. 2007; Henderson et al. 2007). Such complaints are usually considered vertebrogenic or psychosomatic. To a certain extent, the symptoms of DCD are resistant to conventional treatment. Appropriate therapy should be introduced as soon as the diagnosis is established. Sports activities should be integrated within the treatment strategy and team sports are especially recommended. Therapeutic procedures should become a routine part of activities of daily living (ADL) (Poulsen et al. 2008; Schott et al. 2007).

Cerebellar function

The cerebellum is involved in all three levels of integration and matures simultaneously with other parts of the brain. Motor circuits in the brainstem and the cerebellum display a topographic order that relates to specific muscles or muscle groups (Levine et al. 2012). Multiple topographic networks between the sensory system, spinal neurons, the cerebellum, and the cortical system interact to produce coherent movements. The cerebellum plays an important role in muscle tone regulation, uprighting process, and balance maintenance. It helps to regulate the movement's accuracy, including of very precise movements, such as playing musical instruments (Beaton and Mariën 2010). The cerebellum coordinates movements in time and space and plays an important role in cognition (Beaton and Mariën 2010).

The cerebellum develops during ontogenesis. At three months of age, the functional activity in the cerebellum increases substantially (Hadders-Algra 2005; Harry and Chugani 1998) and its maturation continues along with the rest of the brain until adulthood. According to Hadders-Algra, the nervous system obtains its adult configuration at approximately 30 years of age. Based on available research (Grossberg and Paine 2000; Katanoda et al. 2001), we assume that it is especially the maturation of the cerebellar cortex and frontal and parietal cortices that allows for hand motor dexterity that is sufficiently accurate for writing at the age of six. Also, language and cognitive functions are sufficiently developed by this age. All three aspects play a critical role in school education as well as in rehabilitation.

In 1987, Janda introduced the term 'minimal brain dysfunction' (MBD), pointing to the influence of central sensory motor control quality on muscle coordination, noting the effect of biopsychosocial factors in chronic back pain and considering MBD to be an underlying risk factor for developing chronic pain (Janda 1987). According to Janda, MBD can be found in 80% of patients with chronic low back pain, suggesting an organic CNS lesion together with a maladaptation of movement system being the primary cause of chronic pain syndromes. He explained that MBD results in inefficient overflow of muscle activity with subsequent decrease in the ability to perform and adjust fine movements (Page et al. 2010b). Within MBD, Janda distinguished the microspastic syndrome, the disturbed proprioception syndrome, and the cerebellar syndrome. Janda also observed frequent total body asymmetry in MBD individuals and then predicted poorer prognosis in chronic pain syndromes (Page et al. 2010b). We have identified signs of cerebellar dysfunction to be significantly more common in patients with adolescent idiopathic scoliosis (AIS) compared to healthy controls (Kobesova et al. 2013). Therefore, we suggest caution when treating patients with minimal cerebellar dysfunction and recommend that they be screened for signs of AIS purposefully; but also, the other way round, we recommend screening individuals with AIS for signs of cerebellar dysfunction and, if positive, target the rehabilitation treatment accordingly.

Therapeutic strategies to improve sensorimotor integration at cortical level

In patients with poor integration of afferent information (i.e. where poor body image is a key problem), it is advised to integrate body perception training within the rehabilitation programme. We teach the patient to focus on a particular body part with compromised sensory perception. First, with the eyes closed, the patient is instructed to attain the initial position in a segment and then, slowly move the segment while focusing on movement in this segment only. The rest of the body must be relaxed. The patient is instructed to practise isolated movement in one particular segment while fully appreciating the course of the movement, its direction, and range. Any pathological synkinesis or any substitutive patterns need to be avoided. The patient should learn how to isolate movement in one segment only and how to switch between muscle activation and relaxation. The patient learns how to 'read their own body' without visual control. Feldenkrais concept can also be used to train cortical control of movement accuracy and body image (Feldenkrais 1999). Alexander Technique (AT) may also help to train conscious motor and bodily attention (i.e. the AT concept of 'direction') to produce the desired adaptability of muscle tension and to achieve dynamically adaptive elongated posture along the body axis. The emphasis on conscious attention may suggest that higher brain levels contribute to the AT-related increase in tonic modulation (Cacciatore et al. 2011).

Then, visual feedback can be used as the next step to train efficient movement. For example, mirrors can be used to monitor body movements when performing postural exercises. Virtual-reality-based assessment and treatment programmes became recently available for both physical and cognitive rehabilitation. To train balance, mobility, precise extremity movements, cognitive, fitness, and daily living skills, virtual-reality systems have been used mainly in patients after stroke and in cerebral palsy populations (Glegg at al. 2013). Though there is a lack of evidence so far, good results could be expected from modern technologies to train sensorimotor integration in patients with inefficient movements resulting from abnormal gnostic perception.

Concluding thoughts about dynamic neuromuscular stabilization

Assessment of movement patterns is one of the essential evaluation tools in rehabilitation. Many manual medicine textbooks emphasize biomechanical or purely kinesiological aspects with focus on joint shape, its characteristics during movement, muscle strength, or coordination. The relationship between the CNS and movement is often only marginally mentioned. Movement quality is completely dependent on the quality of control functions of the CNS, which intensely develop during the first months and years of human life. Therefore, movement patterns dramatically develop and change during early childhood. The assessment of quality of a child's motor skills allows for an assessment of not only muscle function, but mainly the control function represented by the CNS. The assessment of a child's motor functions in early childhood is considered, by the authors, as a routine component of a basic clinical examination by a neonatologist, neurologist, as well as a pediatrician and general physician. This is important because the quality of movement function that a person 'forms' in early childhood will be 'carried' with them for the rest of their life. Furthermore, motor function, or muscle coordination, plays a role in the formation of the skeleton during growing years.

Early diagnosis, and especially correct therapy to address deviations in motor development, can normalize the later neuromotor–skeletal development, while neglecting even a relatively small deviation in early motor behaviour can result in relatively significant changes in morphological development. Often, a fixation of abnormal movement patterns occurs, which is very difficult to alter in adult age. The basics of clinical assessment of neuromotor functions in childhood should be known by every professional specializing in the movement system.

Acknowledgements

This chapter was supported by the Foundation 'Movement Without Help', Prague, Czech Republic, and by Prague School Rehabilitation (<http://www.rehabps.com>.

References

Abo-Yaqoub, S., Kurjak, A., Mohammed, A.-B., Shadad, A., Abdel-Maaboud, M. (2012) The role of 4-D ultrasonography in prenatal assessment of fetal neurobehaviour and prediction of neurological outcome. *J Maternal Neo Med*, 25, 231–6, doi:10.3109/14767058.2011.568552.

Adib, N., Davies, K., Grahame, R., Woo, P., Murray, K.J. (2005) Joint hypermobility syndrome in childhood. A not so benign multisystem disorder? *Rheumatology*, 44, 744–50, doi:10.1093/rheumatology/keh557.

Angelaki, D.E., Cullen, K.E. (2008) Vestibular system: the many facets of a multimodal sense. *Ann Rev Neurosci* 31, 125–50.

Banaszek, G. (2010) Vojta's method as the early neurodevelopmental diagnosis and therapy concept. *Przeglad Lekarski*, 67, 67–76.

Beaton, A., Mariën, P. (2010) Language, cognition and the cerebellum: grappling with an enigma. *Cortex*, 46(7), 811–20, doi: 10.1016/j.cortex.2010.02.005.

Bonan, I.V., Guettard, E., Leman, M.C., Colle, F.M., Yelnik, A.P. (2006) Subjective visual vertical perception relates to balance in acute stroke. *Arch Phys Med Rehabil*, 87(5), 642–6.

Bos, A.F., Martijn, A., Van Asperen, R.M., Hadders-Algra, M., Okken, A., Prechtl, H.F. (1998) Qualitative assessment of general movements in high-risk preterm infants with chronic lung disease requiring dexamethasone therapy. *J Pediat*, 132, 300–6.

Bouwstra, H., Dijk-Stigter, G.R., Grooten, H.M.J., et al. (2009) Prevalence of abnormal general movements in three-month-old infants. *Early Hum Develop*, 85(6), 399–403, doi:10.1016/j.earlhumdev.2009.01.003.

Bouwstra, H., Dijk-Stigter, G.R., Grooten, H.M.J., et al. (2010) Predictive value of definitely abnormal general movements in the general population. *Develop Med Child Neurol*, 52(5), 456–61, doi:10.1111/j.1469-8749.2009.03529.x.

Bultitude, J.H., Rafal, R.D. (2010) Derangement of body representation in complex regional pain syndrome: report of a case treated with mirror and prisms. *Exp Brain Res* 204(3), 409–18, doi: 10.1007/s00221-009-2107-8.

Byl, N.N.I., Merzenich, M.M., Jenkins, W.M. (1996) A primate genesis model of focal dystonia and repetitive strain injury: I. Learning-induced dedifferentiation of the representation of the hand in the primary somatosensory cortex in adult monkeys. *Neurology*, 47(2), 508–20.

Cacciatore, T.W.I., Gurfinkel, V.S., Horak, F.B., Cordo, P.J., Ames, K.E. (2011) Increased dynamic regulation of postural tone through Alexander Technique training. *Hum Mov Sci*, 30(1), 74–89, doi: 10.1016/j.humov.2010.10.002.

Cakrt, O., Slabý, K., Viktorinová, L., Kolář, P., Jeřábek, J. (2011) Subjective visual vertical in patients with idiopatic scoliosis. *J Vestib Res :Equilib Orient*, 21(3), 161–5, doi:10.3233/VES-2011-0414.

Chugani, H.T. (1998) A critical period of brain development: studies of cerebral glucose utilization with PET. *Prev Med*, 27, 184–8.

Cordo, P.J., Horn, J.L., Künster, D., Cherry, A., Bratt, A., Gurfinkel, V. (2001) Contributions of skin and muscle afferent input to movement sense in the human hand. *J Neurophysiol* 105, 1879–88, doi.org/10.1152/jn.00201.2010.

Cornwall, J., Harris, A.J., Mercer, S.R. (2006) The lumbar multifidus muscle and patterns of pain, *Man Ther*. 2006; 11, 40–5, doi:10.1016/j.math.2005.02.002.

van Dieen, J.H., Cholewicki, J., Radebold, A. (2003a) Trunk muscle recruitment patterns in patients with low back pain enhance the stability of the lumbar spine. *Spine*, 28, 834–41.

van Dieen, J.H., Selen, L.P., Cholewicki, J. (2003b) Trunk muscle activation in low-back pain patients, an analysis of the literature. *J Electromyogr Kinesiol*, 13, 333–51.

Di Russo, F., Taddei, F., Apnile, T., Spinelli, D. (2006) Neural correlates of fast stimulus discrimination and response selection in top-level fencers. *Neurosci Lett*, 408, 113–8, doi:10.1016/j.neulet.2006.08.085.

Edin, B.B., Johansson, N. (1995) Skin strain patterns provide kinaesthetic information to the human central nervous system. *J Physiol*, 487 (Pt1), 243–51.

Ekstrom, R.A. (2008) Surface electromyographic analysis of the low back muscles during rehabilitation exercises. *J Orthop Sports Phys Ther*, 38(12), 736–45, doi:10.2519/jospt.2008.2865.

Feldenkrais, M. (1999) *Awareness through movement*. Harper, San Francisco.

Flor, H., Braun, C., Elbert, T., Birbaumer, N. (1997) Extensive reorganization of primary somatosensory cortex in chronic back pain patients. *Neurosci Lett*, 224, 5–8.

Futagi, Y., Toribe, Y., Suzuki, Y. (2012) The grasp reflex and moro reflex in infants: hierarchy of primitive reflex responses. *Int J Pediat*, 191562, doi:10.1155/2012/191562.

Ghasemi, A., Momeni, M., Jafarzadehpur, E., Rezaee, M., Taheri, H. (2011) Visual skills involved in decision making by expert referees. *Percept Mot Skills*, 112, 161–71.

Gibbs, J., Appleton, J., Appleton, R. (2007) Dyspraxia or developmental coordination disorder? Unravelling the enigma. *Arch Dis Child*, 92, 534–9.

Glegg, S.M., Tatla, S.K., Holsti, L. (2013) The GestureTek virtual reality system in rehabilitation: a scoping review. *Disabil Rehabil Assist Technol*, 2013;9(2):89–111. doi:10.3109/17483107.2013.799236.

Grossberg, S.I., Paine, R.W. (2000) A neural model of cortico-cerebellar interactions during attentive imitation and predictive learning of sequential handwriting movements. *Neural Net*, 13(8–9):999–1046.

Hadders-Algra, M. (2005) Development of postural control during the first 18 months of life. *Neural Plast*. 2005;12(2-3):99–108; discussion 263–72. doi:10.1155/NP.2005.99.

Harris, A.J. (1999) Cortical origin of pathological pain. *Lancet*, 354(9188): 1464–6.

Harry, T., Chugani, M. (1998) A critical period of brain development: studies of cerebral glucose utilization with PET. *Prevent Med*, 27(2), 184–8.

Henderson, S.E., Sugden, D.A., Barmett, A.L. (2007) *Movement Assessment Battery for children: examiner's manual (Movement ABC-2)* (2nd ed). Harcourt Assessment, London.

Hodges, P.W. (2003) Core stability exercise in chronic low back pain. *Orthop Clin N Am*, 34, 245–54.

Imamura, M., Cassius, D.A., Fregni, F. (2009) Fibromyalgia: from treatment to rehabilitation. *Eur J Pain*, 3, 117–22.

Imamura, S., Sakuma, K., Takahashi, T. (1983) Follow-up study of children with cerebral coordination disturbance (CCD, Vojta). *Brain Dev*, 5, 311–4.

Ionta, S., Heydrich, L., Lenggenhager, B., et al. (2011) Multisensory mechanisms in temporo-parietal cortex support self-location and first-person perspective. *Neuron*, 70, 363–74.

Janda, V. (1987) Muscles, central nervous regulation and back problems. In: Korr, I.M. (ed.) *Neurobiological mechanisms in manipulative therapy*. Plenum Press, New York, p. 27–41.

Katanoda, K., Yoshikawa, K., Sugishita, M. (2001) A functional MRI study on the neural substrates for writing. *Hum Brain Mapp*, 13, 34–42.

Kettenmann, B.I., Wille, C., Lurie-Luke, E., Walter, D., Kobal, G. (2007) Impact of continuous low level heatwrap therapy in acute low back pain patients: subjective and objective measurements. *Clin J Pain*, 23(8), 663–8.

Kirby, A., Sugden, D.A. (2007) Children with developmental coordination disorders. *J R Soc Med*, 100, 182–6.

Kobesova, A., Drdakova, L., Andel, R., Kolar, P. (2013) Cerebellar function and hypermobility in patients with idiopathic scoliosis. *Int Muscul Med*, 35(3), 99–105.

Kobesova, A., Kolar, P. (2013) Developmental kinesiology: three levels of motor control in the assessment and treatment of the motor system. *J Bodywork Mov Ther*, doi:10.1016/j.jbmt.2013.04.002.

Kolar, P., Sulc, J., Kyncl, M., et al. (2011) Postural function of the diaphragm in persons with and without chronic low back pain. *J Orthop Sports Phys Ther*, 42(4), 352–62.

Kolber, M. J., Beekhuizen, K. (2007) Lumbar stabilization: an evidence-based approach for the athlete with low back pain. *Strength Cond J*, 29, 26–37.

Krementizer, J.P., Vaughan, H.G., Kurtzberg, D., Dowling, K. (1979) Smooth-pursuit eye movements in the newborn infant. *Child Devel*, 50, 442–8.

Lauche, R., Cramer, H., Haller, H., et al. (2012) My back has shrunk: the influence of traditional cupping on body image in patients with chronic non-specific neck pain. *Forsch Komplementmed*, 19(2), 68–74, doi: 10. 1159/000337688.

Levine, A.J., Lewallen, K.A., Pfaff, S.L. (2012) Spatial organization of cortical and spinal neurons controlling motor behavior. Curr Opin Neurobiol, 22(5), 812–21, doi: 10.1016/j.conb.2012.07.002.

Madeleine, P.I., Prietzel, H., Svarrer, H., Arendt-Nielsen, L. (2004) Quantitative posturography in altered sensory conditions: a way to assess balance instability in patients with chronic whiplash injury. *Arch Phys Med Rehabil*, 85(3), 432–8.

Marras, W.S., Ferguson, S.A., Burr, D., Davis, K.G., Gupta, P. (2004) Spine loading in patients with low back pain during asymmetric lifting exertions. *Spine J*, 4, 64–75.

McGill, S.M. (1998) Low back exercises: evidence for improving exercise regimens. *Phys Ther*, 78, 754–65.

Metcalfe, J.S.,McDowell, K.,Chang, T.Y.,Chen, L.C.,Jeka, J.J.,Clark, J.E. (2005) Development of somatosensory-motor integration: an event-related analysis of infant posture in the first year of independent walking. *Dev Psychobiol*, 46(1),19–35.

Mon-Williams, M., Tresilian, J.R., Wann, J.P. (1999) Perceiving limb position in normal and abnormal control: an equilibrium point perspective. *Hum Mov Sci*, 18, 397–419.

Moreno, F.J., Luis, V., Salgado, F., García, J.A., Reina, R. (2005) Visual behavior and perception of trajectories of moving objects with visual occlusion. *Percept Mot Skills*, 101(1), 13–20.

Moseley, G.L., Wiech, K. (2009) The effect of tactile discrimination training is enhanced when patients watch the reflected image of their unaffected limb during training. Pain, 144(3), 314–9, doi: 10.1016/j. pain.2009.04.030.

Müller, K., Hömberg, V., Lenard, H.G. (1991) Magnetic stimulation of motor cortex and nerve roots in children. Maturation of cortico-motoneuronal projections. *Electroenceph Clin Neurophys*, 81, 63–70.

Nakajima, Y., Einspieler, C., Marschik, P.B., Bos, A.F., Prechtl, H.F.R. (2006) Does a detailed assessment of poor repertoire general movements help to identify those infants who will develop normally? *Early Hum Dev*, 82(1), 53–9, doi:10.1016/j.earlhumdev.2005.07.010.

Page, P., Frank, C.C., Lardner, R. (2010a) Pathomechanics of musculoskeletal pain and muscle imbalance. In: Page, P. (ed.) *Assessment and treatment of muscle imbalance*. Champaign, Human Kinetics, p. 43–55.

Page, P., Frank, C.C., Lardner, R. (2010b) Posture, balance and gait analysis. In: Page, P. (ed.) *Assessment and treatment of muscle imbalance*. Champaign, Human Kinetics, p. 59–75.

Polatajko, H.J., Cantin, N. (2005) Developmental coordination disorder (dyspraxia): an overview of the state of the art. *Semin Pediatr Neurol*, 12, 250–8.

Poulsen, A.A., Ziviani, J.M., Johnson, H., Cuskelly, M. (2008) Loneliness and life satisfaction of boys with developmental coordination disorder: the impact of leisure participation and perceived freedom in leisure. *Hum Mov Sci*, 27, 325–43.

Prechtl, H. (2001) General movement assessment as a method of developmental neurology: new paradigms and their consequences. *Dev Med Child Neurol*, 2001;43:836–842.

Prechtl, H.F., Einspieler, C. (1997) Is neurological assessment of the fetus possible? *Eur J Obstet Gynecol Reprod Biol*, 75, 81–4.

Prechtl, H.F., Ferrari, F., Cioni, G. (1993) Predictive value of general movements in asphyxiated fullterm infants. *Early Hum Dev*, 35, 91–120.

Prechtl, H.F., Hopkins, B. (1986) Developmental transformations of spontaneous movements in early infancy. *Early Hum Dev*, 14, 233–8.

Schott, N., Alof, V., Hultsch, D., Meermann, D. (2007) Physical fitness in children with developmental coordination disorder. *Res Q Exerc Sport*, 78, 438–50.

Schulz, P. (2013) *Videokompendium kinderneurologischer untersuchungen*. Thieme Verlagsgruppe, Stuttgart, p. 96.

Selz, P.A.I., Girardi, M., Konrad, H.R., Hughes, L.F. (1996) Vestibular deficits in deaf children. *Otolaryngol Head Neck Surg*, 115(1):70–7.

Suarez, H.I., Angeli, S., Suarez, A., Rosales, B., Carrera, X., Alonso, R. (2007) Balance sensory organization in children with profound hearing loss and cochlear implants. *Int J Pediatr Otorhinolaryngol*, 71(4), 629–37.

Topp, K.S.I., Byl, N.N. (1999) Movement dysfunction following repetitive hand opening and closing: anatomical analysis in Owl monkeys. *Mov Disord*, 14(2), 295–306.

Vojta, V. (2008) *Die zerebralen bewegungsstörungen im säuglingsalter*. Thieme, Stuttgart, p. 321.

Vojta, V., Peters, A. (2007) *Das Vojta-prinzip* (3rd ed.). Springer, Heidelberg, p. 169.

Vojta, V., Schweizer, E. (2009) *Die entdeckung der idealen motorik*. Pflaum, München, p. 281.

Wander, J.D., Blakely, T., Miller, K.J., et al. (2013) Distributed cortical adaptation during learning of a brain-computer interface task. *Proc Natl Acad Sci USA*, 110(26),10818–23, doi: 10.1073/pnas.1221127110.

Wilson, B.N., Polatajko, H.J., Kaplan, B.J., Faris, P. (1995) Use of the Bruininks-Oseretsky test of motor proficiency in occupational therapy. *Am J Occup Ther*, 49, 8–17.

Zafeiriou, D.I., Tsikoulas, I.G., Kremenopoulos, G.M. (1995) Prospective follow-up of primitive reflex profiles in high-risk infants: clues to an early diagnosis of cerebral palsy. *Ped Neurol*, 13, 148–52.

Zafeiriou, D.I., Tsikoulas, I.G., Kremenopoulos, G.M., Kontopoulos, E.E. (1998) Using postural reactions as a screening test to identify high-risk infants for cerebral palsy: a prospective study. *Brain Dev*, 20, 307–11.

Chapter 9

Hypermobility in adults

Lars Remvig, Birgit Juul-Kristensen, and Raoul Engelbert

Introduction to hypermobility in adults

Joint mobility is a continuous trait that varies with joint location and is strongly influenced by age, gender, and ethnic origin (Remvig et al. 2007). No matter the type of mobility, be it hypo-, normo-, or hypermobility, we anticipate that variation in mobility begins *in utero* as part of the individual's phenotype.

Joint hypermobility (JH) has been known about for centuries, but it has not been until recently (last 50 years) that it has gained a more profound and increasing scientific interest. The reason for that is probably an often observed concomitant presence of JH and musculoskeletal pain, giving rise to the name hypermobility syndrome (HMS) (Kirk et al. 1967). The name was later redefined by an interest group, within the British Society of Rheumatology, as benign joint hypermobility syndrome (BJHS), including more signs than just musculoskeletal complaints (Grahame et al. 2000) (see Table 9.1).

However, hypermobility and pain are also part of the Villefranche criteria for the various types of Ehlers-Danlos syndromes (EDS) (Beighton et al. 1998), as well as the criteria for Marfan syndrome, osteogenesis imperfecta, and other diseases belonging to the group known as hereditary disorders of connective tissue (HDCT).

Clinical characteristics of hypermobility in adults

Normal/abnormal joint movement

According to the American Academy of Orthopedic Surgeons (AAOS), it is not possible to precisely determine mean joint mobility throughout the body (1965). Consequently, the AAOS developed consensus-based estimates, in degrees, derived from statistical means based on reports from four committees of experts.

In general, joint mobility is regarded as a graded phenomenon (Wood 1971), and a consensus has developed that individual joint mobility follows a Gaussian distribution (Allander et al. 1974; Fairbank et al. 1984; Silman et al. 1986). With this in mind, abnormal joint mobility would reflect movements that deviate from the mean with ± two standard deviations (SD), i.e. the general, consensus-based estimates. However, for practical purposes, range of motion (ROM) measurements in degrees are not manageable when testing for generalized JH (GJH). Instead, the Beighton tests that apply a dichotomous principle are widely used (Beighton et al. 1973), although the Rotès-Quérol tests (Rotes-Querol 1957) are more favoured in Spanish- and French-speaking countries. The Beighton tests were described about 40 years ago (Beighton and Horan 1970), but only by photos and short legends to figures (Figure 9.1).

The description was repeated a few years later with minor changes in the photographic presentation (Beighton et al. 1973). However, since then there has been a considerable variation in the descriptions in the literature on how to perform the various tests, and also in the cut-off level for a positive test and in the definition of GJH (Table 9.2).

The Beighton tests, together with the criterion for GJH, have been proven to have high inter-examiner reproducibility in children (Smits-Engelsman et al. 2011), as well as in adults (Bulbena et al. 1992; Juul-Kristensen et al. 2007), and so have the Rotès-Quérol tests (Bulbena et al. 1992). The concurrent validity also seems to be high as a positive Beighton test equals normal mean ROM + 3SD (Fairbank et al. 1984) and as GJH has high correlation to a global joint index (Bulbena et al. 1992). The predictive value of GJH has only been tested in school population studies of children aged 10–14 years. The studies showed that 10-year-old children with GJH and musculoskeletal pain had an increased risk of still having this pain at 14 years of age (El-Metwally et al. 2004, 2005). However, 10-year-old children with GJH and no musculoskeletal pain did not have increased risk of developing musculoskeletal pain at 14 years (El-Metwally et al. 2007).

Hypermobility syndrome versus EDS, hypermobile type (EDS-HT)

The present criteria for these two syndromes—the Villefrance criteria (Beighton et al. 1998) and the Brighton criteria (Grahame et al. 2000)—are, in essence, proposals or recommendations for a classification of two different disease entities. However, there is a considerable overlap in the most important criteria items suggested (Table 9.3).

The inter-examiner reproducibility of diagnosing BJHS by the Brighton criteria is high (Juul-Kristensen et al. 2007) (see Figure 9.2). However, the reproducibility for diagnosing the various EDS entities has never been published, neither has the validity of the criteria sets mentioned and—very important for the clinician—the predictive value of a positive and a negative test result.

Table 9.1 Review of hypermobility syndrome definitions

Publication	Tests and clinical signs		Syndrome criteria
Kirk et al. 1967	Carter & Wilkinson's tests with > 3 positive joint pairs Musculoskeletal complaints (without any other systemic rheumatic disease)		None
Grahame et al. 2000	Major criteria	Minor criteria	BJHS is diagnosed in the presence of: 2 major criteria OR 1 major and 2 minor criteria OR 4 minor criteria 2 minor criteria will suffice where there is an unequivocally affected first- degree relative BJHS is excluded by presence of Marfan or EDS (other than EDS-HT) Criteria major 1 and minor 1 are mutually exclusive, as are major 2 and minor 2
	1. Beighton score ≥4/9 (either currently or historically) 2. Arthralgia for longer than 3 months in 4 or more joints	1. Beighton score of 1, 2, or 3/9 (0–3 if age 50+) 2. Arthralgia ≥3 months in 1–3 joints, or back pain ≥3 months, or spondylosis, spondylolysis/spondylolisthesis 3. Dislocation/subluxation in more than one joint or in one joint on more than one occasion 4. Soft tissue rheumatism ≥3 lesions (e.g. epicondylitis, tenosynovitis, bursitis) 5. Marfanoid habitus (tall, slim, span/height) ratio >1.03, upper/lower segment ratio <0.89, arachnodactyli (+ Steinberg/wrist signs) 6. Abnormal skin: striae or hyperextensibility, thin cutis, or papyraceous scarring 7. Eye signs: drooping eyelids or myopia or antimongoloid slant 8. Varicose veins or hernia or uterine/rectal prolapse	

Data sourced from Kirk, J.A., Ansell, B.M., Bywaters, E.G. (1967) The hypermobility syndrome. Musculoskeletal complaints associated with generalized joint hypermobility. *Ann. Rheum. Dis.*, 26, 419–425.

Data sourced from Grahame, R., Bird, H.A., Child, A. (2000) The revised (Beighton 1998) criteria for the diagnosis of benign joint hypermobility syndrome (BJHS). *J. Rheumatol.*, 27, 1777–9.

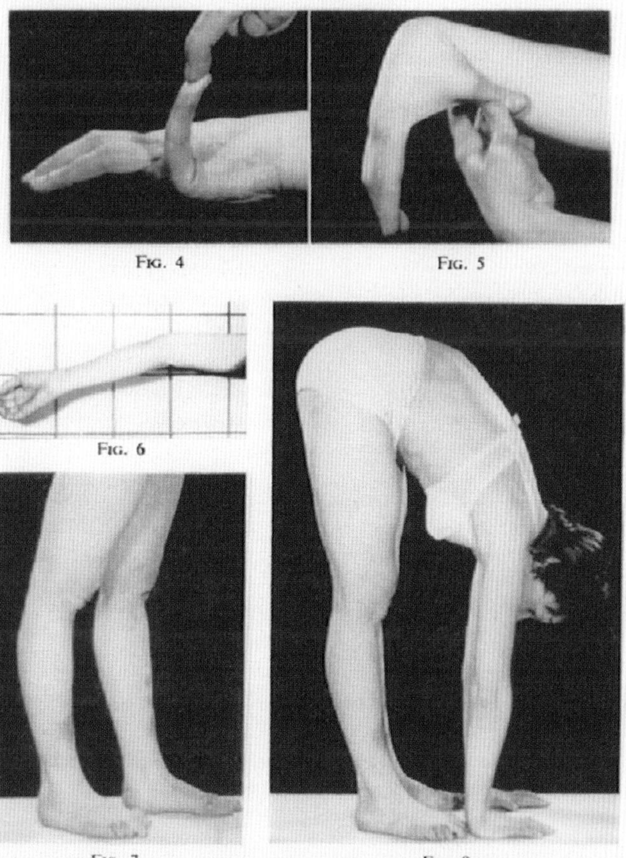

FIG. 4
FIG. 5
FIG. 6
FIG. 7
FIG. 8
Criteria for assessing hypermobility. Figure 4—Hyperextension of the little finger beyond 90 degrees. Figure 5—Passive apposition of the thumb to the flexor aspect of the forearm. Figure 6—Hyperextension of the elbow beyond 10 degrees. Figure 7—Hyperextension of the knee beyond 10 degrees. Figure 8—Forward flexion of the trunk so that the palms of the hands rest easily upon the floor.

Figure 9.1 The original presentation of the hypermobility tests (Beighton et al. 1973).

Reproduced with permission and copyright © of the British Editorial Society of Bone and Joint Surgery "Orthopaedic aspects of the Ehlers-Danlos Syndrome", Beighton P, Horan F, *J Bone Joint Surg Br* August 1969, vol. 51-B no. 3, 444–453.

Table 9.2 Examples of various definitions of GJH, given as number of positive tests in proportion to applied tests

Method	Tests	Definition	Comments
Rotès-Quérol, 1957	3 tests	2/3	Adults
Carter & Wilkinson, 1964	C&W tests	≥3/5	Children, 6–11 years
Beighton (5 tests), 1969	Beighton tests	None	Adults
Rotès-Quérol, 1972	R-Q tests	None	Degré I–IV
Beighton et al. (9 tests), 1973	Beighton tests	None	Twsana Africans
Hospital del Mar Criteria, 1992	Del Mar tests	4–5/10	Gender-dependent
Mikkelsson et al., 1996	Beighton tests	≥6/9	Children
Villefranche criteria, 1998	Beighton tests	≥5/9	Age, gender, ethnicity
Brighton criteria, 2000	Beighton tests	≥4/9	Current or historical

Data sourced from Rotès-Quérol, 1957; Carter & Wilkinson, 1964; Beighton (5 tests), 1969; Rotès-Quérol, 1972; Beighton (9 tests), 1973; Hospital del Mar Criteria, 1992; Mikkelsson et al., 1996; Villefranche criteria, 1998; Brighton criteria, 2000.

Table 9.3 Comparison of important items in the Villefranche criteria for Ehlers-Danlos syndrome (EDS) (Beighton et al. 1998) and the Brighton criteria for benign joint hypermobility syndrome (BJHS) (Grahame et al. 2000)

	EDS classical type	EDS hypermobile type	BJHS
Major criteria	Skin hyperextensibility	Hyperextensible and/or smooth velvety skin	
	Widened atrophic scars		Artralgia for longer than 3 months
	Beighton score ≥5/9	Beighton score ≥5/9	Beighton score ≥4/9
Minor criteria	Smooth, velvety skin	Chronic joint/limb pain	Skin hyperextensibility or papyraceous scarring
	Dislocations/subluxations	Recurring joint dislocations	Dislocation/subluxation
	Positive family history	Positive family history	Positive family history*

* Not a criterion item per se

Data sourced from Beighton et al. 1998 and Grahame et al. 2000.

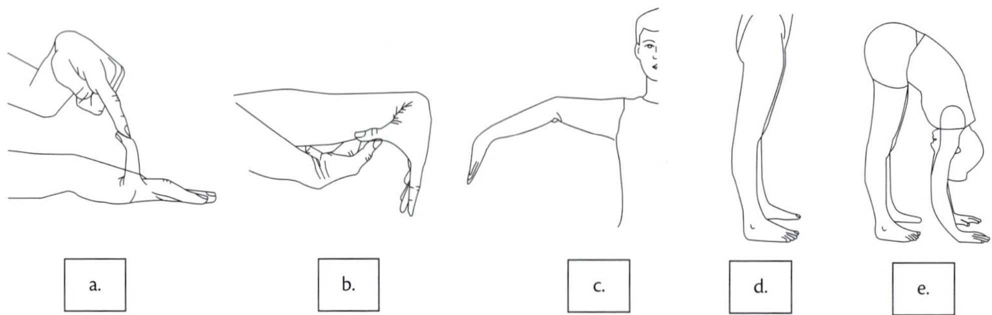

Figure 9.2 Test performance and description of Beighton tests shown to be reproducible (Juul-Kristensen et al. 2007).

(a) With patient seated, ask her/him to place the forearm and hand pronated on the table and to extend, passively, the fifth finger. An extension beyond 90° indicates a positive test.

(b) With patient seated, arm flexed 90° in shoulder, elbow extended 180°, and hand pronated and relaxed, ask the patient to move, passively, the first finger to the volar aspect of the forearm. In the case that the forearm is reached, the test is positive.

(c) With patient standing in front of you, ask her/him to abduct 90° in the shoulder, with relaxed elbow and supinated hand. Support the upper arm with your ipsilateral hand. An extension beyond 10° indicates a positive test.

(d) With patient standing in upright position, turning the side towards you, ask her/him to relax and hyperextend the knee. An extension beyond 10° indicates a positive test.

(e) From a standing position, with her/his feet slightly apart, ask the patient to place his/her hands on the floor, maintaining extended knees. In the case that the palms of the hands can be placed on the floor easily, the test is positive.

Tests (a) to (d) are double-sided, giving in total nine tests.

The overlap in the criteria was already known by the authors when they presented the Brighton criteria: 'From the clinic perspective there is compelling evidence that the hypermobility type of EDS and the BJHS are one and the same' (Grahame et al. 2000), and recently it was recommended to merge the two disease entities into one (Tinkle et al. 2009). However, new knowledge has arisen during the last 10 years which should be taken into account in a revision of the syndrome criteria (Remvig et al. 2011a).

Alterations in motor control in subjects with GJH

It is generally important to differ between adults with non-symptomatic GJH and symptomatic GJH (like, for example, HMS, EDS-HT). Adults with GJH do not necessarily have other problems (e.g. pain or reduced function) than the fact that they are more flexible than their contemporaries. Children and adolescents even seem to perform better than their contemporaries, since they have a better balance (Juul-Kristensen et al. 2009), are better in precision tasks (Remvig et al. 2011b), jump higher (Remvig et al. 2011b; Juul-Kristensen et al. 2012), and are often selected into elite sports, dance, and music playing, partly due to their greater flexibility (Larsson et al. 1993; McCormack et al. 2004). However, that does not quite seem to be the same for the adults, whose stability is actually reduced (Jensen et al. 2013; Juul-Kristensen et al. 2012; Mebes et al. 2008). Whether age accounts for this decreased flexibility is not known. However, it indicates that this condition deteriorates with age.

It is not known when and who will develop pain and reduced function, but since GJH and pain in 10-year-old children is a predictor for repeated non-specific pain and pain in the lower extremities four years after (El-Metwally et al. 2004, 2005), it indicates that when pain has already emerged in childhood, it seems to stay.

Adults with symptomatic GJH, called HMS, are typically seen in the healthcare system, in contrast to adults with non-symptomatic GJH. Pain in HMS may either emerge directly as diffuse and/or joint pain, or indirectly due to mechanical trauma (dislocation, luxation). Since an increased risk of luxation, especially in contact sports, has been found in children as well as in adults with GJH (Pacey et al. 2010), pain in HMS may very often be a consequence of smaller or larger injuries. The body region most often involved is the knee (Konopinski et al. 2012; Pacey et al. 2010), but the shoulder may also be involved (Cameron et al. 2010).

Maximal strength and strength balance

Adults with HMS or EDS-HT (Rombaut et al. 2012; Sahin et al. 2008b) have decreased maximal isokinetic knee extension strength, and those with EDS-HT further have reduced endurance (Rombaut et al. 2012). It is well known that pain is an important inhibitor in maximum voluntary muscle contraction, for example as seen in osteoarthritis (OA) (Ekdahl and Andersson 1989) and in experimental pain (Graven-Nielsen et al. 2002), for which reason reduced strength in HMS and EDS-HT could be due to pain. The reason for reduced strength in EDS-HT has also been ascribed to severe neuromuscular involvements (Voermans et al. 2007, 2009).

Reduced knee strength may also be due to hypermobility alone, as seen in a recent study where women (and also girls at 10 years old) with non-symptomatic GJH had significantly lower maximum isokinetic knee extension strength than their matched contemporaries without GJH (Juul-Kristensen et al. 2012). When tested isometrically though, there was no strength difference (Jensen et al. 2013; Mebes et al. 2008). This means that in the total group (men and women together), adults with GJH do not have reduced maximal strength, neither isokinetically nor isometrically, compared with a matched control group without GJH. However, since adults with GJH have an increased risk of injuries, a normal maximal strength does not seem to protect against injury, and, for example, knee strength balance, called the hamstring/quadriceps-ratio (H/Q-ratio), previously reported to be an important predictor of ligament and muscle injuries (Soderman et al. 2001), may be a more important protecting factor. The H/Q-ratio was actually reduced in adults with HMS and GJH (Juul-Kristensen et al. 2012; Sahin et al. 2008b) when measured isokinetically. Also decreased knee muscle activity balance was seen in adults with GJH during maximum isometric knee extension (Jensen et al. 2013). These different signs of strength and muscle activity imbalance in GJH could result in the increased risk of injuries (like in GJH), and this may not only result in pain but also an increased risk of OA over time (Lohmander et al. 2007).

Several automatic protective motor control strategies for joint stabilization seem to be present in adults with non-symptomatic GJH. This was found, for example, as an increased co-contraction level (muscle activity in both agonists and antagonists of the knee) during submaximal knee extension, correlating positively with the Beighton score, and in normal balance tasks (Ford et al. 2008; Greenwood et al. 2011; Jensen et al. 2013). Further, an increased ability to develop explosive muscle force (rate of force development) during maximum knee extension was seen in women with non-symptomatic GJH, as another protective strategy, due to less stability in the passive structures (Mebes et al. 2008).

Proprioception

Joint instability in patients with EDS-HT could be related to the poorer proprioception as found in adults with EDS-HT and with HMS (Hall et al. 1995; Rombaut et al. 2010; Sahin et al. 2008a). Disturbed sensory feedback mechanisms in subjects with HMS were further confirmed in adolescents, where the reflex in the knee extensors was absent in 47% of 15 patients, compared to none in the healthy controls (Ferrell et al. 2007). However, poor reflexes may be due to the presence of pain, since non-symptomatic adults with GJH seemed to have normal sensory feedback mechanisms (seen as normal proprioception) compared to healthy controls (Jeremiah and Alexander 2010). Further research is however needed on this area.

Proprioception acuity may be improved with training, but only a few studies on HMS have shown this (Ferrell et al. 2004; Sahin et al. 2008a).

Gait

An increased knee joint moment in the sagittal (extensor) and frontal planes (abductor) of 10% and 13% respectively, was seen in adults with GJH (Simonsen et al. 2012). Previous studies have estimated at least a 1% increase in knee abduction moment to increase the risk of OA progression 6.46 times in patients with OA (Andriacchi 2006; Lynn et al. 2007; Miyazaki et al. 2002). Also, adults with EDS-HT walked with significantly decreased step velocity, step length, and stride length, especially combined with cognitive requirements (Rombaut et al. 2011).

Balance

A larger sway in static balance, as seen in non-symptomatic women with GJH, could be due to poorer ability in active stabilization in the frontal plane, where balance is more dependent on passive stabilization (Mebes et al. 2008). In dynamic and thus more challenging balance conditions, non-symptomatic adults with GJH showed less stable trunk segments and less lateral shoulder stability, indicating a less flexible moving pattern. This may compensate for an increased risk of falling (Falkerslev et al. 2013). In adults with EDS-HT, whole body stability or postural control is diminished, and they further reported fear of falling and also had an increased risk of falling, since 95% of these patients fell in the previous year (Rombaut et al. 2011). These results indicate a threat to safety during everyday situations for this patient group.

Physical fitness (endurance)

Adults with HMS and EDS-HT have reduced endurance (in maximum repetitions of knee extension and flexion at 240°/s) (Sahin et al. 2008b; Rombaut et al. 2012). Also, the static endurance test showed that the EDS-HT patients were fatigued twice as fast as controls in the time to maintain a specific posture (Rombaut et al. 2012).

Rehabilitation in generalized joint hypermobility and hypermobility syndrome

General principles

In general, knowledge and perception of the problems that may arise from GJH and HMS are essential. Tailored care in terms of evidence-based diagnostic procedures and clinical expertise is essential in order to construct classification models as well as optimized treatment strategies. So diagnostics and treatment should be founded on evidence-based practice, clinimetrics, and clinical reasoning, eventually leading to sub-classification and treatment strategies.

This requires a shared language, as well as a common framework. In this context, a framework that could be used as the classification for health and health-related domains is the International Classification of Functioning, Disability and Health, known more commonly as the ICF model. The ICF domains are classified from bodily, individual, and societal perspectives by means of two levels: the level of body functions and structure, and the level of activity and participation. Since an individual's functioning and disability occur in a context, the ICF also includes a list of environmental factors (<http://www.who.int/classifications/icf/en>). Although the ICF is frequently used in the provision of healthcare services, it has not been described in detail in adults with GJH, HMS, and EDS-HT.

Intervention, based on clinical decision making, might be effective using the principles of motor learning and training. Reassurance, education, and joint care are cornerstones of treatment strategies (Engelbert and Scheper 2011). For this, a multidisciplinary approach might be indicated, depending on the problems an individual patient will encounter. Treatment has to be tailored to the individual's needs, and where patients encounter problems on more than one domain (psychological, physical, and social), multidisciplinary treatment is recommended (Engelbert et al. 2013).

The motor learning principles as described in a textbook: '1. Use it or lose it, 2. Use it and improve it, 3. Specificity, 4. Repetition, 5. Intensity, 6.Time, 7. Salience, 8. Age, 9. Transference, and 10. Interference' (Schumway-Cook and Woollacott 2010) should be respected, to prolong physiological changes over time. Also, applications of interventions, which should pay respect to transfer and generalization, need attention. This indicates that a standardized programme should enhance the transference and generalization of a task, indicating that tasks or exercises are given in a random order. This also indicates that variation of practices should be performed, meaning that specific tasks or exercises are performed in different contexts.

Treatment strategies should focus on influencing the pathophysiological aspects of GJH and HMS, combined with the individual goals for activities and participation of the individual patient. Although the amount of joint hypermobility cannot be influenced, improving musculoskeletal strength, stability, and coordination, as well as physical fitness should be based on pathophysiological principles.

In general, cardiovascular training and strength training are both important categories of physical fitness. Guidelines for such training for adults are very well described in the position published by the American College of Sports Medicine (ACSM) (Garber et al. 2011). A programme of regular exercise that includes cardiorespiratory, resistance, and neuromotor exercise training, beyond activities of daily living to improve and maintain physical fitness and health, is essential for most adults. The recommended minimal frequency of aerobic training for adults is 3–5 times a week, with a duration of 30–60 minutes of purposeful moderate exercise. The recommended volume for a training session is a minimum of 500–1000 metabolic equivalent minutes per week or a minimum of 2000–7000 step counts per day.

Muscular fitness and its relationship to health has been well established during the past decade (Bird et al. 2011).The recommended frequency for training of muscle strength is 2 or 3 times a week, for each muscle group. The intensity is based on 60–70% of one repetition maximum (RM) (moderate to hard intensity) for novice to intermediate exercisers in order to improve muscle strength.

Neuromotor exercise training incorporates motor skills such as balance, coordination, gait, and agility, and proprioceptive training. Such training is beneficial as part of a comprehensive exercise programme, especially to improve balance, agility, and muscle strength, and to reduce the risk of falls.

Randomized controlled trails

A search in the literature was performed (Pubmed, Cinahl) to find randomized controlled trials (RCTs) focusing on interventions in GJH and HMS in children and adults (Engelbert et al. 2013). Only one randomized controlled study was found on adults, studying knee proprioception and effects of proprioception exercise in adolescent and adult patients with BJHS. To evaluate the proprioceptive sensibility of the knee joint, cases with HMS were randomized into two groups: proprioceptive exercises were undertaken by 15 patients for 8 weeks, and 25 patients were taken as controls and did not receive any treatment. In the HMS group, significant decreases in pain levels were detected in individuals who did exercises compared with those who did not, and also statistically significant improvements were detected in occupational activity for those who engaged in exercise. However, no between-group differences were reported, only within-group differences (Sahin et al. 2008a). Two further uncontrolled studies in adults have been published. Appropriate exercises led not only to symptomatic improvement, but also to demonstrable enhancement of proprioception, although both studies lacked a control group (Barton and Bird 1996; Ferrell et al. 2004).

In children, three RCTs were found (Engelbert and Scheper 2011). One study performed a prospective RCT, comparing a 6-week generalized programme, including muscular strength and fitness training, with a targeted programme aiming at correcting motor control of symptomatic joints. Fifty-seven children, aged 7–16 years, with symptomatic GJH, were randomly assigned to receive a targeted or generalized training programme. The study demonstrated significant and sustained reduction of pain and improved self-reported function when the effects of both groups were combined, but did not detect any difference between the groups (Kemp et al. 2010).

One study of infants referred due to delayed motor development caused by JH and benign hypotonia examined the effect of the frequency of physical therapy (Mintz-Itkin et al. 2009). The study groups comprised 29 infants (8–12 months) who were randomly placed into a monthly or weekly treatment group. No difference in self-reported (by parents or their children) and measured function was found between the two study group scores on the different tests, at all assessment points. However, one exception was the assessment of walking at the age of 15 months, which revealed a clear advantage for the infants who were treated weekly.

In children and adults, further uncontrolled studies of therapeutic strategies have been described in textbooks (Keer and Simmonds 2011; Kerr et al. 2000). The recent topical review reported that joint protection and injury prevention form a major component of a successful rehabilitation programme (Keer and Simmonds 2011). It is suggested that these aims are to be achieved through improving posture, joint stability, and specific motor skills by training with the inclusion of pain-free exercises to enhance proprioception and muscle strength. Also, it was stated that renewed confidence in the joints will lead to resumption of a person's habitual level of physical activity with the benefits of improved physical fitness and well-being. In addition, the review questioned the optimal form of rehabilitation to maintain joint health in HMS (Keer and Simmonds 2011).

Unfortunately, until now, physiotherapy treatment techniques with demonstrated effectiveness are scarce in HMS. Since observations are primarily based on uncontrolled trials, there is a need to be cautious about interpretations of the literature.

As mentioned in the review concerning joint protection and rehabilitation in the adult with HMS, it is not yet known which form the optimal physical rehabilitation programme should adopt. As long as scientific evidence of optimal treatment is lacking (evidence-based), recommendations can only be made based on 'best opinion' (practice -based) (Keer and Simmonds 2011). Transfer of the knowledge of physiological training principles in healthy persons should be performed with care towards patients with HMS, since overuse and triggering musculoskeletal complaints have been reported. Therefore—train as effectively as possible based on clinical reasoning and evidence-based practice/practice-based evidence, but handle with care!

In conclusion, GJH is a condition characterised by decreased muscle strength, stability, and proprioception, in addition to impaired gait pattern, balance, and physical fitness (e.g. endurance). Evidence for treatment is lacking. However, although the amount of JH cannot be influenced, improving musculoskeletal strength, stability, and coordination, as well as physical fitness, is the aim, and should be based on pathophysiological principles.

References

Allander, E., Bjornsson, O.J., Olafsson, O., Sigfusson, N., Thorsteinsson, J. (1974) Normal range of joint movements in shoulder, hip, wrist and thumb with special reference to side: a comparison between two populations. *Int. J. Epidemiol.*, 3, 253–61.

American Academy of Orthopedic Surgeons (AAOS) (1965) *Joint motion. Method of measuring and recording*. AAOS.

Andriacchi, T.P.M.A. (2006) The role of ambulatory mechanics in the initiation and progression of knee osteoarthritis. *Curr. Opin. Rheumatol.*, 18, 514–8.

Barton, L.M., Bird, H.A. (1996) Improving pain by the stabilization of hyperlax joints. *J. Orthopaed. Rheum.*, 9, 46–51.

Beighton, P.H., Horan, F.T. (1970) Dominant inheritance in familial generalised articular hypermobility. *J. Bone Joint Surg. Br.*, 52, 145–7.

Beighton, P., De Paepe, A., Steinmann, B., Tsipouras, P., Wenstrup, R.J. (1998) Ehlers-Danlos syndromes: revised nosology, Villefranche, 1997. Ehlers-Danlos National Foundation (USA) and Ehlers-Danlos Support Group (UK). *Am. J. Med. Genet.*, 77, 31–7.

Beighton, P., Solomon, L., Soskolne, C.L. (1973) Articular mobility in an African population. *Ann. Rheum. Dis.*, 32, 413–8.

Bird, M., Hill, K.D., Ball, M., Hetherington, S., Williams, A.D. (2011) The long-term benefits of a multi-component exercise intervention to balance and mobility in healthy older adults. *Arch. Gerontol. Geriatr.*, 52, 211–6.

Bulbena, A., Duro, J.C., Porta, M., Faus, S., Vallescar, R., Martin-Santos, R. (1992) Clinical assessment of hypermobility of joints: assembling criteria. *J. Rheumatol.*, 19, 115–22.

Cameron, K.L., Duffey, M.L., DeBerardino, T.M., Stoneman, P.D., Jones, C.J., Owens, B.D. (2010) Association of generalized joint hypermobility with a history of glenohumeral joint instability. *J. Athl. Train.*, 45, 253–8.

Ekdahl, C., Andersson, S.I. (1989) Standing balance in rheumatoid arthritis. A comparative study with healthy subjects. *Scand. J. Rheumatol.*, 18, 33–42.

El-Metwally, A., Salminen, J.J., Auvinen, A., Kautiainen, H., Mikkelsson, M. (2004) Prognosis of non-specific musculoskeletal pain in preadolescents: a prospective 4-year follow-up study till adolescence. *Pain*, 110, 550–9.

El-Metwally, A., Salminen, J.J., Auvinen, A., Kautiainen, H., Mikkelsson, M. (2005) Lower limb pain in a preadolescent population: prognosis and risk factors for chronicity—a prospective 1- and 4-year follow-up study. *Pediatrics*, 116, 673–81.

El-Metwally, A., Salminen, J.J., Auvinen, A., Macfarlane, G., Mikkelsson, M. (2007) Risk factors for development of non-specific musculoskeletal pain in preteens and early adolescents: a prospective 1-year follow-up study. *BMC Muscul. Disord.*, 8, 46.

Engelbert, R.H., Scheper, M.C. (2011) Joint hypermobility with and without musculoskeletal complaints: a physiotherapeutic approach. *Int. Musculoskel. Med.*, 33(4), 146–51.

Engelbert, R.H.H., Scheper, M.C., Rameckers, E.A.A., Verbunt, J., Remvig, L., Juul-Kristensen, B. (2013) Children with generalised joint hypermobility and musculoskeletal complaints: state of the art on diagnostics, clinical characteristics and treatment.' Biomed Res Int., Volume 2013, Article ID 121054, 13 pages, http://dx.doi.org/10.1155/2013/121054.

Fairbank, J.C., Pynsent, P.B., Phillips, H. (1984) Quantitative measurements of joint mobility in adolescents. *Ann. Rheum. Dis.*, 43, 288–94.

Falkerslev, S., Baagø, C., Alkjær, T., et al. (2013) Dynamic balance during gait in children and adults with generalised joint hypermobility. Clin Biomech (Bristol, Avon). 2013 Mar; 28(3):318–24. doi: 10.1016/j.clinbiomech.2013.01.006. Epub 2013 Feb 1.

Ferrell, W.R., Tennant, N., Baxendale, R.H., Kusel, M., Sturrock, R.D. (2007) Musculoskeletal reflex function in the joint hypermobility syndrome. *Arthritis Rheum.*, ***57***, 1329–33.

Ferrell, W.R., Tennant, N., Sturrock, R.D., et al. (2004) Amelioration of symptoms by enhancement of proprioception in patients with joint hypermobility syndrome. *Arthritis Rheum.*, 50, 3323–8.

Ford, K.R., van den Bogert, J., Myer, G.D., Shapiro, R., Hewett, T.E. (2008) The effect of age and skill level on the knee musculature co-contraction during functional activities: a systematic review. *Br. J. Sports Med.*, 42, 561–5.

Garber, C.E., Blissmer, B., Deschenes, M.R., et al. (2011) American College of Sports Medicine position stand. Quantity and quality of exercise for developing and maintaining cardiorespiratory, musculoskeletal, and neuromotor fitness in apparently healthy adults: guidance for prescribing exercise. *Med. Sci. Sports Exerc.*, 43, 1334–59.

Grahame, R., Bird, H.A., Child, A. (2000) The revised (Beighton 1998) criteria for the diagnosis of benign joint hypermobility syndrome (BJHS). *J. Rheumatol.*, 27, 1777–9.

Graven-Nielsen, T., Lund, H., Arendt-Nielsen, L., Danneskiold-Samsoe, B., Bliddal, H. (2002) Inhibition of maximal voluntary contraction force by experimental muscle pain: a centrally mediated mechanism. *Muscle & Nerve*, 26, 708–12.

Greenwood, N.L., Duffell, L.D., Alexander, C.M., McGregor, A.H. (2011) Electromyographic activity of pelvic and lower limb muscles during postural tasks in people with benign joint hypermobility syndrome and non hypermobile people. A pilot study. *Man. Ther.*, 16, 623–8.

Hall, M.G., Ferrell, W.R., Sturrock, R.D., Hamblen, D.L., Baxendale, R.H. (1995) The effect of the hypermobility syndrome on knee joint proprioception. *Br. J. Rheumatol.*, **34**, 121–5. Available at: <http://www.who.int/classifications/icf/en>.

Jensen, B.R., Olesen, A.T., Pedersen, M.T., et al. (2013) 'Effect of Generalised Joint Hypermobility on knee function and muscle activation in children and adults.' Muscle and Nerve, 2013 Nov; 48(5):762–9. doi: 10.1002/mus.23802. Epub 2013 Aug 30.

Jeremiah, H.M., Alexander, C.M. (2010) Do hypermobile subjects without pain have alteration to the feedback mechanisms controlling the Shoulder Girdle?' Musculoskelet. Care, 8; 157–163.

Juul-Kristensen, B., Hansen, H., Simonsen, E.B., et al. (2012) Knee function in 10-year-old children and adults with generalised joint hypermobility. *The Knee*, 19, 773–8.

Juul-Kristensen, B., Kristensen, J.H., Frausing, B., Jensen, D.V., Rogind, H., Remvig, L. (2009) Motor competence and physical activity in 8-year-old school children with generalized joint hypermobility. *Pediatrics*, 124, 1380–7.

Juul-Kristensen, B., Rogind, H., Jensen, D.V., Remvig, L. (2007) Inter-examiner reproducibility of tests and criteria for generalized joint hypermobility and benign joint hypermobility syndrome. *Rheumatology(Oxford)*, 46, 1835–41.

Keer, R., Simmonds, J. (2011) Joint protection and physical rehabilitation of the adult with hypermobility syndrome. *Curr. Opin. Rheumatol.*, 23, 131–6.

Kemp, S., Roberts, I., Gamble, C., et al. (2010) A randomized comparative trial of generalized vs targeted physiotherapy in the management of childhood hypermobility. *Rheumatology (Oxford)*, 49, 315–25.

Kerr, A., MacMillan, C., Uttley, W., Luqmani, R. (2000) Physiotherapy for children with hypermobility syndrome. *Physiotherapy*, 86, 313–7.

Kirk, J.A., Ansell, B.M., Bywaters, E.G. (1967) The hypermobility syndrome. Musculoskeletal complaints associated with generalized joint hypermobility. *Ann. Rheum. Dis.*, 26, 419–25.

Konopinski, M.D., Jones, G.J., Johnson, M.I. (2012) The effect of hypermobility on the incidence of injuries in elite-level professional soccer players: a cohort study. *Am. J. Sports Med.*, 40, 763–9.

Larsson, L.G., Baum, J., Mudholkar, G.S., Kollia, G.D. (1993) Benefits and disadvantages of joint hypermobility among musicians. *N. Engl. J. Med.*, 329, 1079–82.

Lohmander, L.S., Englund, P.M., Dahl, L.L., Roos, E.M. (2007) The long-term consequence of anterior cruciate ligament and meniscus injuries: osteoarthritis. *Am. J. Sports Med.*, 35, 1756–69.

Lynn, S.K., Reid, S.M., Costigan, P.A. (2007) The influence of gait pattern on signs of knee osteoarthritis in older adults over a 5–11 year follow-up period: a case study analysis. *The Knee*, 14, 22–8.

McCormack, M., Briggs, J., Hakim, A., Grahame, R. (2004) Joint laxity and the benign joint hypermobility syndrome in student and professional ballet dancers. *J. Rheumatol.*, 31, 173–8.

Mebes, C., Amstutz, A., Luder, G., et al. (2008) Isometric rate of force development, maximum voluntary contraction, and balance in women with and without joint hypermobility. *Arthritis Rheum.*, 59, 1665–9.

Mintz-Itkin, R., Lerman-Sagie, T., Zuk, L., Itkin-Webman, T., Davidovitch, M. (2009) Does physical therapy improve outcome in infants with joint hypermobility and benign hypotonia? *J. Child Neurol.*, 24, 714–9.

Miyazaki, T., Wada, M., Kawahara, H., Sato, M., Baba, H., Shimada, S. (2002) Dynamic load at baseline can predict radiographic disease progression in medial compartment knee osteoarthritis. *Ann. Rheum. Dis.*, 61, 617–22.

Pacey, V., Nicholson, L.L., Adams, R.D., Munn, J., Munns, C.F. (2010) Generalized joint hypermobility and risk of lower limb joint injury during sport: a systematic review with meta-analysis. *Am. J. Sports Med.*, 38, 1487–97.

Remvig, L., Engelbert, R.H., Berglund, B., et al. (2011a) Need for a consensus on the methods by which to measure joint mobility and the definition of norms for hypermobility that reflect age, gender and ethnic-dependent variation: is revision of criteria for joint hypermobility syndrome and Ehlers-Danlos syndrome hypermobility type indicated? *Rheumatology (Oxford)*, 50, 1169–71.

Remvig, L., Jensen, D.V., Ward, R.C. (2007) Epidemiology of general joint hypermobility and basis for the proposed criteria for benign joint hypermobility syndrome: review of the literature. *J. Rheumatol.*, 34, 804–9.

Remvig, L., Kümmel, C., Kristensen, J.H., Boas, G., Juul-Kristensen, B. (2011b) Prevalence of generalised joint hypermobility, arthralgia and motor competence in 10-year old school children. *Int. Muscul. Med.*, 33, 137–45.

Rombaut, L., De, P.A., Malfait, F., Cools, A., Calders, P. (2010) Joint position sense and vibratory perception sense in patients with Ehlers-Danlos syndrome type III (hypermobility type). *Clin. Rheumatol.*, 29, 289–95.

Rombaut, L., Malfait, F., De Wandele, I., et al. (2012) Muscle mass, muscle strength, functional performance, and physical impairment in women with the hypermobility type of Ehlers-Danlos syndrome. *Arthritis Care & Research*, Vol. 64, No. 10, October 2012, pp 1584–1592, DOI 10.1002/acr.21726.

Rombaut, L., Malfait, F., De Wandele, I., et al. (2011) Balance, gait, falls, and fear of falling in women with the hypermobility type of Ehlers-Danlos syndrome. *Arthritis Care Res. (Hoboken)*, 63, 1432–9.

Rotes-Querol, J. (1957) Articular laxity considered as factor of changes of the locomotor apparatus. *Rev. Rhum. Mal. Osteoartic.*, 24, 535–9.

Sahin, N., Baskent, A., Cakmak, A., Salli, A., Ugurlu, H., Berker, E. (2008a) Evaluation of knee proprioception and effects of proprioception exercise in patients with benign joint hypermobility syndrome. *Rheumatol. Int.*, 28, 995–1000.

Sahin, N., Baskent, A., Ugurlu, H., Berker, E. (2008b) Isokinetic evaluation of knee extensor/flexor muscle strength in patients with hypermobility syndrome. *Rheumatol. Int.*, 28, 643–8.

Schumway-Cook, A., Woollacott, M.H. (2010) *Motor control, translating research into clinical practice.* Wolters Kluwer/Lippincott Williams & Wilkins, UK.

Silman, A.J., Haskard, D., Day, S. (1986) Distribution of joint mobility in a normal population: results of the use of fixed torque measuring devices. *Ann. Rheum. Dis.*, 45, 27–30.

Simonsen, E.B., Tegner, H., Alkjaer, T., et al. (2012) Gait analysis of adults with generalised joint hypermobility. *Clin. Biomech*, 27:573–577. doi:10.1016/j.clinbiomech.2012.1001.1008.

Smits-Engelsman, B., Klerks, M., Kirby, A. (2011) Beighton score: a valid measure for generalized hypermobility in children. *J. Pediatr.*, 158, 119–23.

Soderman, K., Alfredson, H., Pietila, T., Werner, S. (2001) Risk factors for leg injuries in female soccer players: a prospective investigation during one out-door season. *Knee Surg. Sports Traumatol. Arthrosc.*, 9, 313–21.

Tinkle, B.T., Bird, H.A., Grahame, R., Lavallee, M., Levy, H.P., Sillence, D. (2009) The lack of clinical distinction between the hypermobility type of Ehlers-Danlos syndrome and the joint hypermobility syndrome (a.k.a. hypermobility syndrome). *Am. J. Med. Gen. Part A*, 149A, 2368–70.

Voermans, N.C., Altenburg, T.M., Hamel, B.C., de Haan, A., van Engelen, B.G. (2007) Reduced quantitative function in tenascin-X deficient Ehlers-Danlos patients. *Neuromuscul. Disord.*, 17, 597–602.

Voermans, N.C., van Alfen, N., Pillen, S., et al. (2009) Neuromuscular involvement in various types of Ehlers-Danlos Syndrome. *Ann. Neurol.*, **65**, 687–97.

Wood, P. (1971) Is hypermobility a discrete entity? *Proc. R. Soc. Med.*, 64, 690–2.

Chapter 10

Somatic dysfunction

Michael L. Kuchera

Definition and underlying concepts of somatic dysfunction

Somatic dysfunction is formally defined as: 'impaired or altered function of related components of the somatic (body framework) system: skeletal, arthrodial, and myofascial structures, and related vascular, lymphatic and neural elements' (Education Council on Osteopathic Principles 2011; WHO 1979). This diagnostic term thus embraces a wide range of relevant clinical findings and conditions. The term broadly encompasses Maigne's 'minor intervertebral derangements' (Maigne and Liberson 1972), Travell and Simons' 'myofascial trigger points' (1999a), Jones' 'tender points' (1981), Maitland's 'locked joint' (1978), and various generic 'manipulable lesions', 'fixations', 'chiropractic subluxations', and 'blockages'. The term 'somatic dysfunction', first coined in 1961 by the Educational Council on Osteopathic Principles (ECOP), replaced the provincial term 'osteopathic lesion'. Somatic dysfunction is now recognized as a valid and codable diagnostic term in the *International Classification of Diseases* (WHO 1979).

The palpable characteristics of somatic dysfunction may be caused by structural or architectural changes (often associated with a loss of range of motion) or by functional aberrations in various somatic tissues associated with recognized physiological and pathophysiological processes. These palpable characteristics are interpreted by various healthcare practitioners to be associated through their anatomical, central nervous system (CNS), or autonomical connections with a particular joint or joints, myofascial structure, subcutaneous tissue or fascia, viscera, or condition (Gilliar et al. 1996). Myofascial trigger points, facet syndromes, and somatovisceral reflex phenomena are all examples of somatic dysfunction discussed in this text on musculoskeletal medicine. In this chapter, however, these specific conditions are not discussed in diagnostic isolation. Instead, a broad conceptual understanding of somatic dysfunction is presented to expand diagnostic and therapeutic options, integrating otherwise disparate approaches to patient complaints.

Certain generalizations apply to somatic dysfunction, its diagnosis, and its treatment. This chapter will address the most important of these generalizations:

- Somatic dysfunction reflects a summation of peripheral and central physiological mechanisms underlying a condition that interferes with maximal health and function.
- Diagnostic testing for somatic dysfunction consists of simple, reproducible palpatory and provocative examinations.
- The four diagnostic criteria for somatic dysfunction are sensory change, tissue texture change, asymmetry, and restriction of motion. These objective findings are summarized by the mnemonic, 'S.T.A.R.'.
- Somatic dysfunction can be subdivided into its physiological characteristics (e.g. acute, chronic); its anatomical location (e.g. cervical, lumbosacral); and/or the specific constellation or pattern of anatomical and physiological characteristics (e.g. acute psoas syndrome, latent sternocleidomastoid myofascial trigger point).
- The severity of somatic dysfunction can be differentiated; graded 'mild', 'moderate', or 'severe'; and recorded to separate background levels of somatic dysfunction from significant 'key' dysfunction.
- *Primary somatic dysfunction* typically responds well to various manipulative medicine approaches, whereas *secondary somatic dysfunction* may respond but recur, respond less well, or fail to respond when addressed by these approaches alone.
- Somatic dysfunction plays a role in a significant number of patient complaints; failure to consider it in diagnosis and treatment overlooks an important underlying pathophysiological process that may limit the ability to obtain optimum health and performance.
- A manual medicine prescription, if indicated, considers individual characteristics of the somatic dysfunction, the patient as a whole, and the skills of the treating physician.
- A number of precipitating and/or perpetuating factors warrant consideration in the diagnosis and treatment of patients with somatic dysfunction.
- Despite the quality of care initially given, recurrent patterns of somatic dysfunction require patient re-evaluation and reconsideration of the patient's present management.

Other chapters in this textbook will address the significance of somatic dysfunction in specific regional disorders (Chapter 27) and physician management strategies (Chapters 50 and 60).

Physiological basis of somatic dysfunction

Physicians practicing in neuromusculoskeletal medicine fields distinguish between peripheral stimuli that can produce pain and the experience of pain itself. The central transmission of noxious stimuli is referred to as *nociception*, the patient's experience as *pain*, and the neuromusculoskeletal reflexes elicited by the nociceptors as being *nocifensive* or *nociautonomic* (Gilliar et al. 1996). The importance of pain itself is variable in the diagnosis and treatment of somatic dysfunction and is often dependent upon the model used by the neuromusculoskeletal practitioner.

Several physiological principles implicated in the production and maintenance of pain and somatic dysfunction require an understanding of both peripheral and central mechanisms. For example, nociception results in local (peripheral) vasodilation and tissue oedema; over time, the central nocifensive and nociautonomic reflexes result in peripheral vasoconstriction, tissue ischaemia, altered sweat gland activity, and other different, but predictable, tissue responses. Thus, local palpatory findings will depend upon the physiological summation of peripheral and central influences.

Substance P plays a role in both peripheral and central processes. Peripherally, up to 90% of substance P produced by sensory neurons is stored and released (as in a paracrine gland) from terminal branches (Pernow 1983). It is pro-inflammatory, and results in vasodilation, hyperalgesia, and oedema (Figure 10.1). Centrally, substance P, performing as a slow-acting neuromodulator, is co-released in the dorsal horn along with other neurotransmitters that are fast acting (Battaglia and Rustioni 1988). These neurotransmitters, in concert, influence the neural plasticity of the dorsal horn leading to segmental spinal facilitation and a shift from acute to chronic pain patterns (Willard et al. 1997).

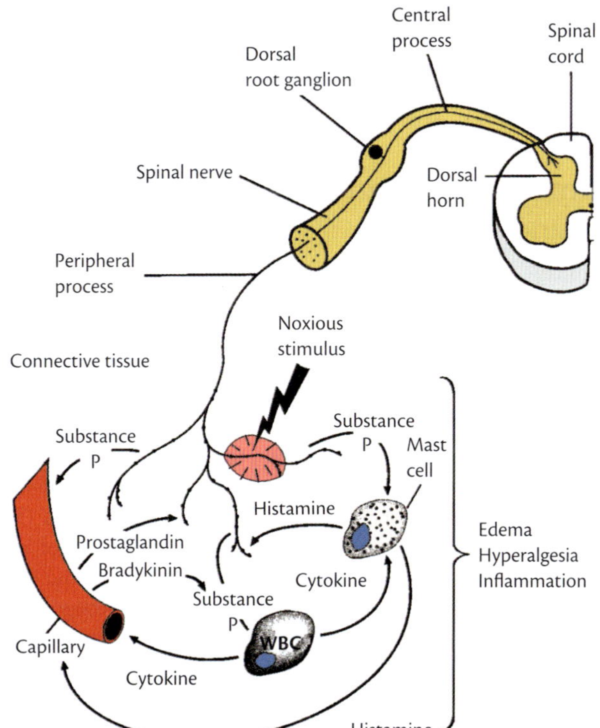

Figure 10.1 Interaction of afferent impulses and immune system. Noxious stimulant initiates secretion of neuropeptides such as substance P from primary afferent fibre. The result is a feedforward cascade of inflammatory events producing oedema and hyperalgesia. (Willard, F. H., Mokler, D. J., Morgane, P. J. Chapter 9. Neuroendocrine-immune system and homeostasis. In Ward, R. C. (ed.). *Foundations for osteopathic medicine* (1997). Williams & Wilkins, Baltimore, MD, pp. 107–35.)

Ultimately, even though the initiating event may have been traumatic, it appears that nociceptive stimuli from local tissues play a major role in initiating the cord-level reflexes that, in turn, alter muscle length, tone, and balance. Other somatic reflexes then play a role in maintaining and organizing these aberrant reflexes. Finally, because of 'cross-talk' by the cord-level segmental circuitry controlling autonomic and visceral functions, the local somatic findings of altered muscle length, tone, and balance are frequently accompanied by segmentally related autonomic and visceral aberrations, completing the symptom complex of somatic dysfunction.

In this manner, the CNS functions both as an 'integrator' that senses and analyses the environment, generating command signals along the motor pathways to muscles and other effectors (Konnitinen et al. 1994), and as an 'organizer', useful in interpreting segmentally related patterns of pain and dysfunction (Korr 1979) (Figure 10.2). The CNS is able to interpret and assign differing priorities to afferent nociceptive stimuli (Dubner and Bennett 1983) with subsequent automatic nocireflexive changes and adaptations largely occurring without conscious awareness (Mitchell and Mitchell 1995). As not all signals from the peripheral nociceptors reach conscious pain, there is a wide variability in pain thresholds and perceived pain intensity, even with the same stimulus in the same person (Cervero 1991). Nonetheless, the barrage of nociceptive stimuli has significant physiological (nociflexive and nociautonomic) ramifications that are capable of manifesting centrally organized peripheral tissue texture abnormalities. At the spinal cord level, these segmental and suprasegmental circuits maintain muscle length and tone and guide reflexes. Ultimately, short-term and chronic alterations in sensory input to the CNS can result in enduring changes in central processing (Patterson and Steinmetz 1986) and recurrent somatic dysfunction (Kuchera 1995).

The physiological impact of somatic dysfunction is not limited to pain and peripheral palpatory changes. In addition to initiating protective reflexes and providing the CNS with warning signs, noxious somatic stimuli influence the release of extracellular messengers from the endocrine–immune axis (Figure 10.3) (Willard et al. 1997). Subsequent increased activity in the hypothalamic–pituitary–adrenal axis results in alteration of levels of adrenal cortical hormones, norepinephrine, and other modulators of homeostasis and immune function. This additional emphasis on the role of somatic dysfunction in disrupting and modulating homeostasis is a major consideration for physicians in neuromusculoskeletal medicine fields who choose to integrate osteopathic concepts.

After differential diagnostic concerns, the primary objective in applying the principles of neuromusculoskeletal medicine is to restore local tissue function while simultaneously promoting central integration of the resultant afferent stimuli from the region. This is intended to bring about optimal biomechanical alignment and function for the individual. Additional long-term objectives seek to optimize tissue level health and to identify and reduce sources of chronic nociception.

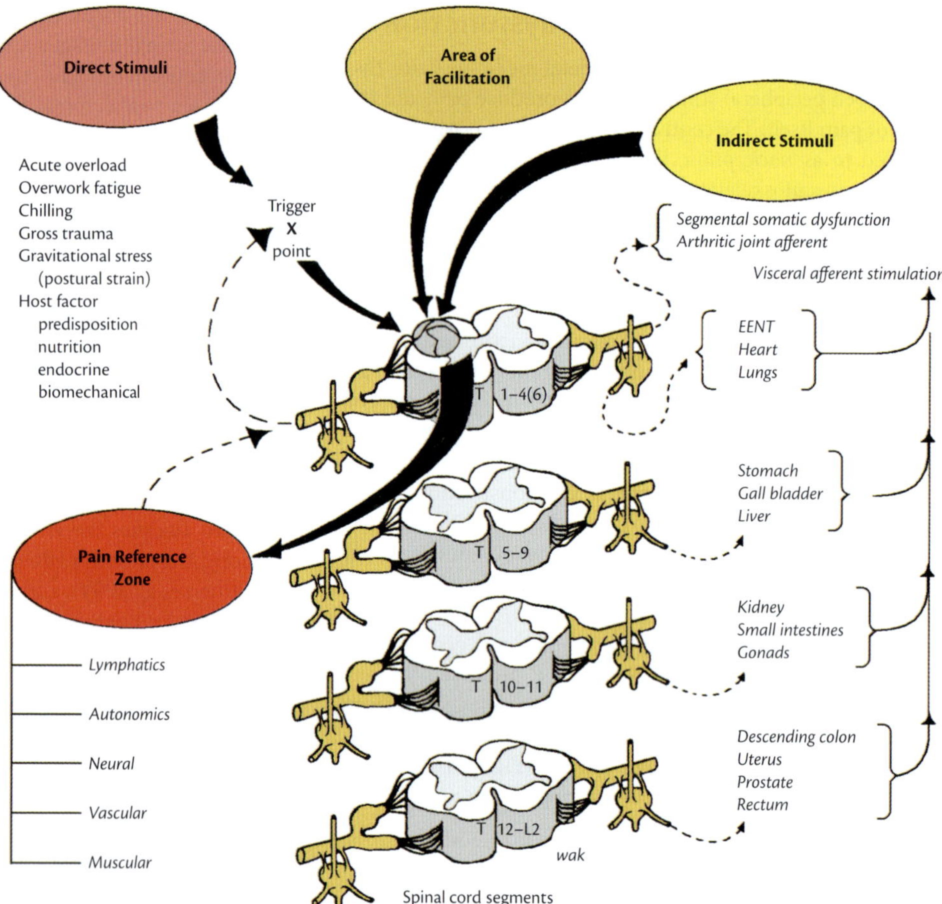

Figure 10.2 Pain reference regions for spinal pain afferent impulses. (Kuchera, M. L. Gravitational stress, musculoligamentous strain, and postural alignment. *Spine: State of the Art Reviews* 1995, 9(2), 463–90.)

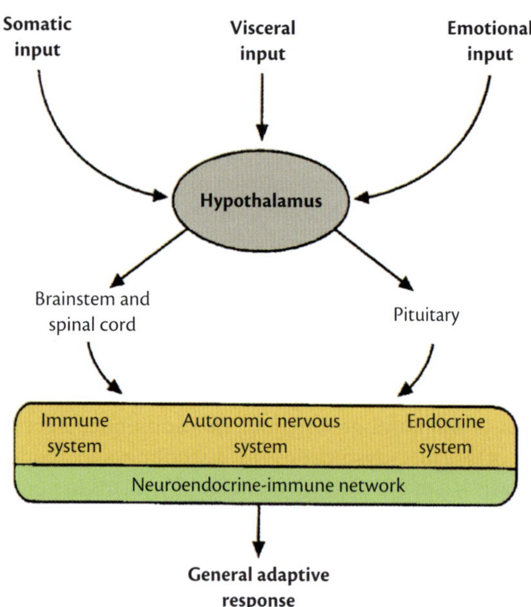

Figure 10.3 Response of neuroimmune network to signals emanating from somatic, visceral or emotional dysfunction. (Willard, F. H., Mokler, D. J., Morgane, P. J. Chapter 9. Neuroendocrine-immune system and homeostasis. In Ward, R. C. (ed.). *Foundations for osteopathic medicine* (1997). Williams & Wilkins, Baltimore, MD, pp. 107–35.)

Examination for and diagnosis of somatic dysfunction

Diagnostic testing for somatic dysfunction consists of simple, reproducible palpatory and provocative examinations. Developing the art of palpation is an asset for any physician, regardless of specialty, but is paramount for physicians specializing in the field of neuromusculoskeletal medicine. Diagnostic palpation is an acquired skill requiring time, patience, and practice. It may be defined as 'the application of variable manual pressure to the surface of the body for the purpose of determining the shape, size, consistency, position, inherent motility, and health of the tissues beneath' (Education Council on Osteopathic Principles 2011). The art of interpreting diagnostic palpation also requires an extensive knowledge base of normal anatomy and physiology, as well as recognition of host variability and pathophysiological connections and manifestations. Early palpatory evidence of underlying pathophysiological change requires a higher level of palpatory skill than that required in palpation of a frank pathological state such as a tumour (Mitchell 1976).

Diagnostic, time-efficient palpation for somatic dysfunction combines screening and scanning surveys of the entire body framework and those specific region(s) indicated by historical and physical findings or the need for a differential diagnosis. Focused layer palpation is then directed at any suspected or identified sites of significance. Rather than going into details about surveying and specific diagnostic palpatory examinations in this chapter, they will be described in other appropriate sections of this text including Chapter 27. The use of *layer palpation* to identify neuromusculoskeletal diagnostic clues in cutaneous, subcutaneous, fascial, muscular, ligamentous, bony, and arthrodial structures has a long history. This process begins with critical palpation of successively deeper body anatomical layers and the physiological interpretation of the findings.

In examining patient complaints, the sites and the scope of palpation are selected according to the physician's knowledge of pain and referred pain mechanisms, structural interconnectedness (including tensegrity—see Chapter 16), and the differential diagnosis that is progressively developed. At each of these sites, physicians trained in neuromusculoskeletal evaluation are initially guided by *S.T.A.R. findings* (see section 'Definition and underlying concepts of somatic dysfunction'). These findings can be interpreted as a diagnosis of local or regional 'somatic dysfunction' and may alert the astute clinician to also evaluate for the presence or absence of other underlying pathophysiological diagnoses within the neuromusculoskeletal and/or visceral systems.

Additional screening and specific tests are often suggested by initial palpatory examination findings. These additional tests should supplement evaluation of the functional ability of potential clinically significant somatic and visceral structures. Test choice should be consistent with accepted professional standards of care and with respect to the neuromusculoskeletal model selected. Deviation from normal structure and function at this level of palpatory evaluation warrants further evaluation of that structure or expanding testing to other related structures. Additional evaluations include neurological or orthopedic tests, or even laboratory, radiographic, and/or electrophysiological testing.

Integration of historical symptoms with the physical examination results in a presumptive diagnosis. The palpatory portion of the physical examination specifically augments differential diagnosis and provides data for guiding decisions regarding the indications, contraindications, and other factors for considering the medical, surgical, and/or manipulative prescription.

S.T.A.R. testing for somatic dysfunction

Sensory change

Sensory change, including neuraesthesia, paraesthesia, or anaesthesia, can be objectively elicited and evaluated in a number of ways. Subjective perception of tenderness, pain and other sensation should also be integrated with these findings. However, pain is a subjective symptom and its presence alone is not an indication of somatic dysfunction. Findings can be quantified in several manners, as can patterns of perceived sensory change and pain. These include progressive layer palpation and provocative testing to elicit pain or altered sensory change in a dermatomal pattern; pain or hyper-reactivity of muscles in isolation or in a myotomal pattern; and sclerotomal sensitivity elicited by applying pressure or stress over ligaments or bony sites. Sensitivity perceived as pain with 4 kg or less of pressure (quantified by the use of a 'dolorimeter') in certain sites (see Chapter 13), is defined by some and interpreted by others as consistent with a fibromyalgia picture (Wolfe et al. 1990).

Sensitivity may also be accompanied by a referred pattern of tenderness, pain or dysesthesia that matches a radicular, sclerotomal, neural, or trigger point pattern. Sensitivity accompanied by different types of tissue texture change is common in tender point systems (Jones et al. 1995; Owens 1963), trigger point diagnosis (Kuchera and McPartland 2002) (see Chapter 58), and other local and regional somatic dysfunction diagnoses. The trigger point pattern is especially likely if the point of sensitivity lies in a taut band that jumps with snapping palpation (Figure 10.4).

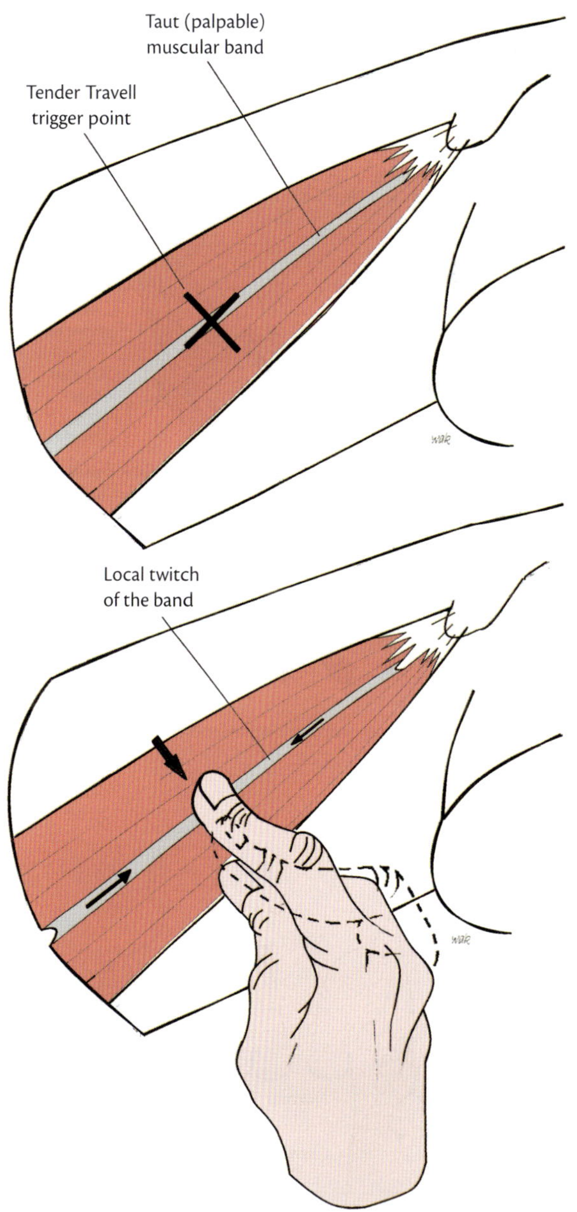

Figure 10.4 Trigger point palpation of local twitch response when manually provoking a local twitch response in a taut band harbouring a myofascial trigger point.

Tissue texture change

Tissue texture considerations include appreciation of moisture (cutaneous humidity), oiliness, dryness, heat or coolness, roughness, as well as the presence or absence of blemishes seen or noted with light palpation (Figure 10.5). Palpation of deeper layers may reveal changes described as subcutaneous swelling, oedema, emphysema, fibrosis, spasm, hypertonicity, flaccidity, atrophy, myofascial points, tumour, nodularity, etc.—each type of tissue texture change having its own different diagnostic consideration. The best way to assess pertinent tissue texture abnormality is by comparing adjacent tissues or the same tissues on the contralateral side. Furthermore, provocative tests for tissue texture change include skin stroking to observe variations in the red reflex (Figure 10.6) and skin rolling (Figure 10.7).

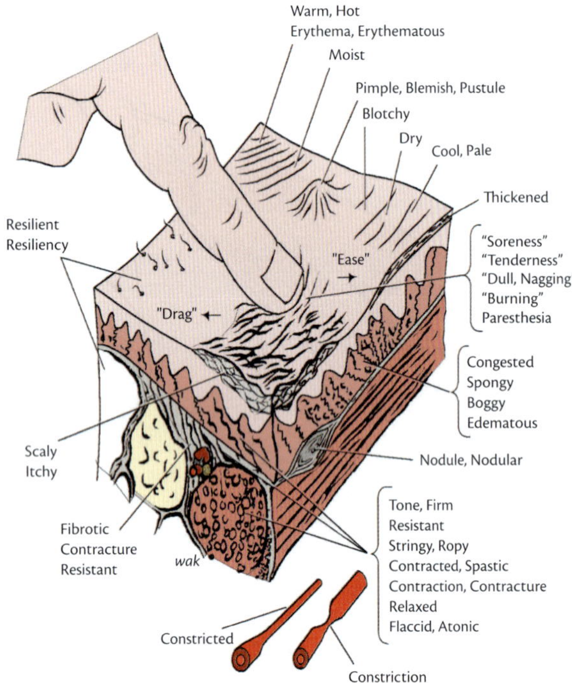

Figure 10.5 Information from palpation of skin and subcutaneous tissues.

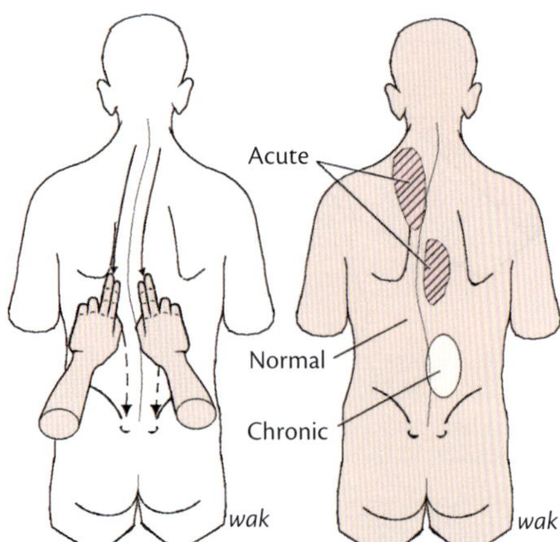

Figure 10.6 Red reflex. Prolonged reddening indicates acute physiology; rapid blanching indicates chronic physiology.

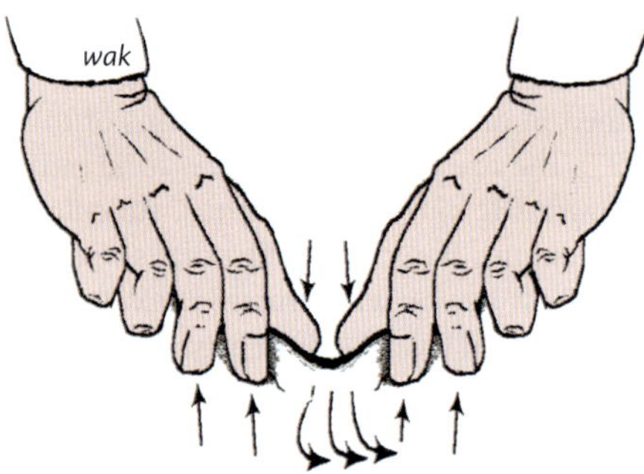

Figure 10.7 Skin rolling to assess for tissue texture abnormality.

Asymmetry

This alone is rarely sufficient for making a specific diagnosis of somatic dysfunction, because true perfect symmetry is rare in humans. Nonetheless, asymmetry of paired structures increases sensitivity for recognition of minor dysfunction or change. Asymmetry of bony landmarks (Figure 10.8) as a screening procedure often provides an early finding suggesting subsequent motion testing.

Restriction of motion

This may be assessed and described in many meaningful, albeit different, ways. The method selected to assess restricted motion and the number of directions tested depends on the structure studied, the patient's condition, and the model used by the examining physician. Restriction of motion can be grossly quantified by total range of motion in degrees (Table 10.1) and compared to established normal ranges or to a corresponding joint in the same individual. Gross motion asymmetry is more often associated with pathological, diseased, or orthopaedic problems in the joint. Somatic dysfunction usually manifests as asymmetry of the minor or gliding motions of the joint and can range from subtle to gross.

Most neuromusculoskeletal medicine physicians will also assess the quality of motion at the barrier to motion—this is called the '*end feel*'. The end feel of an anatomical, a physiological, a pathological, or a dysfunctional barrier (Figure 10.9) will have different palpatory characteristics, warranting different descriptors. Absence of any barrier may indicate pathological change of the restraining structures as occurs in a third-degree ligamentous tear; whereas an abrupt restriction without any normal physiological 'springiness' at the end of motion may indicate differential possibilities ranging from arthrodial somatic dysfunction to osteoarthritis.

Motion restriction in a single plane may be assessed, but combinations of motion restrictions often provide greater diagnostic insights. Combinations of barriers created by certain pathophysiological processes (such as inflammation) create '*capsular patterns*' of restricted motion that are unique to each joint (Table 10.2) (Cyriax and Cyriax 1993).

Both active and passive motion testing provide valuable information. As different anatomical and/or physiological components may be tested using these different methods, active and passive motion testing may provide different motion information in some joints (Figure 10.10). This is also the case in some joints when tested with postural load as opposed to a non-weightbearing supine or prone

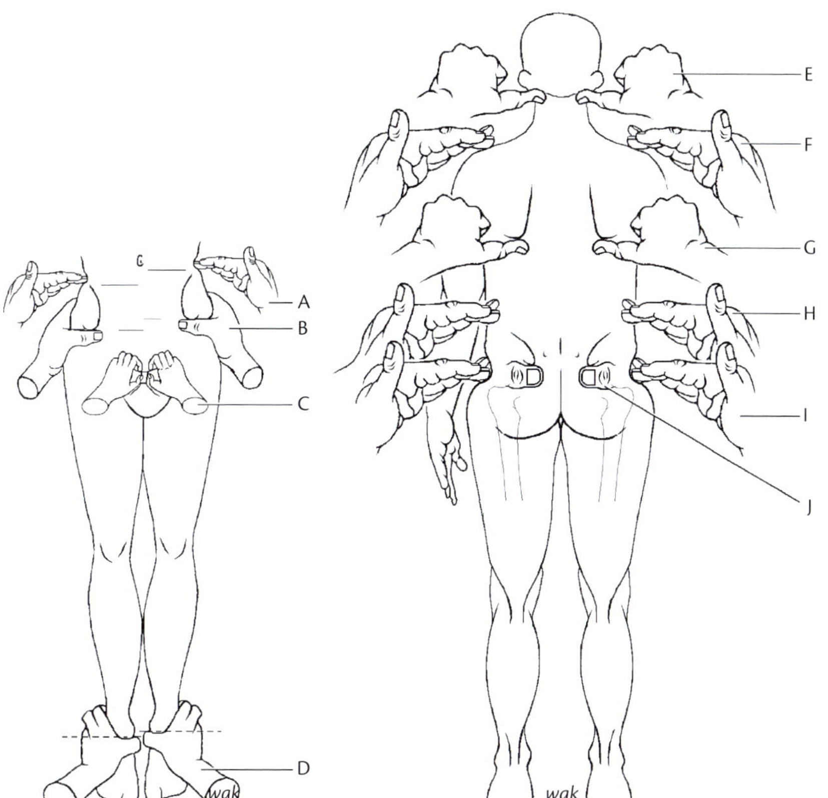

Figure 10.8 Anterior and posterior palpation of horizontal planes.
(A = iliac crests; B = anterior superior iliac spines; C = pubic rami; D= medial malleoli; E = mastoid processes; F = acromioclavicular joints; G = inferior scapular angles; H = iliac crests; I = greater trochanters; J = posterior superior iliac spines.)

position. For these reasons, if reproducibility is desired, it is best to describe the position and form of motion testing used. When the palpatory characteristics and tests used in identifying somatic dysfunction are delineated in this fashion and calibration-training sessions are conducted, reproducibility increases with kappa values (see Chapter 3) in the good to excellent range (Degenhardt et al. 2002a,b; Mense and Simons 2001; Sciotti et al. 2001).

Sensory changes, asymmetry, restricted motion, and tissue texture abnormalities are objective and reliable findings in manual medicine diagnostics. They reflect dysfunction in the anatomical–physiological axis and carry clinical relevance warranting further investigation and consideration of appropriate treatment. Neuromusculoskeletal medicine physicians therefore often use varying combinations of these characteristics to name and/or classify somatic dysfunction in their patient records or in the literature.

Anatomical and physiological classification systems in somatic dysfunction

Somatic dysfunction is often subdivided by its anatomical location (e.g. cervical, lumbosacral); by its physiological characteristics (e.g. acute, chronic); by the specific constellation or pattern of anatomical-physiological characteristics (e.g. chronic psoas syndrome, latent sternocleidomastoid myofascial trigger point); and/or by its order of onset (e.g. primary, secondary). Sometimes it is subdivided by its apparent reflex relationship (e.g. viscerosomatic, somatovisceral, or somatosomatic).

The most obvious system of classifying somatic dysfunction is by its anatomical location. This form of classification names the specific skeletal, arthrodial, or myofascial structure or region where the somatic dysfunction is located. Although simple in its naming, differential diagnosis for anatomically named dysfunction requires a thorough understanding of the functional characteristics and innervation of each of these skeletal, arthrodial, and myofascial structures. Joint inflammation and pathology produce different palpatory findings in different joints (see Table 10.2) and spinal physiological motion mechanics are different in different anatomical regions (Chapter 27).

Pain referral patterns are different for different muscles (Figure 10.11), for different ligaments (Figure 10.12), and for different spondylogenic/sclerotomal reflexes (Figure 10.13). In addition, each of these structures influences motion characteristics; often in a distinctive manner that provides palpatory clues to the source of dysfunction. Somatic dysfunction associated with various regional disorders and their management is subdivided in this manner and presented in Chapters 27 and 50.

Anatomical classification delineating positional and motion aspects may also be used in describing somatic dysfunction. According to the 'Glossary of osteopathic terminology' (Education Council on Osteopathic Principles 2011), the positional and motion aspects of somatic dysfunction are best described using at least one of three parameters:

- position of the body part as determined by palpation and referenced to its adjacent defined structure
- directions in which motions are freer
- directions in which motions are restricted.

Table 10.1 Spinal gross and vertebral unit motion

Craniocervical junction/superior cervical segment

***Physiologic motion*: OA SxRy regardless of sagittal plane; AA limited to discussion of Rx or Ry**

Vertebral unit	Flexion/extension	Sidebending	Rotation
C0 (OA)	10°Flex and 25° extension	3–8° left and 3–8° right	4–6° left and 4–6° right
C1 (AA)	10° total but not typically involved in somatic dysfunction	0–4° but not typically involved in somatic dysfunction	25° left and 25° right

Typical cervical spine

Minimal norms for C0–C7: flexion (60°), extension (75°), SB (45° ea), rotation (80° ea)

Physiologic motion: RxSx regardless of sagittal plane

Vertebral unit	Flexion/Extension		Sidebending		Rotation	
	Range	**Mean**	**Range**	**Mean**	**Range**	**Mean**
C2	5–23	8	11–20	10	6–28	9
C3	7–38	13	9–15	11	10–28	11
C4	8–39	12	0–16	11	10–26	12
C5	3–34	17	0–16	8	8–34	10
C6	1–29	16	0–17	7	6–15	9
C7	4–17	9	0–17	4	5–13	8

Thoracic spine

Minimum norms: flexion (50°), rotation (30° ea)

Physiologic motion: Type I = SxRy with neutral sagittal; Type II = RxSx in extremes of F or E

Vertebral unit	Flexion/extension		Sidebending		Rotation	
	Range	**Mean**	**Range**	**Mean**	**Range**	**Mean**
T1	3–5	4	5	6	5–14	9
T2	3–5	4	5–7	6	4–12	8
T3	2–5	4	3–7	6	5–11	8
T4	2–5	4	5–6	6	4–11	8
T5	3–5	4	5–6	6	5–11	8
T6	2–7	5	6	6	4–11	8
T7	3–8	6	3–8	6	4–11	8
T8	3–8	6	4–7	6	6–7	7
T9	3–8	6	4–7	6	3–5	4
T10	4–14	9	3–10	7	2–3	2
T11	6–20	12	4–13	9	2–3	2
T12	6–20	12	5–10	8	2–3	2

Lumbar spine

Minimum norms: flexion (60°), extension (25°); SB (25° ea)

Physiologic motion: Type I = SxRy within neutral sagittal; Type II = RxSx in extremes of F or E

Vertebral unit	Flexion/extension		Sidebending		Rotation	
	Range	**Mean**	**Range**	**Mean**	**Range**	**Mean**
L1	9–16	12	3–9	6	1–3	2
L2	11–18	14	3–9	6	1–3	2
L3	12–18	15	5–10	8	1–3	2
L4	14–21	17	5–7	6	1–3	2
L5	18–22	20	2–3	3	3–6	5

(Source: AMA 1990; White and Panjabi 1978)

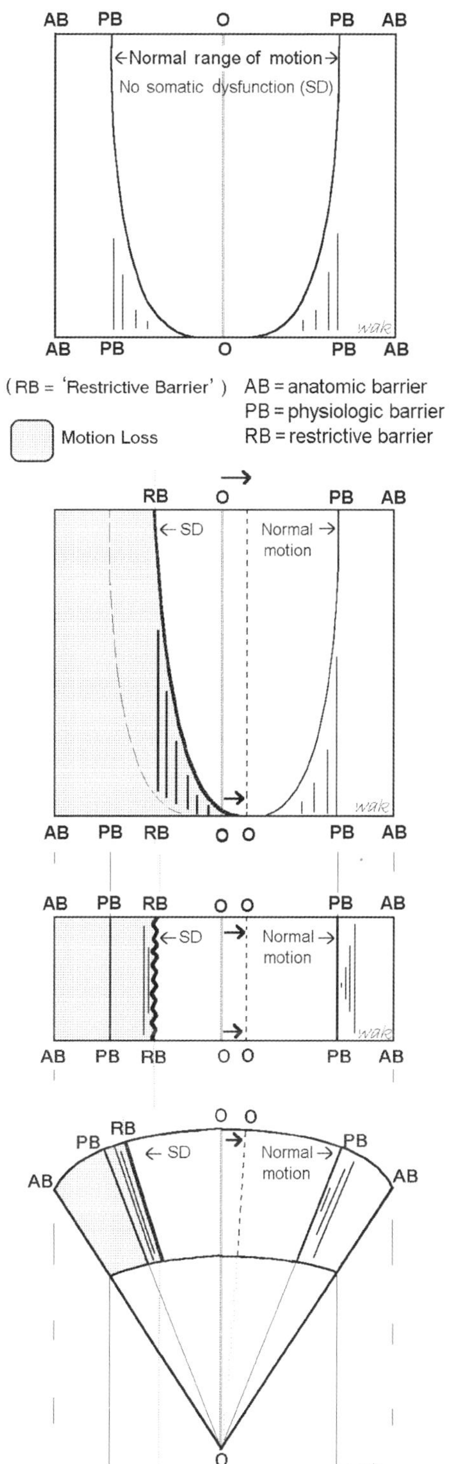

Figure 10.9 Concepts of joint motion in a single plane: end-feel of motion in a normal joint and a joint with somatic dysfunction.

This latter form of classification provides sufficient structure-function descriptors as are needed to formulate specific manual treatments to correct the specific somatic dysfunction named. For example, somatic dysfunction in which the fifth thoracic vertebra permits freer motion towards extension, rotation, and sidebending to the right on the sixth thoracic vertebra could be represented by the standard formula for motion present as T5 ERRSR. This formula could be used to set up indirect method manual treatment—for example, stacking the joint in the direction it prefers to a point of ligamentous balance (Speece et al. 2001). This nomenclature for somatic dysfunction also denotes that the T5 vertebra on T6 is *restricted* in flexion, rotating left and sidebending left. In the Mitchell muscle energy system (Mitchell 1999), T5 ERRSR might be reversed with a direct method manipulative technique designed to create sidebending and rotation to the left along with flexion, thereby re-establishing the lost or restricted motion characteristics. For this same somatic dysfunction, the Maigne star diagram records motion freedom and restriction as shown in Figure 10.14. In Maigne's system, the directions in which the motion is freer are combined with patient subjective responses to constitute his therapeutic 'rule of no pain and free movement' (Maigne and Liberson 1972).

Clinically relevant classification systems should also assist in making diagnostic and/or management choices. Keeping this perspective in mind, underlying physiological characteristics, reflected by tissue texture abnormalities, contribute to an especially valuable system of classification. Tissue texture abnormalities are defined as 'palpable changes in tissues from skin to periarticular structures that represent any combination of the following signs: vasodilation, edema, flaccidity, hypertonicity, contracture, fibrosis; and the following symptoms: itching, pain, tenderness' (Education Council on Osteopathic Principles 2011). Thoroughly understanding the pathophysiological mechanisms associated with each tissue texture abnormality leads to a physiological classification of somatic dysfunction as 'acute' or 'chronic'.

Understanding the different conditions in which somatic dysfunction is acute or chronic is vital to selecting effective treatment strategies ranging from the choice of medication to the choice of a manipulative activating force. Specific acute and chronic characteristics used in the physiological classification of somatic dysfunction appear in Table 10.3 (Kuchera and Kuchera 1994a). Management strategies based on this classification system may be found in Chapter 50.

Yet another classification system used for somatic dysfunction integrates constellations of signs and symptoms recognized as common patterns of dysfunction seen in clinical practice. With time, every practitioner of neuromusculoskeletal medicine will come to recognize common, recurrent patterns that, in turn, increase the efficacy and efficiency of patient management. The most commonly seen and clinically significant group patterns are designated by syndrome names. Such inter- and intraprofessional classifications permit common combinations of signs and symptoms to be discussed quickly and conveniently. In neuromusculoskeletal medicine, common examples include tennis elbow syndrome (Simons et al. 1999b), psoas syndrome (Kappler 1973), theatre (cocktail party) syndrome (Dorman and Ravin 1991), spondylogenic (non-radicular) syndrome (Dvorak et al. 1984), lower or upper crossed syndrome, and other clinical conditions that will be individually addressed as examples throughout this text.

Finally, it should be stated that systems of classification are often mixed as in discussing the 'acute, viscerosomatic L2 FRLSL' vertebral unit somatic dysfunction typically found as part of a 'left psoas syndrome' that is secondary to a left ureteral calculus.

Table 10.2 Somatic dysfunction vs pathology: comparison of palpatory patterns in selected joints (somatic dysfunction vs capsular pattern)

Joint(s)	Somatic dysfunctional pattern	Capsular (pathologic) pattern
Cervical spine (C2–C7)	Sidebending–rotation limitation to same side; free in opposite directions	Flexion usually spared: equal limitation in all other directions
Thoracic spine	Limitation in one direction, freedom in opposite direction (3 planes linked)	Limitation of extension, sidebending and rotation; less limitation of flexion
Lumbar spine	Limitation in one direction, freedom in opposite direction (3 planes linked)	Marked and equal limitation of sidebending; limitation of flexion–extension
Shoulder	Minor motions limited before major motions; minor motions affect quality of major motions; in each pattern of motion, one direction is limited while the opposite direction shows complete freedom of motion	Great limitation of abduction > external rotation limitation > internal rotation limitation
Elbow	Same description as shoulder	Flexion limitation > extension limitation (rotations full and painless except in advanced cases)
Wrist	Same description as shoulder	Flexion limitation = extension limitation; others minimal restriction
Hip	Same description as shoulder	Marked flexion and internal rotation limitations; typically spares adduction and external rotation
Knee	Same description as shoulder	Flexion markedly limited >> extension limitation
Ankle	Same description as shoulder	Plantar flexion limitation >> dorsiflexion limitation
Talocalcaneal joint	Same description as shoulder	Varus limitation progresses until fixation in valgus position
Big toe (1st MTP)	Same description as shoulder	Extension markedly limited >> Flexion limitation

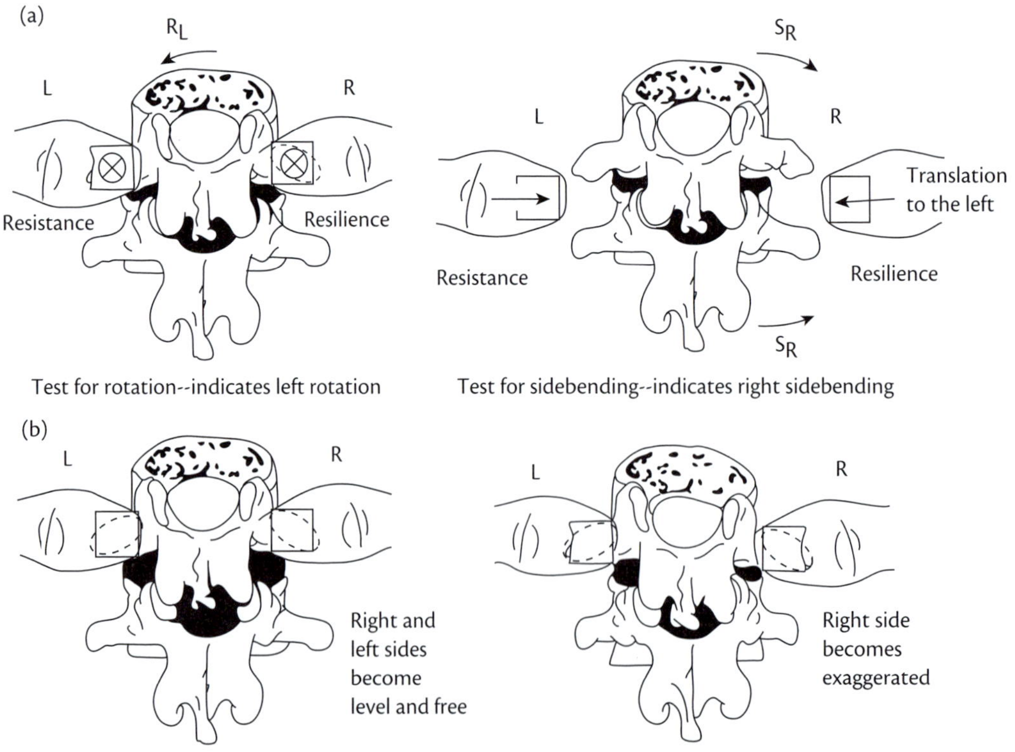

Figure 10.10 Motion testing: (a) passive motion indicates vertebral unit RLSR; (b) active motion indicates FRRSR. (From Kuchera 1995)

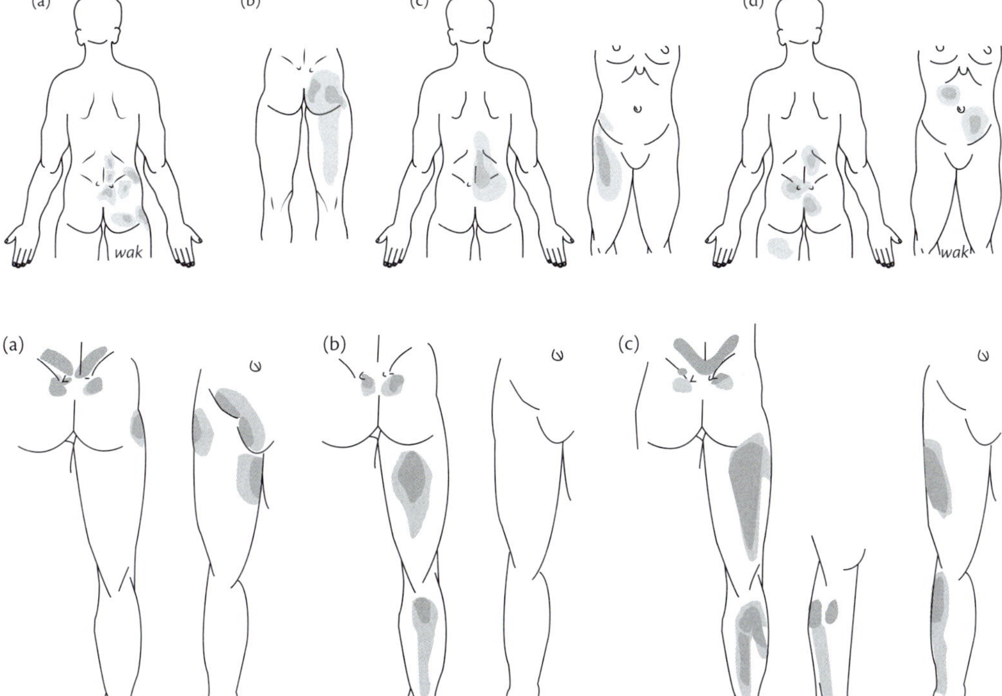

Figure 10.11 Pain referral regions of muscles: (a) quadratus lumborum; (b) piriformis; (c) iliopsoas; (d) rotatores and multifidi muscles.

Figure 10.12 Pain referral regions of ligaments: (a) iliolumbar ligament; (b) sacrospinous and sacrotuberous ligaments; (c) posterior sacroiliac ligament.

Recording severity and significance in somatic dysfunction

Individual S.T.A.R. components can be quantified and recorded. For example, sensory characteristics can be objectively quantified by measuring the amount of pressure needed to elicit pain (using a dolorimeter) or by measuring the distance between stimuli as in a two-point discrimination. These measurements can then be respectively expressed in kilograms or millimetres or clinically interpreted relative to established normative data. In like manner, tissue texture abnormalities, asymmetries, and restriction in motion can also be individually qualified. Each S.T.A.R. component can be numerically scaled and expressed as a number or informally designated as mild, moderate, or severe. Common scales used by musculoskeletal practitioners may combine component evaluations, as in the Krauss-Weber grading of flexibility, strength, and endurance (Table 10.4).

It is also possible to differentiate and record variable grades of severity with respect to somatic dysfunction itself. This is valuable in separating background levels of somatic dysfunction from significant 'key' dysfunction. It is also vital in following treatment outcomes in which somatic dysfunction is specifically or reflexly treated.

Simple method of recording severity using S.T.A.R. characteristics

A simple system using S.T.A.R. characteristics and recording severity from 0 to 3 was defined by the ECOP and adopted as a standard by the Bureau on Health Care Facilities Accreditation of the American Osteopathic Association (AOA) (Figure 10.15 and Table 10.5). The scale shown in Table 10.5 has been adopted by the osteopathic profession in the USA for recording somatic dysfunction severity. As part of their admitting history and physical examination, every patient admitted by a Doctor of Osteopathy (DO) into an AOA-accredited hospital in the USA is required to have an osteopathic musculoskeletal structural examination recorded in the fashion shown in Figure 10.15 or in a specified narrative form.

Background levels of somatic dysfunction exist in almost every individual. Its presence is universal, resulting in few subjects totally free of minimal dysfunction in all anatomical regions. This 'background' level is rarely of clinical significance and is recorded with a '0' on this 0–3 scale, as is the absence of somatic dysfunction. A severity of '1' indicates 'minimal' somatic dysfunction with minor (S.T.A.R.) palpatory findings. At the other end of the scale, a highly significant somatic dysfunction representing extensive and impressive (S.T.A.R.) characteristics, especially involving tissue texture abnormalities and restriction of motion, would be designated 'severe' and documented as a '3'. Severe somatic dysfunction is typically significant and/or symptomatic. The remaining designation of '2' would be more than 'minimal' but less than 'severe'. Typically, clinically relevant, moderate (level 2) somatic dysfunction may or may not be symptomatic.

Primary versus secondary somatic dysfunction

Somatic dysfunction is interpreted and managed consistent with its origin and maintaining factors. If somatic dysfunction originated from direct tissue injury or a somatic stressor, palpable S.T.A.R. characteristics would be consistent with a diagnostic classification of **primary somatic dysfunction**. Somatic dysfunction arising from

Figure 10.13 Sclerotome pain regions.

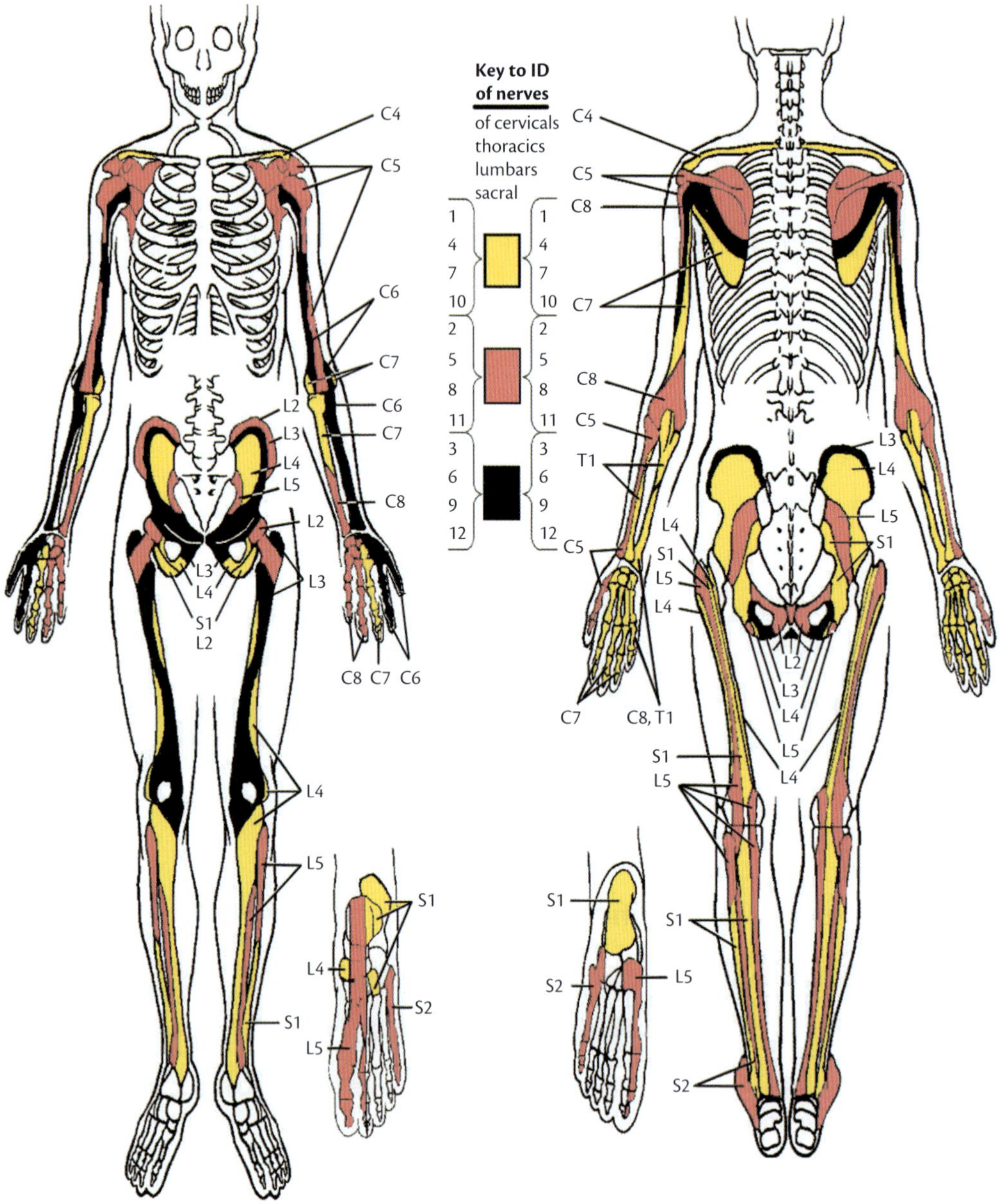

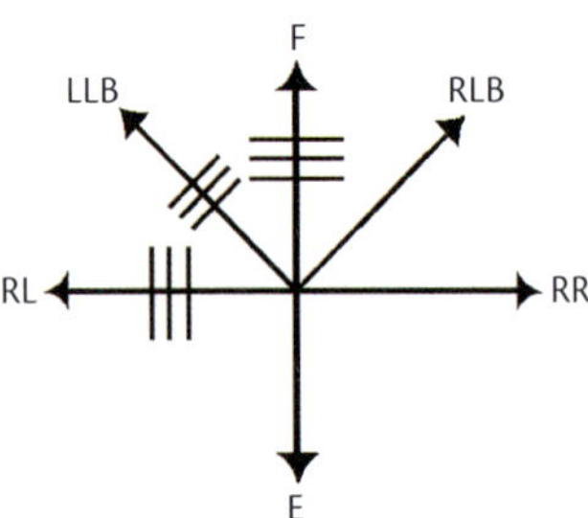

Figure 10.14 Star diagram of Maigne, illustrating the direction in which the patient feels pain. The bars indicate the grade of pain: three bars indicate significant pain, which will correlate with direction of restricted motion. In Maigne's system, manipulation should be considered only when three directions are free of pain when motion is introduced. Somatic dysfunction diagnosis: $E\ R_R S_R$.
(Key: F, flexion; E, extension; RL, rotate left; RR, rotate right; LLB, left lateral bend; RLB, right lateral bend.)

a viscerosomatic or somatosomatic reflex may be classified **secondary somatic dysfunction**. These classifications are parallel to Travell and Simons' classification of trigger points (primary dysfunction) arising from direct somatic stress including trauma, overuse, and chilling and those myofascial points that arise secondary to cardiac, gallbladder, or other visceral indirect stimulus.

Several mechanisms have been proposed and/or documented to explain various aspects of the tissue texture abnormalities and other somatic, visceral, vascular, lymphatic, immune, and neural responses seen in primary and secondary somatic dysfunction (Dvorak et al 1984; Greenman 1984; Korr 1978; Patterson and Howell 1989). Nociceptive levels of somatic dysfunction, especially in severe somatic dysfunction, create segmental spinal facilitation and significant peripheral pathophysiological change (van Buskirk 1990; Willard and Patterson 1991) resulting in significant tissue texture abnormalities. Similarly, many primary visceral afferent fibres affecting the spinal cord have the characteristics of nociceptive fibres. They

Table 10.3 Physiological classification of acute and chronic somatic dysfunction

Acute		Chronic
History	Recent, often an injury	Long-standing
Pain descriptors	Acute, severe, cutting, sharp	Dull, achy; paresthesias (crawling, itching, burning, gnawing)
Vascular	Vessels injured, release of endogenous peptides = chemical vasodilation, inflammation	Vessels constricted because of increased sympathetic tone
Skin	Warm, moist, red, inflamed (via vascular and chemical changes)	Cool, pale (via chronic sympathetic vascular tone increase)
Sympathetics	Systemically increased sympathetic activity contributes some local vasoconstriction (but local effect overpowered by bradykinins resulting in overall local vasodilation due to chemical effect)	Has vasoconstriction due to hypersympathetic tone; regional sympathetic hyperactivity,; systemic sympathetic tone may be reduced towards normal
Musculature	Local increase in muscle tone, muscle contraction, hypertonicity and reactivity, increased tone of the muscle spindle	Decreased muscle tone, flaccid, mushy, limited range of motion because of contracture
Mobility	Range often normal, quality is sluggish	Limited range, with normal quality in the motion that remains
Tissues	Boggy oedema, acute congestion, fluids from vessels and from chemical reactions in tissues	Chronic congestion, doughy, stringy, fibrotic, ropy, thickened, increased resistance, contracted, contractures
Adnexa	Moist skin, no trophic changes	Pimples, scaly, dry, folliculitis, pigmentation (trophic changes)
Visceral	Minimal somatovisceral effects	Somatovisceral effects are common

Source: Kuchera, W. A., Kuchera, M. L. ***Osteopathic principles in practice***, 2nd edn. Greyden Press, Columbus, Ohio, 1994, p. 25

Table 10.4 Modified Krauss-Weber muscle testing

Muscles tested	Patient position	Physician action	Instructions	Interpretation
Test 1: Strength Upper abdominal muscles with psoas action	Supine – hands folded across chest and legs fully extended	At foot of table holding patient feet down	'Curl your head and body off the table.'	Success –30° plus = upper abdominal muscles adequate. 60° to upright = psoas adequate
Test 2: Strength Abdominal muscles without psoas action	Supine – hands folded across chest. Flexed hips and knees; feet flat on the table	At foot of table holding patient feet down	'Curl your body up to the sitting position.'	1. unable – poor muscle strength 2. able with effort – moderate strength 3. without difficulty – strong
Test 3: Strength Lower abdominal muscles	Supine – hands behind the neck and both legs extended	At head of table holding patient shoulders to the table. (Count the 10 seconds during patient effort)	'With your legs straight, lift your feet 10 inches off the table and hold them there for 10 seconds.'	1. unable – poor muscle strength 2. able with effort – moderate strength 3. without difficulty – strong
Test 4: Strength Upper back muscles	Prone – pillow under the abdomen. Legs fully extended: hands clasped behind back.	At foot of the table holding patient hips and legs down. (Count the 10 seconds during patient effort)	'Raise your chest and abdomen off the table and hold that position for 10 seconds.'	1. unable – poor muscle strength 2. able with effort – moderate strength 3. without difficulty – strong
Test 5: Strength Lower back muscles	Prone – pillow under the abdomen. Legs fully extended; hands clasped behind neck	At head of the table holding patient hips and legs down. (Count the 10 seconds during patient effort)	'Without bending your knees, lift both legs off the table and hold that position for 10 seconds'	1. unable – poor muscle strength 2. able with effort – moderate strength 3. without difficulty – strong
Test 6: Strength Spinal flexion and hamstring extensibility	Standing completely upright with feet together and hands to the sides	Stand by the patient and measure distance of patient's fingertips to the floor	'Without bending your knees, bend forward and try to touch the floor.'	<45° = stiff spine. Not to floor = poor hamstring extensibility. Touches floor = good spinal flexion and good hamstring extensibility.
Test 7: Strength Ham-string extensibility	Supine with legs fully extended	Stand by the patient on the side that is to be tested	'Do not use your muscles. Let me raise your legs without your help.'	<60° = loss of hamstring extensibility 80–90° = good extensibility of gluteus maximus >90° = good erector spinae mass extensibility

Source: DiGiovanna, E. L., Schiowitz, S., Dowling, D. *An osteopathic approach to diagnosis and treatment*, 2nd edn. Lippincott-Raven, Philadelphia, 1997, pp. 96–8.

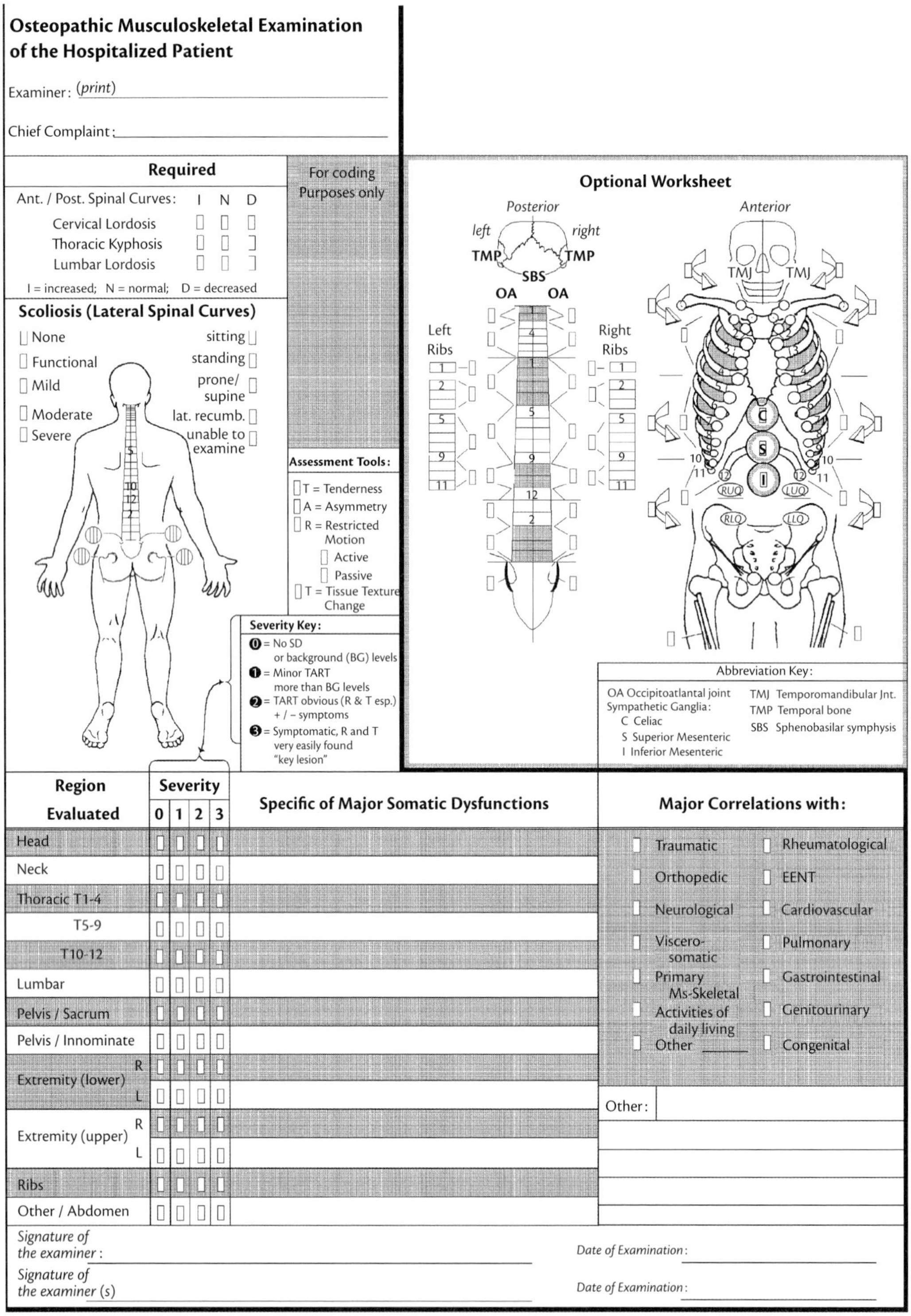

Osteopathic Musculoskeletal Examination of the Hospitalized Patient

Examiner: (print) ______

Chief Complaint: ______

Required | For coding Purposes only

Ant. / Post. Spinal Curves: I N D

	I	N	D
Cervical Lordosis	☐	☐	☐
Thoracic Kyphosis	☐	☐	☐
Lumbar Lordosis	☐	☐	☐

I = increased; N = normal; D = decreased

Scoliosis (Lateral Spinal Curves)

☐ None
☐ Functional
☐ Mild
☐ Moderate
☐ Severe

sitting ☐
standing ☐
prone/supine ☐
lat. recumb. ☐
unable to examine ☐

Assessment Tools:

☐ T = Tenderness
☐ A = Asymmetry
☐ R = Restricted Motion
☐ Active
☐ Passive
☐ T = Tissue Texture Change

Severity Key:

⓿ = No SD or background (BG) levels
❶ = Minor TART more than BG levels
❷ = TART obvious (R & T esp.) + / − symptoms
❸ = Symptomatic, R and T very easily found "key lesion"

Optional Worksheet

Abbreviation Key:

OA Occipitoatlantal joint
Sympathetic Ganglia:
C Celiac
S Superior Mesenteric
I Inferior Mesenteric
TMJ Temporomandibular Jnt.
TMP Temporal bone
SBS Sphenobasilar symphysis

Region Evaluated	Severity 0	1	2	3	Specific of Major Somatic Dysfunctions
Head	☐	☐	☐	☐	
Neck	☐	☐	☐	☐	
Thoracic T1-4	☐	☐	☐	☐	
T5-9	☐	☐	☐	☐	
T10-12	☐	☐	☐	☐	
Lumbar	☐	☐	☐	☐	
Pelvis / Sacrum	☐	☐	☐	☐	
Pelvis / Innominate	☐	☐	☐	☐	
Extremity (lower) R	☐	☐	☐	☐	
Extremity (lower) L	☐	☐	☐	☐	
Extremity (upper) R	☐	☐	☐	☐	
Extremity (upper) L	☐	☐	☐	☐	
Ribs	☐	☐	☐	☐	
Other / Abdomen	☐	☐	☐	☐	

Major Correlations with:

☐ Traumatic	☐ Rheumatological
☐ Orthopedic	☐ EENT
☐ Neurological	☐ Cardiovascular
☐ Viscero-somatic	☐ Pulmonary
☐ Primary Ms-Skeletal	☐ Gastrointestinal
☐ Activities of daily living	☐ Genitourinary
☐ Other ______	☐ Congenital

Other:

Signature of the examiner: ______ *Date of Examination:* ______

Signature of the examiner (s) ______ *Date of Examination:* ______

Figure 10.15 Chart for recording musculoskeletal examination of a hospitalized patient.
(Kuchera, M. L., Kuchera, W.A. (1998) *Osteopathic muscoskeletal examination of the hospitalised patient.* American Osteopathic Association)

Table 10.5 Standardized severity rating for somatic dysfunction

S.T.A.R.		Severity scale	
S	Sensitivity of tissue – i.e. tenderness	0	No SD; or only background level changes
T	Tissue texture changes	1	Minor S.TA.R.; more than background levels
A	Asymmetry	2	S.T.A.R. is obvious (esp. R and T); ± symptoms
R	Restriction of motion	3	Symptomatic; R and T very easily found; this is the 'key lesion'

Source: Kuchera, M. L., Kuchera, W. A. Osteopathic musculoskeletal examination of the hospitalised patient. American Osteopathic Association, 1998.

produce neuropeptides such as substance P and calcitonin gene-related polypeptide and respond to nociceptive stimuli. Some are even capable of eliciting a neurogenic inflammatory response in the surrounding tissue (Dockray and Sharkey 1986; Gilliar et al. 1996). Thus, both somatic and visceral conditions are capable of creating musculoskeletal clues palpable as somatic dysfunction.

Again, primary somatic dysfunction typically responds well to the various management strategies discussed in this text (Part 4) (Chila 2011; Schott 1994) whereas secondary somatic dysfunction responds variably and often recurs (Kuchera and Kuchera 1994b; Simons et al. 1999a) when addressed by these approaches alone.

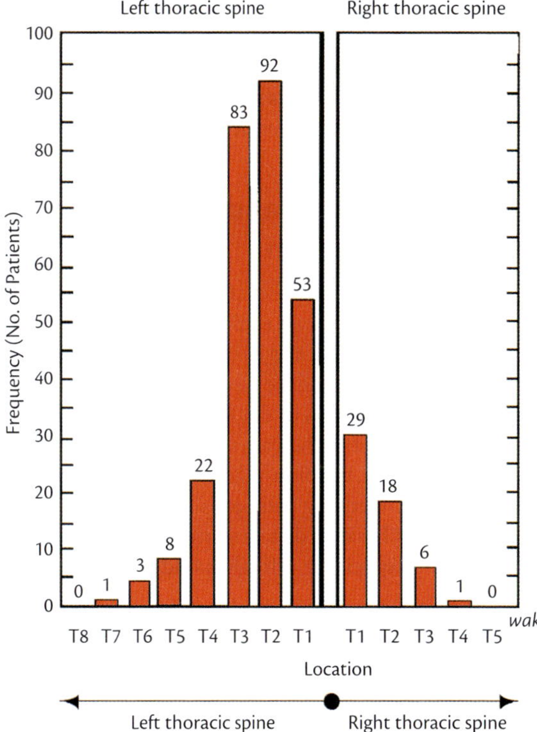

Figure 10.16 Spinal referral pattern for cardiac disorders (n = 94) that correlates well with angiography.
(Kuchera, M.L., Kuchera W.A. *Ostepathic considerations in systematic dysfunction*, 2nd edn, revised (1994) Greyden Press, Dayton, OH.)

Significance of somatic dysfunction in health and 'dis-ease'

Failure to consider somatic dysfunction limits the differential diagnosis and overlooks an important underlying pathophysiological process that may limit optimum health and performance or play a role in patient complaints. The presence of moderate to severe somatic dysfunction in particular spinal patterns correlates with, and thereby augments, the differential diagnosis of a wide range of visceral conditions (Beal 1985; Kuchera and Kuchera 1994b; Smith 1961; Steele 1997). Indeed, irritation of upper thoracic spinal joint receptors simultaneously evokes numerous reflex alterations, including para-vertebral muscle spasm and alterations in endocrine, respiratory, and cardiovascular functions (Wyke 1970).

The cardiovascular system is perhaps the most documented system in which the clinical recognition of somatic dysfunction in health and 'dis-ease' has been demonstrated. Specific palpatory findings of upper thoracic somatic dysfunction (especially affecting left upper thoracic paraspinal tissues) were reported in the *British Medical Journal* as being consistently found in myocardial infarction (Nicholas et al. 1985). Beal (1985) reported 79% specificity of thoracic palpatory findings compared to angiography in coronary artery patients (Figure 10.16). Similarly, Travell and Simons report the palpatory finding of trigger points in the pectoralis major muscles in 61% of 72 patients with cardiac disease (Simons et al. 1999c). These palpatory findings of somatic dysfunction have a completely different pattern than secondary somatic dysfunction associated with patients with gastrointestinal problems (Beal 1985) (Figure 10.16).

Conversely, evidence of somatovisceral reflexes is cited by Travell and Simons. Removal of primary myofascial somatic dysfunction in the pectoralis major muscle on the right, in patients with some forms of supraventricular tachyarrhythmia, 'promptly restores normal sinus rhythm . . . and also can eliminate recurrences of the paroxysmal arrhythmia . . . for a long period of time' (Simons et al. 1999c). Other somatovisceral reflexes are implicated in functional gastrointestinal disorders and from systemic symptoms ranging from asthma to duodenal ulcers to dysmenorrhoea.

In response to a variety of stimuli, homeostatic functions are defensively altered through a series of complex feedback loops that monitor conditions in the peripheral tissues and make local and systemic adjustments as needed. Excessive driving stimuli or dysfunction of the feedback circuits themselves results in decreased compensatory reserve, 'dis-ease', and increased susceptibility to disease. The three primary driving stimuli (stressors) initiating the cascade of chemical messengers first described in Selye's general adaptive response are emotional, somatic, and visceral dysfunction (Willard 1995). These and other stressors create an allostatic load capable of disturbing the individual's normal homeostatic set point (McEwen 1998; Seeman et al. 1997; Sterling and Eyer 1988). Their role and the role that somatic dysfunction specifically plays in disturbing homeostasis through reflex (Denslow 1975) and neuroendocrine-immune (Willard et al. 1997) responses to the inflammation, oedema, and nociceptive biochemical mediators of somatic dysfunction (Willard and Patterson 1991) have been extensively documented and elegantly discussed (Peterson 1979; Willard et al 1997).

Neuromusculoskeletal medicine physicians are capable of assisting the body in maintaining homeostasis by recognizing and modifying any or all of the driving stimuli (stressors). Thus, the education of these practitioners now emphasizes the importance of integrating biopsychosocial, anatomical, and pathophysiological models (ECOP 1999; IFMM 1999). Previously challenged by some musculoskeletal practitioners (Cyriax and Russell 1980), this aspect of neuromusculoskeletal care has most widely been championed by osteopathic physicians of the American school.

Somatic dysfunction and the manual medicine prescription

A knowledgeable physician capable of fully assessing risk:benefit ratios and cost effectiveness is best equipped to direct a manual medicine prescription, if indicated, and its implementation. This is also extremely important for selecting the type of manual method, activating force, frequency, and duration of this form of treatment and its place in the total management of the patient. Individual characteristics of the somatic dysfunction, the biopsychosocial aspects of the patient as a whole, any other underlying pathophysiological processes, and the skills of the treating physician dictate many of these choices. The neuromusculoskeletal physician specifically ponders the following:

- *Goal*: What area or physiological process would benefit from a manual medicine approach? Is there an acceptable risk-to-benefit ratio to consider such an approach?
- *Method*: What forms or techniques of manual medicine are indicated and contraindicated?
- *Dose*: What are the underlying homeostatic reserves of the patient and what duration of treatment administration would provide maximal benefit?
- *Frequency*: How frequently should the manipulation be repeated within the parameters of patient response and cost efficacy?

The manual medicine prescription (Kimberly 1992) takes form after appropriate evaluation and establishment of a working diagnosis by a knowledgeable and skilled physician who then seeks to accomplish a definable therapeutic goal. As with most prescriptive care, in subsequent visits, the patient is re-assessed for symptomatic and physiological change, including a re-examination for somatic dysfunction, before making a decision to re-initiate any subsequent manipulative treatment. Clinical outcomes, patient response to the previous treatment, and visit-specific findings of somatic dysfunction influence the goals, methods, and dose used in follow-up visits and to adjust manipulative frequency decisions.

Limiting factors (Kuchera and Kuchera 1994c) considered in the formulation of a manual medicine prescription and its delivery include:

- *Patient-centred factors* including the knowledge or concern of the patient's ability to respond because of age, sex, size, occupation, dietary or life-activity risk factors, allostatic load (including biopsychosocial stressors), support system, allergies to potential treatment alternatives, and response to similar treatments or modalities given in the past.
- *Disease-centred factors* especially those accompanied by osteoporotic, rheumatological, orthopaedic, neurological, cardiovascular, or oncological change. Even without specific diagnosis, signs or symptoms of other acute or chronic pathophysiological processes affecting the neuromusculoskeletal or related systems must be considered. These conditions often dictate treatment position, the manual medicine method or activation employed, and treatment duration and frequency.
- *Physician-centred factors* including the ability of the physician to accomplish the treatment or to appropriately refer the patient for that form of care. Other factors might include personal stature, training, specialization background, licence limitations, and ability to maintain advances made in the manual medicine field through continuing medical education.

For these reasons, the International Federation of Manual/ Musculoskeletal Medicine (IFMM) and the AOA advocate that only practitioners fully trained in all diagnostic and therapeutic modalities have the total perspective required to make proper manual medicine management decisions in neuromusculoskeletal medicine fields. These management decisions require weighing relative risk-to-benefit ratios as well as the choice and frequency of technique, duration of care, and its potential for integration with other modalities. In workers compensation cases in the USA, physician-level education with core manual medicine training appears to be more cost-effective than management by those employing manual approaches without physician training or physician training without core training in palpatory diagnosis and manual techniques (Figure 10.17) (FCER 1988).

While fully licensed physicians with additional training in the skills of manual medicine diagnosis and treatment are arguably better equipped to take responsibility for the formulation and delivery of the manual medicine prescription, other healthcare providers must continue to be involved. Though they lack the manual medicine physician's perspective to fully identify and weigh risk:benefit ratios, physical therapists and non-physician manipulative practitioners are typically regulated by licensing and other regulating bodies, and may play a role in interdisciplinary management teams. Likewise, although physicians without manual medicine education cannot fully consider relative efficacy or cost effectiveness of manual intervention, they are valuable in interdisciplinary management teams to provide specialty perspectives, consultation, or appropriate referral to those who have additional education in the neuromusculoskeletal medicine field.

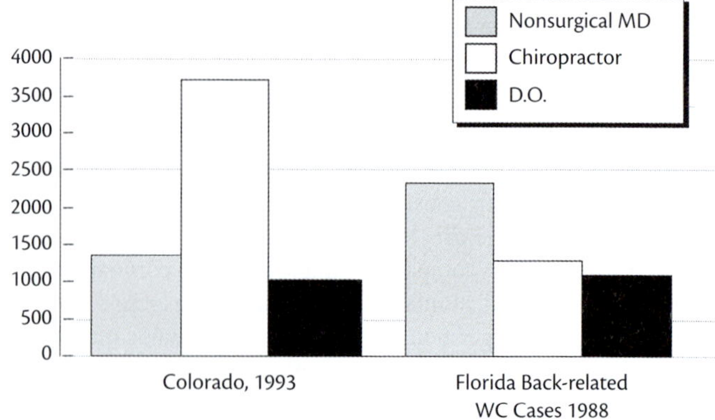

Figure 10.17 Average cost of treatment per patient in U.S. dollars for workmen's compensation cases treated with and without manual medicine techniques by practitioners with differing healthcare degrees and philosophies. (Data compiled by Labor and Industry computers in Florida (FCER 1988, Arlington, Virginia) and Colorado (Tillinghast 1993, Denver, Colorado).)

Precipitating and perpetuating factors in somatic dysfunction

A number of precipitating and/or perpetuating factors warrant diagnostic and treatment consideration in patients with somatic dysfunction. Musculoskeletal physicians (Chila 2011; Simons et al. 1999d) sub-classify precipitating and perpetuating host factors to include mechanical stressors; nutritional, metabolic, and endocrine inadequacies; coexisting radiculopathies, plexopathies, and neuropathies; psychological factors; and chronic infections and infestations.

Mechanical stressors

These are a major consideration in a neuromusculoskeletal practice. Gravitational stress is magnified in a number of postural and structural disorders such as leg length inequality, small hemipelvis, obesity, and accentuation of sagittal plane postural curves (Kuchera 1995). Acute overload or overwork fatigue (Amoronso et al. 1997; Naus et al. 1966; Reynolds et al. 1994) can be aggravated by prolonged exposure to ill-fitting furniture, poor and/or excessive habitual body mechanics, obesity, immobility, repetitive occupational motions, or inappropriate gait mechanics due to pronated or Morton's foot deformity. Direct muscular constriction or trauma, as well as joint micro- and macrotrauma, are precipitating and perpetuating factors for somatic dysfunction. Assessing whole-body postural alignment, analysis of standing postural radiographs, or assessing ergonomic factors in the home or workplace may augment diagnosis. Treatment may require adjunctive use of foot or pelvic orthotics, postural and/or proprioceptive re-education, use of assistive devices, and modification of activities of daily living.

Nutritional, metabolic, and endocrine inadequacies

These preclude the body from using nutritive building blocks, or impair physiological pathways necessary for neuromusculoskeletal function. Travell and Simons note the importance and balance of vitamins B1, B6, and B12, as well as folic acid, vitamin C, calcium, iron, and potassium in the health of myofascial tissues (Simons et al. 1999e). They also note the clinical relevance of conditions such as hypothyroidism and hypoglycaemia that interfere with muscular energy metabolism. Cigarette smoking interferes with myofascial tissue oxygenation and metabolism and is therefore a perpetuating factor for somatic dysfunction and soft tissue healing (Amoronso et al. 1997; Naus et al. 1966; Reynolds et al. 1994; Treiman et al. 2000). Tests for thyroid function, fasting blood sugar, serum vitamin levels, or other blood chemistry profiles may therefore be helpful in diagnosis. Treatment may require pharmacological or dietary strategies as well as patient education. Orthopaedic medicine physicians have empirically seen benefit in nutritionally supplementing patients with the myofascial tissue building blocks, glucosamine and chondroitin sulphate (Deal and Moskowitz 2000).

Radiculopathy or proximal neural entrapment neuropathies

Coexisting radiculopathy or proximal neural entrapment neuropathies have further been implicated in decreasing axoplasmic flow needed to provide trophic factors required in the periphery. This is the mechanism proposed in the so-called 'double-crush' phenomenon (Hurst et al. 1995), leading to increased incidence and symptomatology from more distal somatic dysfunction and neural entrapments. This could also account, in part, for the 10% of patients with carpal tunnel syndrome who are found to have a primary cervical radiculopathy (Upton and McComas 1973). Such diagnoses can usually be made clinically but may require special imaging or neuroelectrodiagnostic studies to localize an anatomical cause or physiological consequence. Treatment may require integration of pharmacological, physical therapeutic, and/or surgical elements.

Psychological factors

As well as arising from chronic pain and dysfunction, these factors perpetuate pain and somatic dysfunction. Thus, suspicion and special questioning may be required to identify those factors interfering with optimum function of the individual. Treatment of underlying anxiety or depression may be required before complete resolution of somatic dysfunction can be accomplished.

Infections and infestations

A variety of viral infections, as well as underlying occult infections and infestations (Simons et al. 1999f) (e.g. *Diphyllobothrium latum, Giardia lamblia, Entamoeba histolytica*), are capable of causing muscle ache and perpetuating myofascial somatic dysfunction. Such a diagnosis might be initiated by the presence of eosinophilia or an elevated white count. Antibiotics, dental care, or other pharmacological intervention for chronic infection may be required before the musculoskeletal findings can be addressed satisfactorily.

The coexistence of many precipitating and perpetuating factors requiring diagnosis and treatment is yet another reason that a broad knowledge base and the capability of ordering and interpreting laboratory, radiographic, nuclear, and neuroelectrophysiological examinations is needed for successful management of neuromusculoskeletal medicine conditions. Treatment requiring integration of pharmacological, physical therapeutic, orthotic, exercise prescription, and surgical approaches is also best coordinated by a physician educated to recognize the indications, contraindications, and relative efficacy of each. Manual diagnostic and treatment techniques alone are rarely sufficient to successfully practice neuromusculoskeletal medicine.

Recurrent patterns of somatic dysfunction

The presence of recurrent patterns of somatic dysfunction, despite quality care, indicates the need for re-evaluation and reconsideration of the existing patient management. Most commonly, recurrent patterns arise from one (or more) of three causes:

- postural compensation
- viscerosomatic referral
- repetitious habitual or occupational posturing and/or motions.

Postural compensation

Patterns of postural compensation occur when gravitational force, acting on individual structures, is biomechanically amplified (Kapandji 1974) in patients who possess a less than ideal postural alignment. Musculoligamentous structures associated with maintenance of posture are, in this manner, subjected to increased strain. When there is viscoelastic deformation of muscle, restraining ligaments,

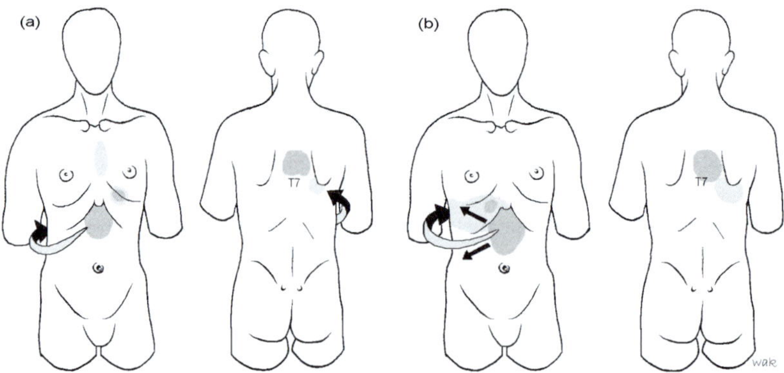

Figure 10.18 Pain patterns: (a) cholelithiasis; (b) gastric ulcer. (Kuchera M.L, Kuchera W.A. Osteopathic considerations in systematic dysfunction, 2nd edn (1994) Greyden Press, Dayton, OH.)

and other connective tissues are unable to resist the stress, neuromuscular reflex activity is automatically and subconsciously initiated to maintain postural equilibrium. Continuous gravitational stress results in various combinations of predictable pathophysiological change (Kuchera 1995), which begins in the connective tissues. It is accentuated and perpetuated by inadequate compensatory mechanisms, including peripheral and central reflexes.

Postural muscles, adapted structurally to function in the presence of prolonged gravitational stress, generally resist fatigue. When their capacity to resist stress is overwhelmed, they become irritable, tight, and shortened. Both structural (anatomical) and functional (physiological and biochemical) changes occur in myofascial structures. They undergo sustained changes in length, and studies (Gossman et al. 1982) suggest that deleterious change is most pronounced in shortened rather than lengthened muscles. New collagen, with a half-life of 10–12 months, realigns the connective tissues in response to stress vectors, thus perpetuating the resultant posture and maintaining biomechanical amplification of gravitational stress. Abnormal stresses, chronically applied to connective tissues, modify their structure and function until they are no longer capable of compensating for the effects of gravitational strain. In an extension of Wolff's law that calcium is laid down along lines of stress, the discovery of bony exostoses and ligamentous calcification may provide radiographic evidence of the stress placed on these soft tissue structures and the fibro-osseous junction.

Thus, when host mechanisms are overwhelmed, signs of gravitational stress appear, including recurrent somatic dysfunction, recurrent myofascial trigger points, postural decompensation, chronic or recurrent strains and sprains, pseudoparesis, and ligamentous laxity. The patient's symptoms include recurrent low back pain, pain referred to extremities, headache, fatigue, weakness, dysfunctional symptoms from various viscera, and other sequelae of neural, vascular, and lymphatic dysfunction resulting from somatic stress. Treatment of the neuromusculoskeletal findings in isolation is often beneficial for short periods of time, but they recur typically with the same underlying patterns of somatic dysfunction.

In general, gravitational stress and the resultant postural effects are most likely to be related to anatomical, histological, physiological, and dysfunctional changes at transitional (junctional) areas of the spine, as these sites are already predisposed to injury and somatic dysfunction. Thus, key patterns of spinal somatic dysfunction commonly occur at the craniocervical, cervicothoracic, thoracolumbar, lumbopelvic, and sacroiliac junctions (Kuchera 1995; Zink and Lawson 1979). The histologic junctional zones created by connective tissue attachments of ligaments, tendons, and joint capsules are also vulnerable to the biomechanical stress of postural decompensation, especially at the site of the fibro-osseous junction of restraining ligaments. The key to efficient diagnosis is to recognize such signs and symptoms as pathophysiological elements of a common musculoligamentous strain pattern caused by gravitational stress.

Viscerosomatic reflex patterns

A second common cause of recurrent patterns of somatic dysfunction may be found in patients with underlying visceral disease or dysfunction. Some of these viscerosomatic reflex patterns, such as those associated with acute appendicitis and gallstones, are widely known and described in a number of texts. Other patterns are less generally known and are described in surgical (Smith 1961) or pain (Cousins 1987) texts written for specialists in those fields. Osteopathic primary care practitioners and specialists in osteopathic manipulative medicine employ these patterns regularly in their practice of neuromusculoskeletal medicine. Regardless of practice type or degree, the finding of specific recurrent patterns of somatic dysfunction in the distribution or combination as shown in Figure 10.18, should prompt the astute neuromusculoskeletal medicine practitioner to consider visceral dysfunction as part of the complete differential diagnosis. A compilation describing the specific role of somatic dysfunction in visceral problems is found in *Osteopathic considerations in systemic dysfunction* (Kuchera and Kuchera 1994b).

Recurrent posturing or repetitious motions

A final cause of recurrent patterns of somatic dysfunction arises from recurrent posturing or repetitious motions associated with habit or occupation. With this in mind, history and an ergonomic evaluation often provide insights to diagnosis and treatment.

Concluding thoughts about somatic dysfunction

Concepts associated with somatic dysfunction pragmatically permit consolidation of many clinically relevant models used in neuromusculoskeletal and manual medicine fields. Building upon anatomical and pathophysiological scientific bases, these concepts can be discussed, explored, and tested. Perhaps even more importantly, neuromusculoskeletal physicians can use 'somatic dysfunction' and associated concepts to communicate with one another. In both situations, palpatory diagnosis and treatment of patients with somatic dysfunction expands the physician's ability to assist patients in their pursuit of function and/or pain relief.

Acknowledgements

The author gratefully thanks his father, William A. Kuchera, DO (professor emeritus), for the design and clarity of all of the line drawings in this chapter.

References

American Medical Association. *AMA guidelines to the evaluation of permanent impairment*, 3rd edn (revised) (1990). AMA, Chicago, IL.

Amoronso, P. J., Reynolds K.L., Barnes J.A., White D.J. *Tobacco and injuries: an annotated bibliography.US Army Research Laboratory technical report ARL-TR-1333.* (1997). US Army Medical Research and Materiel Command: Fort Detrick Fredereick, MD.

Battaglia, G., Rustioni, A. Coexistence of glutamate and substance P in dorsal root ganglion neurons of the rat and monkey. *J Comp Neurol* 1988, 227, 302–12.

Beal, M. C. Viscerosomatic reflexes: a review. *J Am Osteopath Assoc* 1985, 85(12), 53–68.

Beal M. C. Palpatory testing for somatic dysfunction in patients with cardiovascular disease. *JADA* 1983, 82, 73–82.

van Buskirk, R. L. Nociceptive reflexes and somatic dysfunction: a model. *J Am Osteo Assoc* 1990, 90, 792–809.

Cervero, F. Mechanisms of acute visceral pain. *Br Med Bull* 1991, 47, 549–60.

Chila, T. G. (ed.). *Foundations for osteopathic medicine*, 3rd edn (2011). Lippincott, Williams & Wilkins, Baltimore, MD.

Cousins, M. J. Visceral pain. In: Andersson, S., Bond, M., Mehta, M., Swerdlow M (eds). *Chronic non-cancer pain: assessment and practical management* (1987). MTP Press, Lancaster.

Cyriax, J. H., Cyriax, P. J. *Cyriax's illustrated manual of orthopaedic medicine*, 2nd edn (1993). Butterworth-Heinemann, Oxford.

Cyriax, J., Russell, G. *Textbook of orthopaedic medicine: volume 2, treatment by manipulation, massage, and injection*, 10th edn (1980). Baillière Tindall, London, pp. 60–9.

Deal, C. L., Moskowitz, R. W. Nutraceuticals as therapeutic agents in osteoarthritis. The role of glucosamine, chondrotin sulfate, and collagen hydrosalt. *Rheum Dis Clin North Am* 2000, 25(2), 75–95.

Degenhardt, B. F., Snider, K. T., Johnson, J. C., Snider E. J. Interexaminer reliability of osteopathic palpatory evaluation of the lumbar spine. *J Am Osteopath Assoc* 2002a, 102(8), 442.

Degenhardt, B. F., Snider, K. T., Johnson, J. C., Snider E. J. Retention of interexaminer reliability in palpatory evaluation of the lumbar spine. *J Am Osteopath Assoc* 2002b, 102(8), 439.

Denslow J. S. Pathophysiologic evidence for the osteopathic lesion: the known, unknown, and controversial. *J Am Osteopath Assoc* 1975, 74, 315–421.

Dockray, G. J., Sharkey, K. A. Neurochemistry of visceral afferent neurones. *Prog Brain Res.* 1986, 67, 133–48.

Dorman, T. A., Ravin, T. H. *Diagnosis and injection techniques in orthopedic medicine* (1991). Williams & Wilkins, Baltimore, MD.

Dubner, R., Bennett, G. J. Spinal and trigeminal mechanisms of nociception. *Annu Rev Neurosci* 1983, 6, 381–418.

Dvorak, J., Dvorak, V., Drobny, T. *Manual medicine: diagnostics* (1984). Georg Thieme Verlag, Stuttgart, pp. 30–45.

Education Council on Osteopathic Principles. Glossary of osteopathic terminology. In Chila, T.G. (ed.). *Foundations for osteopathic medicine*, 3rd edn (2011). Lippincott, Williams & Wilkins, Baltimore, MD, pp. 1087–110.

Educational Council on Osteophatic Principles (ECOP). *The Core Curriculum in Osteopathic Principles.* Educational Council on Osteopathic Principles of the American Association of Colleges of Osteopathic Medicine: Chevy Chase MD (1999).

FCER/Tillinghast. *Data compiled by labor and industry computers in Florida* (FCER, 1988, Arlington, Virginia) *and in Colorado* (Tillinghast, 1993, Denver, Colorado).

Gilliar, W. G., Kuchera, M. L., Giulianetti, D. A. Neurologic basis of manual medicine. *Phy Med Rehabil Clin N Am* 1996, 7(4), 693–714.

Gossman, M. R., Sahrmann, S. A., Rose, S. J. Review of length-associated changes in muscle. *Phys Ther* 1982, 62, 1799–807.

Greenman, P. E. (ed.). *Concepts and mechanisms of neuromuscular function* (1984). Springer-Verlag, Berlin.

Hurst, L. C., Weissberg, D., Carroll, R. E. The relationship of the double crush to carpal tunnel syndrome (an analysis of 1000 cases of carpal tunnel syndrome). *J Hand Surg* 1995, 10B(2), 202–4.

International Federation of Musculoskeletal/Manual Medicine. *Core education documents, International Federation of Musculoskeletal/ Manual Medicine (IFMM)* (1999). FIMM, Warsage, Belgium.

Jones, L. H. *Strain and counterstrain* (1981). American Academy of Osteopathy, Newark, OH.

Jones, L., Kusunose, R., Goering, E. *Jones' strain-counterstrain* (1995). Jones' Strain-Counterstrain, Inc.: Boise, ID.

Kapandji, I. A. *Physiology of the joints: volume 3* (1974). Churchill Livingstone, New York.

Kappler, R. E. *Role of psoas mechanism in low back complaints. 1973 Academy Yearbook* (1973). AAO Press, Indianapolis, IN, p. 130.

Kimberly, P. E. Formulating a prescription of osteopathic manipulative treatment. In: Beal, M. C. (ed.). *The principles of palpatory diagnosis and manipulative technique* (1992). American Academy of Osteopathy, Newark, OH, pp. 146–52.

Konnitinen, Y. T., Koski, H., Santavirta, S., et al. Nociception, proprioception, and neurotransmitters. In: Bland, J. H. (ed.). *Disorders of the cervical spine*, 2nd edn (1994). W. B. Saunders, Philadelphia, pp. 319–38.

Korr, I. M. Hyperactivity of sympathetic innervation: a common factor in disease. In: Greenman P. E. (ed.). *Concepts and mechanisms of neuromuscular functions* (1984). Springer-Verlag, Berlin. pp 1–8.

Korr, I. M. The spinal cord as organizer of disease processes: the peripheral autonomic nervous system. *J Am Osteopath Assoc* 1979, 79, 82–90.

Korr, I. M. (ed.). *The neurobiologic mechanisms in manipulative therapy* (1978). Plenum Press, New York.

Kuchera, M. L. Gravitational stress, musculoligamentous strain, and postural alignment. *Spine* 1995, 9(2), 463–90.

Kuchera, M. L., McPartland, J. Myofascial trigger points as somatic dysfunction. In: Ward, R. C. (ed.). *Foundations for osteopathic medicine*, 2nd edn (2002). Lippincott, Williams & Wilkins, Baltimore, MD, pp. 1034–50.

Kuchera, W. A., Kuchera, M. L. *Osteopathic principles in practice*, 2nd edn (revised) (1994a). Greyden Press, Columbus, OH. p. 25.

Kuchera, M. L., Kuchera, W. A. *Osteopathic considerations in systemic dysfunction*, 2nd edition (revised) (1994b). Greyden Press, Columbus, OH.

Kuchera, W. A., Kuchera, M. L. *Osteopathic principles in practice*, 2nd edn (revised) (1994c). Greyden Press, Columbus, OH, pp. 297–302.

Maigne, R., Liberson, W. T. *Orthopedic medicine: a new approach to vertebral manipulations* (1972). C. C. Thomas, Springfield, IL.

Maitland, G. D. Acute locking of the cervical spine. *Austral J Physio* 1978, 24, 103–9.

McEwen, B. S. Protective and damaging effects of stress mediators. *New Engl J Med* 1998, 338, 178–9.

Mense, S., Simons, D. *Muscle pain, understanding its nature, diagnosis, and treatment* (2001). Lippincott Williams and Wilkins, Philadelphia, PA.

Mitchell, F Jr. The training and measurement of sensory literacy in relation to osteopathic structural and palpatory diagnosis. *J Am Osteopath Assoc* 1976, 75, 881.

Mitchell, F. L. *The muscle energy manual: vols I–III* (1995–9). MET Press, East Lansing, MI.

Mitchell, F. L., Mitchell, P. K. *The muscle energy manual* (1995). MET Press, East Lansing, MI, p. 33.

Naus, A. et al. Work injuries and smoking. *Industrial Med Surg* 1966, 35, 880–1.

Nicholas, A. S., DeBias, D. A., Ehrenfeuchter, W., et al. A somatic component to myocardial infarction. *BMJ* 1985, 291, 13–7.

Owens, C. *An endocrine interpretation of Chapman's reflexes* (1963 reprint). American Academy of Osteopathy, Indianapolis, IN.

Patterson, M. M., Howell, J. N. (eds). *The central connection: somatovisceral/viscerosomatic interaction* (1989). University Classics, Athens, OH.

Patterson, M. M., Steinmetz, J. E. Long-lasting alterations of spinal reflexes: a potential basis for somatic dysfunction. *Manual Med* 1986, 2, 38–45.

Pernow, B. Substance P. *Pharmacol Rev* 1983, 35, 85–141.

Peterson, B (ed.). *The collected papers of Irvin M. Korr* (1979). American Academy of Osteopathy, Newark, OH.

Reynolds, K. L. et al. Cigarette smoking, physical fitness, and injuries in infantry soldiers. *Am J Preventive Med* 1994, 19, 145–50.

Schott, G. D. Visceral afferent: their contribution to 'sympathetic dependent' pain. *Brain* 1994, 117, 397–413.

Sciotti, V. M., Mittak, V. L., DiMarco, L. Clinical precision of myofascial trigger point location in the trapezius muscle. *Pain* 2001, 93, 259–66.

Seeman, T. E., Singer, B. H., Rowe, J. W., Horwitz, R. I., McEwen, B. S. Price of adaptation—allostatic load and its health consequences: McArthur studies of successful aging. *J Clin Endocrinol Metab* 1997, 157, 2259–68.

Simons, D. G., Travell, J. G., Simons, L. S. *Travell and Simons' myofascial pain and dysfunction: the trigger point manual, vol. 1. Upper half of body* (1999a). Williams & Wilkins, Baltimore, MD.

Simons, D. G., Travell, J. G., Simons, L. S. *Travell and Simons' myofascial pain and dysfunction: the trigger point manual, vol. 1. Upper half of body* (1999b). Williams & Wilkins, Baltimore, MD, pp. 728–42.

Simons, D. G., Travell, J. G., Simons, L. S. *Travell and Simons' myofascial pain and dysfunction: the trigger point manual, vol. 1. Upper half of body* (1999c). Williams & Wilkins, Baltimore, MD, pp. 832–3.

Simons, D. G., Travell, J. G., Simons, L. S. *Travell and Simons' myofascial pain and dysfunction: the trigger point manual, vol. 1. Upper half of body* (1999d). Williams & Wilkins, Baltimore, MD, pp. 178–235.

Simons, D. G., Travell, J. G., Simons, L. S. *Travell and Simons' myofascial pain and dysfunction: the trigger point manual, vol. 1. Upper half of body* (1999e). Williams & Wilkins, Baltimore, MD, pp. 186–220.

Simons, D. G., Travell, J. G., Simons L. S. *Travell and Simons' myofascial pain and dysfunction: the trigger point manual, vol. 1. Upper half of body* (1999f). Williams & Wilkins, Baltimore, MD, pp. 223–5.

Smith, L. A. (ed.). *An atlas of pain patterns: sites and behavior of pain in certain common disease of the upper abdomen* (1961). C. C. Thomas, Springfield, IL.

Speece, C. A., Crow, W. T., Simmon, S. L. *Ligamentous articular strain: osteopathic manipulative techniques for the body* (2001). Eastland Press.

Steele, K. M. Treatment of the acutely ill hospitalized patient. In: Ward, R. C. (ed.) *Foundations for osteopathic medicine* (1997). Williams & Wilkins, Baltimore, MD, pp. 1037–48 (Chapter 75).

Sterling, P., Eyer, J. Allostasis: a new paradigm to explain arousal pathology. In: Fisher, S. Reason, J. (eds). *Handbook of life stress, cognition and health* (1988). Wiley, New York, pp. 629–49.

Treiman, G. S., Oderich, G. S., Ashrafi, A., Schneider, P. A. Management of ischemic heal ulceration and gangrene: an evaluation of factors associated with successful healing. *J Vasc Surg* 2000, 31(6), 1110–8.

Upton, A. R., McComas, A. J. The double crush in nerve entrapment syndromes. *Lancet* 1973, ii, 359–62.

White, A. A., Panjabi, M. M. The basic kinematics of the human spine: a review of past and current knowledge. *Spine* 1978, 3, 12.

Willard, F. H. Neuroendocrine-immune network, nociceptive stress, and the general adaptive response. In: Everett, T., Dennis, M., Ricketts, E (eds). *Physiotherapy in mental health: a practical approach* (1995). Butterworth-Heinemann, Oxford, pp. 102–26.

Willard, F. H., Patterson M. M. (eds). *Nociception and the neuroendocrineimmune connection* (1991). University Classics, Athens, OH.

Willard, F. H., Mokler, D. J., Morgane, P. J. Neuroendocrineimmune system and homeostasis. In: Ward, R. C. (ed.). *Foundations for osteopathic medicine* (1997). Williams & Wilkins, Baltimore, MD, pp. 107–35 (Chapter 9).

Wolfe, F., Smythe, H. A., Yunus, M. B. et al. The American College of Rheumatology 1990 criteria for the classification of fibromyalgia. Report of the Multicenter Committee. *Arthritis Rheum* 1990, 33, 160–72.

World Health Organization. *International classification of diseases, 9th revision, clinical modification (ICD-9-CM)*, 3rd edn (1979). World Health Organization, Geneva.

Wyke, B. D. The neurologic basis of thoracic spinal pain. *Rheum Phys Med* 1970, 10, 356.

Zink, J. G., Lawson, W. B. An osteopathic structural examination and functional interpretation of the soma. *Osteopath Ann* 1979, 7, 12–9.

Chapter 11

Biomechanics and laterality in musculoskeletal medicine: an additional approach?

Sjef Rutte and Jacob Patijn

Introduction to biomechanics and laterality in musculoskeletal medicine

Manual/musculoskeletal (M/M) medicine is characterized, dependent on the hypothesis within a particular school, by different diagnostic and therapeutic approaches. Each of these approaches emphasizes one or more diagnostic aspects of the locomotor system (muscles, fasciae, trigger points) and therapeutic aspects of such as myofascial release, segmental dysfunctions, and postural disturbances. Only in a few M/M medicine publications is body asymmetry integrated into the diagnostic and therapeutic approach of patients with locomotor system pathology (van der Bijl 1986; Ross 2003). A relationship can exist between body asymmetry and both mobility (van der Bijl 1981; Lazenby 2002; Lazenby et al. 2008) and handedness (Lazenby et al. 2008). Biomechanical aspects of body asymmetries can influence preferential motions (van der Bijl 1981, 1986; de Cock 1996; Rutte 2002; van Wylick 2004) which, as such, are dependent on cerebral lateralization integrative processes (Vallortigara and Rogers 2005). In abnormal body asymmetries (for instance, scoliosis), performing preferential motions can become dysfunctional and can even result in pain in one or more areas of the locomotor system of the patient. Diagnostic procedures and treatments, which focus on the aforementioned preferential motion dysfunction, can be an additional approach in M/M medicine (Rutte 2002).

(Bio)mechanics of the human body

In general, Cartesian planes (frontal, sagittal, transverse) are used to define body asymmetry. In daily practice, we generally expect a complete symmetry of the body forms and the left/right range of motions. However, we have to decide whether these asymmetries are normal or related to the complaints and clinical findings of the patient. In addition, we have to estimate whether a relationship exists between the pain experienced by the patient and the diagnosed asymmetry of motion.

In M/M medicine, asymmetry is frequently seen as an abnormal condition of the patient and therefore frequently forms an indication for further examination and/or treatment (Gnat and Saulicz 2008). However, asymmetry of form (Sylvester et al. 2008) (for instance, scoliosis) and function (motion) occurs in 80–90% of asymptomatic and normal subjects (Golomer et al. 2009; Preece et al. 2008; Varela et al. 2003).

It is widely accepted that form and function are mutually dependent and that this dependency can change during ageing or as a consequence of medical conditions. In mechanics, the human body can be seen as a physical mass (see Figure 11.1b), consisting of different constituent parts (see Figure 11.1c). Each of these parts has its own characteristics with respect to mass composition and elasticity. All motions of this mass (the human trunk) in space are also defined according to the three perpendicular Cartesian planes (frontal, sagittal, transverse) (see Figure 11.1a). During motion, different deformations may be demonstrated by different parts, dependent upon the direction of the applied force. For instance, when a patient bends backwards, compression will occur at the dorsal side of his/her trunk. As a logical consequence, the ventral side of the trunk will translate forwards (see Figure 11.2).

As we have labelled the human body with ventral, dorsal, and lateral sides, the motions of the body are always defined according to the three Cartesian planes. The same is true for the deformation and the shifting of the body parts. However, the plane of the primary performed motion of the patient is located outside the three normal Cartesian planes. The qualitative and quantitative characteristics of deformation and shifting will, however, be the same when the motion occurs in the three normal Cartesian planes (see Figures 11.3a and 11.3b). We can translate this mechanical phenomenon into our daily practice of M/M medicine by, for instance, asking a patient to bend forward in combination with a lateral bending. A compression will be observed at the ventral side of the trunk and a simultaneous shift at the dorsal side of the trunk in a plane between the three normal Cartesian planes of the human body (see Figure 11.4) In M/M medicine, this kind of motion is

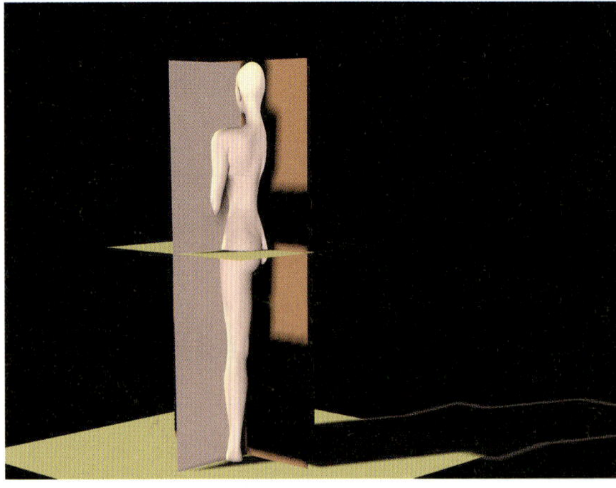

Figure 11.1a Three Cartesian planes: both the sagittal and frontal planes go through the central axis; the transversal (horizontal) plane is perpendicular on the sagittal and frontal plane.
(Reproduced with permission of Marsman Foundation™)

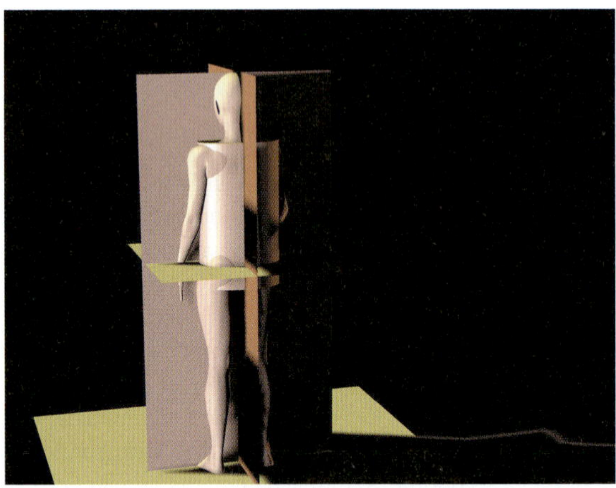

Figure 11.1b The combined motion of forward/lateral flexion occurs in a plane 'b' outside the three normal perpendicular Cartesian planes.
(Reproduced with permission of Marsman Foundation™)

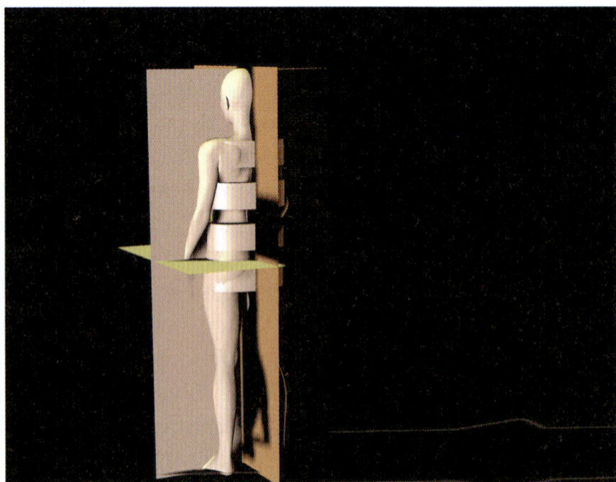

Figure 11.1c After modular division in anatomical segments each segment can move in the same or a different quadrant.
(Reproduced with permission of Marsman Foundation™)

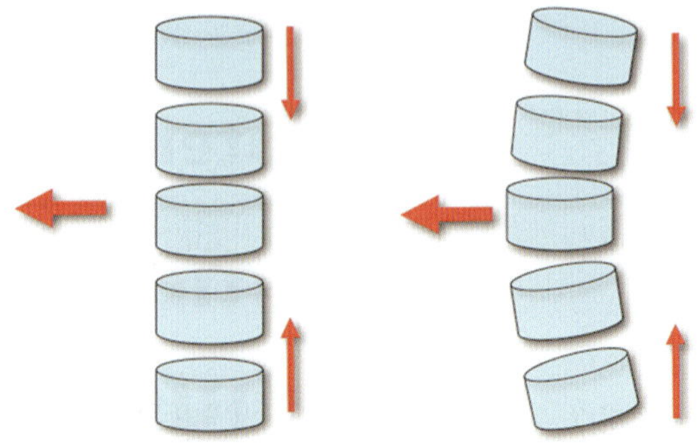

Figure 11.2 Backward bending (in figure to the right) results in compression at the dorsal side of the different modules of his/her trunk. The ventral side of the trunk will translate forwards.
(Reproduced with permission of Marsman Foundation™)

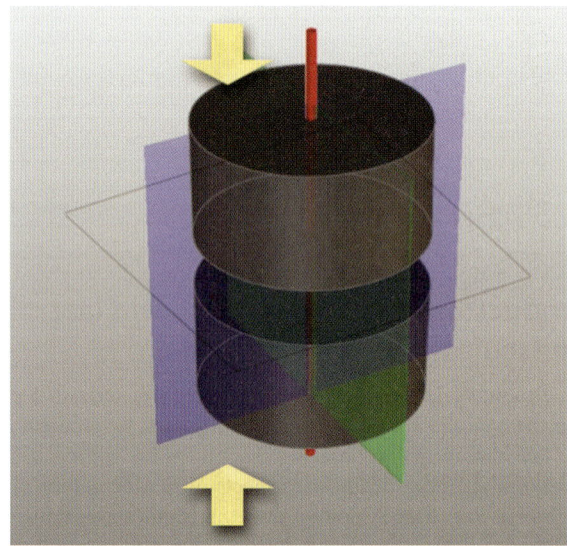

Figure 11.3a Two modules of the trunk in neutral position with three normal Cartesian planes.
(Reproduced with permission of Marsman Foundation™)

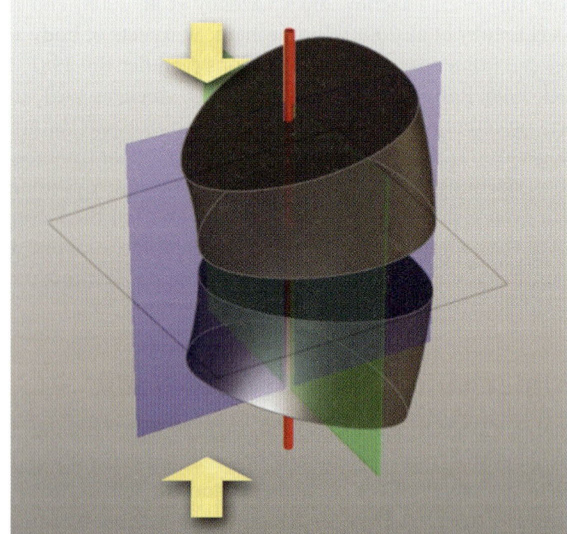

Figure 11.3b Two modules of the trunk during combined lateral/backward flexion. Compression occurs at the left side (yellow arrows) with a simultaneous shifting to the opposite side. Look at the pattern of deformation.
(Reproduced with permission of Marsman Foundation™)

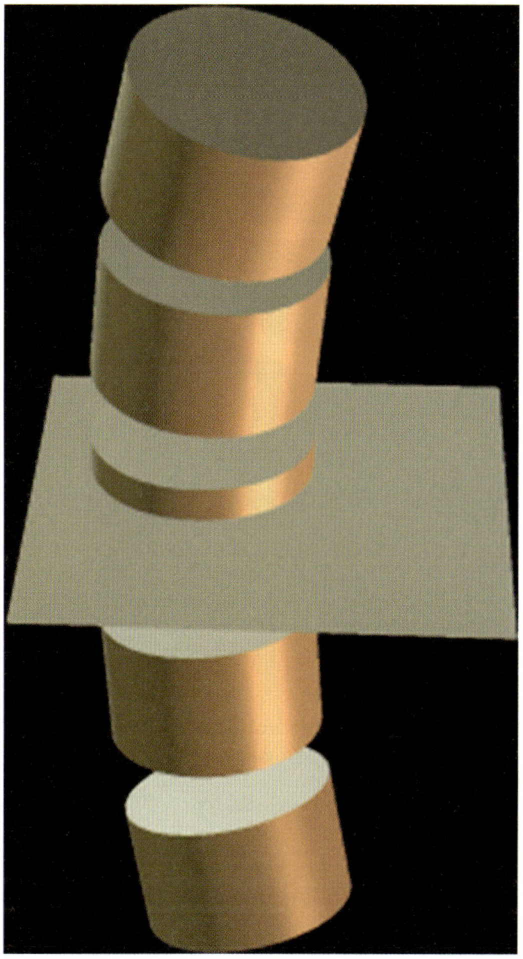

Figure 11.4 Forward bending in combination with a lateral bending of the modules of the trunk: compression will be observed at the ventral side of the trunk with a simultaneous shift at the dorsal side of the trunk in a plane between the three normal Cartesian planes.
(Reproduced with permission of Marsman Foundation™)

named a combined forward/lateral flexion. In addition, the contralateral rotation of, for example, the spinal vertebrae or pelvic ring is only defined in the transverse plane (Lewit 2009). From a mechanical point of view, the combined motion of forward/lateral flexion occurs in a plane (see Figure 11.1b; plane 'b') outside the three normal perpendicular Cartesian planes. No rotation occurs, for instance, of a vertebra in the transverse plane.

M/M medicine should always be considered in combined and Cartesian-planes- related motions. This way of thinking forms the base for certain three-dimensional treatment strategies in M/M medicine (Rutte et al. 2012). If we apply the aforementioned proposed mechanical point of view, we only have to treat in the single diagonal plane of ventral compression and dorsal shifting (see Figure 11.4).

Lateralization and preferred motion of the human body

In daily life, many functions performed by the limbs (handedness, footedness) have an asymmetrical character. In the central nervous system, functions such as talking and calculating are located in one hemisphere. This phenomenon is known as cortical lateralization (Ooki 2014). Both in human beings and animals, lateralization is defined as unilateral dominance of sensory and/or motor function (Heyne and all 1999; Manns and Ströckens 2014; Dittmar 2002). The exact epigenesis of cortical lateralization is not clear. Genetic predisposition can play a role (Annett 1999; Crow 2010; McManus 2004; Medland et al. 2006). Additionally, an adaptive behavioural phenomenon plays a role in the lateralization (Schaafsma et al. 2009). Different chromosomal loci are probably involved in the genetic background of handedness (McManus et al. 2013). Based on genome studies, it has been suggested that the same mechanism that explains handedness is also responsible for left/right body asymmetry (Brandler and Paracchini 2014; McManus et al. 2013)

In the human body, many asymmetric postural positions and motion patterns exist. For instance, when we are crossing our arms or legs, each individual person always performs these motions in the same way. Also in snow boarding, there is a distinction between being a regular or a goofy, reflecting a preferred posture to optimize our body equilibrium. Eye dominance is important in shooting while pointing at the target.

Lateralization, such as left/right handedness, can result in an asymmetric motion pattern (Sainburg 2005). Compared to normal subjects, patients with a brachialgia of their dominant arm will grasp a teacup from the table according to a completely different motion pattern. This means that not only asymmetric form is decisive for an asymmetric motion, but also cortical cognitive pain processes can play a prominent role. If the patient grasps the teacup with his/her normal non-dominant hand, you will find a clearly different motion pattern too, which is of course completely normal. In M/M medicine, diagnostic procedures do not focus on these normal preferred motion patterns.

Summarizing, asymmetric motion patterns can both be normal and abnormal in patients with pain originating from the locomotor system.

Preferential mass mechanics method (PMMM)

Both aspects (mass mechanics and lateralization) can be combined in a different diagnostic and therapeutic approach to a patient with pain originating from the locomotor system. This approach can be integrated in the daily practice of M/M medicine. The combination of mass mechanics and lateralization is called the preferential mass mechanics method (PMMM). PMMM is not referred to as a mono-therapeutic approach, but has to be used complementary to the diagnostic and therapeutic arsenal of the practitioner in M/M medicine. For instance, if a patient shows repeatedly reoccurring complaints and clinical findings after several treatments of regular M/M medicine, one can consider the PMMM approach.

History of the preferential mass mechanics method

In 1979, the American osteopath Zink (Ross 2003) noticed that some of his patients showed patterns of asymmetry in form and in different parts of the body. In 1981, the Dutch osteopath van der Bijl developed a diagnostic model that was based on three aspects: anatomical asymmetries, findings by lateralization tests, and a calculation of sub-centres of gravity of the different parts of the body (van der Bijl 1981) The sub-centres of gravity were related to a deformation of a certain part of the body. Based on his experience with patients, many different and unique patterns could be defined and categorized in different individual models. His treatment aimed to repair patients' passive movements or their own individual models (van der Bijl 1986). The Dutch manual physiotherapist Marsman simplified the van der Bijl method by reducing the enormous number of lateralization tests to only eight (Rutte 2002). Later, mass mechanics was integrated into the method of Marsman and a new relationship was defined with kinematics and central neurophysiological processes such as lateralization (Rutte 2001, 2002; Rutte et al. 2012; van Wylick 2004).

Preferential mass mechanics method in practice

In daily practice, PMMM mainly focuses on the trunk of the patient with respect to deformation during stance and different motions. The trunk is seen as a central mass with attached extremities and head and is divided into different disc-shaped modules (see Figure 11.5). Each disc-shaped module has its own heterogeneous content (skin, soft tissue organs, nerves). Lateralization (handedness) will influence the deformation of the different disc-shaped modules according to the principle of compression/shift (see Figure 11.6). During the preferred motion patterns, derived from lateralization, the disc-shaped module will be further deformed according to the principle of compression/shift. Translated, for example, to the human trunk in the sagittal plane in stance, the different disc-shaped modules of the trunk will each be deformed differently because of the influence of the lateralization phenomenon (see Figure 11.6).

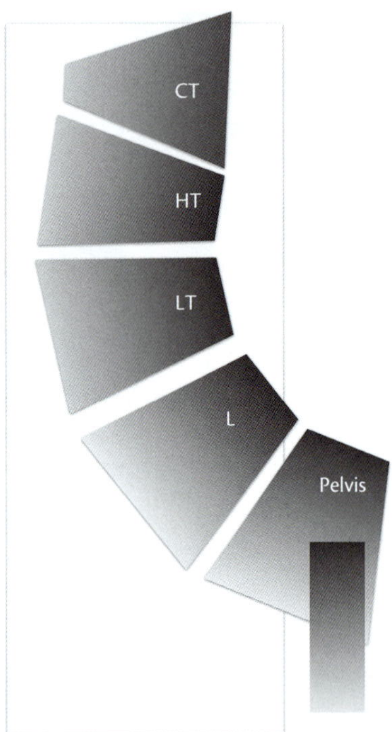

Figure 11.6 Lateralization (handedness) will influence the deformation of the different disc-shaped modules of the trunk according to the principle of compression/shift.
(Reproduced with permission of Marsman Foundation™)

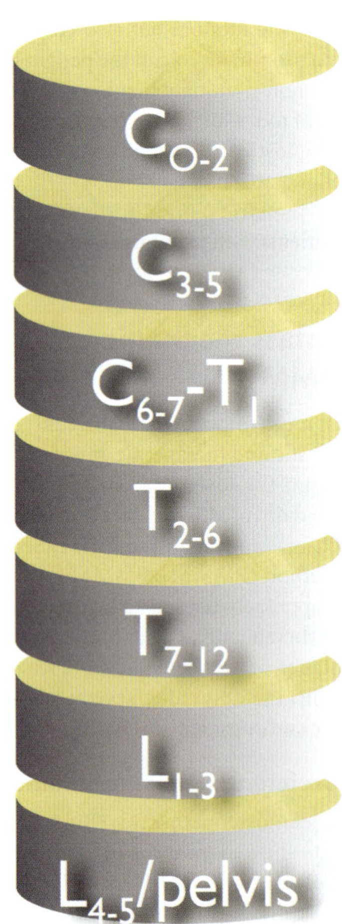

Figure 11.5 Modular division of the trunk into different anatomical regions.
(Reproduced with permission of Marsman Foundation™)

During forward flexion, the most upper module with a ventral compression and dorsal shift enables more forward flexion. In contrast, the caudal module restricts the forward flexion. The opposite will occur in backward flexion. In this case, the most upper module will be the restrictive one. Of course, this phenomenon will take place in any plane of motion and will show a difference in the range of motion out of the neutral position.

In PMMM, eight lateralization tests are performed to objectify the asymmetrical functions of disc-shaped modules of the trunk (Rutte 2001). The patient personally performs these eight standard tests (see the section 'PMMM tests' that follows). The results of the different tests will be influenced by the direction of the motion performed within the test and the pre-existent lateralization that is further affected by the existence of a medical condition.

PMMM tests

The PMMM tests are an integrative part of a standard diagnostic procedure that consists of a proper medical history, a neurological examination, and diagnostic tests used in M/M medicine. Eight PMMM tests are defined to gain an impression of the lateralization aspects of a patient and his/her preferred motions. Secondly, control tests are used to verify lateralization aspects by performing passive general ranges of motion (ROM) of the trunk and to detect ROM abnormalities.

Most of the eight PMMM tests are derived from conditions in the general medical field, sport, or daily life. Seven of the eight tests are not related to handedness and are called 'functional asymmetry' tests (Ogah et al. 2012). The results of the eight PMMM tests are constant for each patient during their life (Ogah et al. 2012). The reproducibility agreement for the eight tests is good, illustrated by kappa values ranging from 0.78–1.00 as a measure for interobserver agreement (van Wylick 2004).

PMMM test 1: eye dominance

Eye dominance is defined as the preferred eye that is used when a subject looks at a target in the sagittal plane. In this case the 'hole in card' method is used to examine the eye dominance (Li et al. 2010). The patient holds a small card with a hole straight before his eyes at a half-arm distance. He/she is asked to look through the hole in the direction of a fixed point (see Figure 11.7) The patient is asked to alternately close one eye. If the dominant eye is closed, the fixed point will disappear.

PMMM test 2: eye phoria

Eye phoria is a vergance disturbance or ocular malalignment of fusion. In this case, the Maddox rod test (Giles 1959), is used. This test uses a handheld device consisting of a series of parallel cylinders that converts a point source of light into a line image (see Figure 11.8). With this test, esophoria or exophoria can be established by demonstrating, respectively, a convergence or divergence between the eyes.

The red rod is placed in front of one of the eyes of the patient. Both eyes of the patient are opened and the patient is asked to fix on a light at a distance of 5 metres located at a horizontal plane through the eyes. By looking through the horizontal-oriented parallel cylinders of the rod, the patient will see a vertical red line located on the left or right side of the light. The degree of convergence is related to horizontal gazing and the head position in forward and backward flexion (de Cock 1996; Procianoy and Procianoy 2008; Rutte 2001).

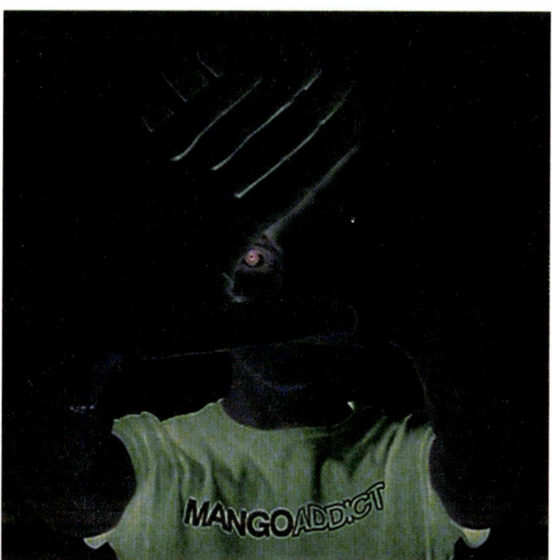

Figure 11.7 Eye dominance test: subject holds a small card with a hole, straight before his/her eyes on a half-arm distance. She/he is asked to look through the hole in the direction of a fixed point.
(Reproduced with permission of Marsman Foundation™)

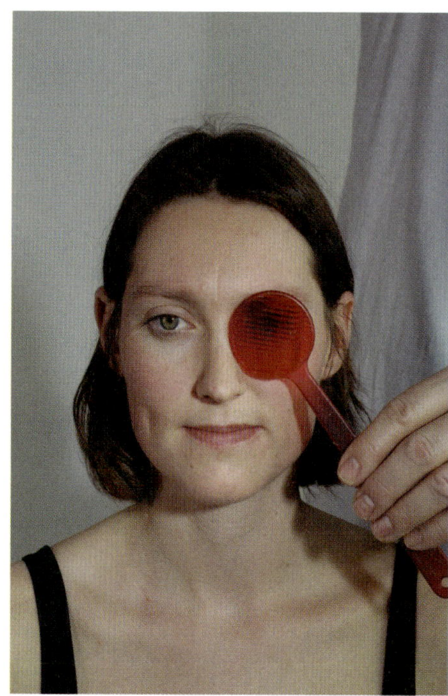

Figure 11.8 Maddox rod test: handheld device consisting of a series of parallel cylinders that converts a point source of light into a line image.

PMMM test 3: handedness sweep test

The way a person brooms, shovels, or sweeps is indicative for his/her handedness. The sweep test is a bi-manual procedure whereby a person places one hand halfway down the broom handle and the other hand on the end of the handle (Annett 2013). The first hand acts as a fulcrum. The second hand is able to manipulate the sweep. The manipulating hand is mostly the dominant hand (see Figure 11.9).

PMMM test 4: crossing arms or arm folding test

The crossing arms or arm folding test refers to preference of a person to fold one forearm over the other in his/her most comfortable way (see Figure 11.10). In contrast with the sweeping test, the arm folding test has no relationship to handedness and is seen as a preferred motion (Ogah et al. 2012). There is probably a genetic base for the way people fold their arms (McManus and Mascie-Taylor 1979; Reiss 1998; Wiener 1932).

PMMM test 5: hand clasping test

In the hand clasping test, one thumb is always positioned above the other one (Kalichman et al. 2008) The other fingers are crossed depending on the position of the thumbs (see Figure 11.11). The hand clasping test has no relationship to handedness and is seen as a preferred motion (Ogah et al. 2012).

PMMM test 6: climbing stairs test

In this test, climbing the first step of a staircase is evaluated. The patient stands in front of a staircase and is asked to spontaneously climb the stairs (see Figures 11.12a and 11.12b). The first foot that a patient uses to start climbing the stairs is called the preferential foot (Rutte 2002).

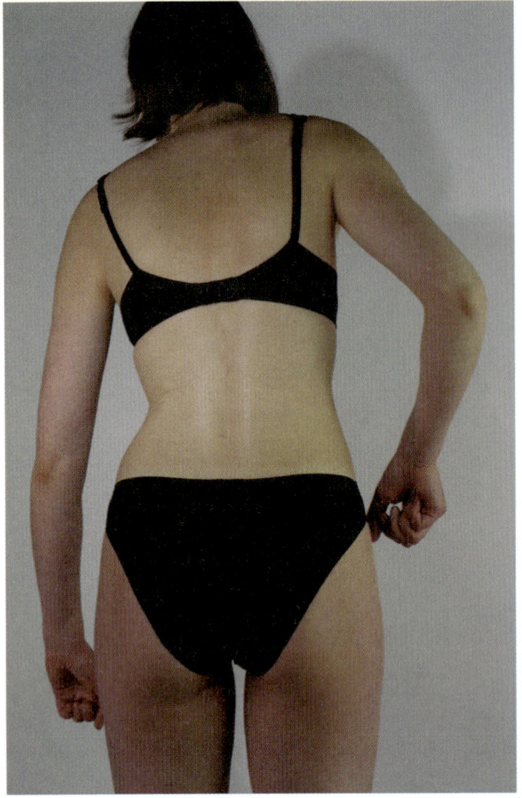

Figure 11.9 Handedness sweep test: in this case, the left hand is placed halfway down the broom handle and the right hand is on the end. The right hand is the dominant hand.

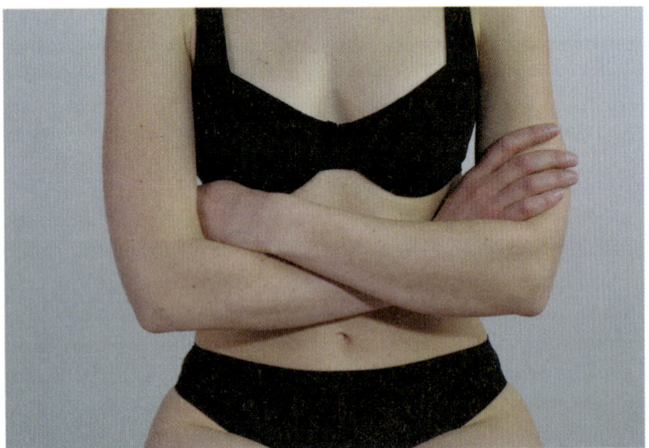

Figure 11.10 Crossing arms or arm folding test: preference of a subject to fold one forearm over the other in his/her most comfortable way.

PMMM test 7: stepping backward test

The stepping backward test can be performed in two ways. One can ask the patient to take one step backwards or ask him/her to complete the backward stepping in one 360° rotation along the vertical axis (Heinen et al. 2012; Lenoir et al. 2006) (see Figure 11.13). The first foot he/she uses is a preferential motion.

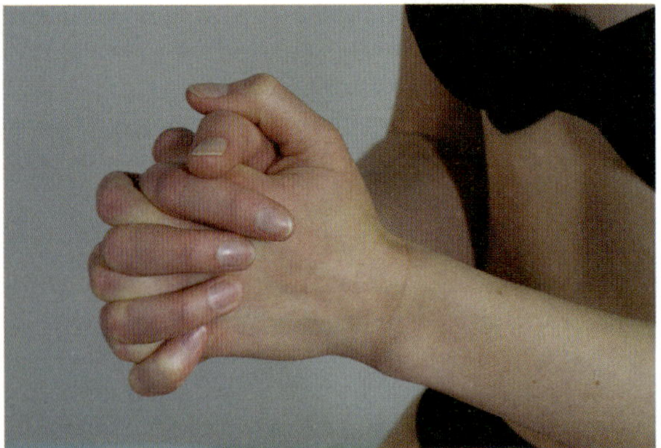

Figure 11.11 Hand clasping test: preference of a subject to put one thumb always above the other thumb.

PMMM test 8: crossing legs test

The crossing legs test has the same properties as the arm folding test in the sense of degree of comfort. The crossing legs test can be performed in both the sitting and supine position (see Figure 11.14). One leg will be crossed over the other one. The leg of which its hip is the most externally rotated, indicates the preference of a patient to perform his leg crossing (Eligar 2011; Reiss 1995).

Based on the results of the eight PMMM tests, one can predict findings of passive performed motions in different areas of the locomotor system (van Wylick 2004). Therefore, after performing

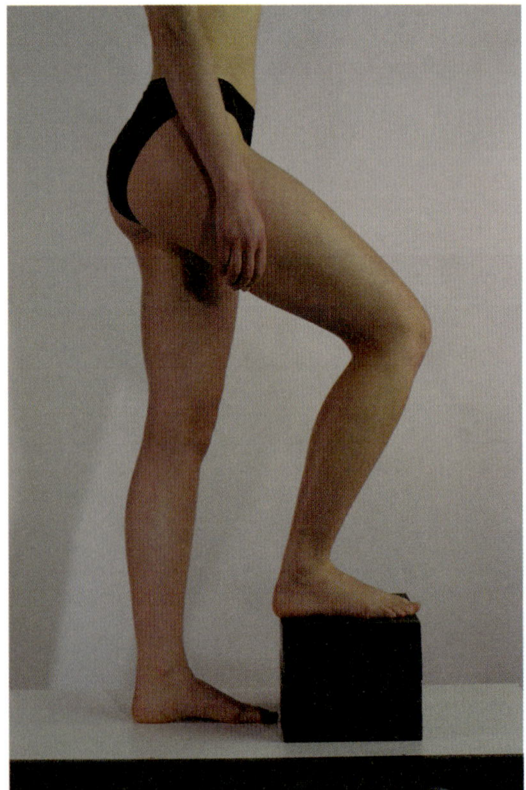

Figure 11.12a Climbing stairs test: subject is asked to spontaneously climb the stairs. The first foot which a patient uses to start climbing the stairs is called the preferential foot.

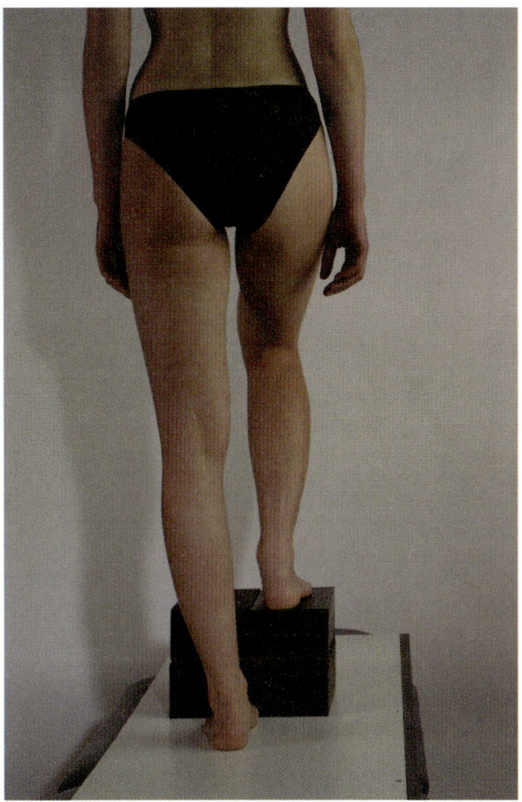

Figure 11.12b *(continued)*

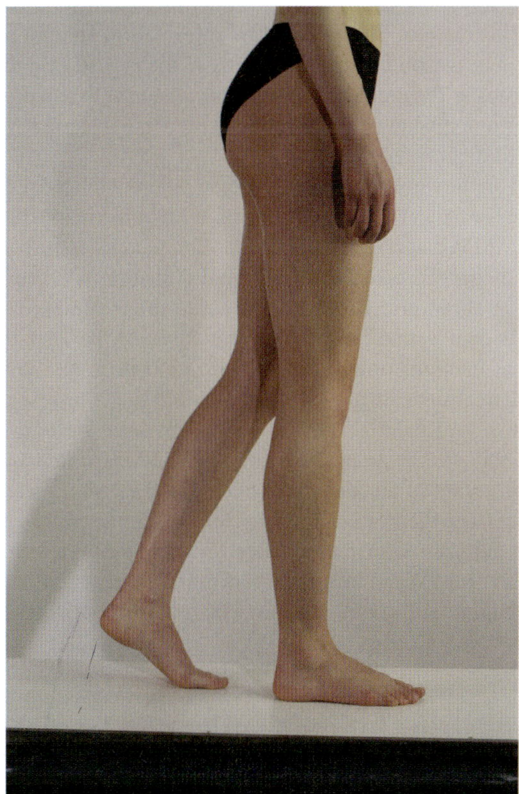

Figure 11.13 Stepping backward test: subject is asked to take one step backwards and/or asked to complete the backward stepping in one 360° rotation along the vertical axis.

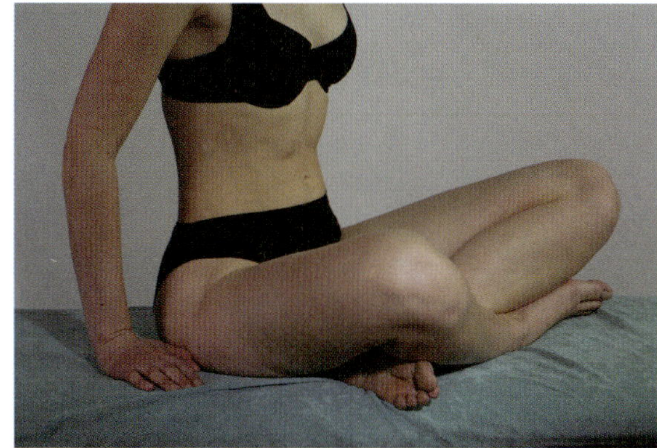

Figure 11.14 Crossing legs test (in sitting position): the leg of which its hip is the most exorotated, indicates the preference of a patient to perform his/her leg crossing. In this example, the right hip is the most exorotated.

these tests, a number of control tests are conducted to confirm the findings of the PMMM tests and to find abnormalities in the preferred motion (van Wylick 2004).

As an example of a control test of the 'sweep', the passive lateral flexion of the trunk is presented (see Figure 11.15). If, in a sweep test, a patient holds the left hand halfway down the broom handle and the right hand at the end of it, one expects that the combination of left lateral flexion and forward flexion will have a larger range compared to the non-preferred right-sided performed motion. At the same time, it becomes clear that more compression of the thoracic part of the trunk is possible on the preferred side of sweeping.

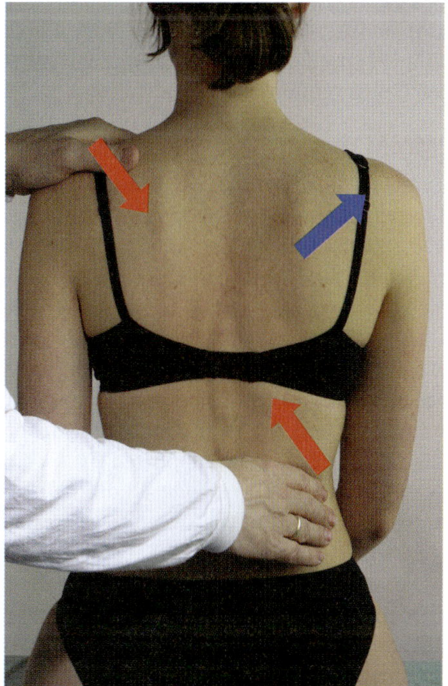

Figure 11.15 Control test for the handedness sweep test: the left hand performs passive left lateral flexion; the right hand fixates at the level of the twelfth rib on the right side. The motion is performed in the frontal plane.

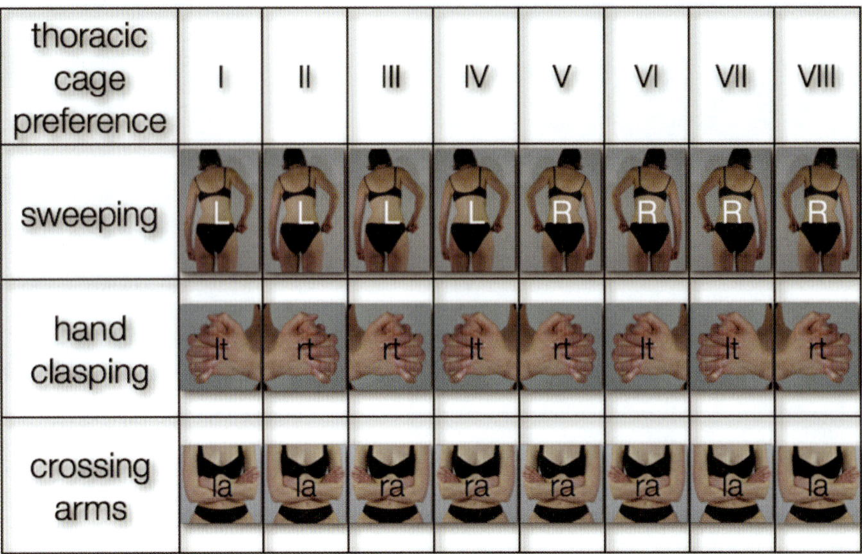

Figure 11.16 Eight different patterns (**I–VIII**) based on three PMMM tests; sweeping test, hand clasping test, and crossing arms test. Sweeping is performed to the left (**L**) or right (**R**). In the hand clasping test, the left (**lt**) or right (**rt**) thumb is on top. In the arm crossing test, the right arm (**ra**) or left arm (**la**) is on top.

Simultaneously, a shift will occur on the opposite (non-preferred) right side.

Based on the results of eight PMMM tests, selections of two or more PMMMs can be made. Dependent upon the number of selected PMMM tests, different patterns can be defined. In the case of a selection of three PMMM tests, $2^3 = 8$ different possible patterns (vertical rows) can be defined, as seen in Figure 11.16. Each of these patterns has a unique combination of test results. Of course, different patterns can be defined in the cervical, pelvic, and lumbar region too.

Based on the findings of the eight PMMM tests, the control tests, and the concluded specific PMMM pattern of the patient, possible PMMM-related interventions can be indicated.

Specific PMMM therapeutic interventions

The primary goal of PMMM interventions is to restore the disturbed and restricted preferred found motion. The results of the eight PMMM tests and their control tests provide information on which region of the trunk (cervicothoracic, upper thoracic, lower thoracic, lumbar/pelvic) has to be treated. Passive mobilizations in the direction of the preferred motion, whether or not combined with isometric mobilization, can be performed. Passive mobilizing treatment can be used to improve the compression component and the shift component of the preferred motion. This therapy is always supported by specific exercise instructions to the patient and is focused on the restricted preferred motion. For instance, if the sweep test is restricted in the preferred direction to the left, passive mobilization through the right shoulder, under fixation at the level of the twelfth rib, can be applied (compression component). On the other hand, the patient can be asked to perform a lateral flexion against resistance combined with a passively performed translation to the opposite side (shift component). In addition, the patient is instructed to exercise, at home, the active left lateral flexion against resistance.

Integrating PMMM in M/M medicine

For the practitioner in M/M medicine, PMMM has to be used as an additional diagnostic and therapeutic approach. In the case of a patient with complaints of localized pain in the locomotor system, the diagnostic phase consists of different phases. First of all, and probably most importantly, a proper medical history has to be taken. This medical history provides information about a possible diagnosis or reason for the complaints of the patient or a differential diagnosis. The medical history is completed with a neurological examination, diagnostic procedures as used in M/M medicine, and a PMMM diagnostic procedure.

Based on the whole diagnostic process, different diagnoses have to be made—a regular medical diagnosis, a M/M medicine diagnosis, and a PMMM diagnosis (preferred motion pattern disturbances).

Both diagnostic procedures and final diagnoses will provide information about priorities with respect to the treatment policy of the individual patient. There may, for instance, be an indication for spinal manipulation and/or mobilization prior to the specific PMMM treatment. It may also be possible that the first priority is a regular treatment, such as a local injection to treat an inflammation, followed by M/M medicine and/or PMMM interventions. Most important of all, and independent of the order of treatment modalities, the therapy is always started with a test treatment.

For a clinician who mainly uses M/M medicine-related treatment, the PMMM can be an alternative if this treatment fails and/or the patient shows an unexplained reoccurrence after several treatment sessions.

Summarizing biomechanics and laterality in musculoskeletal medicine

Although lateralization and mass mechanics play an essential role in the function of the locomotor system, they are not well integrated in the M/M medicine way of thinking. Every patient has his/her own preferential motion patterns for many daily actions. As a logical consequence, it is understandable that disturbances of the performance of these preferred motions can interfere with the daily activities of the patient and can form one of the reasons for the development of pain in one or more regions of the locomotor system.

Evidence for efficacy as an additional therapeutic approach is not yet available. On the other hand, and most importantly, the characteristic diagnostic tests of PMMM have proven to be reproducible (van Wylick 2004). Reproducible test procedures enable us to define homogeneous patient populations for future efficacy studies and, in addition, provide teachers in educational systems of M/M medicine with transferable tests for instructing their students.

PMMM is not meant to be a stand-alone approach or a new 'school' within M/M medicine. Lateralization and mass mechanics are not new concepts as such. Many fundamental studies have been performed in the field of lateralization and mass mechanics and have been integrated into medical disciplines such as neurology and orthopaedic surgery. PMMM can be added to the diagnostic and therapeutic arsenal of already known approaches within M/M medicine such as trigger points, myofascial release, deep postural system, and osteopathy.

Most importantly, PMMM provides the practitioner of M/M medicine with an additional tool and way of thinking to approach his/her therapy-resistant patient.

References

Annett, M. (1999). Eye dominance in families predicted by the right shift theory. *Laterality*, 4(2), 167–72.

Annett, M. (2013). *Handedness and brain asymmetry*. Hove, East Sussex Psychology Press. Ebook.

Van der Bijl, G. (1981). *'Manipulations' from alpha till omega*. Manipulaties van alpha tot omega. Utrecht, Stichting school voor manuele therapie, 78 p.

Van der Bijl, G. (1986). *Het individuelle funktiemodel in de manuele therapie*. De Tijdstroom, Lochem.

Brandler, W. M., Paracchini, S. (2014). The genetic relationship between handedness and neurodevelopmental disorders. *Trends in Molecular Medicine*, 20(2), 83–90. doi:10.1016/j.molmed.2013.10.008.

de Cock, J. J. (1996). *Begrippen van manuele therapie systeem Van der Bijl*. De Tijdstroom, Utrechts.

Crow, T. J. (2010). A theory of the origin of cerebral asymmetry: epigenetic variation superimposed on a fixed right-shift. *Laterality: Asymmetries of Body, Brain and Cognition*, 15(3), 289–303. doi:10.1080/13576500902734900.

Dittmar, M., 2002. Functional and postural lateral preferences in humans: interrelations and life-span age differences. Human biology; an international record of research, 74(4), pp.569–585.

Eligar, R. C. (2011). The laterality of handedness, foot preference and foot overlapping. *Journal of Clinical and Diagnostic Research*.

Gaymans, R. (2004). Manuele geneeskunde en manuele therapie. tigweb.nl, 20(1), pp.142–157.

Gnat, R., Saulicz, E. (2008). Induced static asymmetry of the pelvis is associated with functional asymmetry of the lumbo-pelvo-hip complex. *Journal of Manipulative and Physiological Therapeutics*, 31(3), 204–11. doi:10.1016/j.jmpt.2008.02.012.

Golomer, E., Rosey, F., Dizac, H., Mertz, C., Fagard, J. (2009). The influence of classical dance training on preferred supporting leg and whole body turning bias. *Laterality*, 14(2), 165–77. doi:10.1080/13576500802334934.

Heinen, T., Jeraj, D., Vinken, P., Velentzas, K. (2012). Rotational preference in gymnastics. *Journal of Human Kinetics*, 33(-1). doi:10.2478/v10078-12-0042-4.

Heyne, F. Heyne, B., Pester, H. (1999) *Lateralisations-Asymmetrien: Natur, Kultur und Geschlecht*. Ergebnisse einer Langzeit-Longitudinalstudie. Zeitschrift für Humanontogenetik Heft 2/;S. 39–50.

Giles, G. H. (1959), The Maddox-Rod Phenomenon. AMA Archives of Ophthalmology. 1959;62(5):917. doi:10.1001/archopht.1959.04220050177028.

Kalichman, L., Korostishevsky, M., Kobyliansky, E. (2008). Laterality indices in the Chuvashian population. *Anthropologischer Anzeiger; Bericht Über Die Biologisch-Anthropologische Literatur*, 66(4), 409–18.

Lazenby, R. (2002). Skeletal biology, functional asymmetry and the origins of 'handedness.' *Journal of Theoretical Biology*, 218(1), 129–38.

Lazenby, R. A., Cooper, D. M. L., Angus, S., Hallgrímsson, B. (2008). Articular constraint, handedness, and directional asymmetry in the human second metacarpal. *Journal of Human Evolution*, 54(6), 875–85. doi:10.1016/j.jhevol.2007.12.001.

Lenoir, M., van Overschelde, S., De Rycke, M., Musch, E. (2006). Intrinsic and extrinsic factors of turning preferences in humans. *Neuroscience Letters*, 393(2–3), 179–83. doi:10.1016/j.neulet.2005.09.061.

Lewit, K. (2009). Manipulative therapy: Musculoskeletal medicine. Edinburgh: Elsevier/Churchill Livingstone.

Li, J., Lam, C. S. Y., Yu, M., et al. (2010). Quantifying sensory eye dominance in the normal visual system: a new technique and insights into variation across traditional tests. *Investigative Ophthalmology & Visual Science*, 51(12), 6875–81. doi:10.1167/iovs.10-5549.

Manns, M., Ströckens, F. (2014). Functional and structural comparison of visual lateralization in birds—similar but still different. *Frontiers in Psychology*, 5, 206. doi:10.3389/fpsyg.2014.00206.

McManus, C. (2004). Right hand, left hand: the origins of asymmetry in brains, bodies, atoms and cultures. Available at: < http://www.books.google.com>.

McManus, I. C., Davison, A., Armour, J. A. L. (2013). Multilocus genetic models of handedness closely resemble single-locus models in explaining family data and are compatible with genome-wide association studies. *Annals of the New York Academy of Sciences*, 1288, 48–58. doi:10.1111/nyas.12102.

McManus, I. C., Mascie-Taylor, C. (1979). Hand-clasping and arm-folding: a review and a genetic model. *Annals of Human Biology*. 6(6):527–58

Medland, S.E. et al., 2006. Handedness in twins: joint analysis of data from 35 samples. Twin research and human genetics : the official journal of the International Society for Twin Studies, 9(1), pp.46–53.

Ogah, I., Stewart, E., Treleaven, M., Wassersug, R. J. (2012). Hand clasping, arm folding, and handedness: relationships and strengths of preference. *Laterality: Asymmetries of Body, Brain and Cognition*, 17(2), 169–79. doi:10.1080/1357650X.2010.551126.

Ooki, S. (2014). An overview of human handedness in twins. *Frontiers in Psychology*, 5, 10. doi:10.3389/fpsyg.2014.00010.

Ross, E. P. (2003). The common compensatory pattern: its origin and relationship to the postural model. Am Acad Osteopath J, (Chapter 22), pp. 176–205.

Preece, S. J., Willan, P., Nester, C. J., Graham-Smith, P., Herrington, L., Bowker, P. (2008). Variation in pelvic morphology may prevent the identification of anterior pelvic tilt. *The Journal of Manual & Manipulative Therapy*, 16(2), 113–7.

Procianoy, E., Procianoy, L. (2008). Prevalence of horizontal deviation pattern changes with measurements in extreme gazes. *Eye (London, England)*, 22(2), 229–32. doi:10.1038/sj.eye.6702588.

Reiss, M. (1995). A study of leg-crossing in a German sample. *Anthropologischer Anzeiger; Bericht Über Die Biologisch-Anthropologische Literatur*, 53(3), 263–8.

Reiss, M. (1998). Arm folding—an overview. *Anthropologischer Anzeiger; Bericht Über Die Biologisch-Anthropologische Literatur*, 56(2), 163–78.

Rutte, S. (2001). *Method by Marsman*. Haarlem Marsman Foundaton, pp. 1–15.

Rutte, S. (2002). *A theory about the Marsman method*. Marsman Stichting, Haarlem.

Rutte, S., Fievet, D.,. (2012). *Shoulder function explained by the Marsman theory (Le membre supérieur en Marsman)*. Sauramps Médical ISBN 13: 9782840237730

Sainburg, R. L. (2005). Handedness: differential specializations for control of trajectory and position. *Exercise and Sport Sciences Reviews*, 33(4), 206–13.

Schaafsma, S. M., Riedstra, B. J., Pfannkuche, K. A., Bouma, A., Groothuis, T. G. G. (2009). Epigenesis of behavioural lateralization in humans and other animals. *Philosophical Transactions of the Royal Society of London Series B, Biological Sciences*, 364(1519), 915–27. doi:10.1038/sj.ejhg.5201048.

Sylvester, A. D., Kramer, P. A., Jungers, W. L. (2008). Modern humans are not (quite) isometric. *American Journal of Physical Anthropology*, 137(4), 371–83. doi:10.1002/ajpa.20880.

Vallortigara, G., Rogers, L. J. (2005). Survival with an asymmetrical brain: advantages and disadvantages of cerebral lateralization. *The Behavioral and Brain Sciences*, 28(4), 575–89—discussion 589–633. doi:10.1017/S0140525X05000105.

Varela, J. M. F., Castro, N. B., Biedma, B. M., Da Silva Domínguez, J. L., Quintanilla, J. S., Muñoz, F. M., et al. (2003). A comparison of the methods used to determine chewing preference. *Journal of Oral Rehabilitation*, *30*(10), 990–4.

Vanwylick, Harm. (2004). Voorkeursbewegingen: voorkeur of afkeur? NVOM Bilthoven, ed. Ned Tijdschr Man Gen, (2), pp. 16–21.

Wiener, A. S. (1932). Observations on the manner of clasping the hands and folding the arms. *American Naturalist*, 66(705 (Jul-Aug)), pp. 365–370.

Chapter 12

Muscles in the pathogenesis of musculoskeletal disorders

Vladimir Janda †

The role of muscles in the pathogenesis of musculoskeletal disorders

Although muscles represent the only active tissue that protects the joints, and joints and muscles together form a functional unit, the importance of muscle–joint correlation remains widely underestimated or misunderstood in clinical practice. Even in musculoskeletal medicine, muscles are not considered as an essential factor in the pathogenesis of pain of the musculoskeletal system. These facts are mirrored in the insufficiently precise evaluation of muscle function and in too many unproven treatment programmes. Ironically, active muscle is commonly viewed from a passive aspect, such as various myofascial syndromes and/or trigger points.

One of the first who systematically stressed the importance of muscles in the pathogenesis of low back pain was Hans Kraus. In the 1950s and early 1960s, he noticed that some weakness of the trunk muscles could be demonstrated in about 80% of patients with low back pain (Kraus 1970). Kraus was also one of the first, if not the first, who stressed not only muscle weakness but also muscle tightness in an era when the concept of muscle imbalances was not yet known. Kraus also noticed that dysfunction of the musculoskeletal system starts to develop during childhood. To elucidate this situation he introduced the *Kraus–Weber test* for screening muscle dysfunction (both weakness and tightness) in children. Although more than 50 years old, this test is still valuable.

The role of muscles in pain syndromes of the musculoskeletal system can be considered from several aspects:

- the role of muscles in an acute pain syndrome, both in the pathogenesis as well as in treatment
- the role of muscles in development of chronic pain syndromes
- the role of muscles as a predisposing cause for joint dysfunction
- the role of muscles in prevention of recurrences of acute pain syndromes
- the improvement of muscle function as a basis for a rational treatment programme
- alteration of muscle function in reaction to joint dysfunction, and vice versa.

Muscles in acute pain syndromes

Probably the most important factor that contributes to an acute pain syndrome is the increased tone in a muscle which has anatomical or functional relation to the joint in dysfunction (joint blockage). Generally speaking, the joint blockage is in itself painless. It is commonly the added presence of increased muscle tone to the joint dysfunction that leads to a noticeably painful condition. This fact is often ignored, as detailed evaluation of muscle tone is too rarely carried out. This is indeed surprising, as most (if not all) therapeutic techniques used to treat acute pain syndromes are designed to normalize the increased muscle tone.

Increased muscle tone or hypertonicity are still an obscure clinical entities. Although muscle tone changes can be found in almost every patient, there is no accepted consensus of definition either of muscle tone or of its increase. This is true even for a clinical syndrome such as spasticity.

In musculoskeletal medicine, we have to deal with increased muscle tone that develops as a result of dysfunction (but not a structural lesion) of different levels of the nervous system. These types of hypertonicity are usually described as muscle spasm, although the terminology is not unified and different authors use different terminology for the same phenomenon. Certainly the term 'spasm' should not be confused with 'spasticity'.

From the clinical point of view, muscle tone is a combination of at least two phenomena: shortening of contractile muscle fibres and changes of viscoelasticity, i.e. of the connective tissue of the muscle. Both changes are closely associated with alteration of the irritability threshold of motor units. In musculoskeletal disorders, we have to deal with both types of increased muscle tone, although under different conditions.

Clinical assessment of muscle tone

The clinical assessment of muscle tone is poorly validated and almost always subjective, as all evaluation techniques are non-specific and measure not only the tension of muscle fibres but of all tissue including the skin and subcutaneous tissue. Practical evaluation of muscle tone is currently by deep layer palpation using the examiner's proprioceptive perception.

At least five types of pathologically increased muscle tone can be clinically differentiated in the functional pathology of the motor system. Each can appear separately or in combination. The differential diagnosis is of paramount importance as this may influence the therapeutic result. These five types of increased muscle tone (Janda 1990) may occur due to:

- dysfunction of the limbic system
- dysfunction on the spinal cord segmental level, evidently due to altered function of the interneurons
- impaired coordination of motor unit activation which may finally result in trigger points
- irritation through pain from the musculoskeletal system as well as from the viscera
- muscle tightness (which, however, is more a result of altered elasticity and will be discussed later in the description of muscle imbalance).

The evaluation of muscles can be performed in several ways:

- Evaluation of individual muscles in relation to the joint in dysfunction. This concerns mainly palpation and assessment of muscle spasm and inhibition (muscle pattern), trigger points, and other myofascial syndromes.
- Evaluation of tight and weakened muscles within the framework of muscle imbalance which results in altered biomechanics of the joints, faulty transmission of load across the joint, faulty afferentation from the joint receptors, and ultimately impaired function of joints, with pain as a consequence.
- Evaluation of simple movement patterns in which the main interest is concerned with fine muscle coordination and the sequence in which the main muscles are activated.

Whereas evaluation of muscle spasm should be, as a rule, part of the examination of an acute pain syndrome, evaluation of muscle imbalance and movement patterns is reliable only when the acute episode has subsided and the patient is pain free or almost so.

Treatments for muscle hypertonicity

To decrease muscle hypertonicity due to limbic dysfunction, a locally oriented treatment is generally fruitless. The treatments of choice are techniques oriented to psychological status, such as the autogenic training of Schulze, Alexander technique, some yoga techniques, or even the Feldenkreis approach. Various techniques are available to decrease the other types of hypertonicity, most of them based on principles of postfacilitation inhibition, muscle relaxation, and finally muscle release. However, the details of the treatment technique vary according to the type of hypertonicity. A detailed description is beyond the scope of this chapter, although the differences in technical performance of the therapeutic procedures are quite substantial and may greatly influence the therapeutic effect.

The length of the effect of postfacilitation inhibition techniques varies. It should therefore be considered as an initial treatment that should be followed by an attempt to improve the function of the whole motor system, such as muscle balance or movement patterns.

Muscle imbalance

Muscle imbalance should be considered as one of the principal factors that adversely influence the biomechanics of a joint and contribute to the deterioration of joint function. Muscle imbalance describes the situation in which some muscles become inhibited and weak, while others become tight, lose their extensibility, and become overactive. Moderately tight muscles are usually stronger than normal; however, in the case of pronounced tightness, a decrease of muscle strength occurs. This decrease of muscle strength is called *tightness weakness* (Janda 1993). The principal problem of a tight muscle is not so much the shortening of contractile muscle fibres but rather the altered elastic properties of the connective tissue within the myofascial unit and the decreased irritability threshold of the tight muscle.

The tendency for some muscles to develop weakness or tightness does not occur randomly. Instead, typical patterns of muscle imbalance can be described. The important point is that the development of muscle imbalance follows typical rules that vary individually by degree, but not which muscle will develop tightness or inhibition. Therefore these patterns can be predicted clinically, and this enables the introduction of preventative measures.

Muscles that are tightness-prone are: triceps surae, rectus femoris, hamstrings, thigh adductors, iliopsoas, tensor fasciae latae, quadratus lumborum, pectoralis major and minor, paraspinal extensors, upper trapezius and levator scapulae, and sternocleidomastoid. Less evident tightness-prone muscles are the suprahyoids, in particular the digastric, masseter, and temporalis. In the upper extremity, the flexor muscles are tightness-prone.

On the other hand, muscles that are basically inhibition- or weakness-prone are the dorsiflexors of the foot, vastus medialis, gluteus maximus, medius, and minimus, some abdominal muscles, lower stabilizers of the scapula, deep neck flexors (scaleni, longus colli), and deltoid. In the upper extremity, the extensor muscles are inhibition- prone.

Although muscle imbalance as a systemic response of different muscle groups has been recognized for several decades, there are still some controversies, and some muscles are almost ignored. Thus, for example, we do not have enough knowledge about the differentiation between the abdominal muscles. Evidently, the recti are more inhibition-prone whereas the obliqui often have a tendency to become over-activated. Another muscle which escaped attention for a long time is the transversus abdominis, which is now considered as an important postural muscle (Richardson et al. 1999). Similarly, the importance of the latissimus dorsi is often underestimated and its postural role is uncertain.

Although muscle imbalance involves the whole body, it develops gradually and predictably either in the pelvic region, where we speak of the pelvic or distal crossed syndrome, or in the shoulder girdle/neck region, where we speak of the proximal or shoulder girdle crossed syndrome (Janda 1979). If it starts to develop in the pelvic/hip region and spreads out to the upper part of the body, we speak of the *distoproximal development* of muscle imbalance. If it starts to develop in the shoulder/neck area first and gradually spreads out into the distal part of the body, we speak of the *proximodistal generalization* of muscle imbalance.

There is a correlation between the type of generalization of muscle imbalance and clinical symptoms. Patients with proximodistal generalization suffer first from shoulder–neck problems, whereas those with distoproximal development suffer more from back pain. It is interesting that if the muscle imbalance starts to develop in children, it usually follows the proximodistal direction. This corresponds with clinical experience, as symptoms of neck origin such as school headache are much more frequent in children than low back pain (Gutmann 1984).

Proximal crossed syndrome

The proximal crossed syndrome is characterized by development of tightness of the upper trapezius, levator scapulae, sternocleidomastoid, and pectorals and, on the other hand, inhibition of the deep neck flexors (scaleni) and lower stabilizers of the scapula (serratus anterior, rhomboids, middle and lower trapezius). Topographically, when the inhibited and tight muscles are connected, they form a cross. This type of muscle imbalance results in an altered posture of the upper body. A typical forward position of the head can be found, which results in overstress of three critical segments, i.e. the cervicocranial junction, the cervicocervical transition— the segments C4 and C5, and finally T4 where neck flexion starts. The shoulders are elevated and protracted, altering the resting position of the scapula. This results in an altered position of the axis of the glenoid fossa, which runs more perpendicularly. This increases stresses on the joint capsule and decreases the stability of the joint. As a consequence, altered movement patterns in the shoulder–neck region will develop. This situation can be considered as a predisposing factor for development of typical pain syndromes arising from this region (Janda 1994).

All these changes are not only mirrored in an altered posture but also influence the quality of movements of the whole body, most importantly of gait.

Distal crossed syndrome

Tightness of the hip flexors and trunk erectors and inhibition and weakness of the gluteal and abdominal muscles characterize the distal crossed syndrome. Again, a connection of tight and inhibited muscles forms a cross. This imbalance results in an anterior pelvic tilt, increased flexion of the hips, and a compensatory hyperlordosis. Again, the result is overstress not only of the hips but of the low back as well.

Layers syndrome

In addition to these two syndromes, a layers (stratification) syndrome can be recognized. This syndrome is in principle a combination of the two previous syndromes and can be considered as a response of the muscular system to a long-lasting dysfunction. This development generally means a poor prognosis, and less satisfactory therapeutic results can be expected (Janda 1979). The diagnosis of this syndrome is quick and easy, but important. When the standing patient is observed from the back, the shape of the body looks as if it is composed of layers of bricks. From the bottom, the hamstrings are as a rule hypertrophied and tight, the gluteal muscles hypotonic and loosely hanging and often even atrophied. The paraspinal extensors in the low back area may be atrophied forming a typical groove in the level of lumbar segments, in particular L5–S1. This seems to be paradoxical, as these muscles are usually tightness-prone. Although not confirmed experimentally, this groove may be a result of atrophy of the multifidus, as described by Richardson et al. (1999). This hypotrophied layer is followed by a hypertrophied layer of muscles in the thoracolumbar junction. This hypertrophy is usually associated with segmental hypomobility at the same level. The interscapular area usually shows a marked hypotrophy which can be recognized as flattening of this region. This hypotrophy is frequently associated with shoulder protraction as a result of imbalance between weakened lower stabilizers of the scapula on one hand and shortened pectorals on the other hand. The most proximal layer is formed by a hypertrophied upper trapezius and levator, mostly together with shortened deep neck extensors. Altogether the result is an altered shape of this area, clinically described as *gothic shoulders*.

From the front this syndrome is less pronounced. The most striking appearance is hypotonic abdominal rectis, whereas the obliques are shortened. This can be seen as a deepening along the lateral edge of the recti.

Evaluation of movement patterns in the muscle system

Evaluation of movement patterns is of a paramount importance, as it gives important information about the quality of function of the motor system and in particular of central nervous system (CNS) motor regulation. The more it is understood that function and dysfunction of joints depends on the quality of motor control, the clearer it becomes that movement pattern evaluation is important.

The term 'movement pattern' describes a chain of conditioned and unconditioned motor reflexes that become fixed. Repetition of movement causes this chain to become fixed. Once fixed, the patterns are difficult to change. Borrowing computer language, the patterning process can be compared to the software, whereas the anatomical pathways are the hardware.

Evaluating movement patterns helps us to estimate the degree of inhibition of muscles that are inhibition- prone. Rather than estimating individual muscle strength or weakness, our focus is to determine to what extent, if at all, the particular muscle is included in a specific functional chain.

Basic movement patterns

For diagnostic purposes, in musculoskeletal medicine, six basic movement patterns are used, which cover the main segments of the body (Janda 1996). The first three movement patterns are related to gait (hip extension, hip abduction, curl-up (sit-up) from the supine position); the others relate to the movements of the shoulder girdle and head (head flexion, prone push-up, and shoulder abduction).

Hip extension

This is an important part of the gait cycle. Full hip extension allows minimum anterior tilt of the pelvis in walking and thus reduces the demands and stresses of the low back. The pattern is tested in a prone position. Only the last 10–15° are examined. The most important muscles observed are hamstrings, gluteus maximus, and lumbar and thoracic spinal erectors. The ideal sequence of muscle activation in this chain is: ipsilateral hamstrings, followed by activation of the ipsilateral gluteus and then contralateral lumbar and thoracolumbar erectors. A first sign of an impaired pattern is when the ipsilateral spine erectors precede the activation of the contralateral side. This results in decreased stability of the pelvis and increased anterior pelvic tilt, with overstress of the low back as a consequence. The next step in development of pathology is an increased activity of the thoracolumbar spine erectors and delay of activation of the gluteus maximus, which may in extreme cases even result in its inhibition and inactivity. In patients with chronic low back pain, this inhibition (pseudoparesis) is one of the most frequent pathological findings of the muscle system (Janda 1985).

Hip abduction

Hip abduction and the estimation of the quality of function of the hip abductors is another important evaluation as it gives important information about the stabilization of the pelvis in one leg stance and thus about the degree of lateral shift of the pelvis and overstress on the low back segments in the frontal plane. Tested in a side-lying position, the patient abducts the leg and the sequence of three major muscles is estimated. The ideal sequence is gluteus medius, followed by activation of the tensor fascia lata and the stabilizing role of the quadratus lumborum. The pathological pattern shows the prevalence of the tensor fascia lata, whereas the activity of the gluteus medius is delayed or even absent. In this situation, instead of pure hip abduction, a combined movement composed of hip abduction, flexion, and external rotation, and usually pelvic rotation, produces the movement. This mechanism is described as a tensor mechanism of hip abduction. A worse scenario occurs when the movement is initiated by phasic activity of the quadratus lumborum. In this case, instead of stabilizing the pelvis, the pelvis is shifted up and overstresses the low back.

Curl-up from the supine position

This is used to estimate the interplay between the abdominal muscles and the iliopsoas. The estimation of this relationship is important as the tendency is for the abdominal muscles to weaken whereas the iliopsoas is usually strong and tight. The more active the iliopsoas is, the weaker the abdominals become, which again results in an unwanted overstress of the lumbar segments. The psoas paradox is a situation whereby the functional axis of the tight iliopsoas is shifted beyond the axis of the spine and the muscle, by bilateral action instead of functioning as a flexor of the spine, becomes an extensor of the spine, increasing the lumbar lordosis and the pressures on the lumbar segments.

The test is performed from the supine position. The subject performs an active plantar flexion against the operator's resistance, slight knee flexion pressing the heels toward the plinth. In addition, contraction of the buttocks can be added. During curl-up, the range of motion is stopped when the pelvis starts to tilt forward. The normal range is elevation of the thoracic area (at the level of the inferior angle of the scapula) about 5 cm from the plinth.

Push-up

This gives valuable information about the stabilization of the scapula. Stabilization of the scapula is essential for performance of all movements of the upper extremity. The dysfunctional movements indirectly overstress the cervical spine. Under ideal conditions, the stabilization of the scapula during the push-up should be perfect, i.e. the scapula should not move except at the end of the range of movement, when scapula protraction and abduction normally occurs. Under pathological conditions, the scapula is shifted into adduction or elevation (or both), and in the most severe situation, scapula winging occurs.

When considering muscle function and/or dysfunction in relation to musculoskeletal disorders, we mainly think in terms of muscle weakness of some muscle groups or of muscle shortening in a muscle imbalance syndrome. It has gradually become clear that a chronic pain syndrome is a result of impaired programming of movement or impaired central nervous motor control which has caused impaired coordination between various muscle groups.

As already mentioned, muscles represent the only active tissue which can protect the joints. The question remains, however, as to what are the mechanisms which enable the muscles to protect the joint. It is evident now that the strength of the muscle does not give protection to the joint. Strengthening programmes do not influence the frequency of recurrences of acute pain, so it is necessary to look at other possibilities. Muscle imbalance is definitely one of them. Ekstrand (1982) has shown convincingly, in a series of studies on a group of soccer players, that those who were imbalance-prone suffered almost 10 times more frequently from soft issue injuries than those who maintained a reasonably good muscle balance. When he introduced a training programme oriented towards reducing muscle imbalance, the frequency of soft issue injuries dropped to average. As a result of these observations, Ekstrand concluded that the best way to prevent soft tissue sport injuries is to restore a reasonably good muscle balance. Similarly, much back pain can be compared to a soft tissue injury and one can make a similar conclusion about treatment.

Muscle balance is not, however, to be considered as the only protective factor. Probably the greatest danger for a joint injury is an uncontrolled or poorly controlled movement in a joint beyond its physiological movement barrier. In such cases, the protective function of the muscles is to prevent an excessive range of movement. This depends on the ability of the CNS to activate the necessary number of motor units quickly. In other words, one of the important protective functions of muscles is an improvement of the motor unit firing pattern. The ability of the muscle to activate its motor units fast, and thus to achieve the required intensity of muscle contraction, seems to be the most essential process. Achieving such a fast activation of motor units is a substantial part of a rational exercise programme and seems to be the most effective way to prevent recurrences of acute pain syndromes.

Speed of motor unit firing is thus considered as an important aspect of the role of muscles, not only in treatment but also in the pathogenesis of many pain syndromes.

Muscle patterns and joint dysfunction

The concept of muscle patterns in relation to joint dysfunction is rather new, although it has been known for a long time that a dysfunction or a structural lesion of a joint is associated with changes in muscles that cross the particular joint. These changes, however, were considered to be a reaction of an isolated muscle. Probably the best known example is a vastus medialis wasting associated with knee pathology. Today it is known, however, that these muscle reactions do not just occur in an isolated muscle but involve a group of muscles in a typical pattern. The muscular reaction is not only inhibition, atrophy, and weakness but also muscle spasm. This is true not only for the peripheral joints but for the spinal joints as well. Thus in a joint movement restriction (blockage), we can find that some intrinsic muscles develop spasm whereas others develop inhibition. As these muscles are small and positioned deeply, it is difficult to estimate exactly which muscles respond in which way. This knowledge would facilitate, in particular, the treatment of segmental instability and improve long-term results of mobilization/manipulation of the segment.

In musculoskeletal medicine, probably the most important pattern is that associated with the dysfunction of the sacroiliac joint. On the blocked side, there is spasm in the piriformis and iliopsoas and inhibition of the gluteus maximus. The contralateral side develops inhibition of the gluteus medius and minimus. As a sacroiliac dysfunction is in principle a pelvic torsion, a concurrent shearing tension in the pubic symphysis occurs, evidently resulting in irritation of the lower quadrants of the abdominal recti and thus their spasm and tenderness.

The question remains as to which comes first—the muscle or the joint dysfunction. However, improvement of the muscle pattern may—although there are exceptions—correct the joint dysfunction. More investigation in this area is necessary, but improvement of the muscle pattern often can lead to the correction of the joint dysfunction.

Concluding thoughts about muscles in the pathogenesis of musculoskeletal disorders

The purpose of this chapter is to highlight the enormous importance of muscles in the pathogenesis of musculoskeletal conditions and the need to analyse muscles in much greater detail. This is the case not only in relation to trigger points but also in terms of function. The analysis of function/dysfunction of a single muscle is important, but the coordinated activity of the whole muscle system is in many situations more critical. Any change of position of a joint, active or passive, normal or pathological, is immediately followed by changes within the muscular system. Any change in the CNS is also associated with changes in the muscle system. Muscles can thus be considered as being at a crossroads, where any function, either in the periphery or in the CNS, is mirrored. Muscles therefore belong to one of the most overstressed systems of the body. We are not always aware that even a mental activity is associated with changes in the muscle system.

In addition, muscles should not be understood only as effectors but as an important source of kinesthetic information. This information regulates the function of the CNS which in turn works out the movement patterns and our motor behaviour in general. This fact should be reflected in the treatment of musculoskeletal disorders, such as improvement of proprioception and activation of structures that regulate posture and equilibrium (such as the cerebellar and vestibular system), as well as activation of the brainstem structures (using primitive locomotion).

References

Ekstrand, J. (1982) *Soccer injuries*. Medical Dissertation No. 130, Linkoping University, Sweden.

Gutmann, G. (1984) *Die halswirbelsäule*. G. Fischer Verlag, Stuttgart.

Janda, V. (1979) Die muskulären hauptsyndrome bei vertebragenen beschwerden. In: Neumann, H. D., Wolff H. D. (eds) *Theoretische fortschritte und praktische erfahrungen der manuellen medizin*. Konkordia Verlag, Bühl-Baden.

Janda, V. (1985) Pain in the locomotor system—a broad approach. In: Glasgow, E. F., Twomey, L. T., Scull, E. R., Kleyhans, A. M., Idzak R. M. (eds) *Aspects of manipulative therapy*. Churchill Livingstone, Melbourne.

Janda, V. (1990) Differential diagnosis of muscle tone in respect of inhibitory techniques. In: Paterson, J. K., Burn, L. *Back pain*. Kluwer, Dordrecht.

Janda, V. (1993) Muscle strength in relation to muscle length, pain and muscle imbalance. In: Harms-Ringdahl, K. (ed) *Muscle strength*. Churchill Livingstone, Edinburgh.

Janda, V. (1994) Muscles and motor control in cervicogenic disorders' assessment and management. In: Grant, R. *Physical therapy of the cervical and thoracic spine*, 2nd edn. Churchill Livingstone, New York.

Janda, V. (1996) Evaluation of muscle imbalance. In: Liebenson, C. (ed.) *Rehabilitation of the spine*. Williams and Wilkins, Baltimore, MD.

Kraus, H. (1970) *Clinical treatment of back and neck pain*. McGraw-Hill, New York.

Richardson, C., Jull, G., Hodges, P., Hides, J. (1999) *Therapeutic exercise for spinal segmental stabilization in low back pain*. Churchill Livingstone, Edinburgh.

Chapter 13

Fibromyalgia—a discussion of a diagnostic concept

Jens Foell

We endlessly renegotiate – and we are forced to renegotiate – our notion of reality as our language and our life develops.

Hilary Putnam Sense, nonsense, and the senses: an inquiry into the powers of the human mind. *The Journal of Philosophy* 1994; 91(9):445–517.

Fibromyalgia—essentialism, social constructionism, and classificatory looping

Why does the question of what constitutes reality arise frequently in the context of fibromyalgia? (Harris and Clauw 2006) There is no doubt about the reality of the pain experience and its consequences for those suffering from widespread pain in combination with disturbances of body functions, low mood, and anxiety, but there is controversy about fibromyalgia as a medical diagnosis (Gordon 2003; Wolfe 2009). Similar issues exist in the field of biological psychiatry (Adriaens and De Block 2013). Sceptics see the label 'fibromyalgia' as a medical fad and claim that it is a virtual disease (Hadler 2003). They assume that

> a certain therapeutic domain creates a syndrome in a person with non-specific aches and pains with a tendency to somatise, and with insufficient coping behaviour. In that case we may describe it as the phenotypic iatrogenesis of fibromyalgia. So it is not a disease but also not a constructed syndrome.
>
> Hazemeijer I, Rasker JJ. Fibromyalgia and the therapeutic domain. A philosophical study on the origins of fibromyalgia in a specific social setting. *Rheumatology* 2003; 42(4):507–15.

The opposite position argues that altered nervous system processes in those suffering from chronic pain can be visualized and it is legitimate to say that the brain is in a state of disease in these cases (Abeles et al. 2007; Dadabhoy et al. 2008; Tracey and Bushnell 2009). Measurable deviations from the norm are present in systems regulating autonomic processes like sleep and heart rate variability and can act as biomarkers (Ablin et al. 2009).

Consultations about widespread pain in the locomotion system in combination with mood disturbances, fatigue, and dysfunctions in several organ systems are commonly regarded as difficult (Butler et al. 1999; Jackson and Kroenke 1999). The symptoms may or may not be reported in conjunction by the patient, who may or may not be invited to 'tell the whole story' (Ring et al. 2005). The symptoms may or may not be coded as 'syndrome', a pattern of symptoms indicative of a unifying underlying disease process by the clinician (Jordan et al. 2004). Depending on the setting of the consultation, the cultural background of the participants, and organizational characteristics of the healthcare agency, the formulation for the presented problem may vary (Escobar and Gureje 2007; Kanaan et al. 2012). 'Medically unexplained symptoms', 'somatization', or 'depression' may be the diagnostic vignettes for a heterogeneous set of symptoms with affective, visceral, somatic, and cognitive components. Fibromyalgia is one of them.

The International Classification of Diseases (ICD10) can be seen as a live museum of medical tools. Some are outdated, but not in use; some are relatively new. Fibromyalgia is new. Is 'fibromyalgia' an object or an idea? Ian Hacking distinguishes between classifications of an interactive kind and a natural kind. Natural kinds are not aware of being classified. This is not the case with interactive kinds, social phenomena. Human behaviour and human relationships respond to the way they are categorized (Hacking 1999). In educational literature, this is known as the 'Pygmalion' effect; in the context of fibromyalgia, we are interested in the interactive 'looping' effect of the term. This includes feed forward characteristics ('what is the effect of labelling a person with the diagnosis "fibromyalgia"?') and feed back functions ('how does the concept "fibromyalgia" change in response to being used in clinical contexts?').

The politics of labelling fibromyalgia as a disease

Diagnoses are the basis of transactions in the healthcare industry. They legitimize the boundaries of knowledge domains, form the basis of service remuneration as diagnosis-related groups (DRGs), and guide treatments which should take place (Martin and Singer 2003). In a biomedical framework, they are characterized by the presence of a disease, the aberration from a normal physiological state (Boorse 1975). This seems to lead to a sphere of value-free observations of natural kinds. Exactly this assumption has been questioned.

Medical history is rich in social values expressed through medical diagnoses (Rosenberg 2002). Increasing fragmentation of medical knowledge, expressed in diagnoses, led also to questioning its utility for complex situations, as seen in geriatrics and in rehabilitation medicine (Tinetti and Fried 2004).

The act of establishing a diagnosis can be seen as the duty of the clinician. It can also be seen as an interactive process between the clinician and the patient. Huibers and Wessely explored the challenges of labelling a condition with high impact on people's lives and few consequences for clinical service delivery using chronic fatigue syndrome as their exemplar (Huibers and Wessely 2006). They propose the following elements for a successful management strategy:

- seek an active alliance with the patient
- explore the meaning of suffering, complaints, and predefined illness beliefs
- acknowledge suffering but discourage the sick role or maladaptive illness beliefs
- provide accurate information but be restrictive with implicit prognoses that fuel illness beliefs
- provide simple advice aimed at the necessity to balance rest and activity
- empower the patient to take an active, responsible role in recovery, without inducing blame or guilt.

Table 13.1 Diagnostic criteria for diagnosing fibromyalgia syndrome (American College of Rheumatology 2010) after Wolfe (2010)

Widespread pain index	Score (one for each tick)	Symptom severity (circle one for each option A–D)	0	1	2	3
Shoulder girdle left		A Fatigue	No problem	Mild	Moderate	Severe
Shoulder girdle right						
Upper arm left						
Upper arm right						
Lower arm left		B Waking up unrefreshed in the morning	No problem	Mild	Moderate	Severe
Lower arm right						
Hip (buttock, trochanter) left						
Hip (buttock, trochanter) right						
Upper leg left		C Cognitive symptoms ('fibro-fog')	No problem	Mild	Moderate	Severe
Upper leg right						
Lower leg left						
Lower leg right						
Jaw left		D Number of somatic symptoms	None	Few	Moderate	Many
Jaw right						
Chest						
Abdomen						
Upper back		Score				
Lower back						
Neck						
Total widespread pain index (WPI) (0–19)		**Total somatic symptom score(SS)** (0–12)				

Criteria 1, 2, and 3 are needed for diagnosis of fibromyalgia syndrome:

1) Either widespread pain index (WPI) >7 and somatic symptoms (SS) >5 or WPI 3–6 and SS >9

2) Symptoms at similar level for more than three months

3) No alternative explanation for the pain

Adapted from 'The American College of Rheumatology Preliminary Diagnostic Criteria for Fibromyalgia and Measurement of Symptom Severity', Wolfe, F. et al. (2010). *Arthritis Care and Research* 62(5): 600–10. Copyright © 2014 Wiley.

Fatigue and chronic widespread pain are part of a pool of symptoms which also includes dizziness, nausea, difficulties concentrating, forgetfulness, headaches, restlessness, bloating, or the sensation of having a lump in the throat. Several 'meta-diagnoses' such as 'functional somatic syndromes', 'bodily distress syndrome', 'somatization disorder', or 'idioms of distress' are in use for this symptom pool (Bushnell and Mayer 2009; Crombez et al. 2009; Fink and Rosendal 2008; Hinton and Lewis-Fernández 2010; Landa et al. 2012). Fibromyalgia is one of these 'meta-diagnoses' (Eriksen and Risør 2013). However, the status of fibromyalgia syndrome as a disease is contested amongst doctors (Album and Westin 2008; Tikkinen et al. 2012). Table 13.1 shows the diagnostic criteria for fibromyalgia syndrome.

Historical overview of fibromyalgia

The princess of 'The princess and the pea' is the stereotypical sufferer from the nineteenth-century condition, neurasthenia. She is very delicate. Her reduced pain pressure threshold (a pea under 18 duvet covers) is a sign of her higher social status. Aesthetic refinement was thought to go hand in hand with being physically delicate, in contrast to the assumed robustness of lower-class labourers. Rest cures were the chosen remedy. In contrast, the contemporary stereotypical fibromyalgia sufferer is a woman of low socioeconomical status and low educational attainment, in her post-reproductive life period, with exposure to present or past events of physical or emotional hurt.

The classification of widespread somatic pain associated with polysymptomatic distress has undergone various modifications over the years (see Table 13.2). A common theme is the tenderness of somatic tissue, which appears in the prefix 'fibre'. Sterile inflammation was thought by Gowers in 1903 to be the pathological mechanism accountable for the stiffness and tenderness of the tissue, hence the 'itis' associated with the fibres. Subsequently, the concept was modified and, in the absence of any features of inflammation, the 'itis' was dropped and replaced by the term for aching of the muscles, 'myalgia'. Fibromyalgia as a medical diagnosis was coined in 1990 (Wolfe et al. 1990). Initially, the necessary criteria to attach this diagnostic label to patients included a combination of patient-reported symptoms and the validation of pressure pain tenderness in 18 standardized body locations as physical interaction. In view of the poor specificity and low reliability of the tender point count, the requirement for a diagnostic (or therapeutic) touch-based interaction was removed in 2010 (Wolfe et al. 2010). Current diagnostic criteria rely solely on patients' self-report. They are calculated by combining the amount of painful body regions with the severity of somatic symptoms.

Fibromyalgia as a relatively new diagnostic label is not used with ease by doctors across cultures and specialisms. It is mostly applied in secondary care in rheumatology and pain medicine, also in physiotherapy, and by other actors in the realm of musculoskeletal medicine. The concept arose in the United States from the intersecting interests of patient associations, of the pharmaceutical industry, and of a group of clinicians (Grob 2011). Fibromyalgia has, like chronic fatigue syndrome (CFS), 'orphan status' among the family of diseases—it may be part of confidently used diagnostic labels in some professions, but this does not lead to the delivery of a therapy addressing the causes of the disease. Therapy does not have a home or ownership. This may be related to the fact that drug treatment alone has limited efficacy and multidimensional interdisciplinary treatment is expensive, cumbersome, and difficult to organize.

Table 13.2 Timetable of the evolution of fibromyalgia (after Wolfe 2013)

Neurasthenia	-	1868–1930	Similar to current fibromyalgia: pain, mental fatigue, and myriad other symptoms
Fibrositis	Gowers	1903	Primarily a local condition, with local symptoms including pain and stiffness
Fibrositis	Freyberg	1951	Predominantly a generalized condition
Fibrositis	Graham	1953	Pain, stiffness, and soreness
Fibrositis	Traut	1965–68	Fatigue, poor sleep, headache, colitis, tender points and anxiety
Fibrositis	Smythe-Moldofsky	~1976	Sleep is causal, and tender point counts are diagnostic, widespread aching, very high tender point count (11/14), requirement for specific tender point count, and generalized or widespread pain
Fibrositis	Yunus	1981	Symptoms important, only <25% tender points needed, pain or aching in only three areas
Fibrositis	Goldenberg, Bennett, Wolfe	1980–89	Similar to Smythe-Moldofsky, but only ~60% tender points needed
Fibromyalgia	Wolfe et al. ACR 1990 criteria	1990	11/18 (61%) tender points, widespread pain
Fibromyalgia	Wolfe et al. ACR 2010 criteria	2010	Many painful body regions and high levels of somatic symptoms, fatigue, unrefreshed sleep, cognitive symptoms, can be seen as a continuum

ACR = American College of Rheumatology

Reprinted by permission from Macmillan Publishers Ltd: *Nature Reviews Rheumatology*. Wolfe, F. and B. Walitt (2013). Culture, science and the changing nature of fibromyalgia. Copyright 2015.

Fibromyalgia: consequences of its diagnostic label

What are the consequences? Fibromyalgia as a concept has the capacity to include all the aforementioned components of the symptom pool. The concept is firmly rooted in a neurophysiological model. Functional imaging and immunological investigations demonstrate changes on the molecular level, supporting the idea of fibromyalgia as a disease affecting the pain-processing system (Gur and Aktayoglu 2008; Paiva et al. 2008; Sarzi-Puttini et al. 2010). It can be explained to those who suffer from chronic pain as a maladaptive process (Arthritis Research UK 2013). 'The pain sensation takes place as a product of the interaction between neurophysiological processes, social contexts and cultural meaning' (Wilkinson 2005).

What is the effect of having received a diagnostic label which could reduce illness uncertainty, but without a treatment addressing causative mechanisms? Secondary research using General Practitioner primary care (GP) databases demonstrated a reduction in hospital-based care (Annemans et al. 2008), but qualitative research did not demonstrate increased coping strategies and highlighted the need to negotiate the meaning of this concept in conversations, including with patients and staff alike (Lempp et al. 2009; Undeland and Malterud 2007). A systematic review of pain neurophysiology education (PNE) for chronic low back pain found very low-quality evidence for pain, physical function, psychological function, and social function (Clarke et al. 2011). A metasynthesis of qualitative research into the lived experience of being diagnosed with fibromyalgia highlighted the difficulties of living with an intrusive invisible condition. Patients are reported to frame their experience in a biomedical framework, which potentially could legitimize their suffering with biomedical tests (Sim and Madden 2008), but these tests are absent. Changes in peripheral and central pain processing pathways have been demonstrated in experimental biomedical research, but are not available for the public at large. Central sensitization as a concept makes sense for clinicians with neurophysiological background knowledge, but cannot be measured with biomarkers in individual patients (Yunus 2007). Diagnoses are still based on patient self-report, classified by biomedical experts using arbitrary criteria.

Treatments for fibromyalgia

The general consensus is to conceptualize fibromyalgia as an umbrella term or phenomenological end point of different processes starting at various entry points—adverse childhood experiences, viral infections, inflammatory conditions, traumata, and affective disorders (Clauw 2009). It can also be seen as the end point in the spectrum of polysymptomatic distress (Haeuser et al. 2009).

Fibromyalgia is known as a condition which is associated with high healthcare resource usage (Annemans et al. 2009; Berger et al. 2007; Horndasch 2009). Multidisciplinary treatment is advocated in European and American guidelines (Carville et al. 2008). Combining pharmacological with non-pharmacological approaches is necessary. Non-pharmacological approaches include exercises, education, and dietary interventions—this could be called, euphemistically, lifestyle management or, in a more dramatic way, a change of life. A meta-analysis of randomized trials of cognitive behavioural therapy (CBT) states that CBT can be considered to improve coping with pain and to reduce depressed mood and healthcare-seeking behaviour in patients diagnosed with fibromyalgia (Bernardy et al. 2010).

The multifaceted character of the condition, with an essential psychological component and the association with social disadvantage, introduces complexity in the relationship between intervention and outcome. This includes patient factors such as multimorbidities and network factors such as management by several organizations (Peek et al. 2009; Sturmberg 2012). It is not astonishing that different guideline development groups from different organizations with diverging professional backgrounds come to diverging conclusions about the weighting of research evidence (Häuser et al. 2010).

At present, there are various approaches to treating fibromyalgia, ranging from web-based CBT to mind–body therapies (Wang et al. 2010; Williams et al. 2010). It is very difficult to come to valid conclusions about treatment recommendations if treatment packages, study populations, observation periods, and therapy settings differ as much as they do in this case.

The sequence of the letters B, P, and S

Our reference model is the biopsychosocial (BPS) model (Engel 1977). In this section, I argue that under the surface of being a comprehensive model which takes social, biological, and psychological factors into account, it is a battleground for conflicts about ownership, moral conduct of personhood, accountability, and responsibility (Kirmayer 1988). It can be compared to a board game, with differently labelled sections—'BIO', 'PSYCHO', and 'SOCIAL'. The stakes of pains are placed, shifted, transferred between these sections. The participants in the therapeutic encounter have different, at times diverging or conflicting, interests. In line with the dominance of the biomedical model and specificity theory, placing the stakes of pain in the 'BIO' section has the highest power. It is the location to essentialize the problem (Adriaens and De Block 2013). This also exempts the patient from moral questions. Linking the problem to mental health, formulations starting and including the word 'psyche' may carry suggestions of stigma, blame, or guilt in some cultures.

The sequence of the components in the word 'biopsychosocial' indicates a hierarchy of importance. In the context of the welfare state, a biomedical formulation for distress—the establishment of a disease state—is key to accessing services via healthcare systems. This places the stakes right in the biological sphere. The dilemma of the BPS model lies in the fact that it is still located in a biomedical power relationship (Armstrong 1987). It is governed by interventions which can be done TO the person, IN the organism, by such as invasive procedures or giving drugs. It is rooted in the method of the patho-anatomical correlation, which aims to find structural lesions as cause for the impairment in body function. In contrast, approaches geared to the psychosocial domain aim at improving adaptive work, facilitating behavioural change (Thygeson et al. 2010). Social interventions are outside the power and competency of healthcare practitioners. They are able to assess the influence, but are very limited in changing the environment. Medico-legal dimensions (e.g. access to benefits or successful resolution of compensation claims) are often the highest context in the assessment of a pain state. Tissue damage has high value; maladaptive behaviour after a traumatic event is clinically an important predictive factor, but difficult to assess and judge in a medico-legal context. The most difficult factor is the evaluation of environmental or biographical factors, the fertile ground in which maladaptive responses are likely to develop to some degree. Some authors call these environmental factors which perpetuate pain behaviours and pain states, 'perverse incentives' (Loeser 1999).

Central and peripheral therapeutic targets in fibromyalgia

The old debate about central and peripheral therapeutic targets finds another podium in the concept of fibromyalgia. Chronic low back pain is debated as a problem of the end organ or altered central nervous processing (Apkarian et al. 2009; Roussel et al. 2013). What is the end organ in fibromyalgia? Focal tenderness on palpation in discrete points in muscles, tendons, and entheses, alongside diffuse generalized aching, is a core feature of fibromyalgia. Myofascial trigger points have been identified as sources of nociception in muscle tissue. Their treatment requires identification by mainly palpation, although they have been visualized in imaging studies using magnetic resonance imaging (Chen et al. 2007).

Are fibromyalgia and myofascial pain syndrome separate entities or simply different points on a continuum including peripheral and central aspects? (Bennett and Goldenberg 2011; Gerwin 2005) Does the diagnosis depend on what the clinician is looking for? (Aronoff 1998) One viewpoint sees fibromyalgia as a predominantly central condition with different tissue texture as a component. Manual therapy has a small role in this scenario (Lewit 2011). The opposite position sees an overlap between myofascial trigger points and the tender points in fibromyalgia (Ge 2010). Myofascial trigger points as peripheral pain generators can exacerbate altered central processes (Ge 2006; Ge et al. 2009). Whether a trigger point may be active or latent may be related to descending inhibition processes (Hocking 2010). Proving the effectiveness of either hands-on approaches (such as dry needling for myofascial trigger points) or psychological approaches (such as CBT) may legitimize their inclusion in third-party-funded care packages. In this case, it raises the question of the position of hands-on therapies in the therapeutic arena. Treatment of myofascial trigger points as peripheral targets has been shown to yield positive effects on fibromyalgia, demonstrated by the reduction of aching joints, decrease of analgesia consumption, and decrease of pressure pain threshold (Affaitati et al. 2011).

Being able to reproduce the pain a patient experiences is a very powerful tool in the therapeutic alliance. Identifying myofascial trigger points as peripheral pain generators can do that. Musculoskeletal healthcare practitioners are bound by default to use the modality of touch with more attention to detail than other practitioners. Touch is a powerful communication tool in the interaction with patients complaining of pain in their locomotor system (Gallace and Spence 2010). It is located in the intimate space and invites attachment (Wyschogrod 1981). It enables direct access to the locus of distress and suggests the possibility of bypassing the difficult and tedious process of creating a mutual understanding of the explanation model for the findings. Karel Lewit, a pioneer in musculoskeletal therapies, conceptualizes palpation as a diagnostic modality which can bypass the subjectivity of the patient, just like imaging (Lewit 2011). However, this dimension remains a challenge in encounters about conditions affecting the mental and physical sphere.

Fibromyalgia as a condition with a significant component of an emotional need state, challenges the boundaries of the therapeutic relationship (Davies et al. 2009). Cure as an end point for the therapeutic intervention is an unrealistic expectation. Unsustained and partial pain relief is realistic. This leaves musculoskeletal practitioners in a delicate and ambiguous position. The conversation about boundary setting, about when and how to accept pain, and working *with* pain instead of *against* pain to reduce suffering is a difficult conversation to have (Wilson et al. 2009).

Using hands-on therapies in the context of chronic disease management is an underexplored area, but this is exactly the challenge of using touch-therapies in the management of fibromyalgia. Favouring a predominantly peripheral approach, by focusing on reducing the nociceptive barrage from trigger points, risks neglecting other important factors such as lifestyle modification or changing the attitude towards the problem. On the other hand, favouring a predominantly central approach, by treating sufferers like 'brains in jars' and adding psychotropic medication to the pickling liquid, risks neglecting the body as subject of the lived experience of suffering (Edwards 1998).

At present, there is no reliable way of both identifying fibromyalgia subgroups and delivering tailored treatments. Multicomponent treatments promoting self-management strategies are recommended in current guidelines (Rahman et al. 2014).

Summary of fibromyalgia as a diagnostic concept

Generalizing functional pain disorders are common. Their prevalence rates vary according to research methodology, classification criteria, and sample selection between 1% and 35% (Mansfield 2013; Ospina and Hartstall 2002). Fibromyalgia syndrome is currently considered to represent the severe end of a continuous spectrum of polysymptomatic distress. The diagnostic labels in use to deal with this 'symptom pool' have changed over time and according to culture. Recent progress in basic science and epidemiology changed the understanding of mechanisms on the molecular and the societal level which favour the emergence of persisting widespread pain. Fibromyalgia as a concept organizes this knowledge within a biopsychosocial framework. Despite ongoing controversies, it is established in the biomedical realm. This makes it useful for secondary research or health service planning, if it is used for coding purposes.

Fibromyalgia is, despite the progress in understanding the molecular mechanisms of chronic pain, not associated with effective therapies. 'Cure sometimes, relieve often, comfort always' summarizes an ethical stance of what to do with patients, of what to expect from treatments (Rakel 2000). 'Comfort always' would be comparable with 'small effect sizes' in current terminology (Nüesch et al. 2013). It means that both clinicians and patients ought to let themselves into a longstanding relationship—a relationship which includes the acceptance of only partial and unsustained symptom relief. Care instead of cure is the prevailing paradigm.

Clinical coding or codifying suffering is a political and moral act. It has to take the consequences of this act into account. It is performed within a relationship of stakeholders with at times conflicting interests (Bedson et al. 2004). Coding serves the interest of establishing an accurate information infrastructure for public health purposes. It also is a document of the interaction between clinician and patient and serves the purpose of establishing a therapeutic alliance. Taking these aspects into consideration, we argue that 'fibromyalgia' as a diagnostic label has to be used wisely, with a view towards the consequences it has. Meta-qualitative research demonstrates how labels can both validate or invalidate the patient experience. This has to be seen as a process, not as an individual act (Toye et al. 2013). In musculoskeletal care, it means that the place of hands-on therapies in pain management strategies deserves particular attention. Care instead of cure is the motto.

Touch-based therapies put the therapist in a privileged position. Careful assessment of the musculoskeletal complaint can at times reproduce the patient's pain, which can generate a sense of being understood without having to resort to words. Touch is a powerful interpersonal modality to establish trust. Trust is essential for the therapeutic alliance. In this sense, I argue that touch-based therapies, with their implicit reciprocity, are at least a powerful tool to build a therapeutic relationship, which is essential for the holding work required in a chronic pain condition like fibromyalgia. Whether fibromyalgia as a concept is able to assert authority over the pool of symptoms indicating either central sensitization (in a neurophysiological framework) or aesthetic resistance (in an anthropological framework) remains to be seen (Eriksen et al. 2013; Yunus 2008).

In the absence of effective therapies, as the consequence of a diagnosis, and with the presence of multiple psychological symptoms with potential moral implications and the strong association with social disadvantage, the controversy about the utility of the 'F' word is likely to continue. Nevertheless, it offers the opportunity to give a name to a bothersome condition of polysymptomatic distress. This name can be a tool to measure the prevalence of widespread pain in the population at large. On an individual basis, it has the potential to reduce clinical uncertainty.

References

Abeles AM, Pillinger MH, Solitar BM, Abeles M. Narrative review: the pathophysiology of fibromyalgia. *Annals of Internal Medicine*. 2007; 146(10):726–34.

Ablin J, Buskila D, Clauw D. Biomarkers in fibromyalgia. *Current Pain and Headache Reports*. 2009; 13(5):343–9.

Adriaens PR, De Block A. Why we essentialize mental disorders. *Journal of Medicine and Philosophy*. 2013; 38(2):107–27.

Affaitati G, Costantini R, Fabrizio A, Lapenna D, Tafuri E, Giamberardino M. Effects of treatment of peripheral pain generators in fibromyalgia patients. *European Journal of Pain*. 2011; 15:61–9.

Album D, Westin S. Do diseases have a prestige hierarchy? A survey among physicians and medical students. *Social Science & Medicine*. 2008; 66:182–8.

Annemans L, Le Lay K, Taïeb C. Societal and patient burden of fibromyalgia syndrome. *PharmacoEconomics*. 2009; 27(7):547–59

Annemans L, Wessely S, Spaepen E, et al. Health economic consequences related to the diagnosis of fibromyalgia syndrome. *Arthritis & Rheumatology*. 2008; 58(3):895–902.

Apkarian AV, Baliki MN, Geha PY. Towards a theory of chronic pain. *Progress in Neurobiology*. 2009; 87(2):81–97.

Armstrong D. Theoretical tensions in biopsychosocial medicine. *Social Science & Medicine*. 1987; 25(11):1213–8.

Aronoff GM. Myofascial pain syndrome and fibromyalgia: a critical assessment and alternate view. *The Clinical Journal of Pain*. 1998; 14(1):74–8.

Arthritis Research UK Primary Care Centre. *Musculoskeletal core skills*. Chesterfield: Arthritis Research UK in collaboration with RCGP; 2013.

Bedson J, McCarney R, Croft P. Labelling chronic illness in primary care: a good or a bad thing? *British Journal of General Practice*. 2004; 54(509):932–8.

Bennett R, Goldenberg D. Fibromyalgia, myofascial pain, tender points and trigger points: splitting or lumping? *Arthritis Research & Therapy*. 2011; 13(3):117.

Berger A, Dukes E, Martin S, Edelsberg J, Oster G. Characteristics and healthcare costs of patients with fibromyalgia syndrome. *International Journal of Clinical Practice*. 2007; 61(9):1498–508.

Bernardy K, Füber N, Küllner V, Hüuser W. Efficacy of cognitive-behavioral therapies in fibromyalgia syndrome—a systematic review and metaanalysis of randomized controlled trials. *The Journal of Rheumatology*. 2010; 37(10):1991–2005.

Boorse C. On the distinction between disease and illness. *Philosophy and Public Affairs*. 1975; 5(1):49–68.

Bushnell MC, Mayer EA. Functional pain syndromes: presentation and pathophysiology. In: Mayer EA, Bushnell MC (ed.) Seattle: IASP Press; 2009.

Butler CC, Evans M, Welsh P, General practice discussion group T. The heartsink patient revisited. *British Journal of General Practice*. 1999; 49:230–3.

Carville SF, Arendt-Nielsen S, Bliddal H, et al. EULAR evidence-based recommendations for the management of fibromyalgia syndrome. *Annals of the Rheumatic Diseases*. 2008; 67(4):536–41.

Chen Q, Bensamoun S, Basford JR, Thompson JM, An K-N. Identification and quantification of myofascial taut bands with magnetic resonance elastography. *Archives of Physical Medicine and Rehabilitation*. 2007; 88(12):1658–61.

Clarke CL, Ryan CG, Martin DJ. Pain neurophysiology education for the management of individuals with chronic low back pain: a systematic review and meta-analysis. *Manual Therapy*. 2011; 16(6):544–9.

Clauw DJ. Fibromyalgia: an overview. *The American Journal of Medicine*. 2009; 122(Supp. 12):S3–S13.

Crombez G, Beirens K, Van Damme S, Eccleston C, Fontaine J. The unbearable lightness of somatisation: a systematic review of the concept of somatisation in empirical studies of pain. *Pain*. 2009; 145(1–2): 31–5.

Dadabhoy D, Crofford L, Spaeth M, Russell IJ, Clauw D. Biology and therapy of fibromyalgia. Evidence-based biomarkers for fibromyalgia syndrome. *Arthritis Research & Therapy*. 2008; 10(4):211.

Davies KA, Macfarlane GJ, McBeth J, Morriss R, Dickens C. Insecure attachment style is associated with chronic widespread pain. *Pain*. 2009; 143(3):200–5.

Edwards S. The body as object versus the body as subject: the case of disability. *Medicine, Health Care and Philosophy*. 1998; 1(1):47–56.

Engel G. The need for a new medical model: a challenge for biomedicine. *Science*. 1977; 196(4286):129–36.

Eriksen T, Risør M. What is called symptom? *Medicine, Health Care and Philosophy*. 2013: 1–14.

Eriksen T, Kirkengen A, Vetlesen A. The medically unexplained revisited. *Medicine, Health Care and Philosophy*. 2013; 16(3):587–600.

Escobar JI, Gureje O. Influence of cultural and social factors on the epidemiology of idiopathic somatic complaints and syndromes. *Psychosomatic Medicine*. 2007; 69(9):841–5.

Fink P, Rosendal M. Recent developments in the understanding and management of functional somatic symptoms in primary care. *Current Opinion in Psychiatry*. 2008; 21(2):182–8.

Gallace A, Spence C. The science of interpersonal touch: an overview. *Neuroscience & Biobehavioral Reviews*. 2010; 34(2):246–59.

Ge H. Prevalence of myofascial trigger points in fibromyalgia: the overlap of two common problems. *Current Pain and Headache Reports*. 2010; 14:339–45.

Ge HY, Fernandez-de-Las-Penas C, Rendt-Nielsen L. Sympathetic facilitation of hyperalgesia evoked from myofascial tender and trigger points in patients with unilateral shoulder pain. *Clinical Neurophysiology*. 2006; 117(7):1545–50.

Ge HY, Nie H, Madeleine P, Anneskiold-Samsøe B, Graven-Nielsen T, Arendt-Nielsen L. Contribution of the local and referred pain from active myofascial trigger points in fibromyalgia syndrome. *Pain*. 2009; 147(1–3):233–40.

Gerwin RD. A review of myofascial pain and fibromyalgia—factors that promote their persistence. *Acupuncture in Medicine*. 2005; 23(3):121–34.

Gordon DA. Fibromyalgia—real or imagined? *The Journal of Rheumatology*. 2003; 30(8):1665.

Grob GN. The rise of fibromyalgia in 20th-century America. *Perspectives in Biology and Medicine*. 2011; 54(4):417–37.

Gur A, Oktayoglu P. Status of immune mediators in fibromyalgia. *Current Pain and Headache Reports*. 2008; 12(3):175–81.

Hacking I. *The social construction of what?* Cambridge, Massachusetts and London, England: Harvard University Press; 1999, p. 261.

Hadler NM. 'Fibromyalgia' and the medicalization of misery. *The Journal of Rheumatology*. 2003; 30(8):1668–70.

Haeuser WINF, Schmutzer GABR, Bruehler ELMA, Glaesmer HEID. A cluster within the continuum of biopsychosocial distress can be labeled as fibromyalgia syndrome. Evidence from a representative German population survey. *The Journal of Rheumatology*. 2009; 36(12):2806–12.

Harris R, Clauw D. How do we know that the pain in fibromyalgia is 'real'? *Current Pain and Headache Reports*. 2006; 10(6):403–7.

Häuser W, Thieme K, Turk DC. Guidelines on the management of fibromyalgia syndrome—a systematic review. *European Journal of Pain*. 2010; 14(1):5–10.

Hazemeijer I, Rasker JJ. Fibromyalgia and the therapeutic domain. A philosophical study on the origins of fibromyalgia in a specific social setting. *Rheumatology*. 2003; 42(4):507–15.

Hinton D, Lewis-Fernández R. Idioms of distress among trauma survivors: subtypes and clinical utility. *Culture, Medicine and Psychiatry*. 2010; 34(2):209–18.

Hocking MJL. Trigger points and central modulation—a new hypothesis. *Journal of Musculoskeletal Pain*. 2010; 18(2):186–203.

Horndasch S. Hohe inanspruchnahme des gesundheitswesens durch fibromyalgiepatienten. *Schmerz*. 2009; 23(1):70–1.

Huibers MJH, Wessely S. The act of diagnosis: pros and cons of labelling chronic fatigue syndrome. *Psychological Medicine*. 2006; 36(07): 895–900.

Jackson JL, Kroenke K. Difficult patient encounters in the ambulatory clinic: clinical predictors and outcomes. *Archives of Internal Medicine*. 1999; 159(10):1069–75.

Jordan K, Porcheret M, Croft P. Quality of morbidity coding in general practice computerized medical records: a systematic review. *Family Practice*. 2004; 21:396–412.

Kanaan RA, Armstrong D, Wessely SC. The function of 'functional': a mixed methods investigation. *Journal of Neurology, Neurosurgery & Psychiatry*. 2012; 83(3):248–50.

Kirmayer LJ. Mind and body as metaphors: hidden values in biomedicine. In: Lock M, Gordon D. (ed.) *Biomedicine examined*. Dordrecht: Kluwer; 1988.

Landa A, Peterson BS, Fallon BA. Somatoform pain: a developmental theory and translational research review. *Psychosomatic Medicine*. 2012; 74(7):717–27.

Lempp H, Hatch S, Carville S, Choy E. Patients' experiences of living with and receiving treatment for fibromyalgia syndrome: a qualitative study. *BMC Musculoskeletal Disorders*. 2009; 10(1):124.

Lewit K. Fibromyalgia and palpation. *International Musculoskeletal Medicine*. 2011; 33(1):34–.

Loeser JD. Economic implications of pain management. *Acta Anaesthesiologica Scandinavica*. 1999; 43(9):957–9.

Mansfield K. *Identifying chronic widespread pain in primary care—a medical record database study*. (Doctor of Philosophy thesis). Keele: Keele University; 2013.

Martin D, Singer P. A strategy to improve priority setting in health care institutions. *Health Care Analysis*. 2003; 11(1):59–68.

Nüesch E, Häuser W, Bernardy K, Barth J, Jüni P. Comparative efficacy of pharmacological and non-pharmacological interventions in fibromyalgia syndrome: network meta-analysis. *Annals of the Rheumatic Diseases*. 2013; 72(6):955–62.

Ospina M, Harstall C. Prevalence of chronic pain: an overview. Edmonton: Alberta Heritage Foundation for Medical Research; 2002.

Paiva E, Mariano da Costa E, Scheinberg M. Fibromyalgia: an update and immunological aspects. *Current Pain and Headache Reports*. 2008; 12(5):321–6.

Peek CJ, Baird MA, Coleman E. Primary care for patient complexity, not only disease. *Families, Systems & Health*. 2009; 27(4):287–302.

Putnam H. Sense, nonsense, and the senses: an inquiry into the powers of the human mind. *The Journal of Philosophy*. 1994; 91(9):445–517.

Rahman A, Underwood M, Carnes D. Fibromyalgia. *BMJ*. 2014; 348.

Rakel RE. Compassion and the art of family medicine: from Osler to Oprah. *The Journal of the American Board of Family Practice*. 2000; 13(6): 440–8.

Ring A, Dowrick CF, Humphris GM, Davies J, Salmon P. The somatising effect of clinical consultation: What patients and doctors say and do not say when patients present medically unexplained physical symptoms. *Social Science & Medicine*. 2005;61(7):1505–15.

Rosenberg CE. The tyranny of diagnosis: specific entities and individual experience. *Milbank Quarterly*. 2002; 80(2):237–60.

Roussel NA, Nijs J, Meeus M, Mylius V, Fayt C, Oostendorp R. Central sensitization and altered central pain processing in chronic low back pain: fact or myth? *Clinical Journal of Pain*. 2013; 29(7):625–38.

Sarzi-Puttini P, Atzeni F, Cazzola M. Neuroendocrine therapy of fibromyalgia syndrome: an update. *Annals of the New York Academy of Sciences*. 2010; 1193(1):91–7.

Sim J, Madden S. Illness experience in fibromyalgia syndrome: a metasynthesis of qualitative studies. *Social Science & Medicine*. 2008; 67(1): 57–67.

Sturmberg JP. Caring for people with chronic disease: is 'muddling through' the best way to handle the multiple complexities? *Journal of Evaluation in Clinical Practice*. 2012; 18(6):1220–5.

Thygeson M, Morrissey L, Ulstad V. Adaptive leadership and the practice of medicine: a complexity-based approach to reframing the doctor–patient relationship. *Journal of Evaluation in Clinical Practice*. 2010; 16(5):1009–15.

Tikkinen KAO, Leinonen JS, Guyatt GH, Ebrahim S, Järvinen TLN. What is a disease? Perspectives of the public, health professionals and legislators. *BMJ Open*. 2012; 2(6).

Tinetti ME, Fried T. The end of the disease era. *The American Journal of Medicine*. 2004; 116(3):179–85.

Toye F, Seers K, Allcock N, et al. Patients' experiences of chronic non-malignant musculoskeletal pain: a qualitative systematic review. *British Journal of General Practice*. 2013; 63(617):e829–e41.

Tracey I, Bushnell MC. How neuroimaging studies have challenged us to rethink: is chronic pain a disease? *The Journal of Pain*. 2009; 10(11): 1113–20.

Undeland M, Malterud K. The fibromyalgia diagnosis—hardly helpful for the patients? *Scandinavian Journal of Primary Health Care*. 2007; 25(4): 250–5.

Wade D. Complexity, case-mix and rehabilitation: the importance of a holistic model of illness. *Clinical Rehabilitation*. 2011; 25(5):387–95.

Wang C, Schmid CH, Rones R, et al. A randomized trial of Tai Chi for fibromyalgia. *New England Journal of Medicine*. 2010; 363(8):743–54.

Wilkinson I. *Suffering—a sociological introduction*. Cambridge: Polity; 2005, p. 189.

Williams DA, Kuper D, Segar M, Mohan N, Sheth M, Clauw DJ. Internet-enhanced management of fibromyalgia: a randomized controlled trial. *Pain*. 2010; 151(3):694–702.

Wilson D, Williams M, Butler D. Language and the pain experience. *Physiotherapy Research International*. 2009; 14(1):56–65.

Wolfe F. Fibromyalgia wars. *The Journal of Rheumatology*. 2009; 36(4):671–8.

Wolfe F, Clauw DJ, Fitzcharles M-A, et al. The American College of Rheumatology preliminary diagnostic criteria for fibromyalgia and measurement of symptom severity. *Arthritis Care & Research*. 2010; 62(5):600–10.

Wolfe F, Smythe H, Yunus M, et al. The American College of Rheumatology 1990 criteria for the classification of fibromyalgia. *Arthritis & Rheumatism*. 1990; 33:160–72.

Wyschogrod E. Empathy and sympathy as tactile encounter. *Journal of Medicine and Philosophy*. 1981; 6(1):25–43.

Yunus MB. Central sensitivity syndromes: a new paradigm and group nosology for fibromyalgia and overlapping conditions, and the related issue of disease versus illness. *Seminars in Arthritis and Rheumatism*. 2008; 37(6):339–52.

Yunus MB. Role of central sensitization in symptoms beyond muscle pain, and the evaluation of a patient with widespread pain. *Best Practice & Research Clinical Rheumatology*. 2007; 21(3):481–97.

Chapter 14

Myofascial pain syndrome: a bogus construct

John Quintner and Milton Cohen

Myofascial pain syndrome: the clinical problem

Patients present to their clinicians complaining of pain felt within soft tissues, usually voluntary muscles, in which regions of tenderness and firmness can be detected. Palpation of these regions, which have been evocatively termed 'trigger points,' is reported to reproduce the pain of which they complain. The face validity of this assertion is compelling and has generated a widely but uncritically accepted clinical model, that of 'myofascial pain' (MP). Allied to this is a therapeutic industry that claims success for treatment directed to 'trigger points'. However, the scientific basis of myofascial pain syndrome (MPS) has not been established. Furthermore, there is neither consensus on diagnosis of MP nor evidence for efficacy of therapy directed to 'trigger points' that cannot be attributed to a placebo (contextual) effect.

It is remarkable that the previous statement can be made in an age of such sophisticated techniques for investigating presumed somatic pathology. It is equally astonishing that the logical errors inherent in MPS continue to be ignored by its proponents.

This chapter does not seek to deny the phenomena of muscle pain and tenderness in the absence of an obvious or discernable source of local nociception. Rather, an examination of the tenets of MPS as an explanation for those phenomena finds that it lacks both scientifically valid evidence and logically consistent argument. A replacement for the bogus construct of MPS is necessary, to advance knowledge and enhance patient care.

The assertions of myofascial pain syndrome

MPS falls within the framework of biomedical reductionism wherein a direct cause and effect relationship is said to exist between the complaint of pain felt in bodily tissues and pathological changes in those tissues.

The MPS model is best summarized, in the words of one of its creators, as a 'complex of sensory, motor and autonomic symptoms that are caused by myofascial trigger points' (Simons 1990). In turn, trigger points (TrPs) were defined as 'spots of exquisite tenderness and hyperirritability in muscles or their fascia, localised in taut, palpable bands' (Simons 1990). In other words, MP is caused (*sic*) by painful loci in myofascial tissues—a classical circular argument. Irrespective of this fallacy of logic, the scientific validity of MPS turns on whether this set of assertions does in fact explain and predict the natural processes that underlie localized pain. Determination of these matters is dependent upon the available empirical evidence as to the reliability of TrP examination, and whether there are objective findings that would substantiate the pathological basis of TrPs.

Historical evolution of the MPS model

In the early years of the last century, the eminent British neurologist, Sir William Gowers, proposed the term 'fibrositis' for a condition that he thought responsible for the clinical presentation described here (Gowers 1904). His proposal was in fact dual: that pain might originate from focal lesions within or near voluntary muscles, *and* that the 'pathology' was low-grade inflammation occurring in and spreading within connective tissues, which could then in some way 'compromise' afferent nerves that terminate in the interstitial tissue between the muscle fibres and innervate muscle spindles (Gowers 1904; Travell and Rinzler 1952).

According to Gowers, the main features of 'fibrositis' were the presence in soft tissues (fat, musculo-tendinous structures, and nerve sheaths) of localized 'trigger points' that were tender and from which pain could radiate or apparently be induced elsewhere (Copeman 1936). The phenomenon was thought to be secondary to recent or previous infections (Copeman 1943). When palpable, these points were referred to by Stockman in 1920 as 'fibrositic nodules' (Stockman 1920).

During the late 1930s, Kraus (cited by Simons 1975) postulated that palpable muscle hardenings could set up a reflexly induced increase in muscle tension resulting in a 'pain–reflex–pain self-perpetuating cycle' that could be disrupted by ethyl chloride sprayed onto the overlying skin or by local injections. What was termed the 'vicious circle' hypothesis was favoured by pioneers in pain theory.

In 1952, Travell and Rinzler announced that pain felt in voluntary muscles could be 'myofascial' in origin (Travell and Rinzler 1952). They proclaimed that such 'trigger areas in myofascial structures can maintain pain cycles indefinitely'. In a concise description of their hypothesis (Simons and Travell 1981), and in their highly influential book, Travell and Simons formalized the construct of 'myofascial pain arising from trigger points' (Travell and Simons 1983).

TrPs were described in exactly the same way as were fibrositic nodules. They could potentially develop within every voluntary muscle and in multiple locations within a given muscle. Travell and Rinzler (1952) had determined patterns of referred pain for 32 muscles and, based on their collective observations, compiled anatomical charts of TrPs. They also stated that TrPs varied in location from person to person. Lewit (1979) aptly noted that the diagrams had 'sometimes been chosen arbitrarily, there being no accepted standard'.

Less well remembered, Travell and Simons (1983) claimed that TrPs could be found in other somatic tissues (i.e. non-myofascial TrPs) including skin, scar tissue, fascia, ligaments, and periosteum, as had been initially proposed by Gowers and others. These non-muscular TrPs were not included in their diagrams and have since been overlooked. The 'trigger point' was now held to be a site of focal hypertonicity within muscle, with a local aetiology, and in need of direct treatment.

MPS was then defined by Travell and her co-workers as comprising two essential components: (i) the TrP—a localized area of tenderness or hyperirritability deep within voluntary muscle; and (ii) a predictable discrete zone of deep aching pain, which could be located in the immediate region of, or remote from the TrP, and which was worsened by palpation of the TrP (Travell and Simons 1983).

Described as being located within palpable 'taut bands' (another unsubstantiated phenomenon), TrPs were purported to represent shortened ('contractured'—Dommerholt 2011) muscle fibres. The taut bands were said to be a potential source of peripheral nerve entrapment (Travell and Simons 1983). On 'snapping' palpation or needling of a TrP, a local twitch response could be elicited (termed the 'jump' sign), which was said to be accompanied by an 'irritable' electromyographic response (Travell and Simons 1983). A muscle containing a TrP exhibited both antalgic inhibition when tested for its strength and an intolerance to passive stretch. Muscles that were adjudged as 'normal' exhibited neither taut bands nor local twitch responses, and when subjected to pressure were not associated with pain experienced remotely. This left Travell and Simons with a dilemma: how best to explain the development of TrPs in seemingly 'normal' muscles.

To solve this problem, Travell and Simons invented the concept of the 'latent' TrP, which was said to be a site of tenderness within a muscle, unassociated with spontaneous pain but having the potential to be activated by any one of a myriad of factors residing within or without the body (Travell and Simons 1983). When explaining the tendency for initial localized muscle pain to become widespread, they claimed that 'active' TrPs could in some mysterious way self-propagate to become 'secondary' TrPs in other muscles and even to 'metastasise' throughout the bodily musculature. Travell and Simons also described, in considerable detail, the various techniques of physical therapy designed to 'deactivate' these purportedly offending lesions within muscles and thereby disrupt the 'vicious cycle', with the expectation of relieving the pain for which they were held to be responsible.

Critical examination of the empirical evidence on which myofascial pain syndrome is based

Reliability of TrP examination

Because the identification of individual putative TrPs is entirely a clinical matter, it is important to investigate the reliability of the palpatory findings that are their claimed diagnostic criteria.

In all the studies that have reported on inter-examiner reliability related to TrP localization, the examiners were given the muscle within which to palpate (trapezius or rotator cuff), with or without an accompanying 'diagnosis' (Bron et al. 2007; Lucas et al. 2009; Myburgh et al. 2011; Sciotti et al. 2001). Extensive training, coupled with the use of an algometer, led to examiner agreement in only one study (Lucas et al. 2009). However, when blinded as to 'diagnosis', those who claimed expertise in the field of MP were unable to detect putative TrPs in the majority of subjects diagnosed as MPS (Myburgh et al. 2011). There was virtually no inter-examiner reliability for either putative TrPs or taut bands. Other studies have also reported poor inter-examiner diagnostic reliability (Hsieh et al. 2000: Lew et al. 1997), and have concluded that the published studies are of poor methodological quality (Myburgh et al. 2008).

An extensive review identified the use of at least 19 different sets of diagnostic criteria for the MPS/TrP syndrome, reporting that consistency and consensus on case definition were both lacking (Tough et al. 2007). This same study reported that the majority of studies had utilized the criterion of a 'tender point in a taut band' and the predicted pattern of pain referral. The other criteria, as formulated by Travell and Simons, were used less commonly. The review's authors concluded that until reliable diagnostic criteria had been established, 'there is a need for greater transparency in research papers on how a case of MTrP (sic) pain syndrome is defined, and claims for effective interventions in treating the condition should be viewed with caution.' (Tough et al. 2007)

A similar study found that the diagnosis of MPS from putative TrPs was based on a clinical test of unknown reliability and validity and that there was no accepted reference standard: 'On the basis of the limited number of studies available, and significant problems with their design, reporting, statistical integrity, and clinical applicability, physical examination cannot currently be recommended as a reliable test for the diagnosis of TPs.' (Lucas et al. 2009)

At least three problems were identified that would confound further research: the inclusion of inappropriate (i.e. asymptomatic) cases; the impossibility of determining diagnosis with anatomical precision; and the uncertainty of assessment of TrP resolution after treatment (Lucas et al. 2009). The authors concluded that high-quality studies were needed to address these issues.

In summary, well-designed scientific inquiry has shown that physical examination cannot be relied upon to diagnose a condition that is said to be defined by that physical examination. That is, the pathognomonic criterion for making the 'diagnosis' is unreliable. How then can this putative entity be sustained and inform specific treatment?

The search for a lesion

Much research has been performed to determine whether there are pathological findings that would explain the 'trigger point' phenomenon. All have been performed under the a priori assumption that local pathology exists within muscle.

Anatomical studies

The first histological analysis of 'fibrositic nodules' reported inflammatory hyperplasia with numerous fibroblasts, serous or serofibrinous exudation, and thickening of the walls of the small blood vessels and nerve sheaths (Stockman 1913). No data were presented: only a discussion wherein the author concluded that the essential pathological changes in 'fibrositis' were confined to the white fibrous tissue (fascia) in connection with the muscles, joints, and peripheral nerves. However, these findings were not confirmed in another study, although it was reported that tender muscles contained increased extracellular fluid, consistent with oedema, with few other signs of inflammation (Brendstrup et al. 1957). The authors concluded that this increase, and the resulting turgor, could explain the observed finding of mechanical tenderness. This argument is reasonable, but only by invoking the mechanism of neurogenic inflammation (see the section 'Replacing the construct of myofascial pain syndrome with scientifically testable biological explanations').

In the German literature, the term 'myogelosis' is used to describe a painful change in muscle structure, and has been presented as being analogous to TrPs (Windisch et al. 1999). Samples taken from unfixed cadavers, following judgement of areas that were 'harder' than others, were reported as showing altered histology, but this allowed no correlation with tenderness, and therefore no conclusions relevant to the present discussion can be made.

In another study, heterogeneous myopathic changes were found in muscle biopsies taken from patients with tender muscles (Filosto et al. 2007). However, the significance of these abnormalities is unknown, since the biopsies were not reported as having been taken from a TrP. Importantly, the authors believed that the electromyographic techniques used to diagnose these changes were problematic due to a lack of test–retest relationship data, even for the same observer.

Tissue biochemistry

In a series of experiments (Shah et al. 2005, 2008), micro-dialysis was used to sample tissue fluid within, and near to, a palpated trigger zone, in patients with a diagnosis of TrPs in their trapezius muscles and in normal pain-free subjects. Samples were taken from the following regions: normal (no pain, no TrP), active (pain and TrP detected), and latent (no pain, TrP detected). Samples were also taken from uninvolved gastrocnemius muscles.

Elevated levels of calcitonin gene-related peptide (CGRP), substance P (SP), norepinephrine, TNF-1 alpha, IL-1, and IL-6, and low pH were reported in the muscles of patients in pain. While these findings were heralded by many as proof of the existence of TrPs, there are multiple problems with their interpretation. Mense (2009) pointed out that it is premature to suggest that any or all of these substances are responsible for localized pain. This altered biochemical milieu is consistent with not only inflammation due to tissue damage, but also with that of neurogenic inflammation, where the pathology is not necessarily to be found in the site being sampled (Chiu et al. 2012).

As the authors acknowledge, the very act of data collection could have influenced their results. It was not canvassed whether or not the pro-inflammatory substances were present *before* the mechanical stimulus of the examiner's finger was applied in order to identify the TrP. However, of critical importance were the reported findings of increased levels in *uninvolved, control muscle areas* compared with non-painful control subjects. These findings are consistent with a systemic increase in the general 'inflammatory state' of these patients, as compared with people free of pain.

Electromyographic studies

Electrophysiological studies of putative TrPs are equivocal: one study failed to provide electromyographic (EMG) evidence of ongoing denervation or focal muscle spasm (Durette et al. 1991). By contrast, another reported spontaneous EMG activity (i.e. end-plate noise and spikes) in regions considered TrPs, in patients with chronic tension headache and pericranial muscle tenderness (Hubbard and Berkoff 1993).

Simons et al. (2002; Simons 2001) addressed the question whether end-plate noise and spikes arise from 'normal' end plates. TrP assessment was performed on 25 patients who met the American College of Rheumatology's 1990 criteria for fibromyalgia (Wolfe et al. 1992) and eight pain-free subjects in whom 'latent' TrPs had been identified by manual palpation of taut bands and characteristic referral of pain (*sic*). The authors concluded that end-plate noise is not restricted to TrPs and therefore could not be considered an absolute diagnostic criterion. There are obvious problems with this study design, as the researchers conflated the TrPs of MPS and the 'tender points' of fibromyalgia, another issue that has not been resolved (Bennet and Goldenberg 2011). Moreover, they failed to explain the significance of 'characteristic referral of pain' in patients who were pain-free prior to the examination. An alternate interpretation of these EMG findings is that the investigators were recording insertional and spontaneous activity (i.e. end plate noise) from single muscle fibres generated by the activation of intramuscular nerve terminals irritated by the needle (Katirji 2012).

Imaging

Magnetic resonance elastography was employed to test the hypothesis that localized increases in muscle tone were responsible for the clinical finding of taut bands wherein TrPs are said to be located (Chen et al. 2007). Seven patients with a three-year history of 'myofascial pain' associated with the presence of a taut band in the upper trapezius muscle were examined. The authors reported identification of a signature chevron-like pattern, with its leading edge coincident with the physician-identified taut band. In fact, the authors 'begged the question' as to the underlying cause of their patient's pain (i.e. a TrP), failed to describe the diagnostic criteria that they used, and did not comment on the putative relationship of a 'taut band' to a TrP. A subsequent study of eight subjects, four of whom were said to have myofascial pain and four who did not, is open to the same criticism (Chen et al. 2008).

TrPs were conflated with tender points during imaging of the anterior abdominal wall of 10 patients (Niraj et al. 2011). The points in question appeared as a 'mixed echoic area in the rectus abdominis muscle that *became prominent* on injection of local anaesthetic solution' (italics by authors). A number of possible explanations for these findings were offered, but it was conceded that the findings could have been coincidental. One would reasonably expect that any solution injected into a muscle would be visible upon ultrasound imaging. Moreover, the image presented is consistent with the usual sonographic appearance of the linea alba (Gokhale 2006).

Forty-four patients with acute cervical pain and at least one TrP identified by palpation in the upper trapezius were evaluated using sonoelastography and Doppler imaging (Ballyns et al. 2011). These TrPs were pronounced as either 'active' (spontaneously painful) or 'latent' (painful on palpation but not associated with spontaneous pain). Imaging demonstrated sites deemed to be taut bands and TrPs, although the appearance of these two was identical and therefore not consistent with clinical impressions or current thinking. Unfortunately, there were no control subjects. It is therefore possible that similar sites would be found in pain-free muscles. This is a fatal flaw in the research design, and the results cannot be further interpreted until normative studies are performed.

In a preliminary study, it was suggested that the observed increase in the volume of the vascular compartment and an increase in outflow resistance could be explained by local vasoconstriction due to inflammation, muscle contracture at the TrP compressing the capillary/venous bed, or to externally applied pressure from using the ultrasound transducer during imaging (Sikdar et al. 2010). The possible relationship between a constricted vascular bed and an enlarged vascular volume to evoked pain on palpation 'is yet to be fully understood'.

Animal models of trigger points

Animal models that might inform pathophysiology in humans must have similarities that are relevant and acceptable to others in the field. For TrP research, there remains no such model.

Normal canine muscles were examined and biopsied in an attempt to correlate palpated taut bands with morphological and histological changes, respectively (Simons and Stolov 1976). The findings were negative in all respects—not surprisingly given that there was no evidence of any pain or pathological condition present in the dogs prior to these studies. Of note however was the following quote: 'One gained the impression that rubbing palpation produced a transient contraction which could be primarily responsible for the sensation of a hardness palpated in the dog muscles.' This is the myotatic reflex, which correlates to the 'twitch response' or 'jump sign,' also evocable on palpation of any normal human muscle.

Based upon the conjecture that 'latent MTrP (i.e. tender, but not spontaneously painful) can be identified in almost all skeletal muscles of normal adults' (Travell and Simons 1983), a rabbit model of TrPs was proposed (Chen et al. 2008; Hong and Torigoe 1994). In this model, normal rabbit leg muscles were palpated until they exhibited a myotatic reflex (when both awake and anaesthetized). Such muscles were considered to contain taut bands and, by assumption, TrPs. A number of papers (Chen et al. 1998, 2008; Hong and Torigoe 1994; Hsieh et al. 2011; Kuan et al. 2002) have since been published using this 'model'. However, there was no experimental intervention performed in an attempt to model a TrP in these normal rabbits. There was no behavioural indication of pain or related distress, nor any attempt to assay these critical facets that one would require for a relevant model. The initial study was designed with a faulty premise—that normal muscles in rabbits respond in the same way as painful muscles in humans. Therefore, this model cannot inform postulated pathophysiological mechanisms underlying this or any other human disorder.

Studies of delayed onset muscle soreness (DOMS) have been modelled using eccentric exercise to cause symptoms, in both humans and animals. Although DOMS has only been related to TrPs in one paper (Itoh et al. 2004), such a model was proposed as relevant to MPS (Hayashi et al. 2011). The experiment relating the two was performed in humans, and involved the use of eccentric exercise of the flexor digitorum of the middle finger. Following the development of DOMS, the muscles were palpated and tested, revealing a tender, taut band. However, since the muscle itself is a band, relating the description to TrPs is meaningless. The relevance of DOMS to TrPs remains unclear, much less established. Since almost every human has suffered DOMS, if there was a close causal relationship, it would follow that every human would have at some time developed TrPs, and MPS. Clearly this is not the case.

Myofascial pain syndrome: hypotheses of underlying pathophysiology

In 1991, it was concluded that the proposed 'vicious-circle' models 'have to be considered as working hypotheses rather than explanations of known mechanisms' (Mense 1991). The vast majority of studies published in this area over the 20 years since then have continued to assume the 'truth' of the theory of myofascial TrPs, despite the absence of any empirical basis for them.

Some workers (Mense et al. 2001) suggested that the available electrodiagnostic evidence (i.e. spontaneous electrical activity and spikes at active loci) was consistent with dysfunctional neuromuscular end plates being responsible for the development of putative TrPs. It was announced that 'the critical TrP abnormality now appears to be a neuromuscular dysfunction at the motor endplate of an extrafusal muscle fiber' (Mense et al. 2001, p. 240). These authors suggested that an excessive release of acetylcholine from such end plates was responsible for the 'taut band' phenomenon and that these bands could produce muscle ischaemia, apparently by compressing adjacent capillaries supplying the muscle. This compression can then precipitate an 'energy crisis' in the relevant working muscle, which responds by releasing pro-inflammatory molecules, thereby activating nociceptive neurons.

In their reviews of theories of TrP aetiology, other workers discussed evidence that both low-level static muscle contraction and eccentric and sub-maximal concentric contractions could result in skeletal muscle damage (Bron et al. 2007; Dommerholt 2011). Other possible mechanisms canvassed by them included acute muscle overload and direct trauma to muscle. Presumably, such damage could set the scene for the development of taut bands.

However, the validity of this paradigm (i.e. correlating end-plate activity or noise with pain arising from the TrP) became suspect when it was reported that injection of botulinum toxin A in the region of a TrP had no effect on pain intensity or mechanical pain thresholds, but did significantly reduce motor end-plate activity and EMG interference pattern (Qerama et al. 2006). Others have supported the 'motor end plate' and the 'energy crisis' theories (Gevirtz 2006; Giamberardino et al. 2011b; Huguenin 2004; Niddam et al. 2008). These post-hoc conjectures are consistent with both local and remote pathogeneses. The latter of the two, which as we will see has better support in the biomedical literature, is rarely considered.

Evidence from 'treatment' of 'trigger points'/myofascial pain syndrome

Considerations when assessing effectiveness of treatment of MPS/TrP

It is possible for treatment to be 'accidentally' effective, despite it being based on false theoretical foundations. The fallacy known as *post hoc ergo propter hoc* (after this therefore because of this) has already been mentioned. In this case, the treatment administered may well have had beneficial effects for reasons other than the direct action of the therapist.

There are occasions when a lack of real improvement can be obscured by an observer's 'confirmation bias', here defined as the natural human inclination to interpret information that supports pre-existing expectations. In this case, irrespective of its truth value, a hypothesis is more likely to be confirmed than to be found wrong (MacCoun 1998). The propensity to confirmation bias can be explained by the natural inclination to avoid an unpleasant psychological state (known as cognitive dissonance) and to reject research findings that contradict one's hypothesis (Nickerson 1998). A similar bias is that known as 'expectation bias'. Here, the researcher's expectations of a study's outcomes leads to the publication of data that are in agreement with the expectations, with the 'playing down' of data that appear to conflict with them.

However, more common explanations for improvement (at least in the short term) following treatment include counter-irritation, a multiple-modality treatment approach, non-specific effects, the natural history of the particular problem being treated, and regression to the mean. These factors can all be relevant to the self-reported experience of pain.

As previously hypothesized, peripheral nerve tissue is a more likely source of ongoing nociceptive input (Quintner and Cohen 1994). Should this be the case, it would not be surprising that a counter-irritative noxious stimulus applied in the region where pain is experienced would elicit a transient reduction in pain intensity by recruiting those higher-order brain regions responsible for anti-nociception (Goffaux et al. 2007; Sprenger et al. 2011; Willer et al. 1999).

Specific modalities of treatment

Non-invasive therapy interventions that have been advocated include 'spray and stretch,' transcutaneous electrical stimulation (TENS), massage, and more recently, high-power ultrasound (Unalan et al. 2011). Invasive treatments have included local injections of anaesthetic agents, injection of corticosteroids, injections of botulinum toxin, needle acupuncture, and dry needling (Lavelle et al. 2007).

The factor that most of these therapies have in common is that they elicit pain at the site of their application (i.e. they are noxious stimuli). This would suggest a common mechanism of action—that of analgesia induced by counter-irritation, defined as the application of a competing noxious stimulus (Piche et al. 2009).

Systematic reviews of treatment

In their systematic review of treatment of 'trigger point pain,' Cummings and White were unable to find evidence that needling therapies have any specific efficacy beyond that expected from treatment with a placebo (2011). A review of 1517 studies reported that only seven were of high enough quality for meaningful analysis. These studies gave limited evidence that dry needling of TrPs was associated with a treatment effect compared with standard care. They commented on limited sample sizes, uncertainty as to whether TrPs were the sole cause of pain, as well as technical issues such as the variability in the location of TrPs and in the depth of needle insertion. The studies also varied in the intervals between treatment and the overall number of sessions of treatment. Finally, measurement of outcomes was applied at different times in different studies.

Rickards reached a similar conclusion and commented that the strength of evidence for any treatment should be considered as limited (2006). He surmised that a few of the treatments studied may be effective. However, whether or not they actually address the proposed pathological entity or some other processes is impossible to determine. Another review commented on the heterogeneity of the populations being treated, reporting that there were no widely accepted standard diagnostic criteria for MPS (Annaswamy et al. 2011). Not surprisingly, this author concluded that there is insufficient evidence to support the use of most interventions being advanced.

A systematic review that located 21 randomized controlled trials (RCTs)—with 12 eligible for consideration and only five of these suitable for inclusion—reported that the current evidence does not support the use of botulinum toxin A injections in the region of trigger points (Ho and Tan 2007). As for other such reviews, they reported that the data were limited and that the patient populations were heterogeneous.

One may therefore conclude that the various problems identified by Simons have yet to be resolved (Simons 2004). Within the constraints of MPS theory, well-performed systematic reviews have been unable to determine whether or not the various modalities of therapy (physical and pharmacological) that have been advocated are effective. If there is no consensus on diagnosis and none on consequent treatment, the most appropriate resolution of Simons' problems is to discard the TrP conjecture.

The fundamental errors in myofascial pain syndrome

The attractiveness of the MP model lies in its assertion that the TrP is a discrete and identifiable site of nociception within voluntary muscle. However, as we have already shown, this assertion lacks both empirical and experimental supporting evidence.

The vast majority of studies and meta-analyses do not support the assertion that focal treatment of putative TrPs is effective. Most papers are fraught with poor study design, making it difficult to place confidence in the results. The best interpretation is that such treatment is likely to reflect contextual effects rather than a rationally targeted influence on pathogenesis.

Despite the lack of evidence, some opinion leaders have continued to espouse the MPS model (Giamberardino et al. 2011b) and in so doing, may have failed to appreciate the important distinction that lies between a conjecture and a theory.

Conjecture versus theory

A conjecture is an opinion or a conclusion that is based on incomplete evidence. Less formally, a conjecture is a guess or a speculation. Similarly, an hypothesis or, more correctly in this (medical scientific context), a *working* hypothesis, is a proposed explanation made on the basis of limited evidence as a starting point for further investigation. Testable claims that seem to be true can be deduced from a conjecture or hypothesis but it needs to be remembered that such claims have yet to be proven or disproved (Pólya and Bowden 1977).

By contrast, a theory is generally accepted to be the accurate explanation of an observed phenomenon because it has undergone extensive testing. However, because that which is being observed is always 'theory-laden,' an independent observer can have no neutral or unalloyed access to a realm of pure 'facts' derived from observations (Grayling 1999). Hence there is always the strong possibility of bias.

Evidence that the concept has been embedded in modern literature includes the recent conjecture that 'peripheral pain generators' can reside within muscles (i.e. myofascial tissues), and be responsible not only for spontaneous pain but also for the initiation and maintenance of profound changes within the central nervous system (known as central sensitization) (Ge 2010; Giamberardino et al. 2011a). On this same basis, TrPs have been held responsible for the syndrome of widespread pain known as fibromyalgia (Alonso-Blanco et al. 2011; Ge 2010; Gerwin 2005; Giamberardino et al. 2011a; Staud et al. 2009; Wang et al. 2012).

Comprehensive refutation of the myofascial pain syndrome model

On both scientific and logical grounds, the theoretical model of 'myofascial pain' has been refuted. This argument turns partly on the absence of anatomical or physiological evidence to support the concept of 'trigger points.' Furthermore, the literature consistently reveals no lasting effect of treatments directed to putative TrPs.

However, we emphasize that the facts and discussion presented do not deny the existence of the clinical phenomena with which so many patients present. Rather, our intention here is to apply scientific discipline in an important field of clinical practice and research that has stagnated due to its reliance upon a flawed basic tenet.

Replacing the construct of myofascial pain syndrome with scientifically testable biological explanations

Proponents of MP theory have overlooked the possibility that sensitivity of apparently discrete foci within muscle may well be a *consequence* of nociceptor activation elsewhere, as had been proposed earlier (Elliott 1944). In 1938, Kellgren reported a critical observation: that carefully targeted injections of hypertonic saline into tissues such as voluntary muscle, interspinous ligaments, periosteum, and cancellous bone could induce not only referred pain but also local, and hence referred, tenderness (Kellgren 1938a,b). The distribution of pain arising from stimulation of such deep somatic structures presented as 'a gradual transition from pain which is confined to a spot in the region of the structure stimulated, to a diffuse pain (poorly localized) of full segmental distribution.'

Kellgren also reported that pain intensity in the areas of referred pain induced by saline injections into remote muscle did not diminish when those areas were anaesthetized (Kellgren 1977). By contrast, other investigators have reported that referred pain can be modulated by anaesthetizing such areas (Arendt-Nielsen and Svensson 2001). These contradictory results may be explained by the relative completeness of the anaesthetic block, which was not controlled in either study. However, when all afferent input from the area of injection was blocked (sympathetic and somatic plexus blocks), the phenomenon of referred pain still occurred, implying that no peripheral input from the tissues in the region of referred pain was necessary to explain the remaining ongoing pain (Feinstein et al. 1954).

Although the neurophysiological mechanisms for referred pain are still the subject of investigation (Arendt-Nielsen and Svensson 2001) (and there have been no studies of referred tenderness), the theories of convergence projection and convergence facilitation had both been advanced at the time of Travell and Simons' initial publication (Keele 1957). Their failure to consider this line of research was scientifically inexcusable. Furthermore, Travell and Simons' dogmatic statement that pain arising in peripheral nerve tissue was always associated with clinical evidence of neurological deficit and with electrodiagnostic evidence of nerve fibre damage is demonstrably false (Dyck 1990); especially as such methods cannot evaluate the small-diameter axons that carry nociceptive information.

In 1994, Quintner and Cohen proposed that the phenomenon currently called 'trigger point' could be an area of what was then called secondary (referred) hyperalgesia occurring in muscles that are structurally and physiologically unimpaired (Quintner and Cohen 1994). Since this time, research has accrued that essentially supports this hypothesis, allowing a more scientifically based, and testable, model for the development of focal muscle hypertonicities to be formulated. The question arose: from which structure(s) might such pain be referred?

Nerve inflammation as a source of pain was first discussed in the nineteenth century (Player 1821). Neuritis can have mechanical, traumatic, infective, immune, metabolic, and toxic aetiologies (Logigian et al. 1993; Pentland and Donald 1994; Torkelson et al. 1988), and can occur as an extension of other disease processes (Dyck et al. 2000; Rattananan et al. 2014; Zager et al. 1998), the involved nerve being an 'innocent bystander.'

Inflammation induces two key changes in nociceptor axons innervating muscle and other non-cutaneous structures (Bove 2009; Bove et al. 2003; Dilley and Bove 2008; Dilley et al. 2005):

i) Some axons become mechanically sensitive to pressure and movement, correlating clinically with movement-induced pain.

ii) Some axons become responsive to the inflammatory milieu, correlating clinically with ongoing (spontaneous) pain.

These neurophysiological events are sufficient to explain the pain reported by patients diagnosed with 'TrPs', the poor reliability of palpation, the findings of pro-inflammatory chemicals in the local milieu, and most importantly, the lack of response to treatments directed to the muscle presumed to be at fault.

Inflammation of a peripheral nerve will cause axonal mechanical sensitivity and initiate spontaneous activity of a proportion of deep innervating neurons considered to be nociceptors. These well-documented pathophysiological events account for movement-induced and spontaneous pain perceived in non-cutaneous structures. It is important to understand that no matter where the sensory axon is activated, the perception of sensation will be projected to the structure that is innervated. For example, if the dorsal scapular nerve were sufficiently inflamed anywhere along its anatomical path, such as where it passes across the scalene muscles, pain would be perceived in the rhomboid and levator scapulae muscles, which it innervates. However, could this pathophysiology explain a focal muscle contraction, or tenderness in the innervated area?

Virtually all peripheral nerves carry sensory, sympathetic, and motor axons, and inflammation has effects on all three components. When an axon is activated, the action potentials propagate in both directions. In peptidergic sensory axons, this efferent activity causes the release of a number of neuropeptides into the innervated area, inducing tissue changes termed neurogenic inflammation (Daemen et al. 1998; McMahon et al. 1984). While neurogenic inflammation alone does not sensitize nociceptors in humans or rats (Reeh et al. 1986; Schmelz et al. 1994, 1996), it can lead to muscle oedema (Daemen et al. 1998). Chemical sampling from areas deemed to be TrPs is consistent with neurogenic inflammation.

The effect of neuritis on motor axons has not been studied. Afferent nociceptor activity will lead to reflex muscle contraction that outlasts the stimulus (Woolf and Wall 1986). It has also been reported that palpation of allodynic nerves elicits electrical activity in their innervated muscles (Hall and Quintner 1996). Both of these phenomena could be reflected clinically as focal muscle contraction. It would be expected that the extent of this contraction would have some concordance with the number of affected axons. It is also possible that the reflex muscle contraction far outlasts the initial neuritis; although experimental neuritis did not lead to substantial gross muscle contraction evidenced by persistent hindlimb flexion (Wallas et al. 2003), strong nociceptive stimuli and nerve injury can do so (Anderson and Winterson 1995; Hanning et al. 1992). However, extensive observations in humans have shown that pain from persistent nociceptor activity leads to decreased motor function to the involved muscles as a whole, proposed to be due to effects on central motor control (Lund et al. 1991). The proposed model recognized the possibility of reflex muscle contraction. Pilot studies are underway to determine if neuritis and selective nerve lesions augment motor neuronal activity.

Taken together, these known mechanisms could explain the formation of tender, focal muscle hypertonicities, as well as the formation of non-muscular tender points, as were initially described many decades ago. It is not necessary to invoke any pathophysiological process at the site of perceived pain or tenderness. This mechanism of somatic referred or radiating pain may explain the patterns of spatial and temporal pain propagation (i.e. said to be attributable to 'secondary,' 'satellite,' and 'metastasizing' TrPs). Some of the other clinical features (i.e. intolerance to stretch of muscles purported to contain TrPs, the 'twitch' response, hypoesthesia, and disturbances of vasomotor and sudomotor function) seem better explained as phenomena that are accompaniments of peripheral neural inflammation and pain (Quintner and Cohen 1994).

It is clear that not all axons are affected during experimental neuritis, and factors that dictate which and how many axons become sensitive are unknown. It follows that the site of the afferent activity and other changes would vary depending on which axons were affected, predicting the observed lack of agreement regarding the location of symptomatic spots. These mechanisms are also consistent with the reported lack of efficacy of clinical treatments applied directly to these areas, since such treatments are addressing epiphenomena and not the site(s) of aetiopathogenesis. Above all, this hypothesis is amenable to scientific inquiry, whereas the TrP hypothesis has been refuted.

Acknowledgement

We are indebted to our colleague, Associate Professor Geoffrey Bove, for his assistance in sourcing and evaluating the research behind this chapter.

References

Alonso-Blanco C, Fernandez-de-las-Penas C, Morales-Cabezas M, Zarco-Moreno P, Ge HY, Florez-Garcia M. Multiple active myofascial trigger points reproduce the overall spontaneous pain pattern in women with fibromyalgia and are related to widespread mechanical hypersensitivity. *Clin J Pain* 2011; 27:405–13.

Anderson MF, Winterson BJ. Properties of peripherally induced persistent hindlimb flexion in rat: involvement of N-methyl-D-aspartate receptors and capsaicin-sensitive afferents. *Brain Res* 1995; 678:140–50.

Annaswamy TM, De Luigi AJ, O'Neill BJ, Keole N, Berbrayer D. Emerging concepts in the treatment of myofascial pain: a review of medications, modalities, and needle-based interventions. *Phys Med Rehabil* 2011; 3:940–61.

Arendt-Nielsen L, Svensson P. Referred muscle pain: basic and clinical findings. *Clin J Pain* 2001;17:11–19.

Ballyns JJ, Shah JP, Hammond J, Gebreab T, Gerber LH, Sikdar S. Objective sonographic measures for characterizing myofascial trigger points associated with cervical pain. *J Ultrasound Med* 2011; 30:1331–40.

Bennett RM, Goldenberg DL. Fibromyalgia, myofascial pain, tender points and trigger points: splitting or lumping? *Arthritis Res Ther* 2011; 13:117.

Bove GM. Focal nerve inflammation induces neuronal signs consistent with symptoms of early complex regional pain syndromes. *Exp Neurol* 2009; 219:223–7.

Bove GM, Ransil BJ, Lin HC, et al. Inflammation induces ectopic mechanical sensitivity in axons of nociceptors innervating deep tissues. *J Neurophysiol* 2003; 90:1949–55.

Brendstrup P, Jespersen K, Asboe H. Morphological and chemical connective tissue changes in fibrositic muscles. *Ann Rheum Dis* 1957; 16:438–40.

Bron C, Franssen J, Wensing M, Oostendorp RA. Interrater reliability of palpation of myofascial trigger points in three shoulder muscles. *J Man Manip Ther* 2007; 15:203–15.

Chen Q, Basford J, An KN. Ability of magnetic resonance elastography to assess taut bands. *Clin Biomech* 2008; 23:623–9.

Chen Q, Bensamoun S, Basford J, Thompson J, An K. Identification and quantification of myofascial taut bands with magnetic resonance elastography. *Arch Phys Med and Rehabil* 2007; 88:1658–61.

Chen JT, Chen SM, Kuan TS, Chung KC, Hong CZ. Phentolamine effect on the spontaneous electrical activity of active loci in a myofascial trigger spot of rabbit skeletal muscle. *Arch Phys Med Rehabil* 1998; 79:790–4.

Chen KH, Hong CZ, Kuo FC, Hsu HC, Hsieh YL. Electrophysiologic effects of a therapeutic laser on myofascial trigger spots of rabbit skeletal muscles. *Am J Phys Med Rehabil* 2008; 87:1006–14.

Chiu IM, von Hehn CA, Woolf CJ. Neurogenic inflammation and the peripheral nervous system in host defense and immunopathology. *Nat Neurosci* 2012; 15:1063–7.

Copeman WS. A clinical contribution to the study of the fibrositic nodule. *Ann Rheum Dis* 1943; 3:222–6.

Copeman WS. Treatment of fibrositis. *Brit Med J* 1936; i:1219–20.

Cummings TM, White AR. Needling therapies in the management of myofascial trigger point pain: a systematic review. *Arch Phys Med Rehabil* 2001; 82:986–92.

Daemen MARC, Kurvers HAJM, Kitslaar PJEH, et al. Neurogenic inflammation in an animal model of neuropathic pain. *Neurol Res* 1998; 20:41–5.

Dilley A, Bove GM. Resolution of inflammation induced axonal mechanical sensitivity and conduction slowing in C-fiber nociceptors. *J Pain* 2008; 9:185–92.

Dilley A, Lynn B, Pang SJ. Pressure and stretch mechanosensitivity of peripheral nerve fibres following local inflammation of the nerve trunk. *Pain* 2005; 117:462–72.

Dommerholt J. Dry needling—peripheral and central considerations. *J Man Manip Ther* 2011; 19:223–7.

Durette MR, Rodriquez AA, Agre JC, Silverman JL. Needle electromyographic evaluation of patients with myofascial or fibromyalgic pain. *Am J Phys Med Rehabil* 1991; 70:154–6.

Dyck PJ. Invited review: limitations in predicting pathological abnormality of nerves from the EMG examination. *Muscle Nerve* 1990; 3:371–5.

Dyck PJB, Engelstad J, Norell J, et al. Microvasculitis in non-diabetic lumbosacral radiculoplexus neuropathy (LSRPN): similarity to the diabetic variety (DLSRPN). *J Neuropathol Exp Neurol* 2000; 59:525–38.

Elliott FA. Aspects of 'fibrositis'. *Ann Rheum Dis* 1944; 4:22.

Feinstein B, Langton JNK, Jameson RM, Schiller F. Experiments on pain referred from deep tissues. *J Bone Joint Surg* 1954; 36:981–97.

Filosto M, Tonin P, Vattemi G, et al. The role of muscle biopsy in investigating isolated muscle pain. *Neurology* 2007; 68:181–6.

Ge HY. Prevalence of myofascial trigger points in fibromyalgia: the overlap of two common problems. *Curr Pain Headache Rep* 2010; 14:339–45.

Gerwin RD. A review of myofascial pain and fibromyalgia—factors that promote their persistence. *Acupunct Med* 2005; 23:121–34.

Gevirtz R. The muscle spindle trigger point model of chronic pain. *Biofeedback* 2006; 34:53–6.

Giamberardino MA, Affaitati G, Fabrizio A, Costantini R. Effects of treatment of myofascial trigger points on the pain of fibromyalgia. *Curr Pain Headache Rep* 2011a; 15:393–9.

Giamberardino MA, Affaitati G, Fabrizio A, Costantini R. Myofascial pain syndromes and their evaluation. *Best Pract Res Clin Rheumatol* 2011b; 25:185–98.

Goffaux P, Redmond WJ, Rainville P, Marchand S. Descending analgesia—when the spine echoes what the brain expects. *Pain* 2007; 130:137–43.

Gokhale S. Sonography in identification of abdominal wall lesions presenting as palpable masses. *J Ultrasound Med* 2006; 25:1199–209.

Gowers WR. Lumbago: its lessons and analogues. *Brit Med J 1904*; i:117–21

Grayling ACG. Theory ladenness (of observation). In: Bullock A, Trombley S. (eds) *The new Fontana dictionary of modern thought* (3rd edn). London: HarperCollins Publishers, 1999: 868.

Hall T, Quintner J. Responses to mechanical stimulation of the upper limb in painful cervical radiculopathy. *Aust J Physio* 1996; 42:277–85.

Hanning S, Mokler DJ, Winterson BJ. Persistent hindlimb flexion is associated with an experimental mononeuropathy. *Soc Neurosci Abstr* 1992; 18:286.

Hayashi K, Ozaki N, Kawakita K, et al. Involvement of NGF in the rat model of persistent muscle pain associated with taut band. *J Pain* 2011; 12:1059–68.

Ho KY, Tan KH. Botulinum toxin A for myofascial trigger point injection: a qualitative systematic review. *Eur J Pain* 2007; 11:519–27.

Hong CZ, Torigoe Y. Electrophysiological characteristics of localized twitch responses in responsive taut bands of rabbit skeletal muscle fibers. *J Musculoskel Pain* 1994; 2:17–43.

Hsieh YL, Chou LW, Joe YS, Hong CZ. Spinal cord mechanism involving the remote effects of dry needling on the irritability of myofascial trigger spots in rabbit skeletal muscle. *Arch Phys Med Rehabil* 2011; 92:1098–105.

Hsieh CY, Hong CZ, Adams AH, et al. Interexaminer reliability of palpation of trigger points in the trunk and lower limb muscles. *Arch Phys Med Rehabil* 2000; 81:258–64.

Hubbard DR, Berkoff GM. Myofascial trigger points show spontaneous needle EMG activity. *Spine (Phila Pa 1976)* 1993; 18:1803–7.

Huguenin LK. Myofascial trigger points: the current evidence. *Phys Ther Sport* 2004; 5:2–12.

Itoh K, Okada K, Kawakita K. A proposed experimental model of myofascial trigger points in human muscle after slow eccentric exercise. *Acupunct Med* 2004; 22:2–12.

Katirji B. Clinical neurophysiology; clinical electromyography. In: Daroff RB, Fenichel GM, Jankovic J, Maziotta J. (eds). *Bradley's neurology in clinical practice, vol. 2* (6th edn). Philadelphia: Elsevier Saunders, 2012: 394–420.

Keele KD. *Anatomies of pain*. Springfield: Charles C Thomas (Publisher), 1957: 132–74.

Kellgren JH. A preliminary account of pain arising from muscle. *Brit Med J* 1938a; i:325–7.

Kellgren JH. On the distribution of pain arising from deep somatic structures with charts of segmental pain areas. *Clin Sci* 1938b; 4:35–46.

Kellgren JH. The anatomical source of back pain. *Rheumatol Rehabil* 1977; 16:3–12.

Kuan TS, Chen JT, Chen SM, Chien CH, Hong CZ. Effect of botulinum toxin on endplate noise in myofascial trigger spots of rabbit skeletal muscle. *Am J Phys Med Rehabil* 2002; 81:512–20.

Lavelle ED, Lavelle W, Smith HS. Myofascial trigger points. *Anesthesiol Clin* 2007; 25:841–51.

Lew PC, Lewis J, Story I. Inter-therapist reliability in locating myofascial trigger points using palpation. *Man Ther* 1997; 2:87–90.

Lewit K. The needle effect in the relief of myofascial pain. *Pain* 1979; 6:83–90.

Logigian EL, Shefner JM, Frosch MP, et al. Nonvasculitic, steroid-responsive mononeuritis multiplex. *Neurology* 1993; 43:879–83.

Lucas N, Macaskill P, Irwig L, Moran R, Bogduk N. Reliability of physical examination for diagnosis of myofascial trigger points: a systematic review of the literature. *Clin J Pain* 2009; 25:80–9.

Lund JP, Donga R, Widmer CG, et al. The pain adaptation model: a discussion of the relationship between chronic musculoskeletal pain and motor activity. *Can J Physiol Pharmacol* 1991; 69:683–94.

MacCoun RJ. Biases in the interpretation and use of research results. *Annu Rev Psychol* 1998; 49:259–87.

McMahon SB, Sykova E, Wall PD, et al. Neurogenic extravasation and substance P levels are low in muscle as compared to skin the rat hindlimb. *Neurosci Lett* 1984; 52:235–40.

Mense S. Algesic agents exciting muscle nociceptors. *Exp Brain Res* 2009; 196:129–37.

Mense S. Considerations concerning the neurobiological basis of muscle pain. *Can J Physiol Pharmacol* 1991; 69:610–6.

Mense S, Simons DG, Russell IJ. *Muscle pain: understanding its nature, diagnosis and treatment*. Philadelphia: Lippincott, Williams & Wilkins, 2001.

Myburgh C, Larsen AH, Hartvigsen J. A systematic, critical review of manual palpation for identifying myofascial trigger points: evidence and clinical significance. *Arch Phys Med Rehabil* 2008; 89:1169–76.

Myburgh C, Lauridsen HH, Larsen AH, Hartvigsen J. Standardized manual palpation of myofascial trigger points in relation to neck/shoulder pain: the influence of clinical experience on inter-examiner reproducibility. *Man Ther* 2011; 16:136–40.

Nickerson RS. Confirmation bias: a ubiquitous phenomenon in many guises. *Rev Gen Psychol* 1998; 2:175–220.

Niddam DM, Chan RC, Lee SH, Yeh TC, Hsieh JC. Central representation of hyperalgesia from myofascial trigger point. *Neuroimage* 2008; 39:1299–306.

Niraj G, Collett BJ, Bone M. Ultrasound-guided trigger point injection: first description of changes visible on ultrasound scanning in the muscle containing the trigger point. *Br J Anaesth* 2011; 107:474–5.

Pentland B, Donald SM. Pain in the Guillain-Barre syndrome: a clinical review. *Pain* 1994; 59:159–64.

Piche M, Arsenault M, Rainville P. Cerebral and cerebrospinal processes underlying counterirritation analgesia. *J Neurosci* 2009; 29:14236–46.

Player RP. On irritation of the spinal nerves. *Quart J Sci* 1821; 12:428.

Pólya G, Bowden L. *Mathematical methods in science* (revised edn). Washington DC: Mathematical Association of America, 1977.

Qerama E, Fuglsang-Frederiksen A, Kasch H, Bach FW, Jensen TS. A double-blind, controlled study of botulinum toxin A in chronic myofascial pain. *Neurology* 2006; 67:241–5.

Quintner JL, Cohen ML. Referred pain of peripheral neural origin: an alternative to the 'Myofascial Pain' construct. *Clin J Pain* 1994; 10:243–51.

Rattananan W, Thaisetthawatkul P, Dyck PJ. Postsurgical inflammatory neuropathy: A report of five cases. *J Neurol Sci* 2014; 337:137–40.

Reeh PW, Kocher L, Jung S. Does neurogenic inflammation alter the sensitivity of unmyelinated nociceptors in the rat? *Brain Res* 1986; 384:42–50.

Rickards LD. The effectiveness of non-invasive treatments for active myofascial trigger point pain: a systematic review of the literature. *Int J Osteopathic Med* 2006; 9:120–36.

Schmelz M, Schmidt R, Ringkamp M, et al. Limitation of sensitization to injured parts of receptive fields in human skin C-nociceptors. *Exp Brain Res* 1996; 109:141–7.

Schmelz M, Schmidt R, Ringkamp M, et al. Sensitization of insensitive branches of C nociceptors in human skin. *J Physiol Lond* 1994; 480: 389–94.

Sciotti VM, Mittak VL, DiMarco L, Ford LM, Plezbert J, et al. Clinical precision of myofascial trigger point location in the trapezius muscle. *Pain* 2001; 93:259–66.

Shah J, Danoff J, Desai M, et al. Biochemicals associated with pain and inflammation are elevated in sites near to and remote from active myofascial trigger points. *Arch Phys Med and Rehabil* 2008; 89:16–23.

Shah JP, Phillips TM, Danoff JV, Gerber LH. An in vivo microanalytical technique for measuring the local biochemical milieu of human skeletal muscle. *J Appl Physiol* 2005; 99:1977–84.

Sikdar S, Ortiz R, Gebreab T, Gerber LH, Shah JP. Understanding the vascular environment of myofascial trigger points using ultrasonic imaging and computational modeling. *Conf Proc IEEE Eng Med Biol Soc* 2010:5302–5. doi: 10.1109/IEMBS.2008.4650480.

Simons DG. Review of enigmatic MTrPs as a common cause of enigmatic musculoskeletal pain and dysfunction. *J Electromyogr Kines* 2004; 14:95–107.

Simons DG. Do endplate noise and spikes arise from normal motor endplates? *Am J Phys Med Rehabil* 2001; 80:134–40.

Simons DG. Muscular pain syndromes. *Adv Pain Res Ther* 1990; 17:1–41.

Simons DG. Muscle pain syndromes, Part I. *Amer J Phys Med* 1975; 54:289–311.

Simons DG, Stolov WC. Microscopic features and transient contraction of palpable bands in canine muscle. *Am J Phys Med* 1976; 55:65–88.

Simons DG, Travell JG. Myofascial trigger points, a possible explanation. *Pain* 1981; 10: 106–9.

Simons DG, Hong CZ, Simons LS. Endplate potentials are common to midfiber myofacial trigger points. *Am J Phys Med Rehabil* 2002; 81:212–22.

Sprenger C, Bingel U, Buchel C. Treating pain with pain: supraspinal mechanisms of endogenous analgesia elicited by heterotopic noxious conditioning stimulation. *Pain* 2011; 152:428–39.

Staud R, Nagel S, Robinson ME, Price DD. Enhanced central pain processing of fibromyalgia patients is maintained by muscle afferent input: a randomized, double-blind, placebo-controlled study. *Pain* 2009; 145:96–104.

Stockman R. A discussion on fibrositis. *Proc R Soc Med* 1913; 6:36–9.

Stockman R. *Rheumatism and arthritis*. Edinburgh: W Green & Son, 1920.

Torkelson SJ, Lee RA, Hildahl DB. Endometriosis of the sciatic nerve: a report of two cases and a review of the literature. *Obstet Gynecol* 1988; 71:473–7.

Tough EA, White AR, Richards S, Campbell J. Variability of criteria used to diagnose myofascial trigger point pain syndrome—evidence from a review of the literature. *Clin J Pain* 2007; 23:278–86.

Travell J, Rinzler SH. The myofascial genesis of pain. *Post-Grad Med* 1952; 11:425–34.

Travell JG, Simons DG. *Myofascial pain and dysfunction: the trigger point manual*. Baltimore: Williams and Wilkins, 1983.

Unalan H, Majlesi J, Aydin FY, Palamar D. Comparison of high-power pain threshold ultrasound therapy with local injection in the treatment of active myofascial trigger points of the upper trapezius muscle. *Arch Phys Med Rehabil* 2011; 92:657–62.

Wallas TR, Winterson BJ, Ransil BJ, et al. Paw withdrawal thresholds and persistent hindlimb flexion in experimental mononeuropathies. *J Pain* 2003; 4:222–30.

Wang C, Ge HY, Ibarra JM, Yue SW, Madeleine P, Arendt-Nielsen L. Spatial pain propagation over time following painful glutamate activation of latent myofascial trigger points in humans. *J Pain* 2012; 13:537–45.

Willer JC, Bouhassira D, Le Bars D. Neurophysiological bases of the counterirritation phenomenon: diffuse control inhibitors induced by nociceptive stimulation. *Neurophysiol Clin* 1999; 29:379–400.

Windisch A, Reitinger A, Traxler H, et al. Morphology and histochemistry of myogelosis. *Clin Anat* 1999; 12:266–71.

Wolfe F, Simons DG, Fricton J, et al. The fibromyalgia and myofascial pain syndromes: a preliminary study of trigger points inpersons with fibromyalgia, myofascial pain syndrome and no disease. *J Rheumatol* 1992; 19:944–51.

Woolf CJ, Wall PD. Relative effectiveness of C primary afferent fibers of different origins in evoking a prolonged facilitation of the flexor reflex in the rat. *J Neurosci* 1986; 6:1433–42.

Zager EL, Pfeifer SM, Brown MJ, et al. Catamenial mononeuropathy and radiculopathy: a treatable neuropathic disorder. *J Neurosurg* 1998; 88:827–30.

Chapter 15

Neurodynamics: when and why?

Toby Hall and Kim Robinson

Introduction to neurodynamics

Mobilization of the nervous system is an integral part of modern manual therapy, based on the seminal cadaveric and clinical studies in the 1970s by Robert (Bob) Elvey, who sadly passed away while the authors were writing this chapter. Bob Elvey was a gifted clinician and educator who inspired many orthopaedic manipulative therapists around the world, including the authors, forging cutting-edge developments in clinical practice.

The early enthusiasm for mobilization of the nervous system was partly disseminated by presentations at manual therapy conferences (Elvey 1978), journal articles (Butler and Gifford 1989; Elvey 1979), and textbooks (Butler 1991; Elvey 1985). This was a time when evidence-based practice in manual therapy was very much in its infancy, when learning was experiential rather than scientifically based. There were no randomized controlled trials to report on the efficacy of mobilization of the nervous system. Without these evidence-based guidelines, the appropriate use of such mobilization techniques could not be determined and is only now being better understood.

In those early years, the focus was on the mechanical aspects of mobilization; indeed, the median nerve neurodynamic test was called the 'brachial plexus tension test' (Elvey 1979) and the whole concept called 'adverse mechanical tension in the nervous system' (Butler 1989). The thought process was that nerves became mechanically shortened, under tension, scarred, or adherent in some way and needed stretching to improve. This mechanical focus was very much regretted by Bob Elvey (Elvey 1998) and David Butler (Butler 1998) reflecting on their original publications. Unfortunately, there is still the persistent focus, among some, on adverse mechanical tension as a cause of pain (Anandkumar 2013; Walsh 2012). The authors firmly believe that, instead, the focus should be the neurophysiological affects on pain arising from neural tissue pain disorders.

Dysfunction of the nervous system is well recognized as an important contributing factor to many chronic musculoskeletal pain conditions. For example, our research group found that 75% of people with low back related leg pain had symptoms attributed to a neural tissue disorder (Schäfer et al. 2011). Clinically, mobilization of the nervous system is a commonly used tool to manage patients with such disorders. However, it seems that not all neural pain disorders respond to such management (Ellis and Hing 2008). For example, carpal tunnel syndrome is the most common peripheral neuropathy, yet a systematic review failed to find convincing evidence of significant therapeutic effects for the use of neural mobilization to manage this condition (Medina McKeon and Yancosek 2008). Another study (Scrimshaw and Maher 2001) failed to find any benefit for neural mobilization after spinal fusion, discectomy, or laminectomy. In a third example, this time for patients with symptoms of chronic cubital tunnel syndrome (ulnar neuropathy at the elbow), there was no added benefit of neural mobilization for a control group at 6-month follow-up.

Considering this evidence, it might seem that we should abandon neural mobilization, as it does not seem to be effective. However, as revealed in this chapter and Chapter 56, patient and technique selection is paramount when considering neural mobilization. In the aforementioned studies investigating the treatment of carpal tunnel syndrome, subject selection was poor, inducing a 'washout effect' whereby some patients who are not suitable for the intervention did badly, thus reducing the overall effect of the therapy in the whole group. In the post-surgical study, both patient and treatment selection were inappropriate. Finally, in the cubital tunnel study, sustained nerve stretching techniques were prescribed. We argue, and the evidence confirms, these stretching techniques are not effective.

In contrast to these three reports, a recent study has demonstrated the positive benefits of neural mobilization, compared to a keep active approach, for patients with cervicobrachial pain and specific features of neural tissue dysfunction (Nee et al. 2012), collectively described as peripheral nerve sensitization (PNS). To explain this disparity in treatment response requires an understanding of the basic mechanisms underlying neuropathic and nociceptive pain. This chapter will explore the underlying basis for pain arising from neural tissue disorders, and describe a treatment-based classification system to identify three broad sub-groups of patients with such disorders. Each can be identified with careful clinical examination and each requires a different management approach. It is our contention, with supporting evidence, that only the sub-group of neural pain disorders diagnosed as PNS should be managed with neural mobilization techniques. Management of each sub-group is discussed in Chapter 56.

Pain arising from neural tissue disorders

In the evaluation of pain and the various types of 'pain patterns' that may accompany disorders of the spine and limbs, it is essential for the clinician to keep an open mind with respect to judging the source of pain. Although symptoms such as tingling, burning, pins and needles, and numbness are generally viewed as indicative of a pathological condition affecting neural tissue, pain in isolation may be very difficult to analyse in terms of tissue of origin. Pain may be of the following distinct types or of a variable combination:

1 Musculoskeletal local and referred pain

2 Visceral local and referred pain

3 Neuropathic local and referred pain

Determining the source of symptoms has important implications for correctly localizing treatment, particularly from a manual therapy perspective. The phenomenon of referred pain is an added complexity when trying to identify the source of symptoms (Jinkins 2004). A wise manual therapist once said that the topography and nature of referred pain in any one person is inadequate as a single factor in differential diagnosis of both the tissue involved and the segmental level (Grieve 1994). In addition, there is substantial confusion and a blurring of terminology when describing patients with referred limb pain (Bogduk 2009).

Referred pain

Two types of referred pain are recognized: musculoskeletal referred pain and radicular referred pain. *Musculoskeletal referred pain* is pain perceived in an area remote from its site of origin, but usually within the same spinal segment (Bonica and Procacci 1990) and is explained by afferent impulses from different regions converging upon the same viscerosomatotopic neurons in the central nervous system. This then causes mental projection of pain to the region corresponding with the spinal nerve (Jinkins 2004).

There is wide variation between individuals in the patterns of musculoskeletal referred pain, as well as much overlap from different anatomical structures. See, for example, the patterns of referred pain from intervertebral discs, muscles, and facet joints (April et al. 2002; Cooper et al. 2007; Dwyer et al. 1990a,b; Fukui et al. 1996; Grubb and Kelly 2000; Schmidt-Hansen et al. 2006; Windsor et al. 2003). In addition, the presence of central sensitization has a marked influence on referred pain, making it virtually impossible to identify the pain source (Curatolo et al. 2006).

Radicular pain is pain perceived in a dermatomal distribution, arising from compromise of the dorsal root ganglion or the nerve root (Bogduk 2009). It is important to remember that projecting limb pain may also be caused by damage to peripheral nerve trunks proximal to their peripheral distribution (Bogduk and McGuirk 2002). Examples of projected pain with segmental distribution are the pain of radiculopathy, caused by herpes zoster, intervertebral disc prolapse, or other diseases involving the nerve trunk before it divides into its major peripheral branches. Examples of projected pain with peripheral nerve distribution include trigeminal neuralgia, occipital neuralgia, and meralgia paraesthetica.

It has been traditionally taught to distinguish between radicular pain and musculoskeletal referred pain by the distal extension of the pain in the limb (Bogduk 2004, 2009). This is a tempting over-simplification, as it has been demonstrated that patients with typical symptoms consistent with radicular pain, extending down the whole limb, had similar neurological deficits to those with pseudoradicular pain where symptoms were only proximal (Freynhagen et al. 2007).

Neuropathic pain

Traditionally, pain is divided into either nociceptive or neuropathic (Backonja 2003). Nociceptive pain arises from trauma or inflammation of musculoskeletal structures, whereas neuropathic pain is defined by the International Association for the Study of Pain (IASP) as pain caused by a lesion or disease of the somatosensory system (Jensen et al. 2011). Of particular interest to this chapter is the distinction between nociceptive pain and peripheral neuropathic pain, although separating the two can be difficult on a theoretical (Bennett 2006) and clinical (Markman et al. 2004) level. Further complication arises in radicular pain where both nociceptive pain and neuropathic pain typically coexist. However, we emphasize the clinical importance of differentiating between peripheral neuropathic pain and nociceptive pain as we believe each condition requires a different treatment approach and each has a differing prognosis (Hans et al. 2007). For example, a recent survey of more than 21,000 people in the German general population reported that 4% suffered back pain with a neuropathic component (Schmidt et al. 2009). Costs associated with managing these patients were 67% higher than those with nociceptive pain only.

Patients with positive features of neuropathic pain (spontaneous pain, paraesthesia, dysaesthesia, allodynia, and hyperalgesia) respond less favourably to manual therapy (Jull et al. 2007), particularly neural mobilization (Nee et al. 2013; Schäfer et al. 2011), highlighting the importance of early identification of patients with neuropathic pain.

The fundamental cause of peripheral neuropathic pain is damage to the nervous system itself, but it is interesting that nerve damage does not always cause pain (Zusman 2008). Indeed, it has been suggested that less than 10% of sudden or gradual onset peripheral nerve injuries develop significant pain (Marchettini et al. 2006) On the other hand, minor nerve injury, which may be difficult to detect clinically, is capable of causing severe pain (Bove et al. 2003; Dilley et al. 2005; Greening et al. 2005). Complex regional pain syndrome is a good clinical example where minor nerve trauma causes severe, even lifelong, pain (Rho et al. 2002).

Peripheral nerve sensitization

The neuritis model may be a physiological explanation for pain arising from minor nerve damage (Zusman 2008). The sensory supply to the peripheral nervous system is the nervi nervorum, which form a sporadic plexus in connective tissue layers of peripheral nerves (Bove and Light 1995, 1997). There is evidence of the protective function of the nervi nervorum, as they respond to excessive stretch and focal pressure of the nerve they innervate (Bove and Light 1997; Zochodne 1993). These findings reflect the clinical situation where responses are only reported in normal people when neural tissue is stretched or compressed excessively (Hall and Quintner 1996). However, once inflamed, the sensitized nervi nervorum may be a source of nociception even during small movements. The pain associated with this perineural form of neuritis is better classified as nociceptive as it does not involve damage of the nervous system per se (Zusman 2008). This is an important distinction, particularly when considering the use of neural mobilization techniques, as will become apparent later in this chapter.

In addition to the perineuritis model just outlined, it has been suggested that a milieu of inflammatory mediators (from damaged or diseased adjacent tissues) may penetrate through the various connective tissue layers, breaching the endoneurium to the axons themselves (Eliav et al. 1999). Physiological changes of the nerve tissue occur, which are consistent with neuropathic pain (Bennett 2006; Zusman 2008). Cytokines, including IL-6 and IL-1b among others, appear to be factors involved in this process (Eliav et al. 2009). Inflamed axons demonstrate mechanosensitivity (Bove et al. 2003; Dilley et al. 2005; Eliav et al. 1999) but appear to conduct normally (Dilley et al. 2005), betraying the cardinal sign of neuropathy which is altered axonal conduction and neurological deficit. In more aggressive forms of inflammation, structural nerve damage does occur with associated changes in nerve conduction (Gazda et al. 2001; Kleinschnitz et al. 2005). Thus, there appears to be a sliding scale of nerve injury associated with different degrees of nerve inflammation. It has also been suggested that chronic focal nerve inflammation inducing ongoing C fibre discharge may also explain the development of complex regional pain syndrome (Bove 2009).

Not all nerve fibres develop axonal mechanical sensitivity, but a proportion of A-delta and C fibres do. Most responsive mechanosensitive fibres fire to only 3% stretch (Dilley et al. 2005), which is likely to occur during everyday limb movements such as rising from a chair and walking. The mechanisms underlying mechanosensitivity of axons are complex but are believed to involve disruption to axoplasmic flow and axonal transport at the inflamed site (Dilley and Bove 2008a,b). In addition to these changes, ion channel expression is also altered, resulting in a change in type and density of ion channels produced by the cell body (Campbell and Meyer 2006; Costigan and Woolf 2000). The result is that some axons generate impulses to mechanical stimuli when they would normally not. Collectively, mechanosensitization of axons and nervi nervorum following nerve inflammation is referred to as peripheral nerve sensitization (PNS). This may be identified through careful clinical examination of neurodynamic tests seeking hyperalgesic responses to nerve lengthening and nerve palpation.

The aforementioned finding of axonal mechanosensitivity following induced nerve inflammation provides a possible pathophysiological explanation for the frequent clinical finding of peripheral nerve trunk mechanosensitivity in a range of musculoskeletal disorders (Nee and Butler 2006). It also explains why nerve inflammation can cause pain in the absence of significant fascicular damage. For example, in subjects with mild/moderate features of cubital tunnel syndrome, only 24% of patients were found to have altered axonal conduction (Svernlov et al. 2009). In people with low back pain, radicular pain is present in 65% of subjects (Freynhagen et al. 2006b), but the incidence of radiculopathy is up to 10 times less than the incidence of low back pain in the same population (Ernat et al. 2012; Schoenfeld et al. 2012).

Clinically, it is often found to be the case that radicular symptoms are associated with sciatic nerve mechanosensitivity or from musculoskeletal referred pain from sensitized facet joints or intervertebral discs, rather than true radiculopathy. Similarly, the clinical case of ongoing posterior thigh pain following hamstring muscle injury is all too familiar to the sports therapist. Such ongoing pain may be explained by a variety of factors, but the identification of sciatic nerve mechanosensitivity should be a priority for assessment. Assessment might include the 'slump' (Figure 15.1) and 'straight leg raise' (SLR) test (Figure 15.2), with various sensitizing manoeuvres to selectively stress the sciatic nerve. Palpation of the sciatic nerve (Figure 15.3) and its terminal branches would also be helpful in differential diagnosis. Assessment would also include evaluation of various musculoskeletal structures capable of generating posterior thigh pain.

Once it has been established that PNS is the source of symptoms, management then may include neural mobilization in the form of exercise or passive mobilization techniques. The aim of this approach is to gradually desensitize the peripheral nervous system to a more normal mechanosensitive state, thereby relieving pain and improving function. See Chapter 56 for more details.

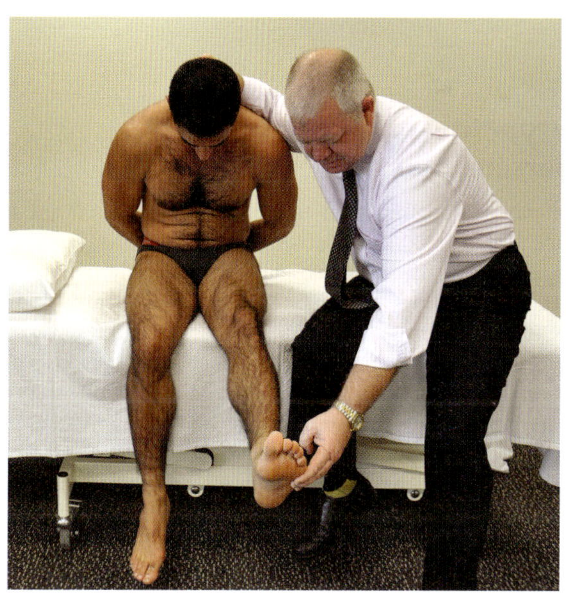

Figure 15.1 Slump test.

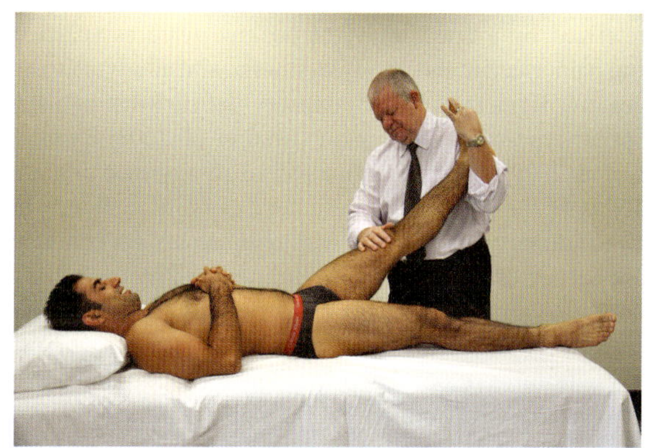

Figure 15.2 Straight leg raise test.

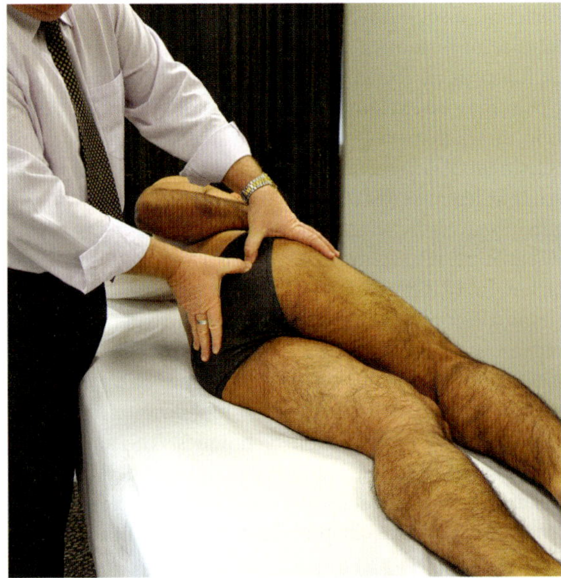

Figure 15.3 Palpation of the sciatic nerve.

Neuropathic pain with sensory hypersensitivity

Peripheral neuropathic pain occurs following significant nerve damage (Treede et al. 2008) arising from infections, vascular and metabolic disease, neurotoxins, autoimmune insult, radiation, and genetic abnormalities (Zusman 2008). Consequently, spontaneous C-fibre input from such injury may drive central sensitization (Woolf 2004). Indeed, stimulus-independent, spontaneous pain is a common feature of this form of pain. In addition, through a process of altered gene transcription, A fibres behave more like C fibres, and non-noxious input now drives central sensitization (Decosterd et al. 2002). Under these circumstances, the normally innocuous stimuli of light touch, joint movement, or muscle contraction produce or maintain central sensitization, sensory hypersensitivity, and ongoing pain (Campbell and Meyer 2006). There is a wide range of changes to the central and peripheral nervous system that can explain this form of neuropathic pain, defined as neuropathic pain with sensory hypersensitivity (NPSH) (Schäfer et al. 2011), which lies towards the extreme end of the neuropathic pain continuum.

Pain associated with NPSH is usually chronic and disabling and characterized by a specific set of positive features (particularly burning pain, electric shocks, dysaesthesia, and allodynia to brush) and negative signs (particularly sensory deficits) distinguishing it from other types of chronic pain (Attal et al. 2008; Baron 2009; Baron et al. 2009). Positive features occur in response to increased excitability of the central and peripheral nervous system, whereas negative features are associated with reduced axonal conductivity. The prevalence of moderate to severe neuropathic pain has been estimated, by survey, to be up to 5% in the general population (Bouhassira et al. 2008). It would appear that patients who present with these features respond poorly to any form of manual therapy, including exercise (O'Connell 2013), or even medical intervention (Finnerup et al. 2007). Hence, early identification is essential for appropriate management.

Screening tools have been developed to aid identification of this form of neuropathic pain and include the Neuropathic Pain Questionnaire (Galer and Jensen 1997), the Douleur Neuropathique 4 (DN4) (Bouhassira et al. 2005), the Leeds Assessment of Neuropathic Symptoms and Signs (LANSS) (Bennett 2001), Pain DETECT (Freynhagen et al. 2006a), ID Pain (Portenoy 2006), and the Standardized Evaluation of Pain (StEP) (Scholz et al. 2009). Each tool characterizes neuropathic pain by the presence of positive and negative symptoms and signs and attempts to identify the presence of neuropathic pain in a different way. For example, ID Pain is purely subjective (Portenoy 2006), whereas the LANSS and DN4 consist of a questionnaire regarding pain description, together with items relating to the bedside clinical examination. The sensitivity and specificity of each questionnaire have been summarized elsewhere (Hall and Elvey 2009). Considering each tool seeks to identify neuropathic pain, it would be logical to assume that they can be used interchangeably, but this may not be the case and further refinement of these tools is required (Walsh et al. 2012).

As NPSH appears to be caused by abnormal afferent processing of sensory information in the central nervous system, then management should be directed at the processing of afferent input and not at mobilization of the nervous system. Management is discussed in Chapter 56.

Compressive neuropathy

Previously in this chapter, we suggested that the majority of nerve trauma or damage does not cause symptoms. For example, in a sample of asymptomatic people of mean age 65, over 30% had magnetic resonance imaging (MRI) evidence, while 52% had electrodiagnostic evidence, of stenosis (Haig et al. 2006). Hence, clearly not all nerve damage is associated with pain. Clinically however, we find some patients have significant radiological and clinical signs of compression neuropathy (CN), correlated with significant pain but with an absence of positive features, and such patients test negative on neuropathic screening tools (Moloney et al. 2013; Schäfer et al. 2011, 2013; Tampin et al. 2013). These patients fit the IASP criteria for neuropathic pain and definite neuropathic pain according to published guidelines (Treede et al. 2008). However, patients with CN appear to respond differently to manual therapy when compared with patients with NPSH, presumably because of different underlying pain mechanisms.

The classic example of CN is lumbar stenosis associated with osteoarthritic or degenerative change. Osteophytes, as well as ligamentum flavum and other soft tissue hypertrophy, progressively compress nerve roots, causing symptoms to develop gradually over time. Although pain is not always a feature of nerve root compression (Kjaer et al. 2005; Macnab 1972; Olmarker et al. 1989; Wiesel et al. 1984), radicular pain in the absence of inflammation of the nerve root is presumably due to chronic compression, causing hypoxia and vascular compromise and subsequent damage of axons within the nerve root. Under these circumstances, there may be minimal evidence of axonal mechanosensitivity on clinical tests that lengthen the nerve (Amundsen et al. 1995; Olmarker et al. 1989) and minimal positive symptoms (Schäfer et al. 2009).

Patients with nerve root or peripheral nerve compression typically present with pain associated with movement or postures that further compress those structures. In the classic example of cervical foraminal stenosis, spine extension and ipsilateral lateral flexion or rotation, either in a single plane or when combined, are typically provocative. These movements further reduce the space around the nerve root (Takasaki et al. 2009) and are the basis for Spurling's test. For these movements to compress neural structures, there must be a reduction in the volume of the nerve space to begin with, which usually occurs through some degenerative process or space-occupying lesion.

Nerve conduction loss is confirmed by the clinical evaluation of deep tendon reflexes, muscle power, skin sensation tests, and vibration perception. In addition to these typical clinical findings, radiological and electrodiagnostic evidence of CN consistent with the clinical findings would also be informative. Imaging by itself is not that useful in diagnosis; rather, the combination of all these factors is likely to improve diagnostic accuracy (Haig et al. 2007).

Apart from compression of the median nerve in the carpal tunnel, symptomatic peripheral nerve compression in the periphery is relatively rare. For example, ulnar nerve compression at the elbow is the second most common CN, but occurs in only 25 cases per 100,000 person years (Mondelli et al. 2005)—a very rare event. In contrast, CN in the spine is more common. In one survey of 77 patients with low back related leg pain attending a German pain clinic, approximately 25% of cases were classified as CN (Schäfer et al. 2008). The identification of such conditions is based on a thorough clinical examination, with particular emphasis on the neurological examination. Table 15.1 outlines a grading system for the identification of neuropathic pain with features of CN, and is founded on evidence-based guidelines (Treede et al. 2008). If all four criteria are met, a definitive diagnosis of neuropathic pain can be made and the source of nerve compression of musculoskeletal origin identified to rule out other forms of nerve damage such as diabetic neuropathy. Logically, it would follow that if a nerve is compressed, treatment options may include manual decompression techniques. This approach is discussed in Chapter 56.

An outline of the classification process is shown in Figure 15.4. Reliability and preliminary validity of this classification system has

Table 15.1 A grading system for the identification of compression neuropathy (Treede et al. 2008)

	Criteria	Explanation
1	Pain with a distinct neuroanatomically plausible distribution	A region corresponding to a peripheral innervation territory in the CNS
2	A history suggestive of a relevant lesion or disease affecting the peripheral or central somatosensory system	The suspected lesion is associated with pain, in a manner consistent for the condition
3	Demonstration of the distinct neuroanatomically plausible distribution of pain by at least one confirmatory test	Neurological signs concordant with the distribution of pain; may be supplemented by laboratory and objective tests for subclinical abnormalities
4	Demonstration of the relevant lesion or disease by at least one confirmatory test	Confirms the presence of the suspected lesion, such as imaging studies (MRI, etc.)

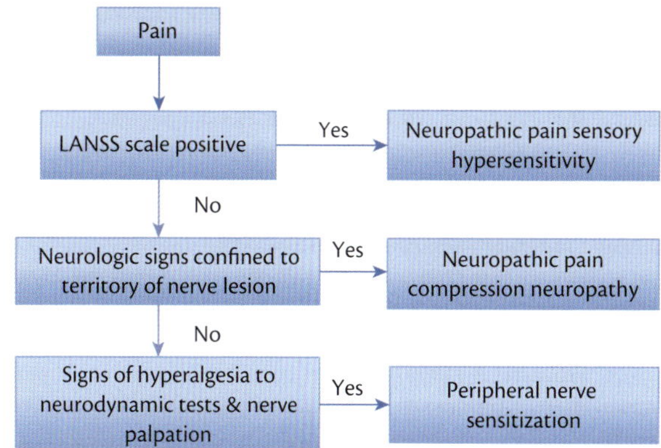

Figure 15.4 Hierarchical classification of neural tissue pain disorders.

been demonstrated (Schäfer et al. 2008, 2009a,c, 2011, 2013); however, much further validation is required.

Concluding thoughts about classification of neural tissue disorders

Mobilization of the nervous system is a maturing aspect of manual therapy, but its implementation must be carefully considered to be effective. A rationale for classification of neural tissue pain disorders into sub-groups, with the goal of identifying potential patients suitable for neural mobilization, has been given, based on neurophysiology and pain mechanisms. To determine which category the patient falls into requires a comprehensive examination process. As the classification system is hierarchical and groups mutually exclusive, the order of diagnosis should be NPSH, CN, PNS, and musculoskeletal pain. In the absence of NPSH (LANSS score >12), the next priority is CN, based on evidence of significant neurological deficit. Thirdly, diagnosis of PNS is based on an absence of NPSH and CN, but in the presence of signs of mechanosensitive neural tissue. This is the group most likely to respond to neural mobilization techniques. Finally, in the absence of any of the features in the previous three criteria, patients would be classified as having musculoskeletal pain.

References

Amundsen, T., Weber, H., Lilleas, F., Nordal, H., Abdelnoor, M., Magnaes, B. (1995). Lumbar spinal stenosis: clinical and radiologic features. *Spine* 20(10):1178–86.

Anandkumar, S. (2013). Kinesio tape management for superficial radial nerve entrapment: a case report. *Physiother Theory Pract* 29(3):232–41.

April, C., Axinn, M., Bogduk, N. (2002). Occipital headaches stemming from the lateral atlanto-axial (C1–2) joint. *Cephalalgia* 22:15–22.

Attal, N., Fermanian, C., Fermanian, J., Lanteri-Minet, M., Alchaar, H., Bouhassira, D. (2008). Neuropathic pain: are there distinct subtypes depending on the aetiology or anatomical lesion? *Pain* 138(2):343–53.

Backonja, M.M. (2003). Defining neuropathic pain. *Anesth Analg* 97(3): 785–90.

Baron, R. (2009). Neuropathic pain: a clinical perspective. *Handb Exp Pharmacol* 194: 3–30.

Baron, R., Tolle, T.R., Gockel, U., Brosz, M., Freynhagen, R. (2009). A cross-sectional cohort survey in 2100 patients with painful diabetic neuropathy and postherpetic neuralgia: Differences in demographic data and sensory symptoms. *Pain* 146(1–2):34–40.

Bennett, G.J. (2006). Can we distinguish between inflammatory and neuropathic pain. *Pain Res Manage* 11(suppl A):11A–15A.

Bennett, M. (2001). The LANSS Pain Scale: the Leeds assessment of neuropathic symptoms and signs. *Pain* 92(1–2):147–57.

Bogduk, N. (2004). *Clinical anatomy of the lumbar spine*. Melbourne, Churchill Livingstone.

Bogduk, N. (2009). On the definitions and physiology of back pain, referred pain, and radicular pain. *Pain* 147(1–3):17–19.

Bogduk, N., McGuirk, B. (2002). *Causes and sources of chronic low back pain. Medical management of acute and chronic low back pain. An evidence based approach*. Amsterdam, Elsevier: 115–25.

Bonica, J.J., Procacci, P. (1990). General considerations of acute pain. In: Bonica, J.J. (ed.) *The management of pain*. Philadelphia, Lea and Febiger,: 59–79.

Bouhassira, D., Attal, N., Alchaar, H., et al. (2005). Comparison of pain syndromes associated with nervous or somatic lesions and development of a new neuropathic pain diagnostic questionnaire (DN4). *Pain* 114(1–2): 29–36.

Bouhassira, D., Lanteri-Minet, M., Attal, N., Laurent, B., Touboul, C. (2008). Prevalence of chronic pain with neuropathic characteristics in the general population. *Pain* 136(3):380–7.

Bove, G.M. (2009). Focal nerve inflammation induces neuronal signs consistent with symptoms of early complex regional pain syndromes. *Exp Neurol* 219(1):223–7.

Bove, G., Light, A. (1995). Unmyelinated nociceptors of rat paraspinal tissues. *J Neurophys* 73:1752–62.

Bove, G., Light, A. (1997). The nervi nervorum: missing link for neuropathic pain? *Pain Forum* 6(3):181–90.

Bove, G.M., Ransil, B.J., Lin, H.C., Leem, J.G. (2003). Inflammation induces ectopic mechanical sensitivity in axons of nociceptors innervating deep tissues. *J Neurophysiol* 90(3):1949–55.

Butler, D.S. (1989). Adverse mechanical tension in the nervous system: a model for assessment and treatment. *Austral J Physiother* 35(4):227–38.

Butler, D.S. (1991). *Mobilisation of the nervous system*. Melbourne, Churchill Livingstone.

Butler, D. (1998). Commentary: adverse mechanical tension in the nervous system: a model for assessment and treatment. In: Maher, C. (ed.) *Adverse neural tension revisited*. Melbourne, Australian Physiotherapy Association: 33–5.

Butler, D.S., Gifford, L. (1989). The concept of adverse mechanical tension in the nervous system. Part one: testing for 'dural tension'. *Physiotherapy* 75(11):622–8.

Campbell, J.N., Meyer, R.A. (2006). Mechanisms of neuropathic pain. *Neuron* 52(1):77–92.

Cooper, G., Bailey, B., Bogduk, N. (2007). Cervical zygapophysial joint pain maps. *Pain Med* 8(4):344–53.

Costigan, M., Woolf, C.J. (2000). Pain: molecular mechanisms. *J Pain* 1(3 Suppl):35–44.

Curatolo, M., Arendt-Nielsen, L., Petersen-Felix, S. (2006). Central hypersensitivity in chronic pain: mechanisms and clinical implications. *Phys Med Rehabil Clin N Am* 17(2):287–302.

Decosterd, I., Allchorne, A., Woolf, C.J. (2002). Progressive tactile hypersensitivity after a peripheral nerve crush: non-noxious mechanical stimulus-induced neuropathic pain. *Pain* 100(1–2):155–62.

Dilley, A., Bove, G.M. (2008a). Disruption of axoplasmic transport induces mechanical sensitivity in intact rat C-fibre nociceptor axons. *J Physiol* 586(2):593–604.

Dilley, A., Bove, G.M. (2008b). Resolution of inflammation-induced axonal mechanical sensitivity and conduction slowing in C-fiber nociceptors. *J Pain* 9(2):185–92.

Dilley, A., Lynn, B., Pang, S.J. (2005). Pressure and stretch mechanosensitivity of peripheral nerve fibres following local inflammation of the nerve trunk. *Pain* 117(3):462–72.

Dwyer, A., Aprill, C., Bogduk, N. (1990a). Cervical zygapophyseal joint pain patterns I: A study of normal volunteers. *Spine* 15(6):453–7.

Dwyer, A., Aprill, C., Bogduk, N. (1990b). Cervical zygapophyseal joint pain patterns II: A clinical evaluation. *Spine* 15(6):458–61.

Eliav, E., Benoliel, R., Herzberg, U., Kalladka, M., Tal, M. (2009). The role of IL-6 and IL-1beta in painful perineural inflammatory neuritis. *Brain Behav Immun* 23(4):474–84.

Eliav, E., Herzberg, U., Ruda, M.A., Bennett, G.J. (1999). Neuropathic pain from an experimental neuritis of the rat sciatic nerve. *Pain* 83(2):169–82.

Ellis, R.F., Hing, W.A. (2008). Neural mobilization: a systematic review of randomized controlled trials with an analysis of therapeutic efficacy. *J Man Manip Ther* 16(1):8–22.

Elvey, R. (1978). *Passive intervertebral movement*. Inaugral Conference of the Manipulative Therapists' Association of Australia (Sydney, Australia).

Elvey, R. (1979). Brachial plexus tension tests and the pathoanatomical origin of arm pain. In: Idczak, R. (ed.) *Aspects of manipulative therapy*. Melbourne, Lincoln Institute of Health Sciences: 105–10.

Elvey, R.L. (1985). Brachial plexus tension tests and the pathoanatomical origin of arm pain. In: Glasgow, E.F., et al. (ed.) *Aspects of manipulative therapy*. Melbourne, Churchill Livingstone: 116–22.

Elvey, R. (1998). Commentary: treatment of arm pain associated with abnormal brachial plexus tension. In: Maher, C. (ed.) *Adverse neural tension revisited*. Melbourne, Australian Physiotherapy Association: 13–7.

Ernat, J., Knox, J., Orchowski, J., Owens, B. (2012). Incidence and risk factors for acute low back pain in active duty infantry. *Mil Med* 177(11):1348–51.

Finnerup, N.B., Otto, M., Jensen, T.S., Sindrup, S.H. (2007). An evidence-based algorithm for the treatment of neuropathic pain. *Med Gen Med* 9(2):36.

Freynhagen, R., Baron, R., Gockel, U., Tolle, T.R. (2006a). PainDETECT: a new screening questionnaire to identify neuropathic components in patients with back pain. *Curr Med Res Opin* 22(10):1911–20.

Freynhagen, R., Baron, R., Tolle, T., et al. (2006b). Screening of neuropathic pain components in patients with chronic back pain associated with nerve root compression: a prospective observational pilot study (MIPORT). *Curr Med Res Opin* 22(3):529–37.

Freynhagen, R., Rolke, R., Baron, R., et al. (2007). Pseudoradicular and radicular low-back pain—a disease continuum rather than different entities? Answers from quantitative sensory testing. *Pain* 135(1–2):65–74.

Fukui, S., Ohseto, K., Shiotani, M., et al. (1996). Referred pain distribution of the cervical zygapophyseal joints and cervical dorsal rami. *Pain* 68(1):79–83.

Galer, B.S., Jensen, M.P. (1997). Development and preliminary validation of a pain measure specific to neuropathic pain: the Neuropathic Pain Scale. *Neurology* 48(2):332–8.

Gazda, L.S., Milligan, E.D., Hansen, M.K., et al. (2001). Sciatic inflammatory neuritis (SIN): behavioral allodynia is paralleled by peri-sciatic proinflammatory cytokine and superoxide production. *J Peripher Nerv Syst* 6(3):111–29.

Greening, J., Dilley, A., Lynn, B. (2005). In vivo study of nerve movement and mechanosensitivity of the median nerve in whiplash and non-specific arm pain patients. *Pain* 115(3):248.

Grieve, G.P. (1994). Referred pain and other clinical features. In:Boyling, J.D., Palastanga, N. (eds) *Grieves modern manual therapy*. Edinburgh, Churchill Livingstone: 271–91.

Grubb, S.A., Kelly, C.K. (2000). Cervical discography: clinical implications from 12 years of experience. *Spine (Phila Pa 1976)* 25(11):1382–9.

Haig, A.J., Geisser, M.E., Tong, H.C., et al. (2007). Electromyographic and magnetic resonance imaging to predict lumbar stenosis, low-back pain, and no back symptoms. *J Bone Joint Surg Am* 89(2):358–66.

Haig, A.J., Tong, H.C., Yamakawa, K.S., et al. (2006). Spinal stenosis, back pain, or no symptoms at all? A masked study comparing radiologic and electrodiagnostic diagnoses to the clinical impression. *Arch Phys Med Rehabil* 87(7):897–903.

Hall, T., Elvey, R.L. (2009). Evaluation and treatment of neural tissue pain disorders. In: Donatell, R., Wooden, M. (eds) *Orthopaedic physical therapy*. New York, Churchill Livingstone.

Hall, T., Quintner, J. (1996). Responses to mechanical stimulation of the upper limb in painful cervical radiculopathy. *Austral J Physiother* 42(4):277–85.

Hans, G., Masquelier, E., De Cock, P. (2007). The diagnosis and management of neuropathic pain in daily practice in Belgium: an observational study.' *BMC Pub Health* 7:170.

Jensen, T.S., Baron, R., Haanpaa, M., et al. (2011). A new definition of neuropathic pain. *Pain* 152(10):2204–5.

Jinkins, J. (2004). The anatomic and physiologic basis of local, referred and radiating lumbosacral pain syndromes related to disease of the spine. *J Neurorad* 31:163–80.

Jull, G., Sterling, M., Kenardy, J., Beller, E. (2007). Does the presence of sensory hypersensitivity influence outcomes of physical rehabilitation for chronic whiplash? A preliminary RCT. *Pain* 129(1–2):28–34.

Kjaer, P., Leboeuf-Yde, C., Korsholm, L., Sorensen, J.S., Bendix, T. (2005). Magnetic resonance imaging and low back pain in adults: a diagnostic imaging study of 40-year-old men and women. *Spine* 30(10):1173–80.

Kleinschnitz, C., Brinkhoff, J., Sommer, C., Stoll, G. (2005). Contralateral cytokine gene induction after peripheral nerve lesions: dependence on the mode of injury and NMDA receptor signaling. *Brain Res Mol Brain Res* 136(1–2):3–8.

Macnab, I. (1972). The mechanism of spondylogenic pain. In: Hirsch, C., Zotterman, Y. (eds) *Cervical pain*. New York, Pergamon Press: 89–95.

Marchettini, P., Lacerenza, M., Mauri, E., Marangoni, C. (2006). Painful peripheral neuropathies. *Curr Neuropharmacol* 4(3):175–81.

Markman, J., Dukes, E., Siffert, J., Griesing, T. (2004). Patient flow in neuropathic pain management: understanding existing patterns of care. *Europ J Neurol* 11:135–6.

Medina McKeon, J.M., Yancosek, K.E. (2008). Neural gliding techniques for the treatment of carpal tunnel syndrome: a systematic review. *J Sport Rehabil* 17(3):324–41.

Moloney, N., Hall, T., Doody, C. (2013). Sensory hyperalgesia is characteristic of nonspecific arm pain: a comparison with cervical radiculopathy and pain-free controls. *Clin J Pain*. 29(11):948–956

Mondelli, M., Giannini, F., Ballerini, M., Ginanneschi, F., Martorelli, E. (2005). Incidence of ulnar neuropathy at the elbow in the province of Siena (Italy). *J Neurol Sci* 234(1–2):5–10.

Nee, R., Butler, D.S. (2006). Management of peripheral neuropathic pain: integrating neurobiology, neurodynamics, and clinical evidence. *Phys Ther Sport* 7:36–49.

Nee, R.J., Vicenzino, B., Jull, G.A., Cleland, J.A., Coppieters, M.W. (2012). Neural tissue management provides immediate clinically relevant benefits without harmful effects for patients with nerve-related neck and arm pain: a randomised trial. *J Physiother* 58(1):23–31.

Nee, R.J., Vicenzino, B., Jull, G.A., Cleland, J.A., Coppieters, M.W. (2013). Baseline characteristics of patients with nerve-related neck and arm pain predict the likely response to neural tissue management. *J Orthop Sports Phys Ther* 43(6):379–391

O'Connell, N.E., Wand, B.M., McAuley, J., Marston, L., Moseley, G. L. 2013. Interventions for treating pain and disability in adults with complex regional pain syndrome. *Cochrane Database Syst Rev*, 4, CD009416.

Olmarker, K., Rydevik, B., Holm, S., Bagge, U. (1989). The effects of experimental graded compression on blood flow in spinal nerve roots. A vital microscopic study on porcine cauda equina. *J Orthop Res* 7:817–23.

Portenoy, R. (2006). Development and testing of a neuropathic pain screening questionnaire: ID Pain. *Curr Med Res Opin* 22(8):1555–65.

Rho, R.H., Brewer, R.P., Lamer, T.J., Wilson, P.R. (2002). Complex regional pain syndrome. *Mayo Clin Proc* 77(2):174–80.

Schäfer, A., Hall, T., Briffa, K. (2009a). Classification of low back-related leg pain–a proposed patho-mechanism-based approach. *Man Ther* 14(2):222–30.

Schäfer, A., Hall, T.M., Briffa, K., Ludtke, K., Mallwitz, J. (2008). *QST profiles of subgroups of patients with low back related leg pain—do they differ?* International Association for the Study of Pain, Glasgow.

Schäfer, A., Hall, T.M., Briffa, K., Ludtke, K., Mallwitz, J. (2009b). *Changes in somatosensory profiles in subgroups of patients with sciatica after 4 weeks of manual therapy—an observational cohort study*. International Association for the Study of Pain, Glasgow; IASP Press.

Schafer, A.G., Hall, T.M., Rolke, R., Treede, R.D., Ludtke, K., Mallwitz, J., Briffa, K. N. 2014. Low back related leg pain: an investigation of construct validity of a new classification system. *Journal of Back Musculoskeleton Rehabilation* 27:409–18.

Schäfer, A., Hall, T.M., Ludtke, K., Mallwitz, J., Briffa, N.K. (2009c). Interrater reliability of a new classification system for patients with neural low back-related leg pain. *J Man Manip Ther* 17(2):109–17.

Schäfer, A., Hall, T., Muller, G., Briffa, K. (2011). Outcomes differ between subgroups of patients with low back and leg pain following neural manual therapy: a prospective cohort study. *Eur Spine J* 20(3):482–90.

Schmidt, C.O., Schweikert, B., Wenig, C.M., et al. (2009). Modelling the prevalence and cost of back pain with neuropathic components in the general population. *Eur J Pain* 13(10):1030–5.

Schmidt-Hansen, P.T., Svensson, P., Jensen, T.S., Graven-Nielsen, T., Bach, F.W. (2006). Patterns of experimentally induced pain in pericranial muscles. *Cephalalgia* 26(5):568–77.

Schoenfeld, A.J., Laughlin, M., Bader, J.O., Bono, C.M. (2012). Characterization of the incidence and risk factors for the development of lumbar radiculopathy. *J Spinal Disord Tech* 25(3):163–7.

Scholz, J., Mannion, R.J., Hord, D.E., et al. (2009). A novel tool for the assessment of pain: validation in low back pain. *PLoS Med* 6(4):e1000047.

Scrimshaw, S.V., Maher, C.G. (2001). Randomized controlled trial of neural mobilization after spinal surgery. *Spine (Phila Pa 1976)* 26(24):2647–52.

Svernlov, B., Larsson, M., Rehn, K., Adolfsson, L. (2009). Conservative treatment of the cubital tunnel syndrome. *J Hand Surg Eur* 34(2):201–7.

Takasaki, H., Hall, T., Jull, G., Kaneko, S., Iizawa, T., Ikemoto, Y. (2009). The influence of cervical traction, compression, and spurling test on cervical intervertebral foramen size. *Spine (Phila Pa 1976)* 34(16):1658–62.

Tampin, B., Slater, H., Briffa, N.K. (2013). Neuropathic pain components are common in patients with painful cervical radiculopathy, but not in patients with nonspecific neck-arm pain. *Clin J Pain* 29: 846–56

Treede, R.D., Jensen, T.S., Campbell, J.N., et al. (2008). Neuropathic pain: redefinition and a grading system for clinical and research purposes. *Neurology* 70(18):1630–5.

Walsh, M.T. (2012). Interventions in the disturbances in the motor and sensory environment. *J Hand Ther* 25(2):202–18; quiz 219.

Walsh, J., Raby, M., Hall, T. (2012). Agreement and correlation between the self-report Leeds assessment of neuropathic symptoms and signs and Douleur Neuropathique 4 questions neuropathic pain screening tools in subjects with low back-related leg pain. *J Man Physiol Therap* 35:196–202.

Wiesel, S.W., Tsourmas, N., Feffer, H.L., Citrin, C.M., Patronas, N. (1984). A study of computer-assisted tomography: 1. The incidence of positive CAT scans in an asymptomatic group of patients. *Spine* 9:549–51.

Windsor, R.E., Nagula, D., Storm, S., Overton, A., Jahnke, S. (2003). Electrical stimulation induced cervical medial branch referral patterns. *Pain Phys* 6(4):411–8.

Woolf, C.J. (2004). Dissecting out mechanisms responsible for peripheral neuropathic pain: implications for diagnosis and therapy. *Life Sci* 74(21):2605–10.

Zochodne, D. (1993). Epineural peptides: a role in neuropathic pain. *Canad J Neurol Sci* 20:69–72.

Zusman, M. (2008). Mechanisms of peripheral neuropathic pain: implications for musculoskeletal physiotherapy. *Phys Ther Rev* 13(5):313–23.

Chapter 16

Tensegrity: the new biomechanics

Stephen M. Levin

The 'design' of plants and animals and of traditional artifacts did not just happen. As a rule both the shape and materials of any structure which has evolved over a long period of time in a competitive world represent an optimization with regard to the loads which it has to carry and to the financial or metabolic cost.

(Gordon 1978, p. 303)

Anomalies of the standard lever model in biomechanics

If we accept the precepts of most present-day biomechanical engineers, a 100-kg weight lifted by your average competitive weightlifter will tear his erector spinae muscle, rupture his discs, crush his vertebrae, and burst his blood vessels (Gracovetsky 1988). Even the less daring sportsperson is at risk: a 2-kg fish dangling at the end of a 3-metre fly rod exerts a compressive load of at least 120 kg on the lumbosacral junction. If we include the weight of the rod and the weight of the torso, arms, and head, the calculated load on the spine would easily exceed the critical load that would fracture the lumbar vertebrae of the average man. This would make fly fishing an exceedingly dangerous activity. Pounded by the forces of the runner striking the ground, with the first metatarsal head acting as the hammer and the ground as the anvil, the soft sesamoids would crush. A batter striking a baseball traveling at 100 mph (160 km/h) will be sheared from the ground, spikes and all. A hockey player striking a puck will be propelled backwards on the near-frictionless ice, as for every action, there is an equal and opposite reaction.

There is more to ponder. The brittleness of bones is about the same in a mouse as it is in an elephant, as the strength and stiffness of bones is about the same in all animals. For animals larger than lions, for example horses, jumping on their slender limbs would smash their bones with any leap (Gordon 1988). According to the linear mechanical laws that dominate biomechanics thinking, the mass of an animal must be cubed as its surface area is squared, so an animal as large as an elephant will be crushed by its own weight. The large dinosaurs could never have existed, let alone be a dominant species for millions of years. Biological tissues work elastically at strains that are about a thousand times higher than strains that ordinary technological solids can withstand. If they behaved as most non-biological materials do, with each heartbeat, the skull should explode as the blood vessels expand and crowd out the brain; urinary bladders should thin and burst as they fill; and the pregnant uterus should burst with the contractions of delivery.

Not only mechanical but also physiological processes would be inconsistent with linear physics. Pressure within a balloon decreases as it empties. Following the same physics, the systolic pressure should decrease as the heart empties—but, of course, it increases. We could never get the air out of our lungs or empty our bladders or bowels. If we functioned as columns and levers, our centre of gravity is too high and our base is too small and weak for ordinary activities. When swinging an axe, sledgehammer, golf club, or fishing rod, our centre of gravity would fall outside our base and we would topple over. We could not lift a shovel full of dirt. The os calci is a very soft bone. Our heels should crush from the superincumbent load and could not sustain the load of a gymnast dismounting a high bar. The 'iron cross' position (Figure 16.1), attainable by any competent gymnast, would tear him/her limb from limb unless she/he defied the cosine law taught in every basic physics course which, in effect, states that the forces pulling on a rope strung between two poles become infinite as the rope becomes straight.

When confronted by these anomalies, biomechanical engineers either ignore the problem or go to great and circuitous lengths to try to justify the results. However, these explanations rarely stand the test of scientific scrutiny or even good sense. According to bioengineers, living organisms are modelled like skyscrapers (Schultz 1983). There are serious inconsistencies that test this model. The base of a skyscraper is always stronger than its top. It is dependent on gravity to hold it together. It cannot be flipped over or even tilted very far as the internal shear created would tear it apart. Its joints must be rigidly welded. Biological hinges are freely moving, not rigidly welded. We are not constructed like skyscrapers with our base firmly and forever rooted to the ground and held in place by the force of gravity. Animals balance on flimsy supports. How does flamingo—a long, thin strut, with a near frictionless hinge in the middle—hold up the bird? (Figure 16.2) Most biological organisms that are upright, including plants, have a top half that is heavier

(a)

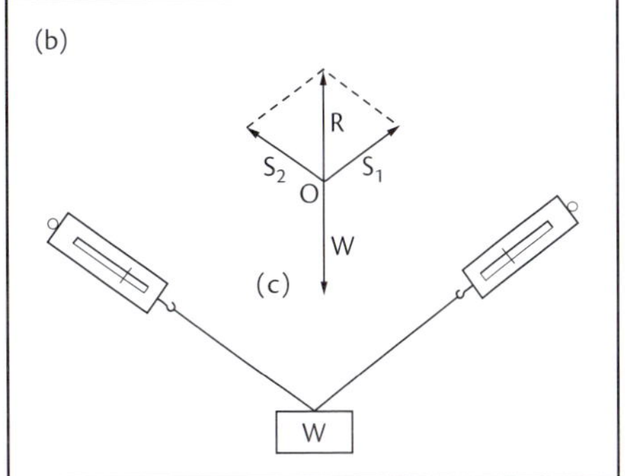

Figure 16.1 Gymnast's 'iron cross' position.

than the base. Stone walls and skyscrapers, but not flamingos, are, necessarily, thicker at their base. If our centre of gravity falls outside our base, we are not torn apart by internal shear forces, as happens to columns of stone. Biological structures exist independent of gravity. They are omnidirectional structures that can exist and adapt to water, land, air, and space.

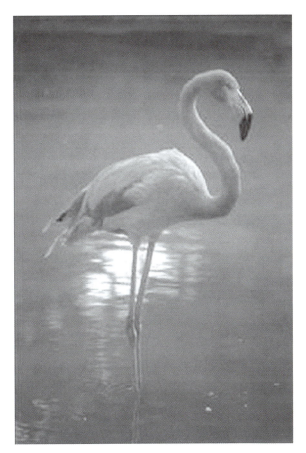

Figure 16.2 The slender leg of a flamingo.

Structural evolution of biological organisms

Certainly, no natural laws are broken. It is just that bioengineers usually consider only Newtonian mechanics as their basis for calculations (see Box 16.1). Biological materials are non-Hookean and non-Newtonian behaving physical structures and we cannot use Hookean and Newtonian laws to understand the material behaviour of biological organisms. Hookean and Newtonian materials

Box 16.1 Newtonian mechanics

Hooke's law: For any given material that obeys Hooke's law, the slope of the graph, or the ratio of stress to strain, will be constant. Biological tissues.

Euler's formula: P =„$^2E/L^2$, where P is the load at which a column will buckle and E is the Young's modulus of the material. The taller the column, the weaker and less stable it is. Very tall columns will bend of their own weight. If the Empire State Building had the same proportions as a stalk of wheat, it would be less than 2 m wide at its base. The spinal ligament should buckle under a load of only 2 kg, which is less than the weight of a person's head.

Galileo's square–cube law: As the surface area of a structure squares, its volume cubes. Eventually, it will crush of its own weight. If we use calculations based on Newtonian mechanics and known tissue strengths, the maximum size of a land-based animal can be no more than a modern elephant. Many dinosaurs far exceeded these weights, which leads to the conclusion that either large dinosaurs did not exist, or their tissues were much stronger, or Galileo's law does not apply to large animals.

Poisson's ratio: If you stretch an elastic material, it gets thinner. If you compress the material, it bulges out. The ratio of these changes in material is Poisson's ratio, which is a constant in most building materials. For engineering materials, the ratio lies between 0.25 and 0.5 and cannot exceed 0.5. However, biological materials usually have a ratio greater than 0.5 and may approach unity.

behave in a linear, additive fashion. Biological materials behave non-linearly or non-additively, and are not predictable using Hookean and Newtonian mechanics (Gordon 1978). As pointed out by Gould (1989), the combined action of any of the parts yields something other than the sum of the parts, and new properties or synergies emerge. What is clearly needed is a new model to replace the post and beam, column and lever, Hookean and Newtonian model that now dominates the thinking of biomechanics.

The military maxim of 'never stand when you can sit, never sit when you can lie down, never stay awake when you can be asleep' applies to nature's ways. Evolution is an exercise in optimization. The solution requiring the least energy will eventually happen, and once it happens, that solution will become the norm. Nature has a predilection for using and reusing whatever works, and works with the least amount of energy expenditure. Patterns and shapes in nature will evolve to their fittest form (Stevens 1974), with the tightest fit, and least energy expenditure. Nature also functions in a 'minimum inventory, maximum diversity' mode, trying to make do with the least amount of basic material to gain the maximum effect (Pearce 1978). DNA is constructed with just four nucleic acids and most of the DNA material of a lowly worm is repeated in the human genome. These genes are then used as templates to construct larger proteins, larger proteins add to other proteins, and so on.

The development of biological structure—whether organelles packed in a cell, cells packed in tissues, tissues packed in organs, or organs packed in organisms—is always in a 'closest packed' environment (Figure 16.3). The same is true of fish eggs in water, bee eggs in a hive, embryos in eggs, and fetuses *in utero*. Structural evolution of biological organisms will, therefore, obey the physical laws of 'triangulation' and 'closest packing' (Figure 16.4) that apply to

(a)

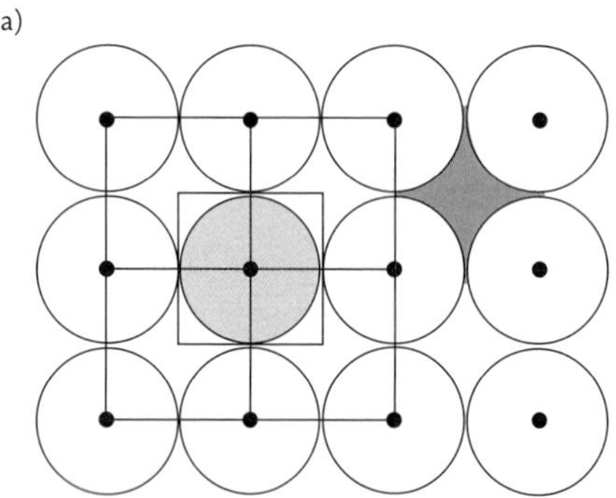

(b)

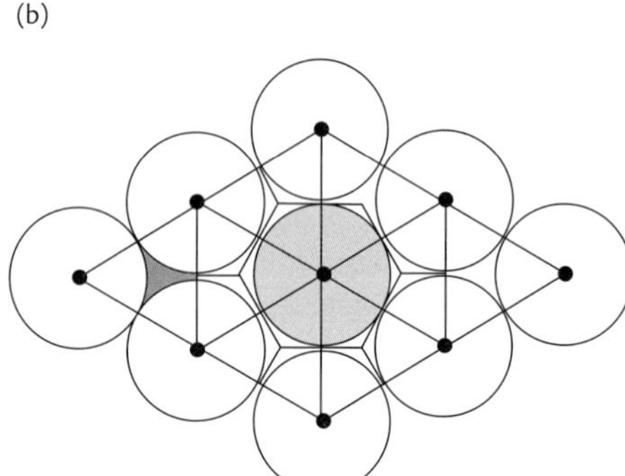

Figure 16.3 'Closest packed' environment.

(a)

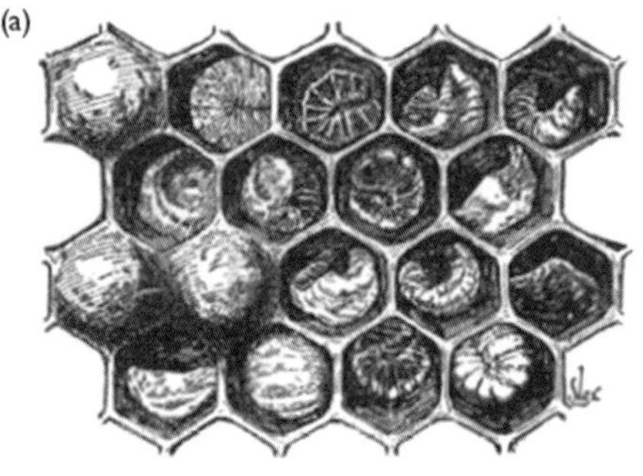

(b)

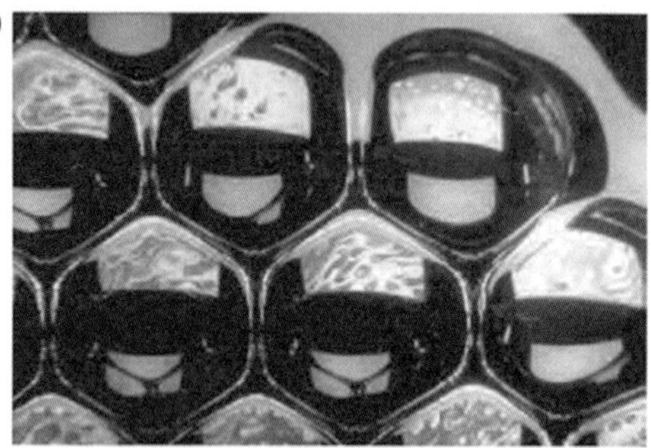

(c)

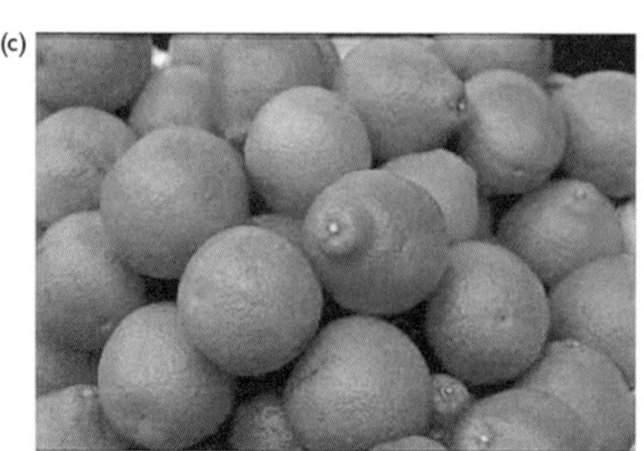

(d)

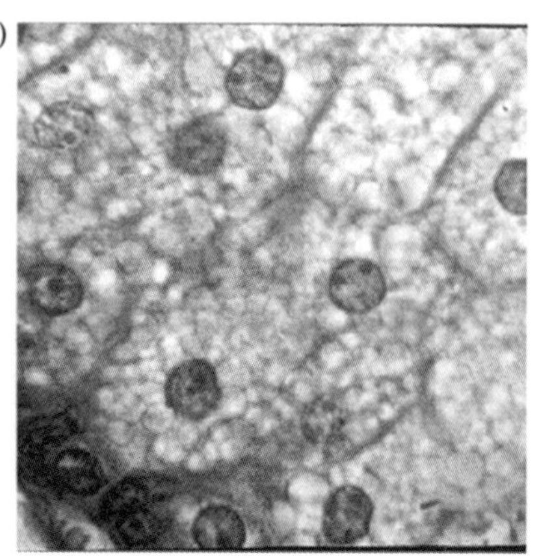

Figure 16.4 Physical laws of triangulation and closest packing.

structures filling space such as soap bubbles, grains of sand on a beach, oranges in a crate, molecules of water in a drop, or boulders on a mountain. In closest packing, there is a balance of the external forces of molecules, sand grains, droplets, cells, etc. crowding each other and the internal forces of the structure being crowded pushing out to keep from being crushed. This balance of forces assumes the least energy-consuming relationships.

The developing mammalian fetus is initially adapting to the closest-packed compressive forces *in utero* (Figure 16.5). Biological tissue adapts to the forces applied by getting stronger and developing specialized structures and tissues to resist those forces (Carter 1991; Wolff 1892). It is remarkable that the fetus, developing to resist the omnidirectional pressure within the uterus, can then resist the asymmetrical and very high compressive forces of delivery through the birth canal, and then instantly adapt to a completely new environment.

Initially adapting to and balancing compressive forces from without, so as not to get crushed, the fetus now has to resist the expanding forces from within, without exploding. With each heartbeat and breath, the newborn should blow up like a balloon. It is not a wine skin, taking its shape from the unconstrained and unorganized fluid within, and neither are any cells that maintain their shape, closest-packed, within the structure or completely removed to an open space environment. The outer container, the skin, does not contain the contents like the walls of a cylinder; the restraint of the explosive forces within comes from deep within the structure itself.

The same is true of cells, tissues, and organs. The chondrocyte has to balance the internal pressures with its external loads; otherwise, it would crush or explode. The chondrocytes in the knee joint must be contained when unloaded but instantly able to withstand the crushing loads of a full-back running down the field. Cartilage tensile strength is 30 times weaker than bone; muscle tensile strength, 1000 times weaker than tendon. Cartilage should shear right off the bone and muscles should tear with only minimal tendon pulls, unless the loads are distributed through the tissues. We know, from Darwinian theory and Wolff's law, that cartilage and muscle are as strong as they need to be. There must be some distribution and dispersing of loads in biological structures. There is a hierarchy of individual closest-packed structures—from sub-cellular, to cellular, to tissue, to organ, to organism—that are interdependent of and, at the same time, independent of one another. These structures must evolve consistent with Darwinian concepts and must be self-generating, omnidirectional, independent of gravity, and minimally energy consuming.

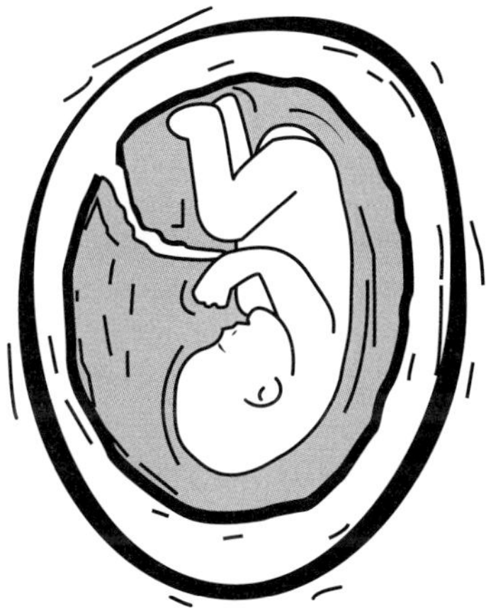

Figure 16.5 In the uterus, the fetus adapts to compressive forces.

To understand the evolution of biological structures, we must understand how nature fills space. Two-dimensional space filling is an exercise in triangulation. The triangle is the simplest, most stable, and least energy-requiring polygon. It will not deform even with flexible corners (vertices) as long as the sides remain connected, straight, and at the same length. Square-frame constructs are unstable and will deform into a parallelogram and eventually flatten to a pancake (Figure 16.6). They require rigidly fixed corners to maintain themselves. A structure that has all joints that are flexible must be fully triangulated. When we fit together six equilateral triangles, arranged around a point in a plane, they form a hexagon. Closest-packed hierarchical arrays of triangles in self-generating hexagons fill a planar space (Figure 16.7). If we pack equal-sized discs, such

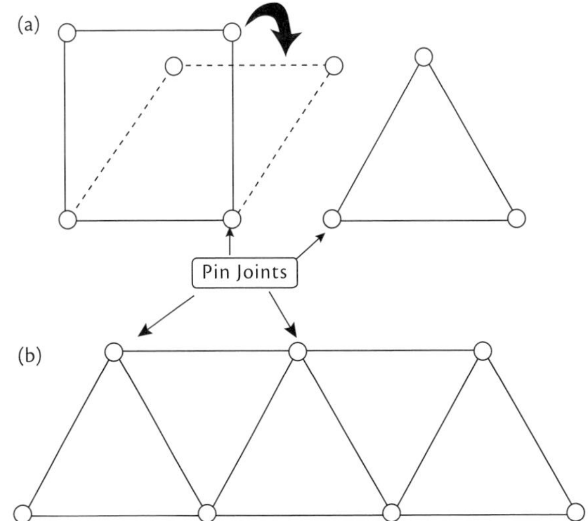

Figure 16.6 Square-frame constructs will deform and eventually flatten to a pancake.

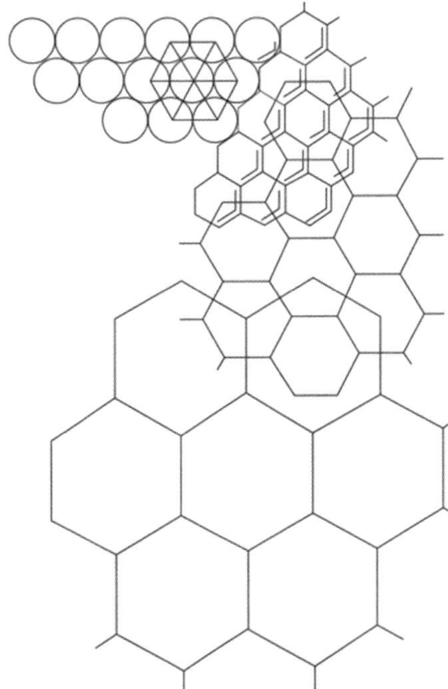

Figure 16.7 Closest-packed hierarchical arrays of triangles in self-generating hexagons fill a planar space.

as coins, into a planar space, their centres form equilateral triangles and assume the same relationship. This is the least energy-requiring arrangement of structure in two-dimensional space, familiar as the cross section of a beehive.

Hexagons, however, will not enclose three-dimensional space. In the three-dimensional world in which we live, pentagons and hexagons are mathematical concepts with only two dimensions. In three dimensions, they can only exist as part of some stable three-dimensional structure—a tetrahedron, octahedron, or icosahedron, which are the only fully triangulated regular polyhedra (Figure 16.8). To do that, the geometry changes a bit. Five equilateral triangles will form a bowl with its perimeter, a pentagon. When you continue to add triangles in a closest-packed environment, they curve back on it and become a hollow closed space. Twenty planar triangles fit together as an icosahedron, perfectly enclosing the space. This configuration, too, has self-generating properties (Figure 16.9). This is one of the Platonic regular convex polyhedra, of which there are only five, which were known to the Greeks and other early mathematicians. All convex polyhedrons are some combination, permutation, or higher frequency of these five basic polyhedrons. Only three of the five are fully triangulated and, therefore, least energy-requiring structures. They are the tetrahedron with four sides, the octahedron with eight sides, and the icosahedron with twenty sides. Water molecules, silicone molecules, carbon molecules, and methane molecules are all tetrahedrons. Twelve pentagon faces will enclose space as a dodecahedron. However, a dodecahedron is an unstable frame structurally, as is the cube. Using the commonly utilized hexagonal (cube) modelling for finite-element analysis would not reflect the structural integrity of the tissue: tetrahedral modelling is more consistent with the way biological structure forms and behaves (Figure 16.10).

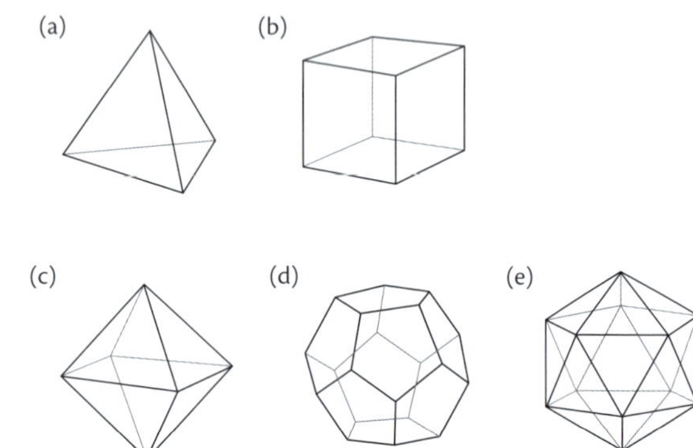

Figure 16.8 Tetrahedrons, octahedrons, and icosahedrons are the only fully triangulated regular polyhedrons.

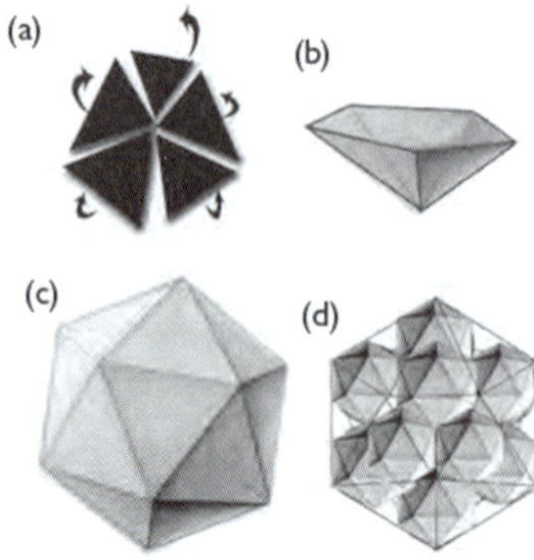

Figure 16.9 An icosahedron has self-generating properties.

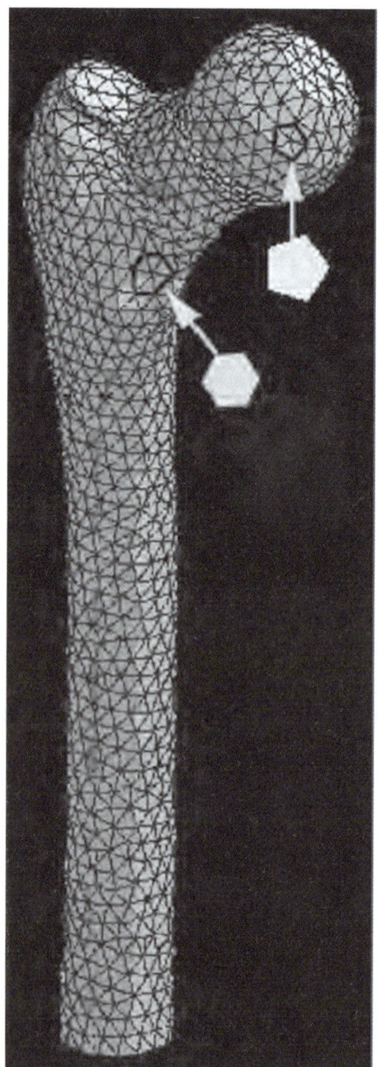

Figure 16.10 Tetrahedral modelling is consistent with biological structure.

Filling the interiors of the hollow polyhedrons must follow the same closest packing laws. Closest packing twenty tetrahedrons around a point in three-dimensional space will create an icosahedron, just as six triangles create a two-dimensional hexagon (see Figure 16.9d). Twelve equal-sized icosahedrons closest pack to form another icosahedron, joining at their five-fold symmetrical (pentagonal) edges. The centre is a hollow, somewhat smaller, icosahedral-shaped vacuole. As fractals (Mandelbrot 1983), sharing faces and edges and intersecting one another, just as soap bubbles do, they will form an infinite array of interlinked, hierarchical, stable structures functioning as a whole or as subsets of icosahedrons.

The icosahedron and its special qualities

The icosahedron has many things going for it. In addition to its self-generating properties and its ability to enclose three-dimensional space, it is mathematically the most symmetrical

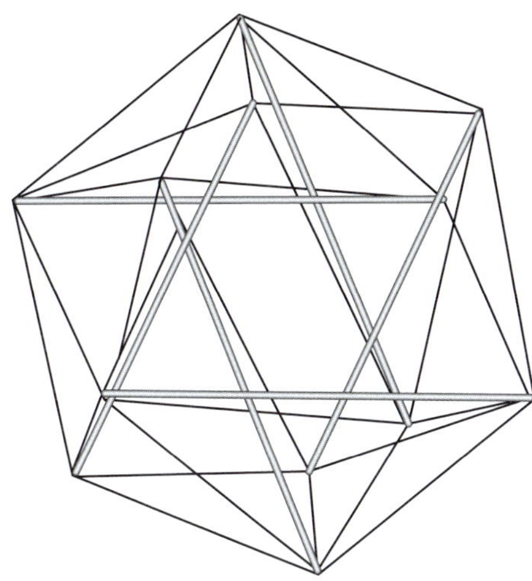

Figure 16.11 The rods do not pass through the centre of the icosahedron but are slightly eccentric and pass each other without touching (see text).

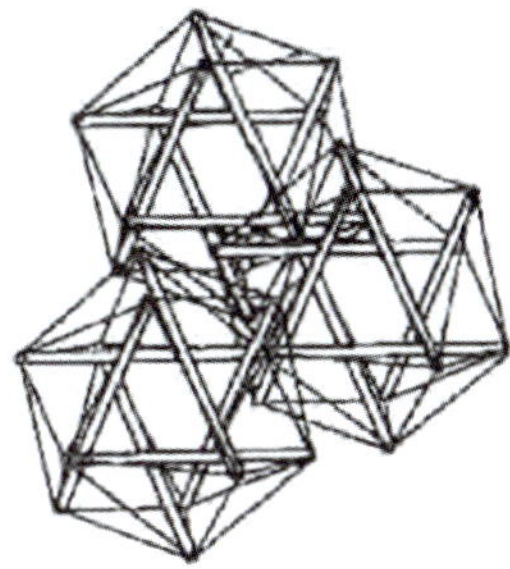

Figure 16.12 The tensegrity icosahedron as a fractal generator.

structure and is omnidirectional in form and function. It has the largest volume for surface area of the regular polyhedra, and larger structures are only higher-frequency icosahedrons. The icosahedron has 30 edges and 12 vertices with 20 sides. If the edges are rigid, then pressure at any point transmits around the 30 edges, putting some under pressure and others under tension, in a regular pattern. The 12 vertices each have three edges that come together at that corner. Some of these edges are under tension and some under compression, depending on the vector of force applied to the structure. The compression load can be transferred away from the outside of the structure by connecting the vertices opposite to one another by rigid, compression-bearing rods. These rods do not pass through the centre of the icosahedron but are slightly eccentric and pass each other without touching (Figure 16.11). These compression rods are now joined at the icosahedral vertices by a continuous tension shell with all the edges on the outside of the icosahedron under tension, the 'tensegrity' icosahedron. These, too, can form infinite arrays, and the tensegrity icosahedron can be a fractal generator (Mandelbrot 1983) (Figure 16.12).

Structural origins of biotensegrity

Tensegrity, a word coined by Buckminster Fuller (1975) to describe continuous-tension discontinuous- compression structures, was applied to constructs designed by Kenneth Snelson (Snelson 2002) and Fuller. Examples of these structures are Snelson's Needle sculpture at the Hirshhorn Museum, Washington DC (Figure 16.13),

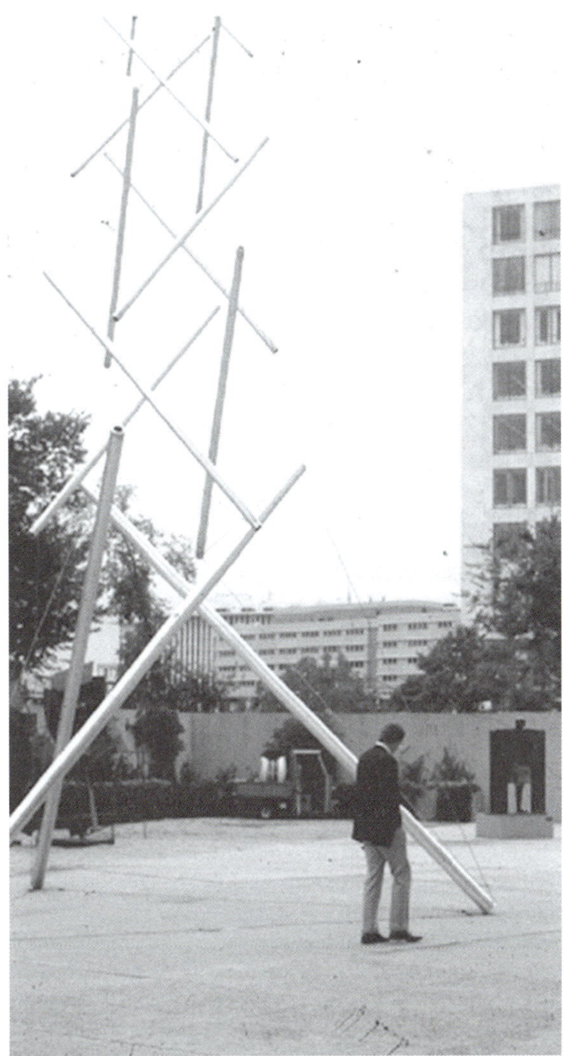

Figure 16.13 Snelson's 'Needle' sculpture, Hirshhorn Museum, Washington DC.

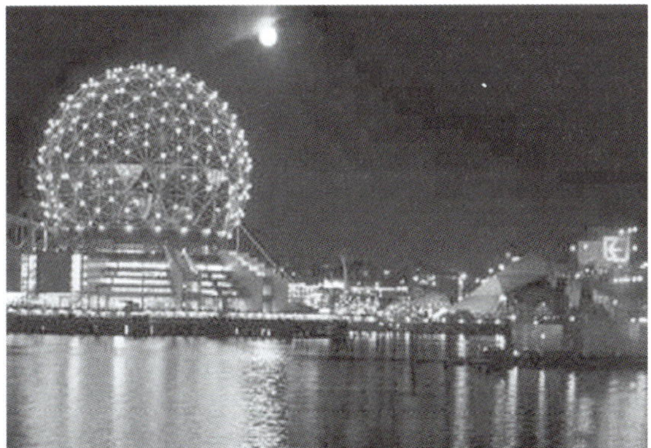

Figure 16.14 Fuller's geodesic domes.

Fuller's now ubiquitous geodesic domes (Figure 16.14), and the wire-spoke bicycle wheel. Biotensegrity is the application of tensegrity principles to biological structures. The tension or tensegrity icosahedron is a pre-stressed, semi-rigid structure constructed of tension and compression members where none of the compression units compress each other. Instead, they 'float' within the tension outer skin. Just as the single icosahedron can have either an exo- or endoskeleton, the linked, hierarchical structure can internalize its compression components, and the whole structure can behave as a single icosahedron. As you can see, what happens is that a hierarchy of icosahedrons creates itself, balancing the external forces and internal forces as a self-generating structure.

A bicycle wheel exemplifies the differences between a tensegrity and a non-tensegrity structure

The dandelion puffball (Figure 16.15) is easily recognized as a tensegrity structure. The bicycle wheel is the most common, easily recognizable, non-biological tensegrity structure. The mechanics of a wagon wheel and a bicycle wheel are completely different (Figure 16.16). A wagon wheel transmits the wagon load to the ground through the axle, compressing the spoke between it and the ground. The spoke has to be strong enough to withstand the full weight of the wagon; it gets no help from the other spokes which, at that moment, sustain no load. Besides the compressive loads, internal shear is created within the spoke. The intervening rim acts as the pedestal of the columnar spoke and has to be equal to the task of being crushed by the full weight of the wagon load. As the wheel rotates, it vaults from spoke to spoke. Halfway through the transfer of compressive load from one spoke to the next, the rigid rim acts as a lever, creates bending moments, and has to be strong enough to withstand the additional loads. At any one moment, the structures are locally loaded and the remaining elements can be stripped away without seriously compromising the structural integrity. (The wheel just could not roll on.)

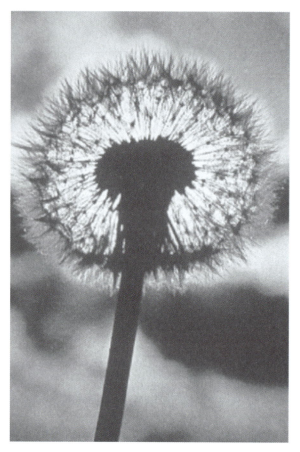

Figure 16.15 Dandelion puffball.

In a bicycle wheel, the hub is suspended, hanging from the topmost spoke. This would cause the thin, weak rim to buckle. It is kept from buckling by the other wire spokes constantly pulling in on the rim to keep it round. All the spokes are under constant and equal tension. The tensions are preset, and do not vary with the load. The wheel is an integrated structure, with each spoke depending on every other to share the load at all times. The compression of the ground to the rim is distributed through the tension spokes to the hub. Therefore, there is no direct compression link between the load on the bicycle frame and the ground reaction force. The bicycle is suspended off the ground in a tension spoke network, hanging like a hammock, and the same system works equally well in a unicycle, bicycle, or tricycle. In a cycle wheel, the hub and rim

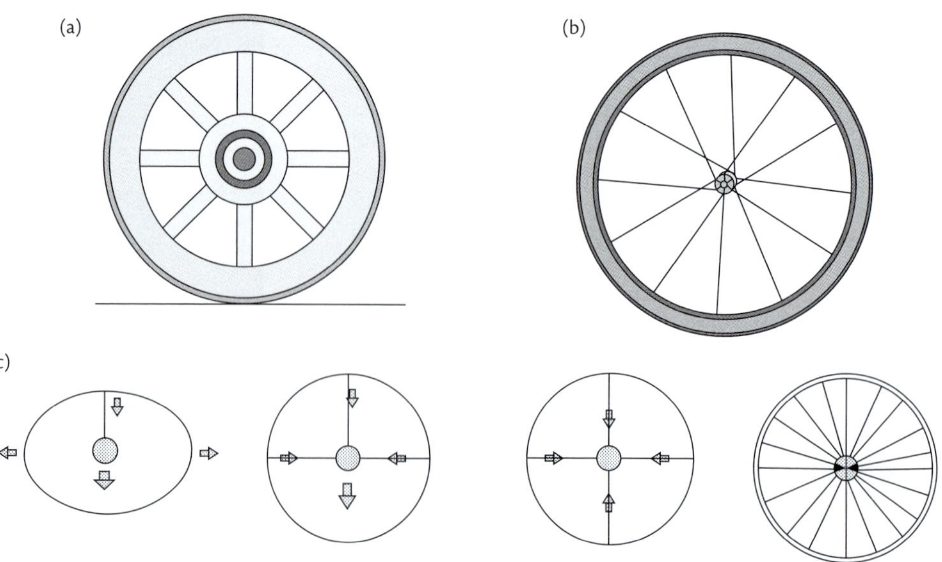

Figure 16.16 The mechanics of a wagon wheel and a bicycle wheel.

are compression elements kept apart by tension spokes. There are no bending moments in the tension spokes, which are prestressed, under constant tension. The cycle wheel exists only as an integrated structure. One spoke will not hold up under the weight of the load.

Once constructed this way, the tension elements remain in tension and compression elements remain under compression, no matter what the direction of force or point of application of the load. It makes no difference where you compress the rim of the cycle wheel; the load is equally distributed through the spokes to the hub. The rim of the bicycle is a geodesic, connecting the many points of the spoke attachments: the more spokes, the rounder it gets. If the narrow rim is expanded to a sphere by creating great circle bands around the hub, then the outer, exoskeleton of the geodesic sphere is rigidly fixed to the central hub and transmits load to or away from that hub by the tension spokes.

Some mechanics peculiar to tensegrities

As already noted, in some tensegrity structures, the compression elements can be internalized and the tension elements externalized to create an endoskeleton using the same mechanics, with the outer skin under tension and the inner skeleton intertwined in the tension network. The structure is truly omnidirectional. It never has to change tension elements to compression elements, or vice versa, to resist the compressive forces from without or the explosive forces from within, no matter from which direction the load is applied. Loads applied to the surface of linear, Hookean structures create a dimple right under it. Loads applied to a point on the skin of a tensegrity icosahedron are distributed evenly around all the edges in tension and across the floating rods under compression. Since load applied to the surface is distributed uniformly over the entire surface, instead of flattening and spreading out, the whole structure starts to compress and the tension icosahedron uniformly becomes smaller and more compact with the compression rods approximating each other more closely. The internal pressure of the icosahedron increases as it becomes more compressed, and it does so as a factor of the square of the radius. The graph of this relationship is a J-shaped curve that represents a non-linear stress–strain relationship. This is radically different from the Hookean, linear behaviour of most non-biological materials and structures (Figure 16.17). In Hookean structures, for each increment of stress, there is a proportional strain until the point of elastic deformation just before it breaks. Hookean structures weaken under load. In the tensegrity structures, there is rapid deformation with the initial load but then the structure stiffens and becomes more rigid and stronger.

How biologic tissues behave like tensegrity structures

This J-shaped non-linear curve is also a characteristic response of biological tissues, from cells to spines. Tug on your lip and you will note that as you tug the skin is loose at first and then becomes stiffer and effects larger and larger areas of skin. The cells under the heel could not sustain crushing loads of the runner without this type of elasticity, as they would burst. This behaviour is true not only of the skin; it also then connects deeper, eventually reaching right down to the bone. The process is reversed when any pressure is applied to the skin, as through the sole of the foot, with the soft tissues resisting the compressive force by tension, just as does the wire spoke, and then distributing it through the compressive-bearing bones.

The importance of the J-shaped non-linear response of biological tissue and the difference between the soft tissue mechanics of biological materials and structures cannot be overemphasized. The rigid materials used in non-biological constructs generally operate at elastic strains in the region of 0.1%. Rarely, they may strain, that is deform to the point to which they can fully recover, to 10 times that amount. Conceivably, they can go to elastic strains of 20% but, at that level, Hookean material reaches the level at which its chemical bonds would explode. Biological tissues commonly operate at strains of 50–100% or more, often 1000 times greater than those of conventional engineering materials. Neither do they behave like rubber, which has an S-shaped stress–strain curve and is characterized by bursting at its elastic limit and aneurysm formation (that would not do well in arteries). The elastic behaviour of biological tissue when initially stressed is comparable to the surface of a liquid at low and moderate strains. It then rises in its very characteristic, non-Hookean, J-shaped response. Mathematically, this is the only sort of elasticity that is completely stable under the fluid pressures at high strains found in blood vessels, alveoli, bladders, bowels, muscles, uteri, and most other biological soft tissues (Gordon 1978). The properties imparted by this curve are flexible and tough.

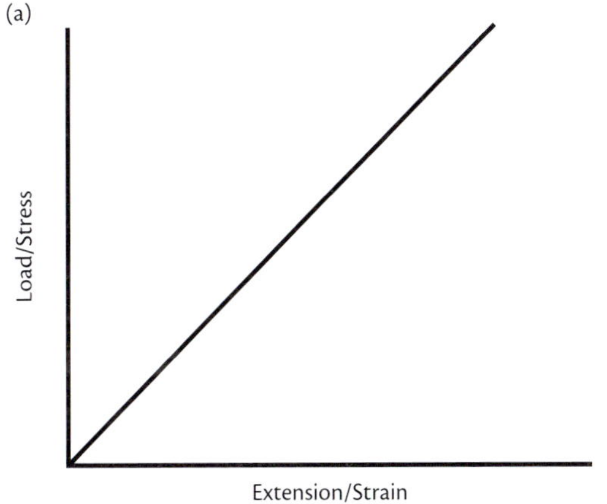

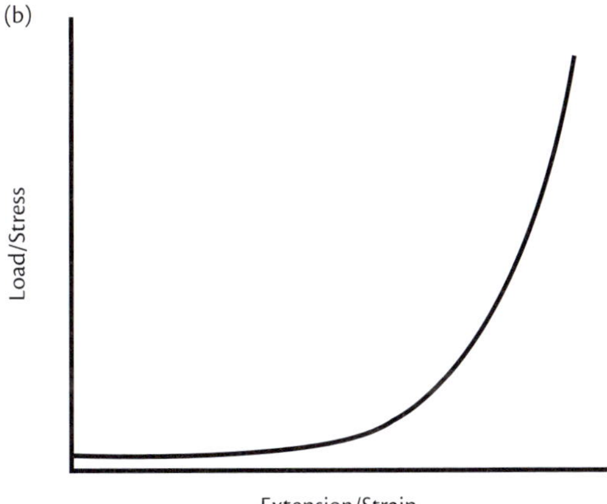

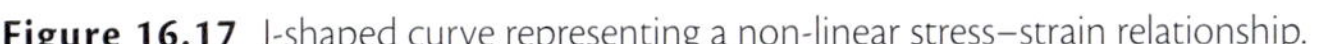

Figure 16.17 J-shaped curve representing a non-linear stress–strain relationship.

With this configuration, biological tissue is unlikely to fracture, explode, or be prone to aneurysm formation. Tendons and bone can store large amounts of energy and return it like a spring, in leaps and bounds. The model usually used to approximate this type of behaviour is the so-called 'viscoelastic' behaviour of biological tissues. This is a complicated and rather contrived behaviour that puts the response of a Hookean elastic material parallel with the response of a Newtonian-behaving fluid, like water, and those, then, in series with another Hookean body. Modelling life's behaviour would be simplified if there were a naturally occurring structure, such as the tensegrity icosahedron, that nature could use for its constructs.

Biological tissues are pre-stressed, with the J-curve never zeroing out, so that there is always a balance of dynamic forces acting on the structure. Often, compression and tension roles can be reversed in these types of structure, but the sum function may remain the same. To appreciate these qualities, consider a pneumatic tyre or a balloon, which are also pre-stressed structures. The walls of the pneumatic structures are prevented from collapsing by the collision of molecules of gas within it pushing on all surfaces equally. The pressure in a tyre is the same whether the car is on a hydraulic lift or sitting on the ground. Sitting there, the tyre seems a little flat. To get a more efficient roll, you can put in more air or heat up the gas inside the tyre, creating more energy in the tyre and more collisions of molecules on the walls. The friction on the road does just that. It is the balance of the internal energy of the gas and the external elastic energy of the tyre wall, which is under tension, that defines its functional capabilities. It reacts to its load but is not dependent on it. In a wire-spoke wheel, the spokes pull the rim towards the centre. Until an adequate number of spokes are properly placed, the spokes cannot be tightened. Once at that point (the minimum number is 12), the wire wheel behaves as the pneumatic tyre does, only in reverse. Instead of the gas molecules pushing out, the spokes pull the rim towards the centre; the tension is inside and the compression is outside. This shows how the tension and compression elements can be reversed, but still perform similar functions.

Over the years, I (Levin 1982, 1986, 1995, 1997) and others (Ingber 1997, 2000; Ingber and Jamieson 1985; Stamenovic et al. 1996; Wang et al. 1993, 2001; Wildy and Home 1963) have proposed a new model for biological structures based on the concept of tensegrity. In vertebrates, the skeleton would be the compression element within a highly organized soft-tissue construct, rather than the frame supporting an amorphous soft-tissue mass. The same organization occurs at the cellular level with the cytoskeleton and the, anything but amorphous, cytoplasm. Tensegrity structures are omnidirectional, independent of gravity, load-distributing and energy-efficient, hierarchical, and self-generating. They are also ubiquitous in nature, once you know what to look for. They can be used to model biological structures, from viruses to vertebrates and their systems and subsystems. They are fully triangulated and, therefore, least energy-consuming systems, that are stable even with flexible hinges. The tensegrity icosahedron can be linked in an infinite array in hierarchical systems and fractal constructs that can function together in unison, acting as an icosahedron no matter what its shape. It can be considered the finite structural element and used as a building block for all biological structures. Its non-linear stress–strain curve is a characteristic, and even defines biological tissues (Gordon 1988). The tensegrity model is now gaining wide acceptance as a model for biological mechanics (Ingber 1998) and is very useful in understanding the mechanisms of action in orthopaedic medicine.

The shoulder modelled as a biotensegrity structure

The principle of tensegrity modelling can be well demonstrated in the shoulder, which is the joint complex least successfully modelled using Newtonian mechanics. In multi-segmented mathematical shoulder models, rigid beams (the bones) act as a series of columns or levers to transmit forces or loads to the axial skeleton. Forces passing through the almost frictionless joints must, somehow, always be directed perfectly perpendicular to the joints, as only loads directed at right angles to the surfaces could transfer across frictionless joints. Loads transmitted to the axial skeleton would have to pass through the moving ribs, or the weak jointed clavicle and then through the ribs.

As the arm circumducts in any plane, it inscribes the rim of an imaginary wheel (Figure 16.18). The arm becomes the spoke that transfers the load, at the hand, to the axial skeleton. Present models conceptualize the upper extremity as the spoke of a wagon wheel (Figure 16.16). This is a classic Newtonian construction with columns, beams, levers, and fulcrums, with resulting bending moments and torque. The bones of the arm are envisioned as the rigid spokes but, although there is a bony articulation at the glenohumeral joint that might be able to transfer compressive loads from the arm to the scapula, there is no rigid, compressive, load-bearing structure between the scapula and the axial skeleton, nor is there a suitable fulcrum. In a linked-lever system, a seamless continuum of compression elements is necessary. Bone must compress bone. The almost frictionless joints would require forces to be always directed at right angles to the joint; otherwise, the bone would slide right out of the joint. The scapula is not anatomically situated to transfer loads through the ribs to the spine. Even if it were, the ribs could not take these loads and act as levers to connect to the spine.

The ribs themselves, by shape, position, and connection, are not structurally capable of transferring these loads. The clavicle is in no shape to transfer loads, either. It is a crank-shaped beam that connects the scapula to the sternum by a small, mobile joint that could not transfer compressive loads of any significant magnitude (Figure 16.19). Cats do not have articulating clavicles, but they can run

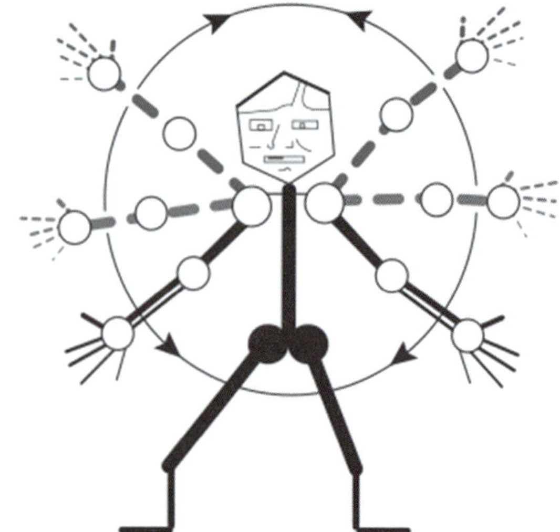

Figure 16.18 As the arm circumducts, it inscribes the rim of an imaginary wheel.

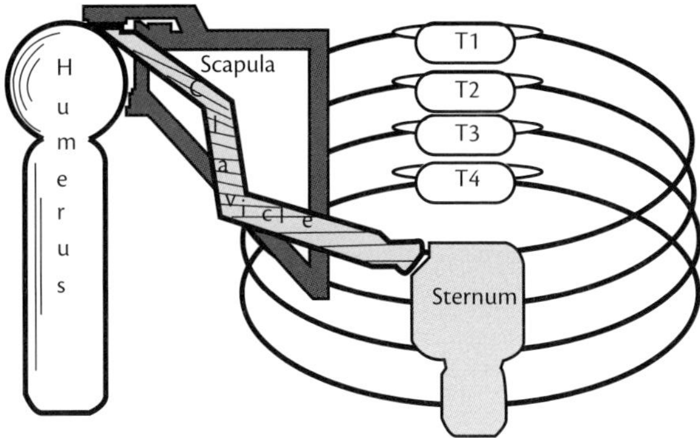

Figure 16.19 The clavicle connects the scapula to the sternum by a small, mobile joint.

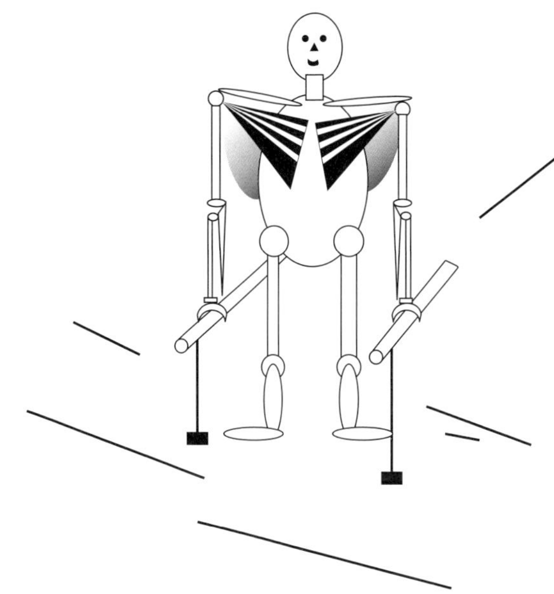

Figure 16.20 Grant's tension model.

and climb with the best of us creatures. The scapula of quadrupeds and bipeds hangs on the thorax by a network of muscles, and all the moment and compression forces generated in the arm must be transferred to the axial skeleton through these soft tissues. A rope cannot withstand compressive loads, nor can it function as a lever, and neither can muscle or tendon. A wagon wheel, which depends on rigid, compressive, load-bearing spokes to transfer loads, is not a suitable analogy for shoulder girdle mechanics. If we use a wire cycle wheel tensegrity structure as our model, the shoulder is readily modelled and takes into account all the necessary factors in joint modelling. If we consider the scapula functioning as the hub of a tensegrity structure, then the forces coming from the spoke-like arm could be transferred to the axial skeleton through the soft tissues rather than the circuitous and imposing linked levers of the bones.

A bicycle wheel tensegrity model is mechanically more efficient than a spoked wagon wheel model. In a wagon wheel, only one or two spokes are sustaining loads at any one time. The spoke must be rigid and strong enough to withstand the entire weight thrust upon it. It gets no help from its neighbours. The rim of the wagon wheel must also be strong enough to withstand these crushing loads directly at the point of contact with the road. In a wire wheel, forces are distributed, all the elements act in concert, and all the spokes contribute all the time. The rim is part of the system and the compressive load, directed at a point, is taken by the entire rim. Tensegrity structures are fully triangulated and, therefore, there are no bending moments in these structures, just tension and compression, and, therefore, significantly less loads to be reckoned with. Tensegrity structures are omnidirectional load distributors. The tension elements always remain in tension and the compression elements always remain in compression, no matter in what direction the loads are applied. This is not so in a column or a lever which is rigidly oriented to resist a load from a specific direction. As the loads in tensegrity structures are distributed all the time, each structural element can be lighter.

Grant (1952) used a tension model to suspend the body, hammock-like, between gymnastic parallel bars (Figure 16.20). However, hammock-like suspension is unidirectional. Turn the hammock or suspension bridge over and not only does everything fall out of the hammock or off the road, but the hammock or road also collapses. A tensegrity structure is omnidirectional in form and function and can be used right side up, upside down, or any position in between, and still maintain its form, its structural integrity, and its ability to transmit loads. When modelling a shoulder as a tensegrity structure, the bones that 'float' in the tension network of soft tissue are only being compressed. There are no moments at the joints because the structure is fully triangulated. In this model, the shoulder becomes inherently stable and changes position only when one of the elements of the triangle is shortened or lengthened, just as changing the tension in a wire spoke will distort the wheel. The continuous tension present in the soft tissues stabilizes the joints at each moment. Therefore, considerably less energy is needed to 'stabilize' the joints.

The scapula, suspended in the 'spokes' of the attached muscles and soft tissue, could function as a stable base for the arm. It could also transfer loads to the 'rim' of vertebrae through these same spokes. With the scapula as a hub in a tensegrity system, loads are transferred from the arm to the spine via the large amount of available muscle and ligaments, through a stable yet easily mobilized, omnidirectional, low-energy-requiring system that would utilize lighter, less bulky parts and accommodates global motion and stability. This contrasts with a multi-segmented articulated column model that is inherently unstable and has high energy requirements. In multi-segmented systems, with each change of direction of load, new mechanics must be established. The tensegrity model is readily visualized when modelling scapular mechanics, since there are really no suitable compressive load-bearing joints that can connect the scapula to the spine.

Muscles, as well as all other soft-tissue elements in the body, are always under some tension—they are pre-stressed. It is the tone of the muscle that holds us upright, keeps our jaw from dropping, and our scapulas from sliding off our chest wall, as we do these things when the electromyograph (EMG) is electrically silent (Basmajian 1962), meaning there is no active contraction of the muscles. The tone of the muscles and the stored elastic energy in the soft tissues must be regarded as stabilizers and as motors, to understand the forces that control stability and mobility in the body. The transfer of forces in the body could possibly be through these already tense soft-tissue elements.

The glenohumeral articulation may appear, at first, to be a more traditional compressive load-bearing joint. However, for the joint to be stable, forces must be directed at right angles (normal) to the joint, since the cartilaginous surfaces are essentially frictionless. The glenohumeral joint is a multi-axial ball-and-socket joint. The head of the humerus is larger than the glenoid fossa, and the surfaces are incongruous ovals and not true spheres. There is no bony structural stability and the joint is loosely packed, with a great deal of play between the surfaces. There are very few positions of the arm in which the humeral head directs its compressive forces normal to the glenoid fossa. Usually, the forces are directed almost parallel to the joint surface. Since there is a change in direction of forces, in order to transfer forces to the scapula, the glenohumeral joint must function much like the universal joint of an automobile drive shaft. As Fuller (1975) points out, the universal joint is analogous to the wire wheel as a basic tensegrity system. It relies on the differentiation of tension and compression for its effectiveness. The soft tissues, the capsule, ligaments, and muscles act as the connecting pins of a universal joint. Both the scapulothoracic and the glenohumeral joints may be modelled, efficiently and easily, as tensegrity-structured joints. Modelling the shoulder as a rigid, multi-segmented lever is a struggle.

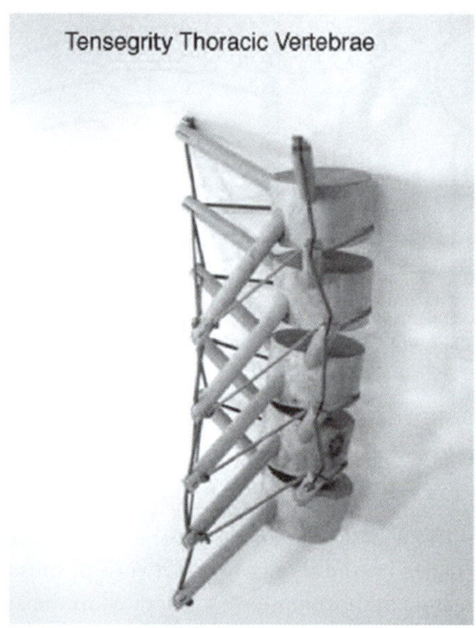

Figure 16.21 Sculptures modelled from tensegrity units.

Matching tensegrity and biological dynamics

Movement is an integral part of animal life, and even the strongest trees sway in the wind. A multi-linked Hookean mechanical structure would move just as you would expect a machine to move, with robotic jerkiness, because of the very nature of Hookean elastic materials. Hookean material has very abrupt transition from stress to unstressed, lending itself to jerky movements, and hence the need for dampening springs with shock absorbers on automobiles. Tensegrity structures restore their full elastic energy more slowly; for example, bent grass returning to its normal, upright stance. Tensegrity structures move as a unit. Tighten one tension member and a ripple of movement runs through the entire structure, be it one cell or billions. The highly integrated flowing movement of the simplest and smallest to the most complex and largest organism is not possible with Hookean systems. Whales and walruses leave no wake, ships and submarines do. The free-flowing integrated movement of a bee buzzing, a bat on the wing, a baboon swinging, and a ballet dancer *en pointe* cannot be matched by any mechanical device. Flemons (2002) and others have modelled sculptures from tensegrity units (Figure 16.21) that demonstrate how these structures move in a flowing transition from one configuration to the next.

Elastic structures store energy when deformed, and the energy is released as they return to their original shape. Much of the movement is with stored elastic energy. Stress, and the resultant strain, stores energy within the system. In bone and tendons, this energy can be quite substantial, and when modelled as tensegrity structures, even more impressive because of its non-linearity and the resulting initial explosive force that automatically smoothes out as it reaches its resting state. Once an icosahedron reaches its resting point (which, unlike Hookean material, is pre-stressed), it will non-linearly resist the overreach recoil. This makes for smooth, flowing movements like a pendulum swinging back and forth. Owing to its collagen matrix, live bone has the springiness of a vaulter's pole, and when the icosahedrons are compressed and released, they put bounce in each step.

The linkages of icosahedrons are similar to organic chemical linkages. There can be one, two, or three bonds between linked icosahedrons, and this imparts varying stability between the links. The joints would be very rigid with three-bond linkage and less so with fewer links. A tree most likely has triple bonding. The double tie-bar hinge arrangement in the knee is an example of a typical two-bar link, with the crossed cruciate ligaments under tension imparting rotations and translations, and the stored energy of the ligaments assisting in knee flexion and extension. If the spine were linked in such a system, movement would cascade up and down the structure like a toy 'Jacob's ladder' (Figure 16.22).

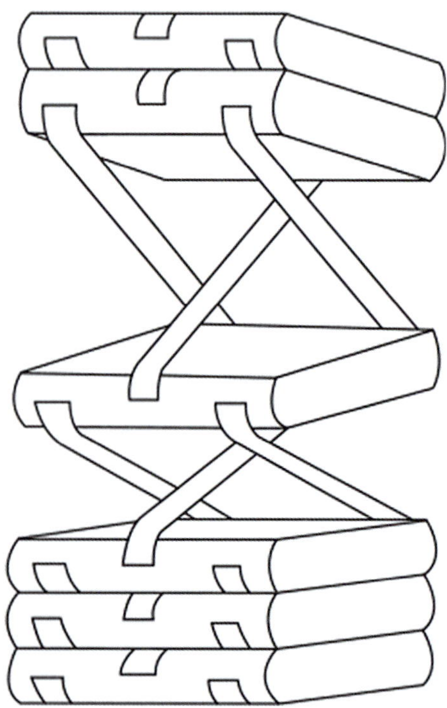

Figure 16.22 The spine modelled as a toy 'Jacob's ladder'.

Concluding thoughts about tensegrity as a model for biologic structures

It is an engineer's job to understand, simplify, and offer predictability when dealing with structures. Imprecise natural processes can only be subjected to approximate descriptions. As Toffler (1984) says:

> While some parts of the universe may operate like machines, these are closed systems, and closed systems, at best, form only a small part of the physical universe. Most phenomena of interest to us are, in fact, open systems, exchanging energy or matter, (and, one might add, information), with their environment. Surely biologic and social systems are open, which means that the attempt to understand them in mechanistic terms is doomed to failure.

Biological structures are chaotic, non-linear, complex, and unpredictable by their very nature. The new sciences of chaos (Gleick 1988; Prigogine and Stengers 1984) and complexity (Waldrop 1992) are needed to explain and understand biological structural mechanics.

Tensegrity structures have unique characteristics that parallel the structural requirements of biology. The giant leap from Newtonian to tensegrity models in biological modelling can be taken in small hops. Cells are tensegrity structures. Ingber, in a series of experiments, has proved that the cytoskeleton is a tensegrity structure and it is connected to the nucleus hub, which is also a tensegrity structure. Pulling on the cell wall, distorting its skin, has a direct effect on the nucleus and shows that they are structurally connected through the cytoskeleton. Clathrins (sub-cellular structures) are geodesic domes, and geodesic domes are tensegrity structures. Actin, the contractile element of muscle, and leukocytes, are arranged as geodesic domes. Viruses are icosahedra, which are the lowest frequency geodesic dome. *Radiolaria, Volvox*, insect eyes, pith, dandelion puffballs, and blowfish are all geodesic domes. Carbon-60, ubiquitous in the universe, is a self-generating geodesic dome (Kroto 1988). Unlike Hookean structures, the mechanics of geodesic domes are non-linear. As the structure is compressed, it uniformly shrinks, increasing its internal pressure non-linearly. The heart, alveoli, bladder, arteries, and all other hollow vesicles within the body do the same. Bone, discs, muscles, and ligaments, individually and as composites, behave non-linearly. In terms of mechanics and physiology, biological tissues behave in the same way as tensegrity structures.

As already noted, from the physicalist and biomechanical viewpoint, as well as according to Darwinian theory, the evolution of structure is an optimization problem (Pearce 1978). At each step of development, the evolving structure optimizes so that it exists with the least amount of energy expenditure. At the cellular level, the internal structure of the cells, the microtubules, together with the cell wall, must resist the crushing forces of the surrounding milieu and the exploding forces of its internal metabolism. Following Wolff's law, the internal skeleton of the cell aligns itself in the most efficient way to resist those forces. An hierarchical construction of an organism would use the same mechanical laws that are behind the building of the most basic biological structure, to generate the more complex organism. Not only is the beehive an icosahedron, so also is the bee's eye.

Of the known tensegrity structures, the tension icosahedron has particular attributes that make it the most suitable for biological musculoskeletal modelling (Levin 1986). Icosahedral tensegrity structures are self-organizing space frames that are hierarchical and evolutionary (Kroto 1988). They will build themselves, conforming to the laws of triangulation, close packing, and, in biological constructs, Wolff's law and Darwinian evolutionary concepts. In the model we have used, the scapula, fixed in space by the tension of its muscles, ligaments, and fascial envelope, functions as the connecting link between the spine and the upper arm, ontogenetically directed not only by phylogenetic forces but also by the physical forces of embryological development. Wolff and Thompson state that the structure of the body is essentially a blueprint of the forces applied to these structures. Carter theorizes that the mechanical forces *in utero* are the determinants of embryological structure that, in turn, evolves to fetal and then newborn structure.

What is obvious in the shoulder joint is equally efficient and functional in all other joints of the body, from the cellular level on upwards. It makes no evolutionary sense to create different mechanical models for each species, or for each cell, each tissue, each joint, each position in space, or for each activity (from swimming in the water to walking on land, swinging from trees, or flying in the air) when there is one mechanical model that does it all, efficiently and with the least energy expenditure. The biotensegrity model does all this, in any direction and under any conditions.

References

Basmajian, J. V. (1962) *Muscles alive—their function revealed by electromyography*. Williams & Wilkins, Baltimore, MD.

Carter, D. R. (1991) Musculoskeletal otogeny, phylogeny, and functional adaptation. *Journal of Biomechanics*, 24, 3–16.

Flemons, T. (2002) <http://intensiondesigns.com>.

Fuller, R. B. (1975) *Synergetics*. Macmillan, New York.

Gleick, J. (1988) *Chaos*. Penguin, New York.

Gordon, J. E. (1978) *Structures: or why things don't fall down*. De Capa Press, New York.

Gordon, J. E. (1988) *The science of structures and materials*. W. H. Freeman, New York.

Gould, S. J. (1989) Gratuitous battle. *Civilization*, 87.

Gracovetsky, S. (1988) *The spinal engine*. Springer-Verlag, New York.

Grant, J. C. B. (1952) *A method of anatomy*. Williams and Wilkins, Baltimore, MD.

Ingber, D. E. (1997) Tensegrity: the architectural basis of cellular mechanotransduction. *Annual Review of Physiology*, 59, 575–99.

Ingber, D. (1998) The architecture of life. *Scientific American*, 278, 48–57.

Ingber, D. E. (2000) The origin of cellular life. *Bioessays*, 22, 1160–70.

Ingber, D. E., Jamieson, J. (1985) Cells as tensegrity structures. Architectural regulation of histodifferentiation by physical forces transduced over basement membrane. Academic Press, New York.

Kroto, H. (1988) Space, stars, C60, and soot. *Science*, 242, 1139–45.

Levin, S. M. (1982) Continuous tension, discontinuous compression, a model for biomechanical support of the body. *Bulletin of structural integration*. Rolf Institute, Boulder, CO, pp. 31–3.

Levin, S. M. (1986) The icosahedron as the three-dimensional finite element in biomechanical support. *Proceedings of the Society of General Systems Research Symposium on Mental Images, Values and Reality. International Conference on Mental Images, Values, and Reality, SGSR 30th Annual Meeting, Philadelphia*, I, G14–26.

Levin, S. M. (1995) *The importance of soft tissues for structural support of the body*. Hanley & Belfus, Philadelphia, PA.

Levin, S. M. (1997) Putting the shoulder to the wheel: a new biomechanical model for the shoulder girdle. *Biomedical Sciences Instrumentation*, 33, 412–7.

Mandelbrot, B. B. (1983) *The fractal geometry of nature*. W. H. Freeman, New York.

Pearce, P. (1978) *Structure in nature as a strategy for design*. MIT Press, Cambridge.

Prigogine, I., Stengers, I. (1984) *Order out of chaos: man's new dialogue with nature*. Bantam Books, London.

Schultz, A. B. (1983) *Biomechanics of the spine. Low back pain and industrial and social disablement*. Back Pain Association, London: 20–5.

Snelson, K. (2002) <http://www.kennethsnelson.net/>.

Stamenovic, D., Fredberg, J. J., Wang, N., Butler, J. P., Ingber, D. E. (1996) A microstructural approach to cytoskeletal mechanics based on tensegrity. *Journal of Theoretical Biology*, 181, 125–36.

Stevens, P. S. (1974) *Patterns in nature*. Little, Brown & Co., Boston.

Toffler, A. (1984) Science and change. In: I. Prigogine, I. Stengers (eds.) *Order out of chaos: man's new dialogue with nature*. Bantam Books, London, pp. xi–xxxi.

Waldrop, M. M. (1992) *Complexity*. Penguin, London.

Wang, N., Butler, J. P., Ingber, D. E. (1993) Mechanotransduction across the cell surface and through the cytoskeleton. *Science*, 260, 1124–7.

Wang, N., Naruse, K., Stamenovic, D., et al. (2001) Mechanical behavior in living cells consistent with the tensegrity model. *Proceedings of the National Academy of Sciences of the USA*, 98, 7765–70.

Wildy, P., Home, R. W. (1963) Structure of animal virus particles. *Progressive Medical Virology*, 5, 1–42.

Wolff, J. (1892) *Das gesetz der transformation der knocchen*. Hirschwald, Berlin.

Chapter 17

The fascioligamentous organ

Thomas Dorman †

Introduction to the fascioligamentous organ

An understanding of the dynamic function of the fascioligamentous organ is a most important conceptual requirement in musculoskeletal medicine. Clinicians who understand the function of the organ they are about to treat are self-evidently much more likely to plan treatment well.

Most soft-tissue injuries presenting with pain, such as back pain, neck pain after a whiplash accident, tennis elbow, sprains of the knees, etc., are due to a localized failure of the *fascioligamentous organ*. This organ encompasses the whole body and constitutes approximately 6% of its make-up. Concentrations of connective tissue in certain areas were given specific names by the early anatomists. Examples include the ligamentum nuchae in the posterior part of the neck, or the posterior sacroiliac ligaments (about which much more later) in the low back. We should maintain in our minds, however, an image of the fascioligamentous organ *as a whole*. It is a continuous structure, and no amount of emphasis is redundant in making this point. Much of this book deals with specific 'lesions' in specific areas—a reductionist approach. No criticism of this approach is implied in this section; it is essential in analysing specific problems. Contrariwise, a holistic view of the fascioligamentous organ of our bodies is also necessary. It is particularly important when a reductionist approach is not successful, such as when having to treat a somatic dysfunction in one location repeatedly, or failing to correct an area of recurrent sprain and inflammation by repeated topical steroid injection. It is in this context that a holistic point of view is likely to yield a fresh analysis and thence a fresh therapeutic approach.

Recent research has demonstrated the unique qualities of the human pelvis as a major anatomical device for the purpose of walking. This perspective has shed much light on the role of ligaments as organs for the storage and release of elastic energy. The fascioligamentous organ transfers the forces of tension through the whole body. It is best thought of as a tensegrity system. For psychological reasons which are not entirely clear to me, it is a characteristic of the human mind that it can easily visualize the transfer of forces through columns, beams, lintels, and cantilevers, but we have difficulty in visualizing the transfer of forces diffusely through a tensegrity model (see Chapter 16). Nevertheless, experience teaches us that the concepts of the tensegrity model are not only germane to understanding the function of our own bodies, but indispensable when analysing its dysfunction. To help with this psychological difficulty I will use a single example. Automobiles travel reliably on soft material. The air and the rubber constituting the tyre and the inner tube of a wheel are each insufficient to support our vehicles, but the integrated function is something we have come to take for granted.

This is a simple model because it is non-hierarchical. A multitude of subdivisions or septa between the compartments in a hierarchical tensegrity system provides certain integrated qualities to what are inherently weak structures, giving them combined strength. This is how organic systems work, and certainly how our own bodies function. From the point of view of the orthopaedic physician, training oneself to think in these terms is invaluable. It affords the tools that allow the practitioner to analyse clinical problems in orthopaedic medicine effectively, and hence make productive therapeutic plans.

Role of elastic tissue in the human pelvis

Fish and snakes advance by waves of lateral contraction and relaxation of groups of muscles within metamers. Reptiles with four legs maintain this mode of locomotion. Their body weight is supported directly on the ground. Quadruped walking of mammals is more complex. The organism alternately supports body quadrants over the swing leg, requiring greatly increased coordination and balance because the body is no longer on the ground. The complexity of the nervous system and the size of the brain parallel the increased intricacy of locomotion and coordination.

Though passive dynamic walking calls for little action from the nervous system (McGeer 1990), biped walking represents another increment in complexity. The static support of any structure on legs calls for at least three points of support, a possibility in the quadruped stance. Biped locomotion, on the other hand, is predicated on balance and coordination with continuous movement. Perhaps this is the reason for the additional increase in size of the human brain (Sinclair and Leakey 1986).

Evolutionary consideration of human posture

Since Charles Darwin's (1871) proposal of a common ancestral origin for *Homo sapiens* and humanoids, it has been assumed that the human biped posture is an evolutionary development from a more primitive quadruped one. The absence of a confirmatory paleontological link after 140 years of research should now raise the consideration that bipedal locomotion and the upright stance represent an earlier, or intrinsic, characteristic of *Homo sapiens* (Berge and Kasmierczak 1986; Brown et al. 1985; Hasegawa et al. 1987). Though it might appear heretical to some contemporary readers, the suggestion that mechanical and gravitational influences have contributed to morphological ontogeny and, by implication, to phylogeny is neither new (Thompson 1961, Berg 1969), nor passé (Carter 1987). In this context, it might be interesting to consider the anatomy, comparative anatomy, and physiology of walking in the human frame as not necessarily closely analogous to quadruped walking.

The physiology of walking

Studies on the efficiency of locomotion have recorded a paradox (Alexander and Jayes 1983). Oxygen consumption in human running is substantially less than calculated from the work done. (It has also been shown that various forms of terrestrial locomotion have similar energy economics; Cavagna et al. 1977). Although a large bibliography has accumulated on gait, the 'research front' (Vaughn 1982) has been on instrumentation based on electromyography and the use of dynamic imaging modalities for comparison of normal and abnormal gait in various conditions. Just as there has been little interest in the anatomy of the pelvic ring in general and the sacrum in particular, so has there has been a deficiency in analysis of the role of these structures in locomotion (Gracovetsky 1988). There has been an interesting suggestion recently that the anatomy of the human pelvis has evolved, teleologically speaking, to accommodate efficient walking rather than parturition (Abitbol 1987, 1988a). The width of the pelvis in the oldest humanoid skeleton has also been given this significance (Rak 1991).

It is 'advantageous' for the bipedal organism to conserve energy during locomotion. Conservation can take several forms.

Walking: a pendulum

A pendulum conserves energy. The analogy of a large pendulum in a grandfather clock might serve as a first approximation. The kinetic energy is stored in the upswing, as gravitational energy, to be released after the pendulum momentarily stops at the inertia point. A small amount of energy is imparted to the pendulum with each swing, the additional push being just sufficient to compensate for the loss by friction. By this means, the clock (with its pendulum) re-uses the swing energy time and again, kinetic and gravitational energy alternating, recycling.

On observing a walking man, the analogy acquires flesh (Alexander 1975), and this contrasts with the relative inefficiency of quadruped walking (Abitbol 1988b). The efficiency of stride length and speed of walking have been evaluated by means of studying oxygen consumption (Inman et al. 1981). There is an optimal speed of walking for each individual, which can be predicted by physical measurements (Holt et al. 1991). It is suggested here that these observations support the analogy with a pendulum (see Figure 17.1). First, walking begins as a controlled fall, then, as the pelvis hitches up on the stance leg and the swing leg departs from the ground, the leg gains momentum at first and decelerates before heel contact. The first acceleration occurs from

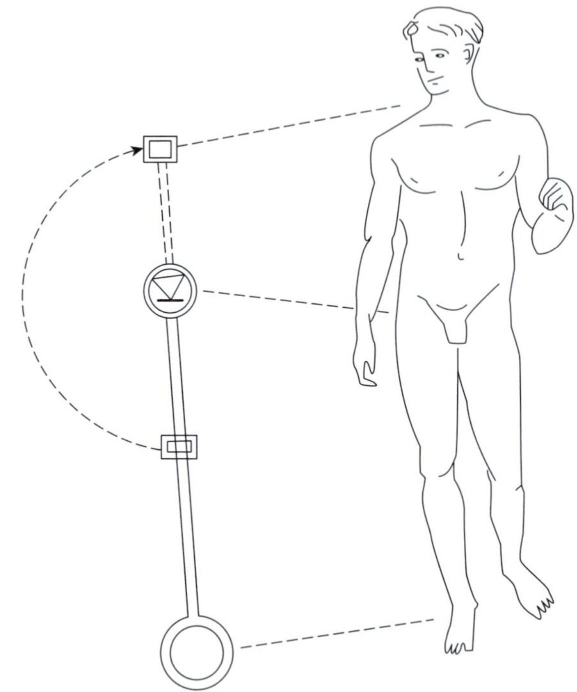

Figure 17.1 Walking: a pendulum.

the controlled fall forward and the deceleration occurs at the end of the swing. Was the decelerating energy dissipated as heat? We now know from some previous studies that, at least in human running, there is some storage or reutilization of energy (Alexander 1975). It is my impression that the kinetic energy of the decelerating leg is transferred, in part, into forward locomotion (every force is opposed by an equal and opposite force; Newton's third law of motion). The upper end of the swing leg, being attached to the pelvis and thence to the trunk, transmits forward locomotion to the body with deceleration. This can be observed in gait-analysis studies, as there is uneven acceleration of the trunk during forward progression.

The body wobbles backwards and forwards during forward walking. In order to appreciate this wobble, which is superimposed on the overall advancement, it is advantageous to subtract the average forward movement. The easiest way to appreciate this is to watch a person walking on a treadmill. This wobble is thought to represent the cyclic intake and dissipation of kinetic energy in synchrony with the pendular movement of the legs.

We know that walking is more efficient than running (Cavagna 1978; Pierrynowski et al. 1980).

Trunk bobbing

During normal walking, the head (and body) move up and down in the equivalent of a sinusoid wave. What is the fate of the gravitational energy dissipated on the down slope? It is proposed that this energy is, by and large, not converted to heat, and thus lost, but stored in the 'walking machine'. Part of it is transmitted to forward locomotion, a fall off the stance leg. Part is transmitted into elastic tissues such as, for instance, the collagen of the ligaments reinforcing the anterior aspect of the hip joint. In long strides, just before the rear leg is converted from a stance to a swing leg, tension can be sensed in the front of the hip. This stretch—elastic energy—is, of course, promptly released again as the stance leg begins to swing. In fact, it contributes to the acceleration of the swing leg together with the gravitational contribution mentioned earlier.

In this context, it is interesting to note that it is more efficient to carry a weight on the head than in a back pack (Maloiy et al. 1986): presumably the weight on the head does not interfere with the vertical 'clockwork mechanism' we are discussing here.

Elastic energy

The storage of elastic energy has been recognized and taken for granted by the keepers of physiological knowledge within the medico-scientific establishment since the turn of the century.

Respiration

Inspiration is the result of active contraction of intercostal muscles and the diaphragm; the chest expands. The initial phase of expiration is passive, the elastic chest wall collapsing to a smaller volume. Forced expiration calls for muscle action contracting the chest to a smaller volume. The neutral position is known in fact to represent a dynamic neutrality because the lungs, when observed outside the rib cage, collapse to an even smaller volume. The vacuum in the pleural space (sometimes called negative pressure, erroneously) stops them from collapse. So the neutral position of the chest in the intact organism represents a greater degree of pulmonary expansion than would be spontaneous for the lungs alone. On the contrary, the chest wall itself is pulled inwards by the elasticity of the lungs proper, so its resting posture is more contracted than would be the case without the inward pull of the lungs. The balance, therefore, is a dynamic equilibrium. In this instance, the elasticity of the rib cage is balanced by the elasticity of the lungs. The breathing organism needs only shift the balance to and fro a little for the bellows to work.

The analogy with a pendulum comes to mind again, but a better analogy is that of the coiled balance spring of a watch escapement. It was the invention of Christiaan Huygens (1629–1695), a Dutch watchmaker, who was first able to store elastic energy in a spring, where formerly clockmakers could only use the gravity pendulum. So it is that as we advance our understanding of the walking machine, another analogy from the clockmaker's trade is brought into service. Where else in the body, we might ask, is elastic energy stored in each step? It would, speaking teleologically again, be advantageous for the walking machine to use the spring-storage model as extensively as possible.

Joint capsules as stores of elastic energy

Anyone can confirm the storage of elastic energy in the ventral ligaments of his/her interdigital joint capsule by stretching a finger backwards and releasing it. From watching the cycle of walking, it seems that elastic energy is stored (as mentioned earlier) in the anterior part of the hip capsule (not only by extension but also by internal rotation of the femur). In this context, note the alignment of the main collagenous fibres in the anterior portion of the hip joint: they are stretched by this movement. Next, the posterior ligaments of the knee, the so-called ligament of Valois; in the foot, the plantar aponeurosis, as well as the ligaments of the deep arches of the foot are all stretched at the end of the stance phase and all release energy as the limb begins its swing.

Fasciae

I use the term fasciae to describe the sheets of connective tissue made up predominantly of woven collagen fibres which in a previous generation were referred to as surgical fasciae and intermuscular septae. Ligaments are connective tissue structures which bind bone to bone. Tendons are connective tissue structures which bind muscle to bone (and occasionally muscle to muscle, as in the digastric or omohyoid muscles). Fasciae are flat sheets of collagenous material which bind other elements of the musculoskeletal system to each other and traverse the body widely (Macintosh and Bogduk 1990). The aphorism of old anatomists that 'the fascia is continuous' is worth repeating.

Storage of elastic energy

A ballerina in the fifth position winds up each leg in external rotation, so tension is created between them. Each is wound up, so to speak, in an opposite direction on the pelvis. When the ballerina initiates the pirouette with a slight muscle-induced knee extension, she releases the stored energy which is converted to a vertical jump. In dancing circles, this force has been recognized since before the days of Diaghilev. In this example, where is the elastic energy stored? It is quite plain that some of it is stored in the foot (as in the case of the posterior stance leg discussed earlier), some is stored in the medial collateral ligaments of the knee, and some in the anterior ligaments of the hip joint. However, anyone who assumes this position, to test it, will sense the tension in the enveloping fasciae of calf and thigh. A crouched runner in a start position similarly stores energy in his calf, although a lot of this elasticity is stored in the triceps surae. Hitherto, conventional wisdom has ascribed the functions of wrapping and compartmentalization to fascia. We now know that fascia has the additional function of the *storage of elastic energy* (Vleeming et al. 1989).

Locus of energy storage

As far as I have been able to understand, it seems that the storage of elastic energy has been imputed to the muscles since early research on locomotion (Cavagna et al. 1964; Thys et al. 1972), and even recent authoritative researchers have assigned a role in elastic storage merely to the tendons of muscles (Alexander 1991). It seems, however, that this ascription has been arbitrary. The contractile elements of muscles (i.e. the actin and myosin) are not inherently elastic; the storage is therefore much more suitably ascribed to collagen and elastin (i.e. the fascial component of the myofascial structures) and to ligaments proper.

In the case of the spring ligament of the foot, it is easy to understand how the talus is supported by elastic tension between calcaneum and navicular. The weight of the body, transmitted via the talus, stretches the spring ligament, which releases its energy to the uprising foot. In the final analysis, it can be reasonably assumed that the energy is stored in electrostatic forces in the outer electron shells of the stretched atoms making up the collagen molecules and strands, right inside the spring ligament (Nimni 1997).

As a final example, contemplate a discus thrower who has wound up his/her torso just before starting the swing that will eventually transmit all his/her elastic, muscular, and kinetic energy into the flying discus. Can an analysis be made of the exact locus of the stored elastic energy at that moment? For that matter, in the case of the coiled watch spring in the mechanical wristwatch escapement,

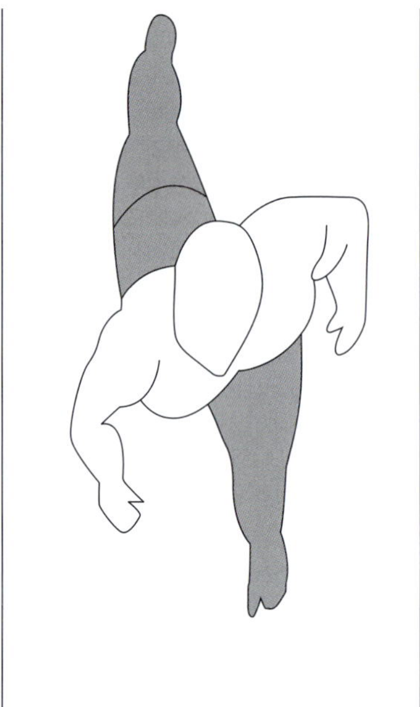

Figure 17.2 Elastic energy: alternating synchrony.

can an analysis be made of where in the spring the elastic energy is stored? In both cases, the answer has to be that the energy is stored diffusely in the whole structure. (It is intuitively understandable that it is not rational to ascribe the storage of a small amount of energy in the spring to a group of molecules at one end of it, and it is proposed here that to a certain extent this analogy can be taken into the body's fascia.) Just as the fascia is anatomically continuous, it is proposed here that so it is with the stored energy. The storage is diffuse. We should start thinking of the connective tissue as an organ for energy storage.

Torque

The arms swing alternately and synchronously with walking. In fact, the upper girdle rotates back and forth with each step. The angular momentum and acceleration are proportionate to the speed of walking. A horological analogy is available. The store of energy in a horizontal circular (so-called) pendulum, which is really a flywheel torqued on a suspensory spring, was invented in the Black Forest in 1881 and serves as the basis for the famous 400-day clock. Though not suspended, the upper girdle functions the same way. Torque is stored in the spine (and a little gravitational energy in the rising and falling arms). It is a common experience that with the arms bound, or the upper girdle restrained with a haversack frame, walking is fatiguing, chaffing, and inefficient. Measurements of oxygen consumption when the torso is in a brace have confirmed this impression (Inman 1966). It is also apparent that the pelvic girdle swivels with each step, in time with the swing leg, and in alternating synchrony with the upper girdle (see Figure 17.2). We now know that elastic energy is stored in the pelvic girdle itself.

The spinal engine: action of the spinal muscles in locomotion

Gracovetsky (1988) has summarized and explained the mechanisms by which the small muscles of the spine convert their contractions into locomotion, and his text is an invaluable reference. Side bending is converted to torque through the 'gearbox' of the zygoapophyseal joints. Finally, pelvic rotation activates the legs. Immobilization of the trunk retards the efficiency of walking (Ralston 1965), as judged by oxygen utilization. Does this represent an interference with the action of the spinal muscles in the 'spinal engine', or does it mean that there is interference with the storage and release of elastic energy (torque) which might enhance the pendular (flywheel) efficiency of the 'walking machine'?

Pelvic dynamics

The opinion once held by scientists that the three pelvic bones are immobile warrants no further comment, except as a reminder that widely held views are not always correct (Weisl 1953, 1955). The relative movement of the ilia versus the sacrum and each other in space, in time, and with the activity of walking in health and disease have been the subject of active study in recent years, and a number of relative movements, axes of rotations, and other dynamics have been suggested. The little research so far available points to variation and differences (Fryette 1954). The presence of movement and the presence of asymmetry are emerging as the norm. All these measurements are based on anatomical observations of the bony parts. The problem is confounded by the complexity of bony geometry, the extraordinary degree of variation, and the extreme difficulty in defining a reference point. Are we perhaps asking the wrong questions? Perhaps we would be better asking questions about the storage capacity of the elastic structures and about hysteresis.

In contemporary podiatry, the role of ligaments in the storage of elastic energy with stepping is gaining acceptance (Dananberg 1992). It can, however, be stated with confidence that the iliac bones move with respect to each other and the sacrum with each step. Asymmetry of the inclination of the pelvis is common (normal in allopathic terminology). It is enhanced in dysfunction and painful conditions and restored towards symmetry with effective healing, whether manual or other (LaCourse et al. 1990).

The relationship of torque at the sacrum to weightbearing with the alternation of stepping in walking has been demonstrated (Stevens 1990), and probably represents the first step in understanding the connection between the passive dynamic walking model of McGeer (1990) and the synchronous flywheel (or rotary pendulum) of the upper trunk, shoulders, and arms, sprung on the elastic spine.

An elastic landscape

If we can allow ourselves, therefore, to look at ligaments and fasciae for a moment only from the perspective of the storage of energy, we should note that ligament tissue is most plentiful in the pelvis. The posterior sacroiliac ligaments are by far the heftiest ligaments in the body. For a while, this observation was dismissed as a pique of nature. Later it was recognized, by analogy (which may have been false analogy) with the quadruped position, that the sacrum is suspended from the ilia and hence the whole weight of the organism is suspended by these ligaments. The strength was attributed to this function. It might be, however, that the function is that of an hierarchical icosahedron, functioning as a whole, so the local concentration of ligament tissue may not necessarily have a role in suspension, after all (Levin 1986a,b). As we now recognize that torque occurs through the sacroiliac joints with each step, perhaps we should regard these massive posterior sacroiliac ligaments as analogous to the mainspring of a clock (the horological analogies are not quite exhausted). There is no reason why a very short but very strong spring should not store a great deal of energy in a small moment. It is, of course, a very small amount of movement that can occur at the sacroiliac joints.

Asymlocation

A universal link in machinery is a unit which transmits forces or torque while allowing free movement in several directions through a series of couplings. As the body has the same requirement, there are connections in the body, consisting of two or more joints usually around one 'universal link' bone, which approximate these models. There are only a few instances in human anatomy where an intervening bone has no muscular or tendinous attachments at all (an example is the lunate at the wrist or the talus at the ankle). In the axial skeleton there are, however, a few instances where one of the bones is almost free of ligament and muscle attachments and is prone to asymlocation, like a universal link. The best examples are the atlas and the sacrum, although the lower lumbar vertebrae (usually the fifth, of course) are also prone to this phenomenon. When asymmetric tensions of the surrounding retaining part, for instance, the lumbodorsal fascia, are present, the universal links are apt to be situated with a degree of asymmetry that exceeds the usual or normal, and can be a source of dysfunction and pain. I have coined the term *asymlocation* to describe this phenomenon.

It seems obvious that the sacrum is suspended from the ilia in the quadruped position. This can be appreciated by viewing the skeleton of any quadruped mammal, or viewing the arrangement in the human model in the quadruped position. What is the function of the sacrum in biped standing? The word 'function' is used here rather broadly to discuss the forces controlling it. As we know, the sacrum has been compared to the keystone of an arch (see Figure 17.4a). The architectural arch is a uniquely stable arrangement. The vertical forces enhance the stability of the masonry. The greater the weight on the arch, the more stable it is. This is so because the adherence of the high-friction surfaces between the stones cut into trapezoid forms is enhanced. Does the sacrum indeed function as a keystone in any circumstance at all?

It is a commonplace observation that humans are a little asymmetric. Not only are the internal organs distributed this way, but some asymmetry seems to be common (normal in allopathic terminology, in the sense that it is usual) in what has been loosely termed the *soma*. For instance, a recent survey of the inclination of the pelvis in healthy athletes has demonstrated that the right ilium is rotated forward, in osteopathic terminology, normally in right-handed individuals versus the left ilium in left-footed people. Anyone taking a class in osteopathic manipulation will have observed other class members, who may be seemingly healthy, to have multiple asymmetries in the pelvis and spine (see Figure 17.3) which are currently termed *somatic dysfunction* (although I am reluctant to using the term 'dysfunction' for what is usual or normal). It is also a common observation in osteopathic and chiropractic circles that when these asymmetries are abolished by manual methods in symptomatic individuals, the dysfunction is often corrected. In this context, dysfunction and disease bear a proximity. What about the 'dysfunction' in the asymptomatic individual? The term 'asymlocation' (Dorman and Ravin 1991) is very helpful here. It seems best suited to describe this circumstance, and it is proposed that when asymlocation is marked, the propensity to pain (dysfunction) is increased. Contrariwise, as the dysfunction of the retaining

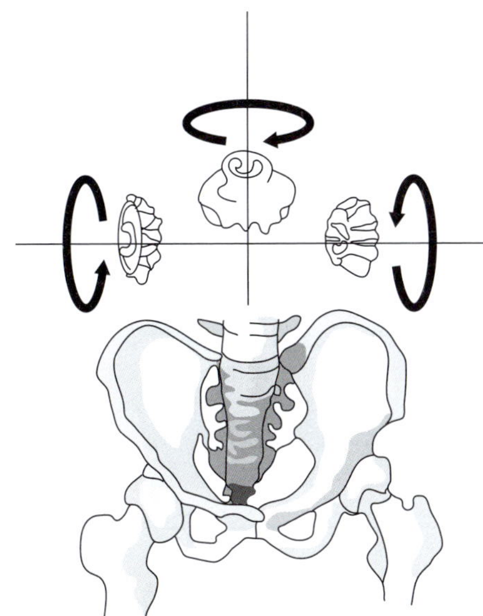

Figure 17.3 Asymlocation of the pelvis.

structures (that is to say, ligaments and fasciae) is healed, asymlocation diminishes.

Perhaps this framework will help bridge the unnecessary gap between osteopathy and allopathic medicine.

The sacroiliac joints as friction absorbers

The irregularities of the auricular surfaces were recognized by early anatomists, and the relation to age defined precisely (Lovejoy et al. 1985), but it is only in recent times that the qualities of the two opposing cartilaginous surfaces of this joint have been demonstrated to function as friction devices. This has been demonstrated in gross anatomy as well as microscopically. These surfaces of the sacroiliac joints can be said, therefore, to function in a manner which is different from that of other synovial joints. They absorb movement by gliding with friction. They encourage stability rather than free movement (Vleeming et al. 1990). It can be easily understood that when forces are acting across these joints in a direction other than pure shear, they are apt to offer a high resistance.

Form and force closure of the sacroiliac joints

The importance of friction in the function of the sacroiliac joints has been conveyed through the introduction of the contrasting concepts of *form closure* and *force closure* (Snijders et al. 1997 (Figure 17.4). Form closure refers to a stable situation with closely fitting joint surfaces. In an idealized model of form closure, weightbearing (and the transfer of other forces) would be achieved through snugly fitting geometrical forms alone. Functional analysis of living joints shows that various mechanical refinements are usually present in each. In the case of the sacroiliac joints, the additional factors are distinct. On first inspection, the sacrum appears to be wedged between the ilia. It has, however, been shown that on standing, the closed kinematic chain is predicated on lateral pressures through the rough surfaces of these joints. This has been termed

(a)

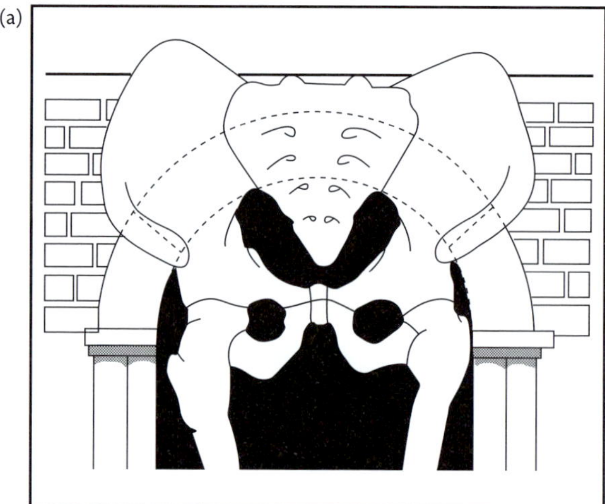

(b)

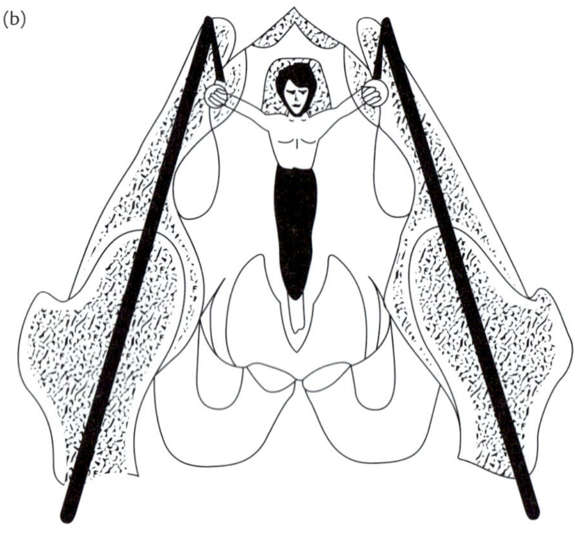

Figure 17.4 Stability of the sacrum in the pelvis (a) as the keystone of an arch and (b) by form and force closure.

force closure. In the sacroiliac joints, both a compressive lateral force and friction are needed to withstand vertical loads. Shear at the sacroiliac joints is prevented by a combination of the specific anatomical features (form closure) and the compression generated by ligaments and muscles acting across the high friction surfaces (force closure) (see Figure 17.4).

Movement and governance of the sacroiliac articulation

A recognition that buttock and leg pain may arise from hypermobility of the joint was raised by Goldthwait and Osgood (1905). Movement of these joints has been accepted since then. Weisl's (1953) work reinforced this understanding. Movement in living humans has been demonstrated stereophotogrammetically (Sturesson et al. 1989) with radiology by the placement of Kirschner wires in the sacrum and ilium (Colachis et al. 1963) and observing the external movement, and through actual measurements of iliac positions with calipers (LaCourse et al. 1990; Pitkin and Pheasant 1936).

Motion at the sacroiliac joints is maintained even in advanced age. Movement of these joints has been recognized in manual medical circles, through methods of palpation, throughout the history of osteopathy (Greenman 1989), and is well established in physiotherapy circles as well (DonTigny 1993; Hesch 1994).The main controlling soft tissue seems to be by the several periarticular ligaments such as the sacroiliac and sacrotuberous ligaments. The capsule of the sacroiliac joint has been shown radiologically to be incomplete in some cases with back pain (Aprill 1992). An analysis of movement at either sacroiliac articulation calls into question movement at the other two joints of the pelvic ring. Although interconnected through the soft tissues, the relative movement of each of the bones versus the others in the three directions of space, let alone the interaction with the fascial tube of the whole organism, creates a three-dimensional puzzle of great complexity. That manual treatment can be beneficial is now official (Schekelle et al. 1991), though the *modus operandi* of the various therapies remains empirical.

What can be said regarding the attendant ligaments and other soft-tissue structures surrounding this joint? What role do any of them have in the governance of function? Interestingly, recent research has shown that the large ligamentous bands, recognized of old in the pelvis, play substantial roles in the governance of the sacrum. Finally, to the extent that there is a model (i.e. most typical pattern of movement round an hypothetical 'axis'), it turns out that the deep posterior interosseous ligaments of the sacroiliac joints play that role (Egund et al. 1978; Sturesson et al. 1989).

Self-bracing forces in the pelvis

The forces acting in the pelvis in the upright biped position are self-bracing. The keystone of the arch, the sacrum (see Figure 17.4a), being wider superiorly, trends downward from the weight of the body, and the traction this applies to the ilia—through the posterior sacroiliac ligaments—tends to bring the ilia into adduction. The wedge shape of the sacrum overall, being wider in front, tends to displace it anteriorly (into the pelvis). A balance occurs between the forward vector and the downward vector. Regardless of the balance, the adducting forces are enhanced through both these vectors. It is plain that the sacrum does not descend into the standing pelvis because of the bracing mechanism and the posterior sacroiliac ligaments. Self-bracing, therefore, is a unique characteristic of the biped human pelvis.

Intuitively, it is understandable that self-bracing applies while we are standing on both legs. Walking, however, consists of one leg support alternating continuously. Hence self-bracing is switched on and off normally in gait. Each sacroiliac joint is locked and unlocked with each step alternately. The joint on the stance side is braced. The demonstration of the production of torque at the sacroiliac articulations with one-legged weightbearing (Stevens 1990) can also be taken to imply the reverse (i.e. the dissipation of the stored (torque) energy into the swing leg with step off). There is a regular transmission of energy back and forth with locomotion, contributing to the efficiency of the 'walking machine'.

Clinical patterns and approach to treatment of back pain: the use of hypothesis

Assuming then that asymlocation and self-bracing are commonly the cause of dysfunction and chronic back pain (recurrent and later becoming continuous), and seeing that objective confirmation from the laboratory is not forthcoming, what can the clinician do about it? From the discussion in this chapter, the question is rhetorical: (1) put it back; (2) keep it back. Hence, the idea that appropriate manipulation to restore symmetry to the pelvis might be followed by ligament refurbishment—*prolotherapy*. This working hypothesis served as the model for the clinical trial of Ongley's technique (Ongley et al. 1987). It is to his clarity of thought that we owe not only an understanding of the mechanisms already discussed, but also the development of the combined technique for treatment. This is perhaps a suitable place to re-emphasize the importance of meticulous diagnosis in orthopaedic medicine. The simple application of a technique of treatment to all patients with back pain, though it will be effective in many, is neither rational nor wise. Not all back pain has one cause.

Points of weakness

A sailor will tell you that in a frayed halyard, the concentration of strain always occurs at the weak point. The weak point itself is always where the rope was damaged first. It is not surprising that clinicians have observed the same phenomenon in the inner lining, the fascia. Just as there are characteristic points of wear for a halyard, so it is that strains in the moving parts of the body tend to concentrate and eventually lead to injuries at internal sites which have patterns. The patterns have mechanical origins which we may or may not be able to analyse mathematically, intellectually, or intuitively. Nonetheless, the clinician recognizes these patterns.

Fascioligamentous tensegrity system

The form of the body is maintained (in part) by tensegrity, as discussed by Steven Levin in Chapter 16. This concept explains how variation in the tension of one component of the system affects the whole. We have already discussed how the pelvic girdle serves as a transmission and differential in locomotion, and how the initiating energy arises in muscles but the transmission is through fasciae and ligaments. The transfer of energy from glycogen to distance in walking is modulated by an escapement analogous to that of a clock in several regards. A major component of the efficient mechanism is in the elastic storage of energy in ligaments and fasciae proportionate to their abundance.

Fault propagation

An example of a typical case might consist of a middle-aged or elderly person who walks, typically, slightly stooped forward and to the right. There is slight compensatory lumbar or thoracolumbar scoliosis to the left. The right ilium is anterior and the right leg slightly externally rotated. On supine examination, one might find a pseudo leg-length discrepancy, the left side being slightly longer, although this is usually easily corrected. There might be a tendency to valgus deformity of the right knee with early osteoarthritic changes and a sprain of the medial coronary and perhaps the medial collateral ligaments. Subsequently, a degree of laxity of the posterior and anterior cruciate ligaments, in that order, will appear. The foot is a little bit flat and the navicular prominent (i.e. there is pronation of the foot). If such an individual is inspected while standing on a glass platform with an illuminated mirror below, unequal distribution of the weight is seen with the person standing. The usual footprint might be maintained on the left, but on the right, pronation is observed and the big toe may not press fully on the glass. When the person walks, the medial step-off syndrome is observed. This will have a tendency to produce a degree of hallux valgus on that side and a hammer-toe on the second and perhaps third toes. The foot will become painful on walking. Partial avulsion of the plantar fascia might develop and a 'spur' detected if a lateral foot radiograph is taken. If this leads to unwise podiatric surgery, the tendency for the fascial strain will be aggravated. If orthotics are used, this will give temporary relief but aggravate the long-term dysfunction of the fascial windlass operating from the dorsolumbar fascia through the whole fascial sleeve of the lower limb, the surgical fascia of the leg onto the foot.

This typical scenario might also arise from an exaggerated forward rotation of the right ilium—asymlocation. The back may or may not be symptomatic at present, and back pain may or may not have been present in the past. The patient may present with a foot problem, a knee problem, or even a problem in the right hip. As the 'walking machine' deteriorates with inefficiency in walking, with increased strain and pressure exerted on the fascial tube, fault propagation might begin to affect the second side. After hip replacement on the first (in this case right) side, the left may be involved, and typically a decade might pass before the same phenomenon appears on the other side.

It goes without saying that early correction of the fault is more productive than an attempted late correction. When permanent stretches occur in the fascia and ligament, as in the example given, restoring the 'walking machine' to a pristine condition is a hopeless proposition. Nonetheless, many of these patients benefit if the primary dysfunction is corrected, and that is more often than not in the pelvis. It must be acknowledged, however, that a dysfunction in the foot can induce the phenomenon of fault propagation retrograde. In other words, the process is interactive.

In conclusion, one should note that the most characteristic and common example of fault propagation in the tensegrity system of the axial skeleton is the phenomenon of pain at one end of the spine appearing 3–6 months after an injury to the other end. I phrase it this way because the initial injury may be in the neck from a whiplash occurrence, or in the low back from a fall on the buttock, or an awkward instance of stooping and lifting with rotation provoking an exaggerated asymlocation—amounting to somatic dysfunction in the pelvis. It is an extraordinarily common observation that individuals suffering from a dysfunction at one end of the spine in due course develop a dysfunction at the other end. Fault propagation through the fascioligamentous tensegrity system is the likely cause.

References

Abitbol, M. (1987) Evolution of the lumbosacral angle. *Am J Physical Anthropol*, 72, 361–72.

Abitbol, M. (1988a) Evolution of the ischial spine and the pelvic floor in the hominoidea. *Am J Physical Anthropol*, 75, 53–67.

Abitbol, M. (1988b) Effect of posture and locomotion on energy expenditure. *Am J Physical Anthropol*, 77, 191–9.

Alexander, R. M. (1975) *Biomechanics*. Chapman & Hall, London.

Alexander, R. M. (1991) Energy-saving mechanisms in walking and running. *J Exp Biol*, 160, 55–69.

Alexander, R. M., Jayes A. S. (1983) A dynamic similarity hypothesis for the gaits of quadrupedal mammals. *J Zool A*, 207, 467–82.

Aprill, C. N. (1992) *The role of anatomically specific injections into the sacroiliac joint in low back pain and its relation to the sacroiliac joint*. Symposium, November 1992, San Diego, CA.

Berg, L. S. (1969) (originally published in Russian in 1922) *Nomogenesis or evolution determined by law*. MIT Press, Cambridge, MA.

Berge, C., Kasmierczak J. B. (1986) Effects of size and locomotor adaptations on the hominid pelvis: evaluation of Australopithecine bipedality with a new multivariate method. *Folia Primatol*, 46, 185–204.

Brown, F., Harris, J., Leakey, R., Walker A. (1985) Early *Homo erectus* skeleton from West Lake, Turkana, Kenya. *Nature*, 316, 788–92.

Carter, R. D. (1987) Mechanical loading history and skeletal biology. *J Biomechanics*, 20(11), 1095–109.

Cavagna, G. (1978) Aspects of efficiency and inefficiency of terrestrial locomotion. In: *Biomechanics VI-A*. University Park Press, Baltimore, MD, pp. 3–22.

Cavagna, G. A., Heglund, N. C., Taylor R. C. (1977) Mechanical work in terrestrial locomotion: two basic mechanisms for minimizing energy expenditure. *Am J Physiol*, 233, R243–61.

Cavagna, G. A., Saibene, F. P., Margaria R. (1964) Mechanical work in running. *J Appl Physiol*, 19/20, 249–56.

Colachis, S. C., Worden, R. E., Bechtol C. O., et al. (1963) Movement of the sacroiliac joint in the adult male: a preliminary report. *Archiv Phys Med Rehabil*, 44, 490–8.

Dananberg, H. J. (1992) Subtle gait malfunction and chronic musculoskeletal pain. *J Orthop Med*, 14(1), 18–25.

Darwin, C. (1871) *The descent of man and selection in relation to sex* (6th edn). London.

DonTigny, R. L. (1993) Mechanics and treatment of the sacroiliac joint. *J Manual Manipulative Ther*, 1(1), 3–12.

Dorman, T., Ravin T. (1991) *Diagnosis and injection techniques in orthopedic medicine*. Williams & Wilkins. Baltimore.

Egund, N., Olson, T. H., Schmid, H., Selvik, G. (1978) Movement in the sacroiliac joints demonstrated with roentgen stereophotogrammetry. *Acta Radiol Diag*, 19, 833–46.

Fryette, H. H. (1954) *Principles of osteopathic technic*. Academy of Applied Osteopathy, Carmel.

Goldthwait, J. E., Osgood R. B. (1905) Essential of body mechanics in health and disease. *Med Surg J*, 152, 593–634.

Gracovetsky, S. (1988) *The spinal engine*. Springer-Verlag, New York.

Greenman, P. E. (1989) *Principles of manual medicine*. Williams & Wilkins, Baltimore, MD.

Hasegawa, M., Kishino, H., Yano, T. (1987) Man's place in hominoidae as inferred from molecular clocks of DNA. *J Mol Evol*, 26, 132–47.

Hesch, J (1994) *The Hesch method of treating sacroiliac joint dysfunction*. 14117 Grand Ave, N. E., Albuquerque, NM.

Holt, K. G., Hamill, J., Andres, R. O. (1991) Predicting the minimal energy costs of human walking. *Med Sci Sports Exer*, 23(4), 491–8.

Inman, V. T. (1966) Human locomotion. *Can Med Assoc J*, 94, 1047–57.

Inman, V. T., Ralston, J. H., Todd F. (1981) *Human walking*. Williams & Wilkins. Baltimore, MD, pp. 62–9.

LaCourse, M., Moore, K., Davis, K., Fune, M., Dorman, T. (1990) A report on the asymmetry of iliac inclination: a study comparing normal, laterality and change in a patient population with painful sacro-iliac dysfunction treated with prolotherapy. *J Orthop Med*, 12, 69–72.

Levin, S. M. (1986a) *Proceedings of the 30th Annual Meeting of the Society of General Systems Research*, Philadelphia, PA, 1, G14–26.

Levin, S. M. (1986b) The ichosahedron as the three-dimensional finite element in biomechanical support. A natural hierarchical system. Presented at the NAAM Annual Meeting, Philadelphia.

Lovejoy, C. O., Meindl, R. S., Pryzbeck, T. R., Mensforth, R. P. (1985) Chronological metamorphosis of the auricular surface of the ilium: a new method for the determination of adult skeletal age at death. *Am J Phys Anthropol*, 68, 15–28.

Macintosh, J. E., Bogduk, N. (1990) Basic biomechanics pertinent to the study of the lumbar disc. *J Man Med*, 5, 52–7.

Maloiy, G. M. O., Heglund, N. C., Prager, L. M., Cavagna, G. A., Taylor, R. C. (1986) Energetic costs of carrying loads: have African women discovered an economic way? *Nature*, 319, 68–9.

McGeer, T. (1990) Passive dynamic walking. *Int J Robotics Res*, 9, 2.

Nimni M. E. (1997) Collagen, structure and function. In: *Encyclopedia of human biology* (2nd edn). Academic Press, New York, pp. 559–74.

Ongley, M. J., Klein, R. G., Dorman, T. A., et al. (1987) A new approach to the treatment of chronic back pain. *Lancet*, ii, 143–6.

Pierrynowski, M., Winter, D., Norman, R. (1980) Transfers of mechanical energy within the total body and mechanical efficiency during treadmill walking. *Ergonomics*, 23, 147–56.

Pitkin, H. C., Pheasant, H. (1936) Sacrarthrogenic telalgia. A study of sacral mobility. *J Bone Jt Surg*, 18, 365–74.

Rak, Y. (1991) Lucy's pelvic anatomy: its role in bipedal gait. *J Human Evol*, 20, 283–90.

Ralston, H. J. (1965) Effects of immobilization of various body segments on the energy cost of human locomotion. *Proceedings of the Second IEA Conference, Dortmund, 1964*. Supplement to *Ergonomics*, p. 53.

Schekelle, P. G., Adams, A. H., Chassin, M. R., Hurwitz, E. L., Phillips, R. B., Brook, R. H. (1991) *The appropriateness of spinal manipulation for low-back pain*. Rand, 1700 Main Street, Santa Monica, CA.

Sinclair A. R. E., Leakey, M. D. (1986) Migration and hominid bipedalism. *Nature*, 324(27), 307–8.

Snijders, C. J., Vleeming, A., Stoeckart, R. (1997) Movement, stability, and low back pain: the central role of the pelvis. Churchill Livingstone, p. 103–13.

Stevens, A. (1990) Side bending and axial rotation of the sacrum inside the pelvic girdle. *Proceedings of the First International Congress on Low Back Pain and the Sacro-Iliac Joint*, San Diego, November.

Sturesson, B., Selvik, G., Udèn, A. (1989) Movement of the sacroiliac joints: a roentgen stereophotogrammetic analysis. *Spine*, 14(2), 162–5.

Thompson, D. W. (1961) (first published 1917) *On growth and form*. Cambridge University Press, Cambridge.

Thys, H., Faraggiana, T., Margaria, R. (1972) Utilization of muscle elasticity in exercise. *J Appl Physiol*, 32, 491–4.

Vaughn, K. (1982) *Biomechanics of human gait: an annotated bibliography*. Dept. Biomedical Engineering, University of Cape Town.

Vleeming, A., Stoeckart, R., Snijders, C. J. (1989) The sacrotuberous ligament: a conceptual approach to its dynamic role in stabilizing the sacroiliac joint. *Clin Biomech*, 4, 201–3.

Vleeming, A., Stoeckart, R., Volkers A. C. W., Snijders, C. J. (1990) Relation between form and function in the sacro-iliac joint. *Spine*, 15(2), 133–6.

Vleeming, A., Van Wingerden, J. P., Dijkstra, P. F., et al. (1992) Mobility in the sacro-iliac joints at high age. In: *The sacroiliac joint: a clinical, biomechanical and radiological study*. Erasmus University, Rotterdam.

Weisl, H. (1953) *The relation of movement to structure in the sacro-iliac joint*. Ph.D. thesis, University of Manchester.

Weisl, H. (1955) The movement of the sacro-iliac joint. *Acta Anat*, 23, 80–91.

Chapter 18

The fascial organ

Thomas Findley

Introduction to the fascial organ

Is fascia an organ? Stedman's dictionary defines an organ as 'any part of the body exercising a specific function (respiration, secretion, or digestion)'. An organ system is a group of anatomical structures that work together to perform a specific function or task. Recognized organ systems are the circulatory system, digestive, endocrine/immune, integumentary, musculoskeletal, nervous, reproductive, respiratory, and urinary. Does that mean we must agree on the function of fascia in order for it to rise to the level of an organ or organ system? Or can we take a structural definition? Is fascia the mechanotransduction system, a body-wide signalling system? (Langevin 2006) Is it part of connective tissues, which also include bone, blood, fat, and cartilage? It certainly does consist of cells of mesodermal origin, embedded in an extracellular matrix. However, as the recent explosion of articles, books, and conferences attest, many people are of the firm opinion that it is more than just a mass of individual cells and fibres.

Regardless of whether one considers fascia an organ, an organ system, or merely structural parts of other organs, we must recognize that there is a collection of structures within this overarching concept. For example, the aortic valve, the cardiac arteries, the myocardium, and the atrium are clearly very different structures in the heart, which is a part of the circulatory system. To describe a new drug's effects on 'the heart' without specifying which structure, or which function (e.g. ejection fraction), would limit our understanding. The evolution of observations by William Withering in 1785 on the herb foxglove to modern use of digitalis for heart failure is a good example. Despite his astute clinical observations and multiple case studies, digitalis was not approved by the Food and Drug Administration (FDA) in the USA until 200 years later, in 1998, after a randomized trial was finally completed (Goldberger and Alexander 2014). Similarly, if we are describing some function, pathology, or the impact of some treatment on 'fascia', we need to specify just which structure or function we mean. General fascial terminological issues have been presented from different viewpoints (Langevin and Huijing 2009; Schleip et al. 2012; Stecco et al. 2013; Wendell-Smith 1997) and regarding cervical (Guidera et al. 2012) or thoracolumbar fascia (Willard et al. 2012). However, whichever system one might choose, more words than 'fascia' are needed for a thorough description.

Any discussion of fascia as an organ must start with the observations on its function made by Dr A.T. Still more than 100 years ago, when he founded the profession of osteopathic medicine (Still 1899). The more we learn, the more we appreciate his conclusion that 'This life is surely too short to solve the uses of the fascia in animal form.' Dr Still spent years studying and experimenting before he opened the American School of Osteopathy in Kirksville in 1892. His philosophy of osteopathy was based upon the concepts of body structure and health maintenance rather than disease. Dr Still recognized the importance of fascia in health, and recent research has shown that many of his ideas about fascia are valid.

Fascia has been gaining increasing interest from physicians and manual therapists. Manual therapy techniques treat the fascial layers by altering density, tonus, viscosity, and the arrangement of fascia (Crane et al. 2012; Pohl 2010; Simmonds et al. 2012). The manual stimulation of sensory nerve endings may lead to tonus changes in muscle. The fascial system is now being recognized as the aetiology of pain and proprioception. Myofascial trigger points are local thickenings of individual muscle fibres that are caused by contractions of a small group of sarcomeres (Mense 2008). Fascia research can help understand aspects of musculoskeletal problems such as myofascial trigger points, low back pain, and fibromyalgia. Connective tissue is also intimately associated with other tissues and organs, so it may influence the normal or pathological processes in a wide variety of organ systems.

The study of fascia best starts with A.T. Still's actual words:

> How to find causes of diseases or where a hindrance is located that stops blood is a great mental worry to the osteopath when he is called to treat a patient. The patient tells a doctor 'where he hurts', 'how much he hurts', 'how long he has hurt', 'how hot or cold he is' . . . An osteopath, in his search for the cause of diseases, starts out to find the mechanical cause. He feels that the people expect more than guessing of an osteopath. He feels that he must put his hand on the cause and prove what he says by what he does; that he will not get off by the feeble-minded trash of stale habits that go with doctors of medicine. By his knowledge he must show his ability to go beyond the musty bread of symptomatology.

Dr Still continued:

> I know of no part of the body that equals the fascia as a hunting-ground. I believe that more rich golden thoughts will appear to the mind's eye as the study of the fascia is pursued than of any other

> division of the body. Nevertheless, one part is just as great and useful as any other in its place. No part can be dispensed with . . . In every view we take of the fascia a wonder appears. The part the fascia takes in life and death gives us one of the greatest problems to solve. It surrounds each muscle, vein, nerve, and all organs of the body. It has a network of nerves, cells, and tubes running to and from it; it is crossed and no doubt filled with millions of nerve-centers and fibers which carry on the work of secreting and excreting fluids vital and destructive. By its action we live and by its failure we die. Each muscle plays its part in active life. Each fiber of all muscle owes its pliability to that yielding septum-washer that allows all muscles to glide over and around all adjacent muscles and ligaments without friction or jar. It not only lubricates the fibers, but gives nourishment to all parts of the body. Its nerves are so abundant that no atom of flesh fails to get nerve- and blood-supply there from.

He further added:

> I write at length of the universality of the fascia to impress the reader with the idea that this connecting substance must be free at all parts to receive and discharge all fluids, and to appropriate and use them in sustaining animal life, and eject all impurities, that health may not be impaired by dead and poisonous fluids. A knowledge of the universal extent of the fascia is imperative, and is one of the greatest aids to the person who seeks the causes of disease. The fascia and its nerves demand his attention, and on his knowledge of them much of his success depends . . . When you deal with the fascia you are doing business with the branch offices of the brain, under a general corporation law, and why not treat these branch offices with the same degree of respect? The doctor of medicine does effectual work through the medium of the fascia. Why should not you relax, contract, stimulate, and clean the whole system of all diseases by that willing and sufficient power you possess to renovate all parts of the system from deadly compounds that are generated on account of delay and stagnation of fluids while in the fascia?
>
> (Still 1899)

Dr Still believed there were four basic principles:

(1) The human body functions as a total biological unit.

(2) The body possesses self-healing and self-regulatory mechanisms.

(3) Structure and function are interrelated.

(4) Abnormal pressure in one part of the body produces abnormal pressures and strains upon other parts of the body.

He recognized early on the connection between structure and function. He specifically described fascia as a covering, with attention to terminology which obscures common origins of individual parts of the fascial system. Fascia assists gliding and fluid flow and is highly innervated. Fascia is intimately involved with respiration and with nourishment of all cells of the body, including those of disease and cancer (Still 1899, 1902, 1910). Let us now examine Dr Still's concepts one by one.

Fascia as a covering

According to Dr Still, fascia

> sheathes, permeates, divides and sub-divides every portion of all animal bodies; surrounding and penetrating every muscle and all its fibers—every artery, and every fiber. (1899, p. 163)

Fascia is connective tissue that surrounds and connects every muscle and organ, forming continuity throughout the body. It is considered to be any dense irregular connective tissue sheet in the human body, including aponeuroses, joint capsules, or muscular envelopes such as the endo-, peri-, and epimysium (Langevin and Huijing 2009). The intramuscular extracellular matrix is composed of the endomysium, perimysium, and epimysium. The epimysium surrounds each muscle. The perimysium divides the muscle into fascicles or muscle fibre bundles. The endomysium is a continuous network of connective tissue that covers individual muscle fibres (Purslow 2002, 2010). Small fascial fibres extend to connect to the cell membrane itself (Passerieux et al. 2006). These layers and their functions are reviewed in detail by Lund (Lund and Cornelison 2013) and Turrina (Turrina et al. 2013).

Gillies (Gillies and Lieber 2011) points out that while these layers may seem distinct in two-dimensional sections, the borders between these three tissues are somewhat arbitrary when viewed as an extensive three-dimensional network, with connective tissue fibres extending both along and across muscle fibres. The middle layer perimysium appears to be continuous with the tendon. This intramuscular connective tissue architecture is not fixed, but shows increased collagen content and decreased organization after a period of immobilization of an extremity (Jarvinen et al. 2002). During growth, the increase in size of the muscle fibres results in increased turnover of the connective tissue. Food scientists are aware that rapid growth of the animal results in more tender connective tissue and increased value when the meat is prepared (Purslow et al. 2012).

Fascia is not isotropic—rather it has different properties when pulled in different directions. Layers of fascia show fibres running in parallel directions, much like reinforced fibres in packing tape. One layer has been observed at a specific orientation of 55° to the layer underneath in the elbow of the human (Stecco et al. 2011) (Figure 18.1), the neck of the cow (Purslow 2010) (Figure 18.2), and the fascia lata of the goat (Pancheri et al. 2014) (Figure 18.3).

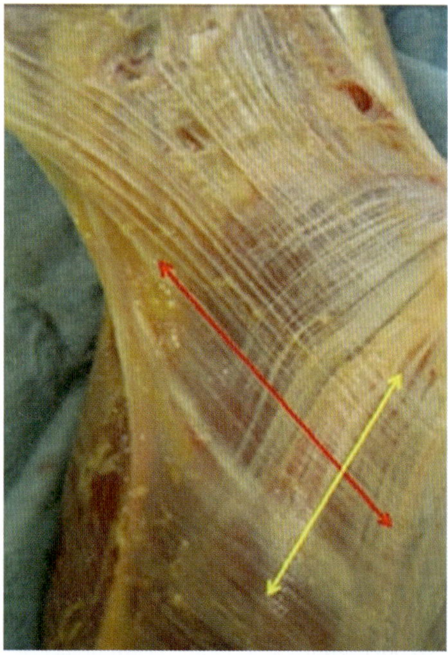

Figure 18.1 Layer of fascia oriented at 55° to the layer underneath in the human elbow.
(Stecco C, Macchi V, Porzionato A, Duparc F, De Caro R. The fascia: the forgotten structure. *Italian Journal of Anatomy & Embryology*. 2011; 116(3):127–38.)

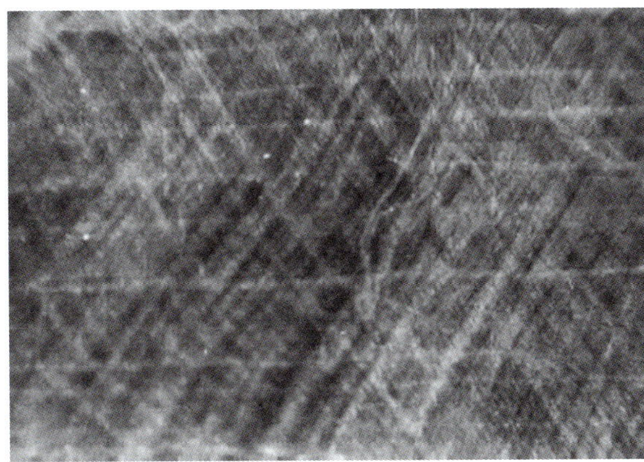

Figure 18.2 Layer of fascia oriented at 55° to the layer underneath in the neck of the cow.
(Purslow PP. Muscle fascia and force transmission. *Journal of Bodywork & Movement Therapies*. 2010; 14(4):411–7.)

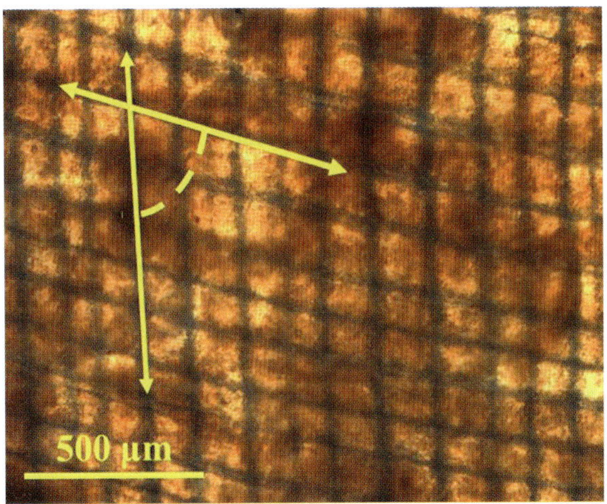

Figure 18.3 Layer of fascia oriented at 55° to the layer underneath in the fascia lata of the goat.
(Pancheri FQ, Eng CM, Lieberman DE, Biewener AA, Dorfmann L. A constitutive description of the anisotropic response of the fascia lata. *Journal of the Mechanical Behavior of Biomedical Materials*. 2014; 30:306–23.)

This remarkable similarity in structure across different parts of the body and different species points to an as yet undetermined functional significance, although fibres of this orientation will allow stretch up to 30% before tensional forces become compressive (Chaudhry et al. 2012). From an engineering perspective, this 55 degree fiber orientation in tubes allows flexibility and resistance to pressure, with neither expansion in diameter or lengthening as the interior pressure increases, and is used in the common garden hose (Vogel 2013).

Dissections and physiological studies have shown that there are fascial connections resulting in myofascial force transmission between adjacent and even antagonistic muscles, with almost 30% of forces transmitted laterally rather than directly to the muscle tendon (Bojsen-Moller et al. 2010; Huijing 1999, 2007; Maas and Sandercock 2008, 2010; Smeulders and Kreulen 2007; Yu et al. 2007; Yucesoy and Huijing 2007). The superficial fascia is a layer of areolar connective tissue or adipose tissue located directly beneath the skin. Fascial limb dissections show the extensive network of fascia throughout the limbs (Stecco et al. 2009).

Deep fascia is tougher and comprises denser connective tissue, containing and separating groups of muscles into well-defined compartments. Fascia plays an ectoskeletal role, creating a functional organization of muscles. Fascia also permeates through compartments, transmitting loads between them (Benjamin 2009). The deep fascia in multiple specimens showed similar structural organization, with ability to adapt to volume variations of muscles during contraction, and to resist high pressure without damage (Stecco et al. 2009).

Fascia as a continuous structure with discontinuous names

Dr Still comments that

> all organs have a covering of this substance, though they may have names to suit the organs, surfaces, or parts spoken of. (1899, p. 166)

The connective tissue that surrounds muscle is not an isolated and independent entity; rather, it is a continuous substance throughout the body. The broad definition of fascia allows fascial tissues to be seen as an interconnected tensional network that adapts its fibre arrangement, length, and density according to local tensional demands. Fascia forms linkages between muscular and non-muscular tissues at several locations in addition to tendon origins and insertions (Yucesoy and Huijing 2007). For example, studies of the Achilles tendon in the foot have shown that the tendon not only attaches to the calcaneus, it is continuous with the plantar aponeurosis over the heel and the fibrous septa of the heel fat pad (Benjamin 2009). Simply pulling or pushing one muscle leads to movement of its neighbouring muscle, showing that muscles are unquestionably linked.

Fascia is traditionally named according to the discrete anatomic structure that it surrounds which obscures its four distinct layers. Fasciae in different regions are named according to their regional anatomy, such as the fascia lata and iliotibial tract, the clavipectoral, axillary, brachial, and thoracolumbar fascia. It is considered to be 'part of' organs or structures instead of a connective tissue continuum throughout the body, which unites and integrates different regions. The naming and studying of fascia in isolation is believed by some to be a 'barrier to understanding the bigger picture of fascial function' (Benjamin 2009).

Dissection methods often start by 'clearing' or 'cleaning' structures from their connective tissue covering. Van der Wal studied the interrelationships of muscle and other structures in the forelimb, using a fascia-sparing dissection technique. He showed that muscular and joint connective tissues are continuous, not separate entities. He found that there are specialized connective tissue structures between muscles and the bone of origin or insertion. This connection, called the 'dynament', can adapt to changes in distance between bones as joints open and close, unlike fixed-length ligaments which can only be of optimal length at one joint angle. The continuity of fascia throughout the body can be attributed to its embryological origin in the mesoderm (van der Wal 2009). Connective tissue provides a structural framework for growth as it develops around structures of the body, continuously adapting and transmitting mechanical and chemical signals to differentiate tissue (Ingber 2003).

The continuum of fascia throughout the body allows it to serve as a body-wide mechanosensitive signalling system (Langevin

2006). Cells in living tissue are anchored to the extracellular matrix through focal adhesions. At these sites, clusters of transmembrane receptors, known as integrins, bind to extracellular matrix molecules on the outside of cells to anchor them in place. These integrins provide a path for mechanical stress to transfer across the cell surface and mediate signals within the cell to modulate growth, remodelling, and viability (apoptosis). Studies have confirmed that mechanical forces on cell surface receptors can immediately alter the organization and composition of molecules in the cytoplasm and nucleus of cells (Chen and Ingber 1999; Ingber 2010). From the moment of conception, the mechanical environment within the embryo is critical to its proper development (Mammoto and Ingber 2010). The extracellular matrix (ECM) plays an essential role in the development of skeletal musculature in the embryo (Thorsteindottir et al. 2011). Furthermore, manual massage applied to the surface of the leg can be traced to effects on underlying cells, with changes in the nucleus and DNA transcription occurring within minutes (Crane et al. 2012).

The amount and composition of the ECM is constantly changing based on the demands on the tissue and mechanical environment (Purslow 2010). Fibroblasts in culture and *in vivo* respond to mechanical loads with measurable effects, such as extracellular calcium influx (through stretch-activated membrane channels), calcium-induced release of intracellular calcium stores, and the release of adenosine triphosphate (ATP). These studies indicate that tissue contraction and relaxation may result in a dynamic, body-wide pattern of cellular activity (Langevin et al. 2010, 2011). Furthermore, the morphology of the embedded fibroblast changes from lamellar to dendritic, depending on the tensional status of the fascial network (Grinnell 2000, 2008).

Fascia is also capable of transmitting electrical signals throughout the body. One of the main components of fascia is collagen. Collagen has been shown to have semi-conductive, piezoelectric, and photoconductive properties *in vitro*. Electronic currents can flow over much greater distances than ionically derived potentials. These electronic currents within connective tissue can be altered by external influences, and cause a physiological response in neighbouring structures (Langevin 2006). However, exploration of the change in bone structures in response to stress (Wolff's law) suggests that fluid flow within tissue is more important than piezoelectric effects (Ahn and Grodzinsky 2009).

Fascia as an organ of gliding

Dr Still notes that fascia

> gives all muscles help to glide over and around all adjacent muscles and ligaments. (1899, p. 164)

All living cells also express some inherent contractility by generating tension within their internal cytoskeleton (Chen and Ingber 1999). Fascia plays a dynamic role in transmitting mechanical tension, and may be able to contract in a smooth, muscle-like manner. *In vitro* studies of human lumbar fascia show that fascia can autonomously contract, hypothesized to be due to the presence of contractile cells within fascia. Fascia contains fibroblasts, which can transform into myofibroblasts which express a gene for alpha-smooth muscle actin (ASMA) and display contractile behaviour (Schleip et al. 2005).

The force generated by skeletal muscle fibres has been shown to spread throughout connective tissue, outside of the skeletal muscle and tendons (Benjamin 2009; Huijing 1999, 2007; Maas and Sandercock 2010). These are known as epimuscular myofascial pathways. Proof of these pathways has been shown by force measurements at the origin and insertion of muscle, as well as the demonstration that length changes in one muscle can affect forces in neighbouring muscles kept at a constant length. These findings suggest that morphologically defined muscle is not the functional unit, as muscle length-force characteristics are variable depending on the conditions of other entities and cannot be considered a fixed property of the muscle. Furthermore, the sarcomere length within a given muscle may not be uniform along its entire length, resulting in the necessity for micro-sliding at and within the muscle fibre level.

Fascia aids muscle contraction by several mechanisms. It links muscles together and to non-muscular structures via the myofascial pathways already described and the direct attachment of muscles into the connective tissue structure around the joint. For example, none of the muscle fibres of the supinator muscle insert directly onto the humeral epicondyle, but go instead to a connective tissue apparatus (van der Wal 2009).

Over 200 *in vivo* hand dissections show the complex network of connective tissue that facilitate sliding adaptation and mobility of structures within the body. Direct and mechanically adaptable multi-microvascular and fibrillar tissue connections between the tendon and the tendon sheath provide vascular access to the tendon. This tissue allows sliding of structures without any dynamic influence on surrounding tissues and can be found everywhere in the body, not just in tendon sheaths (Guimberteau et al. 2010).

Furthermore, even within a single muscle, individual fibres must be able to slide next to each other as the muscle alters shape as it changes length. However, muscle fibres can act in unison by shear force transmission across the very small distance of the endomysium.

Loose connective tissue present between the deep fascia and underlying muscles permits sliding of muscles. This has also been demonstrated by dynamic ultrasound imaging of layers of the thoracolumbar fascia. There is also a layer of lubricating hyaluronic acid between the deep fascia and the muscle, about 100 microns thick (McCombe et al. 2001), which is just at the limit of resolution of newer musculoskeletal ultrasound equipment. Collagen sheets that form layers of connective tissue promote skin sliding and stretching, and allow the skin to maintain its original shape (Benjamin 2009). Fascia plays an important role in separating and organizing muscle groups into compartments. The groups of synergistic muscles are believed to increase the efficiency of muscle contraction, as it has been shown that a small elevation in pressure within each compartment can increase the contractile efficiency of all of the members within the group (Purslow 2002).

Fascia and fluid flow

According to Dr Still, fascia functions by

> secreting and excreting fluid vital and destructive. By its action we live, and by its failure we shrink, swell, and die . . . This connecting substance must be free at all parts to receive and discharge all fluids, if healthy to appropriate and use in sustaining animal life, and eject all impurities that health may not be impaired by the dead and poisoning fluids. (1899, p. 164)

Loose connective tissue harbours the vast majority of the 15 litres of interstitial fluid (Reed and Rubin 2010; Reed et al. 2010). This flows through an ECM which contains cells such as fibroblasts, tumour cells, immune cells, and adipocytes. Interstitial fluid flow can have important effects on tissue morphogenesis, function, cell migration, differentiation, and remodelling, and fibroblast cells embedded in the ECM align themselves perpendicular to the direction of fluid flow. Variations of content of water, ions, and other substances can alter the biomechanical properties of loose connective tissue. The slightest change in fluid flow can alter the shear stress on a cell surface and the biochemical environment of the cell. Interstitial flow regulates nutrient transport to metabolically active cells and plays a crucial role in maintaining healthy tissue. It can also give directional clues to cells by guiding lymphocytes and tumour cells to lymph nodes or towards lymphatic capillaries (Rutkowski and Swartz 2007).

Fluid volume is regulated by interstitial hydrostatic and colloid osmotic pressures, which are constantly readjusting due to alterations in capillary filtration and the lymphatics. Connective tissues can alter transcapillary fluid flux by altering cell tension on dermal fibres which surround the hydrophilic ground substance and prevent its osmotic pressure from drawing fluid out of the capillary. When these fibres relax, this allows glycosaminoglycan ground substance to expand and take up fluid, resulting in oedema formation. After injury, fluid flow can increase almost 100-fold within minutes; most of this is due to the active osmotic pressure of the ECM rather than to capillary leakage (which only increases twofold) (Reed and Rubin 2010; Reed et al. 2010).

Blood flow to skeletal muscle is tightly regulated by its metabolic demands. When muscles contract, the local arterioles rapidly dilate by a mechanism that is not regulated by the skeletal or autonomic nervous system but is, rather, a direct mechanical connection. Tensile forces from contracting skeletal muscle alter the conformation of fibronectin fibrils running from the muscle to the nearby arteriole. This pulls open the nitric oxide receptor and causes local vasodilation (Hocking et al. 2008).

Inelastic fascia can promote lymphatic flow. When muscles contract against a thick, resistant fascia layer, it increases the pressure within a compartment, and permits blood and lymphatic fluid pumping against gravity towards the heart (Benjamin 2009). Compartment syndrome is a painful and potentially limb-threatening condition that occurs when there is an increase in pressure within the deep fascial compartment which impairs blood flow (Benjamin 2009). However, the thick fascia forming the compartment, under normal conditions, results in a rise of compartmental pressures from 15 to 80 mm/Hg with the contraction of just one muscle in the compartment. This raises the contractile efficiency of the other muscles by 15% (Purslow 2002).

Innervation of fascia

Dr Still observed that fascia

> is almost a network of nerves, cells and tubes, running to and from it; it is crossed and filled with, no doubt, millions of nerve centers and fibers . . . Its nerves are so abundant that no atom of flesh fails to get nerve and fluid supply therefrom . . . The cord throws out and supplies millions of nerves by which all organs and parts are supplied with the elements of motion, all to go and terminate in that great system, the fascia. (1899, p. 164–5)

Fascia is richly innervated (van der Wal 2009). Nerves have a three-fascial-layer structure. Endoneurium covers individual axons, perineurium covers bundles of axons, and the epineurium is a thicker layer that covers the perineurium. All layers of the nerve are innervated, and have a plexus of nociceptors (Bove 2008). Fascia contains abundant free and encapsulated nerve endings, and they have been described in the thoracolumbar fascia, the bicipital aponeurosis, and various retinacula (Benjamin 2009). Nerve fibres are found in deep fascia (Bhattacharya et al. 2010). The thoracolumbar fascia (TLF) is densely innervated with different nerve ending distributions in different facial layers. Free sensory nerve endings supply nociceptors. Sensory TLF fibres give input to lumbar dorsal horn neurons, indicating that this may be a source of lower back pain (Tesarz et al. 2011). Similarly, nociceptive fibres originate from crural fascia in rats (Taguchi et al. 2013) and fascial pain endings in humans can be sensitized by local injections of nerve growth factor (Deising et al. 2012).

Fascia plays an important role in proprioception. Muscle spindles are not located uniformly within muscle, but concentrate in areas of force transmission to the fascia surrounding the muscle (van der Wal 2009). A specific pattern of proprioceptor activation occurs when there is fascial tension, and it is directly associated with the deep fascia's relationship to muscle (Benjamin 2009).

Fascia contains several terminal endings of nociceptors, responsible for muscle pain. Nociceptors detect stimuli that are capable of damaging tissue such as mechanical overloading and trauma, and inflammatory mediators such as bradykinin, serotonin, and prostaglandin E2 (Mense 2008). Muscle nociceptors, imaged by light and electron microscopy, were found to be present in all types of tissues within muscle: connective tissue, extrafusal and intrafusal muscle fibres, adventitia of arterioles and venuoles, fat cells, and tendons (Bhattacharya et al. 2010). These nerve endings directly transduce noxious mechanical stimuli. The *in vivo* response of individual mechano-nociceptors is dependent on their physical connection to the ECM (Khalsa 2004).

Fascia beyond A.T. Still

For many years, both amateur and professional athletes have looked to exercise physiologists and trainers for ways to improve and maintain their performance, and avoid injury. Thirty years ago, there was research relating to building muscle strength through concentric and eccentric exercise, with isometric, isokinetic, and isotonic exercises as the building blocks, spaced over various repetitions and intervals. This was followed by research about muscle loss with inactivity, and exercise to combat that loss, made particularly important by the space programme. Muscle biopsies showed slow twitch and fast twitch fibres, with little conversion of fibre types from one to the other. When changes in force generated by muscles were seen in a matter of days, long before there was any demonstrable change in muscle fibre size, this was attributed to changes in the innervations and activation of the muscle. At the end of the day, however, all these studies led to the same conclusion: to improve performance in a specific activity (as opposed to strength in an isolated muscle), the best training is that activity itself, which involves motion of the whole body.

At the same time, models of movement based on muscles and bones were challenged by the reality of motion which could not be explained. In the low back, lumbar fascia needed to be added to the model to account for movement capabilities. The running ability of double-amputee athlete, Oscar Pistorius, has shown that lower-leg muscles are not sufficient or even necessary forces in propelling the human body. Studies of storage of energy in tendon and other connective tissues showed their importance in human gait—it turns out the normal musculoskeletal locomotor system in humans is indeed slightly better (92–95% energy returned from the tendon) than Pistorius's spring-based prostheses (91%), although the mechanics of gait are quite different (Weyand et al. 2009). Additionally, in animals such as the kangaroo, energy storage in tendons is critical in maintaining the repetitive patterns of locomotion (Alexander 2002).

More recently, studies have shown that energy storage in tissues around the shoulder allows the human to throw at speeds over 100 miles an hour, compared to a meagre 20 miles per hour in our closely related primate species. Pre-contraction of the muscle stretches connective tissues, which then explosively release to accomplish a movement for which muscle power alone would be insufficient. While in the leg, large tendons are found in obvious positions to store this energy, this is not the case in the shoulder. Instead, the storage is diffused across a network of as yet undefined tissues, but the 'wind up' for the pitch indicates the whole body is involved (Roach et al. 2013).

The 'fascial organ' consists of a body-wide tensional network of fascia. There is a continuity of fibrils from the ECM, through the integrin receptor and the cell membrane, to the nucleus. Manual massage after exercise can be seen to activate the force conducting pathways to the nucleus, followed within hours by changes in gene transcription (Crane et al. 2012). It is a useful concept to think of the body as a fascial network with connections to muscles and bones, rather than the more traditional view of a musculoskeletal system with fascia connections. This suggests that the contraction of the trunk muscles, prior to use of the superficial muscle slings, may not be just stabilizing the trunk—rather, it may be taking the slack out of core fascial layers to allow 'pre-stretch' and energy storage for release later. Golfers and martial artists know the power in proper trunk rotation.

There are clear differences in mobility of tissues around the joints—with some people being more flexible than others. However, flexibility is not always a uniform function, and the astute clinician will find patients with flexible elbows and tight hamstrings, and vice versa. Indeed, there are some rare muscle disorders characterized by certain tight and other loose joints (Voermans et al. 2009). Stretching results in short-term changes in viscoelastic properties of the muscle and tendons with decreased muscle performance lasting a few minutes (Mizuno et al. 2014). If we return to the notion that fascial tissues store energy for release during activities, we come to the logical conclusion that stretching these tissues to the point where their energy-absorbing properties are permanently altered will result in reduction in energy release and subsequent performance. The mechanical interactions among muscle, tendon, and fascia in humans have developed over many thousands of years to allow us to adapt to a wide range of activities, and we are just beginning to understand these, to be able to direct such adaptation by specific exercises and activities which differ from the final desired task.

Skeletal muscle clearly responds to loading by hypertrophy and other adaptations which increase its capacity for force generation. Extending this concept to connective tissue explores loading in the context of adaptation or overloading pathology. For certain occupations, specific cycles of work/rest can be identified as tolerated or leading to functional loss. Again, task specificity is paramount. Adult tendons show little change or remodelling in the adult, unless there is wound healing to be repaired. To put this into perspective, every two days, there is connective tissue turnover in the tiny fibres connecting a muscle to the nearby arteriole which pull open the nitric oxide receptors and increase blood flow to the contracting muscle (Hocking et al. 2008).

A broad range of physiological and biochemical factors need to be taken into account to understand the basis for the broad spectrum of clinical applications purporting to affect the 'fascial organ'. Some factors are specific to fascia. Others, such as work hardening, are general properties of hardening by plastic deformation which have been used with copper, steel, and other metals for thousands of years.

Guidera et al.'s (2012) paper 'Cervical fascia: a terminological pain in the neck' concisely summarizes:

> There is considerable confusion surrounding the terminology and interpretation of cervical fascia and its associated potential spaces . . . There is a clear need for consistent evidence based definitions and terminology, incorporating results from recent scientific studies using modern anatomical techniques and cross sectional imaging, and clinical investigations.

We would do well to be guided by A.T. Still's insightful clinical observations of fascial functions as we add anatomical precision, using the terms suggested by Langevin (Langevin and Huijing 2009) for specific layers and structures. Also, 'fascia' may graduate from being a connective tissue, a cellular and ECM filler between defined structures, to become regarded as a connective structural system with well-defined functions from the embryo to the adult (and for food scientists, beyond death). In the process, we may learn more about his observations on fascia and respiration and cancer, as we find stem cells located in fascial tissue (Ou et al. 2013) and that the ECM is intimately involved in cancer progression (Lu et al. 2012).

Acknowledgements

This paper is based substantially on previous publications with Mona Shalwala (Findley and Shalwala 2013) and Evan Kwong (Kwong and Findley 2014), and their assistance is gratefully acknowledged. This material is the result of work supported with resources and the use of facilities at the Veteran Affairs New Jersey Healthcare System, East Orange, NJ. The views expressed in this chapter are those of the author and do not necessarily reflect the position or policy of the Department of Veterans Affairs or the United States government.

References

Ahn AC, Grodzinsky AJ. Relevance of collagen piezoelectricity to 'Wolff's Law': a critical review. *Medical Engineering & Physics*. 2009; 31(7): 733–41.

Alexander RM. Tendon elasticity and muscle function. *Comparative Biochemistry & Physiology: Part A, Molecular & Integrative Physiology*. 2002; 133(4):1001–11.

Benjamin M. The fascia of the limbs and back—a review. *Journal of Anatomy*. 2009; 214:1–18.

Bhattacharya V, Barooah P, Nag T, Chaudhuri G, Bhattacharya S. Detail microscopic analysis of deep fascia of lower limb and its surgical implication. *Indian Journal of Plastic Surgery*. 2010; 43(2):135–40.

Bojsen-Moller J, Schwartz S, Kalliokoski KK, Finni T, Magnusson SP. Intermuscular force transmission between human plantarflexor muscles in vivo. *Journal of Applied Physiology*. 2010; 109(6):1608–18.

Bove GM. Epi-perineurial anatomy, innervation, and axonal nociceptive mechanisms. *Journal of Bodywork & Movement Therapies*. 2008; 12(3):185–90.

Chaudhry H, Max R, Antonio S, Findley T. Mathematical model of fiber orientation in anisotropic fascia layers at large displacements. *Journal of Bodywork & Movement Therapies*. 2012; 16(2):158–64.

Chen CS, Ingber DE. Tensegrity and mechanoregulation: from skeleton to cytoskeleton. *Osteoarthritis & Cartilage*. 1999; 7(1):81–94.

Crane JD, Ogborn DI, Cupido C, et al. Massage therapy attenuates inflammatory signaling after exercise-induced muscle damage. *Science Translational Medicine*. 2012; 4(119):119ra13.

Deising S, Weinkauf B, Blunk J, Obreja O, Schmelz M, Rukwied R. NGF-evoked sensitization of muscle fascia nociceptors in humans. *Pain*. 2012; 153(8):1673–9.

Findley TW, Shalwala M. Fascia Research Congress evidence from the 100 year perspective of Andrew Taylor Still. *Journal of Bodywork & Movement Therapies*. 2013; 17(3):356–64.

Gillies AR, Lieber RL. Structure and function of the skeletal muscle extracellular matrix. *Muscle & Nerve*. 2011; 44(3):318–31.

Goldberger ZD, Alexander GC. Digitalis use in comtemporary clinical practice: refitting the foxglove. *JAMA Internal Medicine*. 2014; 174(1): 151–4.

Grinnell F. Fibroblast mechanics in three-dimensional collagen matrices. *Journal of Bodywork & Movement Therapies*. 2008; 12(3):191–3.

Grinnell F. Fibroblast-collagen-matrix contraction: growth-factor signalling and mechanical loading. *Trends in Cell Biology*. 2000; 10(9):362–5.

Guidera AK, Dawes PJ, Stringer MD. Cervical fascia: a terminological pain in the neck. *ANZ Journal of Surgery*. 2012; 82(11):786–91.

Guimberteau JC, Delage JP, Wong J. The role and mechanical behavior of the connective tissue in tendon sliding. *Chirurgie de la Main*. 2010; 29(3):155–66.

Hocking DC, Titus PA, Sumagin R, Sarelius IH. Extracellular matrix fibronectin mechanically couples skeletal muscle contraction with local vasodilation. *Circulation Research*. 2008; 102(3):372–9.

Huijing PA. Epimuscular myofascial force transmission between antagonistic and synergistic muscles can explain movement limitation in spastic paresis. *Journal of Electromyography & Kinesiology*. 2007; 17(6): 708–24.

Huijing PA. Muscle as a collagen fiber reinforced composite: a review of force transmission in muscle and whole limb. *Journal of Biomechanics*. 1999; 32(4):329–45.

Ingber DE. From cellular mechanotransduction to biologically inspired engineering: 2009 Pritzker Award Lecture, BMES Annual Meeting October 10, 2009. *Annals of Biomedical Engineering*. 2010; 38(3):1148–61.

Ingber DE. Mechanosensation through integrins: cells act locally but think globally. *Proceedings of the National Academy of Sciences USA*. 2003; 100(4):1472–4.

Jarvinen TAH, Jozsa L, Kannus P, Jarvinen TLN, Jarvinen M. Organization and distribution of intramuscular connective tissue in normal and immobilized skeletal muscles. An immunohistochemical, polarization and scanning electron microscopic study. *Journal of Muscle Research & Cell Motility*. 2002; 23(3):245–54.

Khalsa PS. Biomechanics of musculoskeletal pain: dynamics of the neuromatrix. *Journal of Electromyography & Kinesiology*. 2004; 14(1):109–20.

Kwong EH, Findley TW. Fascia—current knowledge and future directions in physiatry: a narrative review. *Journal of Rehabilitation Research and Development*. 2014 51(6): 875–884.

Langevin HM. Connective tissue: a body-wide signaling network? *Medical Hypotheses*. 2006; 66(6):1074–7.

Langevin HM, Huijing PA. Communicating about fascia: history, pitfalls, and recommendations. *International Journal of Therapeutic Massage & Bodywork* 2009; 2(4):3–8.

Langevin HM, Bouffard NA, Fox JR, et al. Fibroblast cytoskeletal remodeling contributes to connective tissue tension. *Journal of Cellular Physiology*. 2011; 226(5):1166–75.

Langevin HM, Storch KN, Snapp RR, et al. Tissue stretch induces nuclear remodeling in connective tissue fibroblasts. *Histochemistry & Cell Biology*. 2010; 133(4):405–15.

Lu P, Weaver VM, Werb Z. The extracellular matrix: a dynamic niche in cancer progression. *Journal of Cell Biology*. 2012; 196(4):395–406.

Lund DK, Cornelison DDW. Enter the matrix: shape, signal and superhighway. *FEBS Journal*. 2013; 280(17):4089–99.

Maas H, Sandercock TG. Are skeletal muscles independent actuators? Force transmission from soleus muscle in the cat. *Journal of Applied Physiology*. 2008; 104(6):1557–67.

Maas H, Sandercock TG. Force transmission between synergistic skeletal muscles through connective tissue linkages. *Journal of Biomedicine & Biotechnology*. 2010; 2010:575–672.

Mammoto T, Ingber DE. Mechanical control of tissue and organ development. *Development*. 2010; 137(9):1407–20.

McCombe D, Brown T, Slavin J, Morrison WA. The histochemical structure of the deep fascia and its structural response to surgery. *Journal of Hand Surgery—British Volume*. 2001; 26(2):89–97.

Mense S. Muscle pain: mechanisms and clinical significance. *Deutsches Arzteblatt International*. 2008; 105(12):214–9.

Mizuno T, Matsumoto M, Umemura Y. Stretching-induced deficit of maximal isometric torque is restored within 10 minutes. *Journal of Strength & Conditioning Research*. 2014; 28(1):147–53.

Ou Y, Qu R, Dai J. Experimental biological research on stem cells in fascia tissue. *Journal of Acupuncture & Meridian Studies*. 2013; 6(3):129–33.

Pancheri FQ, Eng CM, Lieberman DE, Biewener AA, Dorfmann L. A constitutive description of the anisotropic response of the fascia lata. *Journal of the Mechanical Behavior of Biomedical Materials*. 2014; 30:306–23.

Passerieux E, Rossignol R, Chopard A, et al. Structural organization of the perimysium in bovine skeletal muscle: junctional plates and associated intracellular subdomains. *Journal of Structural Biology*. 2006; 154(2):206–16.

Pohl H. Changes in the structure of collagen distribution in the skin caused by a manual technique. *Journal of Bodywork & Movement Therapies*. 2010; 14(1):27–34.

Purslow PP. Muscle fascia and force transmission. *Journal of Bodywork & Movement Therapies*. 2010; 14(4):411–7.

Purslow PP. The structure and functional significance of variations in the connective tissue within muscle. *Comparative Biochemistry and Physiology: Part A Molecular Integrated Physiology*. 2002; 133(4):947–66.

Purslow PP, Archile-Contreras AC, Cha MC. Meat Science and Muscle Biology Symposium: manipulating meat tenderness by increasing the turnover of intramuscular connective tissue. *Journal of Animal Science*. 2012; 90(3):950–9.

Reed RK, Rubin K. Transcapillary exchange: role and importance of the interstitial fluid pressure and the extracellular matrix. *Cardiovascular Research*. 2010; 87(2):211–7.

Reed RK, Liden A, Rubin K. Edema and fluid dynamics in connective tissue remodelling. *Journal of Molecular & Cellular Cardiology*. 2010; 48(3):518–23.

Roach NT, Venkadesan M, Rainbow MJ, Lieberman DE. Elastic energy storage in the shoulder and the evolution of high-speed throwing in Homo. *Nature*. 2013; 498(7455):483–6.

Rutkowski JM, Swartz MA. A driving force for change: interstitial flow as a morphoregulator. *Trends in Cell Biology*. 2007; 17(1):44–50.

Schleip R, Jager H, Klingler W. What is 'fascia'? A review of different nomenclatures. *Journal of Bodywork & Movement Therapies*. 2012; 16(4): 496–502.

Schleip R, Klingler W, Lehmann-Horn F. Active fascial contractility: fascia may be able to contract in a smooth muscle-like manner and thereby influence musculoskeletal dynamics. *Medical Hypotheses*. 2005; 65(2):273–7.

Simmonds N, Miller P, Gemmell H. A theoretical framework for the role of fascia in manual therapy. *Journal of Bodywork & Movement Therapies*. 2012; 16(1):83–93.

Smeulders MJC, Kreulen M. Myofascial force transmission and tendon transfer for patients suffering from spastic paresis: a review and some new observations. *Journal of Electromyography & Kinesiology*. 2007; 17(6):644–56.

Stecco A, Gesi M, Stecco C, Stern R. Fascial components of the myofascial pain syndrome. *Current Pain and Headache Reports*. 2013; 17(8):352.

Stecco A, Macchi V, Stecco C, et al. Anatomical study of myofascial continuity in the anterior region of the upper limb. *Journal of Bodywork & Movement Therapies*. 2009; 13(1):53–62.

Stecco C, Macchi V, Porzionato A, Duparc F, De Caro R. The fascia: the forgotten structure. *Italian Journal of Anatomy & Embryology*. 2011; 116(3):127–38.

Still AT. *Osteopathy research and practice*. Kirksville MO: published by the author; 1910.

Still AT. *The philosophy and mechanical principles of osteopathy*. Kansas City MO: Hudson-Eimberlt; 1902.

Still AT. *Philosophy of osteopathy*. Kirksville MO: published by the author; 1899.

Taguchi T, Yasui M, Kubo A, et al. Nociception originating from the crural fascia in rats. *Pain*. 2013; 154(7):1103–14.

Tesarz J, Hoheisel U, Wiedenhofer B, Mense S. Sensory innervation of the thoracolumbar fascia in rats and humans. *Neuroscience*. 2011; 194:302–8.

Thorsteinsdottir S, Deries M, Cachaco AS, Bajanca F. The extracellular matrix dimension of skeletal muscle development. *Developmental Biology*. 2011; 354(2):191–207.

Turrina A, Martinez-Gonzalez MA, Stecco C. The muscular force transmission system: role of the intramuscular connective tissue. *Journal of Bodywork & Movement Therapies*. 2013; 17(1):95–102.

van der Wal JC. The architecture of the connective tissue in the musculoskeletal system—an often overlooked contributor to proprioception in the locomotor apparatus. *International Journal of Therapeutic Bodywork & Massage*. 2009; 4(2):9–23.

Vogel S. Comparative Biomechanics: Life's Physical World 2nd Ed 2013 Princeton NJ: Princeton University Press

Voermans NC, Bonnemann CG, Hamel BCJ, Jungbluth H, van Engelen BG. Joint hypermobility as a distinctive feature in the differential diagnosis of myopathies. *Journal of Neurology*. 2009; 256(1):13–27.

Wendell-Smith CP. Fascia: an illustrative problem in international terminology. Surgical and radiologic anatomy. *Surgical and Radiological Anatomy* 1997; 19(5):273–7.

Weyand PG, Bundle MW, McGowan CP, et al. The fastest runner on artificial legs: different limbs, similar function? *Journal of Applied Physiology*. 2009; 107(3):903–11.

Willard FH, Vleeming A, Schuenke MD, Danneels L, Schleip R. The thoracolumbar fascia: anatomy, function and clinical considerations. *Journal of Anatomy*. 2012; 221(6):507–36.

Yu WS, Kilbreath SL, Fitzpatrick RC, Gandevia SC. Thumb and finger forces produced by motor units in the long flexor of the human thumb. *Journal of Physiology (London)*. 2007; 583(Pt 3):1145–54.

Yucesoy CA, Huijing PA. Substantial effects of epimuscular myofascial force transmission on muscular mechanics have major implications on spastic muscle and remedial surgery. *Journal of Electromyography & Kinesiology*. 2007; 17(6):664–79.

Chapter 19

Pain concepts: chronic pain

Milton Cohen and John Quintner

'Defining' chronic pain

> Chronic pain is a complaint of the vast majority of adults in any developed country. The actions that people take about their pain are of concern because they can lead to heath care consumption and disability. It is no longer adequate to utilise a biomedical model to search for the broken part that will explain the patient's behaviours. Instead, we must look at environmental factors which can perpetuate chronic pain and the associated health care consumption and disability . . . Although tissue damage and nerve injury can lead to chronic pain, most of the disability associated with the complaint of chronic pain cannot be explained by events within the patient's (or claimant's) body. Interpersonal and environmental factors leading to unresolved stress are the major determinants of disability associated with chronic pain.
>
> (Loeser JD. What is chronic pain? *Theoretical Medicine* 1991; 12:213–225.)

> The experience of chronic pain, including the actions taken in the context of this experience, is an interactive process. We do not simply feel pain. The experience of pain emerges from a mix of feelings in the body, thoughts and beliefs in the mind, emotional experiences and our behaviour, as determined by our history and the situation at hand. It is not a process of passive sensory reception and reaction. It is a dynamic process of psychological construction within an equally dynamic process of life activities, as the individual navigates the demands of the social world, demands imposed by the body, and provisions for help and support.
>
> (McCracken L (commentary). Anger, injustice, and the continuing search for psychological mechanisms of pain, suffering and disability. *Pain* 2013; 154:1495–1496.)

These two quotations from eminent pain physicians, twenty-two years apart, exemplify at once the changed paradigm through which the experience of chronic pain should be seen and the clinical and cultural lag that has occurred in how it is seen in advanced societies. That lag is attributable to the extraordinary success of biomedicine in discovering and treating mechanisms of disease on the one hand and the perpetuation of the mind–body dichotomy on the other, so that what cannot be found 'in the body' defaults to responsibilities outside medicine. However, as a textbook of musculoskeletal medicine may not ignore the clinical phenomenon of chronic pain, this chapter will embrace the changed paradigm.

The public health problem

Global estimates of the prevalence of chronic pain (however defined) suggest that 20% of adults will report the experience (Goldberg and McGee 2011). In recent years, there has been increasing recognition that the associated health and societal consequences of such large numbers of people living in pain constitute a huge and almost insoluble public health problem. Apart from obvious comorbid health conditions, such as disturbances of mood, cognition, and sleep pattern, substance abuse, and suicidality, it is now clear that socio-economic factors (poverty, unemployment, homelessness, and lack of social support) are important contributors to the often profound disability of sufferers.

Biomedical framework

The dominant discourse of Western medicine is characterized by two core philosophical tenets, each with two complementary aspects. Firstly, not only are body and mind conceptualized as different and distinct entities but also the physical ('body') dimension, being 'objective' and therefore measurable, is accorded priority over the mental ('mind') dimension, which is 'subjective' and therefore unmeasurable (Crowley-Matoka et al. 2009). The second is the reductionist assumption that all symptoms–including pain–are expressions of a discoverable disease process and that there is a predictable and reliable connection between pathological changes and clinical features. This is complemented by the assumption that knowledge about the properties of parts of a system is sufficient to understand the global behaviour of the whole system.

This primacy of structural pathology located in the body has been the major criterion for discovering disease in Western epistemology, eclipsing functional pathology and relegating to the background behavioural, psychological, and social factors. When applied to the problem of clinical pain, biomedicine posits a predictable—if yet to be discovered—hard-wired relationship between identifiable tissue damage, consequent changes within the brain, and the report of pain.

The implications of this biomedical model of illness are profound. Firstly, the experience of deviation from wellness is demoted to the depersonalized expression of a (structural) disease process. Secondly, the process of clinical diagnosis becomes exclusively reductionist, the only phenomena of interest being those that constitute discrete, linear causal chains. Thirdly, the relationships between such chains are assumed to behave predictably, and to apply universally (Gray 1973).

In effect, this model privileges the ostensibly 'objective' view of the clinician over the sufferer's lived experience of pain. Thus, if there is no discoverable and relevant nociception (the detection and signalling of 'tissue damage', a concept integral to the 'definition' of pain), there can be no 'real' pain. The clinical encounter then resolves as either dismissal of the patient's complaint or an inference of 'psychogenesis' by the clinician (Quintner et al. 2008). This is in effect a reversion to the default tenet of body–mind dualism, defying and confronting the lived experience of pain, which is 'simultaneously and interactively both physical and mental' (Crowley-Matoka et al. 2009).

Biopsychosocial framework

This framework was developed by psychiatrist George Engel (1977a) as an attempt to loosen the constraints of dualism and reductionism and to allow clinicians to embrace aspects of human illness that biomedicine proved unable to contemplate. Engel's proposition retained the assumptions of biomedicine but invited consideration that the experience of illness could be influenced if not determined by psychological, social, and cultural factors.

Engel's model was derived from General Systems Theory (GST) as formulated in the early twentieth century by Viennese theoretical biologists, Ludwig von Bertalanffy and Paul Weiss (Drack and Apfalter 2007). GST holds that organisms are highly organized hierarchical systems, embedded in their respective environments. A perturbation sufficient to cause changes in any one of these systems would evoke changes in any or all of the other systems. Most importantly, the organism itself would produce these changes 'in an effort to stay constant with regard to its outside' (Weiss 1925).

The biopsychosocial framework invited clinicians to collect qualitative and quantitative data in these psychological, social, and cultural domains and to incorporate them into diagnostic and therapeutic processes, thereby arriving at a better understanding of the 'human experience' of disease or, more correctly, of illness. Importantly, these transactions were to take place at the 'two-person' system level, that is, the doctor–patient relationship (Engel 1977b).

Theoreticians in pain medicine were quick to adopt the biopsychosocial framework, as it seemed to fit the growing recognition of pain as an expression of complex interactions between biological, psychological, social, and cultural factors (Aronoff et al. 2000).

Interestingly, from the biological perspective, the Gate Control Theory of Melzack and Wall (1965) had already predicted, based on the plasticity and modifiability of events at all levels within the central nervous system, that whether or not a person perceives and reports pain in response to a particular stimulus would be determined not only by the nature of that stimulus but also by the context within which it is experienced, together with associated memories, emotions, and beliefs (Melzack 1999; Melzack and Wall 1965, 1973).

International Association for the Study of Pain definition and critique

A major outcome of the application of the biopsychosocial approach was the 'official' definition of pain by the International Association for the Study of Pain (IASP) as 'an unpleasant sensory and emotional experience associated with actual or potential tissue damage or described in terms of such damage' (Merskey and Bogduk 1994). This was an advance on the biomedical approach, as it could break the nexus between actual tissue damage and the subjective experience and thus accord legitimacy to the experience of the person in pain.

However, the explanatory notes that accompany the IASP definition contain the rider that '[M]any people report pain in the absence of tissue damage or any likely pathological cause; usually this happens for psychological reasons.' Thus, even this potentially enlightening definition fell back into the circular trap of body–mind dualism, and has inadvertently sanctioned the efforts to seek explanations for a variety of pain syndromes solely from psychosocial factors, from which arises the untestable construct of somatization (Barsky and Borus 1995).

Nonetheless, the biopsychosocial framework generated a number of hierarchical 'models' of pain. First among these was that of Loeser (1980) who proposed four nested hierarchical domains: nociception, pain, suffering, and pain behaviour. Waddell's Glasgow Illness Model was formulated similarly, postulating four domains of interest: physical problem, psychological distress, illness behaviour, and social interactions (Waddell et al. 1984).

Each 'model' explicitly includes the moral dimension of 'suffering' and in fact the only observable domain is the interaction between the person in pain and the surrounding world ('pain behaviour' in Loeser's model; 'illness behaviour' and 'social interaction' in that of Waddell). In each, the clinician was to determine which of the four domains might be 'playing significant roles in the genesis of the person's problem, and then to direct therapies at the appropriate aetiological factors' (Waddell et al. 1984).

This exercise required the clinician not only to differentiate illness behaviour from physical disease but also to detect any mismatch between the amount of demonstrable disease causing pain and the level of disability allegedly caused by the pain. How these crucial decisions were to be made was left entirely to the clinician's discretion, guided by the same arbitrary constructions constrained by dualism.

These approaches pose major theoretical and practical problems. Firstly, the frameworks suggest that pain, suffering, and behaviour are somehow discrete phenomena, whereas in fact the clinician/observer is unable to make such a distinction. Secondly, although nociception may be understood as a specific and quantitative physiological process, the other domains resist such a reductionist approach. Just as the connection between them is undefinable and arbitrary, so is the lived experience of pain not reducible to a neuroscientific explanation. Although these conceptual frameworks imply that there are non-nociceptive influences on pain and behaviour, they neither escape dualism nor solve the unacknowledged 'puzzle of pain' (Melzack and Wall 1973).

The next two decades saw a new trend emerging, with the focus on inferring overarching neurobiological mechanisms for the experience of pain. Flor and Hermann (2004) formulated a 'psychobiological' model of pain, viewing it as a multi-component behavioural response to aversive stimuli. Through prior learning, operant and respondent conditioning, powerful pain memories are formed at all levels of the nervous system, reflecting the dynamic and continuous interplay between various physiological and psychological factors. Once established, such pain memories were said to be capable of maintaining pain even in the absence of peripheral nociceptive input. That is, pain transmutes from being an emergent aversive response into a learned memory that may cause profound reorganizational changes within the nervous system, thus perpetuating itself.

By reconceptualizing pain as a 'homeostatic emotion', Craig (2002) pursued the theme of grounding pain in disturbed bodily function, as one of a number of emotional responses through which the integrity of the body (self) can be maintained in the face of conditions that threaten to disturb its homeostasis. He suggested that pain is not part of the exteroceptive somatosensory system but rather 'part of a hierarchical system of interoception subserving homeostasis, the sense of the physiological condition of the body (interoception) and the subjective awareness of feelings and emotion.'

Craig's formulation was based on the known relationship in humans between activated C-fibres and the conscious perception of pain, and a proposal that slow ongoing spontaneous discharge in C-fibres functions to monitor the physiological condition (metabolic status) of the entire bodily tissues and could be responsible for an individual's subjective awareness of inner body feelings, including emotionality (Craig 2004).

This claim raises two important issues. Firstly, the particular disturbance of homeostasis that gives rise to the experience of pain is quite specific, being signalled only through the summated activation of nociceptors, that is, by tissue damage. Craig is attempting to unify (old) specificity theory with (new) convergence theory, favouring the former. The second and more profound issue is that Craig's hypothesis depends on representationism whereby the nervous system is held to mirror an independent world, which includes a 'thing' called pain and a sensory image of the physiological condition of the body. Not only is this claim untestable, it requires that the organism step outside itself in order to observe its own condition which, as it leads to an infinite regress, would appear to be impossible (Edelman 1992). Furthermore, it would also require what the philosopher Daniel Dennett calls a 'Cartesian Theater', an obscure place in the mind/brain 'where it all comes together' (Dennett 1993).

Possibly because the biopsychosocial initiative is a framework for analysis rather than an explanatory model for the complex phenomenology of pain states, it has tended in practice to default reductionism and dualism (Butler et al. 2004). However, a strong argument remains for clinicians to maintain the program of conceptualization of pain in a sociopsychobiological framework (Carr and Bradshaw 2014).

Dissecting and understanding the biomedical imperative (power and dollars)

In considering the relationship between medicine and the market, Callahan (2009) observes that '[L]eft uncontrolled and unregulated, or allowed to become dominant, the market can be, and often has been, the enemy of solidarity, our human interdependence, and thus indirectly of health as well.' This may well refer to the tension in pain medicine between biomedical therapies such as medications and procedures that have high face validity but little evidence for effectiveness, and the interpersonally intensive multidisciplinary therapies that are more effective and more efficient. The market forces that readily fund the former entrench the biomedical model. This tension between the imperative for rational and ethical pain-related health care and the biomedically driven commercial objectives of the market place (Loeser and Cahana 2013) has been coloured by a relatively new principle: the right of the patient to access pain management (Brennan et al. 2007), even though it is difficult to know how such a right can be legally enforced without prejudicing the patient–clinician relationship (Hall and Boswell 2009).

Those who champion the cause of patient empowerment in health (and pain) care might pay heed to Callahan's concluding remarks:

> But the world of the sick is marked by a loss of strength and independence, by a diminishment of self-management, by a painful dependence upon others. Providing the economic and social goods to well manage that combination of human vulnerabilities has not been a mark of the market anywhere, nor is there any reason to suppose they could or would be. (2009, p. 33)

The 'chronic pain is a disease' debate

The problems with language

Recent attempts (Siddall and Cousins 2004) to classify chronic pain as a diagnosable disease 'in and of itself' have raised important questions of medical language and logic, which are deserving of attention in this chapter.

The philosopher Ludwig Wittgenstein (1953) identified an important principle in relation to nomenclature: 'naming and describing do not stand on the same level: Naming is a preparation for description . . . Naming is so far not a move in the language game anymore than putting a piece in its place on the board is a move in chess.' Pursuing the chess analogy used by Wittgenstein, the act of naming a medical condition (i.e. making a specific diagnosis) only places it on the 'language board' without specifying where it belongs (i.e. in terms of its taxonomy), what are its defining features (the criteria used for diagnosis), and the particular rules (i.e. operational criteria) that might apply to its common usage in medical parlance.

There is yet another important dimension worthy of consideration—that of the context in which language is being used: 'the diagnosis can be understood only as it is used within the contexts or activities that give it meaning. The term is understood by looking at the activities of the profession that uses it, NOT by reference to an object or specific mental process.' (Rosenman and Nasti 2012).

Defining disease

The concept of 'ease' comes from the Old French word *aise* for states of comfort, pleasure, and well-being. 'Dis-ease' refers to those states of being where 'ease' is not the case. However, the current definition of disease does not reflect its lay etymology. Nevertheless, the term 'malaise' (derived from the Old French) is still used by some in medicine.

Dorland's Illustrated Medical Dictionary offers a formal definition of disease: 'any deviation from or interruption of the normal structure or function of any body part, organ, or system that is manifested by a characteristic set of symptoms and signs and whose etiology, pathology, and prognosis may be known or unknown.' (2011) This definition fails to convey the important message that specific diseases are but higher- level abstractions that are consensus-driven within the medical community: 'contemporary medicine and bureaucracy have constructed disease entities as socially real actors through laboratory tests, pathology-defining thresholds, statistically derived risk factors, and other artifacts of a seemingly value-free biomedical scientific enterprise.' (Rosenberg 2002)

Nevertheless, assignment of the term 'disease' hinges upon the presence of 'a characteristic set of symptoms and signs'.

Is pain a disease?

As already mentioned, the IASP defined 'pain' for operational purposes as 'an unpleasant sensory and emotional experience associated with actual or potential tissue damage, or described in terms of such damage' (Merskey and Bogduk 1994).

The IASP definition is unequivocal in identifying pain as an experience or phenomenon, at once both abstract and subjective. Yet, a blanket conferral of disease status upon the symptom 'chronic pain' reifies a complex dynamic experience. We summarize here the argument that the proposition cannot be supported on clinical, pathological, or epistemological grounds (Cohen et al. 2013).

The move to assign disease status to the clinical problem of persistent pain began with Siddall and Cousins (2004) citing 'secondary pathology' within the nervous system induced by altered sensory inputs from the periphery, including anatomical reorganization in nociceptive pathways and alterations in patterns of brain activation and cortical topography found in persistent pain states. In the light of recent knowledge of brain plasticity, this proposition was, in itself, unexceptional. However, their assertion that 'persistent pain does give rise to its own secondary pathology' elevates pain to the status of a causative 'thing', thus constituting the circular argument that pain causes itself.

These authors went further by adducing environmental factors as the 'tertiary pathology' of pain and thus asserted that pain is 'an environmental disease'. Such tertiary pathology was said to include 'factors such as genetic makeup, level of spinal inhibition, psychological status and the societal litigation system.' In effect, this proposition is no different from identifying that non-nociceptive factors may be relevant to the pain experience. However, to label this as 'tertiary pathology' carries the implication that these factors can somehow contribute to a permanently altered nervous system. At the same time, by including 'psychological status' as part of this tertiary pathology, and therefore external to (and acting upon) the body, the argument defaults to the familiar circle of body–mind dualism. Furthermore, what is the pathological basis of the influence, for example, of the 'societal litigation system'?

This proposition appeared to be concordant with the biopsychosocial framework, but the attempt to portray pain itself as a causative 'thing' represented a dramatic return to the linear causality of the biomedical model.

A counter-argument (Siddall 2013) maintains that chronic pain does fulfil the criteria for a disease, as defined earlier in this chapter. This argument turns upon the requirement of 'a characteristic set of symptoms and signs' and it is the phenomenon of central sensitization (an abstract neurophysiological concept embracing 'activity-dependent synaptic plasticity in the spinal cord that generates post-injury pain hypersensitivity') that fulfils this requirement (Woolf 1983, 2011). However, if one were to follow this reasoning, the name of this disease becomes 'central sensitization' rather than 'chronic pain'.

Because pain is an embodied experience, it is logically incorrect (i.e. a circular argument) to assume that the neurophysiological concept (i.e. central sensitization) constitutes in whole or in part, thereof, the phenomenon that has manifested itself (i.e. chronic pain) (Eriksen and Risor 2013).

Bedazzled by technology

Another counter-argument focused on presumed brain pathology that 'defines' pain. The American Association of Pain Medicine Position Paper, citing only one reference, claims that 'research that has demonstrated reduced volumes of neocortical gray matter in patients with chronic back pain' justifies '[t]he evolution of pain from a neurobiologic response ("eudynia") to a neurobiologic disease ("maldynia")' (parentheses added) (Dubois et al. 2009).

In a critical review of 108 neuroimaging reports of human central pain processing, Tracey and Bushnell (2009) set out to 'examine the information from these functional, structural and molecular studies within the framework of a *disease state*' (emphasis added). They conclude, not at all unreasonably, that there is 'substantial functional, anatomical and neurochemical evidence that chronic-pain patients have abnormal brains'. However, they do identify the 'chicken-and-egg' problem inherent in further inference, by asking whether the evidence of 'altered and dysfunctional central nervous system processing' is 'an adaptive response to the constant nociceptive barrage' or constitutes a 'disease like process'.

The claim that the decrease in grey matter in 'pain-processing' areas of the brains of patients with chronic pain is an indication of an underlying pathognomonic process that justifies disease status must be tempered by the absence of 'conclusive data regarding the cause or the consequence of the different cortical and subcortical morphological changes that have been observed in chronic pain states' (May 2011). Reviewing 30 independent studies in 15 chronic pain states, May (2011) concludes, 'it is simply not clear whether the changes described . . . reflect changes due to pain (i.e. nociceptive input) or changes due to the consequences of pain or both'. He points out that changes due to the presence of pain, such as altered physical activity, disturbed social function, and lifestyle effects, as well as the unknown 'impact of pain killers and other medications' may contribute to the observed morphometric findings. He concludes that the 'data of an increase or decrease in gray matter in pain syndromes need to be considered in light of all observations gathered in the past 10 years and probably do not justify a discussion of brain damage or whether the disease (*sic*) is progressive' (May 2011).

This is not to deny the exciting evolving evidence of altered brain function in chronic pain states, especially in those areas known to be involved with processing of nociceptive information, such as the cingulate cortex, insula, temporal lobe, and dorsolateral prefrontal cortex (Tracey and Bushnell 2009). Nor is it to doubt that major knowledge will be gained from this work.

From a definitional standpoint, a disease must be 'manifested by a characteristic set of symptoms and signs', which raises the question of which 'characteristic' clinical features, apart from the complaint of pain, constitute the 'disease' of pain? It is not sufficient to invoke a 'syndrome' or a grouping of symptoms of which pain might be a component, especially when the diversity of conditions associated with pain is considered. Neither on pathological nor on clinical grounds can 'pain' as a 'disease' be justified.

Approach from evolutionary biology

From the viewpoint of evolutionary biology, it has been hypothesized that the experience of pain is but one way in which an animal signals that a perceived stressor is posing an existential threat. Potential 'danger' or 'stress' stimuli can be physical (i.e. tissue damage) or psychological (including environmental), or a combination thereof. Organisms are able to activate evolutionarily conserved stress response systems that are kept under tight control through the mechanism of self-inhibition (Lyon et al. 2011). According to this hypothesis, chronic pain is but one clinical manifestation of undamped stress response system activation. Other manifestations include fatigue, hyperalgesia, mood disturbance, sleep disturbance, and impaired cognition.

Apart from possessing scientific credibility, this hypothesis transcends the body/mind substance dualism that has proven so damaging to so many chronic pain sufferers (Cohen et al. 2011).

Integrated intersubjectivity: the role of the clinical encounter

Why are pain and its ethical treatment so elusive of theory? This question can be addressed by identifying the clinical encounter as the pivotal transaction in pain medicine: the presentation of a person distressed because of a perceived profound threat to their bodily integrity to another person reputed to be learned in the arts (if not also the sciences) of healing. The search for a new theoretical perspective to understand this encounter draws on three vantage points:

i) the central concept of pain as an *aporia* that cannot be accounted for adequately by the biomedical model or in a biopsychosocial framework;

ii) the nature of humans (and indeed other biological systems) as autonomous self-organizing, self-referential, autopoietic units that have different perspectives and needs based on the demands of their particular circumstances (which includes the societies in which they are embedded); and

iii) intersubjectivity or empathy as the natural ground for rapprochement between the world of the clinician and the world of the person in pain in the clinical setting.

Pain experience as an aporia

The lived experience of being human is not linear and indeed is beyond body–mind monism or dualism (Williamson et al. 2005). Pain is not only difficult to express in language but is also ultimately not communicable in these terms: too complex to be apprehended from linear determinism or from a desire to make sense of it. Our attempts to develop explanatory models bounce off a metaphysical brick wall, which constitutes the aporia of pain.

An aporia (from the Greek meaning 'lacking a path, a passage, or a way') is a mystery or puzzle, encompassing the dual problems of not knowing how one has arrived here and not knowing where to go next (Burbules 2000). As it is unlikely that pain can ever be known objectively, the clinician's encounter with the aporia of the patient is often one of uncertainty, discomfort, and doubt. The patient in pain, currently encountering the aporia, presents his/her body to the clinician for investigation and treatment with the quite reasonable expectation that the clinician will be able to 'ground' the lived experience. However, the clinician may also be 'lost', so that both parties lack knowledge and understanding, which leads to a crisis of choice, of action, and of identity (Burbules 2000). The clinician's dilemma can then lead to loss of empathy and even to feelings of resentment towards the person in pain (May 2011).

When confronted with the clinician's dilemma, the patient too is forced to share the same doubt and uncertainty, compounding their discomfort, and with potentially negative epistemic and moral implications for the therapeutic relationship, including stigmatization within the healthcare system (May 2011). The devastating consequences of stigmatization ('social suffering') need to be addressed at both practice and policy levels.

Self-referential biological systems

A critical insight from General Systems Theory is the capacity of a living organism to change itself in response to perturbations in its environment (Gray 1973, Weiss 1925). Chilean biologists Maturana and Varela ((1980) argued that the unique property possessed by living organisms is a particular circular mechanism of spontaneous autonomous activity contained within a semi-permeable boundary, a process which they called autopoiesis, from the Greek meaning 'self-producing'. They defined an 'autopoietic unit' as a particular type of homeostatic system capable of being self-sustaining by virtue of an inner network of reactions (its organization) that regenerate all the system's components (its structure).

Autopoiesis is the continual production by a network of the very components that comprise and sustain the network and its processes of production. In other words, such a system is said to be self-referential (capable of examining itself) and self-organizing (i.e. capable of changing and ordering its internal structure according to local rules) (von Foerster 1960; Luhmann 2003; Luisi 2003).

The critical variable of a living system is its own organization. This is highly negentropic (i.e. operating far from thermodynamic equilibrium): loss of the system's organization results in its death. By contrast, its structure (its various components) changes constantly as the system continues to adapt itself to both predictable and unpredictable disturbances caused by environmental changes.

In higher animals, the nervous system, including ultimately the brain, forms part of this autonomous unity, because its operation is circular or in operational closure. Being an embedded system in continuous structural change, the nervous system has the property of plasticity, which enables it to participate in the process by which the organism and its environment remain in a continuous, inseparable relationship. In this formulation, the brain is not simply a hard-wired computer-like machine that only processes an externally referenced environment. Rather, the brain is both the object of interpretation and the interpreter of its own self-organizing reference (Arbib et al. 1988). In other words, the brain functions as a self-referential system.

When the organism's environment includes another living organism, each triggers changes in the other's structure; such a congruent reciprocal relationship continues for as long as they remain engaged. During that time, the lived body environment of each becomes a unique unitary domain of communication (Maturana and Varela 1980). Importantly, during such interaction each organism conserves its own autopoiesis and compatibility with its environment. However, the result of that interaction is not determined by a stimulus external to the organism but only by the aggregate state of each organism itself at a given moment (Arbib et al. 1988; Lyon 2004).

We argue that the key to understanding pain is found in the role of the self-referential brain embedded in an autopoietic living system. When that living system is a human reporting the experience of pain, we—if we are to be empathically engaged observers—must infer that an important change has occurred in that person's nervous system arising out of an attempt to maintain its autopoietic organization. Sufferers endeavour to elicit from clinicians whatever is needed to assist this process.

Empathy

Although clinician and patient are both excluded from the same aporia (viz. the pain of the 'other'), they interact as two autopoietic autonomous entities, being simultaneously observer and observed. Both come together in a process of exploration. Each is invited to take on the other's questions, problems, and aporia as their own. The domain of this 'level playing field' interaction allows the emergence of the phenomena of intersubjectivity and empathy.

There is a potential neurobiological basis for these phenomena, building on the observation that the knowledge that someone else is currently in pain is sufficient to evoke activity in brain regions associated with the experience of pain. Specifically, such a relationship might be built upon primary involuntary activity of deeply embedded cortical sensorimotor 'mirror' neurons in the observer and the observed (Favareau 2002; Rizzolatti et al. 1999). As Favareau has argued: 'For at the mirror neuron level of organization, the distinction between seer and doer, action and reaction, identity and alterity is— like the "reflection" one finds oneself presented with in front of a full length mirror—a distinction which is impossible to maintain' (Favareau 2002). Clearly that is not a sufficient explanation, but it shows what might happen when neuroscientific findings are interpreted from the point of view of the subject rather than by an observer seeking 'objective' evidence.

The third space concept

The realization of intersubjectivity takes place within what Winnicott termed the 'third space' (1971). In relation to play, the 'third space' is that in which children are able to construct a relevant culture. In the empathetic clinical encounter, clinician and patient seek to carve out a communal public space of signs and understandings created by their respective actions (Favareau 2002).

Achieving change in the clinic

We suggest that both clinician and patient can bring into this space a host of 'baggage' items along with the issue at hand, attempting to make sense of the patient's lived experience of pain. Some of these items are personal, in terms of beliefs, fears, and emotions, but others can be antipathetic, stemming from the culture in which both are deeply embedded (May 2011). However, both are likely to share the belief and expectation that medicine (its scientific component) can provide a firm ground upon which they can both stand during their engagement.

Without a sufficiently negotiated sense-making engagement in this 'third space', the therapeutic encounter can readily default to an imposition of the beliefs and attitudes of the clinician upon the sufferer.

The practicality of implementing such a clinical engagement process is far from straightforward, as shown by the difficulties encountered by those with similar aspirations for various chronic health-related arenas, under the badge of 'chronic disease management' (Bandura 2004). It is now understood that the practices of social systems may need to be changed in order to promote health benefits at a population level (Freil and Marmot 2011; Pilgrim 2008).

Notwithstanding the enormity of the task, there is an urgency for pain medicine, globally, to construct a more ethical basis for its discourse with people in pain—one that utilizes insights from the burgeoning volume of neuroscientific research to an informed scientific methodology. This process will, in itself, tax the resources of the specialty and take some years to implement, but it will bequeath an affirmation to the term 'self-management' that may not only parallel but be the envy of other medical domains. It is an applied ethical challenge but it is also a most propitious time to commence it.

Pain medicine has been challenged to radically reformulate its clinical *modus operandi* (Quintner et al. 2008). If clinicians reframe their conceptual models to incorporate neurobiological insights into the nature of empathy in the clinical encounter, they may be better placed to offer treatment and to recognize the potential for stigmatization of their patients and to assist them towards achieving societal validation and inclusion.

References

Arbib M, P Erdi P, Szentagothai J. Structure, *function and dynamics: an integrated approach to neural organisation*. New York: MIT Press, 1988.

Aronoff, GM, Gallagher RM, Feldman JB. Biopsychosocial evaluation and treatment of chronic pain. In: Raj PP. (ed.) *Practical management of pain* (3rd edn). St Louis: Mosby, 2000, 156–65.

Bandura A. Health promotion by social cognitive means. *Health Educ Behav* 2004; 31:143–64.

Barsky AJ, Borus JF. Somatization and medicalization in the era of managed care. *JAMA* 1995; 274:1931–4.

Brennan F, Carr DB, Cousins M. Pain management: a fundamental human right. *Anaesth Analg* 2007; 105:205–21.

Burbules NC. Aporias, webs, and passages: doubt as an opportunity to learn. *Curric Inq* 2000; 30:171–87.

Butler CC, Evans M, Greaves D, Simpson S. Medically unexplained symptoms: the biopsychosocial model found wanting. *J Roy Soc Med* 2004; 97:219–22.

Callahan D. Medicine and the market. In: Arnold DG. (ed). *Ethics and the business of biomedicine*. Cambridge: Cambridge University Press, 2009, 20–34.

Carr DB, Bradshaw YS. Time to flip the pain curriculum? *Anesthesiology* 2014; 120:12–14.

Cohen ML, Quintner JL, Buchanan D, Nielsen M, Guy L. Stigmatization of patients with chronic pain: the extinction of empathy. *Pain Med* 2011; 12:1637–43.

Cohen ML, Quintner JL, Buchanan D. Is chronic pain a disease? *Pain Med* 2013; 14:1284–8.

Craig AD. How do you feel? Interoception: the sense of the physiological condition of the body. *Nat Rev Neurosci* 2002; 8:655–66.

Craig AD. Human feelings: why are some more aware than others? *Trends Cog Sci* 2004; 8:239–41.

Crowley-Matoka M, Saha S, Dobschka SK, Burgess DJ. Problems of quality and equity in pain management: exploring the role of biomedical culture. *Pain Med* 2009; 10:1312–24.

Dennett D. *Consciousness explained*. London: Penguin Books Ltd.,1993, 21–42.

Dorland WAN. *Dorland's illustrated medical dictionary* (32nd edn). Philadelphia: WB Saunders Company, 2011.

Drack M, Apfalter W. Is Paul Weiss and Ludwig von Bertalanffy's system thinking still valid today? *Sys Res Behav Sci* 2007; 24:537–46.

Dubois MY, Gallagher RM, Lippe PM. (eds). Pain Medicine position paper. *Pain Med* 2009; 10:972–1000.

Edelman G. *Bright air, brilliant fire*. London: Penguin Books Ltd., 1992, 73–80.

Engel GL. The care of the patient: art or science? *Johns Hopkins Med J* 1977; 140:222–32.

Engel GL. The need for a new medical model: a challenge for biomedicine. *Science* 1977; 196:129–36.

Eriksen TE, Risor MB. What is called symptom? *Med Health Care and Philos* 2013. DOI 10.1007/s11019-2-9346-2.

Favareau D. Beyond self and other: on the neurosemiotic emergence of intersubjectivity. *Sign Sys Studies* 2002; 30:57–100.

Flor H, Hermann C. Biopsychosocial models of pain. In: Dworkin RH, Breitbart WS. (eds). *Psychosocial aspects of pain, progress in pain research and management*, vol. 27. Seattle: IASP Press, 2004:47–75.

von Foerster H. On self-organizing systems and their environments. In: Yovits M, Cameron S. (eds). *Self-organizing systems*. London: Pergamon Press,1960, 31–50.

Freil S, Marmot MG. Action in the social determinants of health goes global. *Annu Rev Publ Health* 2011; 32:225–36.

Goldberg DS, McGee SJ. Pain as a global health priority. *BMC Pub Health* 2011;11:770. doi:10.1186/1471-2458-11-770.

Gray W. Ludwig von Bertalanffy and the development of modern psychiatric thought. In: Gray W, Rizzo ND. (eds) *Unity through diversity: a festschrift for Ludwig von Bertalanffy, Part 1*. New York: Gordon and Breach Science Publisher, 1973, 169–83.

Hall JK, Boswell MV. Ethics, law, and pain management as a patient right. *Pain Phys* 2009; 12:499–506.

Loeser JD. Perspectives on pain. In: Turner P. (ed.) *Proceedings of the First World Congress on Clinical Pharmacology and Therapeutics*. London: Macmillan, 1980, 313–6.

Loeser JD. What is chronic pain? *Theor Med* 1991; 12:213–25.

Loeser JD, Cahana A. Pain medicine versus pain management: ethical dilemmas created by contemporary medicine and business. *Clin J Pain* 2013; 29:311–6.

Luhmann N. *Social systems*. Stanford: Stanford University Press, 1995.

Luisi PL. Autopoiesis: a review and a reappraisal, *Naturwissenschaften* 2003; 90:49–59.

Lyon P. Autopoiesis and knowing: reflections on Maturana's biogenic explanation of cognition. *Cybernet Hum Know* 2004; 11:21–46.

Lyon P, Cohen M, Quintner J. An evolutionary stress-response hypothesis for chronic widespread pain (fibromyalgia syndrome). *Pain Med* 2011; 12:1167–78.

Maturana HR, Varela FJ. *Autopoiesis and cognition: the realization of the living*. Dordrecht: Reidel Publishing Co., 1980, 5–58.

May A. Structural brain imaging: a window into chronic pain. *Neuroscientist* 2011; 17:209–20.

McCracken L (commentary). Anger, injustice, and the continuing search for psychological mechanisms of pain, suffering and disability. *Pain* 2013; 154:1495–6.

Melzack R. From the gate to the neuromatrix. *Pain* 1999 Aug; Suppl 6:S121–6.

Melzack R, Wall PD. Pain mechanisms: a new theory. *Science* 1965; 150: 971–9.

Melzack R, Wall PD. *The puzzle of pain*. Harmondsworth: Penguin Books, 1973.

Merskey H, Bogduk N. *Classification of chronic pain*. Seattle: IASP Press, 1994, 210.

Pilgrim D. 'Recovery' and current mental health policy. *Chronic Illn* 2008; 4:295–304.

Quintner JL, Buchanan D, Cohen ML. Katz J, Williamson O. Pain medicine and its models: helping or hindering? *Pain Med* 2008; 9:824–34.

Rizzolatti G, Fadiga L, Fogassi L, Gallese V. Resonance behaviors and mirror neurons. *Arch Ital Biol* 1999; 137:85–100.

Rosenberg CE. The tyranny of diagnosis: specific entities and individual experience. *Milbank Q* 2002; 80:237–60.

Rosenman S, Nasti J. Psychiatric diagnoses are not mental processes: Wittgenstein on conceptual confusion. *Aust NZ J Psychiat* 2012; 46:1046–52.

Siddall PJ. Is chronic pain a disease? *Pain Med* 2013; 14:1289–90.

Siddall PJ, Cousins MJ. Persistent pain as a disease entity: implications for clinical management. *Anesth Analg* 2004; 99:510–20.

Tracey I, Bushnell MC. How neuroimaging studies have challenged us to rethink: is chronic pain a disease? *J Pain* 2009; 10:1113–20.

Waddell G, Bircher M, Finlayson D, Main CJ. Symptoms and signs: physical disease or illness? *Brit Med J* 1984; 289:739–41.

Weiss, PA. Tierisches verhalten als 'systemreaktion'. Die orienterung der Ruhstellungen von Schmetterlingen (Vanessa) gegen licht und schwerkraft. *Biologica Generalis* 1925; 1:165–248.

Williamson, OD, Buchanan DA, Quintner JL, Cohen ML. Pain beyond monism and dualism. *Pain* 2005; 116:169–70.

Winnicott DW. *Playing and reality*. London: Tavistock Publications, 1971.

Wittgenstein L. (trans. Anscombe GEM). *Philosophical investigations*. Oxford: Blackwell, 1953/2001, §67.

Woolf CJ. Central sensitization: implications for the diagnosis and treatment of pain. *Pain* 2011; 152:S2–15.

Woolf CJ. Evidence for a central component of post-injury pain hypersensitivity. *Nature* 1983; 306:686–8.

Chapter 20

Psychological aspects of musculoskeletal pain

Chris J. Main, Paul J. Watson, Peter J. Clough, and Angela E. Clough

This chapter is based on the work of Chris Main and Paul Watson. It includes the more recent developments made by Peter O'Sullivan, David Butler, Lorimer Moseley, and Michael Thacker who have enhanced the evidence base for musculoskeletal clinicians with their work on a cognitive functional approach, using understanding of modern pain biology and neuroscience to enable patients to change their behaviour. Readers are directed to their work for further reading to contextualize musculoskeletal management.

Background to the psychological aspects of musculoskeletal pain

Research into the factors that make musculoskeletal pain likely to become chronic has continued to highlight psychosocial factors. Although the original research related to low back pain, comparable research for other areas of the spine has revealed that similar factors operate there; and there are indications that peripheral areas such as the shoulder are subject to prolongation of pain with adverse psychological and social factors.

Pain is the most common presenting complaint in people seeking the help of a manual therapist. A manual therapist typically attempts to identify the cause of the pain at initial examination. During the clinical interview, the therapist will attempt to establish the mode of onset, the specific characteristics of the pain, and a range of possible precipitating or easing factors including the reported influence of movement. This would include the screening of 'yellow flags' or psychosocial factor screening (e.g. Nicholas et al. 2011). This subjective history-taking interview will be followed typically by a physical examination, including palpation and observation of movement. Reproduction of the pain sensation and/or the identification of abnormality of motion may help to suggest possible pain mechanisms.

The Society of Musculoskeletal Medicine (SOMM) approach is based upon the work of Dr James Cyriax (Atkins et al. 2010) and aimed at a logical assessment to identify the cause of the pain which can, however, be elusive. Even when the therapist feels that the probable cause has been identified, there is no guarantee that the treatment will be successful.

The relationship between pain, physical impairment, and the level of disability is remarkably variable. Research has shown that although these factors are related, the relationships are relatively modest and vary according to the duration of symptoms and clinical subgroups. Consideration of pain mechanisms is now considered to be a first priority for subgrouping. Additional moderators/mediators of pain must also be considered. For example, in the case of whiplash-associated disorders, the presence of substantive and non-abating symptoms of post-traumatic stress has been shown to moderate pain and, as a result, may require specific psychological support (Jull 2012; Sterling et al. 2004; Turk et al. 1996). In chronic back pain in particular, there is frequently little relationship between demonstrable physical impairment and the accompanying degree of functional incapacity or psychological distress (Waddell and Main 1984).

The foundations of pain theory

Although contemporary models of pain include psychological factors, early foundations of pain theories were very different.

Aristotle (384–322 BC) considered pain to be an increased sensitivity in every sensation, particularly touch and pain perception to be felt in the heart. The Aristotelian concept of pain as an affective manifestation—a 'passion of the soul' felt in the heart—prevailed for well over two millennia, despite the conviction of his successors such as Herophilus and Erasistratus that the centre of sensation was located in the brain, and the views of Galen (AD131–200) who established the anatomy of the central and autonomic nervous systems (Hutson 1999).

In the seventeenth century, Descartes (1664) developed the concept of a pain pathway linking the periphery of the body with higher centres in the brain. It led to the specificity theory, in which pain was considered to be a specific sensation independent of the other sensations. Throughout the latter half of the nineteenth century, a specificity theory gained ascendency over a summation theory. By the beginning of the twentieth century, medical opinion had become strongly influenced by the concept of the mind–body dichotomy of Descartes and the Cartesian view of pain as a straightforward response to a physical stimulus. To take account of the known psychological factors that influence pain, the concept of the 'duality of pain' was proposed: the distinct features being neurophysiological (perception of pain) and psychophysiological (reaction to pain) (Hutson 1999). It is acknowledged in research this century that there are a larger number of psychological variables; for example, catastrophizing has been found to be predictive of pain perception and emotional distress (Severeijns et al. 2001; Sullivan et al. 2000) and physical variables (Smart et al. 2012a,b; Thacker and Moseley 2012; Thacker et al. 2009).

The sensory system responsible for mediating pain has been regarded as relatively rigid and straightforward in that any tissue damage was assumed to initiate a sequence of neural events that inevitably produced pain. However, this approach is unable to explain either pain in the absence of tissue damage or variation in pain across individuals with (apparently) the same amount of tissue damage. Individual variation in the perception of pain is frequently attributed to psychological factors, although the nature of such psychological factors is seldom specified.

Therapists may attribute poor outcomes of treatment to incomplete or inadequate assessment, although limitation in therapeutic treatment skills may also be admitted. Possible explanations for the failure of treatment, however, will usually be restricted to those which lie within the boundaries of the therapist's preferred therapeutic model. Much medical and therapeutic education is based on a biomedical model of illness and a specificity theory of pain. This requires that the signs and symptoms are assessed and interpreted in terms of pathology. Once the exact pathology is determined, then a treatment approach is indicated. While such an approach is essential, particularly in the acute stages of the condition, an over-zealous application of this model can lead to the inappropriate classification of patients' problems as physical or psychological. This can lead to suboptimal treatment, the denial of treatment, or referral for psychological or psychiatric intervention. As will be discussed in this chapter, if patients have previously endured painful assessment and treatment, they may be apprehensive about therapy and display guarded movements or apparently exaggerated responses to examination such as palpation or movement. It is important to realize, however, that reaction with a degree of distress to a painful and limiting condition, especially if previous treatment has not been successful, is a normal not an abnormal reaction. Patients presenting with painful conditions and associated loss of function are very rarely psychiatrically ill, and inappropriate referral may simply magnify their distress. In offering a biopsychosocial framework within which to understand therapeutic intervention (Waddell et al. 1984), it is appropriate first to consider the nature of pain.

The multifactorial influences on pain

According to the gate control theory (Melzack and Wall 1965) and its later derivatives (Melzack and Casey 1968), pain perception depends on complex neural interactions in the nervous system where impulses generated by tissue damage are modified both by ascending pathways to the brain and by descending pain suppressing systems activated by various environmental and psychological factors.

Pain is thus not merely the end product of a passive transmission of nociceptive impulses from a receptor organ to an area of interpretation. It is the result of a dynamic process, of perception and interpretation of a wide range of incoming stimuli, some of which are associated with actual or potential harm and some of which are benign but are interpreted and described in terms of damage.

The gate control theory has generated a wide range of research (Melzack 1985, 1986, 1989, 1996; Melzack et al. 1982). The importance from the psychological point of view has been that it produced a testable model of how psychological factors could activate descending pain inhibitory systems, modulate noccep-tive processing, and thereby modulate pain. It has offered a way of integrating concepts of pain behaviour, both as a response to pain and as behaviour that could come under environmental influences and control. The gate control theory has stimulated interest in the role of beliefs about pain, attention to pain, appraisal of its significance, fears about pain, and pain-related coping strategies. The theory has encouraged the investigation of the nature of pain-associated disability and led to the development of biopsychosocial models (Bartz 1999; Borrell-Carrio et al. 2004; Engel 1980, 1988; Waddell and Main 1998a) that have attempted a wide integration of physical, psychological, and social perspectives (Figure 20.1).

In the 35 years since Engel first introduced the biopsychosocial model, it could be made even more robust as a concept by the emergence of two new intellectual trends identified by Borrell-Carrio et al. (2004). Firstly, clinicians can bypass the problematic issue of mind–body duality by recognizing that knowledge is socially constructed and 'mind' and 'body' categories are of our own creation. They are useful in that they focus our thinking and action in a constructive way but we can amend or discard categories as new evidence emerges. Secondly, we can progress beyond multifactorial linear thinking in order to consider complexity theory as a more adequate model for understanding causality, dualism, and participation in care. Complexity theory highlights how, in open systems, it is often very challenging to know all of the contributing impacting influences upon particular health outcomes.

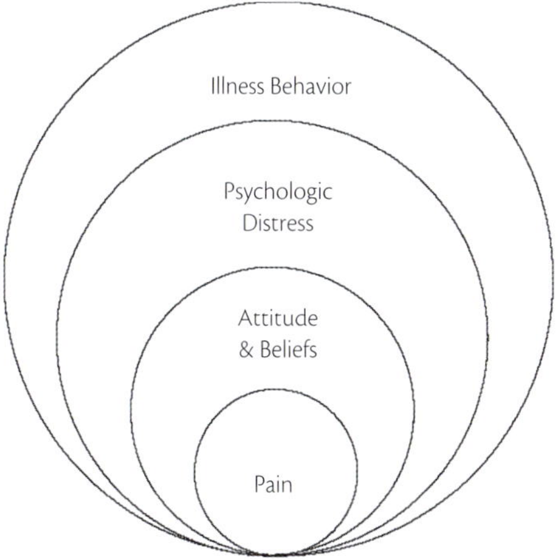

Figure 20.1 The biopsychosocial model of low back pain and disability. (Adapted from Waddell G., Main C. J. 1998c. The back pain revolution. Churchill-Livingstone, Edinburgh, pp. 187–202.)

Models of pain, illness, and disability

A complex chain of events links perception of part of the body as painful and the development of chronic disability. Although the process is multifactorial and not fully understood, a number of key processes seem to be involved. Manual therapy is based on a biomedical understanding of incapacity. The patient's report of pain leads to a pain-focused clinical history with a clinical examination. It has long been considered that chronic pain can only be understood within a biopsychosocial framework (Loeser 1980), but it is now clear that psychological factors are important at an early stage.

The biopsychosocial model of pain and disability

Pain is a symptom, not a sign, and therefore is multiply determined. In specific instances, there may be a clear and specific indication for manipulation, but the dysfunction needs to be understood within a wider model such as the biopsychosocial model of pain and disability (Bartz 1999; Borrell-Carrio et al. 2004; Engel 1980, 1988; Turk 1996; Waddell and Main 1998a; Waddell et al. 1984).

At the heart of the biopsychosocial model is the assumption of an ongoing sensation that is nociceptive in nature or which is perceived by the sufferer as being painful. The patient's cognitions (i.e. what they think and understand about this sensation) will influence their emotional reaction to it. The behaviour demonstrated by an individual at any point in time will be a product of their beliefs and the emotional response to the pain and may, in turn, be influenced (reinforced or modulated) by the social environment in which the behaviour takes place. The model offers a radically different way of understanding the nature of pain-associated incapacity. In understanding manual therapy, it is important to be familiar with the elements from which the biopsychosocial model has been constructed.

Engel's most significant contribution to practice was to broaden the clinician's gaze. His biopsychosocial model was a call to amend our approach and be more flexible to the individual needs and requirements of a more patient-centred approach, in order to better understand the needs of each patient and to explore further the domain of medical knowledge in order to address those needs. The transformation of context may be the reason that illness and healing are now viewed with a much wider perspective and awareness of social context is possibly Engel's most durable contribution to practice (Borrell-Carrio et al. 2004).

Evidence should be communicated in an appropriate manner, with a professional and constructive attitude, in terms the patient can understand and in small, comprehensible pieces, at a pace at which it can be assimiliated. Information overload may have two effects—reduction in comprehension and increasing the emotional distance between the clinician and the patient.

The nature of psychological influences on pain

Fundamental mechanisms

Psychological factors have a wide-ranging impact on the perception of pain and its effects. There is now convincing evidence that central mechanisms can influence the perception of nociceptive signals from the periphery of the body (Woolf 1996). The perception of pain is influenced both by sensory qualities and by the emotional impact (Price et al. 1997). Recent research into experimental pain using positron emission tomography (PET) scanning suggests that individuals may differ in how the brain first reacts to incoming pain signals and leads to the perception of pain (Roland 1993). Perceptual differences in terms of both intensity and aversive response may occur and, as a result, different parts of the brain become 'energized'. It is commonly observed clinically that pain 'feels worse' when patients are feeling tired or depressed. Pain often seems to feel worse during the night when the brain has 'less to do'.

The role of attention and memory

Factors relating to attention are important (Eccleston 1995). Some patients can be taught to distract themselves quite successfully from pain. Research has also shown that individuals differ not only in pain threshold but also in their ability to discriminate pain of different qualities and intensities. The reasons for this are not fully understood. Research into memory of pain suggests, however, that aversive pain memories may have a powerful influence on the perception of new pain stimuli (Price et al. 1997). Psychobiological investigations have demonstrated a wide range of conditioned peripheral and central responses to pain involving both physiological and biochemical events (Flor and Birbaumer 1994). It would appear that the significance of fundamental psychological mechanisms to the perception of clinical pain may be of much more importance than has hitherto been recognized.

Pain, learning, and neuroplastic change

The perception of painful stimuli has been shown to respond to learning (Crombez et al. 1997) and is subject to neuroplastic change (Dubner 1997). Experimental evidence has demonstrated that the brain's response to a painful stimulus, as measured by electroencephalography, and the accompanying report of that pain, can be conditioned in some subjects by the offering of a financial reward. Cross-sectional studies have also demonstrated that the magnitude of response to painful stimuli changes with the duration of chronic pain conditions and may be mediated by attention (Eccleston 1995). In a series of experiments, Flor et al. (1997) demonstrated that patients with chronic low back pain had a significantly greater cortical evoked magnetic field response to pain than normal controls and the difference was greatest when the low back was stimulated. They interpreted this increase in the magnitude of the response as more widespread cortical assembly activation and psychophysiological hyper-reactivity as a result of neuroplastic change.

Butler (2012) suggests a neuroplasticity paradigm. This was well received as a keynote lecture at the International Federation of Orthopaedic and Manipulative Physical Therapists in Quebec, Canada, 2012. A paradigm is an overarching way of thinking, a framework under which clinicians think about, research, and live. Paradigms shift in their importance as understanding changes. Butler proposes four gifts from the neuroplastic paradigm:

1. *Manual therapist as biopsychosocialist*: Clinical trials, expert opinion, textbooks, and bodies such as the World Health Organization (WHO) support a biopsychosocial framework for managing spinal pain. The opposing view of biomedicalism—'find it and fix it'—has served us well and as such is a barrier to change. Butler proposes that biomedicalism fits into biopsychosocialism, but the reverse is not possible. Biopsychosocialism welcomes and embraces biomedical thinking and enhances it further by adding interactions between brain and body, preventative medicine, interdisciplinary

medicine, and psychosocial predictors of chronic problems. Clinicians can indeed manipulate in a biopsychosocial framework; it may be achieved by simply asking the question, 'Why did this person end up as a patient?'.

2. *Manual therapist as brain reinhibitor and sculptor:* Butler (2012) suggests the 'hibitions'—inhibition, disinhibition, and rehinibition—have confused generations of musculoskeletal clinicians. Early restoration of functional movement, reduction of fear to facilitate movement, empowering education, limitation of lingering unhelpful metaphors, mobilization of a body part, and meaningful movement are all potential reinhibitory brain resculpturing techniques.

3. *Manual therapist as immunotherapist:* The immune system is intricately involved in modulating memory, learning, and sensitivity. The immune system is a homeostatic system and its responses range from the learning and activities of the 'resting' immune system to the 'cytokine storms' and immune takeover of severe injury. Higher pro-inflammatory cytokine levels have been shown to be part of some chronic pain states. Manual therapy strategies, including education and movement, could be considered antigenic. Well-known 'immune-healthy behaviours' such as knowledge, meaning in life, appropriate exercise, availability of coping strategies, diet, and even laughter are known pain strategies that may be included into manual therapy.

4. *Manual therapist as linguist:* Neuroplasticity has exposed dated metaphors that require challenging; for example, 'it's just your age'. However, enriching metaphors such as 'motion is lotion' may help with the integration of active exercise. Introduction of positive philosophical metaphors such as 'you are not your thoughts' helps to introduce the concept of mindfulnesss and living in the moment.

In conclusion, together with his four contributory gifts to the neuroplasticity paradigm, Butler (2012) suggests that knowledge makes a profession what it is and that, for many clinicians, to embrace the paradigm may require a cultural shift and an admission that they were not quite right in the past and could do better. Neuroplasticity has already lifted expectations of outcome, and we can refer to 'pain treatment' rather than 'pain management' by engaging patients, where we had little to offer in the past.

Muscle pain, muscle activity, and perception

In a recent study of patients suffering from shoulder pain (Vassiljen and Westgaard 1996), it was suggested that the perception of pain may be better explained by the subjects' perception of muscle tension than by the actual electromyographic activity in the muscle itself. They found, furthermore, that psychologically stressful working conditions and psychological characteristics of individual office workers were significant determinants of whether they reported the perception of muscle tension and pain. In another study of a group of office workers (Vassiljen et al. 1995), a reduction in reported pain was highly correlated with reported reduction in perceived muscle tension, although the reduction in perceived tension was independent of actual electromyographic activity.

In conclusion, therefore, it appears that the perception of pain bears a complex relationship to nociception. A full understanding of this relationship requires consideration of central physiological mechanisms involved in coding the information in the brain, as well as secondary psychological processes affecting perception.

The role of anxiety and depression in pain

Anxiety and depression are two factors which perhaps best characterize the distress of chronic pain sufferers. These features frequently overlap in the individual patient. Manual therapists often deal with patients with significant pain problems that are inextricably linked with anxiety, fears about their condition (and the future), depression about their current pain-associated limitations, and perhaps anger at previous failed management or the attitudes of others to their condition.

Generalized and specific anxiety

Specific anxieties and fears are a common feature of pain patients, particularly when they have not been given a clear explanation for their pain or its likelihood to respond to treatment. Such specific concerns should be distinguished from global or generalized anxiety in which there is no clear focus to the patient's concerns. Widespread longstanding anxiety is sometimes seen in general musculoskeletal practice and may require treatment in its own right. The physician or therapist may treat this, or refer to an appropriate service. The presence of generalized anxiety does not mean, however, that the specific fears and concerns about local musculoskeletal pain and pain-associated incapacity should not be addressed at the first port of call.

Denison et al. (2007) carried out a study to identify and describe subgroups based on self-reported pain intensity, disability, self-efficacy, fear of movement/(re)injury, and catastrophizing in patients with musculoskeletal pain. The profile patterns suggest that different management strategies may be relevant in each subgroup. They concluded that, congruent with the vast literature on fear and anxiety, pain-related fear is associated with catastrophic (mis)interpretations of pain, hypervigilance, increased escape and avoidance behaviours, as well as with intensified pain intensity and functional disability.

Somatic awareness

A subgroup of patients who do not seem to be particularly anxious or fearful but may demonstrate heightened awareness of all sorts of symptoms (Main 1983) clearly exists. This heightened somatic awareness can be indicative of somatic anxiety. Such patients tend to have difficulty in coping with treatment and its side-effects. If sufficiently marked, such preoccupation may need to be understood as a form of hypochondriasis or a somatization disorder for which there are DSM-IV criteria (American Psychiatric Association 1994), and may require psychologically oriented treatment in its own right. Symptoms of such severity are rare, and concern about symptoms is perhaps best understood as a normal phenomenon rather than a psychopathological one (Sullivan and Katon 1993). If such concern is longstanding or marked, it may be considered as a cognitive distortion or misperception. Patients may become preoccupied with bodily sensation of all kinds, and this inevitably focuses attention on painful events. If such specific concerns are accompanied by other features of distress or displays of pain behaviour, the patient may require more psychologically oriented treatment such as a pain management programme (Flor et al. 1992; Main et al. 1992). In treating patients with heightened somatic awareness, it is important for us to offer repeated explanation and reassurance to our patients about the nature of their pain.

Fears

Patients differ in their interpretation of symptoms. The meaning patients assign to physical symptoms is profoundly influenced by their beliefs, assumptions, and so-called 'commonsense explanations' that they may have 'inherited' from influential individuals (whether family, friends, or healthcare professionals) (Cioffi 1991). Amongst the most disabling of such concerns are specific beliefs about hurting and harming (see 'Mistaken beliefs about hurting and harming' in this chapter). These beliefs should always be addressed during assessment and treatment.

The nature of depression

The term 'depression' can be misleading. In common parlance, it is used to refer to a wide spectrum of emotion ranging from the slightly demoralized or fed-up to the suicidal. It is, however, a clearly defined and very serious mental health condition. It is clear that pain patients certainly frequently seem to be demoralized, and many can become clinically depressed. There is a clear link between depression and pain (e.g. Axford et al. 2008; Mossey and Gallagher 2004). It is therefore important to distinguish dysphoric mood from depressive illness for which there are clear diagnostic criteria such as DSM-IV (American Psychiatric Association 1994). It is also important that the therapist screens for depression. For example, Haggman et al. (2004) established a link between depression and the pain prognosis of lower back pain and argued strongly that depression measures should be included in diagnosis and treatment protocols.

Influence of the passage of time

The initial reaction to a painful injury is usually recognized in terms of anxiety, shock, and fear rather than depression (Geisser et al. 1996). With the passage of time, and the failure of treatment, however, a patient's coping skills can become exhausted and depression or anger can become evident. If it is possible to avoid painful activities or compensate successfully by changing activities and routines, then patients are unlikely to become depressed (even with persistence of pain). If, however, the pain is sufficiently severe, cannot be controlled, and, as such, has a widespread effect on a patient's life, then depression is much more likely (Rudy et al. 1988).

Learned helplessness

Pain-associated depression is often best viewed as a form of 'learned helplessness' that can develop after many different types of chronic unresolved stress, including health-related problems. In the context of chronic pain, it is best understood as a psychological consequence of the persistence of pain and its incapacitating effects. If sufficiently severe, it may merit pharmacological treatment in its own right, but can usually best be treated using a cognitive behavioural approach (Gatchell and Turk 1996; Turk et al. 1983), returning a measure of control to the patient over their pain and pain-associated incapacity, and re-establishing their self-confidence.

The influence of anger and frustration with regards to pain

Patients express anger in a number of ways. Anger is often self-evident from the manner and content of the patient's communication. Patients may be disaffected with many aspects of their situation (DeGood and Kiernan 1996). They may be angry about how they have been treated in the past, or may believe that referral for physical treatment may have been undertaken simply because the referring doctor could think of no alternative. Emotional intensity may range from mild annoyance to hostility or even frank aggression.

Patients may be angry about a range of features such as the severity or persistence of their pain and its effect on their daily activities, sleep, sexual functioning, and ability to work. They may also be disaffected by their previous treatment or the socioeconomic consequences of their pain-associated incapacity.

This complex relationship between anger/hostility and adjustment is as yet not well understood. Anger has physiological effects, and persistent anger clouds judgement. It would seem to merit much further investigation, particularly in its influence on compliance and response to treatment (Fernandez and Turk 1995).

Beliefs and coping strategies with regards to pain

Beliefs about pain and outcome of treatment have been identified as key determinants of response to treatment (Waddell and Main 1998c). The term 'cognitive' is frequently taken as being synonymous with 'beliefs', but in fact it has a wider application and has come to refer to a range of factors influencing the perception of pain and response to treatment. It is, therefore, perhaps helpful to distinguish three distinct fields of enquiry (DeGood and Shutty 1992):

- specific beliefs about pain and treatment
- the thought processes involved in judgement or appraisal
- coping styles or strategies.

Each patient is characterized by an individual combination of cognitive features which underpins the appraisal of pain and the response to treatment. The complexity of these interrelationships is indicated in the following quotation:

> Patients who believe they can control their pain, who avoid catastrophizing about their condition, and who believe they are not severely disabled appear to function better than those who do not. Such beliefs may mediate some of the relationships between pain severity and adjustment. (Jensen et al. 1991, p. 249)

Specific beliefs about pain and treatment

Clinically, pessimistic or negative beliefs regarding pain and outcome of treatment are easily recognized. Amongst the most commonly found beliefs are that hurt is synonymous with harm, that pain uniquely determines physical functioning, and that future structural and/or physiological decline is inevitable. Such beliefs not only lead to significant demoralization but also to establishing dysfunctional patterns of behaviour and deconditioning. Such beliefs can also compromise response to therapy and lead to chronic incapacity. Indeed, research has shown that beliefs about the extent to which pain can be controlled appear to be one of the most powerful determinants of adjustment to pain and the development of incapacity (Crisson and Keefe 1988).

Beliefs about control

A recurrent finding in research is the importance of beliefs about the controllability of pain. It is clear that attributions are central to feelings of control. Two seminal pieces of work have tackled this area: Rotter's (1966) work on internal and external locus of control, and Heider's (1944) work on attributions. A number of 'pain locus of control' scales have been developed (Crisson and Keefe 1988; Main and Waddell 1991). In one study, the role of perceived self-control as a factor that mediates pain and depression was explored by Rudy et al. (1988). Although the direct association between pain and depression was minimal, depression developed principally when pain significantly interfered with family, work, and social interactions, and/or existed in conjunction with pessimism about being able to control pain. The issue of 'controllability' may be even more important in relationship to adjustment to pain and incapacity. Optimal adaptation to a chronic condition thus seems to depend on the patient's ability to come to terms with what they can and cannot control.

Pain patients who perceive themselves lacking the capacity to acquire self-management skills might be less persistent, more prone to frustration, and more apt to be non-compliant with treatment recommendations. Hence, some patients might demonstrate adequate understanding of a particular treatment rationale, yet be non-compliant due to their perceived inability to produce the behaviour necessary to follow treatment recommendations (DeGood and Shutty 1992, p. 221). This perspective has two major implications in musculoskeletal medicine:

- Firstly, exercise prescriptions, advice on posture, and graded increase in activity are given to patients to enhance the effectiveness of specific manipulative treatments. The degree to which the patient complies and persists with the recommendations will be determined by their belief in how much personal control they have over their condition.
- Secondly, manual treatment may unwittingly reinforce the patient's perception of lack of control. During 'hands-on' therapies such as manipulation, mobilization, and massage, the doctor or therapist is in control and accepts responsibility for the management of the condition. The patient's role is one of passive acceptance of the therapy. In susceptible individuals, this may foster the belief that they do not have a role in the management of their condition. Recovery is seen as the responsibility entirely of the professional. Over-directing the patient in the resumption of activities, or strict advice to perform only very specific activities and exclude others, may encourage an over-reliance on the therapist. Such a therapeutic relationship may make it extremely difficult, if not impossible, to foster the patient's own self-management skills as part of the therapeutic process. (See Chapter 49.)

The impact of self-efficacy

Patients may believe that they will be unsuccessful in gaining control over pain or re-establishing function. Such beliefs are frequently called self-efficacy beliefs (Bandura 1977; Nicholas et al. 1992). Bandura suggested that people avoid potentially harmful situations not because they experience anxiety but rather that they fear they will be unable to cope. This 'lack of coping' refers to actual behaviour and, perhaps more importantly, the underlying cognitive processes. A relationship between individuals' self-efficacy and their ability to manage pain (whether acute, chronic, or induced) has been found (e.g. Brekke et al. 2003).

Clinical and experimental investigations suggest that perceived coping inefficacy may lead to preoccupation with distressing thoughts and concomitant physiological arousal, thereby increasing pain, decreasing pain tolerance, and leading to increased use of medication, lower levels of functioning, poorer exercise tolerance, and increased invalidism.

A careful line must be drawn between giving good advice and creating a dependent patient. The most useful strategy is to encourage the patient to identify specific activities and goals for increased exercise and incorporate these into a self-management plan.

Mistaken beliefs about hurting and harming

Perhaps the most powerful, yet least acknowledged, cognitive factors are mistaken beliefs about hurting and harming. It is crucial to recognize the role of fear and avoidance as obstacles to rehabilitation after injury (Asmundson et al. 1997). As might be expected, the construct of 'fear avoidance' has both a behavioural and a cognitive component. Behavioural theorists such as Fordyce (1976) explained the development of 'avoidance learning', where successful avoidance of pain established a behavioural pattern which reduced pain but with the cost of maintaining the disability. Vlaeyen et al. (1995) found that fear of movement and re-injury were more related to depressive symptoms and catastrophizing (fearing an inevitable poor outcome) than to pain itself. His model, linking fear, catastrophizing, and avoidance in the development of chronic disability following painful injury, has been widely influential. It is illustrated in Figure 20.2.

A number of new instruments for the assessment of fear and avoidance, such as the Fear Avoidance Beliefs Questionnaire (FABQ) (Waddell et al. 1993) and the Tampa Scale of Kineisiophobia (Kori et al. 1990), have been developed. Evidence from experimental studies in chronic pain patients has demonstrated a close relationship between experimental pain (pressure algometry) and fear of injury. Interestingly, this relationship appears to be independent of the current level of clinical pain (Watson et al. 1996). This has important implications because it suggests that although patients' perception of pain is closely associated with fear in experimental pain situations, there may be much wider influences on patients' rating of clinical pain once it has become chronic. For a manual therapist evaluating a patient, therefore, it is important not be over-reliant on the report of pain intensity without taking the issues of fear and avoidance into account.

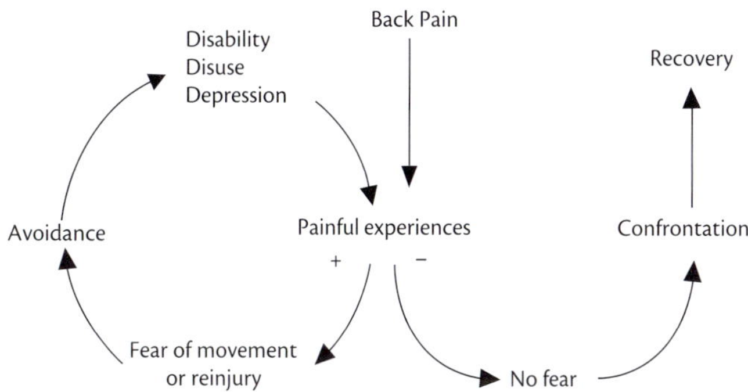

Figure 20.2 Vlaeyen's model of fear of movement and reinjury on back pain. (Adapted from Vlaeyen et al. Fear of movement and (re)-injury in chronic low back pain and its relation to behavioural performance. *Pain*, Vol. 62 (1995), p. 363–372.)

Coping styles and strategies

Active and passive coping strategies

It is also important to consider how people cope with pain. How people react to pain is an important determinant of its future course. Patterns of fear-mediated avoidance behaviour have already been described, but in fact patients use a wide range of behavioural and coping strategies in order to limit the effects of pain. Choice of strategies will depend on patients' beliefs about pain, on their confidence in being able to influence events, and, of course, on their repertoire of coping behaviours. Brown and Nicassio (1987) made the distinction between active and passive coping strategies. Active strategies (e.g. taking exercise) require the individual to take a degree of responsibility for pain management by either attempting to control pain or attempting to function despite pain. Passive strategies (e.g. resting) involve either withdrawal from or the passing on of responsibility for the control of pain to someone else (e.g. the therapist). This distinction is of major importance and key to understanding patients' responses to therapy (Snow-Turek et al. 1996). Both styles can be functional or dysfunctional. In general, active coping strategies have been found to improve coping, reduce pain intensity, and improve recovery rates (Marks et al. 2011).

More specifically, Carroll et al. (2006) performed a large, population-based prospective cohort study of traffic injuries to assess the relationship between pain coping strategies and recovery from whiplash injuries. Those using high levels of passive coping recovered 37% slower than those using low levels of passive coping. However, in the presence of depressive symptomatology, those using high levels of passive coping recovered 75% more slowly than those who coped less passively. In other words, those with depressive symptoms but who used few passive coping strategies recovered four times more quickly than those with depressive symptoms who used high levels of passive coping. They concluded that it was important to obtain early assessment of both coping behaviours and depressive symptomatology.

Appropriate (effective) and inappropriate (ineffective) coping strategies

In the research literature, perhaps the most important distinction is not between active and passive coping per se but between effective (or appropriate) and ineffective (or inappropriate) coping strategies, as assessed, for example, by the Coping Strategies Questionnaire (CSQ) (Rosenstiel and Keefe 1983). This questionnaire identifies both positive (or adaptive) and negative (or maladaptive) coping strategies. Several studies have shown that negative or ineffective coping strategies such as catastrophizing ('fearing the worst') are associated with higher levels of self-reported disability or adjustment (Jensen et al. 1991; Keefe et al. 1989; Main and Waddell 1991). The catastrophizing scale has also shown impressive predictive value for outcome of treatment, particularly in patients with acute low back pain. Burton et al. (1995) and Main and Burton (1995) found that passive coping and, in particular catastrophizing, were highly predictive of disability and pain report at one year in a group of subjects with acute low back pain (less than four weeks' duration).

Coping strategies and adjustment

The relationship between the use of these strategies and psychological adjustment is complex (Jensen et al. 1994). Keefe et al. (1997) demonstrated that perceived daily coping efficacy was associated with greater use of relaxation, redefining of pain, spiritual support seeking with a consequent reduction in pain, negative affect, and enhancement of positive mood. Furthermore, individual judgement of coping effectiveness resulted in lower pain levels on the following day; improvement in mood the following day was also attributed to the use of relaxation strategies. As Turner (1991) points out, however, specific coping strategies are not inherently adaptive or maladaptive. A strategy that is useful at one point in time may be of little value at another, and some strategies may be of benefit if used in moderation but not if used to the exclusion of others. Furthermore, the overall efficacy of coping techniques appears to be moderated by levels of pain intensity and appraisals of perceived pain control abilities (Jensen and Karoly 1992).

It also appears that pain-related coping strategies lead to a reduction of disability only when a high degree of flexibility in goal adjustment was possible (Schmitz et al. 1996). Finally, there has been recent interest in the distinction between emotion-focused coping strategies (which aim to control stress) and problem-focused coping strategies (e.g. reducing maladaptive coping) which are aimed at attempting to relieve or solve the problem more directly. Such strategies are a core component of teaching in most pain management programmes, but are rarely used in acute or subchronic pain situations.

Individual differences and pain: an example

There are clearly a number of individual differences that impact on each person's perceptions of pain. One of these, that is perhaps helpful in tying together the rather disparate strands relating to the psychological aspects of pain, is mental toughness. The model proposed by Clough et al. (2002) incorporates many of the elements that have been associated with different pain perceptions: challenge, commitment, control, and confidence. Levy et al. (2006) showed that mentally tough individuals were better able to cope with pain and displayed more positive threat appraisals. Similarly, Crust and Clough (2005) demonstrated that the mentally tough are better able to cope with physically painful situations. A number of researchers (e.g. Kaisler et al. 2009; Nicholls et al. 2009) have shown that mentally tough individuals are more likely to adopt active coping strategies that have been shown to often be the most effective in dealing with pain.

Conclusion

Patients' cognitive orientations impact on treatment. Some patients are optimistic and self-efficacious, believing that things will turn out for the best and that they have some control over this. Other patients are anxious and fearful, and this impacts on pain perceptions, treatment outcomes, and adherence to treatment regimes.

More specifically, heightened somatic concern or fear may have led to misinterpretation of the patient's symptoms and to a labelling of relatively normal sensations as abnormal if not pathological (Weir et al. 1994). Frequently, apparently unfocused anxiety is based on specific fears of hurting/harming, distorted ideas about the nature of pain and illness, or that the pain will become uncontrollable with progressive and increasing pain-associated incapacity. Individuals high in somatic anxiety have a strong propensity for catastrophizing ('fearing the worst'), and while post-treatment report of catastrophizing is significantly diminished, levels of somatic anxiety are little changed. It may be that in individuals who are somatically focused, it is the degree of catastrophizing that governs emotional and physiological arousal which, in turn, alters pain sensitivity and response to treatment. It is imperative, therefore, that these issues are addressed.

There are a number of different coping approaches adopted by patients. Whilst it is clear that active coping appears to be more helpful, it would be too simplistic to suggest that it is the only one to adopt and develop. It is more useful to think about adaptive and maladaptive coping. Different approaches work for different people. In attempting to maximize patient adherence to treatment recommendations and understand their perceptions of pain, it is important to consider the sorts of coping strategies that individual patients actually use.

Pain behaviour

Range and complexity

There are many different examples of pain behaviour, ranging from the simple to the complex. The classical definition of pain behaviour is 'any and all outputs of the individual that a reasonable observer would characterize as suggesting pain, such as (but not limited to) posture, facial expression, verbalizing, lying down, taking medicines, seeking medical assistance and receiving compensation' (Loeser and Fordyce 1983).

Many such behaviours are crucial in the interaction between patients and those treating them. Patients may communicate pain both verbally and non-verbally. Their expressions of pain may, in turn, produce a range of reactions from the person treating them.

Behavioural mechanisms

Most therapists understand pain behaviour (of whatever sort) simply as a response to pain, and treat it as such. However, since the 1970s, behavioural theorists have investigated the behavioural mechanisms involved in such treatment contexts and it appears that the situation can be much more complex. There are two major perspectives concerning pain behaviour.

Classical conditioning

Within the classical conditioning paradigm (of which Pavlov's experiments with his dogs are perhaps best known), pain behaviour can be viewed simply as an unconditioned response to a pain stimulus (nociception). Through learning, however, conditioning can occur so that fearful patients may begin to show similar responses to situations in which they were injured (the development of fear of hurting and harming can be understood within this paradigm). Not only secondary pain behaviour, but also pain itself, can become conditioned. High-intensity pain can be re-experienced during flashbacks of traumatizing painful injuries. No new injury is occurring, but memory of the circumstances surrounding the injury can reproduce the pain.

Experimental work has demonstrated the conditioning of muscular responses to painful stimuli and to the expectation of a painful stimulus in healthy controls. Flor and Birbaumer (1994) gave electric shocks, paired with an audible tone, to a group of students. The students demonstrated an increase in muscle tension in response to the shock. After a series of trials, the tone alone could elicit the muscular response. The muscular responses were even more pronounced if paired with slides associated with negative emotional states. They also report that the responses were more easily conditioned and took longer to extinguish in those students who reported frequent episodes of neck and shoulder pain, suggesting a susceptibility to conditioned muscular responses.

Operant conditioning

Persistence of pain behaviour can also be understood in terms of its consequences. If the pain behaviour is successful in reducing pain, or leads to pleasant consequences (such as increased attention from a spouse (Romano et al. 1996), absence from a stressful job, or financial compensation), it is likely that the pain behaviour will increase in frequency. The change has been brought about by operant conditioning. Such pain behaviour may have only a small respondent component. Pain behaviours that initially produced an escape from the painful stimulus can produce patterns of complete avoidance. As has been stated elsewhere, 'fear of pain can become more disabling than pain itself' (Waddell et al. 1993). Many such influences can be observed during the course of manual therapy. Successful avoidance of painful activity (such as a painful exercise programme) can inhibit therapeutic progress. Interestingly, patients are often unaware of the mechanisms underpinning their behaviour.

Assessment of pain behaviour

A number of different measures have been developed specifically for the assessment of pain behaviour.

Behavioural rating scales

Behaviourally based interventions require careful assessment, and a number of observation schedules have been developed. Typically, the rater is asked to observe the patient and indicate, on a behavioural rating scale devised for the purpose (Richards et al. 1982), when certain behaviours occur. Such scales are used to rate the videotaped observations, but can also be used to code naturally occurring behaviours. These scales are merely adaptations of observational scales that can be used for many other purposes. The 'diary' format enables the accurate recording of the incidence of such behaviours and their relationships with other events. The information can therefore be used for a 'functional analysis'. Vlaeyen et al. (1987) also used an observational method in which patients were observed over a long period (e.g. during an in-patient rehabilitation programme) and a wide range of pain behaviours were recorded. Although sometimes highly informative, such methods are not practicable in typical out-patient clinical practice. A number of more clinically based instruments have been developed.

The following section of the chapter is abstracted from a review of more commonly used pain behaviour measures in clinical practice (Waddell and Main 1998b). All these tests offer patients an opportunity to communicate about their pain and therefore can be viewed as pain behaviour measures.

Pain drawing test

Pain drawings (manikins) are frequently used in clinics. Patients usually show no reluctance to complete them, and indeed sometimes do so with relish. The drawing indicates where the patient reports pain and other altered sensations. Ransford et al. (1976) originally attempted to distinguish 'non-organic' from 'psychogenic' pain on the basis of drawings. The drawings are evaluated for the extent to which they appear to correspond to a clear anatomical pathway. Widespread patterns, with non-anatomical distributions and the use of all sorts of additional emphasis, are considered indicative of 'psychological overlay' or distress. They should not be over-interpreted. A clearly abnormal pain drawing is almost always indicative of pain-associated distress, and should alert the clinician to the need for a more careful psychosocial assessment. However, 50% of distressed patients produce pain drawings with absolutely no indications of distress (Parker et al. 1995), and so the test is insufficiently sensitive to be recommended as a single screening procedure to identify distress.

Not a test, but an enlightening tool to add to the assessment of a more complex or challenging patient with significant impacting pain, is the inclusion of a patient drawing and their story or yarn. The reader is directed to an enlightening text by Oxford University Fellow and pain scientist, Dr Lorimor Moseley, entitled *Painful yarns* (2007). It is an enlightening, entertaining, and informative way to enhance our integration of concepts within the context of pain biology.

Overt pain behaviour

Keefe and Block (1982) developed the behavioural observation rating test—a 10-minute videotaped analysis of an observation of patients going through a series of movements. Although useful as a research tool, it has been found that clinicians cannot make such ratings reliably without careful training (Waddell and Richardson 1992).

It has also been suggested that naturalistic observation may not allow observation of tasks sufficiently strenuous to precipitate pain behaviour. A task-oriented measure of pain behaviour requiring the patient to perform a series of tasks (such as lifting, carrying, and stair-climbing) has, however, been devised (Watson and Poulter 1997). This measure has proved reliable in a pain management setting and seems to address some of the limitations of the other methods.

Behavioural (non-organic) signs

In clinical practice, the most widely used measure of pain behaviour in patients with chronic back pain is the behaviour (non-organic) signs test (Waddell et al. 1980). The test was devised originally to identify 'non-organic' components in the patient's presentation. The original research led to the development and standardization of seven such behavioural signs:

- superficial tenderness
- non-anatomical tenderness
- simulated axial loading
- simulated rotation
- straight leg raise (under conditions of distraction)
- regional weakness
- regional sensory disturbance.

The method of assessment was carefully standardized. The signs were found to be clearly separable from other physical signs and to correlate highly with measures of psychological distress. They were conceptualized originally as psychological screeners, with the caveat (as with the behavioural symptoms) that isolated signs should not be over-interpreted. The fact that they have been misused and misinterpreted as indicators of malingering has prompted a reappraisal of their use (Main and Waddell 1998a).

Behavioural symptoms

The behavioural symptoms test (Waddell et al. 1984) includes the assessment of five specific symptoms and two clinical history items suggestive of a marked emotional reaction to pain. The five symptoms are:

- pain at the tip of the tailbone
- whole leg pain
- whole leg numbness
- whole leg giving way
- complete absence of spells with very little pain in the previous year.

The two clinical history items are:

- intolerance (or adverse reaction) to many previous treatments
- emergency admission to hospital with simple backache.

As with the pain drawing test, the behavioural symptoms test should not be over-interpreted. Only if the clinician finds three or more such 'symptoms' should the presence of a pain behaviour syndrome be investigated.

Chronic pain (or pain behaviour syndrome)

The persistence of pain can produce wide-ranging and devastating effects on patients (Main and Spanswick 1995). They may display marked and seemingly inappropriate pain behaviour, indicate high levels of distress, and yet have been offered a significant amount of treatment. Such patients frequently require a comprehensive pain management programme (Flor et al. 1992a), although not all can be helped. Such patients are characterized not by isolated or specific indicators of pain behaviour, but by an entire pattern of invalidism. Such presentations are frequently observed in patients involved in litigation (although by no means confined to such situations). Repeated evaluations in an essentially adversarial medicolegal system seem to exacerbate their distress and make assessment even more difficult. We should be aware, therefore, of our patients' economic and occupational contexts, lest there is a significant disincentive for the patient to recover.

Conclusion

In summary, pain behaviour has to be understood in terms of its context. Indeed, pain has been defined as 'an interesting social communication the meaning of which has still to be determined' (Fordyce 1976). This perspective offers a radically different approach to the understanding of the therapeutic mechanisms during therapy compared to the traditional medical model. For the practicing therapist, the most useful aspects of pain behaviour seem to be the observation of guarded movements, the identification of fear-related responses to examination, and the communication of distress.

The role of expectation and influence of previous treatment with regards to pain

The role of patient expectation

Psychological factors influencing response to treatment include patient's expectation, non-specific (placebo) responses to treatment, compliance with treatment (including adherence to treatment protocols), and acceptance of appropriate responsibility for the management of their symptomatology. Patients who have been in pain for a long period of time or who have a recurrent pain problem may have seen several other professionals and received a range of treatments which have proved ineffective.

The adverse influence of failed treatment

Failed treatment can have a profoundly demoralizing effect. The patient may have lost confidence in the likely benefit of any further treatment. They may be concerned that 'something has been missed' (e.g. cancer). They may be significantly disaffected with healthcare professionals, particularly if they feel that they have been misled in terms of likely benefit from treatment or have not been believed, or it has been implied that the problem is 'all in their mind'. Such iatrogenic factors can have a significant influence on a patient's decision to accept treatment or to comply with it (Waddell and Main 1998b).

Implications for the relationship between patient and therapist

The adverse influences of repeated ineffective treatment and differences in diagnosis (as offered by different specialists) have been highlighted. They can lead to significant apprehension about further consultations and demonstrations of pain behaviour in the form of distress and anger (Main and Waddell 1998b). It should be recognized, therefore, that the behaviour demonstrated at initial consultation may have been influenced significantly by previous experiences. This perspective is not just of theoretical importance. Consider a patient presenting with acute low back pain who may have had repeated periods of severe pain on movement in the days before consulting. They may also have had a painful examination by another practitioner (e.g. their GP) and this, in turn, may influence their willingness to move. They may demonstrate muscle guarding (which may be misidentified as involuntary muscle spasm) and appear to be responding excessively to further physical examination. If litigation is involved, unsympathetic assessors attempting to raise doubts about the genuineness of their difficulties may have further confounded the distress.

Psychophysiological responses to pain

Psychophysiological researchers have examined the interaction between mental and physical events in a number of disorders (Turpin 1989), including pain, in which the genesis and maintenance of pain in terms of both central and peripheral mechanisms has been discussed (Flor et al. 1990, 1997).

Underlying the theory of psychophysiological reactivity is the development of a fundamental hyperarousal of the sympathetic nervous system in response to stimuli or stressors. Abnormal psychophysiological reactions to stress and pain have been found in a number of painful conditions. Whether these reactions are the antecedents of the painful condition or merely reactions to it is still unclear, but may be helpful to attempt to differentiate non-specific or generalized responses from more specific reactions that may serve to maintain or exacerbate the pain (Flor et al. 1992). Non-specific reactions to pain are heightened responses in skin sweating, heart rate, and general physiological arousal during painful or stressful conditions. These reactions per se are not normally painful but may serve to increase the perception of pain from a specific source. They may cause pain in conditions where pain is sympathetically maintained, such as complex regional pain syndrome. Specific reactions are themselves algogenic (pain-producing) and serve as a source of nociception in susceptible individuals. For example, site-specific muscle hyper-reactivity has been identified in patients with chronic low back pain and tension headaches, and alterations in vascular flow have been found in some migraine sufferers. The role of muscle activity should be of particular interest to those working in musculoskeletal medicine.

Specific investigations of muscle activity

Flor et al. (1985) identified site-specific hyper-reactivity in patients with chronic low back pain. Increases in surface electromyography readings were demonstrated during a personally relevant stressor. These responses were not demonstrated during an arithmetical control stressor and they did not generalize to other non-painful areas. They concluded that increases in site muscle activity may contribute to pain through increased muscle tension. Site-specific increases in lumbar paraspinal muscle activity in patients with low back pain in response to a tonic pain stressor, the cold pressor test, has been demonstrated by Watson et al. (1998). However, the change in paraspinal activity was not accompanied by a change in back pain report, and so the precise relationship between increases in static muscle activity and a possible myogenic mechanism for pain requires further investigation.

The nature of pain-associated movement abnormalities

The evidence for abnormalities of movement in chronic pain conditions is much more convincing than that for elevated resting baselines. With careful methodology, electromyographic recording of standardized movements can be repeatable and reliable. Patients with chronic low back pain demonstrate different patterns of activity when compared with pain-free controls during movement. Not only that, but the differences in movement can discriminate the patient with back pain from the healthy control with a good degree of sensitivity (Watson et al. 1997a). Changes in these abnormalities have been demonstrated to be more closely related to a change in fear of activity and pain self-efficacy beliefs (the relative confidence that one will be able to perform a movement despite the pain) than the level of clinical pain (Watson et al. 1997b). The clinical significance of these abnormalities, prospectively, still needs to be examined.

Clinical implications: the development of guarded movements

After an injury, there is a natural tendency to guard the injured area to allow for rest and recovery. The development of guarded movements can be understood from both behavioural and cognitive perspectives (as already discussed). Thus, if a patient experiences pain on the performance of an activity, with repeated pain on activity, the muscular guarding responses can become conditioned not only to the performance of the movement but also to the anticipation of the performance of that movement, as the patients anticipate the learned outcome—pain. This respondent conditioning can result in abnormalities of muscle activity which themselves may be implicated in the generation of pain. Guarded movements may become further established through operant conditioning (if the guarded activity is followed by reinforcing events such as displays of increasing concern or sympathy from a spouse or clinician; 'escape' from a painful situation following an invitation to rest; or a financial circumstance which is dependent on continued demonstrations of pain or incapacity). The aforementioned cognitive factors such as fear of further injury or pessimism about being able to achieve an increase in function may also contribute to the development of guarded movements (Main and Watson 1996).

Implications for clinical management of pain

◆ Musculoskeletal assessment places considerable reliance on the accuracy of a patient's self-report of pain and, in arriving at a diagnosis and treatment plan, reported pain intensity is assumed to bear a close relationship to underlying nociception. Perception of pain in experimental situations is influenced by fear, perception of control, and predictability, and it may be more helpful to consider acute pain (or indeed recurrent flare-ups) as a fear-mediated phenomenon.

◆ The rating of chronic clinical pain, however, appears to be affected by a number of other influences and, therefore, its validity as a measure of response to nociception is unclear.

◆ During the course of a clinical examination, the assessor may attempt to arrive at a clinical diagnosis through replication of the patient's pain by palpation of the induction of mechanical stress. There are two problems with this approach: firstly, response to pain provocation (whether palpation or induction of biomechanical stress) can be affected by fear of an adverse outcome (such as pain) and fear of injury; secondly, a patient's global rating of their pain may be widely influenced by factors in addition to nociception.

◆ The musculoskeletal assessment must, therefore, be placed within a biopsychosocial framework. In appraising the patient's response, it may be helpful to incorporate specific assessment of subjectively reported fear or behavioural indicators of fear such as guarded movements or behavioural signs.

◆ Inclusion of screening for yellow flags (ref) to identify psychosocial impacting factors.

◆ Attitude, caring disposition, paternalism, and empathy are all important in pain management—taking Engel`s view that perhaps it is not paternalism that is the problem but practicing as a cold technician rather than a caring healer (Borrell-Carrio et al. 2004; Emanuel and Emanuel 1992; Ubel 2002).

◆ Clinical management may be further enhanced by the use of validated measures in clinical practice; for example, McGill pain questionnaire, Roland Morris disability questionnaire, a quality of life measure like the EQ-5D (recently updated to the EQ-5D-5 L which is being used in a three-year study across the UK in NHS Trust musculoskeletal physiotherapy departments), and Health Anxiety & Depression (HADS).

◆ The introduction of patient education programmes can dispel fallacies, encourage self-management, and improve adherence.

◆ The inclusion of cognitive behavioural therapy/restructuring tends to improve physical function, self- confidence, self-esteem, and social interaction (Critchley et al. 2007).

An integrated person-centred and goal-oriented approach for persistent back pain (PDP), called cognitive functional therapy (CFT), targeting the patient's beliefs and behaviours that drive pain and disability, may be effective (O'Sullivan 2012). Key elements of the CFT approach involve:

- addressing negative beliefs and fear regarding pain and magnetic resonance imaging (MRI) findings
- providing effective multidisciplinary, patient-centred education
- promoting active coping strategies for pain and instilling confidence and hope for change
- facilitating goal-oriented behavioural change regarding, for example, stress management, physical activity, pacing, and diet
- utilizing motivational interviewing techniques
- training mindfulness
- providing feedback which is critical to this process and includes mindfulness of the body–mind responses to pain, movement and its perceived threat, visual feedback with the use of mirrors, video and written instructions
- retraining of maladaptive movements
- targeting 'new' movement behaviours to reduce the threat of the activity and to normalize it
- integration of new behaviours into daily living
- targeted strengthening and conditioning.

A recent randomized controlled trial (RCT) (Fersum et al. 2011) demonstrated that CFT resulted in superior outcomes (reduced pain intensity and episodes, disability, and fear; improved mood; less need for ongoing support; and reduced sick leave) when compared to manual therapy and core stabilization exercises. Trials are continuing.

In manual and musculoskeletal treatments, we are frequently managing the patients' pain behaviour and distress, rather than simply the nociceptive component of their pain. Where musculoskeletal pain has become chronic, it is necessary to rely on the principles of chronic pain management.

References

American Psychiatric Association (1994) *Diagnostic and statistical manual of mental disorders (DSM-IV)* (4th edn). American Psychiatric Association, Washington.

Asmundson, G.G., Norton, G.R., Allerdings, M.D. (1997) Fear and avoidance in dysfunctional back pain patients. *Pain*, 69, 231–6.

Atkins, E., Kerr, J., Goodlad, E. (2010) *Orthopaedic medicine—a practical approach*. Butterworth-Heineman., Oxford.

Averill, P.M., Novy, D.M., Nelson, D.V., Berry, L.A. (1996) Correlates of depression in chronic pain patients: a comprehensive examination. *Pain*, 65, 93–100.

Axford, J., Heron, C., Ross, F., Victor, C.R. (2008) Management of knee osteoarthritis in primary care: pain and depression are the major obstacles. *J Psychosom Res*, 64, 461–7.

Bandura, A. (1977) Self-efficacy: towards a unifying theory of behavioural change. *Psychol Rev*, 84, 191–215.

Borrell-Carrio, F. Suchman, A.L., Epstein R.A. (2004) The biopsychosocial model 25 years later: principles, practice and scientific inquiry. *Ann Fam Med*, 2(6), 576–82.

Brekke, M., Hjortdahl, P., Kvien, T.K. (2003) Changes in self-efficacy and health status over 5 years: a longitudinal observational study of 306 patients with rheumatoid arthritis. *Arthritis Reheum*, 49(3), 342–8.

Brown, G.K., Nicassio, P.M. (1987) The development of a questionnaire for the assessment of active and passive coping strategies in chronic pain patients. *Pain*, 31, 53–65.

Burton, A.K., Tillotson, K.M., Main, C.J., Hollis, S. (1995) Psychosocial predictors of outcome in acute and subchronic low back trouble. *Spine*, 20, 722–8.

Butler, D. (2012) Manual therapy in a neuroplastic world. *J Sports Ther*, 42(10), A17–A21.

Carroll, L.J., Cassidy, J.D., Cote, P. (2006) The role of pain coping strategies in prognosis after whiplash injury: passive coping predicts slowed recovery. *Pain*, 124, 1–2, 18–26.

Cioffi, D. (1991) Beyond attentional strategies: a cognitive-perceptual model of somatic interpretation. *Psychol Bull*, 109, 25–41.

Clough, P.J., Sewell, D., Earle, K. (2002) Mental toughness: the concept and its measurement. In: Cockerill, I. (ed.) *Solutions in sports psychology*. Thompson, London, pp. 32–43.

Crisson, J.E., Keefe, F.J. (1988) The relationship of locus of control to pain coping strategies and psychological distress in chronic pain patients. *Pain*, 35, 147–54.

Critchley, D.J. Ratcliffe, J., Noonan, S., Jones, R.H., Hurley, M.V.(2007) Effectiveness and cost-effectiveness of three types of physiotherapy used to reduce chronic low back pain disability: a pragmatic randomized trial with economic evaluation. *Spine*, 32(14), 1474–81.

Crombez, G., Eccleston, C. Baeyens, F., Eelen, P. (1997) Habituation and the interference of pain with task performance. *Pain*, 70, 149–54.

Crust, L., Clough, P.J. (2005) Relationship between mental toughness and physical endurance. *Percep Mot Skills*, 100, 192–4.

DeGood, D.E., Kiernan, B. (1996) Perception of fault in patients with chronic pain. *Pain*, 64, 153–9.

DeGood, D.E., Shutty, M.S. Jr (1992) Assessment of pain beliefs, coping and self-efficacy. In: Turk, D.C., Melzack R. (eds) *Handbook of pain assessment*. Guilford Press, New York, pp. 214–34.

Denison, E. Asenlof, P., Sandborgh, M., Lindberg, R. (2007).Musculoskeletal pain in primary health care: subgroups based on pain intensity, disability, self-efficacy, and fear-avoidance variables. *J Pain*, 8(1), 67–74.

Descartes, R. (1664) *L'homme*. E. Angot, Paris.

Dubner, R. (1997) Neural basis of persistent pain: sensory specialization, sensory modulation and neuronal plasticity. In: Jensen, T.S., Turner, J.A., Wiesenfeld-Hallin, Z. (eds) *Progress in pain research and management (Proceedings of the 8th World Congress on Pain)*. IASP Press, Seattle, 8, pp. 243–57.

Eccleston, C. (1995) The attentional control of pain: methodological and theoretical concerns. *Pain*, 63, 3–10.

Emanuel. E.J., Emanuel L.L. (1992) Four models of the physician-patient relationship. *JAMA*, 267, 2221–6.

Engel, G. (1980) The clinical application of the biopsychosocial model. *Am J Psychiat*, 137, 535–44.

Engel, G.L. (1988) How much longer must medicine be bounded by a seventeenth century world view? In: White, K.L. (ed.) *The task of medicine: dialogue at Wickenburg*. The Henry Kasiser Family Foundation, Menlo Park, California, pp. 113–36.

Fernandez, F., Turk, D.C. (1995) The scope and significance of anger in chronic pain. *Pain*, 61, 165–75.

Fersum, K.V., O'Sullivan, P.B., Kvale, A., Smith, A., Skouen, J. (2011) *Classification based cognitive functional therapy for the management of non-specific low back pain (NSLBP)—a randomised control trial*. Melbourne International Forum XI: Primary Care Research on Low Back Pain; March 15–18, Melbourne. Australia.

Flor, H., Birbaumer, N. (1994) Acquisition of chronic pain: psychophysiological mechanisms. *Am Pain Soc J*, 3, 119–27.

Flor, H., Birbaumer, N., Turk, D.C. (1990) The psychobiology of chronic pain. *Adv Behav Res Ther*, 12, 47–87.

Flor, H., Braun, C., Elbert, T., Birbaumer, N. (1997) Extensive reorganization of primary somatosensory cortex in chronic back pain patients. *Neurosci Lett*, 224, 5–8.

Flor, H., Fydrich, T., Turk, D.C. (1992) Efficacy of multidisciplinary pain treatment centers: a meta-analytic review. *Pain*, 49, 221–30.

Flor, H., Turk, D.C., Birbaumer, N. (1985) Assessment of stress-related psychophysiological stress reactions in chronic back pain patients. *J Consult Clin Psychol*, 53, 354–64.

Fordyce, W.E. (1976) *Behavioural methods for chronic pain and illness*. Mosby, St Louis.

Gatchell, R., Turk, D.C. (1996) (eds) *Psychological approaches to pain management: a practitioner's handbook*. Guilford Press, New York.

Geisser, M.E., Roth, R.S., Bachman, J.E., Eckert, T.A. (1996) The relationship between symptoms of post-traumatic stress disorder and pain. Affective disturbance and disability among patients with accident and non-accident related pain. *Pain*, 66, 207–14.

Haggman, S., Maher, C.G., Refshauge, K.M. (2004) Screening for symptoms of depression by physical therapists managing low back pain. *Phys Ther*, 84(12), 1157–66.

et al. (2011) A longitudinal study to explain the pain-depression link in older adults with osteoarthritis. *Arthr Care Res*, 63, 1382–90.

Heider, F. (1944) Social perceptions and phenomenological causality. *Psychol Rev*, 51, 358–74.

Hutson, M.A. (1999). *Work related upper limb disorders. Recognition and management*. Butterworth-Heinemann: Oxford

Jensen, M.P., Karoly, P. (1992) Pain-specific beliefs, perceived symptom severity and adjustment to chronic pain. *Clin J Pain*, 8, 123–30.

Jensen, M.P., Turner, J.A., Romano, J.M., Karoldy, P. (1991) Coping with chronic pain: a critical review of the literature. *Pain*, 47, 249–83.

Jensen, M.P., Turner, J.A., Romano, J.M., Lawler, B.K. (1994) Relationship of pain-specific beliefs to chronic pain adjustment. *Pain*, 57, 301–9.

Jull, G.A. (2012) Management of cervical spine disorders: where to now? *J Sports Ther*, 42(10), A3–A7.

Keefe, F.J., Affleck, G., Lefebvre, J., Starr, K., Caldwell, D.S., Tennen, H. (1997) Pain coping strategies and pain efficacy in rheumatoid arthritis: a daily process analysis. *Pain*, 69, 35–42.

Keefe, F.J., Brown, G.K., Wallston, K.A., Caidwell. D.S. (1989) Coping with rheumatoid arthritis pain: catastrophising as a maladaptive strategy. *Pain*, 37, 51–6.

Kori, S.H., Miller, R.P., Todd, D.D. (1990) Kinisophobia: a new view of chronic pain behaviour. *Pain Man*, Jan/Feb, 35–43.

Levy, A., Polman, R., Clough, P.J., Marchant, D., Earle, K. (2006) Mental toughness as a determinant of beliefs, pain and adherence in sport injury rehabilitation. *J Sport Rehab*, 15, 246–54.

Loeser, J.D. (1980) Perspectives on pain. In: Turner, P. (ed.) *Clinical pharmacy and therapeutics*. Macmillan, London, pp. 313–6.

Loeser, J.D., Fordyce, W.E. (1983) Chronic pain. In: Carr, J. E., Dengerik, H.A. (eds) *Behavioural science in the practice of medicine*. Elsevier, Amsterdam.

Main, C.J. (1983) The modified somatic perception questionnaire. *J Psychosom Res*, 27, 503–14.

Main, C.J., Burton A.K. (1995) The patient with low back pain: who or what are we assessing? An experimental investigation of a pain puzzle. *Pain Rev*, 2, 203–9.

Main, C.J., Spanswick, C.C. (1995) Functional overlay and illness behaviour in chronic pain: distress or malingering? Conceptual difficulties in medico-legal assessment of personal injury claims. *J Psychosom Res*, 39, 737–53.

Main, C.J., Waddell, G. (1991) Cognitive measures in pain. *Pain*, 46, 287–98.

Main, C.J., Waddell, G. (1998a) Spine update: behavioural responses to examination: a re-examination: a reappraisal of the interpretation of 'nonorganic signs'. *Spine*, 23, 2367–71.

Main, C.J., Waddell, G. (1998b) Psychologic distress. In: Waddell, G. (ed.) *The back pain revolution*. Churchill Livingstone, Edinburgh, pp. 173–86.

Main, C.J., Watson, P.J. (1996) Guarded movements: development of chronicity. *J Musculo Pain*, 4, 163–70.

Main, C.J., Wood, P.L.R., Hollis, S., Spanswick, C.C., Waddell, G. (1992) The distress assessment method: a simple patient classification to identify distress and evaluate risk of poor outcome. *Spine*, 17, 42–50.

Marks, D.F., Murray, M., Evans, B., Estacio, E.V. (2011). *Health psychology: theory research and practice*. Sage, London.

Melzack, R. (1985) The role of compensation in chronic pain: analysis using a new method of scoring the McGill Pain Questionnnaire. *Pain*, 23, 101–12.

Melzack, R. (1986) Neurophysiological foundations of pain. In: Sternbach, R.A. (ed.) *The psychology of pain* (2nd edn). Raven Press, New York, pp. 1–24.

Melzack, R. (1989) *The challenge of pain* (2nd edn). Penguin, Harmondsworth.

Melzack, R. (1996) Gate control theory: on the evolution of pain concepts. *Pain Forum*, 5, 128–38.

Melzack, R., Casey, K. L. (1968) Sensory, motivational and central control determinants of pain. In: Kenshalo, D.R. (ed.) *The skin senses*. Charles C. Thomas, Springfield, IL, pp. 423–39.

Melzack, R., Wall, P. (1965) Pain mechanisms: a new theory. *Science*, 150, 971–9.

Melzack, R., Wall, P.D., Ty, T.C. (1982) Acute pain in an emergency clinic: latency of onset and descriptor patterns related to different injuries. *Pain*, 14, 33–42.

Moseley, L. (2007) *Painful yarns*. Dancing Giraffe Press, Canberra.

Mossey, J.M., Gallagher, R.M. (2004) The longitudinal occurrence and impact of comorbid chronic pain and chronic depression over two years in continuing care retirement community residents. *Pain Med*, 5, 335–48.

Nicholas, M.K., Linton, S.J., Watson, P.J., Main, C.J. (2011) Early identification and management of psychological risk factors ('yellow flags') in patients with low back pain: a reappraisal. *Phys Ther*, 91(5), 737–53.

Nicholls, A., Polman, R., Levy, A., Backhouse, S. (2009). Mental toughness, optimism, and coping in athletes. *Personal Indiv Diff*, 47, 73–5.

Nicholas, M.K., Wilson, P.H., Goyen, I. (1992) Comparison of cognitive behavioural group treatment and an alternative non-psychological treatment for chronic low back pain. *Pain*, 48, 339–47.

O`Sullivan, P. (2012) A classification-based cognitive functional approach for the management of low back pain. *J Sports Ther*, 42(10_, A17–A21.

Parker, H., Wood, P.L.R., Main, C.J. (1995) The use of the pain drawing as a screening measure to predict psychological distress in chronic low back pain. *Spine*, 20, 236–43.

Price, D.D., Mao, J., Mayer, D.J. (1997) Central consequences of persistent pain states In: Jensen, T.S., Turner, J,A. Weisenfeld-Hallin, Z. (eds) *Progress in pain research and management. (Proceedings of the 8th World Congress on Pain)*. IASP Press, Seattle, 8, 155–84.

Ransford, A.O., Cairns, D., Mooney, V. (1976) The pain drawing as an aid to the psychological evaluation of patients with low back pain. *Spine*, 1, 127–34.

Richards, J.S., Nepomuceno, I.A., Riles, M., Suer, Z. (1982) Assessing pain behaviour: the UAB pain behaviour scale. *Pain*, 14, 393–8.

Roland, P.E. (1993) *Brain activation*. Wiley Liss, New York.

Romano, I.M., Turner, J.A., Jensen, M.P., et al. (1996) Chronic pain patient–spouse behavioral interactions predict patient disability. *Pain*, 63, 353–61.

Rosenstiel, A.K., Keefe, F.J. (1983) The use of coping-strategies in chronic low back pain patients: relationship to patient characteristics and current adjustments. *Pain*, 17, 33–4.

Rotter, J.B. (1966). Generalised expectancies for internal versus external control of reinforcement. *Psychol Mon: Gen Appl*, 80, 609.

Rudy, T. E., Kerns, R.D., Turk, D.C. (1988) Chronic pain and depression: toward a cognitive–behavioral mediation model. *Pain*, 35, 129–40.

Schmitz, U., Saile, H., Nilees, P. (1996) Coping with chronic pain: flexible goal adjustment as an interactive buffer against pain-related distress. *Pain*, 67, 41–51.

Severeijns, R., Vlaeyen, J.W., van den Hout, M.A., et al. (2001) Pain catastrophizing predicts pain intensity, disability and psychological; distress independent of the level of physical impairment. *Clin J Pain*, 17,165–72.

Smart, K.M., Blake, C., Staines, A., Thacker, M., Doody, C. (2012a) Mechanisms-based classifications of musculoskeletal pain: part 1 of 3. Symptoms and signs of central sensitisation in patients with low back (+/- leg) pain. *Man Ther*, 17(4), 336–44.

Smart, K.M., Blake, C., Staines, A., Thacker, M., Doody, C. (2012b) Mechanisms-based classifications of musculoskeletal pain: part 1 of 3. Symptoms and signs of peripheral sensitisation in patients with low back (+/- leg) pain. *Man Ther*, 17(4), 345–51.

Snow-Turek, A.L., Norris, M.P., Tan, G. (1996) Active and passive coping strategies in chronic pain patients. *Pain*, 64, 455–62.

Sterling, M. (2004). A proposed new classification system for whiplash associated disorders: Implications for assessment and management. *Manual Therapy*,9, 60–70.

Sullivan, M., Katon, W. (1993) Focus article: somatization: the path between distress and somatic symptoms. *Am Pain Soc J*, 2, 141–9.

Sullivan, M.J.L., Tripp, D.A., Rodgers, W.M., et al. (2000) Catastrophising and pain perception in sport participants. *J App Sport Psychol*, 12, 151–62.

Thacker, M.A., Moseley, G.L. (2012) First-person neuroscience and the understanding of pain. *Med J Australia*, 196(6), 410–11.

Thacker, M., Moseley, G.L., Flor, H. (2009) Neuropathic pain management is more than pills. *BMJ (Intern Edn)*, 339, b3502.

Turk, D.C. (1996) Biopsychosocial perspective on chronic pain. In: Gatchel, R., Turk, D.C. (eds) *Psychological approaches to pain management: a practitioner's handbook*. Guilford Press, New York, pp. 3–32.

Turk, D.C., Meichenbaum, D.H., Genest, M. (1983) *Pain and behavioral medicine: a cognitive-behavioral perspective*. Guilford Press, New York.

Turk, D.C., Okifuji, A. Sinclair, I.D., Starz, T.W. (1996) Pain, disability and physical functioning in subgroups of patients with fibromyalgia. *J Rheumat*, 23(7), 1255–62.

Turner, J.A. (1991) Coping and chronic pain. In: Bond, M.R., Charlton, J.E., Woolf, C. (eds) *Proceedings of the VIth World Congress on Pain*. Elsevier, New York, pp 219–27.

Turpin, G. (ed.) (1989) *Handbook of clinical psychophysiology*. Wiley, Chichester.

Ubel, P.A. (2002) 'What should I do doc?': some psychogenic benefits of physician recommendations. *Arch Intern Med*, 162, 977–80.

Vassiljen, J.O., Johansen, B.M., Westgaard, R.H. (1995) The effect of pain reduction on perceived tension and EMG recorded trapezius muscle activity in workers with shoulder and neck pain. *Scand J Rehab Med*, 27, 243–52.

Vassiljen, J.O., Westgaard, R.H. (1996) Can stress-related shoulder pain develop independently of muscle activity? *Pain*, 64, 221–30.

Vlaeyen, J.W.S., Kole-Snidjers, A.M.J., Boeren, R.G.B., van Fek, H. (1995) Fear of movement and (re)-injury in chronic low back pain and its relation to behavioural performance. *Pain*, 62, 363–72.

Vlaeyen, J.W.S., van Eek, H., Groenman, N.H., Schuerman, J.A. (1987) Dimensions and components of observed chronic pain behaviour. *Pain*, 31, 65–75.

Waddell, G., Bircher, M., Finlayson, D., Main, C.J. (1984) Symptoms and signs: physical disease or illness behaviour? *BMJ*, 289, 739–41.

Waddell, G., Main, C. (1984) Assessment of severity in low back disorders. *Spine*, 9, 204–8.

Waddell, G., Main, C.J. (1998a) A new clinical model of low back pain and disability. In: Waddell, G. (ed.) *The back pain revolution*. Churchill Livingston, Edinburgh, pp. 223–40.

Waddell, G., Main, C.J. (1998b) Illness behaviour. In: Waddell, G. (ed.) *The back pain revolution*. Churchill Livingston, Edinburgh, pp. 155–72.

Waddell, G., Main, C.J. (1998c) Beliefs about back pain. In: Waddell, G. (ed.) *The back pain revolution*. Churchill Livingston, Edinburgh, pp. 187–202.

Waddell, G. McCulloch, J.A., Kummell, E. Venner, R.M. (1980) Nonorganic physical signs in low back pain. *Spine*, 5, 117–25.

Waddell, G., Richardson, J. (1992) Clinical assessment of overt pain behaviour during routine clinical examination. *J Psychosom Res*, 36, 77–87.

Waddell, G., Somerville, D., Henderson, I., Newton, M., Main, C.J. (1993) A fear avoidance beliefs questionnaire (FABQ) and the role of fear avoidance beliefs in chronic low back pain and disability. *Pain*, 52, 157–68.

Watson, P.J., Booker, C.K., Main, C.J. (1997b) Evidence for the role of psychological factors in abnormal paraspinal activity in patients with chronic low back pain. *J Musculo Pain*, 5, 41–56.

Watson, P.J., Booker, C.K., Main, C.J., Chen, A.C.N. (1997a) Surface electromyography in the identification of chronic low back pain patients: the development of the flexion relaxation ratio. *Clin Biomech*, 12, 165–71.

Watson, P.J., Chen, A.C.N., Booker, C.K., Main, C.J., Jones, A.K.P. (1998) Illness questionnaire: further evidence for its reliability and validity. *Pain*, 58, 377–86.

Watson, P.J., Johnson, T.W., Main, C.J. (1996) *Low back tenderness in CLBP: the influence of pain report and psychological factors*. Paper presented at the 8th World Congress on Pain, Vancouver, Canada.

Watson, P.J., Poulter, M. (1997) The development of a functional task-oriented measure of pain behaviour in chronic low back pain patients. *J Back Musculo Rehab*, 9, 57–9.

Weir, R., Browne, G., Roberts, J., Tunks, E., Gafni, A. (1994) The meaning of differential electromyographic response to experimental cold pressor test in chronic low back pain patients and normal controls. *J Musculo Pain*, 6(2), 51–64.

Woolf, C.J. (1996) Windup and central sensitization are not equivalent. *Pain*, 66, 105–8.

Chapter 21

Placebo theory

Milton Cohen

Introduction to placebo theory

Why should a textbook of musculoskeletal medicine devote a chapter to placebo theory? The doyen of pain medicine, the late Patrick Wall, wrote that the placebo phenomenon 'seems to shake our belief in the reliability of our sensory experience' (1992). Perhaps this arises out of the unpredictability of individual responses to therapy, especially in chronic illness where pathogenesis is uncertain; or perhaps from the recognition that therapies that could not possibly be influencing a known mechanism of disease are nonetheless effective.

Mention of placebo tends to evoke images of charlatanism in practice or of nuisance in research. Indeed, this tainted reputation has tended to persist despite recent advances in understanding of the clinical and, more recently, the biological bases for the placebo phenomenon. In the last three decades, there have been two waves of literature: before 2000, with the textbooks from White et al. (1985) and Harrington (1997) and reviews from Peck and Coleman (1991), Richardson (1994), and Turner et al. (1994) with a psychological bent; and since 2000, the textbook from Benedetti (2008) and reviews from Price et al. (2008) and Finniss et al. (2010) with more neurobiological emphasis.

On placebos, placebo responses, and placebo effects

Despite universal recognition of phenomena attached to the placebo concept, the literature has been dominated by difficulty regarding definitions. This was captured by Gøtzsche (1994) who noted that, while placebos are deliberately used in scientific trials to allow inference of *specific* effect of an intervention, the opposite occurs in clinical practice where an attempt is made to maximize *non-specific* (or placebo) effect. Although a fair reflection, this statement raises the problem of the semantic confusion that permeates the field.

The issue turns on the question, 'To what may apparent responses to therapy be attributed?' Three main processes have been identified:

- Natural history, that recognizes the self-limiting nature of some illnesses or random variations in illness expression. This includes regression to the mean, or the tendency of random variations in measurement to be followed by observations closer to the average (Whitney and Von Korff 1992). Error in measurement itself may also contribute to such observations.
- Specific effects arising out of the characteristic nature of the intervention, such as a drug or a procedure (Turner et al. 1994).
- The so-called 'non-specific' effects of treatment—those that may be associated with the sociocultural context in which a treatment is delivered. These are referred to as placebo effects (Brody 1985) but may not be at all 'non-specific', so that a different conceptualization is required.

A major source of conceptual confusion has been conflation of the terms 'placebo effect' and 'placebo response'. To resolve this confusion, the following explication is offered.

A *placebo* is a substance or procedure that has no inherent power to produce an effect that is sought or expected (Stewart-Williams and Podd 2004). Placebos are used as a 'control' intervention in *experimental* trial situations; however, it is considered unethical to administer a known placebo in a clinical therapeutic situation (unless informed consent has been obtained). In the experimental case, placebos appear to have their own 'pharmacology', with dose–response, time-effect, and side-effect profiles not unlike those of non-placebos (Lasagna et al. 1958).

A *placebo response* is, literally, a response to the administration of a known placebo. That known placebos can exert therapeutic effect is itself a remarkable phenomenon, balanced by the observation that, in certain circumstances, known non-placebo treatments may fail to exert their characteristic effect. The result of administration of a placebo may be detrimental or negative—termed a 'nocebo' response.

A *placebo effect* is a genuine psychological or physiological effect which is attributable to receiving a substance or undergoing a procedure but which is not due to the inherent powers of the substance or procedure (Stewart-Williams and Podd 2004). Because such effects are attributable to the sociocultural context in which a treatment is delivered, in order to avoid confusion, it may be preferable to use the term 'contextual effects' rather than 'placebo/nocebo effects'. Such effects have been studied mainly with respect to pain but are involved in other clinical conditions such as Parkinson's disease (de la Fuent-Fernandez and Stoessl 2002) and depression (Kirsch and Sapirstein 1999).

Two important principles follow:

- Placebo—here termed contextual—effects do *not* require the administration of a placebo.
- A non-placebo treatment will exert *both* a characteristic effect *and* a contextual effect.

Misconceptions regarding the placebo phenomenon

Two major sets of misconceptions permeate the literature on the placebo phenomenon: the fixed-fraction myth and the special mentality myth.

The *fixed-fraction myth* has two aspects: that approximately one-third of the population responds to placebos, and that the extent of that response is also approximately one-third of the response to the active comparison drug (Wall 1992). This myth was perpetuated following a misrepresentation of the pioneering work of Beecher (1959), whose figure of about 35% was the average proportion of placebo responders from 11 studies, among which there was a very large variation. This issue of variation of the placebo response was examined by McQuay et al. (1995) in a review of five randomized, double-blind, parallel-group trials of analgesics in post-operative pain. Individual patients' scores with placebo varied from 0% to 100% of the maximum possible pain relief. Between 7% and 37% of patients given placebo achieved more than 50% pain reduction.

It had been claimed that the placebo response was about 55% of the response to the active treatment, irrespective of the strength of the active drug (Evans 1974). That is, the stronger the drug, the stronger the placebo response. In the study by McQuay et al. (1995), comparison of the mean placebo response with the mean active drug response did produce a regression line with a slope of 0.54—as claimed (Evans 1974)—but with 95% confidence intervals of 0.03–1.08. However, the latter study noted that patient responses were not normally distributed. If median rather than mean responses were used for descriptive purposes, the range of median placebo responses in the five trials surveyed became 2–14%. On average, the median placebo response score was less than 10% of the median active response score, with the slope of the regression line 0.12, with 95% confidence interval of 0.24 to 0.48. This is the expected result if there is no bias in the studies, and dispels the myth that there is a constant relationship between effective analgesic and placebo responses. These fixed-fraction myths can now be seen to have arisen as artefacts of inappropriate statistical description.

The *special mentality myth* also has two aspects: that placebo responders have nothing wrong with them (or, more bluntly, that their apparent response is an hallucination) and that placebo responders suffer some personality defect, such as being 'neurotic', 'suggestible', or 'willing to please' (Wall 1992). Not only are these contentions quite unsupported by the literature (Richardson 1994) but also it has been shown that, under appropriate circumstances, any person can become a placebo responder (Voudouris et al. 1989, 1990). Furthermore, placebo responsiveness itself may not be a consistent characteristic, varying according to time and context (Liberman 1964). Placebo response is not due to psychological pathology in the patient and does not indicate absence of organic pathology.

Mechanisms of placebo responses and contextual (placebo) effects

Most experimental work deals with placebo response, to allow inference of specific effect of an intervention. The greater is the difference between the *verum* (true) response and the placebo response, the more powerful is the intervention, so investigators seek to minimize the latter. This contrasts markedly to clinical practice, where an attempt is made to maximize the contextual (placebo) effect. Studies of *placebo response* in experimental situations have been used as models for understanding *contextual effects* in the clinical arena. The proposed mechanisms can be presented broadly as 'psychological' and 'neurobiological'.

Psychological mechanisms

The main theories include anxiety reduction, conditioning, and expectancy. The apparent tension between these latter two appears to have been resolved, in humans, by learning through association, as proposed in the conditioned placebo model, being mediated by expectancy.

Anxiety reduction

There is little empirical evidence to support reduction in anxiety as a mechanism. Not only is there no consistent finding of trait anxiety in placebo responders, but also state anxiety bore a variable relationship to pain tolerance in a study of placebo analgesia (Richardson 1994). The anxiety reduction hypothesis in the context of pain is complicated by the relationship between pain and anxiety, especially when physiological indices are measured (Gross and Collins 1980). Another consideration is the relationship between anxiety and stress on the one hand and the phenomenon of stress-induced analgesia on the other. It might be expected that (stress-induced) anxiety may in fact reduce pain (Richardson 1994).

Conditioning

The conditioning theory for the explanation of placebo phenomena arises out of the observation of learning through association. Classical conditioning has been induced in animals (Ader 1985; Pavlov 1927) and humans (Voudouris et al. 1985, 1989, 1990). The principle is the linking of an unconditioned stimulus (US), such as an effective drug, that evokes an unconditioned response (UR), with features of the treatment setting, including persons, places, or things, such that those neutral features themselves alone may elicit a component of the UR. Thus, those neutral stimuli become conditioned stimuli (CS) and elicit a conditioned response (CR). Diagrammatically:

i) US ➨ UR

ii) US + CS ➨ UR (conditioning step)

iii) CS ➨ CR

Placebo *responses* can be conditioned in humans. Voudouris et al. (1985, 1989, 1990) performed conditioning trials in which a neutral cream was associated with reduction in experimental iontophoretically induced cutaneous pain. When the same levels of experimental pain were then administered with and without the cream, subjects who had received the conditioning reported a lower response (less pain) with the cream than control subjects. That is:

i) experimental stimulus ➨ pain

ii) lowered stimulus + neutral cream ➨ less pain (conditioning step)

iii) experimental stimulus + neutral cream ➨ less pain

As responses to a placebo can be conditioned by pairing with an experimental stimulus, it follows that responses to a non-placebo may also be modified by pairing with neutral stimuli; that is, a contextual response may be conditioned.

i) non-placebo analgesic in clinical pain	➡	reduction in pain
ii) non-placebo analgesic + white uniform	➡	reduction in pain (conditioning step)
iii) white uniform	➡	some reduction in pain

This model posits that environmental settings (therapists, uniforms, syringes, pills, rituals) that have been associated with ameliorative effects may thereby become conditioned stimuli for the alleviation of symptoms. Similarly, the association of neutral stimuli with aversive stimuli could condition negative or nocebo effects.

The implications of this model are profound (Peck and Coleman 1991; Wickramasekera 1985). Given that learning (or conditioning) is inevitable, the response to a drug, for example, will comprise an UR (non-placebo response) *and* a CR (placebo or contextual effect). This provides one basis for understanding variability in responses between and within subjects: individual learning differences arising out of having experienced particular forms of treatment in particular contexts. Through response generalization, positive and negative CRs may potentiate or attenuate responses to subsequent treatments. It follows that to maintain a strong contextual effect (CR), the treatment environment must be associated regularly with effective treatment. The use of powerful non-placebos will enhance the contextual component of effect; the use of weak non-placebos or placebos will attenuate the non-placebo (UR) component of effect. This is particularly relevant in chronic conditions, where negative contextual effects (nocebo effects) from ineffective therapy may generalize, attenuating responses to a subsequent potent, otherwise effective treatment (unconditioned stimulus), be that a treatment or a treatment provider.

Expectancy

Classical conditioning is considered to be a predominantly non-cognitive process of learning through association. However in humans, it is difficult to exclude a cognitive component, especially one so potentially powerful as expectancy. It is almost axiomatic that the expectations of subject, clinician, and researcher will influence the outcomes of clinical or experimental therapies. Expectation here is synonymous with faith, hope, belief, and confidence, and can interact with desire and emotion (Vase et al. 2003). In this situation, it is important to avoid teleological reasoning: that placebo (contextual) effect occurred because it was expected by the patient.

Like conditioning, expectation is a learned phenomenon, and indeed any distinction between the two may be artificial. There appears to be a reciprocal relationship between expectancy and conditioning, as expectancies may be formed through conditioning and conditioning may be expressed as expectancy. If there is in fact a difference between them, it may be related to (classical) conditioning being attributed to unconscious passive learning of relatively trivial behaviours, whereas expectations are held to arise from conscious cognitive learning. However, examination of conditioned (or, more correctly, conditional) learning suggests that simple stimulus–response associations are an insufficient explanation (Dickenson 1987).

The question arises as to whether expectancies can be formed in the absence of direct experience, that is, through observation, information, or persuasion (Bootzin 1985; Evans 1985; Kirsch 1985). Studies of alcohol ingestion found that when individuals have expectancies that are contrary to the drug's pharmacological effect, their expectancies prevail (Kirsch 1985). By contrast, in their studies of conditioned placebo analgesia, Voudouris et al. (1989, 1990) found that the direct experience of conditioning was more powerful than expectancy through verbal persuasion. In replicating these experiments, however, Montgomery and Kirsch (1997) added the modification of informing one group of subjects that stimulus intensity would be lowered during the 'conditioning' period and thereby eliminated the development of placebo analgesia.

The mechanism of expectancies remains unclear. One proposal suggests that, given that pain and illness are appreciated as aversive events beyond one's control, an expectancy that treatment may exert some control over those events may reduce anxiety, stress, and feelings of being unable to cope. Consistent with that view would be observations that placebos may be most effective in anxious patients (Evans 1985) and that there may be a larger proportion of placebo responders in clinical pain states than in experimental pain states (Beecher 1959). Other learning processes such as past experience and social observation may modulate expectancy and conditioning (Colloca and Benedetti 2006).

Expectancy or conditioning?

Many of the findings in the placebo literature can be explained equally well by either approach (Stewart-Williams and Podd 2004). Montgomery and Kirsch (1997) argued that conditioning trials themselves can be viewed as expectancy manipulations. They claimed that (classical) conditioning is not sufficient, and that expectation of therapeutic effect is necessary for placebo responses. Given that it is unlikely that classical (that is, non-cognitive) conditioning occurs in humans (Dickenson 1987), it seems probable that the learning through association proposed by the conditioned placebo model to explain clinical contextual effects is mediated by expectancy. This was supported by Price et al. (1999) who found that, although classical conditioning may occur, expectancy—whether subtly or overtly induced—was the proximal mediator of placebo analgesic responses. A role for desire for pain relief as a contributor to those responses was not supported.

An integrative view is that some instances of conditioning may be mediated by the creation or adjustment of an explicit expectancy, while in other cases, the link between a conditioning stimulus and the conditioned response may not be mediated by conscious cognition (Stewart-Williams and Podd 2004). Put another way, most placebo responses are linked to expectancies, and conditioning is one of a number of factors by which these expectancies can be produced and altered (Kirsch 2004). Indeed, there may be only one example in the human literature in which expectancy could not be invoked: conditioned respiratory depression induced by exposure to buprenorphine (Benedetti et al. 1999).

Neurobiological mechanisms

Most research into the neurobiology of the placebo response has concerned the reduction in pain experienced after administration of a placebo. The evolving biochemical and anatomical neural correlates of placebo phenomena promise increased insight into the psychologically determined mechanisms.

Endogenous opioids

The proposition that activation of endogenous opioids may mediate placebo phenomena arose out of the use of the opioid antagonist naloxone, administered in a double-blind design in association with placebo analgesic, in the context of pain after third molar tooth extraction (Levine et al. 1978). Naloxone was shown also to antagonize placebo-induced analgesia in an experimental ischaemic arm pain model (Amanzio and Benedetti 1999) and to affect placebo-induced respiratory depression (Benedetti et al. 1999). The demonstration of higher concentration of endorphins in the cerebrospinal fluid of placebo responders compared with non-responders lends further support for the role of endogenous opioids in placebo analgesia (Lipman et al. 1990).

Other neurotransmitters

Cholecystokinin (CCK) appears to play an inhibitory (anti-analgesic) role in placebo analgesia and to be involved in the opposite of placebo analgesia, nocebo hyperalgesia (Benedetti et al. 2006). These opposing effects of endogenous opioids and CCK have also been shown in mood disorders (Hebb et al. 2005). Dopamine has also been implicated in nocebo hyperalgesia (Scott et al. 2008).

Insights from neuroimaging

Using positron-emission tomography, patterns of brain activation during placebo analgesia were similar to those after exogenous opioid administration (Petrovic et al. 2002), while altered neural activity in opioid-rich areas in the brain has been shown in the course of placebo manipulation in an experimental pain protocol (Zubieta et al. 2005). These findings have been correlated with functional magnetic resonance imaging (Wager et al. 2007).

Implications of placebo theory for musculoskeletal medicine

The major source of theory underlying placebo phenomena has been experimental manipulation of placebo response: that this has mostly focused on analgesia makes discussion highly relevant to musculoskeletal medicine. The challenge is how to apply these inferences from the experimental situation, where the 'treatment' is the neutral partner in the pairing, to the clinical situation, where the environment or context plays that role.

Implications for practice

The expectancy/conditioning models of placebo effect suggest that it is the context of a treatment rather than the patient or the treatment itself that determines a variably significant component of any patient's response. Given that under the right circumstances, anyone might become a placebo responder, the model predicts that every interaction with medical or other therapeutic professionals plays a role in determining the contextual (placebo) component of a person's future response to treatment. The challenge is how these factors can be harnessed to enhance positive contextual (placebo) effects and limit negative contextual (nocebo) effects (Chaput de Saintonge and Herxheimer 1994; Peck and Coleman 1991; Wickramasekera 1985).

Exploitation of positive contextual effects does not extend to the use of known inert treatments (placebos). This raises the ethical question of whether a clinician should institute or persist with treatment that has been shown to be no better than 'placebo'. A recent review of 57 reviews on acupuncture concluded that there was little convincing evidence that the technique is effective in reducing pain. That is, any outcome is attributable to contextual effect only—and may not be without harm (Ernst et al. 2011). While (informed) deception in studies of placebo research raises one set of issues, the question of using a known placebo to elicit contextual effect in clinical practice entails another set of concerns (Miller et al. 2005; Price et al. 2008).

By contrast, the theory predicts that known placebos (as conditioning stimuli) may be of most effect when paired with powerful non-placebos; that is, drug and placebo rather than drug or placebo (Ader 1985). An example is the use of the pain cocktail, where the unconditioned stimulus (the powerful non-placebo) is paired with a neutral conditioning stimulus (the placebo) and then gradually withdrawn. Ethical principles are not violated: patients are informed about the withdrawal but remain unaware of its timing. Thus, it may be possible to achieve the same effect at a lower dosage of the powerful non-placebo.

Irrespectively of ethical considerations concerning the therapeutic use of known placebos, it is not necessary to use a placebo to enhance a contextual (placebo) effect, as a component of the latter involved is in every non-placebo treatment. Choice of size, colour, or route of administration of non-placebo treatments may manipulate response, as may pairing with specific suggestions (Chaput de Saintonge and Herxheimer 1994). Expectancies related to the context of treatment may be enhancing factors, such as the credibility of the therapist, of the therapeutic setting, and of the specific treatment itself, including the credibility of the ritual of administration (Wickramasekera 1985).

Lastly, in this arena of enhancing contextual (placebo) effects is the importance of assessing treatment history, including past experiences of treatments and expectations, as the contextual component of such past interactions may have had a positive or negative effect on the non-placebo component (Voudouris et al. 1985). The high rate of non-compliance suggests that therapists need to assess directly their patients' expectations of the effectiveness of treatment and be prepared to receive and discuss feedback (Peck and King 1986).

The other side of this coin is to limit negative contextual (nocebo) effects. In the context of musculoskeletal medicine, chronic pain conditions are unsuccessfully treated pain problems. Expectancy/conditioning theory predicts that the experience of many and varied unsuccessful treatments may contribute to extinction of the contextual component which, in turn, may attenuate the effectiveness of even powerful non-placebos (Peck and Coleman 1991; Wickramasekera 1985). This consideration implies that therapists should be aware of the effects of over-servicing patients with chronic pain, especially when the treatments used have questionable efficacy and may in fact be pure placebos. As well as contributing to the phenomenon of extinction, the failure of placebo treatments that are believed by the patient to be non-placebo treatments may lead to reinforcement of illness or disability. It follows that the use of known placebos for 'diagnostic' purposes is fundamentally flawed.

Implications for research

The expectancy/conditioning models take into account the experience of the individual and the consequent potential for modifying both the contextual effect of non-placebo treatments and the response to known placebos themselves. In musculoskeletal medicine, with its major clinical feature of pain, an important factor in research design is the choice of appropriate controls (Kleijnen et al. 1994; Peck and Coleman 1991). In pharmacotherapeutic studies, the usual comparison of parallel groups under double-blind conditions fails to control for expectancy. To counter this, a 'balanced placebo' design has been suggested, in which half the subjects are told that they will receive the drug and the other half that they will not. Within each of these two groups, half actually receive the drug and the other half does not. This design generates four groups, to cater for all combinations of drug and expectancies (Marlatt and Roshenow 1980).

The complicated interaction between expectancy and efficacy may also apply to within-subject designs in clinical trials. It has been shown that there is an order effect: placebos administered after effective non-placebos were rated as more effective than when administered before effective non-placebos (Kantor et al. 1966). Modifications of the balanced placebo design have been proposed, to control for such order effects (Koch et al. 1989) and for the expectancies of the administrators of the trial as well as those of the subjects (Rosenthal 1985).

Meta-analysis has added new caveats contingent upon placebo phenomena. In such a review of trials of non-steroidal anti-inflammatory drugs (NSAIDs), no significant difference in response was found between patients receiving an NSAID in comparative studies and those receiving the same NSAID in placebo-controlled studies (Gøtzsche 1993). By contrast, the same NSAID was likely to be rated as less efficacious and associated with fewer withdrawals due to adverse effect when administered in a placebo trial than when administered in a comparative trial (Rochon et al. 1999). These findings were attributed to subjects' knowledge of the type of trial in which they were involved, as predicted by placebo theory. This led to the suggestion that placebo-controlled trials may be more appropriate for evaluation of efficacy and comparative trials may be more appropriate for assessment of adverse effects.

The magnitude of the placebo effect in trials has attracted attention. Traditionally in randomized clinical trials, the placebo condition serves as a control for an active treatment under study. Such studies rarely include a no-treatment group that might control for natural history. In that case, there is no way of knowing whether participants would have improved without the placebo. Indeed, an influential meta-analysis of 114 trials in different conditions in which patients were randomly assigned to either placebo or no treatment found that placebos had no significant pooled effect on subjective or objective binary or continuous outcomes (Hrøbjartsson and Gøtzsche 2001). In the 27 of those trials that involved the treatment of pain, placebo did have a beneficial effect, although a small sample in many cases limited that interpretation (Hrøbjartsson and Gøtzsche 2001; Stewart-Williams and Podd 2004).

However, most studies that address the placebo analgesic effect in its own right do show a distinct difference in pain levels between the placebo condition and the no-treatment natural history condition. This was supported in two meta-analyses, one of 23 studies (from the 27 mentioned in the preceding paragraph) that used placebo as a control condition and one of 14 studies in which placebo analgesia mechanisms themselves were investigated. Magnitudes of placebo analgesic effects were much higher in the latter (mean effect size 0.95) compared with the former (mean effect size 0.15). The authors found also that placebo suggestions combined with conditioning led to a greater placebo analgesia effect than suggestion or conditioning alone (Vase et al. 2002).

To some extent in pharmacotherapeutic research, the introduction of the 'number needed to treat' (NNT) technique in reporting trial results has acknowledged the pervasiveness of contextual effects. Rather than quote a response rate of subjects to a drug, NNT focuses on the number of patients who need to be treated in order for one of them to achieve a successful outcome who would not have done so with placebo (Cook and Sackett 1995). Mathematically, NNT is the reciprocal of the difference between the experimental response rate and the control response rate. A NNT of less than four is considered to reflect an effective therapy. Trial designs that include a no-treatment 'response' rate might change this consideration.

Extension of these principles to studies (as well as to practice) of physical therapy (Gam et al. 1993), to invasive techniques including surgery (Ernst et al. 2011; Johnson 1994), and indeed to psychotherapy (Horvath 1988; Kirsch 2004) poses particular challenges. The often-quoted double-blind study of internal mammary artery ligation for angina pectoris (Cobb et al. 1959) raises the question of contextual effect in all invasive procedures, while the effect of sham ultrasound on pain (and swelling) following wisdom-tooth extraction (Hashish et al. 1988) suggests that non-invasive technology also cannot escape these considerations. In the context of musculoskeletal medicine, there is an onus on researchers (and clinicians) seeking to demonstrate the specific effects of physical therapies to be especially mindful of these implications of placebo theory.

Implications for training

With its assertion of the importance of context, placebo theory embraces the clinical interaction itself and how that may determine expectancies (Shapiro and Morris 1978). Factors include aspects of the doctor or therapist's behaviour such as friendliness; consideration of patients' concerns; provision of time; clear explanations of diagnosis, prognosis, and treatment; enthusiasm for treatment; and the choice of words, gestures, or other non-verbal forms of communication. Consideration of these interactional skills follows from expectancy theory, and it has been argued that they should be accorded as much priority in training as the attaining of medical knowledge (Friedman and DiMatteo 1982). This has been formalized as 'engage, empathise, educate, enlist and end' as components in every patient encounter in order to maximize contextual effects (Jamison 2011).

Conclusions on placebo theory

The phenomenon of placebo or contextual effect pervades all forms of therapy. Placebo phenomena have been addressed more through psychological than neurobiological approaches, although the convergence of these holds much promise. A combination of expectancy and conditioning models provides the greatest explanatory power for these phenomena in the current state of knowledge. Both practitioners and researchers in musculoskeletal medicine need to be aware of the complex interactions that constitute the healing process and to incorporate recognition of contextual factors into their endeavours.

References

Ader R. Conditioned immunopharmacological effects in animals: implications for a conditioning model of pharmacotherapy. In: White L, Tursky B, Schwartz GE. (eds) *Placebo: theory, research, and mechanisms*. London: Guildford Press; 1985, pp. 306–23.

Amanzio M, Benedetti F. Neuropharmacological dissection of placebo analgesia: expectation-activated opioid systems versus conditioning-activated specific sub-systems. *J Neurosci* 1999; 19:484–94.

Beecher HK. *Measurement of subjective responses.* New York: Oxford University Press;1959.

Benedetti F. *Placebo effects: understanding the mechanism in health and disease.* Oxford: Oxford University Press; 2008.

Benedetti F, Amanzio M, Baldi SD, Casadio C, Maggi G. Inducing placebo respiratory depressant responses in humans via opioid receptors. *Europ J Neurosci* 1999; 11:625–31.

Benedetti F, Amanzio M, Vighetti S, et al. The biochemical and neuroendocrine basis of the hyperalgesic nocebo effect. *J Neurosci* 2006; 26:12014–22.

Bootzin RR. The role of expectancy in behaviour change. In: White L, Tursky B, Schwartz GE. (eds) *Placebo: theory, research, and mechanisms.* London: Guildford Press; 1985, pp. 196–210.

Brody H. Placebo effect: an examination of Grünbaum's definition. In: White L, Tursky B, Schwartz GE. (eds) *Placebo: theory, research, and mechanisms.* London: Guildford Press; 1985, pp. 37–58.

Chaput de Saintonge DM, Herxheimer A. Harnessing placebo effects in healthcare. *Lancet* 1994; 344:995–8.

Cobb LA, Thomas GI, Dillard DH, Merendino KA, Bruce RA. An evaluation of internal mammary artery ligation by a double-blind technic. *New Eng J Med* 1959; 20:1115–8.

Colloca L, Benedetti F. How prior experience shapes placebo analgesia. *Pain* 2006; 124:126–33.

Cook RJ, Sackett DL. The number needed to treat: a clinically useful measure of treatment effect. *Brit Med J* 1995; 310:452–4.

Dickenson A. Conditioning. In: Gregory RL. (ed.) *The Oxford companion to the mind.* Oxford: Oxford University Press; 1987, pp. 159–60.

Ernst E, Myeong SL, Choi T-Y. Acupuncture: does it alleviate pain and are there serious risks? A review of reviews. *Pain* 2011; 152:755–64.

Evans FJ. Expectancy, therapeutic instructions and the placebo response. In: White L, Tursky B, Schwartz GE. (eds) *Placebo: theory, research, and mechanisms.* London: Guildford Press; 1985, pp. 215–28.

Evans FJ. The placebo response and pain reduction. In: Bonica JJ. (ed.) *Advances in neurology, Vol 4.* New York: Raven Press; 1974, pp. 289–96.

Finniss DG, Kaptchuk TJ, Miller F, Benedetti F. Biological, clinical, and ethical advances of placebo effects. *Lancet* 2010; 375:686–95.

Friedman HS, DiMatteo MR. (eds) *Interpersonal issues in health care.* New York: Academic Press; 1982.

de la Fuente-Fernandez R, Stoessl AJ. The placebo effect in Parkinson's disease. *Trends Neurosci* 2002; 25:302–6.

Gam AN, Thorsen H, Lønnberg F. The effect of low level laser therapy on musculokeletal pain: a meta-analysis. *Pain* 1993; 52:63–6.

Gøtzsche PC. Is there logic in the placebo? *Lancet* 1994; 344:925–6.

Gøtzsche PC. Meta-analysis of NSAIDs: contribution of drugs, doses, trial design and meta-analytic techniques. *Scand J Rheum* 1993; 22:255–60.

Gross RT, Collins FL. On the relationship between anxiety and pain: a methodological confounding. *Clin Psychol Rev* 1980; 1:375–86.

Harrington A. (ed.) *Placebo: probing the self-healing brain.* Boston: Harvard University Press; 1997.

Hashish I, Feinman C, Harvey W. Reduction of post-operative pain and swelling by ultrasound: a placebo effect. *Pain* 1988; 83:303–11.

Hebb AL, Poulin J-F, Roach SP, Zacharko RM, Drolet G. Cholecystokinin and endogenous opioid peptides: interactive influence on pain, cognition and emotion. *Prog Neuropsychopharm Biol Psychiat* 2005; 29:1225–38.

Horvath P. Placebos and common factors in two decades of psychotherapy research. *Psychol Bulletin* 1988; 104:214–25.

Hrøbjartsson A, Gøtzsche PC. Is the placebo powerless? An analysis of clinical trials comparing placebo with no treatment. *New Eng J Med* 2001; 21:1594–601.

Jamison RN. Nonspecific treatment effects in pain medicine. *IASP Pain Clinical Updates*, XIX(2), 2011.

Johnson AG. Surgery as a placebo. *Lancet* 1994; 344:1140–2.

Kantor TG, Sunshine A, Laska E, Meisner M, Hopper M. Oral analgesic studies: pentazocine hydrochloride, codeine, aspirin and placebo and their influence on response to placebo. *Clin Pharmacol Ther* 966; 7:447–54.

Kirsch I. Conditioning, expectancy, and the placebo effect: comment on Stewart-Willians and Podd (2004). *Psychol Bulletin* 2004; 130:341–3.

Kirsch, I. Response expectancy as a determinant of experience and behaviour. *Amer Psychol* 1985; 40:1189–202.

Kirsch I, Sapirstein G. Listening to Prozac but hearing placebo: a meta-analysis of antidepressant medications. In: Kirsch I. (ed.) *How expectancies shape experience.* Washington DC: American Psychological Association; 1999, pp. 303–20.

Kleijnen J, de Craen AJM, van Everdingen J, Kro L. Placebo effect in double-blind clinical trials: a review of interactions with medications. *Lancet* 1994; 344:1347–9.

Koch GG, Amara IM, Brown BW, Colton T, Gillings DB. A two-period cross-over design for the comparison of two active treatments and placebo. *Statis Med* 1989; 8:487–504.

Lasagna L, Laties VG, Dohan JL. Further studies on the 'pharmacology' of placebo administration. *J Clin Invest* 1958; 37:533–7.

Levine JD, Gordon NC, Fields HL. The mechanism of placebo analgesia. *Lancet* 1978; 3:654–7.

Liberman R. An experimental study of the placebo response under three different situations of pain. *J Psychiatr Research* 1964; 2:233–46.

Lipman JJ, Miller BE, Mays KS, et al. Peak beta-endorphin concentration in cerebrospinal fluid: reduced in chronic pain patients and increased during the placebo response. *Psychopharmacol* 1990; 102:112–6.

Marlatt GA, Roshenow DJ. Cognitive processes in alcohol use: expectancy and the balanced placebo design. In: Mello NK. (ed.) *Advances in substance abuse: behavioural and biological research.* Greenwich CT: JAI Press; 1980, pp. 150–9.

McQuay H, Carroll D, Moore A. Variation in the placebo effect in randomised controlled trials: all is as blind as it seems. *Pain* 1995; 64:331–5.

Miller FG, Wendler D, Swartzman LC. Deception in research on the placebo effect. *PloS Med* 2005; 2:e262.

Montgomery GH, Kirsch I. Classical conditioning and the placebo effect. *Pain* 1997; 72:107–13.

Pavlov I. *Conditioned reflexes.* London: Oxford Press; 1927.

Peck C, Coleman G. Implications of placebo theory for clinical research and practice in pain management. *Theor Med* 1991; 12:247–70.

Peck C, Coleman G. Implications of placebo theory for clinical research and practice in pain management. *Theor Med* 1991; 12:247–70.

Peck C, King NJ Medical compliance. In: King NJ, Remenyi A. (eds) *Health care: a behavioural approach.* New York: Grune & Stratton; 1986, pp. 185–92.

Petrovic P, Kalso E, Petersson KM, Ingvar M. Placebo and opioid analgesia—imaging a shared neuronal network. *Science* 2002; 295:1737–40.

Price DD, Finniss DG, Benedetti F. A comprehensive review of the placebo effects: recent advances and current thought. *Annu Rev Psychol* 2008; 48:33–60.

Price DD, Milling LS, Kirsch I, Duff A, Montgomery GH, Nicholl, SS. An analysis of factors that contribute to the magnitude of placebo analgesia in an experimental paradigm. *Pain* 1999; 83:147–56.

Richardson PH. Placebo effects in pain management. *Pain Reviews* 1994; 1:15–32.

Rochon PA, Binns MA, Litner JA, et al. Are randomized controlled trial outcomes influenced by the inclusion of a placebo group? A systematic review of nonsteroidal anti-inflammatory drug trials for arthritis treatment. *J Clin Epidem* 1999; 52:113–22.

Rosenthal R. Designing, analyzing, interpreting and summarizing placebo studies. In: White L, Tursky B, Schwartz GE. (eds) *Placebo: theory, research, and mechanisms.* London: Guildford Press; 1985, p. 110–36.

Scott DJ, Stohler CS, Egnatuk CM, Wang H, Koeppe RA, Zubieta JK. Placebo and nocebo effects are defined by opposite opioid and dopaminergic responses. *Arch Gen Psychiatry* 2008; 65:220–31.

Shapiro AK, Morris LA. The placebo effect in medical and psychological therapies. In: Bergin AE, Garfield S. (eds) *Handbook of psychotherapy and behavioural change* (2nd edn). New York: John Wiley; 1978, pp. 369–410.

Stewart-Williams S, Podd J. The placebo effect: dissolving the expectancy versus conditioning debate. *Psychol Bull* 2004; 130:324–40.

Turner JA, Deyo RA, Loeser JD, Von Korff M, Fordyce WE. The importance of placebo effects in pain treatment and research. *J Amer Med Assoc* 1994; 271:1609–14.

Vase L, Riley JL, Price DD. A comparison of placebo effects in clinical analgesic trials versus studies of placebo analgesia. *Pain* 2002; 99: 443–52.

Vase L, Robinson ME, Verne GN, Price DD. The contributions of suggestion, desire and expectation to placebo effects in irritable bowel syndrome patients. An empirical investigation. *Pain* 2003; 105:17–25.

Voudouris NJ, Peck CL, Coleman G. Conditioned placebo responses. *J Pers Soc Psychol* 1985; 48:47–53.

Voudouris NJ, Peck CL, Coleman G. Conditioned response models of placebo phenomena. *Pain* 1989; 38:109–16.

Voudouris NJ, Peck CL, Coleman G. The role of conditioning and verbal expectancy in the placebo response. *Pain* 1990; 43:121–8.

Wager TD, Scott DJ, Zubieta JK. Placebo effects on human mu-opioid activity during pain. *Proc Nat Acad Sci* 2007; 104:11056–61.

Wall PD. The placebo effect: an unpopular topic. *Pain* 1992; 51:1–3.

White L, Tursky B, Schwartz GE. (eds) *Placebo: theory, research, and mechanisms.* London: Guildford Press; 1985.

Whitney CW, Von Korff M. Regression to the mean in treated versus untreated chronic pain. *Pain* 1992; 50:281–5.

Wickramasekera I. A conditioned response model of the placebo effect: predictions from the model. In: White L, Tursky B, Schwartz GE. (eds) *Placebo: theory, research, and mechanisms.* London: Guildford Press; 1985, pp. 255–87.

Zubieta JK, Bueller JA, Jackson LR, et al. Placebo effects mediated by endogenous opioid activity on mu-opioid receptors. *J Neurosci* 2005; 25:7754–62.

Chapter 22

Functional disorders of the spine in small children

Heiner Biedermann

Introduction to functional disorders of the spine in small children

In order to understand the adult, we are well advised to look at the child, and even more so at the baby. Close contact with small children and their problems helps us to come to grips with the potential of functional disorders in influencing the long-term development in adults. Internal medicine examines this with laboratory findings or radiological tools—manual medicine looks for patterns of (mal-) function. Most of those active in this field have a tendency to assume laboratory pathologies can only be influenced by biochemical tools (i.e. pharmacologically). Accustomed to the 'gold standard' of double-blinded trials, one disregards any involvement above the biochemical level as 'soft' or 'fuzzy'. From headache to depression, from vertigo to obesity, drugs rule.

Those of us busy in the realm of musculoskeletal medicine know from daily experience about the enormous influence that a well-crafted intervention can have. We know that the change initiated functionally can be documented in changes of laboratory parameters (e.g. blood pressure) (Bakris et al. 2007). We know, too, that this effect depends on several specific factors which render it impossible to turn this into an arbitrarily multipliable product on an industrial scale. The older our patients are, the more we deal with an individual marked and altered by his/her biography. It is impossible to squeeze these cases into a chi-squarable mould—lest we invent scores of scores which, more often than not, do render this complex readily computable, but utterly meaningless.

In small children, we deal with a situation which offers us several advantages:

- Their case history is rather short and clear. Besides the delivery details and some findings from the intra-uterine period, there is not much to consider.
- The other influencing factors are mostly genetic (i.e. information from the family history) and thus reasonably easily identifiable.
- The reaction pattern of infants is much more predictable than in adolescents or adults.
- The positive effects of manual therapy encompass the entire psychosomatic equilibrium, reaching much further often till adult life.

Most physicians specializing in manual medicine are used to dealing with adults. Treating adolescents confronts them with another kind of patient—and small children are even more different. This starts with the mechanical aspect: as the chondral part of the joints is much greater in toddlers, their examination yields haptically quite distinctive sensations. Translating these into meaningful information necessitates more than a tuning down of the situation found in adults. The interaction with small patients starts with the mothers, whose confidence has to be earned first. Only then can one even start to come to grips (in the true sense of the word) with the small patient him/herself. Deep palpation and—finally—the manipulation itself 'feel' different in small children. This is due to the already mentioned chondral domination, but is also aggravated by the much thicker subcutaneous fat stratum, which has a different consistency in adults.

So, we have a patient who is in most cases not overly willing to co-operate, a nervous mother next to us, and a palpation pattern we are not used to—small wonder that many colleagues give up trying faster than they started.

However, treating newborns can be extremely rewarding and, often, just one intervention can change the basic parameters of an individual's development for the decades to come. In the last few years, we were able to compile the data that substantiate these assertions.

The special situation regarding development in small children

As much as 'form follows function' is true for the fully developed individual, 'function determines form' should be the slogan for the years before, and especially during the months after birth. The Swiss biologist, A. Portmann, described babies in their first year as 'living in a social uterus'[1]:

> This is a critical year for the human development, as the maturation is taken out of the well-equilibrated milieu of the mother's womb

[1] A. Portmann (1998): „Das Jahr im ‚sozialen Uterus' ist entscheidend, weil damit das für höhere Säuger normale späte Ausreifen aller Strukturen im gleichmässigen, reizarmen, mütterlichen Medium in eine an Reizen reiche, wechselvolle Sozialwelt verlegt wird. Gerade in diesem der Uteruszeit abgewonnenen Jahr wird die aufrechte Haltung, das Sprechen, das Denken ausgebildet—(. . .) durch eine Kombination von biologischen Reifungsprozessen und sozial bedingten Lernprozessen"

into an extremely stimulating and varied social context. During this time posture, speech and thought are developed by a combination of biological maturation and socially induced learning processes. (Portmann 1998)

This unique situation of developmental potential on one side and extreme vulnerability on the other is the hallmark of these first months. The adequate stimuli and the right internal equilibrium co-operate to lay the foundation of all later sensorimotor, cognitive, and intellectual formation. Function dominates, form is secondary and adapts with extreme flexibility.

Knowledge of this special situation helps in the treatment of older patients, too. The morphological facts established during the first year of life exert a life-long influence on function of the spinal engine (Gracovetsky 1988). A better understanding of the interaction between the genetic predisposition and the individual birth trauma improves the precision with which patients suitable for manual therapy can be selected, as signs of functional disorders in early childhood increase the probability of a relevant influence of similar problems later on in life.

The reason why disturbances at the beginning of neuromotor development exert such a wide-ranging influence lies in the realization that we rarely 'unlearn' an acquired pattern. As Jaques Brel put it in his famous chanson, 'we don't forget anything, we just get used to it'[2]. So, whatever baggage we get saddled with in early childhood can influence our behaviour years and decades later. This makes the understanding of neuromotor development at the beginning of our life so important. The post-natal period is paramount for our understanding of this process, as it is the first moment where we are able to actively and directly influence these developments. A lot of other factors are essential during this time, first of which is the equilibrated and loving atmosphere at the baby's home, with as much bodily contact as possible. To cast the net even wider, one has to evaluate the socio-economic status of the family and its social integration into a local community—also a dimension of well-being often overlooked and/or underestimated.

Even if we were able to take these items into account when evaluating the child's future, we would not be in a situation to do much about it. The big advantage of manual medicine at this age is that it gives us an opportunity to improve the situation of a child without interfering with the other forms of help available and—last not least—without a big investment in time and energy. We are able to help children even in situations where other forms of therapy would not work because the amount of discipline and persistence is not realistically expectable from the families concerned.

The one prerequisite necessary should, in any case, not be forgotten or underestimated: the children have to be brought to somebody for manual therapy first. This implies an awareness of the potential of manual therapy in the parents and/or other adults involved in the upbringing of the children. The clinical patterns where it is worthwhile to send the babies have to be communicated and this has to be done efficiently.

Clinical patterns of vertebrogenic disorders in small children

The leading symptom of vertebrogenic disorders in babies is a fixed and asymmetrical posture. We see two main types of fixed asymmetry: fixed lateroflexion (i.e. the classic 'muscular torticollis') and fixed retroflexion (often confounded with neurological problems).

A wide overlap exists between these two. The symptoms vary according to the main postural imbalance. We have proposed the acronym KISS (Kinematic Imbalances caused by Suboccipital Strain). The risk factors we found in our statistics (Biedermann 1992, 1993) are:

long labour

extraction with vacuum, etc.

twins or triplets

prenatal positional anomalies.

Any combination of these factors is possible. An obliquely positioned fetus has more difficulties in adapting to the contortions of the birth canal, and long labour often results in the use of extraction aids, etc. The common denominator is the mechanical stress exerted on the most vulnerable structures (i.e. the cerebral tissues and the occipito-cervical area with its high density of sensory and transport structures).

KISS I: fixed lateroflexion

Symptoms of KISS I (Figure 22.1) are:

- torticollis
- unilateral microsomia
- asymmetry of the skull

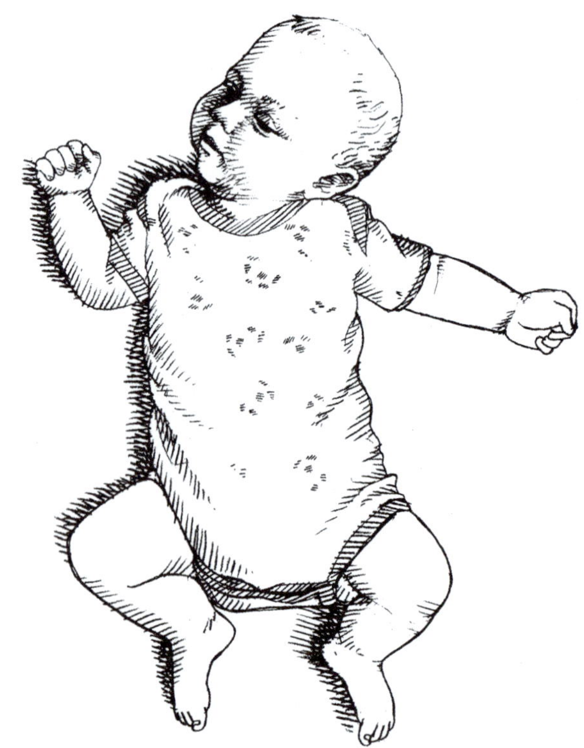

Figure 22.1 In KISS I, the fixed lateroflexion results in a torticollis, which leads to a morphologically relevant asymmetry, starting from the head and encompassing the entire body later on.

[2] 'On oublie rien de rien, on s'habitue, c'est tout'

- C-scoliosis of the neck and trunk
- asymmetry of the gluteal area
- asymmetry of motion of the limbs
- unilateral retardation of motor development.

In KISS I, the fixed lateroflexion results in a torticollis, which leads to a morphologically relevant asymmetry, starting from the head and encompassing the entire body later on.

KISS 2: fixed retroflexion

Symptoms of KISS II (Figure 22.2) are:

- hyperextension (during sleep)
- (asymmetric) occipital flattening
- shoulders pulled up
- fixed supination of the arms
- cannot lift trunk from ventral position
- orofacial muscular hypotonia with aerophagia
- breastfeeding difficult on one side.

These two basic types can overlap, but in most cases, one component is the most relevant, leading the clinical picture.

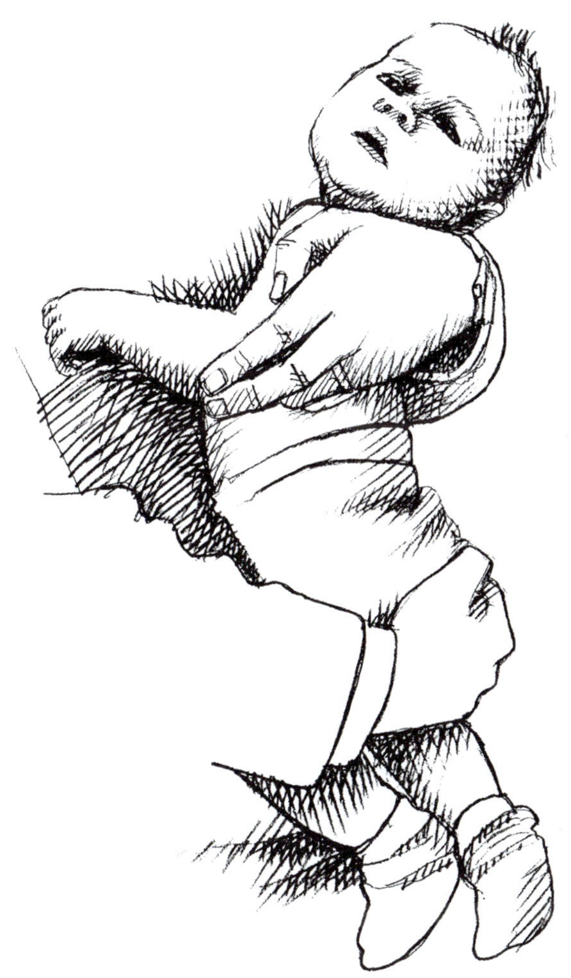

Figure 22.2 KISS II starts with a fixed hyperextension, leading to the flattened back of the head, the protectively raised shoulders.

Pathogenetic model of vertebrogenic problems in small children

The common denominator for functional problems of the spine in newborns is a fixed posture due to pain avoidance. Several factors contribute to the reaction pattern:

- family history (i.e. predisposition for vertebrogenic problems)
- individual pain threshold
- base level of muscular tonus
- degree of trauma intra-utero or during birth
- location of trauma, resulting in different postural preferences
- cultural influences (e.g. dorsal sleeping position to avoid sudden infant death syndrome—SIDS).

The enormous plasticity of the skull and vertebrae results in visible asymmetries after only a few weeks of fixed posture. Function influences form very rapidly indeed, immediately after birth. Often this skull asymmetry is mistakenly considered a primary cause of other problems observed in these babies, leading to the proposition of orthotic correction. We were able to show that this costly manoeuvre is unnecessary, as the cranial asymmetry can be reliably corrected by treating the primary problem, the fixed posture. Symmetric and active movement is the best remedy for cranial asymmetry after the stress of the upper cervical spine is taken care of.

Manual therapy (chiropractics, osteopathy, etc.) is a craft, something one learns by doing and something where the, by now, famous 10,000 hours rule (Ericsson 2008; Ericsson et al. 1993; Gladwell 2008; Sennet 2008) applies unreservedly. During the training of a student, the teacher can give background information, details of 'how to', and guide the hand of the apprentice. However, the difficult part of learning and absorbing whatever needs to be absorbed takes time—the aforementioned timeframe is not the worst guess: 'it seems that it takes the brain as long (as 10,000 hours) to assimilate all that it needs to know to achieve true mastery' (Levitin 2006). So yes, we can give a general idea about the how and how much, but at the end of the day, the eventual success of the manipulation depends to a large extent on the proficiency of the individual caregiver.

After several decades of teaching, it can be said that most beginners overestimate the number of treatments necessary and the force needed, and underestimate the reaction time to a well-placed manipulation. Time and again, we have shown that the maximum effect attainable needs three basics:

- no mechanical irritation to the cervical spine in the days before the treatment
- sufficient time afterwards to let the body react
- the right set-up.

For the vast majority of the babies treated (>90%), one or two sessions sufficed. Those cases where more than two treatments were necessary were more often cases where additional complications arose. The minimal interval between two treatments was five weeks (Biedermann, 1999).

Those mothers who were still breastfeeding reported a more relaxed child. The contact between the child's mouth and the breast was closer and less air was swallowed. Several parents were glad 'to finally be able to hug our baby'. Before treatment, the fixed retroflexion of the child caused the mother to surmise that her baby 'did not want to embrace me'.

In a third of the cases, we have seen a swift and complete recovery; in another third, a slightly less impressive but still satisfactory development; and in the last third, no relevant or only minor changes. This refers to a single treatment with no further accompanying therapy. In combination with other measures, the effects are better, albeit impossible to document as the means used are too diverse (Biedermann 2000, 2003, 2006).

Practical examination and treatment of vertebrogenic disorders in infants

After many years of treating children and newborn we devised a protocol to organize the information- gathering as efficiently as possible:

- Beforehand the families get a questionnaire covering the relevant medical details of the family history, specifics of the delivery and information about the development of the child after birth.
- Before the baby is seen by the therapist, this case history which was compiled by the family is re-examined with the parents by a secretary. Based on this information we decide the need of an X-ray of the cervical spine. In small children (up to 15 months), one anterior/posterior (A/P) view of the cervical spine is sufficient. The lateral view is of limited information, as the babies tend to slump in a sitting position and are very difficult to fixate properly in a lying position. This X-ray plate is examined morphologically and functionally, thus giving a first indication of the postural situation.

After this, the baby enters the examination room, where the case history is re-evaluated once more. Often the parents provide additional information as they have had time to read our questionnaire. We check the items reported by the assistant, supplementing new details. During this time, the baby is on the lap of one of the parents and, by observing the reaction of the infant, we gain additional information about posture, sensorimotor skills, and endurance.

After the end of the dialogue with the parents, we take the baby and verify, by examining the global and segmental movement patterns, if the case history, the plate of the cervical spine, and the manual examination fit the same pattern.

In examining the babies, we first check the tonus and mobility of the extremities. Then, we use a selection of neuro-paediatric procedures (Bobath 1976; Goddard 2002; Herschkowitz et al. 1997; Ratner and Bondarchuk 1990; Ratner and Khaibullina 1991; Vojta and Peters 1992) to test the reflex patterns. These tests give a fairly good idea of the maturity of the baby's sensorimotor development and the symmetry of the reactions to the postural tests. One always has to compromise between completeness of the test and the patience of the little patient, which is in most cases *very* limited. As soon as enough information is assembled to be reasonably sure of the necessity of a treatment, we try to make the transition between the diagnostic and the therapeutic phase as smooth as possible.

The technique we use for the manipulation puts the child in front of the therapist, preferably in a lying position (Figure 22.3). Some children are easier to soothe when half upright as shown in Figure 22.4. In most cases, the impaired range of movement of the occipito-cervical (O/C) junction is the most important problem to tackle. The thrust is moderate (Koch and Girnus 1998) and applied in the interval between forced expiration (i.e. crying) and inspiration. In this split second, the baby *has* to relax and thus only minimal force is needed. Depending on the clinical findings and the

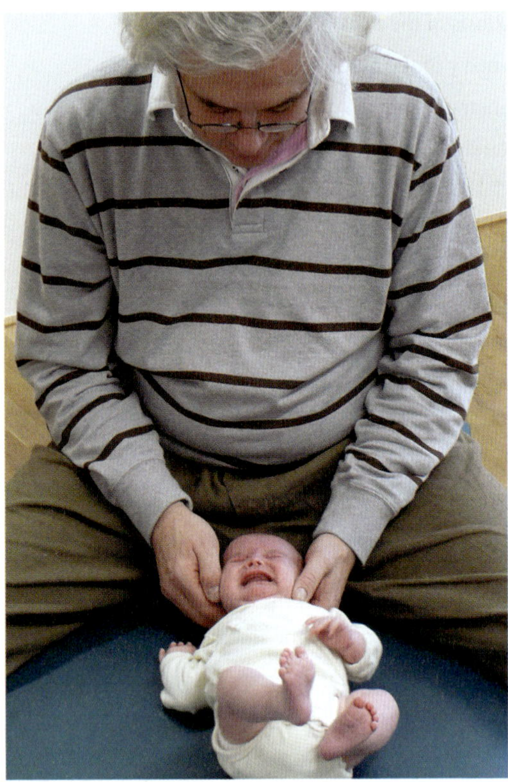

Figure 22.3 The classic positioning of a baby prior to treatment. In most cases, the upper cervical spine is quite sensitive and the infant patient reacts with crying—more reason to explain everything as clearly as possible to the parents beforehand.

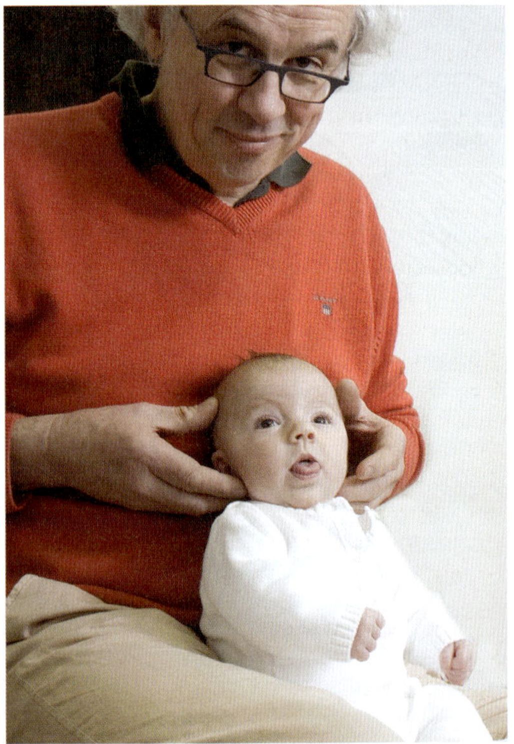

Figure 22.4 Sometimes it is less disturbing for the babies to be treated in a semi-upright position as shown here. Typical is the marked orofacial hypotonia and the clenched fists. The hands of the therapist touch the region C1/C2 (i.e. the transverse process of C1).

functional analysis of the plate of the cervical spine, the direction of the impulse is determined.

We have not encountered any serious side-effects of this therapy in the babies treated according to our specifications (Biedermann 2004a)—40,000 in our own consultations and as many by members of the EWMM[3] in the last 20 years (Schmitz and Ewers 2002).

Radiology in the diagnosis and treatment of vertebrogenic disorders in infants

Any radiography taken for diagnostic purposes has to be justified by the information eventually gained through it. The most commonly held idea about the use of X-ray plates in the diagnosis and treatment of vertebrogenic disorders is to look for morphological changes, especially for contraindications to manual therapy. In these cases, one needs to define a standard, and anything deviating from that standard is considered more or less pathological. This is undoubtedly correct and important—but it is by far not the whole picture. Standard radiographs are not a very convincing tool in the search for tumours or neurodegenerative diseases, which are the most important contraindications for manual therapy with children (Baker et al. 1999; Biedermann 2004b; Lansade et al. 2009; Penning 1978; Swischuk 2002). Osseous malformations are easier to spot on conventional radiographs. At least as important is the role of the functional examination of the radiography in order to fine-tune one's manipulation technique and to improve the precision of the diagnosis.

It seems to be difficult to judge the validity of this assertion in all circumstances. For the purposes of orthopaedic surgery—and even more so in dealing with problems related to the vertebral spine—it is safe to say that whatever non-standard facts can be extracted from a radiological picture (X-ray, computed tomography (CT) scan, magnetic resonance imaging (MRI), etc.), they have to be compared with and validated by the clinical examination. Publications abound which reiterate the well-known (but often ignored) fact that there is no such thing as a radiological diagnosis of, for example, a discus hernia (a clinically relevant hernia, one has to add to avoid useless squabbling). The radiological finding, as such, needs the causal connection with the clinical picture to be validated and only then should it be accepted as a base for clinical decisions. This is especially true in small children, where most of the findings relate to functional peculiarities.

One school of thought takes the obvious and radical consequence to disregard X-ray analysis altogether. 'We do not need radiographs'—this argument is facilitated by the fact that many of those applying manual therapy to the vertebral spine often do not have ready access to radiography, as is the case for most physiotherapists or chiropractors. Departing from the just cause of relativizing the findings of radiological examinations, they extend this argument beyond its breaking point and disregard X-rays altogether, thus losing a valuable source of information.

At birth, many of the features of an adult's X-ray picture of this region are not yet fully developed:

- apophyses are open
- dens axis is not ossified
- much thicker cartilaginous material exists between the bones in the joint areas
- everything is softer, less accentuated (e.g. the angle of the C0/C1 joint is almost horizontal) (Sacher 2004)

The morphology is less easily interpreted, as many of the necessary markers to determine rotation or translation cannot be fixed as precisely as in adults. However, this fuzziness of the radiology reflects only the undetermined state of the biomechanical components.

Differentiation of, for example, the rotational position of the cervical vertebrae, is less precise than in adults, but for most practical purposes, much less relevant for the treatment too. The cushioning influence of the extended peri-articular cartilaginous strata prevents the hard blockages we find in adults.

Combining the functional- and morphological-level spinal radiographs of small children yields an amazing amount of information (see Figures 22.5–22.7) which helps to bolster the diagnosis and make the technique used more precise (Biedermann 2004b). We do

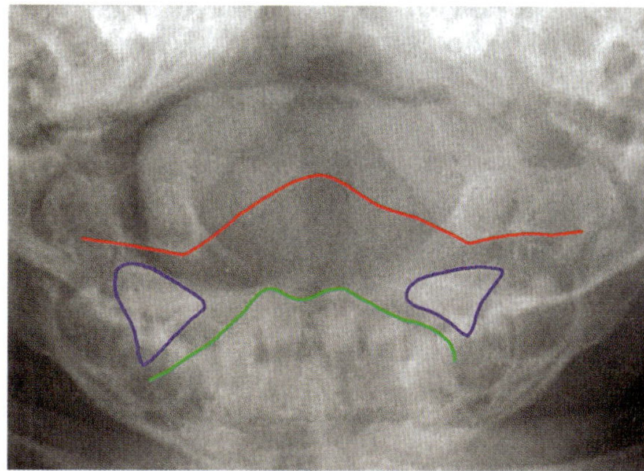

Figure 22.5 This 5-month-old baby shows a fairly typical situation. The condylar angle is—as often during the first months—almost horizontal. In this case, we see a rotation and translation of C1 and C2 relative to the occiput to the left of the radiograph.
(Red: the base of the skull with the condyles; blue: massa lateralis of the atlas; green: joint facet of C2 and the superior articular surfaces; in the middle of C2, the epiphyseal plate between the body of C2 and the dens.)

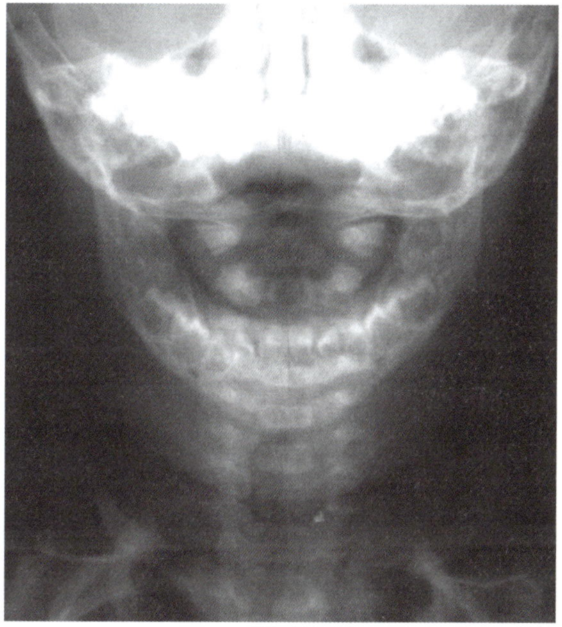

Figure 22.6 Marked asymmetry of the condylar contours. C1 and C2 are shifted to the right relative to the occiput. Morphology, as far as is visible, is normal for the age of 9 months.

[3] EWMM: European Workgroup for Manual Medicine (<http://www.manmed.org>)

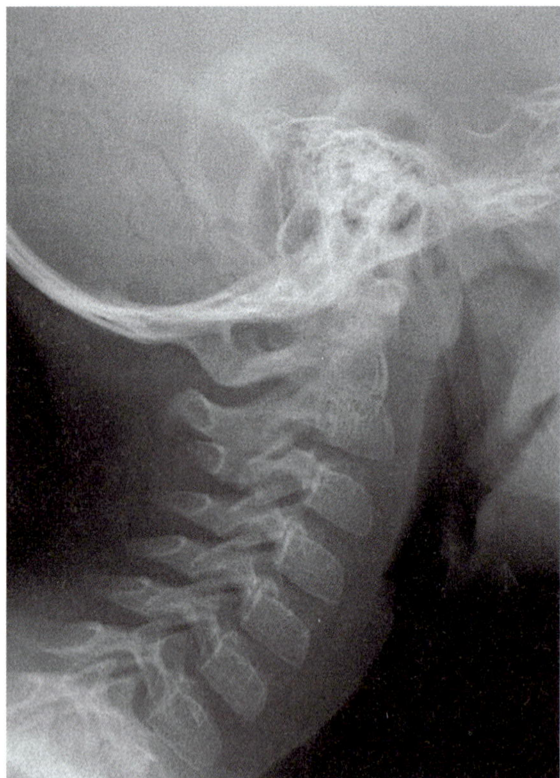

Figure 22.7 Rare but relevant—lateral view of the cervical spine of a 3.5-year-old boy showing fusion of the dorsal portion of C1 with the occiput. These 'hard' morphological findings occur in 8–12% of cases.

not treat without a recent radiograph of the cervical spine, last but not least for forensic reasons, but mostly because of the additional assurance this information furnishes.

Outcome data for treatment of vertebrogenic disorders in infants

In several catamnestic studies, a comparable distribution pattern emerged. As an example, the results of a sample of 256 babies (of a total of 584) treated between May 1994 and April 1995 are presented here (Table 22.1). These data are chosen as we did a follow-up of these children when they were young adults in 2010 (Biedermann 2013).

The clinical picture of babies referred to us is as follows:

> The basic trigger which makes paediatricians send the babies to a specialist in manual therapy is the hypersensitivity of the neck region in combination with a restricted range of movement of the head. Those who already observed the success of manual therapy in cases of colic or feeding problems are looking actively for these signs to help them decide if it is advisable to present these babies to a specialist. Others find it easier to first look for signs of asymmetry before they take manual therapy as a treatment option into account. In both cases, it helps to have the pattern of typical KISS complaints present, even if not all symptoms can be found in an individual case. We experienced the 'KiSS pattern' as a very useful communication tool to facilitate the referral of babies to a specialist. It helps to have an understanding of the structural problem behind a given symptom (i.e. treat a KISS child and get rid of colic or sleeping problems).

The complaint patterns of the babies referred to us depends on the previous experiences of the therapist with manual therapy. In the 1990s, the classical torticollis was dominant (see Table 22.2). These babies were immediately identifiable as in need of help on the mechanical level. Nowadays, most of these children are successfully treated by physiotherapists or osteopaths. Most newborns we see now have already had one or more treatments by those colleagues, with the result deemed insufficient. This implies that our patient group has become more complex, entailing mixed patterns with neurological symptoms (see Table 22.2). The 'simple' KISS I baby (i.e. the classic torticollis neonatorum) has been substituted by a newborn with symptoms of colic and 'reflux'. Table 22.3 shows the composition of main complaints of babies treated in our consultations in 2012.

This changing picture reflects the different perceptions of the parents and the fact that most of the uncomplicated cases are treated by physiotherapists or osteopaths. We rarely see babies who have not received some treatment before presentation. As the cases we treat nowadays are more complex than those seen 10 or 20 years ago, we had expected the outcome to be less favourable. However, this does not seem to be the case. An ongoing audit of babies treated between April and June 2013 showed the same pattern as we had seen before. Roughly 80% of the parents were very content or content with the treatment.

Long-term observations

Screening potential patients for manual therapy helps to check their early development and to decide if there are signs of KISS-related problems during the first year of life. We can show that in these cases, the probability of a positive outcome is higher (Biedermann

Table 22.1 Results of treatment (interviews with parents)

Symptom	(Very) good result after				Improved	No change	Total
	1 day	1 week	2 weeks	3 weeks			
Torticollis	78	28	33	19	40	25	223
Ophistotonos	10	6	5	7	12	5	45
Restless/crying	26	5	6	2	6	7	52
Fixed sleeping posture	16	3	3	6	4	1	33

Biedermann, H., KISS-Kinder: eine katamnestische Untersuchung. In *Manualtherapie bei Kindern*, H. Biedermann, Editor. 1999, Enke: Stuttgart, p. 27–42.

Table 22.2 Spontaneous complaints reported by the parents in 1996 and 2003

	n = 263 1991 (Biedermann 1991)	n = 200 2003 (Biedermann 2004)
Torticollis	89.3%	53.2%
Reduced range of head movements	84.7%	78.3%
Cervical hypersensitivity	76.0%	64.7%
Cranial asymmetry	40.1%	67.6%
Opisthotonos	27.9%	44.8%
Restlessness	23.7%	39.2%
Forced sleeping posture	14.5%	45.7%
Unable to control head movements	9.5%	37.2%
Uses one arm much less than the other	7.6%	12.4%
Breastfeeding problems	—	18.4%

Table 22.3 Composition of main complaints of babies treated in 2012, as reported by the parents

(multiple responses possible)		
Excessive crying, 'colic'	734	44.0%
Fixed posture, asymmetrical movements	622	37.2%
Vomiting, 'reflux'	581	34.8%
Sleeping disorders	451	27.0%
Cranial asymmetry	386	23.1%
Breastfeeding problems	366	21.9%

2005, 2009). This seems to implicate that babies suffering from these symptoms in their first months always have a higher chance to develop vertebrogenic disorders later on. To check this, we used the cohort of our 1995 babies and tried to establish contact with these families 18 years later. During clinical follow-up or by telephone interviews with the families, we learned that the vast majority of these young adults did not have more complaints that the average members of their age group. In some regards (dental malpositioning, ametropia), this group showed markedly less problems (Biedermann 2013).

These findings allow us to conjecture, but they are corroborated by our daily experiences and the communications from other colleagues active in the field. The necessary prospective studies are, regrettably, more often than not impossible to implement in the setting of a walk-in clinic, as control groups are out of reach.

Manual medicine at the different stages of life

Manual medicine is focused on the interaction of biomechanical (mal-)function and the homoeostasis of an individual. Function and form depend on each other. In small children, it is the function which determines, to a big extent, the pathway of the developing morphology. Once we are aware of this, we can find the relics of early dysfunction in adolescents and adults and understand better the constraints imposed on their individual spectrum of functional disorders. After adolescence, the individual's function interacts with the morphology. The older one gets, the more '*form follows function*' is turned into '*function follows form*'. This makes it so difficult to compare the effects of manual therapy, as every therapeutic interaction has to be evaluated on the background of the traumata that the specific patient underwent. In old patients, the situation is different again: here, the decreasing elasticity of the connective tissue limits the efficiency of manipulative manoeuvres. However, these persons are rigid in more than one regard: their values and beliefs are set and altered only with difficulty.

The following schema indicates the numbers of patients, in different age groups, treated in our consultations in 2012, and their specific reaction to functional disorders. In total, there were 6374 patients, treated by three physicians.

Newborns (0–2 years): 1669 patients

'Clean slate', i.e. establishing reaction patterns

Extreme susceptibility to irritation and/or stimulation

Small children (2–6 years): 1337 patients

Subtle reactions

Extreme flexibility

Function determines form

Adolescents and young adults (7–30 years): 1873 patients

Psychosomatic influence dominant

Form and function interact

Robust and subtle reactions equally relevant

Adults (30–55 years): 1143 patients

Case history becomes more and more relevant

Loss of flexibility of muscles and ligaments

Form determines function

Older persons (>55 years): 352 patients

Rigidity of reactions

Inflexible expectation patterns

Robust reactions to manual medicine dominate

Keeping the structural differences between the age groups in mind, we realize that small children are like a laboratory for the impact of manual therapy. We cannot copy and paste these insights onto the therapy of older patients, but the observations of the effects of re-establishing functional normality are valid at all ages. This makes the expertise gained by treating small children even more valuable. We have presented a lot of observations which need to be validated. We learned the hard way how difficult it is to gather the data for such an endeavour, and the workload of the general practitioners (GPs) and the paediatricians is only increasing. So yes, there is an urgent need to push for hard data, but for the time being, we can only campaign for a wider use of manual therapy in small children based on the many thousands of casuistical observations available.

Closing thoughts on functional disorders of the spine in small children

In many cases, manual therapy can alleviate problems of babies and their families. Often the ailments where manual therapy can be of use are not yet considered as caused by vertebrogenic disorders. The KISS pattern we proposed in 1991 (Biedermann 1991) was intended to bridge that gap. Careful evaluation, a frontal radiography of the cervical spine, and the avoidance of superfluous irritation helps in three-quarters of these cases. In the hands of an experienced therapist, this is an easy and safe procedure with quick and positive results.

Two problems persist: the interprofessional communication barrier and the fact that this craftsmanship relies on individual accomplishment. These skills in dealing with patients are being frustrated by the push for institutional standards. Manual therapy uses the 'triad of the intelligent hand'—coordination of hand, eye, and brain (Sennet 2008)—and only an expert has the success rates mentioned in Table 22.1.

Holt's observation of the causes of colic was: 'Pain, temper, hunger, illness, and habit' (1894). They are still valid for most of the functional disorders we see and treat in babies. We can add the dimension of functional disorders of the cervical spine to this list. This addition has the advantage of giving us an easy therapeutic access.

The pathogenetic model we propose (KISS) offers a tool for a better differential diagnosis, a long-term prognostic instrument, and an effective device to communicate with those involved with our potential patients

Even the methodologically imperfect studies on chiropractics (see Vernon 2005) for small children show:

> The evidence suggests that chiropractic has no benefit over placebo in the treatment of infantile colic. However, there is good evidence that taking a colicky infant to a chiropractor will result in fewer reported hours of colic by the parents. In this clinical scenario where the family is under significant strain, where the infant may be at risk of harm and possible long term repercussions, where there are limited alternative effective interventions, and where the mother has confidence in a chiropractor from other experiences, the advice is to seek chiropractic treatment. (Klougart et al. 1989)

Having realized that *less is more*, we can advise all colleagues to refrain from too frequent interventions. Using only one precise manipulation considerably increases the slope of the signal we give and, thus, the effectiveness of the treatment, as this specific intervention is perceived by patient and family more clearly then – e.g. – a whole series of treatments

If this helps to make Darwin's observation come true, so much the better: 'So again when young children are just beginning to cry, an unexpected event will sometimes suddenly turn their crying into laughter, which apparently serves equally well to expend their superfluous nervous energy.' (Darwin 1899)

Acknowledgements

Bettina Küsgen, Howard Vernon, and Jens Foell helped considerably by reading the text and suggesting improvements in form and content.

References

Baker, C., Kadish, H., Schunk, J. Evaluation of pediatric cervical spine injuries. *Am J Emerg Med*, 1999, 17(3):230–4.

Bakris, G., et al. Atlas vertebra realignment and achievement of arterial pressure goal in hypertensive patients: a pilot study. *J Hum Hypertens*, 2007, 21(5):347–52.

Biedermann, H. Kopfgelenk-induzierte Symmetriestörungen bei Kleinkindern. *Kinderarzt*, 1991, 22:1475–82.

Biedermann, H. Kinematic imbalances due to suboccipital strain. *J Man Med*, 1992, 6:151–6

Biedermann, H. Das Kiss-Syndrom der Neugeborenen und Kleinkinder. *Manuelle Medizin*, 1993, 31:97–107.

Biedermann, H. KISS-kinder: eine katamnestische Untersuchung. In: Biedermann, H. (ed.) *Manualtherapie bei Kindern*. Stuttgart: Enke; 1999, p. 27–42.

Biedermann, H. Primary and secondary cranial asymmetry in KISS-children. In: von Piekartz, H., Bryden, L. (eds) Craniofacial dysfunction and pain. Manual therapy, assessment and management. London: Butterworth & Heinemann; 2000, p. 46–62.

Biedermann, H. Upper cervical manipulation for infants and children with the KiSS- syndrome. In: *World Federation of Chiropractic's 7th Biennial Congress, 2003*. Orlando, Florida: WFC; 2003.

Biedermann, H. Examination and treatment of the cervical spine in children. In: Biedermann, H. (ed.) *Manual therapy in children*. Churchill Livingstone: Edinburgh; 2004a, p. 334.

Biedermann, H. Functional radiology of the cervical spine in children. In: Biedermann, H. (ed.) *Manual therapy in children*. Churchill Livingstone: Edinburgh; 2004b, p. 215–34.

Biedermann, H. Manualmedizin bei (Klein-)Kindern: Kooperation zwischen Neuropädiatrie und Manualmedizin. *Man Med*, 2005, 43:111–5.

Biedermann, H. KISS-Syndrom—ein Geburtstrauma? *Hebammen-Zeitschrift*, 2006, 10:27–31.

Biedermann, H. Phase transitions: how the functional pathology of the vertebral spine influences the morphological development in children. In: *World Federation of Chiropractic's 10th Biennial Congress, 2009*. Montreal, Canada: WFC; 2009, p. 34–76.

Biedermann, H. Küsgen, B. Langzeit-beobachtungen nach KiSS—Behandlung im säuglingsalter. *Man Med*, 2013, 51.

Bobath, B. *Abnorme Haltungsreflexe bei Gehirnschäden*. Stuttgart: Thieme

Darwin, C. *The expression of the emotions in man and animals*. New York: Appleton; 1899, p. 254.

Ericsson, K.A. Deliberate practice and acquisition of expert performance: a general overview. *Acad Emerg Med*, 2008, 15(11):988–94.

Ericsson, K.A., Krampe, R.T., Tesch- Römer, C. The role of deliberate practice in the acquisition of expert performance. *Psychol Rev*, 1993, 100:363–406.

Gladwell, M. *Outliers: the story of success*. New York: Little, Brown & Co.; 2008, p. 320.

Goddard, S. *Reflexes, learning and behaviour*. Eugene, OR: Fern Ridge Press; 2002, p. 181.

Gracovetsky, S.A. *The spinal engine*. Wien, New York: Springer

Herschkowitz, N., Kagan, J., Zilles, K. Neurobiological bases of behavioral development in the first year. *Neuropediatrics*, 1997, 28(6):296–306.

Holt, L.E. *The care and feeding of children: a catechism for the use of mothers and childrens' nurses*. New York: Appleton; 1894.

Klougart, N., Nilsson, N., Jacobsen, J. Infantile colic treated by chiropractors: a prospective study of 316 cases. *J Manip Physiol Therap*, 1989, 12:281–8.

Koch, L.E., Girnus, U. Kraftmessung bei Anwendung der Impulstechnik in der Chirotherapie. *Man Med*, 1998, 36(1):21–6.

Lansade, C., et al. Three-dimensional analysis of the cervical spine kinematics: effect of age and gender in healthy subjects. *Spine*, 2009, 34(26):2900–6.

Levitin, D. *This is your brain on music*. Upper Saddle River, NJ: Pearson; 2006, p. 272.

Penning, L. *Normal movements of the cervical spine. AJR Am J Roentgenol*, 1978, 130(2):317–26.

Portmann, A. *Biologie und Geist*. Göttingen: Edition Nereide; 1998, p. 336.

Ratner, A., Bondarchuk, S.V. Neurologic evaluation of unconditioned reflexes in the newborn. *Pediatriia*, 1990, 4:38–41.

Ratner, A., Khaibullina, F.G. Zadachi i vozmozhnosti usovershenstvovaniia pediatrov po detskoi nevrologii. (Goals and possibilities of advanced training of pediatricians in pediatric neurology). *Pediatriia*, 1991, 3:83–5.

Sacher, R. Die Postnatale Entwicklung des frontalen Kondylen-Gelenkachsenwinkels C_0/C_1. *RöFo*, 2004, 176(6):847–51.

Schmitz, H., Ewers, J. EWMM workshop Antwerpen. *Man Med*, 2002, 40:253–4.

Sennet, R. *The Craftsman*. Yale: Yale University Press; 2008, p. 324.

Swischuk, L. *Imaging of the cervical spine in children*. New York: Springer; 2002, p. 140.

Vernon, H. The treatment of headache, neurologic and non-musculosceletal disorders by spinal manipulation. In: Haldeman, S. (ed.) *Principles and practice of chiropractic*. McGraw-Hill: New York; 2005, p. 167–82.

Vojta, V., Peters, A. *Das Vojta-Prinzip*. Berlin: Springer; 1992.

PART 3

Regional disorders

Chapter 23

Clinical examination

David Knott

General observations during consultation with a patient

These are generally made when the patient first enters the room and is greeted by the clinician. Impressions of their facial attitude (happy, sad, anxious, tired, etc.) along with any abnormalities of gait are noted. In particular, are such observations found to be consistent with the history subsequently obtained? As well as general appearance, common observations could include apparent tiredness from sleep disturbance or a sad or depressed/anxious appearance in those with spinal pain. At the other extreme is the rare but striking *la belle indifference* of conversion disorder (formerly known as hysteria). Here, the patient appears cheerful and unconcerned whilst describing and displaying (apparently) severe or serious symptoms and signs. Any obvious deformity or postural abnormality, or limbs held in protective 'antalgic' postures should be noted.

Verbal (subjective) history during consultation with a patient

After basic introductions and pleasantries, the patient should ideally be allowed to tell his or her own story without interruption from the examiner. Studies have shown that, on average, a doctor will interrupt the patient after a mere 18 seconds! The practicality of this approach will, to some extent, depend upon patient, examiner, and circumstances. While some patients are better historians than others, the majority will tell their story (and, in some cases, effectively give you the diagnosis) if allowed the chance. By listening carefully, the clinician can not only discover the history in terms of the condition as presented, but may well also discover underlying beliefs and fears which may have a great bearing on the management. This initial presentation of the story by the patient can then be followed by appropriate questions from the examiner, ideally 'open' to start with and then more targeted to 'complete the story' and obtain other information that may be relevant to the diagnosis and/or treatment options. Following this pattern in the time-challenged environment of general practice is far from easy but should be attempted.

It is always useful to have a routine framework for a history, although this can of course be varied as necessary. For example, it would be usually appropriate and essential to take a longer and more thorough history in cases of spinal pain than in one of thumb joint arthritis. One such suggested framework for history taking is as follows:

- **Age**—some conditions tend to be age-specific (and maybe sex-specific), or at least more likely to occur within these specific groups. For example:
    - Children do not commonly present with musculoskeletal problems and so the clinician needs to be alert to the possibility of more serious pathology, to specific childhood ailments (Perthes' disease, for example), and, sadly, also for any suggestion of child abuse. Congenital and developmental problems and trauma are more commonly presented in children than in later life. Accidents and trauma are also relatively common in children.
    - Young adults are more likely to be subject to either trauma or overuse injuries from work, sport, or leisure activities. Some spinal conditions such as scoliosis may present for the first time in adolescence.
    - 'Middle age'—the exact definition of which can vary with the age of the examiner!—is the commonest age group to present with onset of spinal problems such as prolapsed intervertebral discs and also many connective tissue problems such as tendonopathy. This is an age when the connective tissues are becoming less robust, the owner of them perhaps less fit in general, and yet still having/wishing to use them repetitively in work or leisure activities.
    - In old age, degenerative conditions, especially spinal and peripheral joint arthritis, will predominate, although trauma will potentially have more serious consequences than in the young. Fractures at hip, wrist, and vertebra are all more common. Cancers, both primary and secondary, and other systemic diseases become more common with increasing age.
- **Occupation**—what is the patient's job? Do you know what the job actually entails? If not, ask the patient. Does it involve repetitive actions with a risk of overuse injury, or is it physically demanding with risks of injury or premature degeneration in tissues? Does it involve adopting sustained and mechanically inadvisable postures?

- **Leisure activities**—especially sports, that may be relevant. If sporting, which sport? At what level is it undertaken? Is participation regular or episodic? Does the patient take part in any training, etc.?
- **Onset of symptoms**—was the onset sudden or gradual? If sudden, what happened, and if an injury, what was the nature of it? With knee and shoulder injuries, for example, what was the position of the joint?
- **Duration of symptoms**—is the presentation acute, subacute, or chronic? If chronic, have symptoms been continuous or intermittent? Overall, allowing for short-term variability, is the condition getting better or worse?
- **Site of pain (symptoms) and any spread**—are symptoms unilateral or bilateral? Upper body or lower? Is any spread consistent with recognized dermatome patterns? Referral of pain and neurological symptoms is typically unilateral and distal; the distance of the referral is commonly proportional to the degree of inflammation or irritability of the injury/problem.
- **Behaviour of symptoms**—what is the nature of the pain? Is it aching, burning, stabbing, etc.? What makes it better? Or worse? Does posture affect the pain? Can they sleep? Pain that is affected by posture and that is intermittent is generally benign and often mechanical. Pain that is continuous, not affected by posture, and present through the night can potentially mean serious disease, especially if progressive.
- **Other symptoms**—if the main symptom is pain, are there any others? Especially ask about neurological symptoms such as numbness, paraesthesiae, and weakness, or giving way. Any abnormality of bladder and bowel function should be sought in cases of spinal pain, as well as changes in perineal sensation. Other symptoms such as weight loss or night sweats can be more worrying and should be enquired about as appropriate.
- **Treatment**—that has been given so far. If drugs—which ones and what dosage? Did they help? If injections—where and by whom? Did they help and if so, for how long? If physiotherapy—exactly what did that consist of and did it help? Any other treatments such as osteopathy, chiropractic, acupuncture, etc.? Have any *investigations* been done? If so, what and where and are the results known/available?
- **Current medication**—both for the condition in question and for any other medical problems. In particular, ask about:
    - Current use of *analgesics, non-steroidal anti-inflammatories*, or *neuropathic pain medications*. Dosage? Regular or 'as needed'? Increasing or decreasing?
    - *Corticosteroids*—reason for taking them, dosage, and duration. Remember the possibility of osteoporosis with longer-term steroid therapy, although hopefully this will be less of a problem now with greater awareness on the part of prescribers and the use of prophylactic bone-protective therapy.
    - *Anticoagulants*—reason for taking them, but mainly as they will impact upon treatment options (especially warfarin and clopidogrel). They will generally be regarded as contraindications for manipulation and some injections.
    - *Chemotherapy and other immunosuppressive therapy*—reason for taking it. If cancer, is that relevant to the diagnosis? Chemotherapy may adversely affect the immune system, increasing the possibility of infection following injection treatment, for example, influencing treatment decisions.
- **Allergies to drugs**—especially those which may be used in treatments such as steroids, non-steroidal anti-inflammatory drugs, and local anaesthetics, and also possibly contrast media. Sometimes patients need careful questioning about this as they may describe side-effects as allergies.
- **Past medical history**—ask especially about other relevant orthopaedic issues, as well as medically important conditions such as diabetes, thyroid disease, heart disease, past operations and cancers, bleeding tendencies, etc. Psoriasis may be relevant if they have arthritis.
- **Family history**—this can be relevant, especially in some cases of arthritis and back pain (e.g. rheumatoid arthritis, ankylosing spondylitis).
- **Social history** (as relevant)—problems within the home/school/work environment or relationship problems can significantly affect the presentation, as can unresolved grief over deaths/relationship breakdowns, etc. Financial problems and compensation/litigation issues can also be relevant and can adversely affect both presentation and prognosis.

Whilst the history will normally be obtained from the patient themselves, family members or friends may volunteer additional useful history. This can be particularly helpful if the patient is an unreliable historian—as in dementia, for example. It also may give a truer picture in the case of patients who play down (or exaggerate) the extent of their problem.

Objective physical examination as part of the patient consultation

A full description of an individual region-specific physical examination is beyond the scope of this chapter—the reader is advised to consult one of the many excellent volumes detailing this, such as that by Atkins et al. (2010). However, we may consider the general underlying principles of an effective and time-efficient physical examination. Different clinicians will tend to develop their own style and pattern of examination, but it is again useful to have a routine framework that can be adapted to the particular case in question. A suggested framework could be:

- **Inspect** the relevant body part and adjacent/related parts of anatomy looking particularly for:
    - *Any bony deformity*—limb length inequality, asymmetry, spinal curvatures, obvious bony enlargement or deformity, etc.
    - *Colour changes*—redness, blueness, pallor, bruising. This is more likely to be seen at superficial sites (e.g. hand or foot), and less likely at deep ones (e.g. hip).
    - *Muscle wasting*—from disuse or neurological problem, or occasionally muscle disease. This tends to be more common at some sites—e.g. quadriceps wasting in knee problems, thenar eminence wasting in advance carpal tunnel syndrome—than at others.
    - *Swelling(s)*—of the affected joint/tendon/bursa/etc. or as an incidental finding in the vicinity (lipoma, ganglion, etc.).

After inspection, it may be appropriate to briefly examine any other body areas that may be the source of the patient's symptoms through referral of pain or neurological symptoms. For example, the cervical spine should be examined in cases of shoulder pain and some other upper limb conditions, and the hip examined in cases of knee pain. Usually, a brief 'screening' examination is sufficient—if suspicion of referred symptoms is raised, then a more thorough examination should be made.

- **Palpate**—for heat, swelling, and synovial thickening—all suggestive of an inflammatory process. (However, not at this stage for tenderness—that comes later.) This is generally only for more superficial sites. For heat, compare with the other limb and use the back of the hand as it tends to be more sensitive than the palm. Synovial thickening can most easily be appreciated by palpation along a joint line.
- **Move**—the affected part. It is suggested that the selective tension approach, as suggested by Dr James Cyriax (1982), is both logical, productive, and time-efficient. This system involves three sets of movements—active, passive, and resisted:
  - **Active**—where the patient moves the limb/joint and the examiner observes and notes the range obtained, symmetry between sides, (apparent) pain produced, and, sometimes, specific features such as a painful arc during the movement. It is also useful for giving an impression of the patient's willingness to move the joint and can give some insight into cases in which psychological features may be prominent. It can be performed at any joint but is more useful at some sites (e.g. spine, shoulder) than at others (hand, knee)—perhaps because psychological factors tend to be more common in the former areas, and so, in the interests of time efficiency, active movements should probably be reserved for examination of these sites.
  - **Passive**—the patient relaxes completely (not always easy to achieve!) and the examiner moves the joint. It is important to achieve a full range of movement for the joint concerned—to achieve end range—and the examiner is looking for any pain produced, the range achieved, and the feeling imparted to the examiner's hands at the end of range (the 'end feel'). The examiner should position his body and hands to optimum effect and try to involve only one joint. For peripheral joints, it is customary to examine the normal side (assuming it is normal) first as patients vary considerably in the range of movement of their joints. Passive movements are mainly testing non-contractile structures (although a passive movement may also stretch a relaxed contractile unit and sometimes produce symptoms).

  There are various '*end feels*' to be perceived at the end of range. For the majority of joints, this will be *elastic*, but other findings are possible, as described by Cyriax and shown in Table 23.1.

  If a reduced range of movement is detected (as compared to the patient's other side—assuming that to be normal), then the pattern of the reduction is useful. Cyriax described the '*capsular pattern*'—a consistent and reproducible pattern of reduced joint movement that suggests that the pathology is either arthritis or capsulitis. By implication, a reduction in range of movement in a different (non-capsular) pattern implies pathology in other tissues within or adjacent to the joint such as ligament, cartilage, tendon, muscle, or bursa. The capsular pattern: (i) is joint-specific—differing for each joint; (ii) is variable in degree of reduction with the severity of the pathology; (iii) does not differentiate between different causes of arthritis.

Table 23.1 Cyriax's findings

Finding (end feel)	Implication
Elastic	Normal at most locations, the degree of elasticity varies between joints and individuals and generally tends to decrease with increasing age
Hard	Normal at some sites (e.g. elbow extension, where bone on bone contact limits movement) but would be abnormal if found where it should be elastic (as in shoulder external rotation, for example)
Soft	Normal at some sites—knee flexion, elbow flexion—where soft tissue on soft tissue limits movement
'Springy'	Differs from elastic—think of a small piece of rubber stuck in the hinge of a door preventing closing and causing a 'bounce'—suggests a loose body or displaced cartilage
'Empty'	Not really an end feel at all but means that the patient actively prevents the examiner reaching the end of range because of anticipated severe pain—implies serious (or at least more severe/ irritable) pathology in or around that joint

Reprinted from Textbook of Orthopaedic Medicine, Cyriax J 1982 (Bailliere Tindall).

  The different patterns for each joint must be learned, but as an *aide-memoire*, if one can visualize the changes observed in old age (arthrosis) or those of a deforming arthritis, such as untreated rheumatoid, then the restrictions imposed as part of a capsular pattern will be the same.

- **Resisted**—the joint is held in a mid-range position and the examiner resists attempted movements. At most joints, we are trying, as far as possible, to test individual muscles or groups of muscles. Again, positioning of body and hands is important to achieve good mechanical advantage and test maximal contraction. This will be particularly so with a small examiner and a large/strong patient, if smaller lesions are not to be missed. Because the joint is held in mid-range and not allowed to move, theoretically, only contractile structures are tested. The contractile unit consists of the muscle belly, the tendon, and the teno-osseous junction. Sometimes, resisted tests will need to be repeated to bring out more minor symptoms. Resisted testing may be omitted at some sites (spinal, for example) unless the history suggests they are likely to be useful.

  With resisted testing, various findings are possible. These, with their significance, are detailed in Table 23.2.

Table 23.2 Significance of resisted testing findings

Finding	Implication
Strong and painless	Normal
Strong and painful	Small/mild pathology in contractile unit
Weak and painful	Large/severe pathology in contractile unit
Weak and painless	Neurological problem; complete tendon/ muscle tear
All movements painful/weak	Severe pathology or 'yellow flag'
Painful on repetition	Small pathology; possibly vascular insufficiency

- **Palpate again**—but this time for tenderness. Hopefully, a diagnosis will have been reached by this time, and the object of the palpation is now to localize the pathology within the tissue. With a contractile unit lesion, for example, the tenderness may be found at the teno-osseous junction, within the body of the tendon, at the musculo-tendinous junction, or within the body of the muscle. This will enable treatment to be applied accurately and may also affect the choice of treatment to be used.
- **Neurological examination** (where appropriate)—will usually be with spinal cases, but possibly also for suspected peripheral nerve problems. Power, sensation, and reflexes will be tested, along with additional tests such as plantar response. Usually, a fairly basic sensory screen will be adequate but this can be extended and refined where appropriate. A good knowledge of the dermatomes and myotomes is important to be able to link findings to symptoms, and also to the results of any subsequent investigations such as neurophysiology or spinal magnetic resonance imaging (MRI) scans. Differing texts will disagree to some extent over these, but commonly accepted patterns of dermatomes and myotomes are shown in Figure 23.1 and Table 23.3.
- **Additional tests**—are not done routinely but may be used to confirm or clarify a diagnosis if this is not clear ('impingement tests' at the shoulder, for example). There are a great number of additional tests, especially at the shoulder and the knee—often with confusing names, and that may well be performed differently by differing clinicians. The examiner is advised to become familiar with a limited number of generally useful tests and then to have a reference, such as that by Hattam and Smeatham

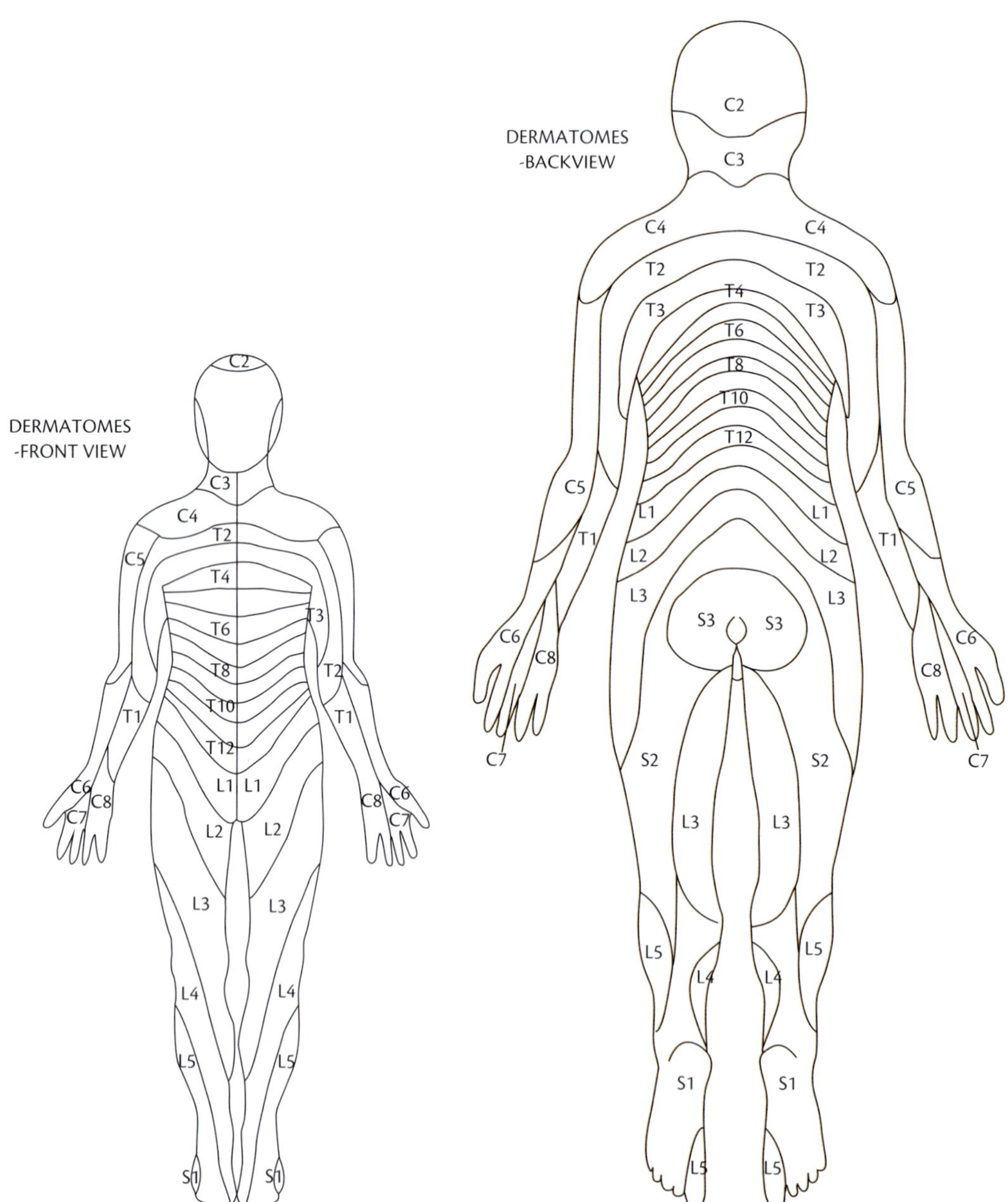

Figure 23.1 Commonly accepted patterns of dermatomes.

Table 23.3 Commonly accepted patterns of myotomes

Common myotomes	Mainly	Also some
Shoulder elevation	C3,4, spinal accessory XI	
Shoulder abduction	C5	C4,6
Shoulder external rotation	C5	C6
Shoulder internal rotation	C5,6	
Elbow flexion	C5,6	
Elbow extension	C7	C6,8
Wrist extension	C6	C7,8
Wrist flexion	C7	C6,8,T1
Finger adduction	T1	C8
Thumb adduction	C8	T1
Hip flexion	L1,2	L3
Hip extension	S1,2	L5,S3
Hip abduction	L4,5,S1	
Hip adduction	L3,4	L2
Knee flexion	L5,S1	S2
Knee extension	L3,4	L2
Ankle dorsiflexion	L4	L5
Ankle plantarflexion	S1	S2
Foot eversion	L5,S1	L4
Hallux extension	L5,S1	L4

Table 23.4 Examples of additional tests (for shoulder)

Observations:	Face, attitude, etc. Arm may be held in protective antalgic posture.
Inspection:	Spinal curves, especially postural attitude of neck and shoulders. Maybe raised/dropped shoulder. Muscle wasting in trapezius, deltoid, infraspinatus. Very occasionally, swelling with large joint or bursa effusion.
Palpation:	Would not usually palpate as heat, swelling, and synovial thickening all unlikely (deep joint).
History:	Not always that helpful—but ask about trauma or overuse. If trauma, think of rotator cuff tear or secondary capsulitis or labral tear. Radiation of pain into arm—how far down. Question about night-time discomfort. Any neurological symptoms in arm? Any history suggesting instability? Other history—e.g. diabetes (capsulitis more common). Had physiotherapy and/or injections already?
Examination:	Active, passive, and resisted, + /− extra tests (see Figures 23.2–23.5)
Palpation:	For tenderness—if diagnosis is tendon pathology, you can palpate for site in tendon; can palpate acromioclavicular (AC) joint line.
Investigations:	Not often needed, but consider X-ray and/or ultrasound or occasionally MRI.

(2010), available for the less commonly used tests. This volume also reviews the evidence for commonly used tests and, in particular, their sensitivity and specificity.

In the majority of cases, a diagnosis will by now have been reached and treatment may be planned and carried out. If necessary however, further investigation may be requested at this stage—to confirm or refine a diagnosis, or to rule out serious pathology. Details of such further investigations can be found elsewhere in this book.

This whole process of the physical examination can summarized with an example—the shoulder—as illustrated in Figures 23.2–23.5 and in Table 23.4.

'Red flags' as possible indicators of serious disease

Some aspects of the history and/or examination may raise the possibility of more serious disease, and may prompt further investigation to rule out pathology such as fracture, infection, or cancer. Some red flags may indeed prompt immediate referral to specialist services rather than awaiting investigation—cauda equina symptoms or signs in cases of low back pain, for example. The type of symptoms that could raise concern include:

- Age—children under 16; new onset back pain in the elderly.
- Trauma—if, for example, fracture or significant neurological injury is likely.
- Unremitting pain—which continues throughout the night and is not affected by rest or change in posture.
- Progressive symptoms—which are either getting progressively worse week by week, or getting rapidly worse day by day, or are spreading in an anatomical sense to cover a wider area of reference and that could represent an enlarging or worsening pathology. Conversely, symptoms that are static over a long period of time, or that are intermittent, while annoying for the patient, are less likely to be serious.
- Additional generalized symptoms—such as weight loss, sweating at night, fever, or feeling generally unwell.
- Past medical history—of previous cancer, for example, especially if of a type known to more readily metastasize to bone (more common with cancers of the breast, bronchus, thyroid, kidney, prostate).

Signs could include:

- Severe tenderness—much more than expected (although this could also be a 'yellow flag'—to be discussed) could be suggestive of infection, fracture, or cancer. It can also be found in benign but very 'irritable' conditions such as gout.
- Severely restricted movement—again, if much more than expected and is consistent and/or widespread, affecting more than one movement or tissue. An example might be Cyriax's 'sign of the buttock' in which both straight leg raising and hip flexion are severely restricted and very painful, resulting in an 'empty end feel' as previously mentioned. In such cases, serious pathology in or around the hip or pelvis should be considered.
- Generally ill; cachexic; wasted appearance.

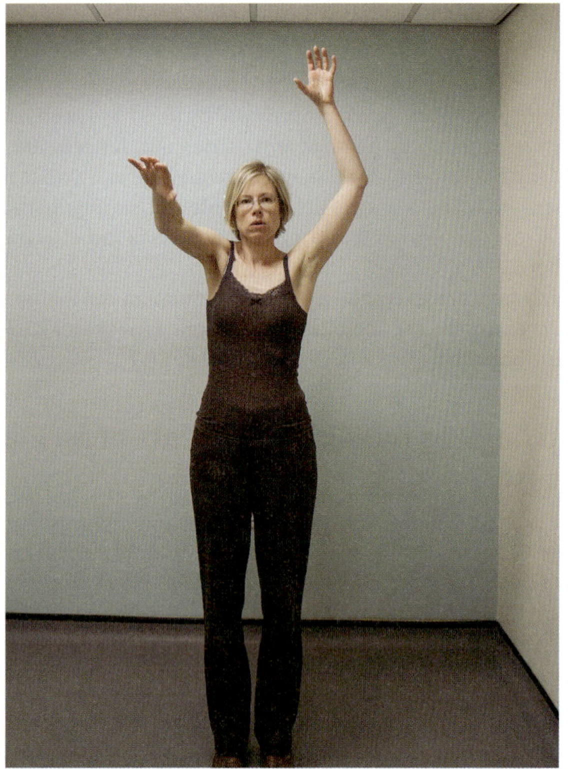

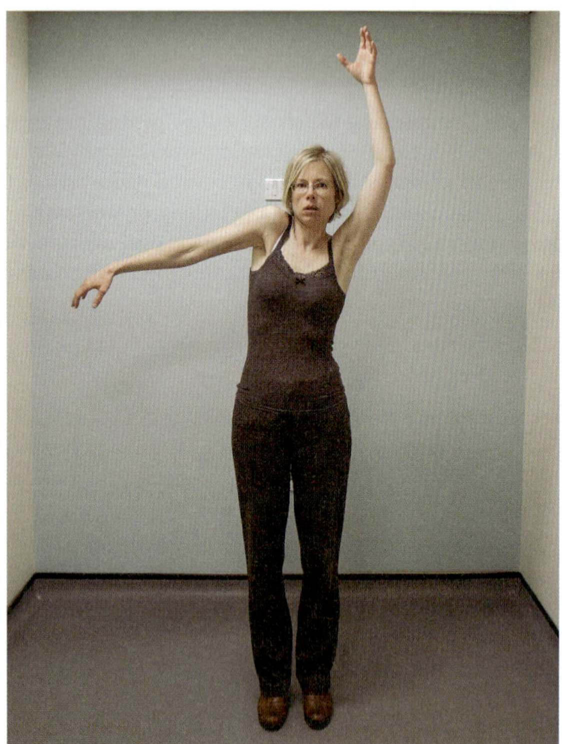

Figure 23.2 Active movements—elevation and abduction. Looking for range, pain, *willingness* (as the shoulder is considered an 'emotional joint'), and maybe a painful arc.

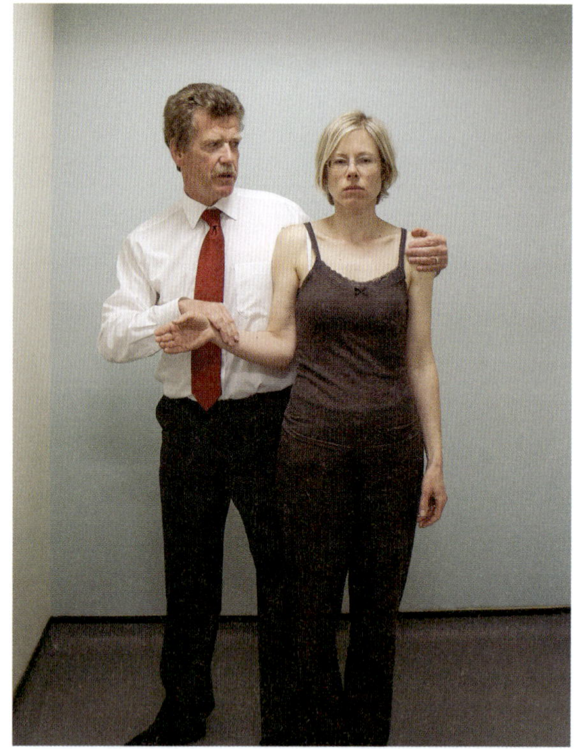

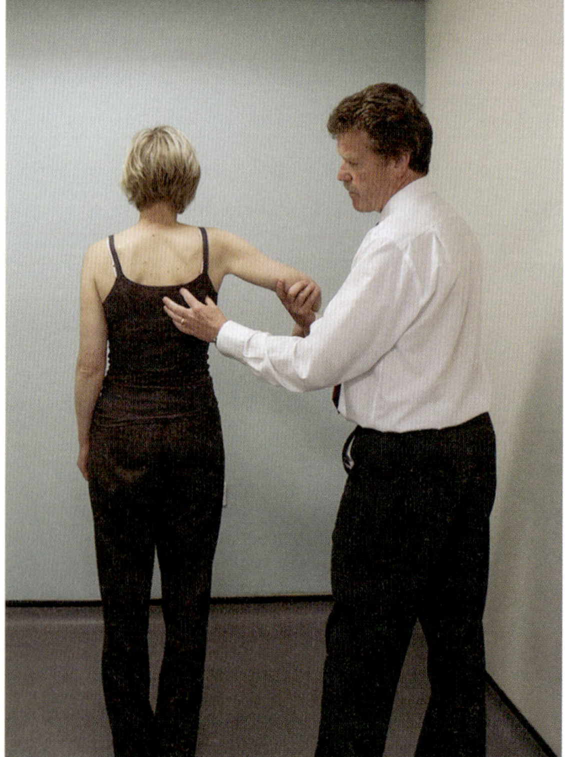

Figure 23.3 Passive movements—external rotation, abduction, and internal rotation. Looking for pain, range, and 'end feel'.

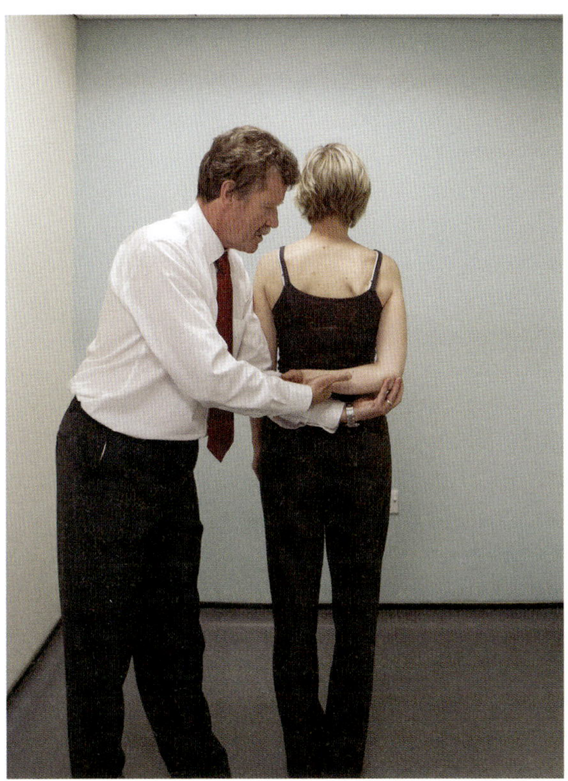

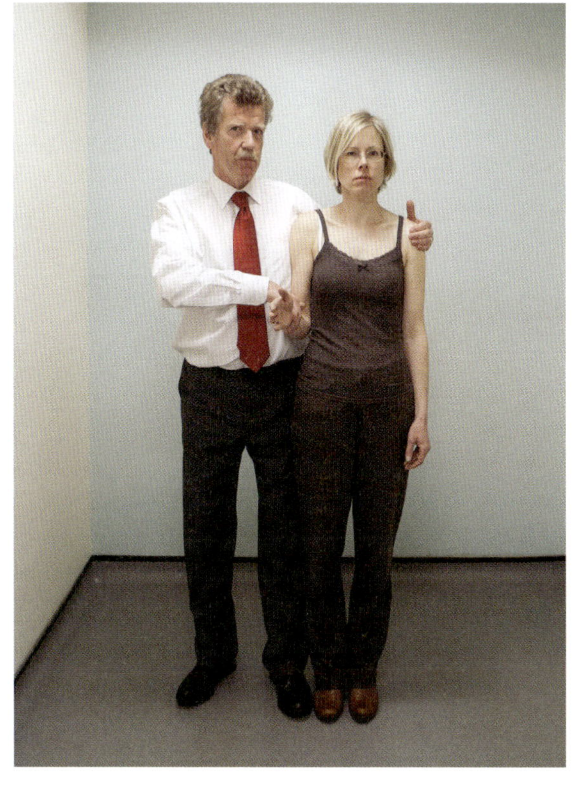

Figure 23.3 (*continued*)

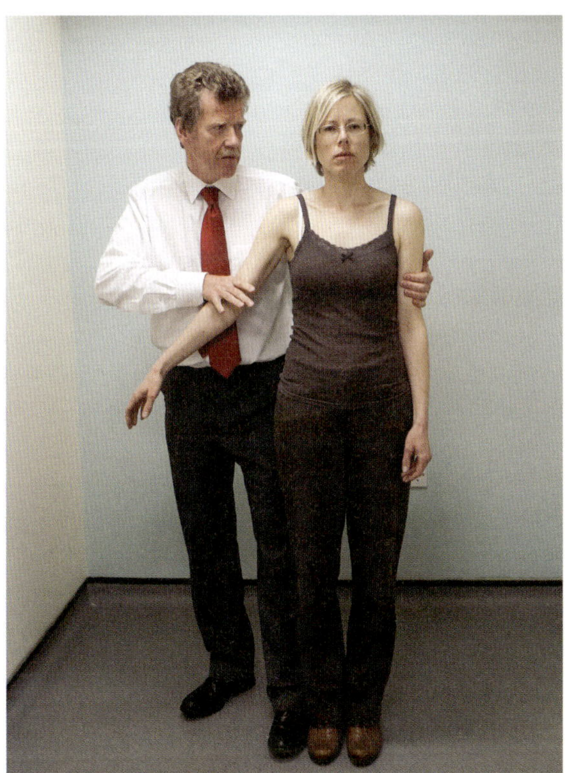

Figure 23.4 Resisted movements—abduction, internal and external rotation, elbow extension and flexion, and finally, adduction. Looking for pain and power.

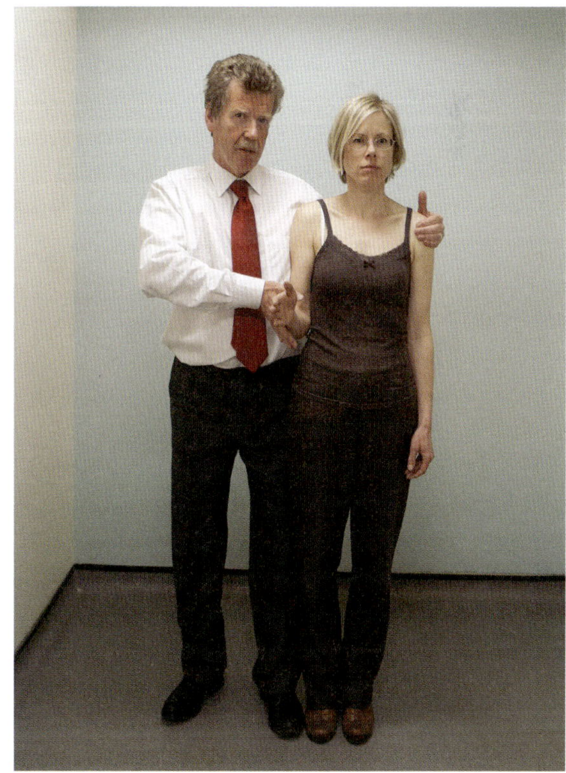

Figure 23.4 (*continued*)

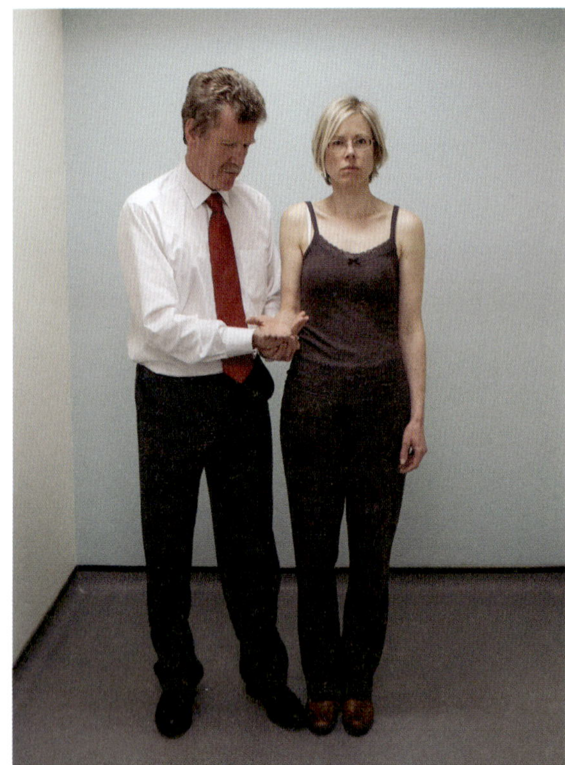

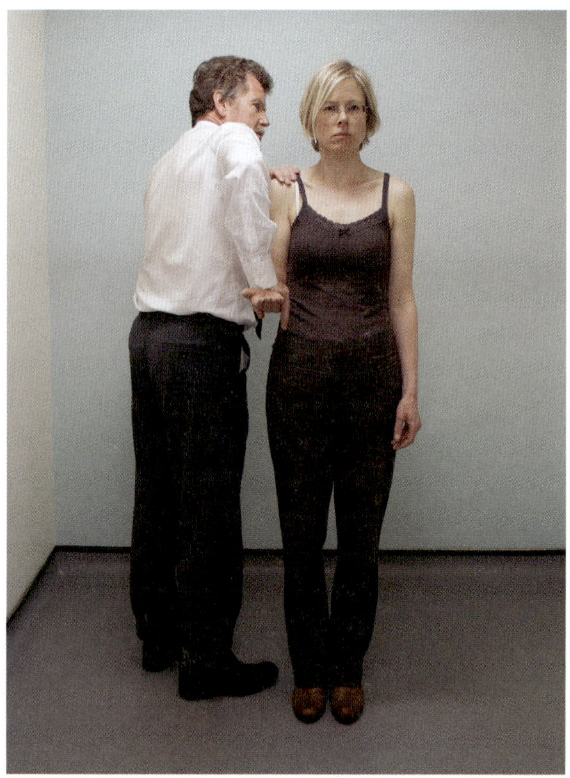

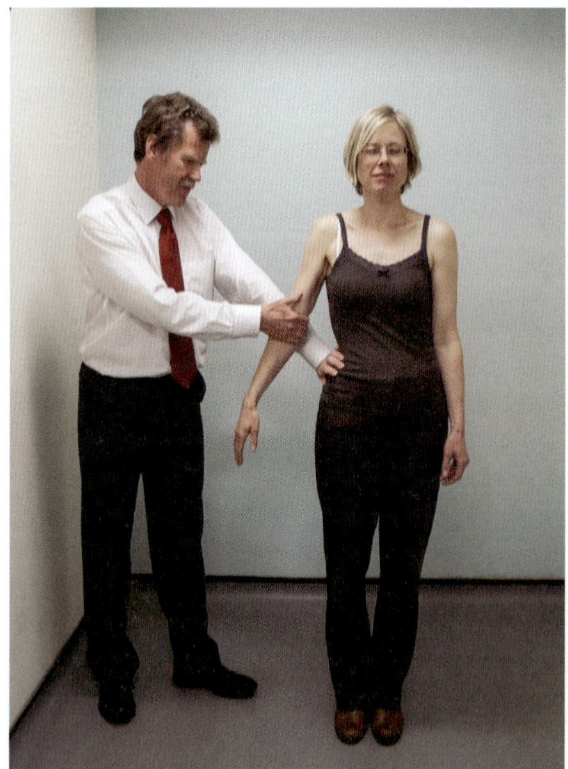

Figure 23.4 *(continued)*

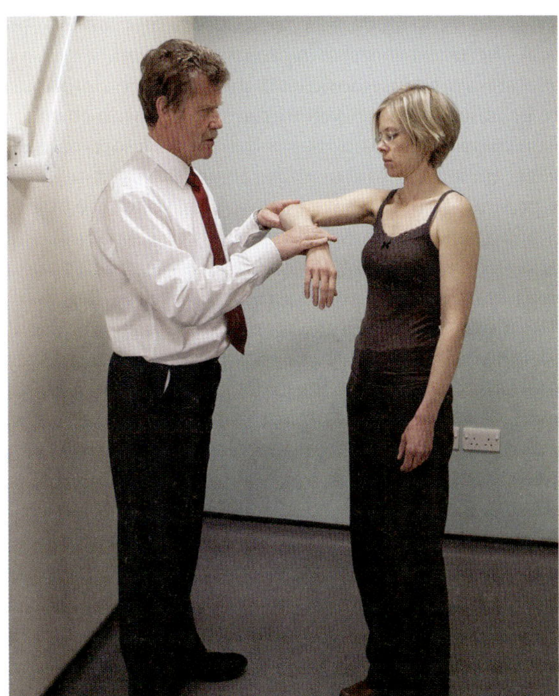

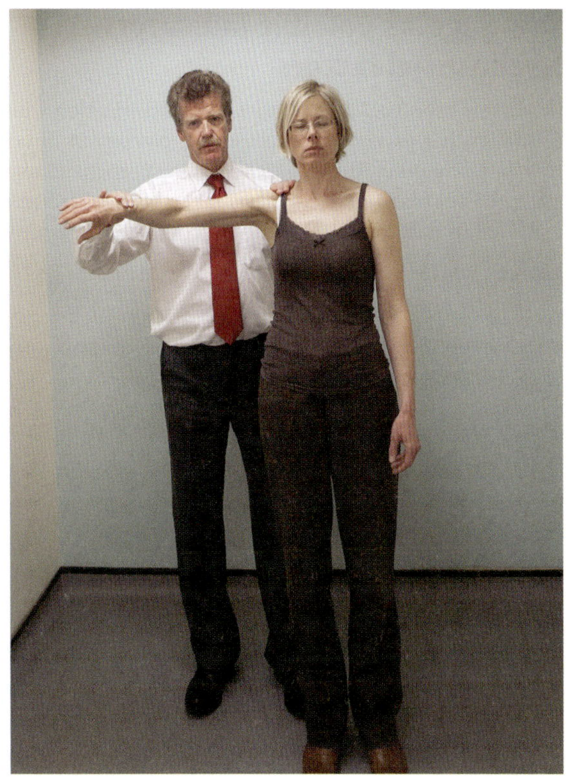

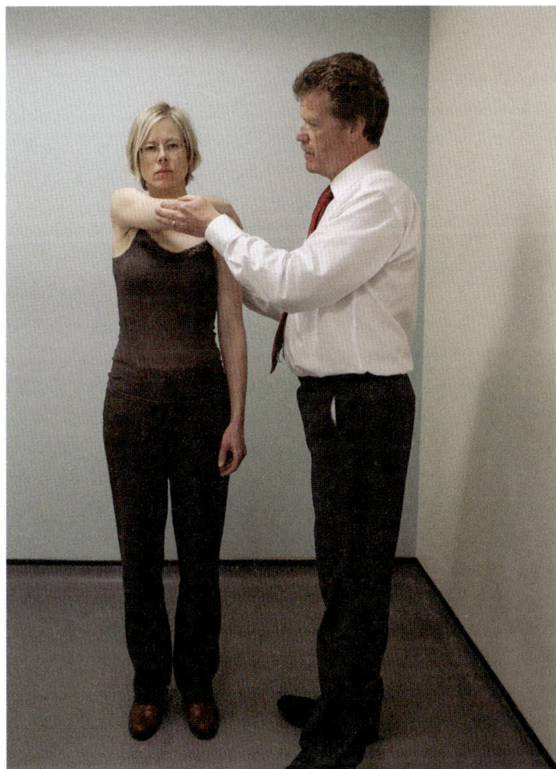

Figure 23.5 Extra tests—for example, Hawkins-Kennedy, 'empty can', and 'scarf'.

'Yellow flags' as possible indicators of psychosocial factors

Similarly, some aspects of the history and/or examination will raise the possibility that psychosocial factors are playing an important part in the presentation. This does tend to affect prognosis and will also affect the approach that should be taken with regard to management. 'Yellow flag' items in the history could include:

- A history that is inconsistent and changes with time or has symptoms that are mutually incompatible
- Bizarre symptoms which do not have any rational physical basis
- Significant compensation and/or litigation issues
- Attitudes and beliefs to their problem—guilt, catastrophization, for example
- Problems with relationships at home, work, school; family or friends who are either under- or over-supportive
- Pre-existing mental health issues or certain personality types, especially those involving depression and/or anxiety

'Yellow flag' signs could include:

- Unwillingness (or over-willingness) to be involved and co-operate with the examination
- Incompatible findings—such as an apparent inability to flex the lumbar spine or achieve any significant straight leg raise, yet with the ability to sit upright on the couch with legs straight out in front
- 'Juddering'—the alternating resisting and giving way of a tested limb

However, do remember that patients do not always present typically—beware the bizarre *but consistent* patient.

Some areas of musculoskeletal medicine are notoriously liable to be influenced by psychosocial factors—with chronic pain, and especially spinal pain, being the most important, and 'yellow flags' are a way of recognizing the presence of such factors. Many papers and books have been written about the biopyschosocial approach to medicine in general, and back pain in particular. Gordon Waddell (2004) has done much of the pioneering work in this field. Failure to recognize yellow flags and then take them into account in the management plan will result in a considerably reduced chance of a successful outcome. Although an experienced clinician will usually have little difficulty if picking up these signs and symptoms through verbal and non-verbal cues, more reliable and consistent results, especially with less experienced clinicians, may be obtained with the use of specific screening tools such as the STarT Back Tool developed by Keele University (and available at: <http://www.keele.ac.uk/sbst/>). Identification, at an early stage, of patients with a strong psychosocial component to their presentation will enable them to receive more appropriate management and, hopefully, more rapid improvement.

References

Atkins E, Kerr J, Goodlad EA. (2010) *Practical approach to orthopaedic medicine* (3rd edn). Churchill Livingstone.

Cyriax J. (1982) *Textbook of orthopaedic medicine*. Bailliere Tindall, London.

Hattam P, Smeatham A. (2010) *Special tests in musculoskeletal examination*. Churchill Livingstone.

Waddell G. (2004) *The back pain revolution*. Elsevier Health Sciences.

Chapter 24

Investigative techniques

David Knott

Introduction to investigative techniques

Unlike some other areas of medicine, musculoskeletal conditions often produce symptoms and signs that render a diagnosis possible without further investigation. With a thorough, logical history and clinical examination, a diagnosis should be possible in the majority of musculoskeletal cases. In order to be able to commence treatment promptly and also to avoid unnecessary expense and use of resources, over-investigation is to be avoided. However, sometimes further investigation may be deemed appropriate. This may be to:

- establish or confirm a diagnosis if this is not clear enough to confidently proceed with treatment—to clarify the type of an arthritic joint(s), for example
- assess the degree of severity of, or to refine a known diagnosis if this may make a difference to the type of treatment selected—particularly, for example, if surgery is contemplated or possible
- confirm or exclude serious pathology in 'red flag' cases if, for example, there is a suspicion of cancer, fracture, infection, or a serious underlying medical condition.

Ideally, we would wish an investigation to identify 100% of patients with a given condition (i.e. 'not miss any— no false negatives') and not to falsely identify any patients who do not have the condition ('no false positives'). Unfortunately, most investigations fall short of this ideal to varying degrees. Any given investigation can be said to have a certain sensitivity and specificity. These parameters may be defined as:

Sensitivity is the proportion of true positives that are correctly identified by the test.

Specificity is the proportion of true negatives that are correctly identified by the test.

A highly specific test is unlikely to give a false positive result: a positive result is therefore likely to be a true positive. A sign or symptom with very high specificity can be described as pathognomonic for that condition. In contrast, a sensitive test rarely misses a condition, so a negative result should be reassuring (that the disease tested for is absent). For example, in one study, magnetic resonance imaging (MRI) scanning at the shoulder for suspected tears of the glenoid labrum had a sensitivity of 89% (i.e. identified 89 out of 100 true cases) and a specificity of 100% (did not show any tears that were not present) (Shellock et al. 2001).

A wide variety of potential investigations are available to the musculoskeletal clinician, although local circumstances and access policies will often limit the choice. For our purposes, investigations can be conveniently grouped into:

1. Imaging tests
2. Blood tests
3. Other tests

Imaging tests in musculoskeletal medicine

Imaging techniques are the most widely used investigations in most musculoskeletal (MSK) medical practice. They can yield useful information but must be used logically and appropriately for reasons of cost, logistics, and patient safety. Guidelines are available to help with decision making, such as those from the Royal College of Radiologists (2007), available in both printed and electronic formats. Modern computer-based digital imaging systems enable X-rays to be viewed from any location, with an internet connection giving much greater convenience and speed of results than with previous film-based systems. It also highlights the advisability of MSK clinicians acquiring sufficient skills to interpret such images for themselves rather than having to wait for the report from the hospital radiologist.

Increasingly, it is common for patients to request X-rays and MRI scans to 'find the cause of their symptoms'. This is especially true with cases of spinal pain. Frequently, such requests are prompted by information obtained from the media or the internet, and sometimes recommendations have been given by other health professionals. However, the clinician must remain focused on the clinical need for such investigation and, in particular, as to whether it will materially affect the diagnosis or treatment of the patient. Although the usual reasons to justify investigation are those listed at the start of this chapter, we must acknowledge that there will be occasions when investigation has a role in reassurance and 'moving the patient on'. In such cases, however, the clinician must ensure that the patient is subsequently given an accurate and appropriate interpretation of the findings and their relevance to the patient's symptoms. As far as possible, a realistic but positive view should be given—terms such as 'crumbling spine' are not helpful and are to be avoided!

X-rays

X-rays are widely available and relatively inexpensive. The potential for their medical use was realized by American physiologist Walter Bradford Cannon within a short time of their discovery by Roentgen in 1895. They are now used widely throughout the world. Radiation scientists at the Health Protection Agency have estimated that about 46 million medical and dental X-ray examinations were carried out across the UK in 2008, an increase of 10% since 1997. About 67% of the procedures were carried out in NHS hospitals while 26% were performed by dentists.

X-rays do involve the use of ionizing radiation that for some examinations, for example, lumbar spinal views, can be considerable (Table 24.1). A recent Health Protection Agency (HPA) study revealed that the average annual radiation dose to each member of the public from all diagnostic X-rays has increased from 0.33 millisieverts (mSv) in 1997, the last time a detailed frequency survey was completed, to 0.4 mSv. Most of the increase is due to the growth in the number of higher-dose computed tomography (CT) examinations. Medical X-rays remain the largest single artificial source of radiation exposure for the UK population. The average radiation dose from all sources of ionizing radiation remains about 2.7mSv per person year and medical X-rays contribute 15% of this total. However, according to the HPA—'Despite the increased use of diagnostic X-rays in medicine in the UK, the average dose to the population is still considerably lower than in comparable countries'. The HPA has calculated that there are small but real risks from medical X-ray examinations; for example, X-rays of hips/pelvis/lumbar spine probably give a risk of developing cancer of between 1:10,000 and 1:100,000 (Wall et al. 2011).

Think carefully before requesting X-rays in younger people and especially in women of childbearing age. Although the dosage of X-rays used diagnostically is not thought likely to cause harm to the fetus, it is generally best to avoid X-rays, especially those involving the abdomen, in pregnancy, unless there is a clear and unavoidable need.

X-rays are principally used when bony pathology is suspected, as in fracture, dislocation, arthritis, or metastasis. They can also sometimes provide 'circumstantial evidence' of related soft-tissue disease as in impingement syndromes at the shoulder. Although a single X-ray is usually sufficient to help achieve a diagnosis, a repeat film after an interval of 10–14 days may be needed in some cases of suspected fracture—e.g. metatarsal or scaphoid—as changes may not show on a film taken soon after injury. If in doubt, a radionucleotide bone scan, or a CT scan, can help here. In addition, repeat X-rays taken after appropriate intervals can help to show whether a degenerative condition is progressing or not, and at what rate.

It must be remembered that findings on X-ray examination do not always correlate with the clinical symptoms presented by the patient. Patients pressing for X-rays do not always realize this. It is common, for example, to see degenerative changes in spinal X-rays in individuals with no back pain, just as it is to find normal X-rays in those with back pain. Similarly, congenital anomalies around the lumbosacral junction are relatively frequent and may not be relevant to the problem being treated. Even if such findings prove to be relevant to the diagnosis, they do not necessarily lead to an alteration in the treatment plan. One study showed that out of 1200 cervical spine X-rays, only one led to a change in management of the case (Heller et al. 1983).

Clinicians need to complete request forms carefully and legibly, giving an adequate history, asking any specific questions for a radiologist to answer, and also requesting specific views, as appropriate, if these are not 'routine' for that body part. In the lower limb, for example, it is usually most productive to have weight-bearing X-rays and these may not always be done unless specifically requested. If it is not clear which is the most appropriate investigation for a patient's clinical circumstances, or if an investigation is deemed urgent, most radiologists are helpful and willing to advise.

Table 24.1 Relative radiation dosages for some common examinations

	Relative radiation dosage (Hart and Wall 2002)
Chest X-ray (single PA film)	1
Peripheral joint (most)	0.5
Cervical spine	5
Hip	20
Pelvis	35
Lumbar spine	50
CT scan lumbar spine	400–500

MRI scans

The theory behind MRI scanning had its origin in the 1950s but it was not until 1977 that Damadian, Minkoff, and Goldsmith performed the first MRI body scan of a human being. After overcoming further technical issues, MRI scanners began to appear for routine clinical use in the 1980s. MRI scanning is much more widely available now than in the past. The scanner applies a strong magnetic field across body tissues and this field is rapidly turned on and off, and varied. The magnetic field affects the protons of the hydrogen atom nuclei in differing tissues to differing extents. Recording the responses and then computer manipulation of the data can produce detailed images that can demonstrate contrast between the different tissues. Basic views—commonly known as t-1 and t-2—are adequate for most purposes. They differentiate between the appearance of body fat and water in different ways. Sometimes, it is necessary to inject contrast media (gadolinium) to produced enhanced MRI views, especially in the investigation of cancers and when it is useful to demonstrate vascular details, and also in cases of post-operative fibrosis.

Most MRI scanners are large, expensive, fixed machines situated in hospitals. The patient lies still within the 'tunnel' of the machine whilst the scan is performed. Although non-invasive, some patients find the noise, confined environment, and need to remain still and supine for prolonged periods hard to cope with. Open MRI scanners are better suited to claustrophobic patients but these machines are less widely available and more expensive for the NHS. Smaller, more portable machines have been developed for MRI of the limbs. In addition, MRI can be applied in certain situations to allow movements during the examination (real-time MRI) or to aid some minimally invasive procedures (interventional MRI).

MRI does not use ionizing radiation and is therefore generally considered safer and preferable to CT scanning where possible. It is not known to have any definite adverse affects excepting the potential of moving loose, or potentially loose metal during the examination, and to have possible effects on some implanted electrical devices. It is not known to be harmful in pregnancy but, as a precaution, is usually avoided during the first trimester.

There are, therefore, a number of contraindications (CIs) and cautions:

CIs: Pacemakers, defibrillators, and some cardiac reveal devices

Metallic foreign bodies in eyes

Aneurysm clips in brain; some central nervous system (CNS) shunts

Cautions: Pregnancy, especially first trimester (uncertain if totally safe)

Cochlear and other implants

Artificial heart valve

Severe claustrophobia (unless open scanner available)

Other: Metal implants/prostheses—degrades image (less so if titanium)

MRI can give excellent views of soft tissues and is often the investigation of choice for spinal cases where disc and/or nerve root pathology is suspected. Although it is still reasonable and appropriate to treat non-specific low back pain and uncomplicated sciatica on clinical grounds alone, MRI scanning is helpful in more persistent or complicated spinal cases and certainly if surgery is being considered. It is also the most appropriate investigation for patients with suspected intra-articular meniscal or ligament injuries of the knee (see Figures 24.1 and 24.2). Many knee surgeons will now request MRI scan before committing a patient to arthroscopy, even if the symptoms and signs are highly suggestive of meniscal damage. The fine resolution of MRI scanning can be helpful to demonstrate synovitis in early inflammatory arthritis and also at the sacro-iliac joints in suspected ankylosing spondylitis.

By providing good-quality images with a non-invasive, safe technique, MRI has been viewed as a revolution in diagnostics for many conditions. However, MRI scans remain relatively expensive and scarce compared with X-rays and, like X-rays, may show much pathology, especially of a degenerative nature, that is not always relevant to the patient's symptoms. (See Figure 24.3 for a comparative MRI scan and X-ray.) In one study, 20% of asymptomatic individuals aged under 60 had disc protrusions on MRI scan (Brenner

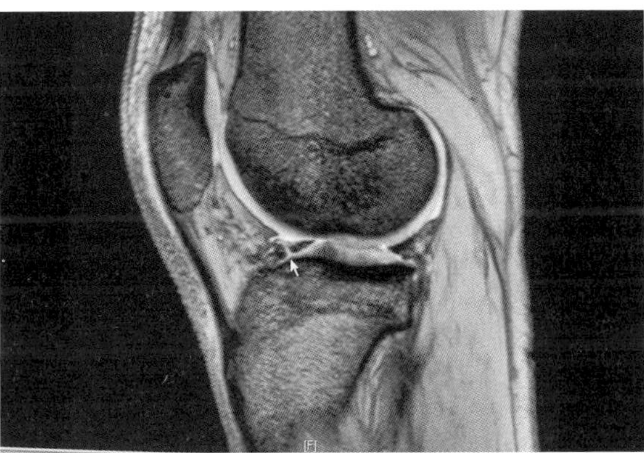

Figure 24.1 Tear (arrowed) in anterior horn of lateral meniscus.

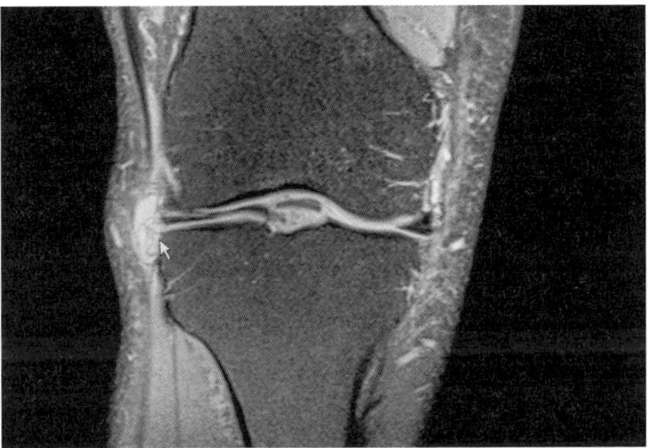

Figure 24.2 Parameniscal cyst (arrowed) associated with meniscal tear.

(a)

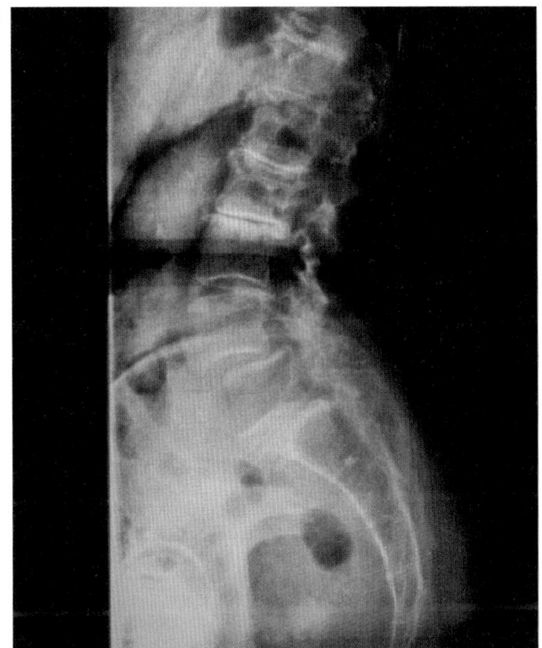

(b)

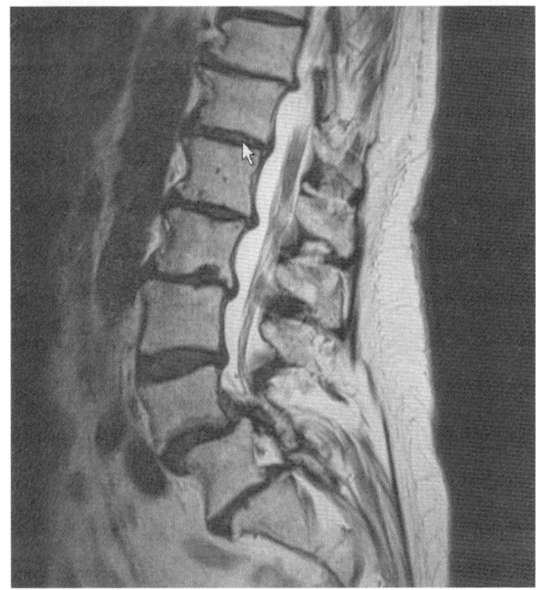

Figure 24.3 Corresponding (a) X-ray and (b) MRI images of a significantly spondylotic lumbar spine with scoliosis, disc, and facet joint degeneration and L4/5 and L5/S1 spondylolistheses.

and Hall 2007) and in another, 76% of 'high risk individuals'—those with physically demanding jobs (but still asymptomatic)—had disc protrusion or extrusion (Laitt et al. 1996). In addition, it is not unusual to find a patient with back and/or leg pain with a normal MRI. Although patients (and some clinicians) find this hard to understand, modern pain theory allows for such pains to exist in the absence of current tissue damage.

CT scans

CT scanners (X-ray computed tomography) were developed in the early 1970s, although much of the theoretical work dates back to the 1950s. Multiple X-ray images are manipulated by a computer to produce clear and accurate two-dimensional cross- sectional images (and now, potentially, three-dimensional images) of both soft tissue and bony pathologies (see Figure 24.4). As with MRI, contrast media may be used to enhance images. They can have a place where an MRI scan is contraindicated (e.g. in a patient with a pacemaker). In addition, because they show bone cortex particularly well, they demonstrate greater detail of bony abnormalities that can be useful in the diagnosis of suspected fractures and some tumours.

Patients will have to lie supine for 10–30 minutes, as for an MRI scan, but not within a tunnel, and so the claustrophobic patient should be able to cope. The dose of ionizing radiation will depend on the area to be scanned and the quality of image required, but can be considerable, and this needs to be borne in mind if repeated scans are considered. For this reason, CT scans are normally avoided in pregnancy and only used after careful consideration in children. There is likely to be a small increase in rates of cancer as a result of current level of CT scanning—it is estimated that 0.4% of current cancers in the USA occur as a result of CT scanning (Brenner and Hall 2007).

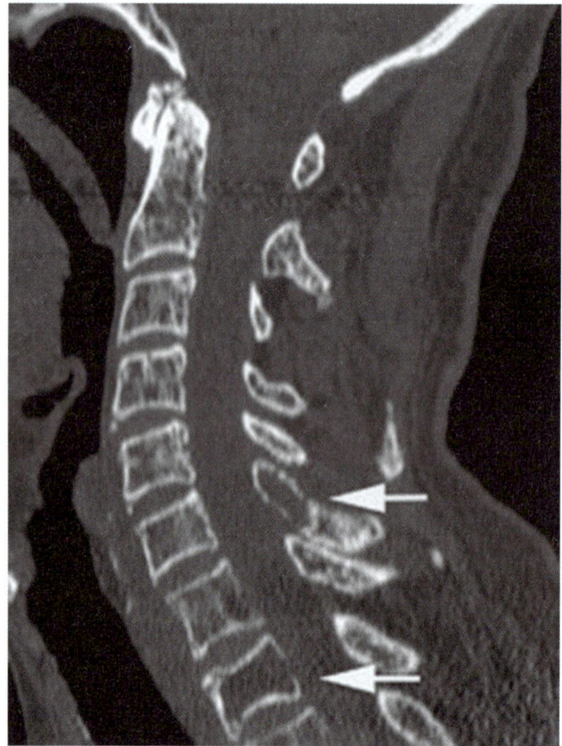

Figure 24.4 Sagittal CT of the cervical spine demonstrating lytic lesions in the posterior elements of C6 and the body of T1 (arrows) in multiple myeloma.

Myelography

This technique became established in the 1920s and for decades was the only diagnostic method that could yield information about soft tissues within the spinal canal. With a myelogram, a radio-opaque dye is introduced into the spinal canal and then X-rays are taken. In the past, it was the investigation of choice in significant radiculopathy and suspected intervertebral disc prolapse. Compared to MRI, it is a prolonged, invasive, and fairly unpleasant procedure involving some discomfort and the possibility of either intra- or post-procedure adverse effects such as allergic reaction and headache. More seriously, there also appears to be a small incidence of adhesive arachnoiditis after myelography (Laitt et al. 1996).

Myelography has a much smaller role in diagnosis since the introduction of MRI, but could still have a role in those patients in whom MRI is contraindicated and a CT scan would not be considered to give adequate information. There are also some clinicians who believe that myelography can deliver a more accurate estimation of spinal stenosis than MRI (Morita et al. 2011). One study showed that nerve root compression in the lateral recess is underestimated by MRI in nearly 30% of surgically confirmed cases, compared to only 5–7% in myelography (Bartynski and Lin 2003).

Discography

Discography is sometimes used to confirm that a certain intervertebral disc is responsible for producing a patient's pain before proceeding to fusion-type surgery. X-ray and MRI scan may well have shown degenerative changes or damage to the disc, sometimes with evidence of instability, but it may still not be clinically clear that this is the cause of the patient's pain. Discography consists of the injection of fluid (usually X-ray contrast media) into the centre of the suspect disc(s) causing an increase in pressure. A normal disc can only accommodate 1–1.5 ml of fluid. The patient is asked whether this causes pain, and if the pain so produced is their usual pain. If so, then it may be expected that fusion surgery across that disc would have a good chance of relieving the patient's pain. Discography will also test the competency of the disc (i.e. whether the injected fluid leaks out through a fissure). Possible complications of the procedure include nerve damage and discitis—a potentially serious infection of the disc. Results of discography must be interpreted with some caution as there can be a high rate of false positives as shown in the study by Carragee et al. (2000).

Isotope bone scans

In an isotope bone scan (bone scintigraphy), a radioactive substance is injected into the body and preferentially taken up by different body tissues—in this case bone. The pattern of subsequent emissions is then detected and images are produced. It reflects the physiology and metabolism of the bone rather than static anatomical structure and the whole body can be scanned at once. Areas of increased blood flow and bone turnover will display as 'hot spots'.

Although bone scans will demonstrate benign pathology such as osteoarthritis, they are useful when more serious diseases are suspected, such as fractures and metastatic malignant disease (although MRI can also provide much useful information in this situation). They are most commonly used in the diagnosis and assessment of suspected bony tumours, infections, and fractures when X-rays have not given sufficient information (see Figure 24.5). A suspicious history could include past cancer, pathological fracture,

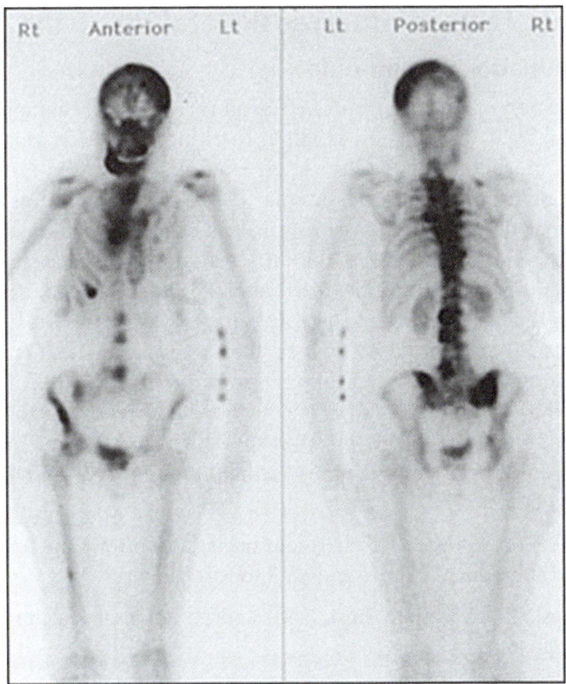

Figure 24.5 Bone scan showing multiple bony cancer secondary deposits throughout the spine.

or unexpectedly raised alkaline phosphatase. Although only minimally invasive, it must be remembered that ionizing radiation is again an issue, and doses tend to be higher than with conventional X-ray examinations.

Ultrasound

Doctor Karl Dussik of Austria published the first paper on medical ultrasonics in 1942, based on his research on transmission ultrasound investigation of the brain; Professor Ian Donald of Scotland subsequently developed practical technology and applications for ultrasound in the 1950s.

Ultrasound scanning is a modality in which high-frequency (20,000 or more vibrations per second) sound waves are passed through body tissues. When these waves encounter a tissue with a greater density, they are reflected back. These reflected waves can then be detected by the ultrasound probe and used to produce an image that can be interpreted. Ultrasound scans can be useful for demonstrating the appearance of soft tissues, both normal and abnormal, especially in such as muscles, tendons, and tendon sheaths. They can also deliver useful information regarding the nature of lumps and swellings, particularly as to whether they are solid or fluid- containing. Furthermore, an ultrasound scan can also demonstrate the presence of increased blood flow in soft tissues in conditions such as synovitis and teno-synovitis, as well as showing the neovascularization of tendinopathy. Images produced are usually clearest when the tissue being investigated is relatively superficial.

Ultrasound also has the advantage that it does not use ionizing radiation and is therefore considered very safe, including in pregnancy. In addition, it allows the relevant body part to be moved during the examination, if appropriate. In the shoulder, for example, this may enable confirmation of suspected tendon impingement as well as clarifying and grading the resulting tendon pathology (see Figure 24.6). In such a case, as well as helping clarify the diagnosis, the result of the ultrasound may well help select those patients who are, or who are not, suitable for particular treatment options such as injection and surgery.

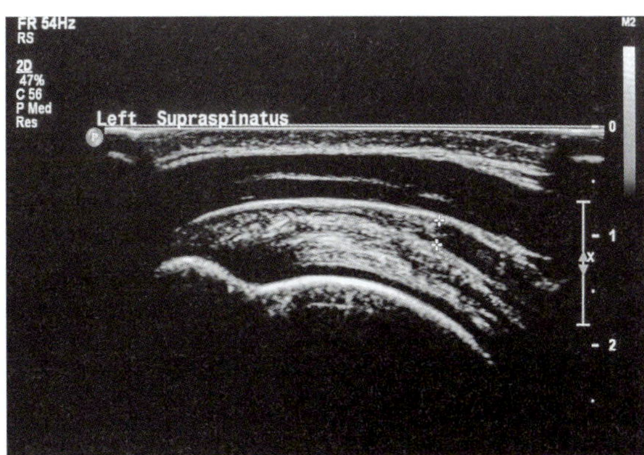

Figure 24.6 Ultrasound of left supraspinatus tendon, also showing thickened subacromial bursa.

Results and their interpretation are highly dependent on the quality of the equipment used and also very much on the skill of the ultrasonographer. In addition, the body morphology of the patient will potentially affect the quality of results obtained—producing good-quality images in the obese or excessively muscled patients can prove difficult for some areas such as the shoulder, and other imaging techniques such as MRI scan may then be preferable.

Unlike most other imaging techniques, ultrasound scanning is a technique that may be learned and performed by the MSK clinician in a clinic setting, often using a portable machine in a wide variety of environments. It can prove a steep learning curve, but many courses and on-line resources are available. In addition to its diagnostic role, an ultrasound machine can also be used as an aid to treatment, such as in the guidance of nerve block and corticosteroid injections. As so often in MSK medicine, the evidence as to whether this produces better results than anatomically guided injections is less than ideal and is often contradictory (Hall and Buchbinder 2004; Naredo et al. 2004).

So which imaging technique is best?

In the spine—it is generally accepted that X-rays are over-used and often contribute little useful or management-changing information. They should be used mainly to diagnose or exclude conditions such as vertebral fracture/collapse, suspected bony metastases, and anatomical abnormalities such as scoliosis and spondylolisis/spondylolisthesis. If spondylolisis is suspected, oblique views should be requested. Flexion and extension views of the lumbar spine can be useful in cases of suspected instability. MRI has become the investigation of choice for intervertebral disc and nerve root pathology, as well as for suspected infections and tumours. CT scanning may be required in some patients and an isotope bone scan may be useful to more fully demonstrate the extent of metastases. A discogram may be required in some patients to decide if surgery would be appropriate.

With peripheral joints—X-ray is usually the first-line investigation to demonstrate and quantify degenerative pathology or anatomical variations. Serial X-rays can demonstrate progression of degenerative changes. If inflammatory disease such as rheumatoid arthritis is suspected, then erosions may be shown on X-rays but these, and associated synovitis, are better and more sensitively demonstrated by either ultrasound scan or MRI. Soft-tissue lesions within, or adjacent to a joint are best demonstrated by either ultrasound or MRI scans—the choice will often be dictated by local facilities and policies, by patient choice, and, occasionally, body habitus.

With other connective tissues—such as muscles, ligaments, and tendons—an ultrasound scan is most commonly used, but MRI may be indicated or preferable in some situations.

Blood tests in musculoskeletal medicine

Blood tests are readily available and are mostly inexpensive. They are commonly used when an inflammatory condition is suspected, and also in 'red flag' cases if infection, malignant diseases, or other serious bony pathology are suspected. In addition, sometimes they can be indicated when neurological symptoms are prominent in a patient's presentation or when there are symptoms or signs of systemic medical disease.

A reasonable 'screen' for suspected inflammatory disease would be to request:

- Full blood count (FBC)
- Erythrocyte sedimentation rate (ESR)
- C-reactive protein (CRP)

ESR and CRP are both useful for screening for inflammation or infection. CRP is generally considered to be more sensitive than ESR and it must also be remembered that ESR tends to increase with age, especially beyond 60 years, whereas CRP is less affected by age (Osei-Bimpong et al. 2007). These inflammatory markers can be useful to both diagnose disease and also to monitor progress and response to treatment. Other tests such as rheumatoid factor (RF), Anti-cyclic Citrullinated Peptide (anti-CCP), and Human Leukocyte Antigen (HLA-B27) status may be indicated if specific rheumatological conditions are suspected. As with imaging, it should be remembered that some of these tests are of low specificity, such as rheumatoid factor, which can be positive in 10–15% of normal individuals. HLA- B27 tissue type is present in 95% cases of ankylosing spondylitis, but also in 8% of the normal population in developed countries.

Other blood tests that may be useful can be seen in Table 24.2.

Table 24.2 Useful blood tests

Blood test	Indications/relevance
Bone chemistry including calcium and alkaline phosphatase	Suspicion of significant bony disease or abnormalities of calcium/parathyroid disease
Protein electrophoresis	If myeloma is suspected
Serum urate	If gout is suspected—but can be normal during an attack
Prostate specific antigen (PSA)	If prostate cancer is suspected
B12 and folate	In some cases with neurological symptoms
Creatinine kinase	If myositis is suspected
Thyroid function (T4, TSH)	If thyroid disease is suspected

Other tests in musculoskeletal medicine

Examination of joint fluid

Aspiration of a joint or bursa effusion is commonly therapeutic, especially if the effusion is large. In clinical practice, this will occur most commonly at the knee. However, aspiration can also have an important diagnostic role. The naked eye appearance of synovial fluid can be reassuring if it is clear and yellow-green, with no more than minor blood streaking, or it can be more worrying if turbid, cloudy, or frankly bloody. If fluid is reassuring to the naked eye, and there are no worrying symptoms, then it is usually discarded without further examination. If it is at all suspicious, then further examination of the fluid in the laboratory may well be indicated, and it may be appropriate to refer the patient at that stage for more specialized acute care. The aspirated fluid can be sent off to the laboratory and examined for signs of:

- Infection—presence of cells and bacteria on direct microscopy and subsequent culture and antibiotic sensitivity
- Crystals—as in gout (uric acid) and pseudogout (calcium pyrophosphate)

Although these are the commonest investigations, many other examinations can be performed upon synovial fluid, although most of these are of little relevance to everyday musculoskeletal practice—a thorough review can be found in the article by Revell (1982).

Neurophysiology

Neurophysiological tests are generally considered safe, although some patients do find them mildly uncomfortable. There are relatively few contraindications or complications but patients with pacemakers, or other implanted electronic devices, will need assessment first to see if they are suitable.

Nerve conduction studies (NCS)

Nerve conduction studies can be useful to confirm compression or disease of peripheral nerves in conditions such as carpal tunnel syndrome (see Table 24.3) or ulnar nerve entrapment, and to assess the severity of the compression—especially if the patient's presentation is not typical. Electrical stimulation of the nerve and recording of the subsequent action potential at a distant site along the same nerve will show increased latency (the time taken for the impulse to travel from the stimulating to the recording point) and probably reduced amplitude in cases of compression. Motor and sensory components can both be assessed (see Table 24.3).

NCS are also helpful to differentiate between neurological symptoms in a limb that may be of either peripheral or radicular origin. This can be particularly useful in patients with both nerve root and peripheral nerve pathology—so-called 'double crush' situations. In the double crush syndrome, as postulated by Upton and McComas, the presence of a more proximal lesion does seem to render the more distal nerve trunk more vulnerable to compression. Practice studies have shown that given a more proximal root compression, less involvement of the median nerve across the carpal tunnel was required to produce symptoms. Furthermore, the surgical outcome of carpal tunnel release in this double crush group was poorer (Osterman 1988).

Table 24.3 NCS result from 76-year-old lady with carpal tunnel syndrome—sensory nerve conduction velocities are reduced in digits 1 and 2, absent in 3, but normal in digit 5

Motor Nerve Conduction Study								
Site	Latency (ms)	Amplitude	Area	Segment	Distance (mrts)	Interval (ms)	NCV (m/s)	NCV N.D.
Median & Ulnar. L								
Wrist – APB	7.8ms	1.97mV	8.83mVms	Wrist – APR	60mm	7.80ms		
Forearm – APB	11.84ms	1.93mV	9.12mVms	Wrist – APB – Forearm – APB	180mm	4.04ms	44.6m/s	
Wrist – 2 L	4.94ms	1.35mV	10.01mVms	Wrist – 2 L	100mm	4.94ms		
Wrist-2DIO	2.76ms	2.96mV	9.82mVms	Wrist – 2DIO	100mm	2.76ms		
Wrist – ADM	2.52ms	8.76mV	30.25mVms	Wrist – ADM	60mm	252ms		
Sensory Nerve Conduction Study								
Site	Latency (ms)	Amplitude	Area	Segment	Distance (mrts)	Interval (ms)	NCV (m/s)	NCV N.D.
Median & Ulnar. L								
D1 – Wrist	3.06ms	1.70uV	0.07uVms	D1 – Wrist	8.2mm	3.06ms	26.8m/s	
D2 – Wrist	3 54ms	4.30uV	0.36uVms	D2 – Wrist	115mm	3.54ms	32.5m/s	
D3 – Wrist absent	0ms							
D5 – Wrist	2.14ms	4.50uV	4.81uVms	D5 – Wrist	102mm	2 14ms	47.7m/s	

Electromyography (EMG)

This is the recording of electrical activity within muscles at rest and on either voluntary contraction or electrical stimulation. It is used in the diagnosis of neuromuscular disease. EMG is usually done by inserting fine needle electrodes into the relevant muscles but can sometimes be done using surface electrodes. It is principally used in differentiating between muscle and nerve pathologies in cases of muscle weakness or wasting. Certain conditions, such as myasthenia gravis or muscular dystrophies, can produce characteristic recording patterns. It can also give helpful evidence in cases of suspected motor radiculopathy.

It must be remembered that nerve conduction studies—both the performance and interpretation—rely upon skilled staff, and that they can also yield both false positive and false negative results. In one recent study by Witt et al. (2004), 25% of carpal tunnel syndrome patients had normal NCS and, in addition, the NCS results when positive were not found to help predict the outcome of non-surgical treatment. NCS are less accurate in the early stages of carpal tunnel syndrome and in younger patients (Wilder-Smith et al. 2006).

Readers wishing to know more about neurophysiology testing are referred to the excellent article by Mallik and Weir (2005).

References

Bartynski WS, Lin L. Lumbar root compression in the lateral recess: MR imaging, conventional myelography, and CT myelography comparison with surgical confirmation. *Am J Neurorad* 2003; 24(3):348–60.

Brenner DJ, Hall EJ. Computed tomography—an increasing source of radiation exposure. *N Engl J Med* 2007; 357(22):2277–84.

Carragee EJ, Tanner CM, Khurana S, et al. The rates of false-positive lumbar discography in select patients without low back symptoms. *Spine* 2000; 25:1373–81.

Hall S, Buchbinder R. Do imaging methods that guide needle placement improve outcome? *Ann Rheum Dis* 2004; 63:1007–8.

Hart D, Wall BF. (2002) *Radiation exposure of the UK population from medical and dental X-ray examinations.* National Radiological Protection Board, Oxfordshire.

Heller, C.A. et al. Value of X-ray examinations of the cervical spine. *BMJ* 1983; 287:1276–8.

Laitt R, Jackson A, Isherwood I. Patterns of chronic adhesive arachnoiditis following myodil myelography: the significance of spinal canal stenosis and previous surgery. *Br J Radiol* 1996; 69:693–8.

Mallik A, Weir A. Nerve conduction studies: essentials and pitfalls in practice. *J Neurol Neurosurg Psychiatry* 2005; 76.

Morita M, Miyauchi A, Okuda S, Oda T, Iwasaki M. Comparison between MRI and myelography in lumbar spinal canal stenosis for the decision of levels of decompression surgery. *J Spinal Dis Tech* 2011; 24(1):31–6.

Naredo E, et al. A randomized comparative study of short-term response to blind injection versus sonographic-guided injection of local corticosteroids in patients with painful shoulder. *J Rheumatol* 2004; 31:308–14.

Osei-Bimpong A, Meek JH, Lewis SM. ESR or CRP? A comparison of their clinical utility. *Haematology* 2007 Aug; 12(4): 353–7.

Osterman AL. The double crush syndrome. *Orthop Clin North Am* 1988; 19(1):147–55.

Revell PA. *Examination of synovial fluid. Bone and joint disease.* Springer-Verlag 1982.

Royal College of Radiologists (RCR). *Making best use of clinical radiology services.* RCR 2007. Available at: <http://www.rcr.ac.uk>.

Shellock FG, Bert JM, Fritts HM, et al. Evaluation of the rotator cuff and glenoid labrum using a 0.2-Tesla extremity magnetic resonance (MR) system: MR results compared to surgical findings. *J Magn Reson Imaging* 2001; 14:763–70.

Wall BF, et al. (2011) *HPA-CRCE-028. Radiation risks from medical X-ray examinations as a function of the age and sex of the patient.* Health Protection Agency, Centre for Radiation, Chemical and Environmental Hazards Chilton, Didcot Oxfordshire.

Wilder-Smith E, et al. Diagnosing carpal tunnel syndrome—clinical criteria and ancillary tests. *Neurology* 2006; 2(7).

Witt, J.C. et al. Carpal tunnel syndrome with normal nerve conduction studies. *Muscle Nerve* 2004; 29(4):515–22.

Chapter 25

Musculoskeletal injections

Hany Elmadbouh

Introduction to musculoskeletal injections

Musculoskeletal injections are commonly performed by practitioners from different disciplines including rheumatology, orthopaedics, musculoskeletal medicine, sports medicine, pain management, general practice, physiotherapy, and radiology.

Pain is one of the most frequent causes of loss in productivity with an annual cost estimated at approximately $225 billion in the United States alone (Stewart et al. 2003a). Musculoskeletal pain accounts for more than 50% of the estimated loss (Stewart et al. 2003b). Approximately 13% of the annual cost of reductions in productivity related to health problems is caused by pain (Stewart et al. 2003a). Interventions aimed at limiting the decrease in productivity can produce a return of approximately $3 for every dollar spent in reducing absences from the workplace (Aldana 2001). This highlights the economic importance and strong social impact of the growing use of low-cost interventions for pain relief (Robotti et al. 2013).

Most joint and soft tissue injections can be performed via the visualization and direct palpation of anatomical landmarks to guide appropriate needle placement. However, blind injections are potentially inaccurate and carry the risk of accidental needling or drug delivery to non-target structures, and this could be dangerous and potentially fatal.

Many injections are given using only anatomical landmarks and although there has been an increase in the use of ultrasound-guided injections, particularly by rheumatologists, it is the interventional radiologists who use image guidance without exception in their work. Perhaps the primary reason for the increased use of image guidance has been the improved technology. Better visualization of anatomy yields greater confidence to undertake procedures that were previously thought to be dangerous or impossible. Improvements in the speed of image acquisition and display and the development of 3-D technology are changing the way that procedures are performed and making new procedures possible.

Ultrasound has become an increasingly valuable tool for guiding musculoskeletal interventions due to improvements in probes and image-processing software. Ultrasound offers the added advantage of portability, low cost, availability, and use of non-ionizing radiation.

Image-guided joint and soft tissue injections can also be performed under computer tomography (CT), fluoroscopy and, more recently, magnetic resonance imaging (MRI). In general, the majority of injections are performed using ultrasound or fluoroscopy which is more readily available and more cost-effective than CT. The exception is spinal injections which are more readily and safely done under CT guidance. The choice of the imaging modality may be dependent on availability, the expertise of the clinician performing the injection, the characteristics of the patient, and the clinical problem.

In general, ultrasound is used for soft tissue injections, fluoroscopy for superficial bone lesions and joint injections, and CT (with or without CT fluoroscopy) for spine injections. Recently, CT-integrated fluoroscopy equipment has become available. This has allowed a combination of CT-like imaging co-registered with live fluoroscopy, and 3-D imaging with needle guidance in one unit. This combination allows more advanced image-guided procedures involving complex angled approaches not possible with standard CT alone.

Image guidance of musculoskeletal injections offers a number of advantages. An initial diagnostic examination helps to confirm the indication/contraindication of the procedure. With image guidance, it is possible to plan an accurate and safe access route. Image-guided procedures are less painful than blind injection. The accurate needle and treatment positioning may potentially lead to better clinical outcome.

Evidence for the accuracy of landmarked versus image-guided injections

In recent years, there has been a great increase in the number of investigations into the accurate placement of musculoskeletal injections. A search on Pubmed using the term 'accuracy of intra-articular injection' revealed 70 studies in the 60 years from 1948–2008 and 104 publications in the last five years from 2008–2013.

A number of studies have reported on the accuracy of landmark-guided joint and soft tissue injection techniques and some have explored the relationship of the accuracy of these 'blind' (as opposed to image-guided) injections to clinical outcomes. An accuracy of more than 80% for landmark-guided joint and soft tissue injections at multiple sites has been reported (Koski et al. 2006). This included the subacromial space, knee, and the thumb carpometacarpal joint (Esenyel et al. 2003; Jackson et al. 2002; Luc et al. 2006; Pollard et al. 2007; Rutten et al. 2007; Toda and Tsukimura 2008), while the hip joint was successfully injected in 78% of cases (Ziv et al. 2009).

In other studies, landmark-guided injection of the subacromial space had low success rates of 27–70% (Eustace et al. 1997; Kanga et al. 2008; Yamakado 2002). There is a 40% chance for acromioclavicular joint injections to be in the joint if performed by landmarks alone, and the routine use of image intensification guidance has been recommended for this injection (Bisbinas et al. 2006). The glenohumeral joint proved to be particularly difficult to inject accurately using landmark guidance in three studies, with success rates of 27–52% (Hegedus et al. 2010; Jacobs et al. 1991; Sethi et al. 2005). In a study of landmark-guided thumb carpometacarpal joint injections, the needle was incorrectly placed in 42% of cases, and needling of osteoarthritic joints was particularly challenging (Helm et al. 2003). See Figures 25.1 and 25.2.

Blind hip injections had a success rate of 51–65%. Obese patients, patients with severe arthritis and severe narrowing of the joint space, and those with flexion deformities were the majority of failed cases. The authors proposed that hip injections (see Figure 25.3) should be carried out under imaging guidance (Dikici et al. 2009: Kurup and Ward 2010). The trochanteric bursa was successfully injected only 45% of the times in one study (Cohen et al. 2009).

The feasibility and accuracy of ultrasound-guided injections have been shown in multiple studies including the subacromial bursa (Yamakado 2002), radiocarpal joint (Lohman et al. 2007), the carpal tunnel (Grassi et al. 2002), trigger finger (Bodor and Flossman 2009), hip (Micu et al. 2010; Smith et al. 2009), knee (Im et al. 2009), Achilles and patellar tendons (Fredberg et al. 2004), and the foot and ankle (Reach et al. 2009).

However, there is a significant learning curve and time commitment for the acquisition of the ultrasound skills that are also highly operator-dependent with moderate to good inter-observer reliability (Le Corroller et al. 2008).

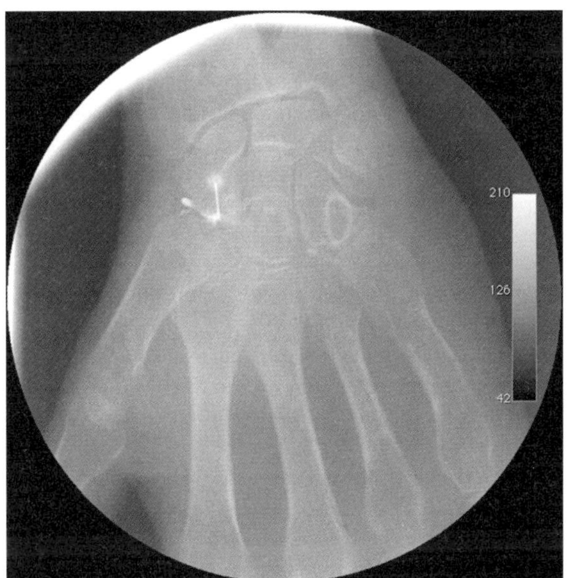

Figure 25.1 Fluoroscopic-guided injection of the scaphoid-trapezium joint in a patient with osteoarthritis.

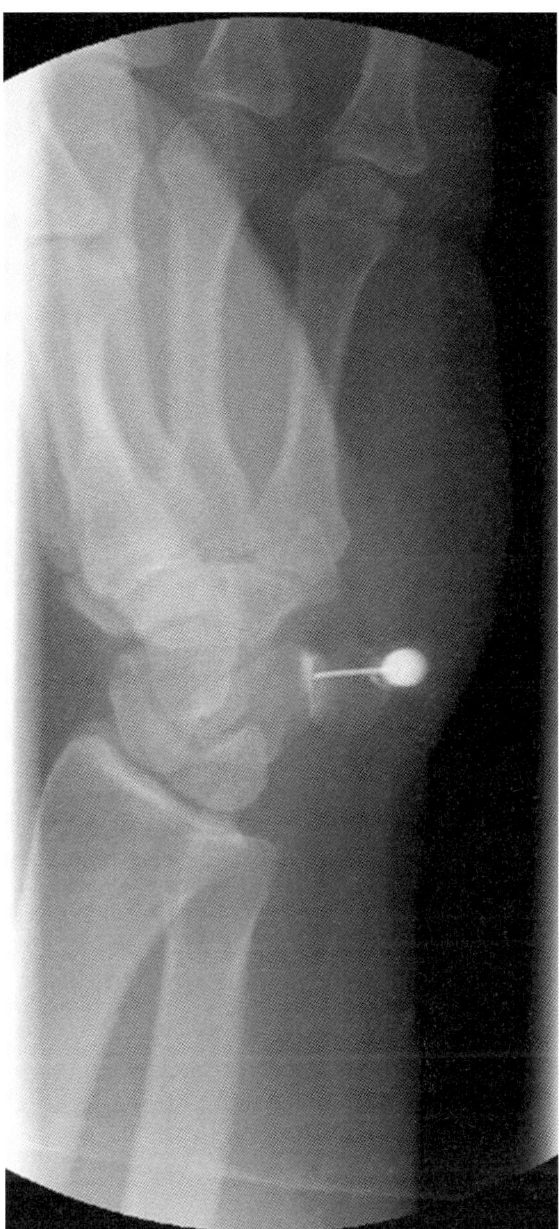

Figure 25.2 Fluoroscopic-guided injection of the triquetrum-pisiform joint in a patient with suspected joint pain.

A study comparing blind versus ultrasound-guided aspirations found successful aspirations in 25% versus 100% for the shoulder, 40% versus 95% for the knee, 20% versus 100% for the ankle joint, and 0% versus 100% for small joints (Zingas et al. 1998). Another study involving the puncture of 13 extremities and 34 axial lesions, found an accuracy in the USA of 98% (Rubens et al. 1997). Raza et al. carried out a study on aspiration of metacarpophalangeal and proximal interphalangeal joints and found a blind clinical accuracy of 59% and an accuracy in the USA of 96% (Raza et al. 2003). Jones et al. conducted a study in which 109 patients received blind intra-articular injections. Even for two commonly injected joints (i.e. shoulder and knee), the accuracy of blind injection was only 25% and 70%, respectively (Jones et al. 1993).

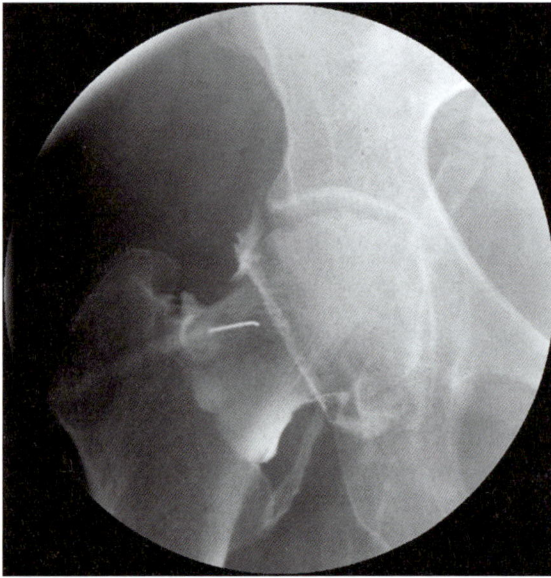

Figure 25.3 An 82-year-old with suspect hip joint pain. Anterior approach with the needle inserted targeting the lateral third of the upper femoral neck. Calcification of the iliopsoas tendon is noted.

Because of the complex anatomy of the foot articulations, with many different joints within a small anatomical region, this is one area where image-guided injections have routinely been used (Khosla et al. 2009; Khoury et al. 1996; Lucas et al. 1997; Mitchell et al. 1995; Saifuddin et al. 2005; Wiewiorski et al. 2009). Fluoroscopy is the most commonly used imaging modality (see Figure 25.4) but CT is suggested for patients with severe osteoarthritis or disorganization of bones and joints from previous trauma (Saifuddin et al. 2005; Wiewiorski et al. 2009).

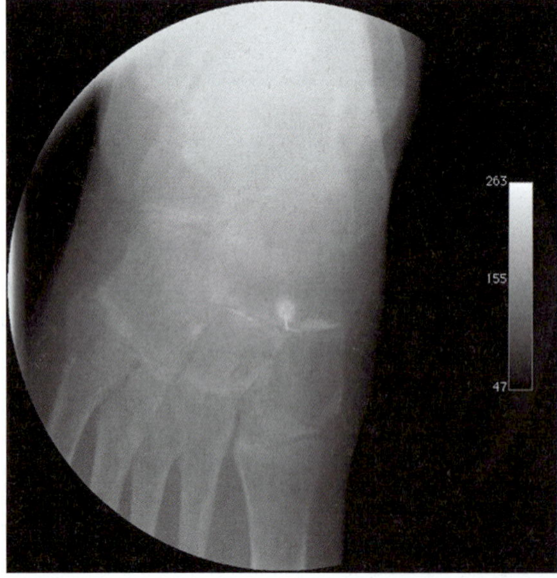

Figure 25.4 Fluoroscopic-guided injection of the navicular-cuneiform joint in a patient with rheumatoid arthritis.

Does accuracy improve the clinical outcome of musculoskeletal injections?

The key question is whether guided injections, irrespective of greater potential for accuracy, produce a significantly different clinical outcome from those using anatomical landmarks (Hall and Buchbinder 2004).

In one study of painful joint injections, relative to conventional blind methods, ultrasound-guided injections resulted in a reduction in procedural pain and absolute pain scores at two weeks. It also increased detection of effusion by 200% and volume of aspirated fluid by 337% and, the authors concluded, significantly improved clinical performance and outcomes of guided injections compared with conventional landmark guidance (Sibbitt et al. 2009).

In a study comparing joint and soft tissue aspiration using clinical landmark technique and ultrasound-guided technique, the guided technique greatly improved the rate of diagnostic synovial fluid aspiration, particularly in small joints, with important implications for accurate administration of local steroid therapy (Balint et al. 2002). In a study of blind glenohumeral injections, about half were not intra-articular, but there was improvement in all subjects for pain and self-reported function at four weeks post-injection, irrespective of accuracy (Hegedus et al. 2010).

In a study of rheumatoid arthritis patients, one third of landmark-guided injections were inaccurate and, although ultrasound guidance significantly improved the accuracy of joint injection, it did not improve the short-term outcome of joint injection (Cunnington et al. 2010). A study of subacromial injection for impingement compared shoulder abduction following blind and ultrasound-guided injection in a group of 40 patients and found a significant superior improvement in abduction in the group treated with ultrasound-guided compared to blind injection (Chen et al. 2006).

A study of trochanteric bursa injections found that guidance does not improve outcomes compared to blind injection (Cohen et al. 2009). There were similar findings for sacro-iliac joints injections (Hartung et al. 2010). A study on the outcome of plantar fasciitis did not show any difference between ultrasound-guided injections and conventional injection (Kane et al. 2001).

In a study of 68 patients, knowledge of the ultrasound findings led clinicians to change their clinical decision regarding local corticosteroid injection in 82% of cases (D'Agostino et al. 2005). Moreover, the patient global assessment of therapy was superior in the group knowing the ultrasound results at three months. On the other hand, a study on suprascapular nerve block for chronic shoulder pain comparing CT-guided injection and conventionally blind placement found no difference in the clinical outcome (Shanahan et al. 2004).

Surprisingly, in a study of trigger finger injections, when the injection was placed in the tendon sheath, there was a 47% good response, while a subcutaneous injection resulted in a 70% good response. This suggests that accurate intra-sheath injection offers no advantage over superficial subcutaneous injection in the treatment of trigger digits (Taras et al. 1998). In some cases, a good therapeutic response may be experienced when an attempted joint or tendon sheath injection resulted in peri-articular or peri- tendinous deposition. This suggests that total accuracy of needle placement may not be essential to a satisfactory outcome (Pollard et al. 2007; Taras et al. 1998).

The mechanism of local corticosteroid action is not well understood. A local action and/or a systemic effect by diffusion of the steroid suspension into blood vessels or the surrounding anatomical structures could explain its therapeutic effect, even when the injection does not reach the target tissue.

There are only a few double-blind randomized controlled trials of intra-articular versus systemic corticosteroid injection therapy for the treatment of any inflammatory arthropathies. The superior clinical efficacy of joint injection therapy has been reported only recently. In one randomized study, patients with polyarticular disease who were treated with intra-articular injections of triamcinolone demonstrated significantly better pain control and range of motion than did those who were treated with the same total dosage of mini-pulse systemic steroids. Patient evaluation of disease activity, tender joint count, blood pressure, side-effects, physician contacts, and hospital visits were significantly better for those treated with intra-articular steroids (Furtado et al. 2005). The second study demonstrated that intra-articular injection with glucocorticoids was superior to its systemic use for the management of monoarticular synovitis in rheumatoid patients. The intra-articular approach showed better results in terms of local inflammatory variables and improvement evaluation by the patient and physician (Konai et al. 2009). No significant differences in short-term outcomes were found between local ultrasound-guided corticosteroid injection and systemic injection in rotator cuff disease (Ekeberg et al. 2009; Koes 2009).

There is a tendency in the current literature to emphasize the positives and highlight marginal benefits and not to delve too deeply into the duration of any benefits or issues related to cost effectiveness of image-guided versus blind injections. Until there is good evidence that image-guided injections used in routine practice are both clinically effective and cost-effective compared with blind injection, it would be reasonable to conclude that most soft tissue and joint injections can be given using an anatomical landmark approach.

Image guidance for musculoskeletal injections is particularly useful in the following conditions:

- When the diagnosis is confirmed but conventional landmark-guided injection/aspiration has failed.
- When the purpose of the injection is primarily diagnostic, rather than therapeutic, particularly for surgical planning.
- In very obese patients with difficulty in palpation of the landmarks.
- In the small joints of the hands and feet and in severely deranged joints.
- Spinal injections.
- When correct placement is essential (e.g. in research studies).
- When monitoring the effect of the treatment (Filippuccil et al. 2004; Terslev et al. 2003).

Indications and contraindications for musculoskeletal injections

Injections can be used to treat a condition, to provide a pain-free window for other treatment such as rehabilitative therapy, or to provide episodic pain and symptom relief (see Table 25.1). In general, injections can be within the joint space (intra-articular), around the joint space (periarticular), or within specific soft tissue structures.

Table 25.1 Common indications for musculoskeletal injections

Arthropathic joints
Acute and chronic capsulitis
Acute and chronic bursitis
Chronic tendinopathy and tenosynovitis
Tendon nodule
Trigger finger or thumb
Suprascapular nerve
Lateral cutaneous nerve (meralgia paraesthetica)
Carpal tunnel syndrome
Plantar digital neuritis (Morton's neuroma)
Nerve root blocks
Epidural
Acute plantar fascia
Masses and cysts

Musculoskeletal interventional procedures can be performed in patients treated with aspirin if the needles are 18 gauge or less (Hegedus et al. 2010; Jackson et al. 2002). Clopidogrel (anti-platelet), some non-steroidal anti-inflammatory drugs (naproxen, pyroxicam), and antidepressant drugs (serotonin re-uptake inhibitors) have an anti-platelet effect similar to that of aspirin and may affect blood coagulation. In patients receiving prophylactic low-dose heparin therapy, the injection procedure must be carried out according to the heparin injection schedule, whereas the procedure is contraindicated in patients who receive full-dose heparin therapy and in patients who receive anti- vitamin-K drug therapy.

Corticosteroids are absolutely contraindicated in patients with infections, glaucoma, cataracts, and some psychiatric diseases (see Table 25.2). In case of osteoporosis or severe hypertension, steroids should be avoided or used only in limited amounts (Jones et al. 1995). Diabetic patients should be told to check blood glucose every day for a week in case of significant hyperglycaemia.

Table 25.2 Absolute contraindications to intra-articular injections

Uncontrolled diabetes
Overlying soft tissue infection/dermatitis
Joint infection (steroid injection)
Bacteraemia
Intra-articular including osteochondral fracture
Severe joint destruction
Joint prosthesis
Known hypersensitivity to intra-articular agent
Uncontrolled bleeding disorder

Table 25.3 Relative contraindications to intra-articular injections

Diabetes
Severe immunodeficiency
Anticoagulation therapy
Poor response to prior injections
Psychogenic pain

For other drugs that are used in musculoskeletal injection (phenol, lidocaine or other anaesthetics, radiological contrast agents, sodium hyaluronate, and polidocanol), the specific precautions and contraindications related to each drug must be followed.

See Table 25.3 for a summary of relative contraindications for intra-articular injections.

Musculoskeletal injection technique: general considerations

Patient preparation

- Take history, examine patient, and confirm clinical diagnosis.
- Perform diagnostic ultrasound if ultrasound is used for guidance.
- Exclude absolute or relative contraindications.
- Discuss all treatment options, injection procedure, and possible side-effects.
- Check for allergy to drugs.
- Obtain and record informed consent.
- Place the patient in a comfortable position with easy access to the injection site.

Drug selection

- Decide on the drugs to be used.
- Determine the dose of drug/s; use the minimal effective dose and volume.
- Check drug names, strengths, and expiry dates.

Assemble consumables

- Appropriate size in-date sterile syringe.
- Sterile in-date green 21 G needle for drawing up.
- Sterile in-date needle of correct length for infiltrating.
- Alcohol swab or iodine skin preparation.
- Cotton wool/gauze and skin plaster.
- Waste bin and sharps box.
- Spare syringe and sterile container if aspiration likely.

Site preparation

- Identify the structure to be injected.
- Mark injection site with skin marker or the end of fresh needle cap.
- Clean skin with suitable preparation (see Table 25.4).

Injection process

- Wash hands with cleanser for 1 minute and dry well with paper towel.
- Draw up accurate dose of drugs to appropriate-sized syringe using 21 G green needle.
- Attach needle of correct length to the syringe.
- Inject the target structure.
- Apply plaster unless allergic.
- Record drug names, doses, batch numbers and expiry dates, advice and warnings given.
- Ensure patient waits for 30 minutes after injection.
- Reassess patient and record results.

Image-guided musculoskeletal injection techniques

The guidance technique used for musculoskeletal injections should be both precise and safe. The choice of technique depends on the experience and preferences of the clinician, the body habitus and

Table 25.4 Mechanism and spectrum of activity of antiseptic agents commonly used for pre-operative skin preparation and surgical scrubs

Scrubs	Mechanism of action	Gram + bacteria	Gram – bacteria	MtB	Fungi	Virus	Rapidity of action	Residual activity	Toxicity	Uses
Alcohol	Denature proteins	E	E	G	G	G	Most rapid	None	Drying, volatile	SP,SS
Chlorhexidine	Disrupt cell membrane	E	G	P	F	G	Intermediate	E	Ototoxicity Keratitis	SP,SS
Iodine iodophores	Oxidation/substitution by free iodine	E	G	G	G	G	Intermediate	Minimal	Absorption from skin with possible toxicity Skin irritation	SP,SS
PCMX	Disrupt cell wall	G	F*	F	F	F	Intermediate	G	More data needed	SS
Triclosan	Disrupt cell wall	G	G	G	P	U	Intermediate	E	More data needed	SS

Abbreviations: E, excellent; F, fair; G, good; Mtb, mycobacterium tuberculosis; P, poor; PCMX, parachlorometaxylenol; SP, skin preparation; SS, surgical scrubs; U, unknown.
Data from Larson 1988
* Fair, except for pseudomonas spp.; activity improved by addition of chelating agent such as Ethylenediaminetetraacetic acid.

condition of the patient, the nature of the intervention, and the availability of the equipments.

Ultrasound is an excellent guidance technique, especially for superficial interventions on soft tissues or in the paediatric population. It has the advantages of multi-planar as well as real-time imaging, but it is very operator-dependent and not suitable if the target is obscured by bone or air-filled structures.

Fluoroscopy provides real-time guidance for joint injection. It allows a three-dimensional view, which can be important in complex procedures of the spine such as vertebroplasty.

CT provides very precise guidance for bone, joints, as well as in soft tissues. CT fluoroscopy allows real-time imaging but only in a thin plane (usually 1–10 mm). The radiation dosage of CT fluoroscopy is relatively high compared to conventional fluoroscopy.

MRI has been used for the guidance of musculoskeletal injections. It has no ionizing radiation. MRI guidance can deliver a very precise three-dimensional real-time image. MRI-compatible needles (needles using non-ferromagnetic materials like titanium, carbon) are needed. The main limitation, however, lies in both the high costs and the availability of interventional MRI equipment (open MRI magnets) and interventional material (non-ferromagnetic devices). Moreover, MRI-guided procedures are time-consuming. With improvements in interventional MRI systems, MRI may become the modality of choice for guidance of certain musculoskeletal interventional procedures.

Sonographic technique

The choice of the transducer depends on the depth of the structure being injected (for deep structures, it may be necessary to use a convex low-frequency transducer, while for superficial structures, a linear high-frequency probe is always used). The transducer should be appropriately disinfected and covered with a sterile probe cover, and the gel used should also be sterile.

There are two approaches to guide the needle with ultrasound. The indirect method uses skin marking, for which the ultrasound is used to locate the area to be injected. The skin is marked and the depth of target is measured. Injection is done using the markings for guidance and the correct position of the needle is confirmed by ultrasound. The second method is the direct one, in which ultrasound is used to locate the target and the needle is advanced under direct visualization in real time to ensure accurate placement.

Needle advancement can be done free-hand or with the aid of needle guides mounted on the transducer. These devices allow the operator to guide the needle along a predetermined track visualized on the monitor. During the procedure, the transducer should be manipulated with the non-dominant hand and the needle with the dominant hand. This maximizes both sensitivity and precision. Needle selection will vary based on the depth of the structure being imaged. The gauge will depend on the dimensions of the structure. Longer, smaller-bore needles are more likely to deviate from the planned trajectory, thus rendering the procedure more difficult.

Once the target structure has been reached, a small bolus of normal saline can be injected under direct sonographic visualization to confirm that the needle has been correctly positioned. When the position has been verified, the chosen drug can be injected.

Musculoskeletal injection agents and procedures

There are an increasing number of injectable substances. These can be divided into several groups on the basis of their structural characteristics or mechanisms of action (see Table 25.5).

The effects of musculoskeletal injections may be related to one or more of the following mechanism of actions (see Table 25.6):

- Anti-inflammatory drugs; cortisone; and local anaesthetics
- Neo-vascularization (and neo-innervation) disruption:
  - Disrupting vessels at the point of entrance into tendon
  - Mechanical stripping
  - Hydrodissection (brisment/hydrostatic decompression)
  - Sclerosing agent injection
  - Electrocoagulation (radio-frequency treatment)
- Tendon repair: creating an inflammatory reaction and growth factors
  - Dry needling (fenestration)
  - Autologous blood injection
  - Plasma-rich platelet injection
- Prolotherapy: injection of an irritant substance (hyperosmolar dextrose) to initiate a local inflammatory response
- Lavage/barbotage of calcific tendinopathy
- Cyst aspiration

Local anaesthetics

These drugs act by blocking the sodium-specific ion channels on neural cell membranes causing a reversible block to the nerve conduction. Small nerve fibres carrying pain and autonomic function are more sensitive than thick motor fibres. The peak arterial plasma concentration develops within 10–25 minutes following the

Table 25.5 Common injectable musculoskeletal substances and procedures

Local anaesthetics
Corticosteroids
Hyaluronans
Autologous substances (blood and platelet-rich plasma)
Sclerosants, phenol/polidocanol
Prolotherapy
Ozone
Normal saline
Dry needling
Percutaneous hydrostatic decompression
Percutaneous lavage
Electrocoagulation
Cryotherapy
Vertebroplasty/kyphoplasty

Table 25.6 Mechanism of action of musculoskeletal injections

Anti-inflammatory
Neovascularization and neoinnervation
Mechanical stripping
Hydrodissection
Lavage/barbotage
Cyst aspiration

injection, so observation for a minimum of 30 minutes after the injection is recommended if significant volumes are used (BNF 2010).

The use of local anaesthetic during the injection makes the procedure well tolerated by the patient and increases the confidence of the patient in the treating clinician. Immediate pain relief following the injection helps to establish the diagnosis (Crawford et al. 1998; Khoury et al. 1996), differentiate local from referred pain (Ines and da Silva 2005; Rifat and Moeller 2002; Tallia and Cardone 2003), and confirm the correct positioning of the needle. In cases of joint injection, increasing the injectable volume by the addition of the local anaesthetic may help to spread the steroid around the joint surface (Ines and da Silva 2005) and with stretching of the joint capsule with disruption of adhesions (Buchbinder et al. 2004; Jacobs et al. 1991).

Local anaesthetics vary widely in their strength, duration of action, and toxicity. Those most commonly used for joint and soft tissue injection (see Table 25.7) are:

- Lidocaine hydrochloride (lignocaine hydrochloride): the most widely used local anaesthetic, it acts more rapidly than others. Its effects occur within seconds and duration of action is about 30 minutes.
- Marcain (bupivacaine) has a slow onset of action (about 30 minutes for full effect) but the duration of block is up to 8 hours.

There is no evidence of any long-term benefit from using bupivacaine instead of lidocaine (Sölveborn et al. 1995).

Side-effects

Local anaesthetics may cause significant adverse effects to the central nervous and cardiovascular systems if inadvertently injected intravascularly (MacMahon et al. 2009). Local adverse effects of joint injections include chrondrolysis, particularly if administered with vasoconstrictors (MacMahon et al. 2009). Injection of corticosteroid concurrently may ameliorate this effect (MacMahon et al. 2009). 0.5% ropivacaine (Naropin) has been shown to be less toxic to human articular chondrocytes *in vitro* compared with 0.5% bupivacaine (Piper and Kim 2008).

Corticosteroids

The commonly used injectable corticosteroids are synthetic analogues of the adrenal glucocorticoid hormone cortisol (hydrocortisone): methyl prednisolone acetate; triamcinolone acetonide; betamethasone acetate/sodium phosphate; and dexamethasone sodium phosphate.

There is variability in the solubility of the different preparations of corticosteroids, due to relative content of esters. Dexamethasone and betamethasone sodium phosphate are water soluble and more rapidly absorbed by cells, having a rapid onset of action but reduced duration (Jacobs et al. 1991). Of particular note, other substances are contained within the corticosteroid preparation, including preservatives (usually benzyl alcohol) and a drug vehicle (polyethylene glycol), which may rarely cause allergic reactions.

There is anecdotal evidence that mixing steroid and local anaesthetic can cause aggregation of the corticosteroid crystals. However, a study by Benzon et al. (2007) has shown that corticosteroid crystals retain their shape and size when mixed with lignocaine or iodinated contrast agents.

Mechanism of action

The clinical effects of steroids result from several different mechanisms of action. Steroids suppress the inflammation in cases of inflammatory (Anon 2004; Coombes and Bax 1996; Franz and Burmester 2005; Gossec and Dougados 2004; Kirwan and Rankin 1997; af Klint et al. 2005) and degenerative (Creamer 1997; Jones and Doheryt 1996; Kirwan and Rankin 1997) arthropathy. Intra-articular corticosteroids reduce synovial blood flow (Caldwell 1996), lower the local leukocyte and inflammatory modulator response (Lavelle et al. 2007), and alter local collagen synthesis (Wei et al. 2006).

Corticosteroids may have a chondroprotective effect by acting directly on the cartilage metabolism or other effects not related to its anti-inflammatory response (e.g. promotion of articular surfactant production) (Creamer 1997; Cutolo 1998; Hills et al. 1998; Jubb 1992; Larsson et al. 2004; Pelletier and Pelletier 1987; Pelletier et al. 1994; Raynauld 1999; Verbruggen 2006; Weitoft et al. 2005, 2008).

Tendon pain in cases of tendinopathy may not be due to inflammation (tendinitis) or structural disruption of the tendon fibres (tendinosis) but might instead be caused by the stimulation of nociceptors by chemicals such as glutamate, substance P, and chondroitin sulphate released from the damaged tendon (Gialanella and Prometti 2011; Johansson et al. 1990). Corticosteroids (and possibly local anaesthetics) may inhibit release of these noxious chemicals and/or the local nociceptors. *In vitro*, corticosteroids have also been shown to inhibit the transmission of pain along unmyelinated C-fibres by direct membrane action (Johansson et al. 1990). The pain relief of steroids could also partially relate to the reduced

Table 25.7 Local anaesthetics for musculoskeletal injections

Drug	How supplied	Dosage	Onset of action (minutes)	Duration of action (hours)
Bupivacaine (Marcaine)	0.25%, 0.5%, and 0.75%	0.25% and 0.5% solutions generally used for joint injection; 1–2 ml mixed with corticosteroid	30	8
Lidocaine (Xylocaine)	0.5%, 1%, 1.5%, 2%, and 4%	1% and 2% solutions generally used for joint injection; 1–2 ml mixed with corticosteroid	1 to 2	1

formation of fibrosis, which indirectly increases the mobility of structures like tendons and reduces friction-related pain. However, there are no direct improvements on the functional aspects of the disorder being treated and the disability it causes (Gialanella and Prometti 2011).

Preparations and dosage

There is little systematic evidence to guide corticosteroid selection for therapeutic injections. Most recommendations are based on a combination of clinical experience and personal preference. Only modest differences have been demonstrated between these drugs, and none is significantly superior to the others (Bellamy et al. 2006) (see Table 25.8).

Side-effects

Side-effects from corticosteroids are uncommon and when they do occur are usually mild and transient (Habib et al. 2010; Kumar and Newman 1999; Nichols 2005). Serious local side-effects are rare (Habib et al. 2010).

Post-injection flare of pain

The incidence varies between 2% and 10% (Gaujoux-Viala et al. 2009; Kumar and Newman 1999), usually after soft tissue injection and rarely following joint injection (108). Flocculation/precipitation of the steroid/local anaesthetic mixture may be related to the post-injection flare of pain (Cole and Schumacher 2005). This side-effect is more common with mythylepredsinolone and could be related to the preservative in the drug preparation rather than the steroid itself (Pullar 1998). Transient synovitis following joint injection may occur, with an early increase in the joint stiffness after the procedure (Helliwell 1997).

Post-injection flare may develop within hours and can last 2–3 days. If severe, this flare may be difficult to distinguish from sepsis. The prevalence of post-injection flare is 2–25% (Brown et al. 1953; Friedman and Moore 1980; Hollander et al. 1961) and does not predict a poor response to therapy (Berger and Yount 1990; Hollander et al. 1961; Kendall 1963).

Skin changes

Subcutaneous atrophy and/or skin depigmentation (Basadonna et al. 1999; Berger and Yount 1990; Brown et al. 1953; Cole and Schumacher 2005; Friedman and Moore 1980; Gaujoux-Viala et al. 2009; Helliwell 1997; Hollander et al. 1961; Kendall 1963; Pullar 1998; Reddy et al. 1995) and soft tissue calcification (Gray et al. 1981) can occur. In a meta-analysis of shoulder and elbow injections, 'skin modification' had a frequency of 4% (Gaujoux-Viala et al. 2009). Skin changes are more likely in dark-skinned patients and when a superficial lesion is injected. Local atrophy appears within 1–4 months after injection and proceeds to resolution 6–24 months later, but may take longer (Cassidy and Bole 1966).

Bleeding or bruising

This may occur at the injection site, especially in patients with deranged blood coagulation, possibly more frequently in patients taking warfarin, aspirin, or oral non-steroidal anti-inflammatory drugs (NSAIDs) with significant anti-platelet activity (e.g. naproxen).

Steroid arthropathy

There is a good evidence of the association of osteonecrosis and oral corticosteroid administration (Nichols 2005) but almost all the reports linking injected steroids with accelerated non-septic joint destruction are anecdotal, and mainly relate to joints receiving huge numbers of injections (Cameron 1995). There is no evidence supporting the promotion of osteoarthritis progression by steroid injections (Mahler and Fritsch 1992.). Repeat injections into the knee every three months seem to be safe over two years (Raynauld et al. 2003).

Tendon rupture and atrophy

Tendon and facial ruptures are reported complications of injection in the treatment of athletic injuries (Fredberg 1997; Nichols 2005). Tendon (Mahler and Fritsch 1992; Shrier and Godron 1996; Smith et al. 1999) and facial rupture (Acevedo and Beskin 1998; Saxena and Fullem 2004) or atrophy (Fredberg 1997) following steroid treatment has been published. The issue of steroid-associated tendon rupture remains controversial (Acevedo and Beskin 1998; Mahler and Fritsch 1992; McWhorter et al. 1991; Shrier and Gordon 1996), disputed (Read 1999), anecdotal (Mair et al. 2004; Nichols 2005; Smith et al. 1999), and not well supported in the literature (Mahler and Fritsch 1992). However, it is widely accepted that repeated injections of steroids into load-bearing tendons carries the risk of rupture (Mottram 1996). The risk of tendon rupture is highest with

Table 25.8 Corticosteroids for musculoskeletal injections

Drug	Common concentration (mg/ml)	Common equivalent dose (mg)	Relative anti-inflammatory potency	Solubility (% wt/vol)	Approx. duration of action (days)	Dosage (joint size)
Methylprednisolone acetate (Depomedrol)	40 or 80	40	5	Intermediate solubility 0.0014	8	Large 20–80 mg Small 4–10 mg
Triamcinolone acetonide (Kenalog)	10 or 40	40	5	Intermediate solubility 0.004	14	Large 5–15 mg Small 2.5–5 mg
Triamcinolone hexacetonide (Aristospan)	20	40	5	Intermediate solubility 0.0002	21	Large 10–40 mg Small 2–6 mg
Dexamethasone acetate (Decadron-LA)	8	8	25	Low	8	Large 2–4 mg Small 0.8–1 mg
Dexamethasone sodium(Decadron)	4 or 8	8	25	Low	6	Large 2–4 mg Small 0.8–1 mg

Large joints include the shoulder, hip, knee, and ankle joints.
Small joints include the metacarpophalangeal, metatarsophalangeal, interphalangeal, and temporomandibular joints.
The dose for medium joints such as the elbow and wrist, bursa, ganglion, and tendinopathy is generally somewhere between the dose of the large and small joints.

soft tissue injections around the Achilles tendon and plantar fascia (Acevedo and Beskin 1998). However, in the treatment of the Achilles tendon, low-dose peritendinous steroid injections appear to be safe (Gills et al. 2004) and peritendinous steroid injections have not been shown to be associated with an increased risk of rupture (Read 1999). Following the injection, the patient should rest from strenuous activity for 6–8 weeks (Shrier and Godron 1996). Bilateral injections should be avoided as they may have a systemic effect in conjunction with the local effect, further weakening the tendon (Hugate et al. 2004).

Sepsis

Joint sepsis is the most serious complication of steroid injection treatment (Hughes 1996); it may be lethal (Yangco et al. 1982), but occurs rarely (Charalambous et al. 2003; Habib et al. 2010). The incidence of post-injection infection is as low as 0.01–0.03% (Acevedo and Beskin 1998; Basadonna et al. 1999; Berger and Yount 1990; Brown et al. 1953; Cameron 1995; Cassidy and Bole 1966; Charalambous et al. 2003; Fredberg 1997; Friedman and Moore 1980; Gills et al. 2004; Gray et al. 1981; Hollander et al. 1961; Hugate et al. 2004; Hughes 1996; Kendall 1963; Mahler and Fritsch 1992; Mair et al. 2004; McWhorter et al. 1991; Mottram 1996; Raynauld et al. 2003; Read 1999; Reddy et al. 1995; Saxena and Fullem 2004; Shrier and Gordon 1996; Smith et al. 1999; Yangco et al. 1982). Infection occurred in only 1 in 17,000–162,000 patients when joint and soft tissue injections were performed as an 'office' procedure (Acevedo and Beskin 1998; Cameron 1995; Cassidy and Bole 1966; Charalambous et al. 2003; Fredberg 1997; Gills 2004; Gray et al. 1981; Hugate et al. 2004; Hughes 1996; Mahler and Fritsch 1992; Mair et al. 2004; McWhorter et al. 1991; Pal and Morris 1999; Raynauld et al. 2003; Read 1999; Saxena and Fullem 2004; Seror et al. 1999; Shrier and Gordon 1996; Smith et al. 1999; Yangco et al. 1982). Soft tissue infections and osteomyelitis can also occur after local soft tissue injection (Grayson 1998; Jawed and Allard 2000). Infection was most common in children and the elderly. Underlying risk factors were reported in one fifth of cases, the most frequent being a prosthetic joint (11%). Others risk factors included haematological malignancy, joint disease or connective tissue disorder, diabetes, oral steroid therapy, chemotherapy, presence of an intravenous line, intravenous drug abuse, and post-arthroscopy (Ryan et al. 1997). Steroid injection may delay presentation of sepsis by 6–12 days (Gosal et al. 1999).

Joint infection has also been reported as occurring between 4 days and 3 weeks after injection (Grayson 1998).

Facial flushing

This is probably the commonest systemic side-effect with a reported incidence between 5% (Anon 1995) and 1% (Gray and Gottlieb 1982). It may occur within 24–48 hours after the injection and may last 1–2 days.

Deterioration of diabetic glycaemic control

Following steroid injection, the blood sugar levels may show a modest rise for up to a week, rarely longer. When larger doses of corticosteroid than recommended are used or multiple injections are given over a few consecutive days, this may lead to a more prolonged (up to 3 weeks) elevation of blood sugar.

Uterine bleeding (pre- and post-menopausal)

The exact mechanism is unknown but intra-articular steroid treatment causes a temporary but considerable suppression of sex steroid hormone secretion in women (Mens et al. 1998; Weitoft et al. 2008).

Suppression of the hypothalamic–pituitary axis

This occurs following intra-articular and intra-muscular injection of corticosteroids (see Table 25.9) (Lazarevic et al. 1995; van Tuyl and Slee 2002) but usually appears to be of no significant clinical consequence (de Vos et al. 2010).

Anaphylaxis

Severe anaphylactic reactions to local anaesthetic injections are rare, but can be fatal (Ewan 1998). Anaphylactic reactions to corticosteroid injections are extremely rare and are probably a reaction to the stabilizers that the drug is mixed with, rather than the drug itself (Beaudouin et al. 1992; de Vos et al. 2010).

Hyaluronans

Hyaluronan (HA, previously known as hyaluronic acid) is a large, linear glycosaminoglycan and a major non-structural component of both the synovial and cartilage extracellular matrix. It is also found in synovial fluid and is produced by the cells (type B synoviocytes or fibroblasts) lining layer of the joint. These molecules produce a highly viscoelastic solution that is a viscous lubricant at low shear (during slow movement of the joint, e.g. walking) and an elastic shock absorber at high shear (during rapid movement, e.g. running).

As well as conferring viscoelasticity, the other key roles of HA in the joint are lubrication and the maintenance of tissue hydration and protein homeostasis through the prevention of large fluid movements by functioning as an osmotic buffer. HA is also considered a physiological factor in the trophic status of cartilage. It has a very high water binding capacity; one gram dissolved in physiological saline occupies three litres of solution (NICE 2008; Uthman et al. 2003). HA has analgesic properties, which are related to its direct inhibition of nocioceptors and its ability to bind substance P (a pain mediator) (Tagliafico et al. 2011).

The rationale for joint injection therapy was to replace the normal physiological properties lost to the osteoarthritic joint as a consequence of the associated reduction in the volume and quality of hyaluoronic acid, a concept known as viscosupplementation.

Table 25.9 Complications of intra-articular corticosteroid injections

Immediate side-effects (within 1–2 hours)
Pain at the injection site
Bleeding or bruising
Syncope
Facial flushing
Anaphylaxis
Vasovagal reaction
Nerve injury
Delayed side-effects
Disturbed diabetic control
Post-injection flare of pain
Subcutaneous atrophy and/or skin atrophy and depigmentation
Steroid arthropathy
Septic arthritis

Commercial preparations of HA have the same structure as endogenous hyaluronic acid, although cross-linked molecules (known as hylans) were later engineered in order to obtain greater elastoviscosity and intra-articular dwell-time (NICE 2008). There are a number of commercial preparations available. Hyalgan has a lower molecular weight and is licensed as a medicinal product; it is injected once weekly for 5 weeks and is repeatable no more than 6-monthly. Synvisc has a higher molecular weight and is licensed as a medical device; it is injected once weekly for 3 weeks, repeatable once within 6 months, with at least 4 weeks between courses.

A systematic review and meta-analysis has concluded that from baseline to week 4, intra-articular corticosteroids appear to be relatively more effective for pain than intra-articular hyaluronic acid. By week 4, both therapies have equal efficacy, but beyond week 8, HA has greater efficacy (Bannuru et al. 2009). A Cochrane review also suggests that the pain relief with HA therapy is achieved more slowly than with steroid injections, but the effect may be more prolonged (Bellamy et al. 2006).

Some commercial HAs are licensed for use in the hip joint. One systematic review concluded that HA injection for hips should only be used under careful supervision and only in those cases where other treatments have failed (Fernandez-Lopez and Ruano-Ravina 2006). A second systematic review concluded that despite the relatively low level of evidence of the included studies, HA injection performed under fluoroscopic or ultrasound guidance seems to be effective, and appears to be safe and well tolerated, but cannot be recommended as standard therapy in the wider population (van den Bekerom et al. 2008a). A third review concluded that this therapy seems to be a valuable technique that may delay the need for surgical intervention, with no difference between products, but further studies are necessary (van den Bekerom 2008b).

The use of HA injections in other joints is under investigation (Blaine et al. 2008; Brander et al. 2010; Heyworth et al. 2008; Nyska et al. 2003; Schumacher et al. 2004; Tagliafico et al. 2011).Encouraging but inconclusive results have been observed for the treatment of shoulder, carpometacarpal, and ankle osteoarthritis (Abate et al. 2010).

Side-effects

The toxicity of intra-articular HA appears to be negligible. No major safety issues have been identified when compared with placebo, but a definitive conclusion is precluded due to sample-size restrictions (Bellamy et al. 2006). They may cause a short-term increase in knee inflammation (Bernardeu et al. 2001). A small percentage may experience a transient mild to moderate increase in pain following injection, and some have a flare with marked effusion.

Hyaluronic acid has some side-effects, including attacks of pseudo-gout, with onset within 24–48 hours after the initiation of treatment, and gastrointestinal bleeding (Fernandez-Lopez and Ruano-Ravina 2006).

Autologous substances (blood and platelet-rich plasma)

The substances include platelet-rich plasma (PRP), autologous blood, and autologous conditioned serum (ACS).

Tendon healing occurs through three overlapping phases (inflammation, proliferation, and remodelling), which are controlled by a variety of growth factors. The blood contains moderate amounts of these growth factors, such as fibroblast growth factor and transforming growth factor. These substances stimulate the production of granulation tissue, which becomes organized and increases the overall resistance of the tendon (Suresh et al. 2006). The rationale for the use of platelet-rich plasma to promote tendon healing is the high content of these cytokines and cells in hyperphysiological doses of platelet-rich plasma. When the platelets reach the site of injury, they release a series of chemokines and growth factors that can stimulate repair processes and block catabolic processes in the tendon (de Vos et al. 2010a). The growth factors continue to act for the next 7 days. It has been suggested that for this reason, a repeat injection should not be required (Samson et al. 2008).

PRP is produced by centrifuging heparinized whole autologous blood, separating the platelets from the other blood components. The platelets are then diluted with normal saline to obtain the required concentration (de Vos et al. 2010a). The benefit of PRP over autologous blood is that the concentration of platelets is four to five times higher.

In a systematic review, all studies showed that injections of autologous growth factor (AGF; whole blood and PRP) in chronic tendinopathy had a significant impact on improving pain and/or function over time. However, the review concluded that there is strong evidence that the use of injections with autologous whole blood should not be recommended due to inadequate number of studies of high methodology and lack of benefit of AGF compared to the control (de Vos et al. 2010b). In a recent double-blind, randomized, placebo-controlled trial of eccentric exercises plus either PRP or saline injection for chronic mid portion Achilles tendinopathy, PRP injection did not result in greater improvement in pain and activity (de Vos at al. 2010a).

Autologous blood has been used in medial epicondylitis (Mishra and Pavelko 2006), lateral epicondylitis (Connell et al. 2006: Mishra and Pavelko 2006), patellar tendinosis (James et al. 2007), and plantar fasciitis (Barrett and Erredge 2004). Platelet gels and PRP are also used in the context of total knee replacement, wound healing, lumbar spinal fusion, and maxillofacial surgical procedures (Samson et al. 2008). Chronic tendonopathies including wrist extensors, flexors, Achilles tendons (and plantar fascia), have been treated with PRP (de Vos 2010b). PRP has also been injected into the knee to encourage the healing of cartilage (Kon et al. 2010).

ACS is derived from incubating the blood with glass beads and spinning the blood down in order to extract the serum, which contains the released growth factor (GF). However, this method produces a lower yield of GF (Creaney and Hamilton 2008).

Side-effects

It has been noted that patients may experience mild or moderate discomfort during the injection, which can be relieved with ice or simple analgesics, such as paracetamol (Samson et al. 2008).

A number of potential risks have been postulated for autologous substances (Creaney and Hamilton 2008). Potential local complications include the induction of excessive fibrosis, due to the presence of TGF-b1 or by concomitant use of non-steroidal anti-inflammatory drugs (NSAIDs). Potential systemic risks include infection (although this is unlikely with autologous substances) and an effect on the serum GF levels (which have been shown to decrease in some small studies) (Banfi et al. 2006).

Sclerosants (phenol/polidocanol)

These are used in patellar tendinosis (Hoksrud et al. 2006), tennis elbow (Zeisig et al. 2008), chronic Achilles tendinosis (Ohberg and Alfredson 2002), Morton's neuralgia (Magnan et al. 2005), and stump neuromata (Gruber et al. 2008). The outcome of these studies shows promising results for the use of sclerosants in Morton's neuroma and painful tendinopathy.

The most common sclerosants used are phenol or polidocanol. Phenol is used for alcoholization of interdigital neuroma via a percutaneous intraneural route and causes a chemical neurolysis (due to its affinity for nerve tissue), causing dehydration and necrosis (Fanucci et al. 2004). Polidocanol is a local anaesthetic agent, which is a licensed drug and used for sclerosis of varicose veins and telangiectasia (Hills et al. 1998). The proposed hypothesis for its beneficial effects in chronic Achilles tendinosis is that the development of neovascularity around the abnormal tendon is associated with abnormal nerve growth at the same site and pain (Kingma et al. 2007). Polidocanol causes sclerosis of these neovessels and reduces pain. However, it is still unproven whether neovascularity is beneficial or detrimental.

Prolotherapy

Prolotherapy entails the injection of any substance that promotes growth of normal or injured cells or tissues; it is a non-pharmacotherapeutic and non-surgical alternative that involves injecting small volumes of an irritant solution into painful ligaments and tendon insertions (enthuses, ligament or tendon attachment site to bone at the fibro-osseous junction), joints, and in adjacent joint spaces, over several treatment sessions (Hauser et al. 2014). This induces fibroblastic hyperplasia, seeking to stimulate connective tissue growth and promote the formation of collagen (Dagenais et al. 2008).

The treatment aims to cause soft tissue inflammation, the opposite objective to corticosteroid injection therapy (Dorman and Ravin 1991), but the histological response may not be different from that caused by saline injections or dry needling procedures (Jensen et al. 2008). The most commonly used irritant is hyperosmolar dextrose.

Prolotherapy is mostly used for back pain (Dagenais et al. 2005, 2007, 2008; Dorman and Ravin 1991; Rabago et al. 2010), including the sacroiliac joint (Cusi et al. 2010). A Cochrane review concluded that there is conflicting evidence regarding the efficacy of prolotherapy for chronic low back pain, and that when used alone, it is not an effective treatment. When combined with spinal manipulation, exercise, and other co-interventions, prolotherapy may improve chronic low back pain and disability. Conclusions were confounded by clinical heterogeneity amongst studies and by the presence of co-interventions (Dagenais et al. 2007).

Prolotherapy has also been tried for peripheral instability (Rabago et al. 2010; Reeves et al. 2000) and in elite kicking-sport athletes with chronic groin pain from osteitis pubis and/or adductor tendinopathy (Topol et al. 2005), chronic groin pain and coccydynia (Khan et al. 2008).

Articular dextrose sclerotherapy for anterior cruciate ligament laxity has also been reported in a small study (Reeves and Hassanein 2003). Intratendinous injection of 25% hyperosmolar dextrose has also been used to treat lateral epicondylitis (Robago et al. 2009), chronic Achilles tendinopathy (Maxwell et al. 2007), and plantar fasciitis (Ryan et al. 2009).

Dry needling

Dry needling is a treatment method in which a needle is placed into the lesion and repeated punctures are performed (see Figure 25.5).

(a)

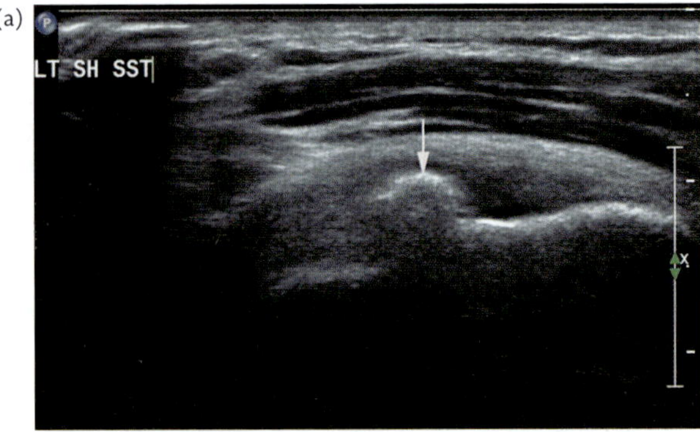

(b)

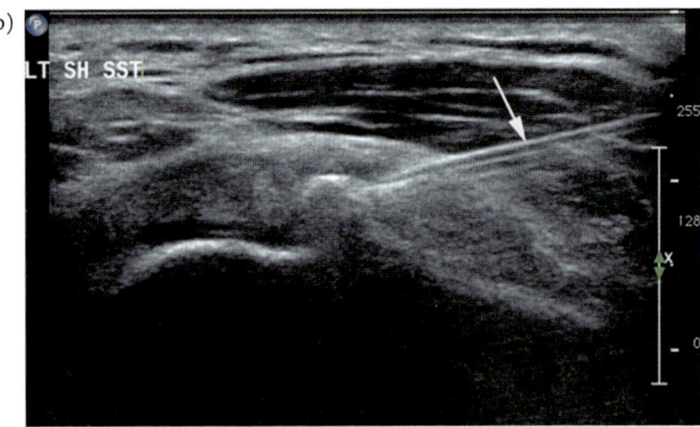

Figure 25.5 Dry needling of rotator cuff calcific tendinopathy in a 51-years old man. (a) Initial transverse ultrasound image of the rotator cuff showing a calcific deposit in the supraspinatus tendon. (b) Transverse ultrasound image of the rotator cuff showing the needle in the supraspinatus tendon calcification.

The aim of this procedure is to form fenestrations which may initiate advantageous bleeding and thus bring about the influx of growth factors (activating healing and regeneration), which leads to granulation tissue formation and increased tendon strength (James et al. 2007).

Dry needling has been used in the treatment of patellar tendinosis (James et al. 2007), lateral epicondylitis (Connell et al. 2006), medial epicondylitis (Suresh et al. 2006), and plantar fasciitis (Bartold 2004). US-guided fine-needle technique for calcified tendinitis of the shoulder was shown to be an effective therapy (Alna et al. 2001).

Percutaneous hydrostatic decompression (brisement)

Brisement has been used in the treatment of Achilles tendinopathy. The Achilles has no tendon sheath but is surrounded by connective tissue (paratenon).

It is postulated that the development of abnormally oriented vessels and nerves in Achilles tendinopathy contributes to pain (Ilum Boesen et al. 2006; Zanetti et al. 2003) and the disruption of these neurovascular structures by brisement is thought to reduce pain. Brisement involves the injection under pressure of dilute local anaesthetic or saline solution between the paratenon and Achilles tendon to break up adhesions (see Figure 25.6). Volume adhesiotomy may be performed using ultrasound guidance to better direct the injection into the paratenon/tendon interspace.

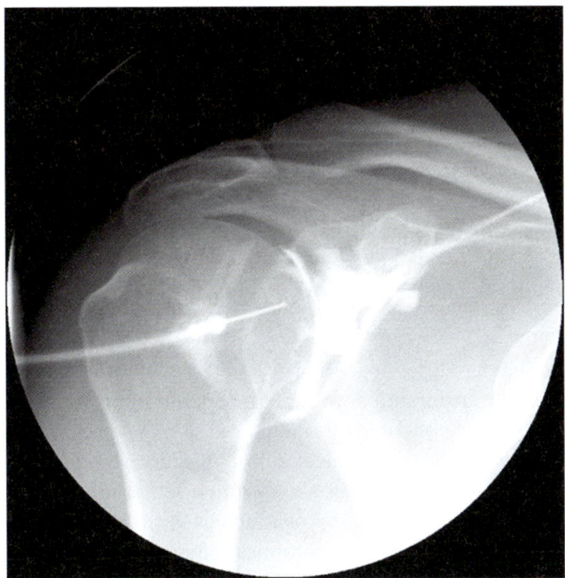

Figure 25.6a Fluoroscopic-guided hydrodilation of the shoulder: initial arthrogram with anterior approach confirms adhesive capsulitis with restricted joint capsule and shallow axillary recesses.

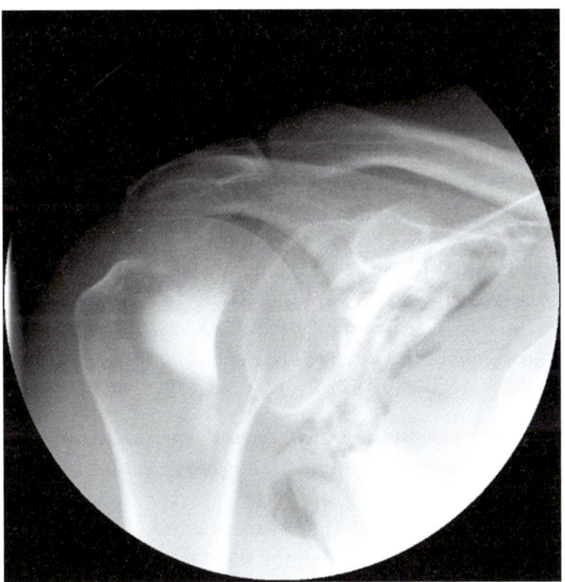

Figure 25.6b Fluoroscopic-guided hydrodilation of the shoulder: after hydrodilation with successful rupture of the joint capsule.

Chan et al. (2008) hypothesized that high-volume ultrasound-guided injection of normal saline around the Achilles tendon would produce local mechanical effects causing neovessels to rupture or occlude. A local anaesthetic and steroid combination was injected between the anterior aspect of Achilles tendon and Kager's fat pad, followed by 40 ml of injectable saline. They found that high-volume injections significantly reduced pain and improved function in 30 patients with chronic Achilles tendinopathy.

The review by Cormick (2009) describes a method using 20 ml of cold 0.9% saline with Celestone (betamethasone) and local anaesthetic, which is injected to strip the paratenon off the tendon. However, the use of steroids, in the context of abnormal tendon, is not advised because of the potential risk of rupture from inadvertent intratendinous injection (Andres and Murrell 2008).

Percutaneous lavage (barbotage)

Percutaneous lavage is synonymous with barbotage or image-guided needle irrigation and aspiration. Aspiration of the intratendinous calcifications is usually performed under direct ultrasound guidance using either a single- or dual-needle technique. In the two-needle technique, a saline solution is injected through one needle and dissolved calcium extracted through the other. If the calciferous material is liquid, it can be aspirated. The procedure was described in a number of review articles (Louis 2008).

Comfort and Arafiles (1978) first performed percutaneous needle aspiration of calcific deposits under fluoroscopic guidance in 1978. In 1995, Farin et al. improved the percutaneous needle aspiration and lavage technique by using ultrasound guidance to accurately and reliably localize calcifications (1995).

A new technique has been described which involves a fine-needle technique (22 G) with lavage of 1% lignocaine, which has led to reduced pain and disability, in a prospective study of 30 patients (Alna et al. 2001). Pain and function were measured using the Shoulder Pain and Disability Index (SPADI) questionnaire, using visual analogue scales. Patients attended a follow-up appointment at a mean of 53 days, where the overall SPADI decreased by 27%, with pain reduced by 30.5% and disability by 23.9%.

There are several non-randomized follow-up studies that show good results of the barbotage; however, a randomized controlled study is lacking. Serafini et al. (2009) have shown improved symptoms at 1 and 3 months and 1 year using this technique.

Ozone

Ozone's high reactivity gives it a short half-life. It can be produced artificially by subjecting diatomic oxygen to a high-voltage electrical discharge.

Its current use in the field of musculoskeletal disorders is mainly confined to the treatment of small joints and localized diseases, such as Morton's neuroma and disorders involving the facet joints of the spine (Al-Jaziri and Mahmoodi 2008) or the temporomandibular joint (Daif 2012), and lumbar disc herniation (Zhang et al. 2013). Although the exact mechanism of action of medical ozone is not completely understood, there are a number of characteristics of this molecule that offer some insights into its mode of action (Lu et al. 2010). Ozone has an effect on the inflammatory cascade by altering the breakdown of arachidonic acid to inflammatory prostaglandins. As a result, by reducing the inflammatory components, there is a subsequent decrease in pain.

In lumbar disc herniation, ozone is a rapid and strong oxidizing agent. The ozone molecule breaks down some of the glycosaminoglycan chains in the nucleus pulposus and reduces their ability to hold water, thereby diminishing the size of the herniation and subsequently contributing to pain relief. In addition, the disc herniation can impinge on the venous and arterial flow and cause phlebostasis and arteriostenosis, which leads to a serious hypoxaemia of the area. By applying the ozone to the herniated site, hyperoxygenation of the area occurs, which reduces the pain.

The stimulation of fibroblastic activity by ozone will result in the initiation of the repair process by stimulating collagen deposition (Rahimi-Movaghar and Eslami 2012; Zhang et al. 2013).

Normal saline

Physiological saline is a 0.9% w/v solution (that is approximately 9 g/l) of NaCl in purified water. Its use in interventional musculoskeletal procedures is related to its ability to dissolve intratendinous calcifications, which leads not only to a reduction of the pain, but also to functional improvement. This technique is used frequently for the treatment of rotator cuff calcifications, but it can be adapted to any site of intratendinous calcification.

Spinal injections

Low back pain is a common and costly medical condition. While low back pain rarely indicates a serious disorder, it is a major cause of pain, disability, and social cost. However, a cause for the back pain can be established in only 15% of all cases (Manchikanti et al. 2010).

Spine injection for the relief of chronic back is one of the most commonly performed procedures. The mechanisms of action are thought to include an anti-inflammatory effect of the corticosteroid, which reduces the inflammatory mediators around the nerve roots and reduces adhesions owing to the volume effect of the injection. Nevertheless, spine injections have drawn a significant controversy regarding efficiency, safety, and relevance. Much of this controversy is due to many studies of poor quality (Arden et al. 2005; Bush and Hillier 1991; Buttermann 2004; Carette et al. 1991, 1997; Jackson et al. 1980; Koes et al. 1995; McQuay and Moore 1996; Riew et al. 2000; Samanta and Beardsley 1999; Samanta and Samanta 2004; Slosar and White 1998; Staal et al. 2008; van Tulder and Koes 2004; Valat et al. 2003; Watts and Silagy 1995).

There is a paucity of well-designed, randomized controlled studies and a lack of statistically significant results. A solid conclusion for the effectiveness of spinal injection therapy is lacking (Riew et al. 2000). NICE, the UK National Institute for Health and Clinical Excellence, recommended that patients with persistent nonspecific low back pain should not be offered injections of therapeutic substances (2009).

Epidural injections are one of the most commonly used invasive interventions in the treatment of low back pain, with or without radicular pain. The goal of the injection is pain relief; at times, the injection alone is sufficient to provide relief, but commonly an epidural steroid injection is used in combination with a comprehensive rehabilitation programme to provide additional benefit.

There is currently little consensus about epidural injections and wide variation in practice (Cluff et al. 2002). There is also no agreement on the most effective approach for lumbar epidural injection (whether to use steroid, local anaesthetic, saline, or a combination) or the exact volume required. Depot steroids are not licensed for spinal use (Ferner 1996; Wildsmith 1996) but are used extensively in epidural injections (Fanciullo et al. 2001). The caudal route of lumbar epidural may require a larger volume but is less likely to cause dural puncture (Abi et al. 2005; Snarr 2007).

A Cochrane review concluded that there is no strong evidence for or against the use of any type of injection therapy for individuals with subacute or chronic low back pain (Staal et al. 2008).

Side-effects

A Cochrane review found minor side-effects such as headache, dizziness, transient local pain, tingling, numbness, and nausea reported in a small number of patients in only half the trials reviewed (Staal et al. 2008).

Increased age, needle gauge, needle approach, needle insertion at multiple interspaces, number of needle passes, volume of injectant, and accidental dural puncture are all significant risk factors for minor haemorrhagic complications (Horlocker et al. 2002).

Minor worsening of neurological function may occur after epidural steroid injection and must be differentiated from aetiologies requiring intervention. New neurological symptoms or worsening of pre-existing complaints that persist for more than 24 hours (median duration of symptoms 3 days, range 1–20 days) might occur after epidural injection (Horlocker et al. 2002).

Accuracy

The lumbar epidural space is accessible either by caudal, interlaminar, or transforaminal routes. The epidural injections are performed with or without image guidance.

Accuracy of blind caudal epidural injections compared with targeted placement has been assessed in a few studies. Successful placement on the first attempt was achieved in 75% of cases. Results were improved when anatomical landmarks were identified easily (88%) and no air was palpable subcutaneously over the sacrum when injected through the needle (83%). The combination of these two signs predicted a successful injection in 91% of attempts (Price et al. 2000).

In another study, blind injections were correctly placed in only two out of three attempts and the success rate was less than half when the operator was not certain. If the patient was obese, the success rate reduced even further. In a third prospective randomized, double-blind trial, the results showed no advantage of spinal endoscopic placement compared with the more traditional caudal approach (Barre et al. 2004; Botwin et al. 2007; Bryan et al. 2000; Dashfield et al. 2005; Price et al. 2000; Stitz and Sommer 1999).

The weight of the patient and intended approach need to be considered when deciding the method used to enter the epidural space. In the non-obese patient, lumbar epidural injections can be accurately placed without X-ray screening, but caudal epidural injections, to be placed accurately, require X-ray screening no matter what the weight of the patient (Price et al. 2000).

Efficacy

Reports of the effectiveness of all types of epidural corticosteroids, irrespective of route of administration, have varied from 18% to 90% (Manchikanti et al. 2010).

A systematic review of epidural corticosteroids for back pain found at least 75% pain relief in the short term (1–60 days) with at least 50% pain relief in the long term (3–12 months) (McQuay and Moore 1996). A randomized, double-blind, controlled trial concluded that lumbar epidural of local anaesthetic with steroid was effective in 86% of patients, and without steroid, in 74% (Manchikanti et al. 2010).

A systematic review indicated positive evidence (Level II-2) for short-term relief of pain from disc herniation or radiculopathy by blind interlaminar epidural steroid injections; there was less strong evidence for long-term pain relief for these conditions and for the short- and long-term relief of pain from spinal stenosis and from discogenic pain without radiculopathy or disc herniation (Conn et al. 2009).

Another review showed the lack of long-term relief of pain of both lumbar and caudal epidural injections (Koes et al. 1995). Yet another showed strong evidence for epidurals in the management of nerve root pain due to disc prolapse, but limited evidence in spinal stenosis (Abi et al. 2005). A multi-centre randomized controlled trial of epidurals for sciatica reported significant relief at 3 weeks but no long-term benefit (Arden et al. 2005).

A significantly greater proportion of patients treated with transforaminal injection of steroid (54%) achieved relief of pain than did patients treated with transforaminal injection of local anaesthetic (7%) or transforaminal injection of saline (19%), intramuscular steroids (21%), or intramuscular saline (13%). Selective guided nerve-root injections of corticosteroids are significantly more effective than those of bupivacaine alone in obviating the need for operative decompression for 13–28 months following the injections in operative candidates. When symptoms have been present for more than 12 months, local anaesthetic alone may be just as effective as steroid and local anaesthetic together (Ghahreman et al. 2010; Ng and Sell 2004; Riew et al. 2000).

When conservative measures fail, one study suggests that nerve-root injections are effective in reducing pain in patients with osteoporotic vertebral fractures and that these patients should be considered for this treatment before percutaneous vertebroplasty or operative intervention is attempted (Kim et al. 2003).

Injection of the sacroiliac joints for painful sacroiliitis appears to be safe and effective. It can be considered in patients with contra-indications or complications with NSAIDs, or if other medical treatment is ineffective (Maugars et al. 1996). However, accurate placement of the drug without the use of imaging is estimated to be successful in only 12% of patients (Hansen 2003).

The choice between giving an epidural injection and nerve-root injection can be aided by laterality of pain; if the pain is clearly on one side in the lumbar area, or radiating down one leg, a nerve-root injection may be effective. If the pain is bilateral or central in the lumbar spine, an epidural may be a better choice. The following are the main indications for epidural and nerve root injections:

- Acute back and/or leg pain where pain makes manipulation impossible to perform
- Chronic back and/or leg pain where conservative treatment has failed
- Prior to considering surgery.

Patients with chronic back pain increased on active extension, suggesting facet joints symptoms, may benefit from facet joint injections.

Lumbar epidural injection is also commonly used to treat pain of spinal stenosis. A retrospective study of patients with spinal stenosis found that 35% of patients had at least 50% improvement. There was a better outcome in patients with spondylolisthesis, single-level stenosis, and those older than 73 years (Barre et al. 2004). Less commonly, spinal injections include injections for coccydinia or sacroiliac joint pain following acute trauma or delivery.

There is a controversy in the literature regarding the optimal imaging technique for spinal injection procedures. While some practitioners prefer blind injections, there are also others who prefer to use image guidance by sonography, MRI, fluoroscopy, or CT for a safe epidural or periradicular needle placement (Carette et al. 1991; Jackson et al. 1980; McQuay and Moore 1996; Riew et al. 2000; Staal et al. 2008). The CT-guided technique is described as fast, safe, and highly accurate in proving appropriate needle placement in epidural injections (Slosar and White 1998) For selective nerve block, CT-guided injections are described to be superior to fluoroscopy-guided for both the visualization and a longer-lasting effect (Staal et al. 2008). Despite the accuracy, the patient's and physician's exposure to radiation in CT-guided interventions remains a serious concern (Artner et al. 2012; Valat et al. 2003). However, a new CT scanning system incorporates several improvements to reduce radiation exposure. Radiation exposure was decreased by as much as 95% relative to other CT scanners currently in use.

Technique

CT-guided injections

The procedure is performed on an out-patient basis. The patient is placed prone on the CT table. A CT scan of the affected level allows precise choice of needle pathway. Radiolucent markers are placed on the skin surface to assist with landmarking of the target structure, and the entry point and pathway are determined.

Epidural injection

After local anaesthesia of the skin, a 22-gauge spinal needle is placed, under CT guidance, via a posterior approach in the epidural space (see Figures 25.7 and 25.8). Once the needle is in the epidural space, air is injected to confirm the extradural position of the needle tip and absence of cerebrospinal fluid (CSF) is verified by aspiration. Then, a long-acting steroid solution mixed with a solution of long-acting local anaesthetic is injected.

Selective nerve block

The patient is placed in the supine position with the head slightly turned away from the side to be injected for cervical nerves injection. For the lumbar area, the patient is placed in prone position.

After local anaesthesia of the skin, a 22-gauge spinal needle is placed near the painful nerve root via a lateral approach under CT guidance (see Figures 25.9 and 25.10). In the cervical area, a soluble long-acting steroid and anaesthetic is injected. For lumbar nerve block, a long-acting steroid solution mixed with a solution of long-acting local anaesthetic is injected. For cervical epidural, a long-acting steroid solution is injected only.

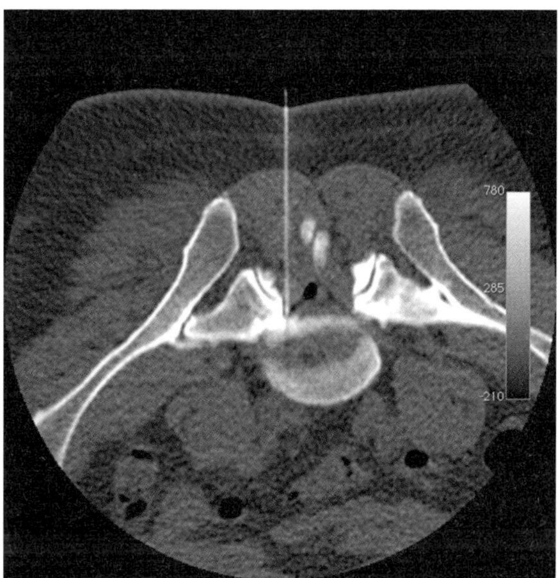

Figure 25.7 A 53-year-old with spinal stenosis. An axial CT image showing a translaminar approach of epidural injection. The position of the needle in the epidural space is confirmed by air injection.

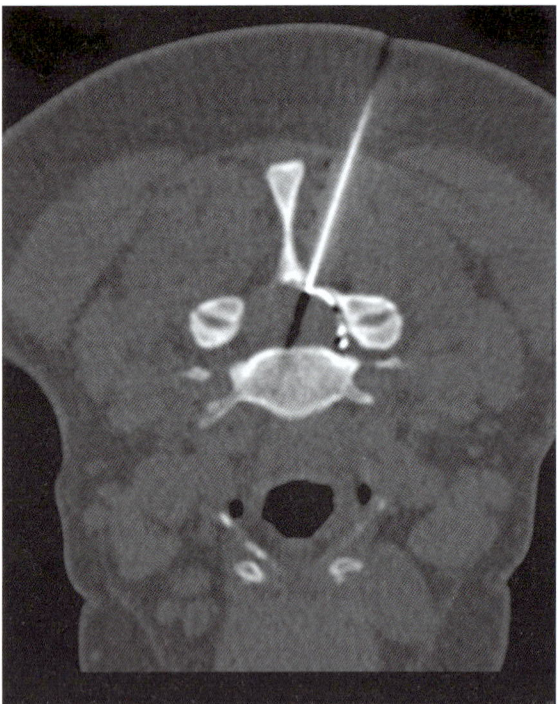

Figure 25.8 CT-guided cervical epidural injection in a patient with bilateral brachalgia. A translaminar approach with the needle position confirmed by contrast injection.

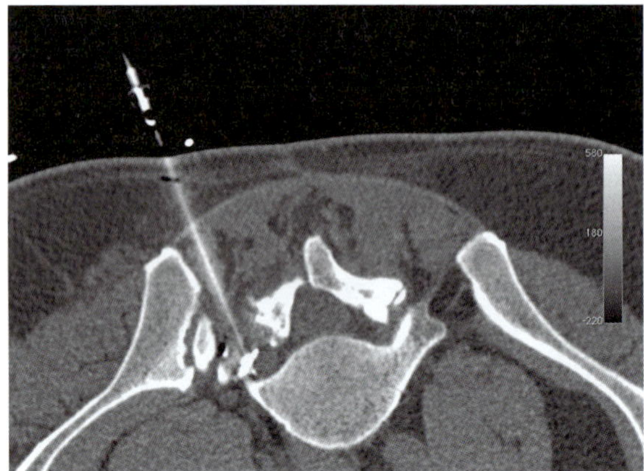

Figure 25.9 CT-guided lumbar selective nerve block. A 50-year-old with right L5 sciatica.

Although rare, a variety of side-effects and technical complications are associated with spinal injections. The most common complications are increased pain (1.1%), pain at the injection site (0.33%), persistent numbness (0.14%), and 'other' (0.80%). Other potential complications include infection, steroid side-effects, dural puncture, post-puncture headache, and neural damage (Cohen et al. 2013; McGrath et al. 2011).

Vertebroplasty

Galibert and Deramend introduced vertebroplasty in France in 1984 for treating haemangiomas at the C2 vertebra (Galibert et al. 1987). Later, vertebroplasty was successfully introduced for

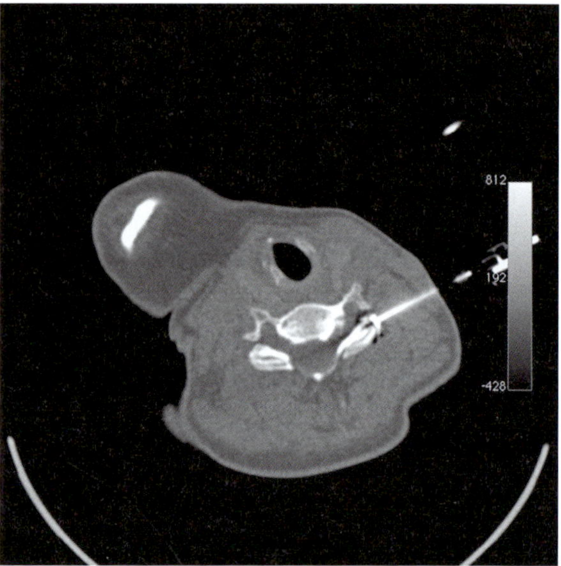

Figure 25.10 CT-guided cervical nerve root injection: a patient with LT C6 brachalgia due to formanial stenosis. An axial CT image showing the position of the needle anterior to the facet joint with injected air outlining the perineural space.

the management of osteoporotic compression fractures (Deramond et al. 1998). From 1984, vertebroplasty has been used to treat vertebral compression fractures caused by myeloma, trauma, and osteoporosis. Balloon kyphoplasty was first performed in 1998. It is a minimally invasive surgical technique that attempts to correct kyphosis secondary to collapsed vertebral bodies (Garfin et al. 2001). Both procedures involve placing needles into fractured vertebral bodies and injecting bone cement under imaging control. They both increase bone strength and reduce the pain caused by the vertebral fracture.

Two randomized controlled trials have indicated that both of the procedures can produce immediate pain relief over conservative treatments (Klazen et al. 2010). The other study, with 24 months of follow-up, reported that kyphoplasty reduced pain and improved function, disability, and quality of life more effectively than non-surgical therapy, without increasing the risk of additional vertebral fractures (Boonen et al. 2011). However, there is controversy over which of the two procedures leads to superior results and long-term outcomes. There is no consensus as to whether kyphoplasty or vertebroplasty is the optimal treatment. Although there are a limited number of randomized controlled trials, several non-randomized controlled trials have been published. For patients with osteoporotic fractures, the data is conflicting (Boonen et al. 2011; Folman and Shabat 2011; Grohs et al. 2005; Hiwatashi et al. 2009; Klazen et al. 2010; Kumar et al. 2010; Liu et al. 2010; Lovi et al. 2009; Movrin et al. 2010; Rollinghoff et al. 2009; Santiago et al. 2010; Schofer et al. 2009; Yan et al. 2011; Zhou et al. 2008).

A meta-analysis and systemic review concluded that quality of the evidence currently available is poor but both vertebroplasty and kyphoplasty are safe and effective procedures for treating osteoporotic vertebral fractures. Kyphoplasty may be superior to vertebroplasty in patients with large kyphosis angles, vertebral fissures, fractures in the posterior edge of the vertebral body, or significant height loss in the fractured vertebrae (Xing et al. 2013).

However, not all evidence is positive for the use of cement augmentation. Two placebo-controlled vertebroplasty studies have sobering results with regard to pain and functional outcome after cement augmentation with vertebroplasty, if compared to a sham operation (Buchbinder et al. 2009; Kallmes et al. 2009). In both studies, the sham procedure included percutaneous needle insertion and opening of polymethylmethacrylate (PMMA)-monomer mixture to simulate the specific odour. The sham-controlled trial by Buchbinder et al. (2009) in 78 patients with MRI-confirmed, fresh, and painful vertebral fractures found no beneficial effect of vertebroplasty when compared to a sham procedure. A very similar study by Kallmes et al. investigating 131 patients found similar results. Both studies were criticized on the basis of methodology and statistical analysis (Baerlocher et al. 2009; Bono et al. 2010; Mathis 2003; Munk et al. 2009).

The randomized controlled trial by Rousing et al. (2009) found no greater improvement in back pain in patients treated with vertebroplasty when compared to medical therapy. Interestingly, they found a significant improvement in the Barthel score after 12 months ($p < 0.02$), indicating improved function (Fisher and Vaccaro 2009).

Owing to the aforementioned results, some practitioners abandoned the use of vertebroplasty (Hasserius et al. 2010; Karlsson et al. 2010), while others are hesitant and question the quality of the sham-controlled vertebroplasty trials (Fisher and Vaccaro 2009; Heini 2010).

Indications and contraindications

Vertebroplasty is indicated in those patients with painful vertebral fractures who fail to benefit from conservative treatment or in cases of severe pain with the patient requiring hospitalization. Patients with pain of longer than three months' duration are less likely to benefit from vertebroplasty (Klazen et al. 2010).

Recently, the National Institute of Clinical Excellence (NICE) has concluded that percutaneous vertebroplasty and percutaneous balloon kyphoplasty without stenting are recommended as options for treating osteoporotic vertebral compression fractures only in people:

- who have severe ongoing pain after a recent, unhealed vertebral fracture despite optimal pain management and
- in whom the pain has been confirmed to be at the level of the fracture by physical examination and imaging.

There are few absolute contraindications to vertebroplasty including patients with bleeding diathesis and those with severe cardiac or respiratory failure precluding safe conscious sedation or general anaesthesia. These patients are considered high risk for clinically significant procedure-related fat embolism (Syed and Shaikh 2007). Infection or fever is also an absolute contraindication. Severe loss of vertebral body height is a relative contraindication, but good results can often be obtained in even severely compressed vertebrae (O'Brien et al. 2000).

Technique

The procedure is performed under fluoroscopic guidance and/or in combination with CT guidance (see Figure 25.11). The patient is placed in the prone position. Sedation is used but general anaesthesia may be required if the patient is in severe pain and difficult to position.

With aseptic technique and following local anaesthesia, an 11G or 13G bone needle is inserted down onto the periosteum overlying the pedicle, aiming for the lateral cortical margin of the pedicle at the 10:00 position on the left and the 2:00 position on the right. A transpedicular approach is the technique of choice. The tip of the cannula is advanced to a point approximately 1 cm posterior to the anterior vertebral body. The PMMA cement is prepared by mixing polymer powder with liquid monomer. Mixing of the powder and liquid leads to exothermic polymerization and then progressive thickening of the paste, which subsequently hardens. Once the cement has a toothpaste-like consistency, the mixture is injected. Continuous screening for cement extravasation during injection is performed.

In balloon kyphoplasty, a tamp (balloon) is inserted into the vertebral body using either a transpedicular or extrapedicular route,

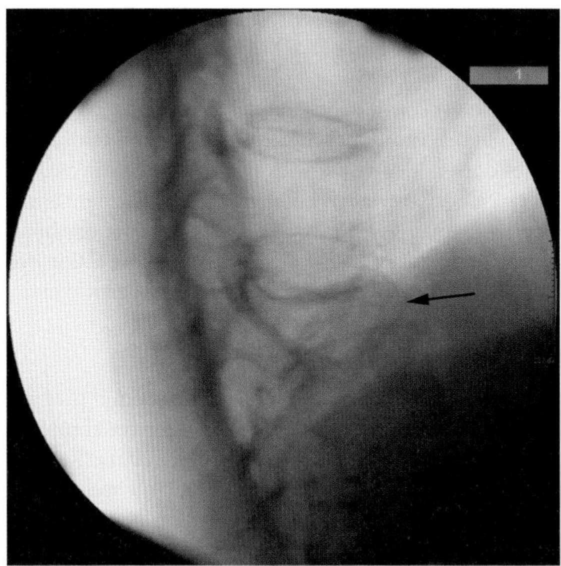

Figure 25.11a A 58-year-old man with acute back pain. Lateral radiograph of the lumbar spine shows T12 vertebra compression fractures.

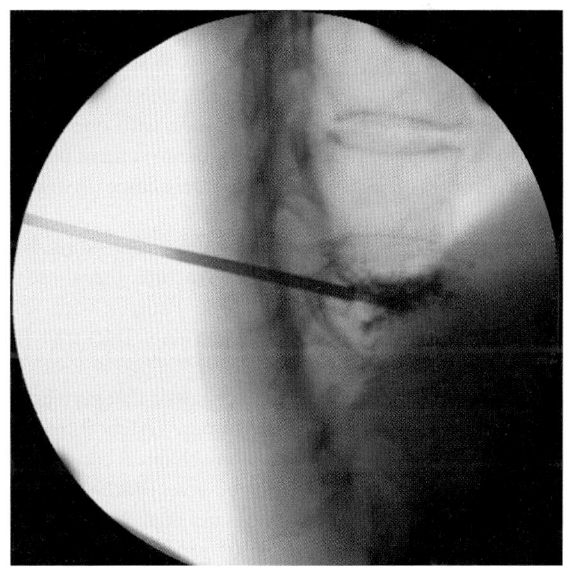

Figure 25.11b Fluoroscopic view during vertebroplasty confirms the proper positioning of the needle and cement injected in the vertebral body.

leading to compression of cancellous bone and creation of a cavity. After removal of the balloon, PMMA is injected to fix and stabilize the fracture.

The volume of cement to be injected at each level for maximal efficacy has not been accurately determined (Belkoff et al. 2001). The pain relief does not correlate with the volume of injected cement (Barr et al. 2000). On average, between 3–5 ml of cement is injected.

The patient remains supine or semi-recumbent for one hour, with monitoring of neurovascular status and wound inspection every 15 and 30 minutes respectively. The patient is then gently mobilized, then discharged home after two hours.

Complications

Complications can occur in both procedures, even if they are very rare. In fact, overall complications are 1–6% for vertebroplasty and about 1.2% for kyphoplasty (Lieberman et al. 2001). Recently, the risk of major complications after vertebroplasty seems to be less than 1% (Phillips 2003). Cement leakage and neurological injuries are reported with both procedures and extravertebral cement leakage represents the major risk of vertebroplasty (40–65%) (Deramond and Mathis 2002; Pateder et al. 2007) and is, generally, clinically asymptomatic (Cortet et al. 1999; Deramond et al. 1998; Garfin et al. 2001; Heini et al. 2000; Peh and Gilula 2005; Zoaeski et al. 2002). Cases of spinal cord and nerve root injuries due to cement leakage have been reported (Adachi et al. 2002; Bhatia et al. 2006; Burton and Mendel 2003; Chen et al. 2006; Kahn and Macdonald 2004; Lee et al. 2002; Lips et al. 1999; Riggs and Melton 1995). Systemic cement embolization is rare, with one study estimating as many as 5% of patients may undergo cement pulmonary embolism (Choe et al. 2004). These are rarely clinically significant (Padovani et al. 1999).

Other complications of vertebroplasty include bleeding, haematoma, infection, pneumothorax, pedicle fracture, thecal sac puncture, and cerebrospinal fluid (CSF) leak. Patients with severely lowered bone mineral density may experience fractured ribs or sternum while the procedure is performed.

Some reports in the literature have suggested that vertebroplasty is associated with a higher incidence of new vertebral fractures at adjacent levels, possibly reflecting a biomechanical consequence of the augmented stiffness of the cemented level (Baroud et al. 2003; Grados et al. 2000; Lin et al. 2004; Mudano et al. 2009). Data from the VERTOS II trial (Klazen et al. 2010), randomizing painful vertebral fractures to conservative treatment or vertebroplasty, showed the incidence of new vertebral fractures between the two groups was not different at 12 months' follow-up, and the only risk factor identified for new vertebral fractures was the number of baseline vertebral fractures. This adds weight to the theory that new vertebral fractures post-vertebroplasty are manifestations of the natural history of osteoporosis rather than reflecting a risk intrinsic to vertebroplasty.

Conclusion to musculoskeletal injections

Almost every aspect of musculoskeletal injections is non-standardized. There is a wealth of anecdotal evidence for the efficiency of the injections but few definitive studies and a rather small number of studies comparing injection therapy with other treatment. The interpretations and conclusions of the reported studies are often contradictory and there is no universal expert agreement, with wide variation in methodology and quality.

Nevertheless, musculoskeletal injections are recommended in national and international guidelines given its relative safety, ease of application in trained hands, and cost effectiveness, plus the frequent lack of convincing systematic evidence for the effectiveness of alternatives. Injection therapy remains the most common therapeutic intervention in rheumatology practice.

In-depth familiarity with the equipment, materials, and techniques are fundamental for safe, effective administration of musculoskeletal injections. It is also equally important to be aware of the current indications for the substances being injected and how they are used and the possible complications of each procedure undertaken.

References

Abate M, Pulcini D, Di Iorio A, et al. Viscosupplementation with intra-articular hyaluronic acid for treatment of osteoarthritis in the elderly. *Curr Pharm Des* 2010; 16(6):631–40.

Abi S, Datt S, Lucas L. Role of epidural steroids in management of chronic spinal pain: systematic review of effectiveness and complications. *Pain Physician* 2005; 8(1):127–43.

Acevedo JI, Beskin JL. Complications of plantar fascia rupture associated with corticosteroid injection. *Foot Ankle Int* 1998; 19:91–7.

Adachi JD, Ioannidis G, Olszynski WP, et al. The impact of incident vertebral and non-vertebral fractures on health related quality of life in postmenopausal women. *BMC Musculoskelet Disord* 2002; 3:11.

af Klint E, Grundtman C, Engström M, et al. Intraarticular glucocorticoid treatment reduces inflammation in synovial cell infiltrations more efficiently than in synovial blood vessels. *Arthritis Rheum* 2005; 52 (12):3880–9.

Aldana SG. Financial impact of health promotion programs: a comprehensive review of the literature. *Am J Health Prom* 2001; 15(5):296–320.

Al-Jaziri AA, Mahmoodi SM Pain killing effect of ozone-oxygen injection on spine and joint osteoarthritis. *Saudi Med J* 2008; 29(4):553–7.

Alna R, Cardinal E, Bureau NJ, et al. Calcific shoulder tendinitis: treatment with modified US-guided fine-needle technique. *Radiology* 2001; 221:455–61.

Andres BM, Murrell GA. Treatment of tendinopathy: what works, what does not, and what is on the horizon. *Clin Orthop Relat Res* 2008; 466:1539–54.

Anon. Articular and periarticular corticosteroid injection. *Drug Ther Bull* 1995; 33(9):67–70.

Anon. Gout in primary care. *Drug Ther Bull* 2004; 42(5):39.

Arden NK, Price C, Reading I, et al. A multicentre randomized controlled trial of epidural corticosteroid injections for sciatica: the WEST study. *Rheumatology* 2005; 44(11):1399–406.

Artner J, Lattig F, Reichel H, Cakir B. Effective dose of CT-guided epidural and periradicular injections of the lumbar spine: a retrospective study. *Open Orthop J* 2012; 6:357–61.

Baerlocher MO, Munk Pl, Liu DM. Trials of vertebroplasty for vertebral fractures. *N Engl J Med* 2009; 361(21):2098.

Balint PV, Kane D, Hunter J, McInnes IB, Field M, Sturrock RD Ultrasound guided versus conventional joint and soft tissue fluid aspiration in rheumatology practice: a pilot study. *J Rheumatol* 2002; 29:2209–13.

Banfi G, Corsi MM, Volpi P. Could platelet rich plasma have effects on systemic circulating growth factors and cytokine release in orthopaedic applications? *Br J Sports Med* 2006; 40:816.

Bannuru RR, Natov NS, Obadan IE, et al. Therapeutic trajectory of hyaluronic acid versus corticosteroids in the treatment of knee osteoarthritis: a systematic review and meta-analysis. *Arthritis Rheum* 2009; 61(12):1704–11.

Baroud G, Heini P, Nemes J, et al. Biomechanical explanation of adjacent fractures following vertebroplasty. *Radiology* 2003; 229(2):606–7.

Barr JD, Barr MS, Lemley TJ, McCann RM. Percutaneous vertebroplasty for pain relief and spinal stabilization. *Spine* 2000; 25(8):923–8.

Barre L, Lutz GE, Southern D, et al. Fluoroscopically guided caudal epidurals for lumbar/spinal stenosis. *Pain Physician* 2004; 7(2):187–93.

Barrett S, Erredge S. Growth factors for chronic plantar fasciitis. *Podiatry Today* 2004; 17:27–42.

Bartold SJ. Plantar heel syndrome: overview and management. The plantar fascia as a source of pain and biomechanics, presentation and treatment. *J Bodywork Move Ther* 2004; 8:214–26.

Basadonna PT, Rucco V, Gasparini D, et al. Plantar fat pad atrophy after corticosteroid injection for an interdigital neuroma: a case report. *Am J Phys Med Rehabil* 1999; 78:283–5.

Beaudouin E, Kanny G, Gueant JL, et al. Anaphylaxis caused by carboxymethylcellulose: report of 2 cases of shock from injectable corticoids. (Article in French.) *Allerg Immunol (Paris)* 1992; 24(9):333–5.

van den Bekerom MP, Lamme B, Sermon A, et al. What is the evidence for viscosupplementation in the treatment of patients with hip osteoarthritis? Systematic review of the literature. *Arch Orthop Trauma Surg* 2008; 128 (8):815–23.

van den Bekerom MPJ, Rys B, Mulier M. Viscosupplementation in the hip: evaluation of hyaluronic acid formulations. *Arch Orthop Trauma Surg* 2008; 128(3):275–80.

Belkoff SM, Mathis JM, Jasper LE, Deramond H. The biomechanics of vertebroplasty: the effect of cement volume on mechanical behavior. *Spine* 2001; 26(14):1537–41.

Bellamy N, Campbell J, Robinson V, et al. Viscosupplementation for the treatment of osteoarthritis of the knee. *Cochrane Database Syst Rev* 2006; (2):CD005321.

Bellamy N, Campbell J, Robinson V, Gee T, Bourne R, Wells G Intraarticular corticosteroid for treatment of osteoarthritis of the knee. Cochrane Database Syst Rev 2006; 19(2):CD005328.

Benzon HT, Chew TL, McCarthy RJ, et al. Comparison of the particle sizes of different steroids and the effect of dilution: a review of the relative neurotoxicities of the steroids. *Anaesthesiology* 2007; 106:331–8.

Berger RG, Yount WJ. Immediate 'steroid flare' from intraarticular triamcinolone hexacetonide injection: case report and review of the literature. *Arthritis Rheum* 1990; 33:1284–6.

Bernardeau C, Bucki B, Liotea F. Acute arthritis after intra-articular hyaluronate injection: onset of effusions without crystal. *Ann Rheum Dis* 2001; 60:518–20.

Bhatia C, Barzilay Y, Krishna M, et al. Cement leakage in percutaneous vertebroplasty: effect of preinjection gelfoam embolization. Friesem T, Pollock R. *Spine* 2006; 31(8):915–9.

Bisbinas I, Belthur M, Said HG,Green M, Learmonth DJ. Accuracy of needle placement in ACJ injections. *Knee Surg Sports Traum Arthrosc* 2006; 14 (8):762–5.

Blaine T, Moskowitz R, Udell J, et al. Treatment of persistent shoulder pain with sodium hyaluronate: a randomized, controlled trial. A multicenter study. *J Bone Joint Surg Am* 2008; 90:5970–9.

Bodor M, Flossman T. Ultrasound-guided first annular pulley injection for trigger finger. *J Ultrasound Med* 2009; 28:737–43.

Bono CM, Heggeness M, Mick C, Resnick D, Watters WC. North American Spine Society: newly released vertebroplasty randomized controlled trials: a tale of two trials. *Spine* 2010; 10(3):238–40.

Boonen S, Van Meirhaeghe J, Bastian L, et al. Balloon kyphoplasty for the treatment of acute vertebral compression fractures: 2-year results from a randomized trial. *J Bone Miner Res* 2011; 26:1627–37.

Botwin K, Brown LA, Fishman M, et al. Fluoroscopically guided caudal epidural injections in degenerative lumbar spinal stenosis. *Pain Physician* 2007; 10(4):547–8.

Brander VA, Gomberawalla A, Chambers M, et al. Efficacy and safety of hylan G-F 20 for symptomatic glenohumeral osteoarthritis: a prospective, pilot study. *Poly Rheumat* 2010; 2(4):259–67.

British National Formulary No 59; Section 15.2. London: BMA/RPSGB; 2010.

Brown EM Jr, Frain JB, Udell L, Hollander JL. Locally administered hydrocortisone in the rheumatic diseases; a summary of its use in 547 patients. *Am J Med* 1953; 15:656–665.

Bryan BM, Lutz C, Lutz GE. Fluoroscopic assessment of epidural contrast spread after caudal injection. *J Orthop Med* 2000; 22(2):38–41.

Buchbinder R, Green S, Forbes A, et al. Arthrographic joint distension with saline and steroid improves function and reduces pain in patients with painful stiff shoulder: results of a randomised, double blind, placebo controlled trial. *Ann Rheum Dis* 2004; 63:302–9.

Buchbinder R, Osborne RH, Ebeling PR, et al. A randomized trial of vertebroplasty for painful osteoporotic vertebral fractures. *N Engl J Med* 2009; 361:557–68.

Burton AW, Mendel E. *Vertebroplasty and kyphoplasty: a comprehensive review.* 2003. Available at: <http://www.ampainsoc.org/pub/%20bulletin/jul03/innol.htm>.

Bush K, Hillier S. A controlled study of caudal epidural injections of triamcinolone plus procaine for the management of intractable sciatica. *Spine* 1991; 16(5):572–5.

Buttermann GR. Treatment of lumbar disc herniation: epidural steroid injection compared with discectomy; a prospective, randomized study. *J Bone Joint Surg Am* 2004; 86:670–9.

Caldwell JR. Intra-articular corticosteroids. Guide to selection and indications for use. *Drugs* 1996; 52(4):507–14.

Cameron G. Steroid arthropathy: myth or reality? *J Ortho Med* 1995; 17(2):51–5.

Carette S, Leclaire R, Marcoux S, et al. Epidural corticosteroid injections for sciatica due to herniated nucleus pulposus. *N Engl J Med* 1997; 336 (23):1634–40.

Carette S, Marcoux S, Truchon R, et al. A controlled trial of corticosteroid injections into facet joints for chronic low back pain. *N Engl J Med* 1991; 325(14):1002–7.

Cassidy JT, Bole GG. Cutaneous atrophy secondary to intra-articular corticosteroid administration. *Ann Intern Med* 1966; 65(5):1008–18.

Chan O, O'Dowd D, Padhiar N, et al. High volume image guided injections in chronic Achilles tendinopathy. *Disabil Rehab* 2008; 30:1697–708.

Charalambous CP, Tryfonidis M, Sadiq S, et al. Septic arthritis following intra-articular glucocorticoid injection of the knee—a survey of current practice regarding antiseptic technique used during intra-articular glucocorticoid injection of the knee. *Clin Rheumatol* 2003; 22: 386–90.

Chen MJ, Lew HL, Hsu TC, et al. Ultrasound-guided shoulder injections in the treatment of subacromial bursitis. *Am J Phys Med Rehabil* 2006; 85:31–5.

Chen YJ, Tan TS, Chen WH, et al. Intradural cement leakage: a devastatingly rare complication of vertebroplasty. *Spine* 2006; 31(12):E379–82.

Choe DH, Marom EM, Ahrar K, Truong MT, Madewell JE. Pulmonary embolism of polymethyl methacrylate during percutaneous vertebroplasty and kyphoplasty. *Am J Roentgenol* 2004; 183(4):1097–102.

Cluff R, Mehio AK, Cohen SP, et al. The technical aspects of epidural steroid injections: a national survey. *Anesth Analg* 2002; 95:403–8.

Cohen SP, Strassels SA, Foster L, et al. Comparison of fluoroscopically guided and blind corticosteroid injections for greater trochanteric pain syndrome: multicentre randomised controlled trial. *BMJ* 2009; 338:b1088.

Cohen SP1, Bicket MC, Jamison D, Wilkinson I, Rathmell JP. Epidural steroids: a comprehensive, evidence-based review. *Reg Anesth Pain Med* 2013; 38(3):175–200.

Cole BJ, Schumacher HR. Injectable corticosteroids in modern practice. *J Am Acad Orthop Surg* 2005; 139(1):37–46.

Comfort TH, Arafiles RP. Barbotage of the shoulder with image-intensified fluoroscopic control of needle placement for calcific tendonitis. *Clin Orthop Relat Res* 1978; 135:171–8.

Conn A, Buenaventura RM, Datta S, et al. Systematic review of caudal epidural injections in the management of chronic low back pain. *Pain Physician* 2009; 12:109–35.

Connell DA, Ali KE, Ahmad M, et al. Ultrasound-guided autologous blood injection for tennis elbow. *Skeletal Radiol* 2006; 35:371–7.

Coombes GM, Bax DE. The use and abuse of steroids in rheumatology. *Rep Rheum Dis (Series 3). Practical Problems (No. 8)* 1996.

Cormick W. Ultrasound, tendon pain and tendon disease: what's new and what's around the corner. Sound effects. *J Aus Sonographers* 2009; 2: 12–5.

Cortet B, Cotten A, Boutry N, et al. Percutaneous vertebroplasty in the treatment of osteoporotic vertebral compression fractures: an open prospective study. *J Rheumatol* 1999; 26(10):2222–8.

Crawford RW, Gie GA, Ling RS, Murray DW. Diagnostic value of intra-articular an- aesthetic in primary osteoarthritis of the hip. *J Bone Joint Surg Br* 1998; 80:279–281.

Creamer P. Intra-articular corticosteroid injections in osteoarthritis: do they work, and if so, how? *Ann Rheum Dis* 1997; 56:634–6.

Creaney L, Hamilton B. Growth factor delivery methods in the management of sports injuries: the state of play. *Br J Sports Med* 2008; 42:34e320.

Cunnington J, Marshall N, Hide G, et al. A randomized, double-blind, controlled study of ultrasound-guided corticosteroid injection into the joint of patients with inflammatory arthritis. *Arthritis Rheum* 2010; 62 (7):1862–86.

Cusi M, Saunders J, Hungerford B, et al. The use of prolotherapy in the sacroiliac joint. *Br J Sports Med* 2010; 44(2):100–4.

Cutolo M. The roles of steroid hormones in arthritis. *Br J Rheumatol* 1998; 37:597–601.

D'Agostino MA, Ayral X, Baron G, et al. Impact of ultrasound imaging on local corticosteroid injections of symptomatic ankle, hind-, and mid-foot in chronic inflammatory diseases. *Arthritis Rheum* 2005; 53:284–92.

Dagenais S, Haldeman S, Wooley JR. Intraligamentous injection of sclerosing solutions (prolotherapy) for spinal pain: a critical review of the literature. *Spine J* 2005; 5(3):310–28.

Dagenais S, Mayer J, Haldeman S, et al. Evidence-informed management of chronic low back pain with prolotherapy. *Spine J* 2008; 8(1):203–12.

Dagenais S, Yelland MJ, Del Mar C, et al. Prolotherapy injections for chronic low-back pain. *Cochrane Database Syst Rev* 2007; (2). Art. No. CD004059.

Daif ET. Role of intra-articular ozone gas injection in the management of internal derangement of the temporomandibular joint. *Oral Surg Oral Med Oral Pathol Oral Radiol* 2012; 113(6):e10–4.

Dashfield K, Taylor M, Clekven J, et al. Comparison of caudal steroid epidural with targeted steroid placement during spinal endoscopy for chronic sciatica; a prospective randomized, double-blind trial. *Br J Anaesth* 2005; 94(4):514–6.

Deramond H, Depriester C, Galibert P, et al. Percutaneous vertebroplasty with polymethylmethacrylate. Technique, indications, and results. *Radiol Clin North Am* 1998; 36:533–46

Deramond H, Mathis JM. Vertebroplasty in osteoporosis. *Semin Musculoskelet Radiol* 2002; 6:263–8.

Dikici F, Balci HI, Ozcakar L, Aksoy C. Evaluation of needle positioning during blind intra-articular hip injections for osteoarthritis: fluoroscopy versus arthrography. *Arch Phys Med Rehabil* 2009; 90 (12):2112–5.

Dorman T, Ravin T. *Diagnosis and injection techniques in orthopaedic medicine.* Baltimore, Maryland: Williams and Wilkins; 1991: 33–4.

Ekeberg OM, Bautz-Holter E, Tveita EK, et al. Subacromial ultrasound guided or systemic steroid injection for rotator cuff disease: randomised double blind study. *BMJ* 2009; 338:a3112.

Esenyel CZ, Esenyel M, Yeşiltepe R. The correlation between the accuracy of steroid injections and subsequent shoulder pain and function in subacromial impingement syndrome. (Article in Turkish.) *Acta Orthop Traumatol Turc* 2003; 37(1):41–5.

Eustace JA, Brophy DP, Gibney RP, Bresnihan B, FitzGerald O. Comparison of the accuracy of steroid placement with clinical outcome in patients with shoulder symptoms. *Ann Rheum Dis* 1997; 56:59–63.

Ewan PW. Anaphylaxis (ABC of allergies). *BMJ* 1998; 316:1442–5.

Fanciullo GJ, Hanscom B, Seville J, et al. An observational study of the frequency and pattern of use of epidural steroid injection in 25,479 patients with spinal and radicular pain. *Reg Anesth Pain Med* 2001; 26(1):5–11.

Fanucci E, Masala S, Fabiano S, et al. Treatment of intermetatarsal Morton's neuroma with alcohol injection under US guide: 10-month follow-up. *Eur Radiol* 2004; 14:514–8.

Farin PU, Jaroma H, Soimakallio S. Rotator cuff calcifications: treatment with US-guided technique. *Radiology* 1995; 195:841–3.

Fernandez-Lopez JC, Ruano-Ravina A. Efficacy and safety of intraarticular hyaluronic acid in the treatment of hip osteoarthritis: a systematic review. *Osteoarth Cart* 2006; 14(12):3106–11.

Ferner RE. Prescribing licensed medicines for unlicensed indications. *Prescribers J* 1996; 36(2):73–8.

Filippuccil E, Farinal A, Carotti M, et al. Grey scale and power Doppler sonographic changes induced by intra-articular steroid injection treatment. *Ann Rheum Dis* 2004; 63:740–3.

Fisher CG, Vaccaro AR. The highest level of evidence in a high impact journal: is this the final verdict? *Spine* 35(15):E676–7.

Folman Y, Shabat S. A comparison of two new technologies for percutaneous vertebral augmentation: confidence vertebroplasty vs. sky kyphoplasty. *Isr Med Assoc J* 2011; 13:394–7.

Franz JK, Burmester G-R. Antirheumatic treatment: the needle and the damage done. *Ann Rheum Dis* 2005; 64:798–800.

Fredberg U. Local corticosteroid injection in sport: review of literature and guidelines for treatment. *Scand J Med Sci Sport* 1997; 7:131–9.

Fredberg U, Bolvig L, Pfeiffer-Jensen M, et al. Ultrasonography as a tool for diagnosis, guidance of local steroid injection and, together with pressure algometry, monitoring of the treatment of athletes with chronic jumper's knee and Achilles tendinitis: a randomized, double-blind, placebo- controlled study. *Scand J Rheumatol* 2004; 33(2):94–101.

Friedman DM, Moore ME. The efficacy of intraarticular steroids in osteoarthritis: a double-blind study. *J Rheumatol* 1980; 7:850–6.

Furtado RN, Oliveira LM, Natour J. Polyarticular corticosteroid injection versus systemic administration in treatment of rheumatoid arthritis patients: a randomized controlled study. *J Rheumatol* 2005; 32:1691–8.

Galibert P, Deramond H, Rosat P, Le Gars D. Preliminary note on the treatment of vertebral angioma by percutaneous acrylic vertebroplasty. *Neurochirurgie* 1987; 33(2):166–8.

Garfin SR, Yuan HAM, Reiley MAM. New technologies in spine. *Spine* 2001; 26(14):1511–5.

Gaujoux-Viala C, Dougados M, Gossec L. Efficacy and safety of steroid injections for shoulder and elbow tendonitis: a meta-analysis of randomised controlled trials. *Ann Rheum Dis* 2009; 68(12):1843–9.

Ghahreman A, Ferch R, Bogduk N. The efficacy of transforaminal injection of steroids for the treatment of lumbar radicular pain. *Pain Med* 2010; 11(8):1149–68.

Gialanella B, Prometti P Effects of corticosteroids injection in rotator cuff tears. *Pain Med* 2011; 12(10):1559–65.

Gills S, Gelbke MK, Matson SL, et al. Fluoroscopically guided low-volume peritendinous corticosteroid injection for Achilles tendinopathy; a safety study. *J Bone Joint Sur Am* 2004; 86:802–6.

Gosal HS, Jackson AM, Bickerstaff DR. Intra-articular steroids after arthroscopy for osteoarthritis of the knee. *J Bone Joint Surg Br* 1999; 81:952–4.

Gossec L, Dougados M. Intra-articular treatments in osteoarthritis: from the symptomatic to the structure modifying. *Ann Rheum Dis* 2004; 63: 478–82.

Gotoh M, Hamada K, Yamakawa H, et al. Increased substance P in subacromial bursa and shoulder pain in rotator cuff disease. *J Orthop Res* 1998; 16:618–21.

Grados F, Depriester C, Cayrolle G, Hardy N, Deramond H, Fardellone P. Long-term observations of vertebral osteoporotic fractures treated by percutaneous vertebroplasty. Rheumatology 2000; 39(12):1410–4.

Grassi W, Farina A, Filippucci E, Cervini C. Intralesional therapy in carpal tunnel syndrome: a sonographic-guided approach. *Clin Exp Rheumatol* 2002; 20 (1):73–6.

Gray RG, Gottlieb NL. Basic science and pathology: intra-articular corticosteroids, an updated assessment. *Clin Orthop Relat Res* 1982; 177:235–63.

Gray RG, Tenenbaum J, Gottlieb NL. Local corticosteroid injection treatment in rheumatic disorders. *Semin Arthritis Rheum* 1981; 10:231–54.

Grayson M. Three infected injections from the same organism. *Br J Rheumatol* 1998; 37:592–3.

Grohs JG, Matzner M, Trieb K, Krepler P Minimal invasive stabilization of osteoporotic vertebral fractures: a prospective nonrandomized comparison of vertebroplasty and bal- loon kyphoplasty. *J Spinal Disord Tech* 2005; 18:238–42.

Gruber H, Glodny B, Bodner G, et al. Practical experience with sonographically guided phenol instillation of stump neuroma: predictors of effects, success and outcome. *Am J Roentgenol* 2008; 190:1263–9.

Guido R, Grazia Canepa M, Bortolotto C, Draghi F. Interventional musculoskeletal US: an update on materials and methods. *J Ultrasound* 2013; 16:45–55.

Habib GS, Saliba W, Nashashibi M. Local effects of intra-articular corticosteroids. *Clin Rheumatol* 2010; 29(4):347–56.

Hall S, Buchbinder R. Do imaging methods that guide needle placement improve outcome? *Ann Rheum Dis* 2004; 63:1007–8.

Hansen H. Is fluoroscopy necessary for sacroiliac injections? *Pain Physician* 2003; 6:155–8.

Hartung W, Ross CJ, Straub R, et al. Ultrasound-guided sacroiliac joint injection in patients with established sacroiliitis: precise IA injection verified by MRI scanning does not predict clinical outcome. *Rheumatology* 2010; 49(8):1479–82.

Hasserius R, Ohlin A, Karlsson M. Vertebroplasty and kyphoplasty—evidence-based methods? *Acta Orthopaedica* 2010; 81(5):521–3.

Hauser RA, Blakemore PJ, Wang J, Stellien D. Structural basis of joint instability as cause for chronic musculoskeletal pain and its successful treatment with regenerative injection therapy (prolotherapy). *Open Pain J* 2014; 7:9–22.

Hegedus EJ, Zavala J, Kissenberth M, et al. Positive outcomes with intra-articular glenohumeral injections are independent of accuracy. *J Shoulder Elbow Surg* 2010; 19(6):795–801.

Heini PF. Vertebroplasty: an update: value of percutaneous cement augmentation after randomized, placebo-controlled trials. *Orthopade*, 2010; 39:658–64 (article in german).

Heini PF, Wälchli B, Berlemann U. Percutaneous transpedicular vertebroplasty with PMMA: operative technique and early results. A prospective study for the treatment of osteoporotic compression fractures. *Eur Spine J* 2000; 9:445–50.

Helliwell PS. Use of an objective measure of articular stiffness to record changes in finger joints after intra-articular injection of corticosteroid. *Ann Rheum Dis* 1997; 56:71–3.

Helm AT, Higgins G, Rajkumar P, Redfern DR. Accuracy of intra-articular injections for osteoarthritis of the trapeziometacarpal joint. *Int J Clin Pract* 2003; 57(4):265–6.

Heyworth BE, Lee JH, Kim PD, et al. Hylan versus corticosteroid versus placebo for treatment of basal joint arthritis: a prospective, randomized, double-blinded clinical trial. *J Hand Surg (Am)* 2008; 33(1):40–8.

Hills BA, Ethell MT, Hodgson DR. Release of lubricating synovial surfactant by intra-articular steroid. *Br J Rheumatol* 1998; 37(6):649–52.

Hiwatashi A, Westesson PL, Yoshiura T, et al. Kyphoplasty and vertebroplasty produce the same degree of height restoration. *Am J Neuroradiol* 2009; 30:669–73.

Hoksrud A, Ohberg L, Alfredson H, et al. Ultrasound-guided sclerosis of neovessels in painful chronic patellar tendinopathy: a randomized controlled trial. *Am J Sports Med* 2006; 34:1738–46.

Hollander JL, Jessar RA, Brown EM Jr. Intra-synovial corticosteroid therapy: a decade of use. *Bull Rheum Dis* 1961; 11:239–40.

Horlocker T, Zahid H, Bajwa ZH, et al. Risk assessment of hemorrhagic complications associated with non-steroidal anti-inflammatory medications in ambulatory pain clinic patients undergoing epidural steroid injection. *Anesth Analg* 2002; 95:1691–7.

Hugate R, Pennypacker J, Saunders M, et al. The effects of intratendinous and retrocalcaneal intrabursal injections of corticosteroid on the biomechanical properties of rabbit Achilles tendons. *J Bone Joint Surg Am* 2004; 86:794–801.

Hughes RA. Septicarthritis. *Rep Rheum Dis(Series3). Practical Problems (No. 7)* 1996.

Ilum Boesen M, Torp-Pederson S, Juhl Koenig M, et al. Ultrasound guided electrocoagulation in patients with chronic non-insertional Achilles tendinopathy: a pilot study. *Br J Sports Med* 2006; 40:761–6.

Im SH, Lee SC, Park YB, Cho SR, Kim JC. Feasibility of sonography for intra-articular injections in the knee through a medial patellar portal. *J Ultrasound Med* 2009; 28(11):1465–70.

Ines LPBS, daSilva JAP. Soft tissue injections. *Best Pract Res Clin Rheumatol* 2005; 19(3):503–27.

Jackson DW, Evans NA, Thomas BM. Accuracy of needle placement into the intra-articular space of the knee. *J Bone Joint Surg Am* 2002; 84:1522–7.

Jackson DW, Rettig AC, Wiltse LL. Epidural cortisone injections in the young athletic adult. *Am J Sports Med* 1980; 8(4):239–43.

Jacobs LGH, Barton MAJ, Wallace WA, Ferrousis J, Dunn NA, Bossingham DH. Intraarticular distension and steroids in the management of capsulitis of the shoulder. *BMJ* 1991; 302:1498–501.

James SLJ, Ali K, Pocock C, et al. Ultrasound guided dry needling and autologous blood injection for patellar tendinosis. *Br J Sports Med* 2007; 41:518–22.

Jawed S, Allard SA. Osteomyelitis of the humerus following steroid injections for tennis elbow. (Letter) *Rheumatology* 2000; 39:923–4.

Jensen KT, Rabago D, Best TM, et al. Early inflammatory response of knee ligaments to prolotherapy in a rat model. *J Orthop Res* 2008; 26(6):816–23.

Johansson A, Hao J, Sjölund B. Local corticosteroid application blocks transmission in normal nociceptive C-fibres. *Acta Anaesthesiol Scand* 1990; 34(5):335–8.

Jones A, Doherty M. Intra-articular corticosteroid injections are effective in OA but there are no clinical predictors of response. *Ann Rheum Dis* 1996; 55:829–32.

JonesA, Regan M, Ledingham L, Pattrick M,Manhire A, Doherty M. Importance of placement of intra-articular steroid injections. *BMJ* 1993:1329–30.

Jubb RW. Anti-rheumatic drugs and articular cartilage. *Rep Rheum Dis (Series 2). Topical Reviews (No. 20)* 1992.

Kahn AN, Macdonald S. Involutional osteoporosis imaging. *Medscape* 2004 (updated 2013). Available at: <http: //www.emedicine.com/RADIO/topic503.htm>.

Kallmes DF, Comstock BA, Heagerty PJ, et al. A randomized trial of vertebroplasty for osteoporotic spinal fractures. *N Engl J Med* 2009; 361:569–79.

Kane D, Greaney T, Shnahan M, et al. The role of ultrasonography in the diagnosis and management of idiopathic plantar fasciitis. *Rheumatology* 2001; 40:1002–8.

Kang MN, Rizio L, Prybicien M, Middlemas DA, Blacksin MF. The accuracy of subacromial corticosteroid injections: a comparison of multiple methods. *J Shoulder Elbow Surg* 2008; 17(Suppl 1):61S–66S.

Karlsson M, Ohlin A, Hasserius R. Could vertebroplasty and kyphoplasty be regarded as evidence-based treatment of osteoporotic vertebral fractures? *Acta Radiologica*, 2010; 51(8):828–31.

Kendall PH. Local corticosteroid injection therapy. III. *Ann Phys Med* 1963; 7:31–8.

Khan KM, Cook JL, Maffulli N, et al. Where is the pain coming from in tendinopathy? It may be biochemical, not structural in origin. *Br J Sports Med* 2000; 34(2):81–3.

Khan SA, Varshney MK, Trikha V, et al. Dextrose prolotherapy for recalcitrant coccydynia. *J Orthopaed Surg* 2008; 16:27–9.

Khosla S, Thiele R, Baumhauer FJ. Ultrasound guidance for intra-articular injections of the foot and ankle. *Foot Ankle Int* 2009; 30:886–90.

Khoury NJ, el-Khoury GY, Saltzman CL, Brandser EA. Intraarticular foot and ankle injections to identify source of pain before arthrodesis. *Am J Roentgenol* 1996; 167:669–73.

Kim D, Yun Y, Wang J. Nerve-root injections for the relief of pain in patients with osteoporotic vertebral fractures. *J Bone Joint Surg Br* 2003; 85(2):250–4.

Kingma JJ, de Knikker R, Wittink HM, et al. Eccentric overload training in patients with chronic Achilles tendinopathy: a systematic review. *Br J Sports Med* 2007; 41–3.

Kirwan JR, Rankin E. Intraarticular therapy in osteoarthritis. *Baillière's Clin Rheumatol* 1997; 11:769–94.

Klazen CA, Lohle PN, de Vries J, et al. Vertebroplasty versus conservative treatment in acute osteoporotic vertebral compression fractures (VERTOS II): an open-label randomised trial. *Lancet* 2010; 376:1085–92.

Klazen CAH, Venmans A, De Vries J, et al. Percutaneous vertebroplasty is not a risk factor for new osteoporotic compression fractures: results from VERTOS II. Am J Neuroradiol 2010; 31(8):1447–50.

Koes BW. Corticosteroid injection for rotator cuff disease. *BMJ* 2009; 338:a2599.

Koes B, Scholten R, Mens J, et al. Efficacy of epidural steroid injections for low back pain and sciatica: a systematic review of randomised clinical trials. *Pain* 1995; 63:279–88.

Kon E, Buda R, Filardo G, et al. Platelet-rich plasma: intra-articular knee injections produced favorable results on degenerative cartilage lesions. *Knee Surg Sports Traumatol Arthrosc* 2010; 18(4):472–9.

Konai MS, Vilar Furtado RN, Dos Santos MF, et al. Monoarticular corticosteroid injection versus systemic administration in the treatment of rheumatoid arthritis patients: a randomized double-blind controlled study. *Clin Exp Rheumatol* 2009; 27:214–21.

Koski JM, Hermunen HS, Kilponen VM, et al. Verification of palpation-guided intra-articular injections using glucocorticoid-air-saline mixture and ultrasound imaging (GAS-graphy). *Clin Exp Rheumatol* 2006; 24(3):247–52.

Kumar K, Nguyen R, Bishop S. A comparative analysis of the results of vertebroplasty and kyphoplasty in osteoporotic vertebral compression fractures. Neurosurgery 2010; 67:s171–s188.

Kumar N, Newman R. Complications of intra- and peri-articular steroid injections. *Br J Gen Pract* 1999; 49:465–6.

Kurup H, Ward P. Do we need radiological guidance for hip joint injections? *Acta Orthop Belg* 2010; 76(2):205–7.

Larson E. Guideline for use of topical antimicrobial agents.. *Am J Infect Control* 1988; 16:253–66.

Larsson E, Harris HE, Larsson A. Corticosteroid treatment of experimental arthritis retards cartilage destruction as determined by histology and serum COMP. *Rheumatology* 2004; 43(4):428–34.

Lavelle W, Lavelle ED, Lavelle L. Intra-articular injection. *Med Clin North Am* 2007; 91(2):241–50.

Lazarevic MB, Skosey JL, Djordjevic-Denic G. Reduction of cortisol levels after single intra-articular and intramuscular steroid injection. *Am J Med* 1995; 99(4):370–3.

Le Corroller T, Cohen M, Aswad R, Pauly V, Champsaur P. Sonography of the painful shoulder: role of the operator's experience. *Skeletal Radiol* 2008; 37 (11):979–86.

Lee BJ, Lee SR, Yoo TY. Paraplegia as a complication of percutaneous vertebroplasty with polymethylmethacrylate: a case report. *Spine* 2002; 27(19):E419–22.

Lieberman IH, Dudeney SM, Reinhardt K, et al. Initial outcome and efficacy of 'kyphoplasty' in the treatment of painful osteoporotic vertebral compression fractures. *Spine* 2001; 26:1631–8.

Lin EP, Ekholm S, Hiwatashi A, Westesson PL. Vertebroplasty: cement leakage into the disc increases the risk of new fracture of adjacent vertebral body. Am J Neuroradiol 2004; 25(2):175–80.

Lips P, Cooper C, Agnusdei D, et al. Quality of life in patients with vertebral fractures: validation of the Quality of Life Questionnaire of the European Foundation for Osteoporosis (QUALEFFO). Working Party for Quality of Life of the European Foundation for Osteoporosis. *Osteoporos Int* 1999; 10:150–60.

Liu JT, Liao WJ, Tan WC, et al. Balloon kyphoplasty versus vertebroplasty for treatment of osteoporotic vertebral compression fracture: a prospective, comparative, and randomized clinical study. *Osteoporos Int* 2010; 21:359–64.

Lohman M, Vasenius J, Nieminen O. Ultrasound guidance for puncture and injection in the radiocarpal joint. *Acta Radiol* 2007; 48 (7):744–7.

Louis LJ. Musculoskeletal ultrasound intervention: principles and advances. *Radiol Clin North Am* 2008; 46:515–33.

Lovi A, Teli M, Ortolina A, Costa F, Fornari M, Brayda-Bruno M. Vertebroplasty and kyphoplasty: complementary techniques for the treatment of painful osteoporotic vertebral com- pression fractures. A prospective non-randomised study on 154 patients. *Eur Spine J* 2009; 18(Suppl 1):95–101.

Lu W, Li YH, He XF. Treatment of large lumbar disc herniation with percutaneous ozone injection via the posterior-lateral route and inner margin of the facet joint. *World J Radiol* 2010; 2(3):109–12.

Luc M, Pham T, Chagnaud C, Lafforgue P, Legre V. Placement of intra-articular injection verified by the backflow technique. *Osteoarth Cart* 2006; 14:714–6.

Lucas PE, Hurwitz SR, Kaplan PA, Dussault RG, Maurer EJ. Fluoroscopically guided injections into the foot and ankle: localization of the source of pain as a guide to treatment—prospective study. *Radiology* 1997; 204:411–5.

MacMahon PJ, Eustace SJ, Kavanagh EC. Injectable corticosteroid and local anaesthetic preparations: a review for radiologists. *Radiology* 2009; 252(3):647–61.

Magnan B, Marangon A, Frigo A, et al. Local phenol injection in the treatment of interdigital neuritis of the foot (Morton's neuroma). *Chir Organi Mov* 2005; 90:371–7.

Mahler F, Fritsch YD. Partial and complete ruptures of the Achilles tendon and local corticosteroid injections. *Br J Sports Med* 1992; 26:7–14.

Mair SD, Isbell WM, Gill TJ, et al. Triceps tendon ruptures in professional football players. *Am J Sports Med* 2004; 32:431–4.

Manchikanti L, Cash KA, McManus CD, et al. Preliminary results of randomized double-blind controlled trial of fluoroscopic lumbar interlaminar epidural injections in managing chronic lumbar discogenic pain without disc herniation or radiculitis. *Pain Physician* 2010; 13(4):E279–E292.

Manchikanti M, Singh V, Falco FJE, et al. Evaluation of effectiveness of lumbar interlaminar epidural injections in managing chronic pain of lumbar disc herniation of radiculitis: a randomized double-blind controlled trial. *Pain Physician* 2010; 13:343–55.

Mangram AJ, Horan TC, Pearson ML, Silver LC, Jarvis WR. Guideline for prevention of surgical site infection, 1999. Hospital Infection Control Practices Advisory Committee. *Infect Control Hosp Epidemiol* 1999; 20:250–78.

Mathis JM. Percutaneous vertebroplasty: complication avoidance and technique optimization, *Am J Neuroradiol* 2003; 24(8):1697–706.

Maugars Y, et al. Assessment of the efficacy of sacroiliac corticosteroid injections in spondylarthropathies: a double-blind study. *Br J Rheumatol* 1996; 35:767–70.

Maxwell NJ, Ryan MB, Taunton JE, et al. Sonographically guided intratendinous injection of hyperosmolar dextrose to treat chronic tendinosis of the Achilles tendon: a pilot study. *Am J Roentgenol* 2007; 189:W215–W220.

McGrath J, Schaefer M, Malkamaki D. Incidence and characteristics of complications from epidural steroid injections. *Pain Med* 2011; 12:726–31.

McQuay HJ, Moore RA. Epidural steroids for sciatica. (Letter). *Anaesth Intensive Care* 1996; 24:284–5.

McWhorter JW, Francis RS, Heckmann RA. Influence of local steroid injections on traumatized tendon properties; a biomechanical and histological study. *Am J Sports Med* 1991; 19(5):435–9.

Mens JMA, De Wolf AN, Berkhout BJ, et al. Disturbance of the menstrual pattern after local injection with triamcinolone acetonide. *Ann Rheum Dis* 1998; 57:700.

Micu MC, Bogdan GD, Fodor D. Steroid injection for hip osteoarthritis: efficacy under ultrasound guidance. *Rheumatology* 2010; 49 (8):1490–4.

Miller FG, Kallmes DF. The case of vertebroplasty trials: promoting a culture of evidence-based procedural medicine. *Spine* 2010; 35(23):2023–6.

Mishra A, Pavelko T. Treatment of chronic elbow tendinosis with buffered platelet-rich plasma. *Am J Sports Med* 2006; 34:1774–8.

Mitchell MJ, Bielecki D, Bergman AG, Kursunoglu-Brahme S, Sartoris DJ, Resnick D. Localization of specific joint causing hindfoot pain: value of injecting local anesthetics into individual joints during arthrography. *Am J Roentgenol* 1995; 164:1473–6.

Mottram DR. (ed.) *Drugs in sport* (2nd edn). London: E & FN Spon; 1996.

Movrin I, Vengust R, Komadina R Adjacent vertebral fractures after percutaneous vertebral augmentation of osteoporotic vertebral compression fracture: a comparison of balloon kyphoplasty and vertebroplasty. *Arch Orthop Trauma Surg* 2010; 130:1157–66.

Mudano AS, Bian J, Cope JU, et al. Vertebroplasty and kyphoplasty are associated with an increased risk of secondary vertebral compression fractures: a population-based cohort study. Osteopor Intern 2009; 20(5):819–26.

Munk PL, Liu DM, Murphy KP, Baerlocher MO. Effectiveness of vertebroplasty: a recent controversy. Can Assoc Radiol J 2009; 60(4):170–1.

Ng LC, Sell P. Outcomes of a prospective cohort study on peri-radicular infiltration for radicular pain in patients with lumbar disc herniation and spinal stenosis. *Eur Spine J* 2004; 13(4):325–9.

NICE/ National Collaborating Centre for Chronic Conditions. *Osteoarthritis: national clinical guideline for care and management in adults (NICE guideline)*. London: Royal College of Physicians; 2008.

NICE/National Collaborating Centre for Primary Care. *Low back pain: early management of persistent non-specific low back pain (NICE guideline CG88)*. NICE; 2009.

Nichols AW. Complications associated with the use of corticosteroids in the treatment of athletic injuries. *Clin J Sport Med* 2005; 15(5):370–5.

Nyska M, Kish B, Shabat S, et al. The treatment of osteoarthritis of the ankle by intra-articular sodium hyaluronate injection. *J Bone Joint Surg Br* 2003; 85:246.

O'Brien JP, Sims JT, Evans AJ. Vertebroplasty in patients with severe vertebral compression fractures: a technical report. Am J Neurorad 2000; 21(8):1555–8.

Ohberg L, Alfredson H. Ultrasound guided sclerosis of neovessels in painful chronic Achilles tendinosis: pilot study of a new treatment. *Br J Sports Med* 2002; 36:173–7.

Padovani O, Kasriel P, Brunner, Peretti-Viton P. Pulmonary embolism caused by acrylic cement: a rare complication of percutaneous vertebroplasty. *Am J Neuroradiol* 1999; 20(3):375–7.

Pal B, Morris J. Perceived risks of joint infection following intra-articular corticosteroid injections: a survey of rheumatologists. *Clin Rheumato.* 1999; 18(3):264–5.

Pateder DB, Khanna AJ, Lieberman IH. Vertebroplasty and kyphoplasty for the management of osteoporotic vertebral compression fractures. *Orthop Clin North Am* 2007; 38(3):409–18.

Peh WC, Gilula LA. Percutaneous vertebroplasty: an update. *Semin Ultrasound CT MR.* 2005; 26:52–64.

Pelletier JP, Pelletier JM. Proteoglycan degrading metalloprotease activity in human osteoarthritis cartilage and the effect of intraarticular steroid injections. *Arthritis Rheum* 1987; 30(5):541–9.

Pelletier JP, Mineau F, Raynauld JP, et al. Intraarticular injections with methylprednisolone acetate reduce osteoarthritic lesions in parallel with chondrocyte stromelysin synthesis in experimental osteoarthritis. *Arthritis Rheum* 1994; 37:414–23.

Phillips FM. Minimally invasive treatments of osteoporotic fractures. *Spine* 2003; 28:S45–S53.

Piper SL1, Kim HT. Comparison of ropivacaine and bupivacaine toxicity in human articular chondrocytes. *J Bone Joint Surg Am* 2008; 90(5):986–91.

Pollard MA, Cermak MB, Buck WR, Williams DP. Accuracy of injection into the basal joint of the thumb. *Am J Orthop* 2007; 36:204–6.

Price CM, Roger PD, Prosser ASJ, et al. Comparison of the caudal and lumbar approaches to the epidural space. *Ann Rheum Dis* 2000; 59(11):879–82.

Pullar T. Routes of drug administration: intra-articular route. *Prescribers' J* 1998; 38(2):123–6.

Rabago D, Slattengren A, Zgierska A. Prolotherapy in primary care practice. *Prim Care* 2010; 37(1):65–80.

Rahimi-Movaghar V, Eslami V. The major efficient mechanisms of ozone therapy are obtained in intradiscal procedures. *Pain Physician* 2012; 15(6):E1007–8.

Raynauld JP. Clinical trials: impact of intra-articular steroid injections on the progression of knee osteoarthritis. *Osteoarth Cart* 1999; 7:348–9.

Raynauld J, Buckland-Wright C, Ward R, et al. Safety and efficacy of long term intraarticular steroid injections in osteoarthritis of the knee. *Arthritis Rheum* 2003; 48:370–4.

Raza K, Lee CY, Pilling D, et al. Ultrasound guidance allows accurate needle placement and aspiration from small joints in patients with early inflammatory arthritis. *Rheumatology* 2003; 42:976–9.

Reach JS, Easley ME, Chuckpaiwong B, Nunley JA II. Accuracy of ultrasound guided injections in the foot and ankle. *Foot Ankle Int* 2009; 30 (3):239–42.

Read MTF. Safe relief of rest pain that eases with activity in achillodynia by intrabursal or peritendinous steroid injection: the rupture rate was not increased by these steroid injections. *Br J Sports Med* 1999; 33:134–5.

Reddy PD, Zelicof SB, Ruotolo C, et al. Interdigital neuroma. Local cutaneous changes after corticosteroid injection. *Clin Orthop Relat Res* 1995; 317:185–7.

Reeves KD, Hassanein K. Randomized, prospective, placebo-controlled double-blind study of dextrose prolotherapy for osteoarthritic thumb and finger (DIP, PIP, and trapeziometacarpal) joints: evidence of clinical efficacy. *J Altern Complement Med* 2000; 6(4):311–20.

Reeves KD, Hassanein KM. Long term effects of dextrose prolotherapy for anterior cruciate ligament laxity. *Altern Ther Health Med* 2003; 9:358.

Riew KD, Yin Y, Gilula L, et al. The effect of nerve root injections on the need for operative treatment of lumbar radicular pain. A prospective, randomised, controlled, double blind study. *J Bone Joint Surg Am* 2000; 82:1589–93.

Rifat SF, Moeller JL. Injection and aspiration techniques for the primary care physician. *Compr Ther* 2002; 28(4):222–9.

Riggs BL, Melton LJ. The worldwide problem of osteoporosis: insights afforded by epidemiology. *Bone* 1995; 17(5):505S–511S

Robago D, Best TM, Zgierska AE, et al. A systematic review of four injection therapies for lateral epicondylosis: prolotherapy, polidocanol, whole blood and platelet-rich plasma. *Br J Sports Med* 2009; 43:471–81.

Rollinghoff M, Siewe J, Zarghooni K, et al. Effectiveness, security and height restoration on fresh compression fractures—a comparative prospective study of vertebroplasty and kyphoplasty. *Minim Invasive Neurosurg* 2009; 52:233–7.

Rousing R, Andersen MO, Jespersen SM, Thomsen K, Lauritsen J. Percutaneous vertebroplasty compared to conservative treatment in patients with painful acute or subacute osteoporotic vertebral fractures: three months' follow-up in a clinical randomized study. *Spine* (Phila Pa 1976) 2009; 34:1349–54.

Rubens DJ, Fultz PJ, Gottlieb RH, Rubin SJ. Effective ultrasonographically guided intervention for diagnosis of musculo-skeletal lesions. *J Ultrasound Med* 1997; 16:831–42.

Rutten MJ, Maresch BJ, Jager GJ, de Waal Malefijt MC. Injection of the subacromial-subdeltoid bursa: blind or ultrasound-guided? *Acta Orthop* 2007; 78(2):254–7.

Ryan MB, Wong AD, Gillies JH, et al. Sonographically guided intratendinous injections of hyperosmolar dextrose/lidocaine: a pilot study for the treatment of chronic plantar fasciitis. *Br J Sports Med* 2009; 43(4):303–6.

Ryan MJ, Kavanagh R, Wall PG, et al. Bacterial joint infections in England and Wales: analysis of bacterial isolates over a four year period. *Br J Rheumatol* 1997; 36:370–3.

Saifuddin A, Abdus-Samee M, Mann C, Singh D, Angle JC. CT guided diagnostic foot injections. *Clin Radiol* 2005; 60:191–5.

Samanta A, Beardsley J. Sciatica: which intervention? *BMJ* 1999; 319:302–3.

Samanta A, Samanta J. Is epidural injection of steroids effective for low back pain? *BMJ* 2004; 328:1509–10.

Samson S, Gerhadt M, Mandelbaum B. Platelet rich plasma injection grafts for musculoskeletal injuries: a review. *Curr Rev Musculoskelet Med* 2008; 1:165–74.

Santiago FR, Abela AP, Alvarez LG, Osuna RM, Garcia MM. Pain and functional outcome after vertebroplasty and kyphoplasty. A comparative study. *Eur J Radiol* 2010; 75:e108–e113

Saxena A, Fullem B. Plantar fascia ruptures in athletes. *Am J Sports Med* 2004; 32:662–5.

Schofer MD, Efe T, Timmesfeld N, Kortmann HR, Quante M. Comparison of kyphoplasty and vertebroplasty in the treatment of fresh vertebral compression fractures. *Arch Orthop Trauma Surg* 2009; 129:1391–9.

Schumacher HR, Meador R, Sieck M, et al. Pilot investigation of hyaluronate injections for first metacarpal-carpal (MC-C) osteoarthritis. *J Clin Rheumatol* 2004; 10(2):59–62.

Serafini G, Sconfienza LM, Lacelli F, et al. Rotator cuff calcific tendonitis: short-term and 10-year outcomes after two-needle US-guided percutaneous treatment-nonrandomized controlled trial. *Radiology* 2009; 252:157–64.

Seror P, Pluvinage P, Lecoq F, et al. Frequency of sepsis after local corticosteroid injection (an inquiry on 1,160,000 injections in rheumatological private practice in France). *Rheumatology* 1999; 38:1272–4.

Sethi PM, Kingston S, Elattrache N. Accuracy of anterior intra-articular injection of the glenohumeral joint. *Arthroscopy* 2005; 21(1):77–80.

Shanahan EM, Smith MD, Wetherall M, et al. Suprascapular nerve block in chronic shoulder pain: are the radiologists better? *Ann Rheum Dis* 2004; 63:1035–40.

Shrier I, Gordon O. Achilles tendon: are corticosteroid injections useful or harmful? *Clin J Sport Med* 1996; 6:245–50.

Sibbitt WL Jr, Peisajovich A, Michael AA, et al. Does sonographic needle guidance affect the clinical outcome of intraarticular injections? *J Rheumatol* 2009; 36(9):1892–902.

Slosar P, White AH. Controversy—the use of selective nerve root blocks: diagnostic, therapeutic or placebo? *Spine* 1998; 20:2253–6.

Smith AG, Kosygan K, Williams H, et al. Common extensor tendon rupture following corticosteroid injection for lateral tendinosis of the elbow. *Br J Sports Med* 1999; 33:423–5.

Smith K, Hurdle MB, Weingarten TN. Accuracy of sonographically guided intra-articular injections in the native adult hip. *J Ultrasound Med* 2009; 28:329–35.

Snarr J. Risks, benefits and complications of epidural steroid injections: case report. *Am Assoc Nurse Anesth J* 2007; 75(3):183–8.

Sölveborn S-A, Buck F, Mallmin H, et al. Cortisone injection with anaesthetic additives for radial epicondylalgia. *Clin Orthop Relat Res* 1995; 316:99–105.

Staal JB, de Bie R, de Vet HCW, et al. Injection therapy for subacute and chronic low-back pain. *Cochrane Database Syst Rev* 2008; (3). Art. No. CD001824.

Stewart WF, Ricci JA, Chee E, Morganstein D, Lipton R. Lost productive time and cost due to common pain conditions in the US workforce. *JAMA* 2003a; 12; 290(18):2443–54.

Stewart WF, Ricci JA, Chee E, Morganstein D. Lost productive work time costs from health conditions in the United States: results from the American Productivity Audit. *J Occup Environ Med* 2003b; 45(12):1234–46.

Stitz MY, Sommer HM. Accuracy of blind versus fluoroscopically guided caudal epidural injection. *Spine* 1999; 24(13):1371.

Suresh SP, Ali KE, Jones H, Connell DA. Medial epicondylitis: is ultrasound guided autologous blood injection an effective treatment? *Br J Sports Med* 2006; 40(11):935–9.

Syed MI, Shaikh A. Vertebroplasty: a systematic approach. *Pain Physician* 2007; 10(2):367–80.

Tagliafico A, Serafini G, Sconfienza LM, et al. Ultrasound-guided viscosupplementation of subacromial space in elderly patients with cuff tear arthropathy using a high weight hyaluronic acid: prospective open-label non- randomized trial. *Eur Radiol* 2011; 21(1):182–7.

Tallia AF, Cardone DA. Diagnostic and therapeutic injection of the shoulder region. *Am Fam Physician* 2003; 67(6):1271–8.

Tallia AF, Cardone DA. Diagnostic and therapeutic injection of the ankle and foot. *Am Fam Physician* 2003; 68(7):1356–62.

Taras JS, Raphael JS, Pan WT, et al. Corticosteroid injections for trigger digits: is intrasheath injection necessary? *J Hand Surg (Am)* 1998; 23:717–22.

Terslev L, Torp-Pedersen S, Qvistgaard E, et al. Estimation of inflammation by Doppler ultrasound: quantitative changes after intra-articular treatment in rheumatoid arthritis. *Ann Rheum Dis* 2003; 62:1049–53.

Toda Y, Tsukimura N. A comparison of intra-articular hyaluronan injection accuracy rates between three approaches based on radiographic severity of knee osteoarthritis. *Osteoarth Cart* 2008; 16 (9):980–5.

Topol GA, Reeves KD, Hassanein KM. Efficacy of dextrose prolotherapy in elite male kicking-sport athletes with chronic groin pain. *Arch Phys Med Rehabil* 2005; 86(4):697–702.

van Tulder M, Koes B. *Low back pain and sciatica (acute and chronic). Clinical evidence concise no. 11.* London: BMJ Books; 2004: 286–91.

van Tuyl SAC, Slee PH. Are the effects of local glucocorticoid treatment only local? *Neth J Med* 2002; 60:130–2.

Uthman I, Raynauld JP, Haraoui B. Intra-articular therapy in osteoarthritis. *Postgrad Med J* 2003; 79:449–54.

Valat J-P, Giraudeau B, Rozenburg S, et al. Epidural corticosteroid injections for sciatica: a randomised, double blind, controlled clinical trial. *Ann Rheum Dis* 2003; 62:639–43.

Verbruggen G. Chondroprotective drugs in degenerative joint diseases. *Rheumatology* 2006; 45(2):129–38.

de Vos RJ, van Veldhoven PLJ, Moen MH, et al. Autologous growth factor injections in chronic tendinopathy: a systematic review. *Br Med Bull* 2010b; 95:63–77.

de Vos RJ, Weir A, van Schie HT, et al. Platelet-rich plasma injection for chronic Achilles tendinopathy: a randomized controlled trial. *JAMA* 13 2010a; 303(2):144–9.

Watts RW, Silagy CA. A meta-analysis on the efficacy of epidural corticosteroids in the treatment of sciatica. *Anaesth Intensive Care* 1995; 23: 564–9.

Wei AS, Callaci JJ, Juknelis D, et al. The effect of corticosteroid on collagen expression in injured rotator cuff tendon. *J Bone Joint Surg Am* 2006; 88(6):1331–8.

Weitoft T, Larsson A, Ronnblom L. Serum levels of sex steroid hormones and matrix metalloproteinases after intra-articular glucocorticoid treatment in female patients with rheumatoid arthritis. *Ann Rheum Dis* 2008; 67:422–4.

Weitoft T, Larsson A, Saxne T. et al. Changes of cartilage and bone markers after intra-articular glucocorticoid treatment with and without post-injection rest in patients with rheumatoid arthritis. *Ann Rheum Dis* 2005; 64:1750–3.

Wiewiorski M, Valderrabano V, Kretzschmar M, et al. CT-guided robotically-assisted infiltration of foot and ankle joints. *Minim Invasive Ther Allied Technol* 2009; 18:291–6.

Wildsmith JA. Routes of drug administration: 6. Intrathecal and epidural injection. *Prescribers J* 1996; 36(2):110–5.

Xing D, Ma JX, Ma XL, et al. A meta-analysis of balloon kyphoplasty compared to percutaneous vertebroplasty for treating osteoporotic vertebral compression fractures. *J Clin Neurosci* 2013; 20(6):795–803.

Yamakado K. The targeting accuracy of subacromial injection to the shoulder: an arthrographic evaluation. *Arthroscopy* 2002; 18(8):887–91.

Yan D, Duan L, Li J, Soo C, Zhu H, Zhang Z. Comparative study of percutaneous vertebroplasty and kyphoplasty in the treatment of osteoporotic vertebral compression fractures. *Arch Orthop Trauma Surg* 2011; 131:645–50.

Yangco BG, Germain BF, Deresinski SC. Case report: fatal gas gangrene following intra-articular steroid injection. *Am J Med Sci* 1982; 283:294–8.

Zanetti M, Metzdorf A, Kundert HP, et al. Achilles tendon: clinical relevance of neovascularization diagnosed with power Doppler US. *Radiology* 2003; 227:556–60.

Zeisig E, Fahlstrom M, Ohberg L, et al. Pain relief after intratendinous injections in patients with tennis elbow: results of a randomized study. *Br J Sports Med* 2008; 42:267–71.

Zhang Y, Ma Y, Jiang J, Ding T, Wang J. Treatment of the lumbar disc herniation with intradiscal and intraforaminal injection of oxygen-ozone. *J Back Musculoskelet Rehabil* 2013; 26(3):317–22.

Zhou JL, Liu SQ, Ming JH, Peng H, Qiu B. Comparison of therapeutic effect between percutaneous vertebroplasty and kyphoplasty on vertebral compression fracture. *Chin J Traumatol* 2008; 11:42–4

Zingas C, Failla JM, van Holsbeeck M. Injection accuracy and clinical relief of the Quervain's tendonitis. *J Hand Surg (Am)* 1998; 23:89–96.

Ziv YB, Kardosh R, Debi R, Backstein D, Safir O. Kosashvili Y. An inexpensive and accurate method for hip injections without the use of imaging. *J Clin Rheumatol* 2009; 15(3):103–5.

Zoaeski GH, Snow P, Olan WJ, et al. Percutaneous vertebroplasty for osteoporotic compression fractures: quantitative prospective evaluation of long-term putcomes. *J Vasc Intervent Radiol* 2002; 13:139–48.

Chapter 26

Endoscopically determined pain sources in the lumbar spine

Martin T.N. Knight

Introduction to endoscopically determined pain sources in the lumbar spine

Aware-state spinal endoscopy has allowed us to develop a patient-sensitive system for precisely identifying the sources of a patient's pain and concepts that often confound conventional precepts of the generation of back, neck, and referred pain. Transforaminal endoscopy allows us to examine and palpate the exiting nerve and foraminal and epidural contents under direct vision, at several levels, and match these findings to the patient's predominant presenting symptoms (PPS).

Patient feedback has taught us that the disc, epidural, foraminal, and extraforaminal structures, once irritated or inflamed, provide axial and referred pain. The mechanisms of pain production centre upon repetitive traction, impaction, or distortion of the tethered nerve more often than of the disc. These discrete pain sources are associated with persistent and disabling pain. The resolution of symptoms by their specific treatment or ablation confirms the significance of such sources. These hitherto under-appreciated sources of pain in the foramen can be treated by reduction of the irritation by postural stabilization, adjunctive anti-inflammatory injections, or endoscopic undercutting of the foramen, removal of scarring and ligaments and mobilization of the nerve without the need for open surgery.

Appreciation of the role of the 'new' foraminal pain sources has assisted in the development of precise conservative and minimally invasive treatment techniques. Their presence may account for the persistence of elusive back pain and sciatica following conventional treatment and may provide the explanation of 'memory' pain, 'illness behaviour', 'instability syndromes', 'chronic joint pain', 'failed back syndromes', and 'failed back surgery syndromes'. The plethora of syndromes built upon indirect methods of examination is a testimonial to our ignorance of the actual source of axial and referred pain. Their successful treatment by transforaminal means endorses their importance as the causal incubus of pain resulting from the sequelae of degenerative disc disease. Transforaminal endoscopic aware-state surgery—foraminoplasty—is a treatment concept that detects the pain foci *in vivo* and offers an effective treatment modality which is specific, discrete, and of low morbidity.

Background to transforaminal endoscopic aware-state surgery

Since 1990, we have used aware-state surgery to detect the pain sources arising from spinal disorders. The therapeutic pathway is termed 'viviprudence' and consists of an evaluation cascade of in-depth questionnaires, postural analysis, extended clinical examination, and weight-bearing radiographs in flexion and extension standing and sitting, magnetic resonance imaging (MRI) scans, and occasionally, computed tomography (CT) or CT/SPECT (single-photon emission computed tomography) scans. This is followed by extended postural restabilization and motor reprogramming physiotherapy for 6–12 weeks, after which persistent debilitating symptoms may merit intervention. If the history is short and the pathology is mild and a SPECT/CT scan is positive, then root blocks and facet joint injections may be tried. Otherwise, in cases of enduring intrusive pain and significant pathology, the intervention takes the form of spinal (foraminal) probing and discography, with foraminal probing being the more valuable. Multiple-point probing serves to pinpoint pain sites at the facet margin, neural margins, annulus, and safe working zone. The safe working zone is a triangular region bounded by the dura or traversing nerve medially, the medial border of the exiting nerve laterally, and the superior endplate margin of the inferior bounding vertebra.

Discography reproduces pain in only 27% of patients with non-compressive radiculopathy, but is valuable in defining the disposition of degeneration within the disc and the integrity of the annulus. Discography defines most leaks and the direction of leakage. The acceptance volume of radio-opaque dye defines the degree of degeneration present.

For those cases where pain is either incompletely reproduced or there is overlap in the symptoms reproduced, we used to rely upon *differential discography* to define the segment mainly responsible for the symptom production. Differential discography uses the intradiscal instillation of methylprednisolone, Omnipaque 240, or bupivacaine to produce amelioration of symptoms for 6–10 days, 12–18 hours, and 5–8 hours respectively to determine the contribution to a symptom complex from each specific segment. However, we subsequently supplemented foraminal probing with neural stimulation using the Neurotherm electro-stimulator. This, in turn, has been superseded by *combination endoscopic minimally invasive spine surgery* in which all the painful levels can now be addressed.

Our experience with aware-state surgery began in 1990, when we performed percutaneous discectomy. The 12.5% annual recurrence rate led us to explore laser disc decompression as a minimalist alternative to treating compressive and non-compressive radiculopathy. In 1992, we developed biportal endoscopic intradiscal discectomy but found that although this technique could address more significant lesions, such as disc extrusion and large focal protrusions, outcome was extremely susceptible to lateral recess stenosis. This led us to develop a method of foraminal decompression termed endoscopic laser foraminoplasty (ELF) which provides the means to explore the epidural, foraminal, and extraforaminal zones as well as effect intradiscal discectomy, all by the posterolateral route and in the aware state. Clinical implementation of uniportal ELF started in 1993 and refined over the years to transforaminal endoscopic lumbar decompression and foraminoplasty (TELDF) with endoscopic intradiscal discectomy or laser disc decompression or gelstix enhancement.

The system of viviprudence and aware-state endoscopic examination has allowed surgeons to address lateral recess stenosis, epidural scarring, osteophytosis, settlement, olisthesis, disc extrusion, spondylolytic spondylolisthesis, 'instability', sequestration, 'failed back syndrome', and 'failed back surgery syndrome'. Our experience of over 7750 interventions has demonstrated numerous unsuspected causes of pain arising in degenerative disc disease (see the section 'Anatomy and pathology of spinal axial and referred pain').

Surgical protocol for transforaminal endoscopic lumbar decompression and foraminoplasty

Patients are consented for a staged multi-interventional TELDF procedure consisting of:

- Spinal (foraminal) probing and discography at suspected levels approached on the side of maximal symptoms. This may be supplemented by neural stimulation with a Neurotherm flexi-probe. The segment with maximal symptoms and pathology would be addressed by TELDF; those with lesser symptoms, by endoscopic decompression; and adjacent levels, by laser disc decompression or gelstix therapy. The treatment of the disc would depend upon the degree of protrusion, internal disruption, and leakage.

- Exploration of extraforaminal, foraminal, and epidural zones' definition of the boundaries of the foramen, clearance of perineural scarring and resection of the superior foraminal ligament; clearance of the safe working zone; undercutting of the foramen; mobilization of the nerve from the disc and inferior pedicle or other structures such as exuberant graft or misplaced cages or prostheses; removal of facet joint, vertebral rim, and shoulder osteophytes. Less degenerate levels would be treated by manual decompression of the foramen with reamers and removal of ligaments and scarring. The intradiscal contents would be treated either by endoscopic intradiscal discectomy through a 3.5 mm portal, laser disc decompression through a 2 mm portal, or gelstix instillation.

- In the past, where symptom reproduction was imperfect, then a differential discogram was performed with the instillation of 2 ml of methylprednisolone at the presumed level. If post-operative observation revealed a reduction of symptoms for 5–10 days, then those affected symptoms could be expected to be modified by TELDF at that level. However, nowadays, in the presence of better equipment, we overcome this problem by addressing several levels with an escalator of interventional severity.

The minimally invasive spine surgeon, unlike conventional surgeons, does not choose an intervention pre-operatively and decide upon discectomy, decompression, or fusion of disc replacement in advance. Rather, the endoscopist aims to find the pain source and treat that discretely and precisely, and relies upon the patient to lead the surgeon to these sources. Spinal foraminal probing differs from discography in that it allows specific probing of the anterior margin of the facet joint, perineural structures, and the disc wall at several points, to reproduce the symptoms. While discography defines the distribution of degeneration within the disc and the acceptance volume, and the presence of annular leaks, it relies upon disturbance of the nerve to reproduce symptoms and is a less sensitive determinator of the index segment for the patient's pain. If discography on a contained disc produces radicular pain, then it usually does this by compressing the nerve. The annulus itself is rarely the source of the patient's PPS. If a leak reproduces the patient's compressive or non-compressive pain, then this identifies the leak as a contributor to that evoked pain. Where foraminal probing reproduces specific pain, then this confirms the foraminal exiting nerve as the source of the pain. Endoscopy subsequently demonstrates the contribution to the pain arising from an inflamed disc, disc pad, and foraminal structures.

Operative technique

Current neurolept (aware-state) analgesia relies upon constantly monitored infusion of remifentanyl and propofal. Patient feedback is essential in these cases where the presence of perineural scarring is often unexpectedly dense and masks the neural structures. A bolus dose of 1.5 g cefuroxime is given at the onset of the operation. The skin and subcutis are infiltrated with local anaesthetic (xylocaine 0.25% 0.75–1.5 mg/kg) with 1:200,000 adrenaline. The optimal entry portal is selected with a radio-opaque jig.

Push-up and leg extension test

The patient is placed prone on the Knight-Sheffield translucent operating table. This allows the pre-operative push-up test to be performed. This consists of extending the arms, hyperextending the lumbar spine, while encouraging the abdomen to sag in the prone position. If this manoeuvre evokes the patient's leg or back pain before surgery, then clearance of the pain at the end of the procedure denotes sufficient clearance of the cause of the pain. Similarly, the patient can be asked to extend the lower leg to reproduce their symptoms and if when repeated at the end of the procedure, the symptoms have been cleared, then this usually indicates a beneficial outcome.

Lasing technique

The foraminal probe is replaced with a guide wire and, under biplanar radiographic control, a 5.6-mm dilator tube is railroaded to the foramen. During the entire procedure, an image intensifier is used at intervals to ensure the correct position of the endoscope and the laser probe. The trocar is removed and an endoscope with an eccentrically placed 4.0-mm working channel is inserted. A side-firing 2.1-mm diameter laser probe with internal irrigation is inserted through the endoscope. The extraforaminal zone and margin of the foramen are cleared. The ascending and descending facet joint surfaces are then excavated and undercut with laser, Kerrisons, trephines, and reamers, thus allowing admission of the endoscope beyond the isthmus of the foramen into the epidural space. Vertebral body and facet joint osteophytes, ligamentum flavum and superior foraminal ligament, perineural and epidural scarring are ablated and the facet joint undercut until the annulus and epidural space are displayed. A radio-frequency probe can be used to supplement haemostasis.

The exiting and transiting nerve roots are mobilized and decompressed medially and laterally until the functional axilla of the root at the apex of the safe working zone is displayed and pulsatility of the nerve is restored.

The nerve is cleared of perineural fibrosis. The bone margin of the superior notch and the superior foraminal ligament are then addressed. Osteophytes along the ascending facet joint and in the superior notch, dorsum of the vertebral margin, and the vertebral shoulder (shoulder osteophytes) are ablated under endoscopic vision. In the presence of a disc protrusion in the epidural or foraminal zone, disc degeneration, or annular collection or leaks, the disc is entered and cleared by laser ablation and manual punches or treated with gelstix.

Anatomy and pathology of spinal axial and referred pain

Experience of over 7750 endoscopic and laser interventions has taught us that the majority of spinal axial and referred pain arises from pathology in the foramen and extraforaminal regions (Figures 26.1 and 26.2) including:

- superior foraminal ligament impingement
- superior facet osteophytosis
- dorsal and 'shoulder' vertebral osteophytes
- facet joint impaction
- facet joint cysts
- pars interarticularis tethering
- safe working zone granulations
- ligamentum flavum infolding
- disc pad inflammation
- posterior longitudinal ligament irritation
- intertransverse ligament and muscle entrapment
- inferior pedicular tethering
- annulus protrusion—extrusions—sequestra
- Lateral and axial stenosis
- annular high-intensity zones and tears
- lateral vertebral osteophytosis
- paravertebral bone graft tethering
- post-fusion and aseptic discitis
- instrumentation neural tethering
- perineural and neural tethering and irritation.

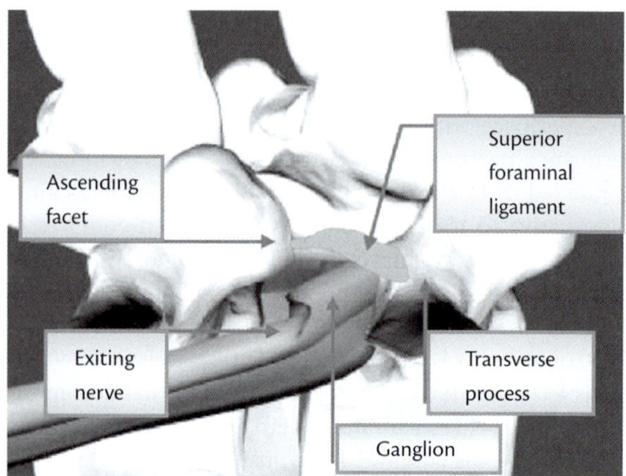

Figure 26.1 Some of the foraminal pathologies demonstrated by endoscopic aware-state evaluation of the foramina via the posterolateral approach.

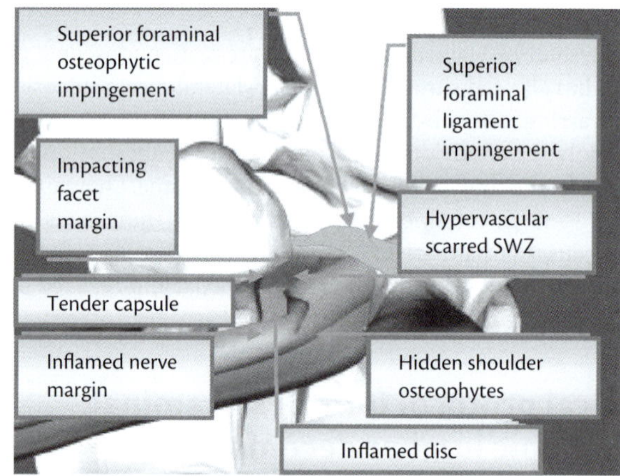

Figure 26.2 Foraminal anatomy and superior foraminal ligament and the impacting ascending facet joint margin deforming the nerve and ganglion.

Superior foraminal ligament impingement

The superior foraminal ligament passes from the ascending facet to the base of the transverse process. As settlement occurs, so this ligament bears down on the exiting nerve, which may become tethered, causing local hyperaemia and irritation of the nerve at that point. This irritation is further aggravated by calcification of the ligament. The ligament is often found adherent to the nerve and the nerve, inflamed and tender at that point. While normal radicular symptoms may be elicited from quiescent sections of the same nerve, the inflamed nerve may produce atypical dysaesthesiae.

Superior facet osteophytosis

As the superior foraminal ligament is resected, so superior notch osteophytes may be displayed in the superior notch adherent to the exiting nerve and produce local inflammation. These osteophytes arise from the superior facet joint margin.

Dorsal and shoulder osteophytes

Osteophytes are covered by a soft tissue cap which increases their compressive effect on adjacent tissues. This effect is worsened by tethering between the osteophyte fibrous cap and the nerve, posterior longitudinal ligament, or dura. Shoulder osteophytes can be found as a peripheral extension of dorsal osteophytes or as individual entities. Causal dorsal osteophytes usually arise from the upper vertebral body margin and produce midline or medial foraminal tethering and inflammation and displacement of the nerve pathway. This tethering or displacement is especially noticeable during flexion. Shoulder osteophytes may also occur on the superior or inferior vertebral margin in the foramen or lateral foramen lying anterior to the nerve and tethering to the same. These are often hidden from view unless an active search is made on the medial or anterior (deep) surface of the nerve. They appear to lie in the pathway of the abutting impacting ascending facet joint and may indeed arise as a consequence of such impaction. The endoscopy cannula can be used to mobilize and retract the nerve while it is separated from the fibrous cap of the osteophyte and subsequently ablated with reamers or laser.

Facet joint impaction

Facet joint impaction arises from the ascending facet joint impacting on the exiting nerve root or the tissues in the safe working zone. The frequent presence of tissues tethering the nerve to the facet margin increases the effect of the impaction as and when disc degeneration leads to overriding of the facet joints during settlement and displacement (olisthesis). The effect is worsened as retrolisthesis and anterior olisthesis occurs. Tethering between the nerve and facet joint needs to be resected and the facet joint needs to be undercut to remove the dynamic impaction. Such dynamic impaction is the mechanism underlying many instances of so-called 'instability'.

Facet joint cysts

These can cause compression on exiting and traversing nerves and can increase in size during activity and can be marsupialized after the foraminal isthmus has been enlarged and traversed.

Pars interarticularis tethering

Pars interarticularis defects cause tethering to traversing and exiting nerve roots. Tethering to the fibrous defect and to the bone of the anterior pars fracture site can be resected and the nerve root mobilized and decompressed. In the presence of anterior displacement, the disc wall is deformed and causes dorsal displacement of the traversing nerve roots; often, in addition, a knuckle of disc wall displaces into the foramen, further compromising the exiting nerve root. Each of these elements can be resected under vision with amelioration of symptoms without the need for fusion.

Safe working zone granulations

Hypervascular tissue consisting of scar, hypervascular veins, and arterioles can be found in the superior and inferior notch and in the safe working zone. These can become engorged, producing stenotic and claudicant symptoms, and may themselves be directly tender when inflamed.

Ligamentum flavum infolding

The ligamentum flavum infolds as disc height is reduced. The infolding crowds the exiting nerve root in the superior notch and in the inferior notch if the nerve is medially displaced. On occasions, the ligamentum flavum may be found to blend with the posterior disc pad and posterior longitudinal ligament. Resection of the ligamentum flavum at these sites serves to decompress the exiting and traversing nerve roots and mobilize same from local tethering. The procedure should be combined with anterior mobilization of the nerve to achieve full mobilization.

The ligamentum flavum may blend with the posterior foraminal ligament which passes from the superior notch, blends with the capsule, and extends to the inferior notch but of itself does not appear to cause compression.

Disc pad inflammation

On the posterior aspect of the disc, a pad of tissue may be found which is thick and contains inflammatory blood vessels and nerves which may be locally tender, in contradistinction to the annulus itself which, if not injected, is often pain-free to probing. Removal may produce immediate relief of local back pain. This may occur in the absence of a posterior collection of dye in the annulus, or a leak, but is more commonly found in association with them.

Posterior longitudinal ligament irritation

The posterior longitudinal ligament may be inflamed and locally tender but is usually found in this state when adjacent tissues such as the disc are inflamed. Local neurolysis and ablation of adjacent inflamed tissues can resolve the inflammation. Probing of the inflamed posterior longitudinal ligament will produce pain arising in territories normally expected to be subtended by both the index and adjacent levels.

Intertransverse ligament and muscle entrapment

The intertransverse ligament and muscle pass on the lateral aspect of the exiting nerve. In the degenerate state, the nerve may be tethered on the lateral aspect to the intertransverse ligament and muscle, causing local inflammation. Alternatively, degenerative loss of disc height may lead to crowding of the exiting nerve by the intertransversus muscle and ligament, so preventing the exiting nerve from escaping the impacting ascending facet. Endoscopic neurolysis and division of the ligament and muscle relieves lateral constraint and assists access and mobilization of the nerve root.

Inferior pedicular tethering

The exiting nerve may be tethered to the external surface of the inferior pedicle especially following previous surgery and prior posterolateral bone grafted fusion. Local endoscopic neurolysis is valuable in mobilizing the nerve root from the pedicle and may be combined with resection of dorsally placed hypertrophic tethering bone graft.

Annulus protrusion—extrusion—sequestration

The annulus may be extruded or protruding into the foramen, lateral foraminal zone, or epidural posterolateral or central zones. Discectomy or resection of the central or posterolateral bulging disc may be appropriate and concur with expected clinical findings, but certain instances are non-contributory. However, protrusions in the lateral foramen may impact on the exiting nerve and produce unexpected clinical signs. The disc protrusion in this area may be surprisingly small, even imperceptible on the MR scan, and yet produce significant impact on the nerve, especially where the nerve is tethered to the disc wall or the foraminal volume is reduced by facet joint hypertrophy or overriding.

In situations of degenerate disc height loss, the wall of the disc may be playing only a limited role in the pathogenesis of symptoms and, under these circumstances, the wall of the disc may be shrunk thermoplastically with the laser, rather than removing and further damaging the degenerate remnants of the disc.

In 68% of cases, intradiscal clearance may be performed without pain. This indicates that in these cases the inosculation of blood vessels and nerves into the annulus had either not been contributory to the symptom complex or was not extensive. Foraminoplasty allows the disc pathology to be treated either as a limited resection (herniectomy) or, where there is an extrusion, for the disrupted disc material to be withdrawn into the disc and then removed posterolaterally. In cases of sequestra, the isthmus of the foramen is opened and the fragment retrieved from the epidural space.

Lateral and axial stenosis

Axial stenosis is often over-diagnosed when, in fact, the problem is more commonly bilateral lateral recess stenosis. The axial claudicant symptoms can be improved by reduction of the axial disc protrusion or osteophytosis, and the lateral recess stenosis cleared by means of foraminoplasty without the postural disturbance of a fusion or interspinous spacer.

Annular tears

The annulus may be the site of intradiscal tears which may breach the annulus either under the posterior longitudinal ligament (subligamentous) or through it (transligamentous), occasioning symptoms according to the point of liberation of the type of breakdown products produced. The most symptomatic are those ejecting breakdown products directly onto the nerve in the foramen. Their effect is amplified where the nerve is tethered adjacent to the exit portal of the tear. The reaction to the leakage may be to lay down perineural scarring, causing adherence of the nerve to the disc, thus impeding movement of the nerve away from the point of leakage during flexion or rotation. The fibrous response may cause encapsulation of the leakage, resulting in containment and concentration of the breakdown products around the nerve. These effects worsen the symptoms and are found in patients with long-lasting pre-operative symptoms.

Clearance of the perineural scarring and mobilization of the nerve should be complemented by opening of the radial tear orifice and removal of debris, often holding the tear open. The course of the tear is often serpiginous, so the route of the tear cannot be fully explored. It is recommended that the nucleus be explored and that degenerate material be removed manually and by laser ablation. The wall of the disc is then treated by thermoplastic annealing. While a high-intensity zone may be an indicator of the pathology, the only sign may be a dehydrated 'black' disc on the MRI scan.

Lateral osteophytosis

Lateral osteophytes displace the exiting nerve root dorsally and into the inferior notch, amplifying compression by the redundant annulus at that point. In addition, the lateral osteophytes can cause displacement of the nerve into the middle section of the foramen, thus displacing the nerve into the path of the impacting facet joint. Partial resection of the osteophytes where they displace the nerve is valuable as part of general undercutting and enlargement of the foramen. This is an important contributor to patients with degenerative scoliosis and allows treatment without the need for fusion because significant progression of the scoliosis is usually deterred by the lateral compensatory osteophytosis.

Paravertebral bone graft tethering

After instrumented or non-instrumented fusion, paravertebral bone graft causes anterior tethering to exiting nerve roots with profound entrapment, often in the presence of a secure and technically correct fusion. Wide neurolysis on the anterior surface of the graft results in nerve root mobilization and resolution of symptoms resulting from tethering caused by such extraforaminal entrapment.

Post-fusion and aseptic discitis

Post-fusion and aseptic discitis manifest as a highly inflamed and tender annulus which can be relieved by manual and laser discectomy under endoscopic control. If clinical suspicion of infection exists, then a fine cannula can be placed intradiscally to insert antibiotics until intravenous conversion is achieved. However, in cases of aseptic discitis, removal of the inflamed disc contents serves to reduce the back pain significantly, with subsequent resolution after a short period of intravenous antibiosis. The role of low-grade infection in the causation of spinal inflammatory pain is the subject of current research.

Instrumentation and neural tethering

Pedicle screw instrumentation can produce neural tethering either by direct impingement of the metalwork or by tethering of the nerve to misplaced metalwork or microfractures of adjacent pedicles. When identified, the former should be treated by endoscopic mobilization of the nerve and removal of the metalwork and the latter should be treated by mobilization of the nerve and chamfering or removal of the displaced fragments.

Perineural tethering and nerve irritation

Perineural tethering may arise as a consequence of direct irritation from a disc protrusion or facet joint impaction or the release of breakdown products. The nerve may be reddened because it is entrapped by an impacting facet joint, osteophytes, and inflamed and engorged hypervascular tissues in the notch. The inflammation may be aggravated by displacement of the nerve by scarring, lateral small knuckles of disc protrusion, and shoulder osteophytes. The nerve may be bound adjacent to annular tears which cause inflammation by direct release of intradiscal breakdown products onto the nerve. The often profound scarring fails to show on the MRI scan and deprives the nerve of its normal pulsatility which, in turn, must impair its functionality.

The exiting or traversing nerve root will produce normal radicular signs with compression. However, the irritated reddened nerve will often produce dysaesthesiae of unexpected distribution. Interestingly, adjacent sections of the nerve not irritated produce symptoms in expected territories. This may explain the cause of persistent symptoms after conventional surgery using conventional guidelines, rather than the results of aware-state feedback which may indicate that the nerve is being irritated at an adjacent and unexpected level—a finding which is noted in about 20% of patients referred to this unit with failed back surgery.

Outcome of endoscopic laser foraminoplasty

The results of ELF (Knight et al. 1999) indicate that this technique provides a minimalist means of exploring the extraforaminal zone, the foramen, and the epidural space, and performing discectomy, osteophytectomy, and perineural neurolysis with encouraging results. It incorporates the prophylactic advantage of foraminal undercutting and provides a promising means of identifying and treating the pain of 'failed back surgery' and back pain and sciatica of indeterminate origin and patients with 'instability'. Done in the aware state, ELF serves to identify and localize the source of pain generation at the time of surgery and the relevance of these findings. It avoids the morbidity associated with open spinal surgery and serves as a useful means of effecting 'keyhole' neurolysis without extensive exploration and fusion. Current improvements in equipment promise wider application and more encouraging results in the future.

Discussion about endoscopially determined pain sources in the lumbar spine

Instability is not a diagnosis but merely a mechanism, the treatment of which requires an understanding of the effects of abnormal micro-movements of the facet joint and disc wall as the disc degenerates, loses disc height and turgor, and the facet joint overrides and hypertrophies. These factors have a repetitive micro-traumatic effect upon the nerve and encourage micro-bleeds and the development of fibrosis and tethering to adjacent tissues and structures. Inflammation and irritation occur in these adjacent structures, with consequent symptoms.

The posterolateral approach conducted in the aware state, with the additional benefit of endoscopic evaluation, has confirmed that the foramen and extraforaminal zone is the source of hitherto poorly appreciated causes of pain, parasthesiae, and neurological deficit. In the foramen, the facet joint is consistently found to be tethered to the nerve and may be tethered to the disc. When there is partial settlement or olisthesis, micro-movements occur which result in abnormal movements and, in particular, impaction between the facet joint and the nerve or bulging disc. This causes irritation and sensitization of the nerve and evoked pain. This nerve compromise arises at the foramen as the nerve leaves the spinal canal; the pain distribution matches that normally attributed to segmental disease at the level above. This leads to misdiagnosis and incorrect indications for conventional surgery.

Other features of the foraminal construct provide unfamiliar causes of symptoms. The superior foraminal ligament may contain small osteophytes. Either individually or in combination, the superior foraminal ligament or the contained osteophytes may impinge upon the exiting nerve root. This is often seen as reddening at the point of impact. Again, the guillotining action of these structures is aggravated by settlement or short pedicles.

The nerve may be tethered directly to the disc which, if inflamed or focally weak at the point of tethering, will be distorted and irritated causing pain in the exiting or, occasionally, the transiting nerve. Again, this would be attributed to the superior segmental level, especially as the MRI scan will not demonstrate small areas of focal annular weakness or tethering to the disc.

After prior surgery or trauma, or in the case of settlement or facet joint hypertrophy, the nerve may be displaced medially or, occasionally, displaced superiorly and laterally. The displacement is then held by perineural scarring. Under these circumstances, the nerve cannot deploy normally into the superior or inferior notches during flexion, extension, and rotation and is vulnerable to impact from the facet joint, a focally distorted or broad-based bulging disc, or a combination of the two.

Shoulder osteophytes occurring on the shoulder of the vertebral rim lie anterior to the exiting nerve and usually arise from the superior vertebral margin in the plane of the impacting facet. They result in tethering of the exiting nerve and local irritation and marked sensitivity. This can occur even in the presence of a successful fusion or conventional decompression and may account for persistent symptoms following technically satisfactory surgery, contributing to the 'failed back surgery' syndrome. Fusion with restoration of disc height can merely drag the exiting more tightly onto the shoulder osteophyte and worsen symptoms.

Conventional discectomy, decompression, or fusion, and height restoration fail to treat, for instance, the nerve tethered to the disc wall or the superior notch and superior foraminal ligament tethering and, indeed, may aggravate it. Endoscopy would determine the presence of such pathology and specifically treat it without the need for extensive conventional surgery such as a fusion and, importantly, preserves postural function.

Tears and leaks are a common source of elusive pain. The distribution of pain depends upon the direction of the leak and its containment around the exiting or transiting nerve or dispersal along and around the posterior longitudinal ligament. Lumbar leakage may produce global dysthaesthesia in the limb, urinary irritation, partial weakness, partial numbness, disproportionate back, buttock, or leg pain, individually or in any combination.

These clinical examinations indicate that in cases of non-compressive radiculopathy or mild compressive radiculopathy, the textbook guidelines to the source of the pain may be seriously misleading. Elusive back pain and referred pain may arise from a variety of sources which may be difficult to determine from clinical examination, X-rays, and scans alone. Spinal foraminal probing and endoscopy, however, do provide a reliable method of identifying pain sources and treating these specifically, accurately, and discretely.

The conventional diagnostician favours an axial diagnosis or a facet joint arthropathy in the causation of back pain, but ignores the adjacent level foramen or the foraminal contents and may, therefore, be addressing the wrong level or the wrong sources of pain at the correct level. In our experience, facet joint injections may be misleading because the steroid injection, rather than affecting the joint itself, is in fact influencing the pathology in the foramen on the anterior aspect of the joint.

The failures of conventional treatment may often arise because the pathology is not in or around the midline or epidural space but, surprisingly, commonly affecting the same nerve as it exits the subjacent foramen.

We pay lip service to the fact that conventional surgery may fail because the incorrect level has been addressed. In fact, it may not just be the wrong level but the wrong structure at that level that has been addressed. Acknowledging the prerequisite to address the correct level, surgeons seem peculiarly reluctant to define the pain site accurately before proceeding to intervention. Aware-state surgery and endoscopy provide an ideal solution to identifying the level and the aetiopathology for cervical and lumbar axial and referred pain.

The inexplicably elevated severity or persistence of symptoms should not be classed as 'illness behaviour' but, rather, should spark a quest to further identify the remaining pain source and treat this specifically. After all, following effective hip or knee replacement in patients with long-term pain, surgeons do not need to resort to concepts such as 'memory pain', 'centrally perpetuated pain', 'coping courses', or 'psychiatric support', because the source of the pain has been effectively eradicated.

Aware-state surgery offers us the opportunity to learn more about the mechanisms of pain arising in the back and neck and referred pain, and to address these by conservative rehabilitation or minimalist surgical intervention. It has already shown us that there are many extremely sensitive pain sources hitherto unappreciated in and about the foramen. I consider that this technique allows us to step forward from diagnostic 'guesstimating' to precise definition of pain sources and to devise specific, discrete, conservative or minimalist treatment. These remedies and the future direction of endoscopic minimally invasive spine surgery are further explored at <http://www.spinal-foundation.org>.

Reference

Knight, M.T.N., Goswami, A.K.D., Patko, J. Endoscopic laser foraminoplasty and aware state surgery: a treatment concept and outcome analysis. *Die Arthroscopie*, 1999, 2, 1–12.

Chapter 27

Regional somatic dysfunction

Michael L. Kuchera

Expertise in the field of neuromusculoskeletal medicine or other specialties which integrate manual medicine provides unique insights into patient care. Knowledge and skills in this discipline insightfully expand the scope of the anamnesis, physical examination, and differential diagnosis. It presupposes extensive, specific knowledge of the regional and systemic structure (anatomy) and function (physiology and kinesiology), integrated with a comprehensive understanding of the patient as a unique individual. It necessitates highly practiced palpatory skills with the ability to diagnose somatic dysfunction and competence in delivering therapeutic modalities to effectively rectify dysfunctions affecting skeletal, arthrodial, and/or myofascial structures. It requires the perspective of a broadly trained physician to perform the examinations needed to establish a differential diagnosis and to fully weigh the indications, contraindications, and risk to benefit ratios of different treatment approaches. At all times, it is tempered by the distinctive patient–physician relationship incorporating the art and compassion of the healthcare professional with an understanding of biopsychosocial, biomechanical, orthopaedic, biophysiological, and neurological models of care.

The knowledge, skill, training, and art of the manual medicine physician are then focused, through a unifying model, philosophy, or perspective, in a safe, time-efficient, and cost-effective manner. Current practitioners of neuromusculoskeletal medicine may practice under a variety of titles denoting their approach to this field. Some are specialists with certification or other recognition in disciplines termed 'physical medicine and rehabilitation', 'musculoskeletal medicine', 'osteopathic manipulative medicine', 'neuromusculoskeletal medicine', or 'orthopaedic medicine'. The American schools of osteopathic medicine integrate this perspective and core manual medicine skills into the pre-doctoral education of all physicians in training, regardless of their eventual specialty. Other physicians obtain core post-graduate training in manual medicine skills and add these skills to an evolving perspective gained through reading and professional interactions with colleagues in one or more of these disciplines.

Although a specialty or school of training may emphasize a different component of the whole neuromusculoskeletal medicine field or even a different explanatory model, each recognizes the value of:

- diagnostic screening and regional and local palpatory examinations to identify somatic dysfunction and neuromusculoskeletal pathophysiology
- safe and effective treatment skills (FIMM 2014), including the ability to select and deliver any of a core of manual medicine techniques used in modifying the neuromusculoskeletal system
- a patient-centred approach requiring an individualized neuromusculoskeletal prescription.

In the USA, independent studies of patients receiving workmen's compensation in several different states compared the cost of management of different musculoskeletal complaints by different types of healthcare practitioners (see Figure 10.17 in Chapter 10). These studies included musculoskeletal problems in each anatomical region and care for each provided by surgical doctors of medicine (MDs) and doctors of osteopathic medicine (DOs), non-surgical MDs and DOs, chiropractors, and physical therapists. Of all practitioners included in this review, only the US-trained DO has an educational combination of core training in manual medicine techniques, unifying philosophy emphasizing the neuromusculoskeletal system, and complete medical training paralleling that of the international musculoskeletal medicine physician. Non-surgical osteopathic physicians with this educational background were the most cost-effective in every anatomical region (Labor and Industry Computers 1988/1993). Such studies suggest that physicians with core training in manual techniques and a unifying philosophical approach to neuromusculoskeletal problems will be more cost-effective than non-physicians employing manual approaches alone. These studies may also suggest the value of a manual medicine education of physicians without such core training to promote cost-effective patient management. Further controlled cost-efficacy studies are warranted.

Applying concepts of somatic dysfunction to regional disorders

This chapter develops the clinical importance of somatic dysfunction in various regions of the body and approaches for recognizing it.

Somatic dysfunction is an umbrella term embracing impaired or altered function of related components of the somatic system (body framework): skeletal, arthrodial, and myofascial structures, and related vascular, lymphatic, and neural elements (ECOP 2011; WHO 1979). Concepts of somatic dysfunction are fully discussed in Chapter 10, and an understanding of those concepts is essential to the clinical value of this chapter.

In keeping with values previously outlined, this chapter describes screening, regional and local palpatory examinations for somatic dysfunction, as well as those patient-centred variables that play a role in individualizing the manual medicine prescription (Dinnar 1980, 1982; Kimberly 1980). For each region, one or more common clinical conditions in which somatic dysfunction plays a major role have been chosen to illustrate the application of these values. Specific treatment of somatic dysfunction in various regions, using manual medicine techniques, is more fully discussed in Chapter 50.

Applying screening, regional and local examinations for somatic dysfunction

A palpatory examination for somatic dysfunction is an integral part of the physical examination in this field of medicine. This examination should not be conducted in isolation, nor tacked on as an afterthought. It is individually designed to evaluate various aspects of the neuromusculoskeletal system on the basis of a careful history and other findings in the general physical examination. In moving towards the differential diagnosis of a patient's complaint, the physician's understanding of pathophysiology, pain generators, referred and reflex pain mechanisms, and the interconnectedness of function and structure direct the site and extent of an appropriate palpatory examination.

Time-efficient examination for somatic dysfunction is best performed in stages, culminating in a final site-specific definition based on the S.T.A.R characteristics (**s**ensory changes, **t**issue texture abnormality, **a**symmetry, and **r**estriction of motion; see Chapter 10) (Degenhardt et al. 2002; Kuchera et al. 1997). Within each stage of the examination, any number of specific tests may be integrated, their particular order being related to the manual medicine model adopted and to the experience and preference of the examining physician.

A multi-stage examination for somatic dysfunction usually progresses from *screening* the patient for initial general impressions, to intermediate *scanning* of body regions identified by the screening process. The scanning process, in turn, identifies specific regions, joints, or tissues to be targeted for the more detailed *local examination* used in differential diagnosis and appropriate for designing an individualized neuromusculoskeletal prescription. Although certain principles apply, each examination is different and evolves from the progressive integration of discovered historical and physical findings unique to the patient being examined. Rarely, if ever, will a physician include all test procedures outlined in this chapter in a single examination.

Neuromusculoskeletal screening, scanning, and local examinations incorporate palpatory test choices according to the musculoskeletal model selected and lead to a peer-accepted standard of care (Chila 2011; Cyriax 1980; Greenman 1996; Lewit 1985; Maigne 1972; Mennell 1960; Simons et al. 1999). Identification of structure or function that deviates from normal at each level of palpatory evaluation invites a differential diagnosis and leads either to further specific testing of that site or to the expansion of testing to other related structures. Findings may eventually warrant additional neurological or orthopaedic tests or even laboratory, radiographical, and/or electrophysiological testing to fully establish a differential diagnosis and to safely and effectively reach an appropriate, individualized manual medicine prescription.

Screening and scanning examinations

According to Greenman (1996, pp. 18–36), a relevant neuromusculoskeletal examination answers the question, 'Is there a problem within the musculoskeletal system that deserves additional evaluation?' Screening examinations of the neuromusculoskeletal system often include observation of general appearance including general health status, presence of systemic disorders, and structural stressors apparent to observation; posture; gross movements and gait. General health status, systemic disorders, and structural stressors significantly affect the progression and form of the examination for somatic dysfunction. Screening for these factors also influences the subsequent intent, type, extent, and prognosis expected from treatment of the patient with musculoskeletal medicine techniques. General appearance provides clues to general health status and the possibility of certain systemic diseases:

- In particular, examination of hair, skin, and nails with respect to tissue texture abnormalities may uncover clues to underlying tissue health. Hair texture and distribution often provide clues to metabolic or endocrine disorders, and a number of rheumatological disorders also present with clues in ectodermal tissues. From a rheumatological perspective alone, the neuromusculoskeletal physician should especially note alopecia, nail pitting or ridging, skin ulcers, psoriasis, photosensitivity, purpura, malar rash, Raynaud's phenomenon, or tightening of the skin (Rubin 1997). Skin turgor in patients who abuse nicotine is quite distinctive, empirically suggesting poor connective tissue health (Amoronso et al. 1997; Naus et al. 1966; Reynolds et al. 1994), and prognosticates a lesser response to otherwise successful strategies for re-establishing neuromusculoskeletal health.
- The patient's general appearance may also suggest certain biomechanical stressors. For example, various types of obesity and pregnancy each alter the distribution of weight with respect to the centre of gravity. Likewise, the presence of a foot with an elongated second ray (Dudley J. Morton foot) is capable of altering the biomechanics of gait. Postural observation provides significant insight into patterns of somatic dysfunction and the inherent capability of that individual to compensate to gravitational stress and strain.

Various other external signs provide clues to systemic disease with associated musculoskeletal ramifications as well as underlying skeletal abnormalities and biomechanical disadvantages. Each can be recognized by careful observation of the patient's appearance.

Generalized postural analysis provides screening information about joints, muscles, and supportive connective tissues subjected to biomechanical stress. Clinically, this is correlated with the discovery of recurrent patterns of somatic dysfunction and myofascial trigger points (TrPs) (Kuchera 1995a). Posture must be examined in the three cardinal planes (Figure 27.1) for rotoscoliotic as well as accentuated or flattened sagittal plane curves. Static postural analysis also provides an opportunity to palpate and assess symmetry of paired anatomical landmarks including mastoid processes, acromion processes, inferior angles of the scapulae, iliac crests, posterior superior iliac spines, and greater trochanters of the femurs (Figure 27.2). The presence of aberrant postural alignment including asymmetrical landmarks may direct a scanning examination of the junctional areas of the spine and postural crossover sites or a local examination of specifically stressed ligaments and muscles

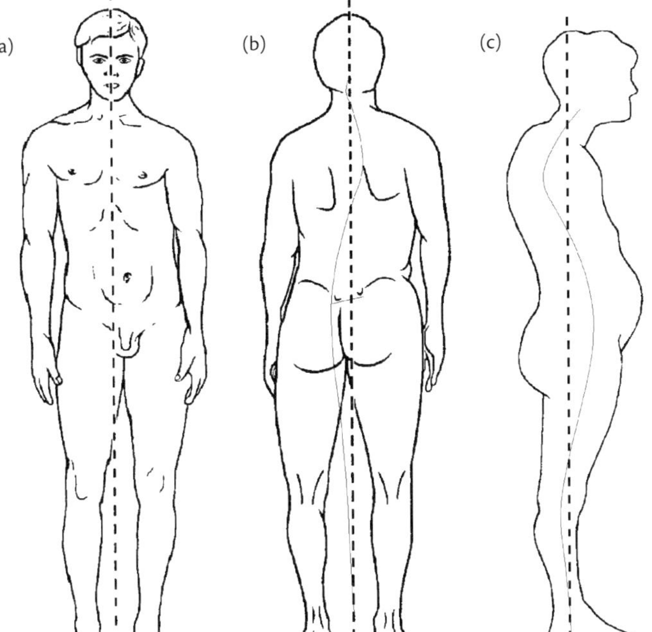

Figure 27.1 Observing posture: (a) anteroposterior; (b) posteroanterior; (c) lateral; (d) cephalocaudad.

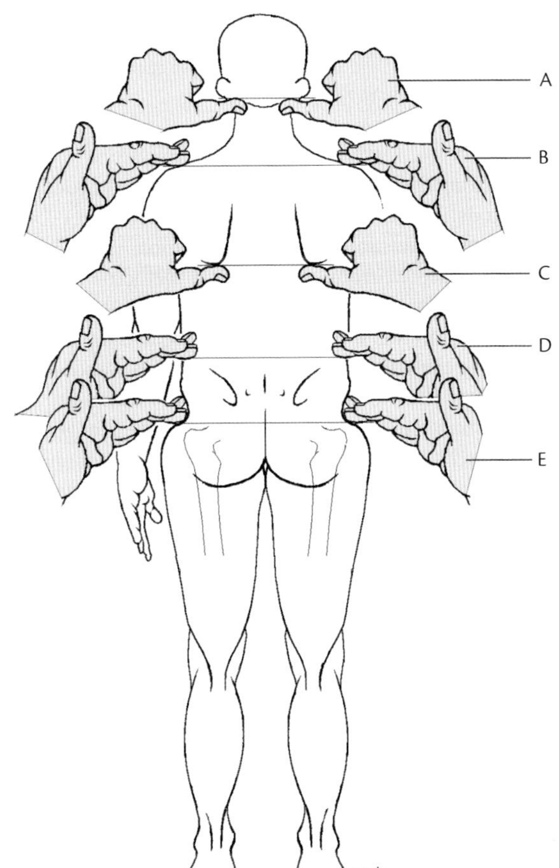

Figure 27.2 Posterior horizontal planes: (A) mastoid processes; (B) acromion processes; (C) inferior angles of the scapulae; (D) iliac crests; (E) greater trochanters of the femur.

(Kuchera and Kuchera 1997). These characteristic sites are well documented (Kuchera 1995b; Peterson 1983; Zink and Lawson 1979) and are discussed with relevance to each region later in this chapter.

Detailed observation of impaired or altered gross movements offers significant insights into the location and tissue type of an underlying somatic dysfunction.

- Gross spinal motion observation easily screens the total range of motion of the cervical, thoracic, and lumbar regions in flexion, extension, side-bending, and rotation (Figure 27.3). It becomes even more informative if, at the end of active regional motion observation, the physician gently continues the passive motion in the direction of the test. This scans for restriction of motion in that particular region and for possible aetiologies for the restriction by evaluating and assessing the characteristic quality of the restrictive barrier.
- Comparing side to side symmetry during a full respiratory cycle and gently palpating over the anterior upper chest and anterolateral lower rib cage may screen gross motion of the chest cage. In particular, observation of passive respiration provides insight into diaphragmatic and thoracic cage function. Normally, passive inhalation by a supine patient creates visible movement all the way down to the pubic region.
- Fully raising both upper extremities from the anatomical position in the coronal plane and turning the backs of the hands together quickly provides functional motion screening of the upper extremities (especially the shoulder girdle) (Figure 27.3).
- Seated and standing flexion tests constitute one style of pelvic screening examination (Figure 27.4). Asymmetrical motion during either flexion test indicates dysfunction localized to one side of the body. Comparison of the two tests can assist in

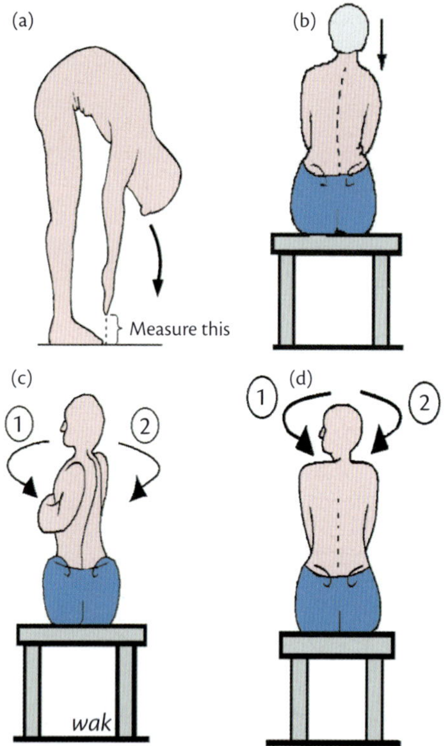

Figure 27.3 Active spinal motion testing: (a) flexion; (b) side-bending; (c) thoracolumbar rotation; (d) cervical rotation.

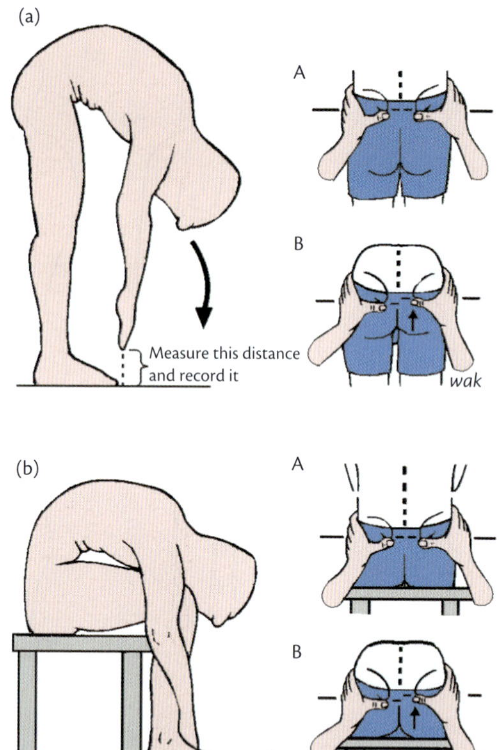

Figure 27.4 (a) Standing and (b) seated flexion tests. Regardless of any asymmetry at the onset (A), each test is noted to be positive (dysfunctional) on the side that moves the farthest and/or continues to move after the opposite side has stopped after completely bending forward (B).

determining whether major restrictors involve the pelvic structures or whether function is affected by structures below the pelvis. Test interpretation will be discussed in the pelvic region of this chapter.

- Examination of the lower extremities often includes both a modification of Patrick's FABERE test (Figure 27.5) screening for hip or sacroiliac dysfunction/pathology as well as an active deep knee-bend squatting test with heels maintained on the floor (Figure 27.6) which screens for strength and mobility of hips, knees, ankle, and feet bilaterally.

Any asymmetry or gross restriction of motion in any of these screening tests warrants further study, including more detailed evaluation for regional or local somatic dysfunction.

Beyond recognizing pathological gaits, the gait analysis portion of the musculoskeletal screening examination provides information about the presence and impact of underlying somatic dysfunction. Gait analysis should assess length, pattern, and symmetry of stride, arm swing, heel strike, toe off, tilting of the pelvis, and shoulder compensatory movements. Additional clues may be obtained by observing the wear patterns of the patient's shoes. Somatic dysfunction is capable of significantly altering the pattern of gait and, over time, may modify central programming enough to maintain the abnormal gait even though there has been a correction or resolution of the somatic dysfunction. Conversely, an improper biomechanical gait, structural change (such as a Dudley J. Morton foot), or anatomically asymmetrical lower extremities will require compensation throughout the body unit. Each alters tensegrity throughout the body and creates recurrent patterns of somatic dysfunction. As the patient walks for you, observe gait for forward head position, a straight lumbar spine, decreased hip flexion during single support phase, flexed knee in mid stance, failure of heel lift, and visible foot pronation during the single support phase. Each of these compensatory motions is a screening *gait marker* (Dananberg 1997), the presence of which warrants further examination.

Those who teach neuromusculoskeletal medicine diagnosis incorporate the above elements in most screening examinations, regardless of the model employed. Their pupils may be taught to approach these elements in a specific order as in standardized '10-step' or '12-step' examinations. This is not so much a requirement as a way of minimizing the number of positional changes made by the patient and preventing the inadvertent omission of one or more of the screening elements. Taught and performed in sequence, most screening examinations are, in fact, quick and efficient diagnostic tools to identify where to look next for neuromusculoskeletal clues, including somatic dysfunction (Mitchell et al. 2002). Nonetheless, the guiding principle that must be addressed in its entirety is the original question, 'Is there a problem within the musculoskeletal system that deserves additional evaluation?' Thus, testing sequence, time needed for the examination, and stated preference of specific tests by teachers of various schools, models, or disciplines are all less important to the neuromusculoskeletal medicine practitioner than answering the screening examination question and proceeding to the next diagnostic level.

Scanning and screening for somatic dysfunction

The definition of a *scanning examination* is 'an intermediate detailed examination of specific body regions which have been identified by findings emerging from the initial screen; the scan (for somatic

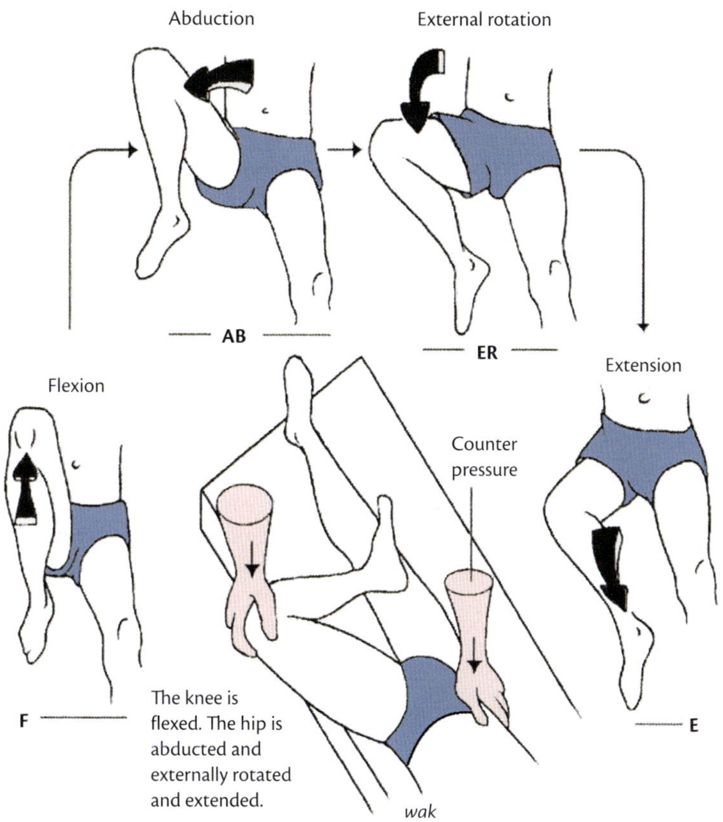

Figure 27.5 FABERE hip test with augmented external rotation to test sacroiliac structures.

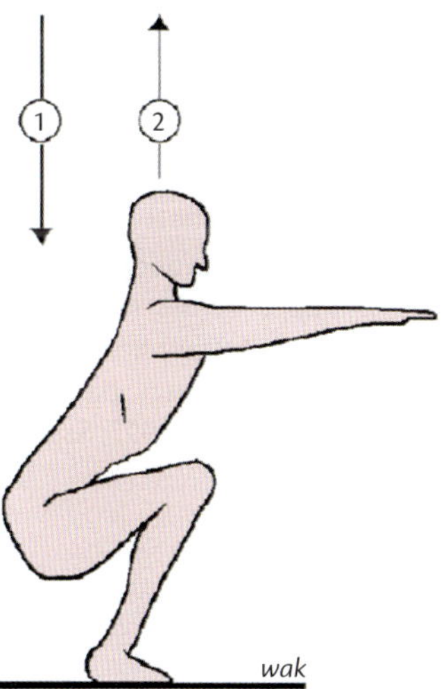

Figure 27.6 Squat test for screening flexion of joints of the lower extremity.

dysfunction) focuses on segmental areas for further definition or diagnosis' (ECOP 2011). According to Greenman (1996, p. 36), a scanning examination simply answers the questions, 'What part of the region and what tissues within the region may be significantly dysfunctional?'

All neuromusculoskeletal scanning examinations will seek to identify one or more of the S.T.A.R. findings in the region. Combinations of these findings constitute the objective diagnostic criteria for local or regional somatic dysfunction but, in isolation, may alert the astute clinician to also evaluate for the presence or absence of other underlying pathophysiological diagnoses.

Directed by the screening and scanning examinations to significant tissue sites, local diagnostic testing for the remaining S.T.A.R. characteristics should be performed to gather the final information needed to formulate an individualized manual medicine prescription.

Tissue texture and layer examination

Most manual medicine clinicians initially scan regions with a quick survey of tissue texture characteristics (Figure 27.7). Typical scanning tests of tissue texture abnormalities include skin drag, red reflex induction, and skin rolling.

- To perform *skin drag* (Figure 27.7a), the fingers pass over the skin with varying degrees of pressure depending upon the information sought. The lightest pressure is used to sense minor variations in skin temperature or sweat gland activity. In the paraspinal regions, increased resistance to lightly dragging the pads of the fingers along the skin in a stroking fashion denotes relative cutaneous humidity; less resistance denotes dryness.
- Significant changes can also be visually monitored in the friction-induced *red reflex* pattern (Figure 27.7b) produced by heavier stroking with the finger pads. Positive skin drag testing is demonstrated by asymmetrical responses in temperature, sweat gland activity, hyperesthesia, drag or ease, and/or the reddening/blanching pattern of the skin.
- *Skin rolling* (Figure 27.7c) is another scanning tool commonly used in the neuromusculoskeletal examination to assess tissue texture abnormalities. A positive finding is the provocation of local tenderness and pain in a dermatomal distribution with tightness

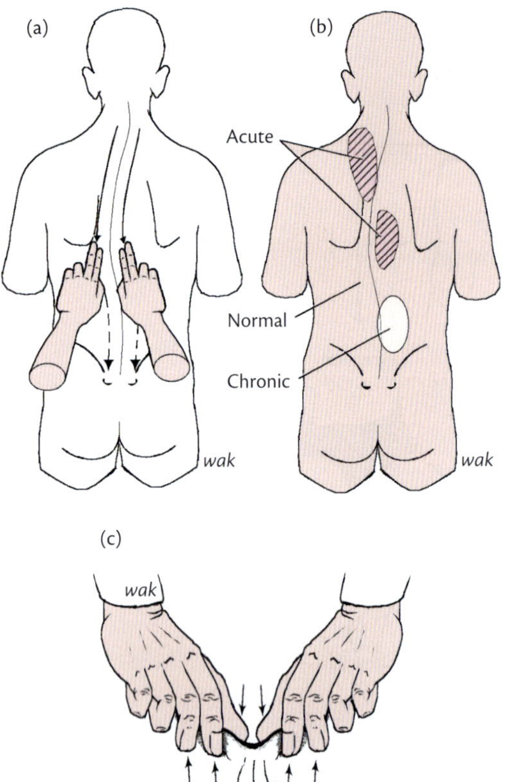

Figure 27.7 Scanning spinal regions: (a) light paraspinal palpation with (b) possible red reflex outcomes—acute showing prolonged reddening response; chronic blanching more rapidly after red reflex; (c) skin rolling.

of the skin and loss of resiliency in the related subcutaneous structures. Small tender nodules may also be identified in or on the deeper fascia using this test. Generally touted as a scanning test, skin rolling can be very segmentally specific (Greenman 1996).

Layer palpation involves increasing pressure over muscles, ligaments, vertebral processes, joint lines, or other clinically relevant structures in each region. It is yet another scanning tool for assessing sensation and tissue texture abnormalities. A positive test involves palpable tissue texture abnormalities, subjective tenderness, and pain provocation over the local structure. Pressure on one site may also elicit a pain referral pattern consistent with that structure. In the case of muscle, contraction or inhibition are palpable reactions to pressure, providing clinically valuable information. In the spinal region, this test, applied to the supraspinal ligaments and over each transverse process, identifies vertebral units requiring further examination (Figure 27.8). Maigne (1972, pp. 84, 268) advocated use of a key instead of a finger to induce pressure over the supraspinal ligaments and, therefore, referred to this test as the 'key test' or 'key sign'. This is not to be confused with the 'key lesion' or 'key somatic dysfunction' (ECOP 2011) discussed extensively in the osteopathic literature.

Myofascial point examination

Layer palpation is also effective in identifying various myofascial points. Three specific types of myofascial points merit specific mention: myofascial TrPs empirically mapped by Travell and Simons (Simons et al. 1999; Travell and Simons 1992); myofascial tender points used in Jones' system of strain–counterstrain (Jones et al. 1995); and myofascial reflex points empirically mapped out by Chapman (Owens 1963).

- **Myofascial TrPs:** Scanning for TrPs involves adequate pressure in flat muscles and pincer grip in certain other muscles to look for the presence of tenderness and tissue texture changes, including a taut muscle band. The subject typically experiences exquisite tenderness that is most prominent over the TrP nodule found in this palpable taut band of muscle. Quickly drawing the finger across this site perpendicular to the taut band (a 'snapping palpation') typically elicits a local muscular twitch response. Pressure on an active TrP site typically elicits ('triggers') or exacerbates a distant pain pattern and occasionally provokes an autonomic response consistent for that muscular TrP. As with most palpatory findings, inter-examiner reliability for TrPs is at its highest when there has been specific training and calibration of the examiners (Mense and Simons 2001). Kappa values (see Chapter 3) have been shown to vary from muscle to muscle, depending on a variety of factors including depth of the muscle palpated and experience of the palpating hand (Gerwin et al. 1997; Sciotti et al. 2001).

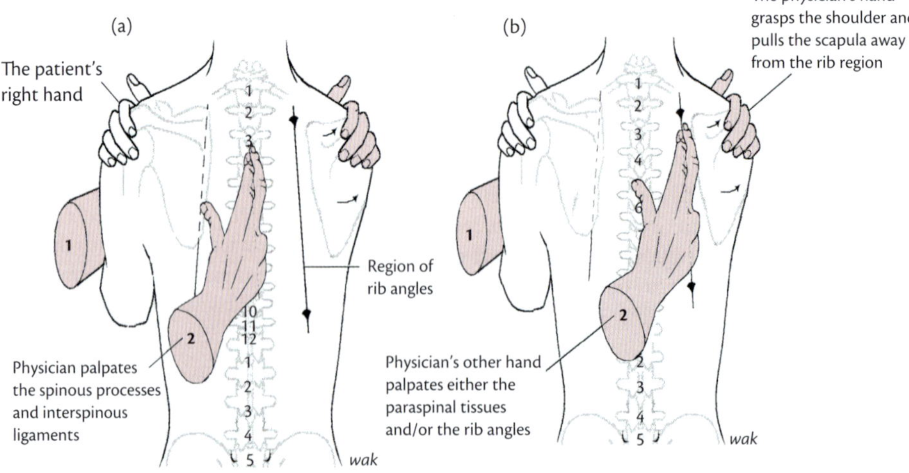

Figure 27.8 (a) Palpating spinal processes; (b) paraspinal and rib angle palpation.

- **Jones' tender points:** Part of Jones' counterstrain diagnostic and therapeutic system, these points are located near bony attachments of tendons or ligaments, or in muscle bellies. They are also discovered through pressure over these sites. Palpably, they are described as small, tense, oedematous, and locally tender areas. Unlike TrPs, they do not trigger pain to some distant site. Careful questioning, however, often uncovers the history of prolonged or awkward shortening of the muscle harbouring the tender point. Both Simons (1991) and Myers (2012) describe significant overlapping locations in the tender point and TrP system maps. Kuchera (2012) points out that each meets the definition of somatic dysfunction and Chaitow (1987) also believes that their distinction is arbitrary. Nonetheless, the empirical diagnostic and manual treatment system described by Jones is easily learned and applied.
- **Chapman's reflex points:** A third myofascial point system of interest is attributed to Chapman (Patriquin 1997). These are correlated with reflex somatic change initiated by dysfunction of viscera (Kuchera 2012; Washington et al. 2003). These points have many of the same palpatory characteristics and tenderness as Jones' points. Therefore, questioning and other physical examination to begin to differentiate between somatic and visceral underlying causes must follow finding a positive tender point in certain locations. Like Jones' and Travell points, Chapman reflex point scanning employs pressure over empirically mapped points of the system. Superimposing maps of the Chapman, Jones', Travell, and even acupuncture systems reveals a significant overlap in location and clinical relevance (Kuchera 2012). The anterior points in the Chapman system (Figure 27.9) are generally much more tender to palpation than posterior points and more likely to be used for viscerosomatic diagnosis than posterior points. Unlike Jones' and Travell points, Chapman points are secondary forms of somatic dysfunction. Patients with Chapman points are less likely to present with primary musculoskeletal complaints and often present with visceral symptoms.

In all three systems, scanning palpation assesses sensation and tissue texture characteristics. Each system of myofascial points is well mapped out and a physician's knowledge of the common tender points for each speeds the diagnostic evaluation and eventual treatment. Differential scanning of a region for TrPs, tender points, and/or viscerosomatic reflex points follows largely from the screening clinical history, presenting complaints, and elicitable mechanism of injury or overuse (see Table 27.1).

Alternatively, a myofascial tender point scan may be initiated because the screening examination revealed variations from ideal posture. Both Travell's and Jones' myofascial points have been associated with articular somatic dysfunction (Kuchera 1997a; Glover and Yates 1997), and their discovery in a scanning process therefore warrants further specific diagnosis. Chapman reflex points are referred from organ dysfunctions, and each organ or group of organs has a differing but predictable pattern of associated articular and soft tissue dysfunction (Kuchera and Kuchera 1994). Conversely, both Jones' tender points and Travell's TrPs are specific diagnoses in themselves, constituting branch points for various therapeutic options where identified.

Regional and segmental scan or screen

The analysis of the systems of myofascial points and articular dysfunction pioneered by various neuromusculoskeletal practitioners

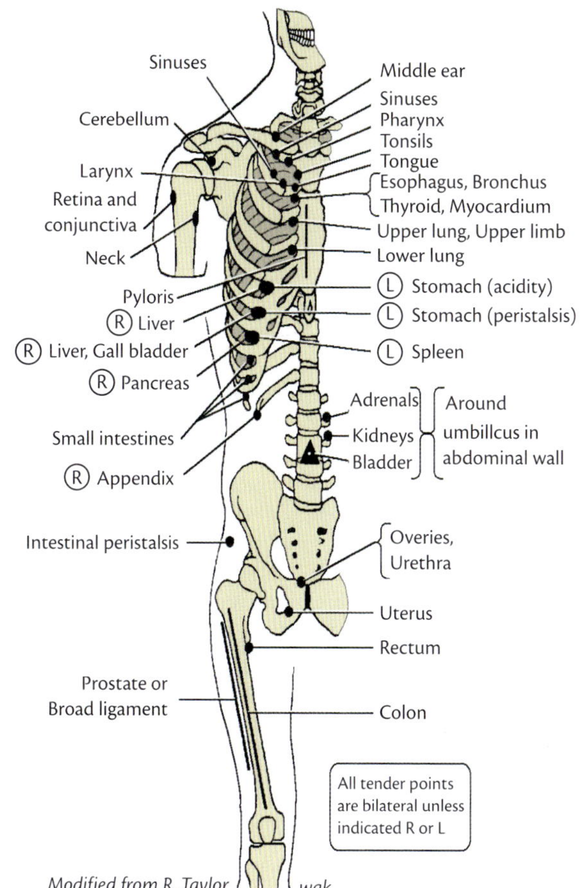

Figure 27.9 Anterior Chapman's points. All are bilateral except where indicated as R for right and L for left. (From Kuchera and Kuchera 1994.)

provides significant clinical insight, regardless of their underlying proposed origin. It reinforces the clinical utility of careful observation and palpation of the musculoskeletal system when looking for clues to differential diagnosis. Each system views the body as an interconnected unit with all parts and systems working together. Each expresses a common goal: the identification and treatment of somatic elements to re-establish normal functional characteristics that promote beneficial changes in the body's homeostatic mechanisms.

Scanning for motion restriction can be quickly and efficiently applied to regions or specific segments. In evaluating transitional regions of the body (craniocervical junction, cervicothoracic junction, thoracolumbar junction, and lumbopelvic junction), the fascial tissues of each junctional region may be manually engaged (Figure 27.10). Each area is rotated and/or translated to the point where the tissues begin to tighten. Fascial drag and ease are noted. Asymmetrical motion characteristics in any region are considered a positive test result. Often, the pattern of restriction from region to region provides as much insight into the underlying dysfunction as the individual regional restriction. Alternating fascial patterns are usually compensatory and may be relatively asymptomatic. Fascial patterns whose regional directions of restriction do not alternate from one transition zone to the next are said to be *noncompensated*, and are often traumatically induced and/or symptomatic (Kuchera 1995c).

Alternating side to side pressures over vertebral transverse processes and/or alternating left–right translational pressures can also

Table 27.1 Suspicious history, physical, or screening examination findings

Region	History	Physical/screening examination
All regions	Significant trauma (e.g. motor vehicle accident or fall)	Pelvic shear somatic dysfunctions
	Recurrent microtrauma (occupational, habitual)	Unlevel sacral base; small hemipelvis and/or short lower extremity
	General aches and/or pain	Postural asymmetry
		Gait disorder
		Dudley J. Morton foot
Head/craniocervical junction	Headaches (any type)	+ Screen/scan tests:
	Dizziness/vertigo/ataxia	Regional S.T.A.R. findings
	Atypical facial pain	Non-parallel mastoid and occipital planes; head, face, jaw, or ear angle asymmetry
	EENT symptoms (e.g. sinus conditions, tinnitus, baroacusis, recurrent otitis media, strabismus diplopia)	Forward-head posture
		Fullness in supraclavicular area
		Asymmetric or low amplitude CRI
	Tooth/jaw symptoms (e.g. tooth pain, bruxism, jaw popping/pain)	Ataxic gait
		Fullness in supraclavicular area
	Asthma	Abnormal cranial nerve testing
	Ataxia, especially with concomitant travel sickness	Sacral somatic dysfunction
		Eustachian tube dysfunction
		Strabismus; extraocular muscle weakness
		Sternocleidomastoid or trapezius TrPs
		High arch palate and narrow dental arch
		Dysfunction/disease of EENT, sinuses, heart, respiratory tract, and/or upper GI system (Kuchera 1998)
Lower cervicals, CT junction, superior thoracic inlet	Headaches (any type)	+ Screen/scan tests:
	Symptoms of EENT, cardiac, pulmonary, or upper	Regional S.T.A.R. findings
	GI disorders	Cervical *pointe sonnette* (cervical doorbell) sign
	Postural dizziness, vertigo, nausea	Mandibular skin-rolling test
	Inertial injury	Maigne key test
	Habitual or occupational accentuated cervical posturing or compression over trapezius muscle(s)	Acromion drop test
		Supine thoracoabdominal passive inhalation observation
		Ataxic gait
	Cervical crepitus, esp. with discomfort	Sternocleidomastoid or trapezius TrPs
	Significant coughing Recurrent or prolonged singultus (hiccoughs)	Neurological findings in upper extremity(ies), esp. aggravated by Valsalva or cervical position
	Upper extremity paresthesias or dysesthesias aggravated by cervical or arm positions	+ Cervical compression test
		+ Upper extremity deep tendon reflexes
	Upper extremity vascular or sympathetic instability symptoms including Raynaud's phenomenon, finger swelling, cold/sweaty palm(s)	Loss of radial pulse with any of several provoking cervical or shoulder positions
		Signs of ENT, heart, and/or respiratory tract disorder (Patterson and Burn 1985)
	Ataxia, especially with concomitant travel sickness	
Thoracics, thoracic cage	History of chest wall trauma or significant motor vehicle accident while wearing a shoulder strap	+ Screen/scan tests: Regional S.T.A.R. findings
	Prolonged use of steroids or NSAIDs	Postural asymmetry; flattened or increased thoracic kyphotic curve; rotoscoliosis
	Chest wall pain, esp. if aggravated by coughing, sneezing, or side-bending	Maigne key test
		Asymmetric 'shingle test' of Kuchera (Kuchera and Kuchera 2012)1
	Chest pain in a dermatomal pattern	Spring test over anterior and lateral rib cage

Table 27.1 (Continued) Suspicious history, physical, or screening examination findings

Region	History	Physical/screening examination
	Visceral symptoms (e.g. gastritis, irritable bowel dysfunction, hypertension, cardiac dysrhythmia, dysmenorrhea), esp. if aggravated by stress	Supine passive inhalation efforts failing to extend to pubic region
		Anterior intercostal Chapman points
		Tender fullness over abdominal collateral ganglion sites
		Pectus excavatum or pectus carinatum
		Skin eruptions in dermatomal pattern
		Quadratus lumborum TrP or spasm
		Puffy fingers or hands
		Objective findings of cardiovascular, gastrointestinal, kidney, lung, ovarian or uterine disorder
Thoracolumbar junction, inferior thoracic outlet, lumbars	History or symptoms of visceral dysfunction originating in the lower urinary system, the descending colon, sigmoid colon, rectum, uterus, or prostate	+ Screen/scan tests:
		Regional S.T.A.R. findings
	Irritable bowel syndrome or a tendency towards constipation when stressed	Postural asymmetry; reduced or increased lumbar lordosis; rotoscoliosis; inability to stand upright or pelvic side-shift
	Recurrent or chronic low back pain	Supine passive inhalation efforts failing to extend to pubic region
	Inability to stand upright; recurrent psoas posturing	Straight lumbar curve on hip drop test
	Systemic congestive phenomena	+ Skin rolling over buttocks (Elkiss et al. 1997)
	Pain, dysesthesia, or other symptoms that radiate from the low back into one or both lower extremities	+ Thomas test for psoas
		Spondylolisthesis drop-off sign
		Short leg syndrome or small hemipelvis
		Palpable quadratus lumborum TrPs, tender iliopsoas points within pelvic brim
		Spinous process spondylolisthesis drop-off sign or a tuft of deep tendon reflex
		+ Lasegue's test (straight leg raising)
		+ Trendelenburg test
		Abnormal LE muscle strength testing
		Objective findings of lower GI or GU disorder; lower lobe pneumonic signs
Lumbopelvic junction, pelvis (sacroiliacs, sacrococcygeal, and pubic symphysis)	Low back pain ± lower extremity radiation	+ Screen/scan tests:
	Postpartum headache, depression or excessive fatigue; other symptom related to pregnancy/postpartum period	Regional S.T.A.R. findings
		Seated and/or standing flexion tests
		Stork test (aka Gillet's or march/stork test)
	Pelvic floor complaints (dyspareunia, prostatodynia, menstrual bloating, haemorrhoids, pelvic floor spasm)	+ Pelvic side shift test
		+ Supine long sitting test
	Enuresis, urinary frequency	+ SI joint stress/spring tests (thigh thrust, cranial shear, sacral thrust, SI gapping)
	Buttock trauma and/or pratfalls	
	Auto accident while bracing lower extremity; pelvic bruising by seat belt	+ Hip rotation test
	Lifting injury in an awkward position	+ Thigh thrust SI stress test (aka posterior pelvic pain provocation test)
	Twisting movements while weight-bearing	+ Yeoman's test
	Onset of problem after sit-ups or falling asleep in a soft recliner	+ Gaenslen's test
		+ Trendelenburg test
		Postural asymmetry; reduced or increased lumbar lordosis; rotoscoliosis; inability to stand upright or pelvic side-shift; unlevel iliac crests, greater trochanters, sacral base
		Spondylolisthesis drop-off sign
		Supine passive inhalation efforts failing to extend to pubic region
		Short leg syndrome or small hemipelvis
		Spinous process spondylolisthesis drop-off sign or a tuft of hair over lumbars

(*Continued*)

Table 27.1 (Continued) Suspicious history, physical, or screening examination findings

Region	History	Physical/screening examination
		Abnormal neurological exam or reduced lower extremity deep tendon reflex
		+ Lasegue's test (straight leg raising)
		+ Trendelenburg test
		Abnormal muscle strength testing
		Objective findings of lower GI or GU disorder; lower lobe pneumonic signs
Lower extremities	Lower extremity pain or dysesthesia with or without low back pain	+ Screen/scan tests:
	'Buckling knee'	Regional S.T.A.R. findings
	Leg cramps	Postural asymmetry
	'Restless legs'	Gait disturbance
	'Growing pains'	Inability to deep squat and return
	Recurrent ankle sprains	Tight, ticklish, tender inguinal area; fullness in popliteal area; fullness around Achilles tendon
	Foot drop	Abnormal sole wear pattern
	History of inappropriate footwear	Coxa and/or genu varus/valgus; increased Q angle; pronated or supinated foot
		Heel spur
		Patellar grind with compression
		Foot calluses, hammertoes, bunions
		Somatic dysfunction T11–L2
		Abnormal neurological exam or reduced lower extremity deep tendon reflex
		+ Lasegue's test (straight leg raising)
		+ Trendelenburg test
		Lower extremity muscle weakness
		+ Tinel's over fibular head
		Abnormal orthopaedic exam (lower extremity)
		+ Patrick-Fabere (aka Figure 4) test with ligament stress
		+ Drawer, pivot-shift, valgus/varus stress tests of knee
		+ Ant. ankle drawer test
Upper extremities	Upper extremity pain or dysesthesia with or without cervical pain Repetitious habitual or occupational upper extremity motion Reduced grip strength	+ Screen/scan tests:
		Regional S.T.A.R. findings
		Postural asymmetry
		Shoulder girdle ROM screen
		Elbow spring tests (extension, valgus, and varus) Posterior axillary fold tissue texture abnormalities Abnormal neurological exam or reduced upper extremity deep tendon reflex
		+ Tinel's at wrist or ulnar groove
		+ Phalen's test
		T2–8 somatic dysfunction
Abdomen	Visceral symptoms (e.g. gastritis, irritable bowel dysfunction, constipation, dysmenorrhoea) esp. if aggravated by stress Inability to stand upright; recurrent psoas posturing Onset of problem after sit-ups or falling asleep in a soft recliner	+ Screen/scan tests:
		Regional S.T.A.R. findings
		Postural asymmetry; flattened or increased thoracic kyphotic curve; rotoscoliosis; psoas posturing
		Supine passive inhalation efforts failing to extend to pubic region
		Anterior intercostal Chapman points
		Tender fullness over abdominal collateral ganglion sites Weakness of abdominal muscle testing
		Recurrent somatic dysfunction of OA–C2, T5–L2, and/or sacroiliac regions
		Objective findings of cardiovascular, gastrointestinal, kidney, lung, ovarian, or uterine disorder

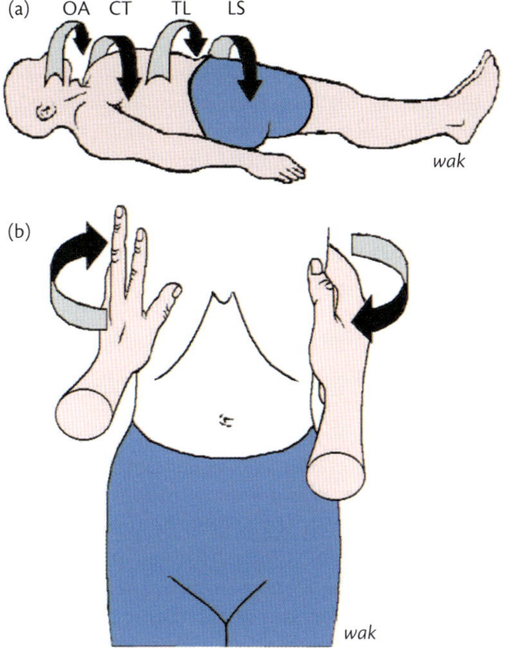

Figure 27.10 (a) Total body fascial pattern with common compensatory pattern (seen in 80% of asymptomatic people) depicted; (b) testing rotation of the fascias at the thoracolumbar region (inferior thoracic outlet), rotation right preference depicted.

be used as a quick scan for segmental restriction of rotation and side-bending motion, respectively (Figure 27.11). A positive scan for vertebral somatic dysfunction reveals restriction in one direction and freedom of motion in the opposite direction. Zygopophyseal tenderness is often elicited on the restricted side (Paterson and Burn 1985, p. 144). Significant regional asymmetrical restriction or tenderness identified in this manner should be examined more completely on a local (segmental) basis.

Another scanning technique for either regional or segmental motion involves springing the test sites. Typically, the heel of the hand or a thumb is gently positioned, depending on the amount of area to be tested. Gradual pressure is applied, compressing soft tissues that overlie the deeper tissues being evaluated. A springing force is then gently applied seeking to assess the quality of the end-feel barrier. A positive *springing test* is recorded if the tissues have an abrupt rather than a physiological resilient end-feel. This form of testing is commonly applied over ribs, vertebral spinous processes, poles of the sacrum, and ASIS (Figure 27.12). Comparing left to right side, a springing test may provide a *lateralization test* for naming dysfunction. In some manual medicine models, elicited tenderness rather than restricted motion constitutes a positive scan test for regional or segmental springing.

Local examinations of vertebral somatic dysfunction

Common principles and methods govern clinically meaningful segmental examinations of the vertebral column. Because of the anatomical structure of typical vertebral units and their articulations, segmental motion characteristics in each region of the spine follow certain general physiological motion parameters (Kuchera 2002). Physiological motion affecting the typical cervical segments C2–7 has been documented to involve coupled side-bending and rotation to the same side in all cervical positions. Conversely, physiological motion in the thoracic and lumbar regions has been shown to depend upon sagittal plane position when the patient's motion occurred. Thoracic and lumbar side-bending and rotation occur to the same side when the vertebral unit facets are engaged, as in extreme forward or backward bending. In the 'easy neutral' positions between these two extremes, side-bending to one side in these regions automatically induces rotation to the opposite side.

In the thoracic and lumbar regions, where sagittal plane position modifies the pattern of coupled motion, two types of somatic dysfunction can be differentiated:

- *Type I somatic dysfunction* occurs when the patient is in the easy neutral position and side-bending and rotation occur to opposite sides, usually in groups.
- In *type II somatic dysfunction*, occurring with significant flexion or extension, rotation and side-bending occur at a single segment and to the same side.

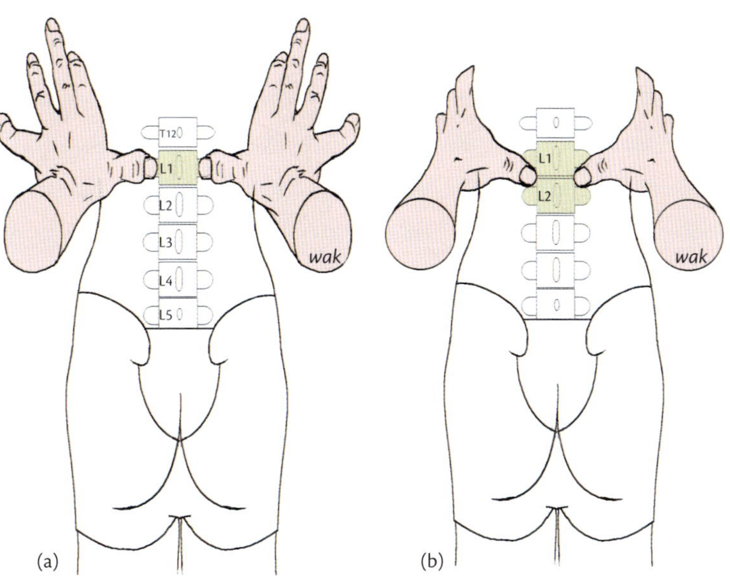

Figure 27.11 Scanning or local tests: (a) testing L1 rotation; (b) testing L1 side-bending. See also figure 27.13a

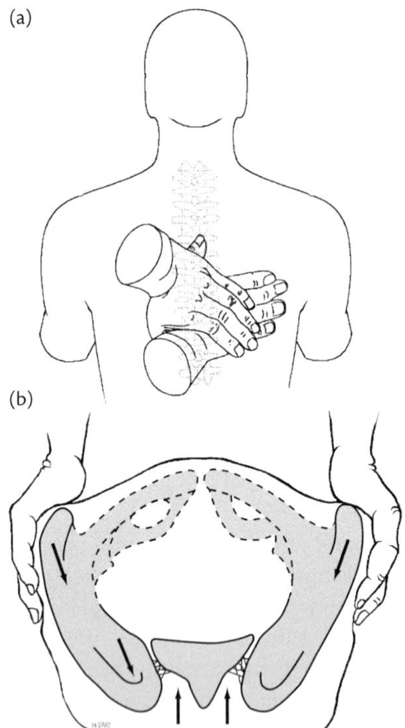

Figure 27.12 (a) Spinal compression for extension screening; (b) ASIS compression test (alternate left then right pressure into respective sacroiliac joint—test is positive on the restricted side.)

In all regions, somatic dysfunction occurring as restricted spinal motion within the physiological range of motion will demonstrate the capability of moving further in the direction associated with initiation of somatic dysfunction and be restricted in the direction that was associated with the starting position.

Generally, type II somatic dysfunctions in the thoracic and lumbar regions are more symptomatic and create more physiological discord by restricting motions associated with normal activities of daily living. For example, consider a situation in which a worker has bent forward enough to significantly engage the facets of his lumbar spine and then tries to move a large box off to the left. If, in the middle of this activity, the box hits a nail in the floor and abruptly arrests the physiological spinal motion that is taking place, the timing or stress might be sufficient to initiate a somatic dysfunction. When the patient tries to return to an upright position, he is likely to experience pain when the somatic dysfunction barrier is reached. That is because this barrier restricts his further backward bending, side-bending right, or rotation right needed to regain his neutral position. Clinically, this discomfort may be provoked every time the patient tries to function in a neutral position. The somatic dysfunction in this example is a type II, single-segment L3 somatic dysfunction. Motion testing would reveal that it prefers to flex, rotate left, and side-bend left.

As previously noted, rotation and/or lateral translation tests may be performed at each level as a scan or used for specific diagnosis of individual spinal levels. To test for the rotational component of somatic dysfunction, the clinician should place the palpating fingers over the left and right articular pillars in the cervical region or over the transverse processes of the thoracic/lumbar vertebral unit in question. Either the patient's active rotation or the physician's induction of passive rotation is used as the physician palpates and assesses the quality of the end-feel of any barrier to motion (Figure 27.13). Additional palpatory information is gained if this is repeated with the spine in both forward-bent and backward-bent positions. In the lateral translation test, assessing side-bending capabilities, the physician places fingertips over the posterolateral aspects of the articular column in the typical cervical region or in the lateral region of the articular facets in the thoracic or lumbar spine. The force is localized to one segmental level and translation is checked in each direction. (Note: translation to the left creates side-bending to the right.) This test can also be performed with the spine in flexion and then repeated in extension. Restriction in left translation (restricted right side-bending) at C5 on C6, worse in extension and coupled with restriction in right rotation, may be

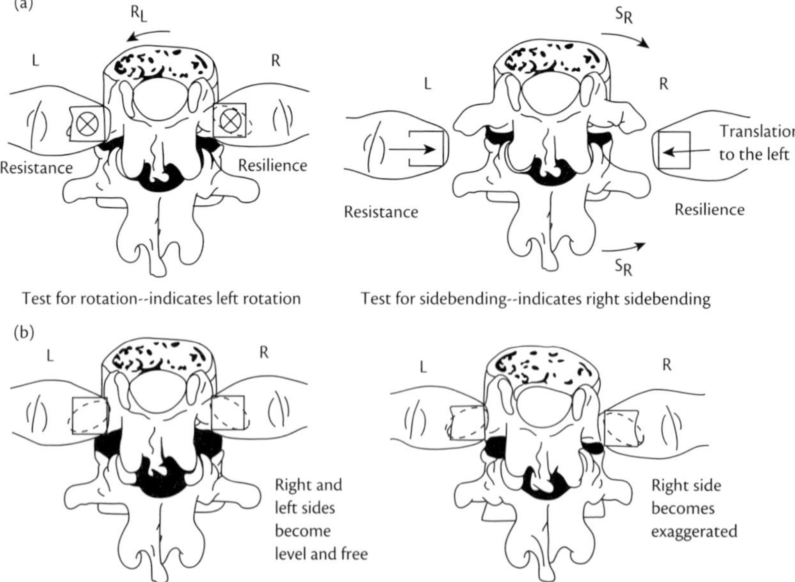

Figure 27.13 Testing for spinal motion: (a) passive testing; (b) active testing.

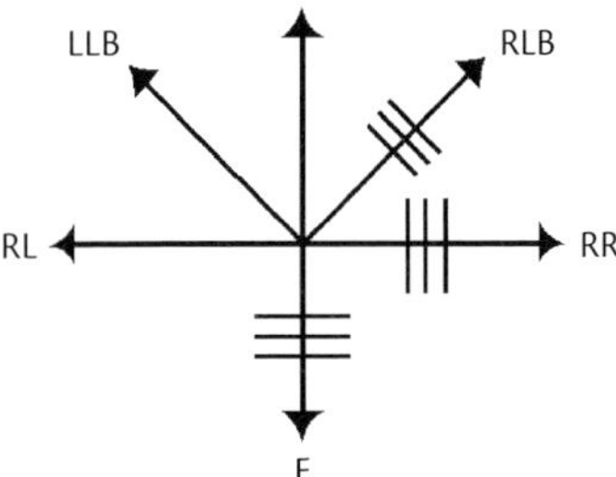

Figure 27.14 Star diagram of Maigne, illustrating the direction in which the patient feels pain. The bars indicate the grade of pain: three bars indicate significant pain, which will correlate with direction of restricted motion. Somatic dysfunction diagnosis: FRLSL. In the Maigne system, manipulation should be considered only when three directions are free of pain when motion is introduced. (Key: F, flexion; E, extension; RL, rotate left; RR, rotate right; LLB, left lateral bend; RLB, right lateral bend.)

recorded as a C5 flexed, side-bent, and rotated left (C5 F RLSL) somatic dysfunction. The Fryette formula for C5 F RLSL somatic dysfunction with pain elicited in the directions where motion is restricted could also be recorded as shown using Maigne's star diagram (Figure 27.14).

Somatic dysfunction overview: indications for specific joint examinations

Clinicians regularly use several of the regional scanning (and some local) examinations for somatic dysfunction described in this chapter as screening examinations. For example, patients presenting with low back pain may be routinely screened with a hip drop test, pelvic side shift test, stork test, and Trendelenburg test. Conversely, screening tests modified to gather more specific information are more properly classified as scanning examinations. Some regional scanning tests, such as skin rolling or palpation for myofascial tender points/TrPs, are easily adapted to provide specific 'local' diagnostic information. The screening, regional scanning, and local tests described in this chapter provide additional insight into the structure and function of various regions or segments of the body.

Appropriately classifying a test as a screening, scanning, or local examination is of little importance compared to properly performing, understanding, and interpreting the information gained. Nonetheless, understanding these artificial classifications helps to shape the eventual patterns of palpatory examination that each manual medicine physician adopts. It also allows physicians and non-physicians to communicate accurately with each other. In the end, the amount of detail sought, its interpretation, and the level of clinical suspicion will influence the selection of any additional examination procedures that will be needed.

With minor adaptations for patient position and consideration of the distinctive regional anatomical variations, the principles, methods, and nomenclature discussed in this overview are applicable in conducting a segmental palpatory examination in every region.

Regional disorders: the role of regional somatic dysfunction

Indications for regional scanning and local palpation of specific somatic regions and their related component parts include the suspicious history, physical, or screening examination findings listed in Table 27.1 (Kuchera and Kuchera 1994; Greenman 1996, p. 166). Although somatic dysfunction plays a significant role in the extremities, this chapter covers only the spinal and pelvic (axial) regions.

Despite the artificial regional grouping of clinical presentations in Table 27.1, regions distant from those that are symptomatic should be considered because of tensegrity principles (Levin 1997) (see Chapter 16) and the body's physiological response as a unit. Compensatory, reflex, and central mechanisms dictate that a change in one region creates dysfunction in adjacent regions. Table 27.2, for example, depicts common combinations of somatic dysfunction associated with common clinical conditions. A single somatic dysfunction (segmental or regional) is unlikely to be the sole cause or consequence of most clinical presentations.

This chapter introduces additional palpatory diagnostic examinations pertinent to each region or condition and applies the diagnostic principles and considerations discussed thus far to conditions commonly encountered in the clinical arena. Considering the number of specific joints and the wide range of clinically relevant conditions, relatively few conditions in each region were selected for presentation. However, each regional part of this section discusses an example of the role of regional somatic dysfunction and at least one neuromusculoskeletal approach to its palpatory diagnosis.

Head and craniocervical junction areas

Regional somatic dysfunction of the head and craniocervical junction initiates a wide range of presenting signs and symptoms, as indicated previously in Table 27.1. Anatomical relationships in this region are capable of significant pain referral as well as autonomic and cranial nerve dysfunction. Furthermore, palpatory diagnostic findings in this section are particularly relevant to common musculoskeletal disorders such as headache and temporomandibular joint dysfunction.

Conversely, examples of reflex relationships between visceral disorders and this region, as discussed in conditions such as sinus disorders (trigeminal reflexes) or gastric disturbances (vagal reflexes), reflect the importance of providing complete differential diagnosis in conjunction with the discovery of somatic dysfunction during the palpatory examination. Diagnosis and manipulative treatment of such secondary somatic dysfunction may provide additional symptomatic care or may even play a role in improving physiological homeostatic mechanisms important in healing (Kuchera and Kuchera 1994; Kuchera and Kuchera 2012).

Certain manual medicine techniques may be inappropriate or contraindicated in some conditions in this region (Kuchera et al. 2002). Therefore, the following should be documented:

- The specific time, mechanism, and extent of head and cervical trauma.
- Prior responses to manual techniques. A history of ataxia, nystagmus, or other significant neurological sequelae to prior manual techniques or cervical trauma may alert the physician to the possibility of a potentially fatal vertebral artery abnormality. (This is discussed further in Chapter 50.)
- Headaches that wake the patient at night, are progressively more severe, or are accompanied by neurological change.
- Evidence or absence of physical findings suggestive of Down syndrome and/or severe rheumatoid arthritis, as these conditions influence manual treatment considerations.

Table 27.2 Examples of multiregional somatic dysfunction complexes in common clinical conditions

Common clinical conditions	Examples of possible associated multiregional somatic dysfunction complexes
Common headache	
(a) left occipitomastoid suture (b) OA = E $S_R R_L$ (c–d) C2–3 = E $R_R S_R$ (e) Travell's points for upper end of semispinalis muscle (f) Travell's points for suboccipital muscle	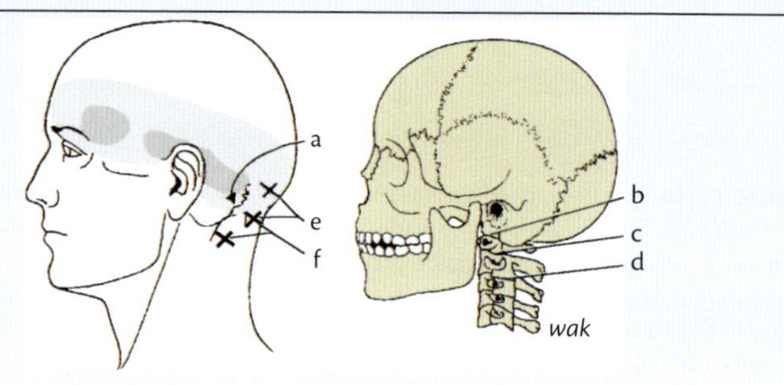
Sternocleidomastoid headache	
(a) right occipitomastoid suture (b) Travell's right sternocleidomastoid TrPs (c) Jones' AC7 point (d) temporomandibular joint dysfunction	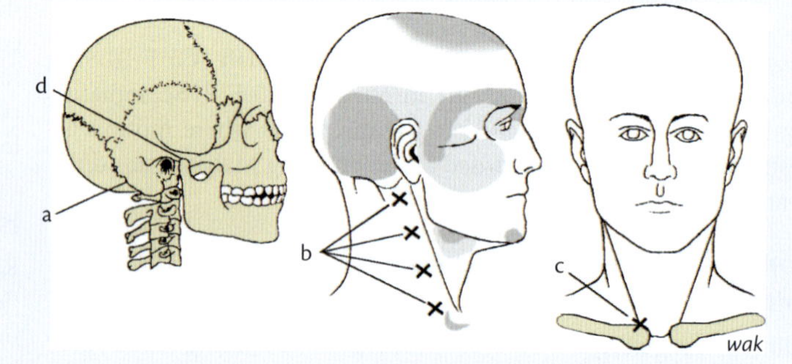
Reactive airway	
(a) extension-type cranium (b, d) left rib 2–3 SD (c) fullness of left supraclavicular region (d) Chapman's point; tender point reference to the bronchus (e) C2 TTC (f) left T1–3 TTC	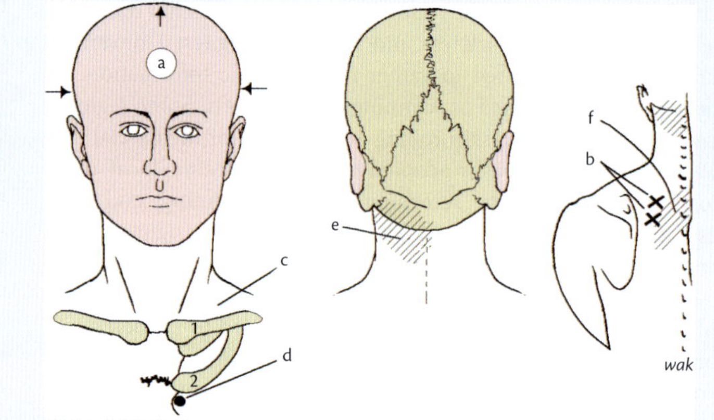
Gastritis	
(a) left C2 TTC (b) left occipitomastoid suture TTC (c) T5 E $R_L S_L$ (d) Travell's external oblique muscle TrP and pain pattern (e) Chapman's stomach and pylorus reflex points (f) celiac ganglion tension (g) epigastric congestion (h) left rib 5 SD (i) postural crossover at T5	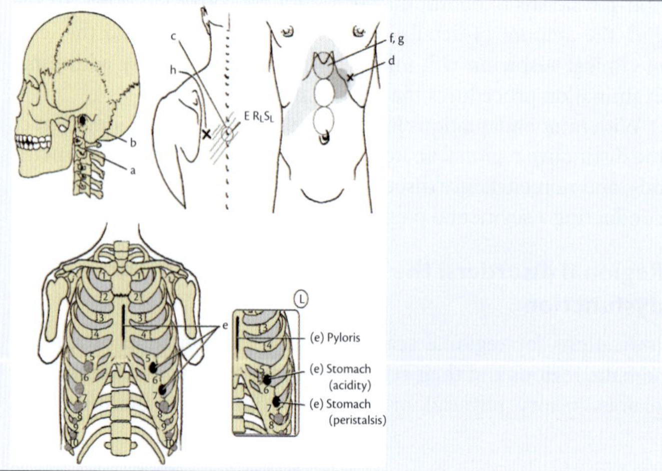

Table 27.2 (Continued) Examples of multiregional somatic dysfunction complexes in common clinical conditions

Common clinical conditions	Examples of possible associated multiregional somatic dysfunction complexes
Irritable bowel dysfunction	
(a) bilateral iliotibial band tenderness and TTC (Chapman's) (b) thoracolumbar SD and TTC (c) left SI TTC (d) post. Chapman's lumbar TTC (low back pain). (e) lower rectus abdominis muscle TrP and pain pattern (f) inferior mesenteric ganglion TTC (g) sigmoid loop palpable	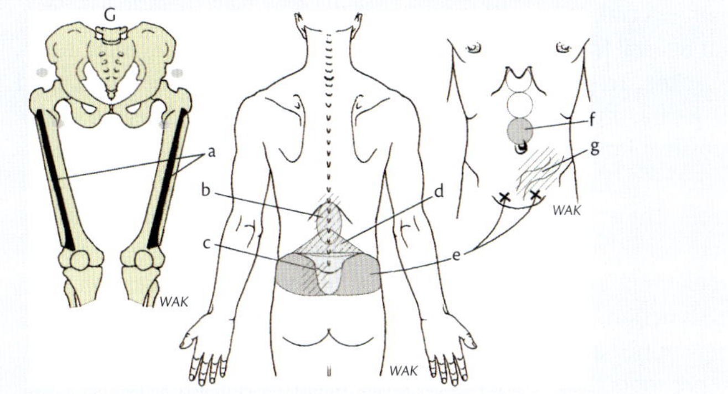
Right carpal tunnel syndrome	
(a) elevated first rib SD (b) thoracic inlet SD (c) right supraclavicular congestion (d) right posterior axillary fold tenderness and TTC (e) generic elbow SD (f) generic wrist SD (g) right paraspinal T2–8 SD (h) scalene TrP and pain patterns of the right arm (i) Jones' CTS points (j) Travell's trigger points: J1, pronator teres; J2, flexor digitorum; J3, flexor carpi radialis; J4, flexor pollicis longus;J5, opponens pollicis	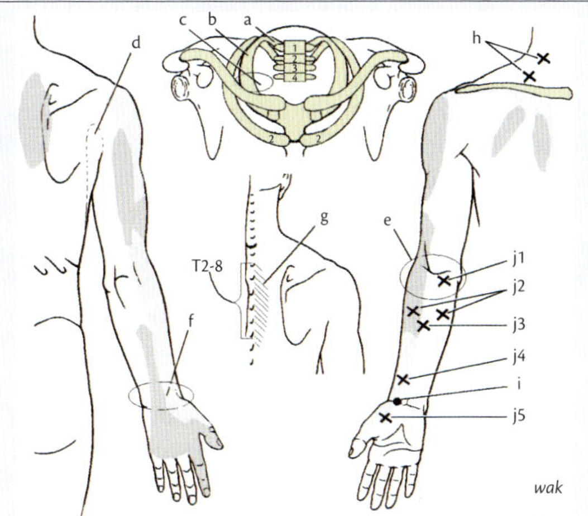
Sprained right ankle	
(a) plantar SD of cuboid and navicular bones (b) posterolateral talus SD (c) externally rotated tibia (d) anteromedial glide of the tibia (e) internally rotated femur (f) posterior right innominate (g) L5 $S_R R_L$ (h) sacrum rotated right on right oblique axis (i) Travell's TrPs	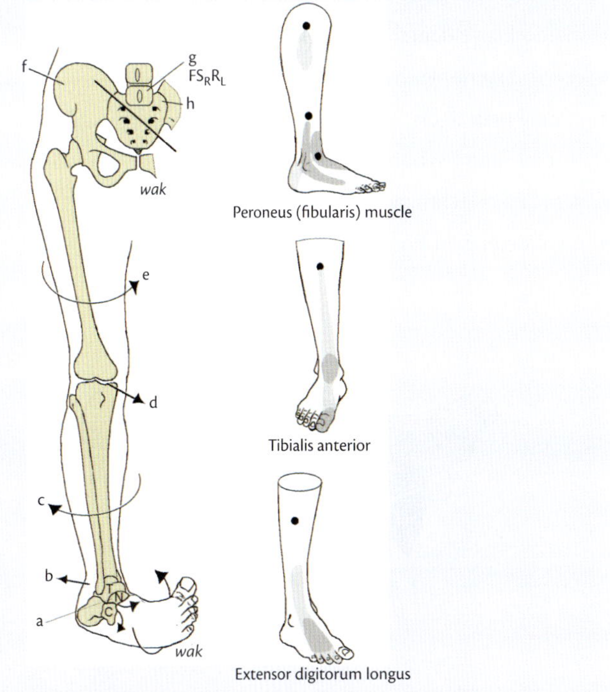

TTC = tissue texture change; TrP = trigger point; SD = somatic dysfunction; CTS = carpal tunnel syndrome; SI = sacroiliac

Head area

Headache is the most common pain-presenting complaint in the USA and among the most frequent complaints of patients presenting for any problem to both generalists and neurologists.

Many structures of the head are pain-sensitive or are capable of pain referral. Pain in this region of the body can result from afferent referral from eyes, ears, sinuses, temporomandibular joint, teeth, pharynx, respiratory tract, heart, and upper gastrointestinal tract as well as musculoskeletal referral from the cervical region. Pain-sensitive intracranial structures include the venous sinuses, the arteries of both the pia-arachnoid and the dura mater, and the dura itself. There are also a number of extracranial structures that are pain-sensitive including skin, myofascial structures, regional articulations, arteries, and the cranial periosteum. Nociception from dysfunction, displacement, or encroachment on these structures is transmitted along cranial nerves V, VII, IX, and X as well as cervical nerve roots from C2 and C3. Even when head pain is not of musculoskeletal origin, secondary somatic dysfunction may result from repeated muscular splinting and positional compensations that the patient makes to reduce pain (Simons et al. 1999, p. 254). Differential diagnoses therefore require evaluation of each of these structures.

Differential diagnosis should attempt to separate life-threatening causes from those that limit quality of life, structural from functional causes, and primary from referred causes. The neuromusculoskeletal physician must be expert at this differential, current in management skills, and have the capability of treating functional causes and sequelae while decreasing pain and increasing the patient's quality of life.

Headache management by physicians trained in neuromusculoskeletal diagnosis and the value of treating related somatic dysfunction in this condition is well established (Kuchera 1998; Paterson and Burn 1985; Simons et al. 1999, pp. 237–77). Other such conditions in this region commonly managed or co-managed by the neuromusculoskeletal practitioner include (Elkiss and Rentz 1997):

- temporomandibular joint dysfunction
- atypical facial pain
- malocclusive dental syndromes
- cervical spine syndromes
- cranial neuralgias
- cranial suture syndrome
- nerve encroachment syndrome
- myofascial pain syndromes.

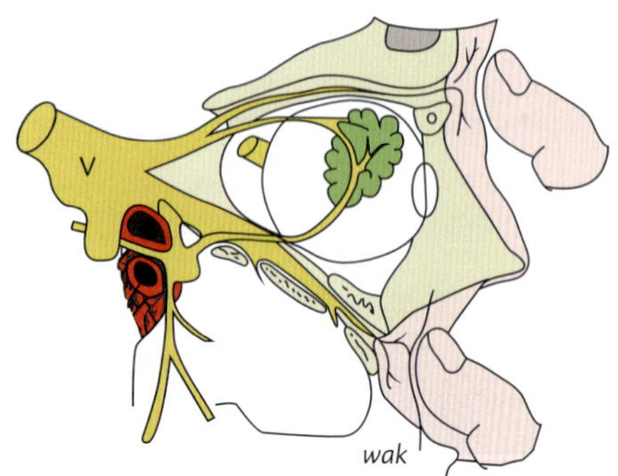

Figure 27.15 Palpation of supraorbital and infraorbital branches of trigeminal nerve for tissue texture change or tenderness.

Each of these conditions deserves careful screening, scanning, and where indicated, local diagnosis and management of regional somatic dysfunction. Regardless of other diagnoses, myofascial pain due to TrPs is likely to contribute to and complicate management of most chronic pain complaints in the region (Simons et al. 1999, p. 256). Specific tissue texture scanning for myofascial tender points and TrPs is, therefore, very productive. In patients presenting with headaches, temporomandibular joint pain and/or dysfunction, atypical facial pain, sinus pain and/or dysfunction, toothache, dental occlusal disharmony, eustachian tube dysfunction, difficulty in swallowing, tinnitus, and/or visual disturbances, Travell and Simons advocate searching for TrPs using pressure over specific cranial muscle sites (Simons et al. 1999, pp. 329–96, 416–31). These authors point out that 'it is important to remember that a systematic and thorough examination of *all* of the head and neck muscles looking for active and latent myofascial TrPs is essential for complete evaluation of any persistent or chronic head and neck pain complaint'.

Greenman also advocates palpating the skull itself, scanning for resiliency in general, noting that normal bone has a characteristic pliability that is lost in the presence of motion restriction (Greenman 1996, p. 166). Pressure applied over the supraorbital or infraorbital foramina (Figure 27.15) often reveals both tenderness and oedematous change when visceral afferents facilitate the trigeminal nerve, as in a case of sinusitis (Kuchera and Kuchera 2012). Pressure can also be applied to scan regional articulations such as the cranial sutures. Scanning palpation of the head region can begin with the application of pressure over or across sutures looking for tenderness and/or tension as well as widening or narrowing of

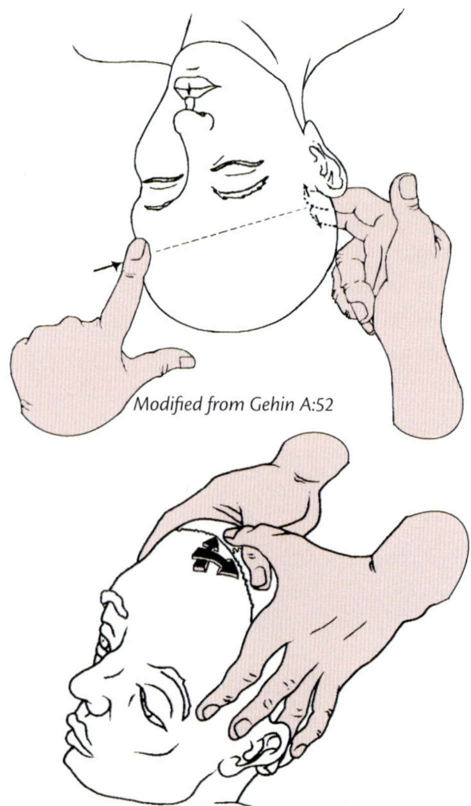

Figure 27.16 (a) Occipitomastoid suture spread with fluid force; (b) V-spread of sagittal suture of skull.
(Gehin, A., Atlas of manipulative techniques for the cranium and face (1985). Eastland Press, Seattle, WA.)

the sutural sites (Greenman 1996, p. 166). This is especially useful in planning treatment for patients with dizziness, posterior headaches, or functional symptoms associated with the upper respiratory, cardiac, or upper gastrointestinal systems. In these patients, there is oedematous tissue texture change over the occipitomastoid suture and it is frequently tender to palpation (Kuchera and Kuchera 2012). Interparietal sutural somatic dysfunction often extends the typical tension headache pattern to include the vertex along the sagittal suture. Patients scanned by applying pressure across a sagittal suture with somatic dysfunction typically experience a pain of 'ice-pick' intensity at the site of the restriction (Figure 27.16).

Examine the temporomandibular joint and the masseter muscles more closely if there is a positive postural screen for anterior head positioning, Dudley J. Morton foot (Simons et al. 1999, p. 337), or short leg syndrome—especially if accompanied by a history of jaw clicking, temporomandibular joint pain, tinnitus, or problems chewing. Asking the patient to open and close the mouth while simultaneously observing and palpating the region may further scan for the aetiology of these latter symptoms. Mandibular opening in an adult should be 40–60 mm (normally admitting a tier of two to three knuckles between the incisor teeth) (Simons et al. 1999, pp. 256–67, 329–48) and should be symmetrical. Watch for jaw deviation and listen or palpate for a click emanating from either joint.

Palpate the lateral poles of each temporomandibular joint by applying pressure with fingertips immediately anterior to the tragus of the ear as well as palpating the retrodiscal tissues by placing fifth digits just inside the ear (Figure 27.17). In a positive scanning examination for dysfunction or pathology, the jaw will deviate and/or be restricted in its range of motion. Deviation is toward the side of a restriction (pathological or dysfunctional) of the temporomandibular joint itself, toward the side of a temporal bone with external rotation somatic dysfunction, and away from an internally rotated temporal bone (Kappler and Ramey 1997, pp. 538–9). Sphenoid dysfunction also may affect the temporomandibular joint through the influence of the sphenomandibular ligament. If asymmetric jaw deviation goes away when the patient opens the mouth with tongue placed high on the hard palate, the lateral pterygoid muscle is often the source of the patient's dysfunction (Simons et al. 1999).

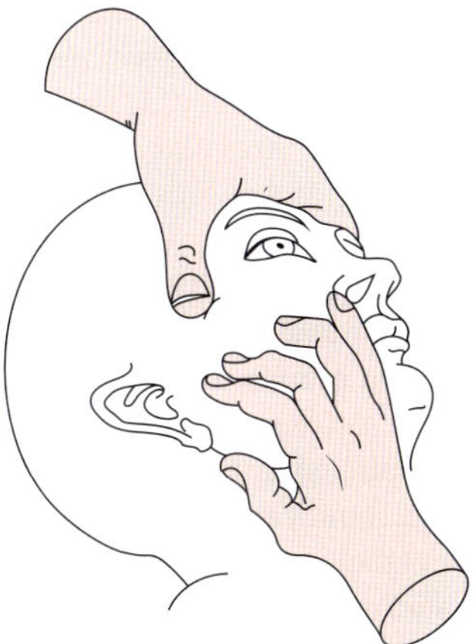

Figure 27.17 Palpation of temporomandibular joint with index finger anterior to the tragus. Note any asymmetry of tracking or clicking as mouth opens and closes.

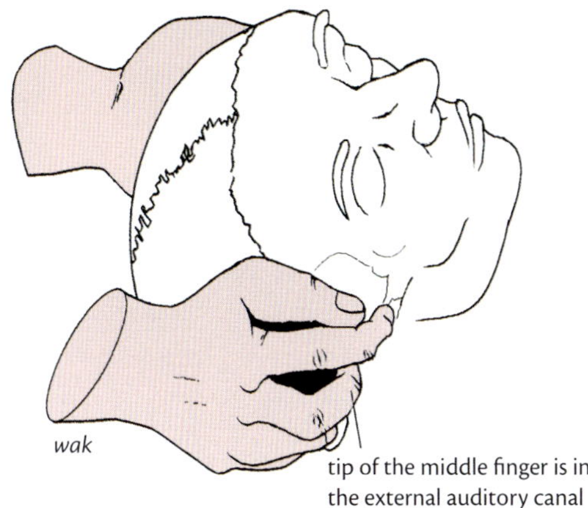
wak
tip of the middle finger is in the external auditory canal

Figure 27.18 Temporal lift.

There are multiple causes for temporomandibular joint dysfunction, and a positive scanning examination of the temporomandibular joint should be followed with local diagnosis for articular somatic dysfunction of the sphenoid, temporal bones, and mandible, and for myofascial somatic dysfunction of the posterior temporalis, lateral pterygoid, masseter, digastric, and buccinator muscles.

The temporal bone has justifiably been named 'the troublemaker of the head' (Magoun 1974) because of its structural and functional connections. A more detailed scan or local diagnosis for temporal bone somatic dysfunction is especially indicated with a patient's history of dizziness or vertigo, strabismus, Bell's palsy, trigeminal neuralgia, headache, swallowing or suckling disorders, otitis media, acute torticollis, and temporomandibular joint dysfunction. In this author's experience, myofascial TrPs in the sternocleidomastoid or trapezius muscles may fail to respond to conventional treatment until dysfunction of the temporal bone (especially at the occipitomastoid suture) is first diagnosed and treated. Magoun claims that functional disorders of the temporal bones may be responsible for affecting 9 of the 12 cranial nerves—excluding only the olfactory, optic, and hypoglossal nerves.

Greenman describes a *temporal lift* scanning examination to assess temporal somatic dysfunction (Greenman 1996, p. 166). With the patient supine, each temporal bone is gently grasped with the middle finger in the external auditory meatus, the thumb and index finger on the superior and inferior aspect of the zygomatic process respectively, and the mastoid process between the fourth and fifth digits (Figure 27.18). In the scan, each temporal is gently pulled toward the vertex and then allowed to settle back to its neutral position. A positive scan for dysfunction is indicated by restriction in joint play on one or both sides. This same hand position (the temporal hold) is used for specific diagnosis of either internal or external rotation somatic dysfunction of a temporal bone (Magoun 1976; Kuchera and Kuchera 2012).

Scanning or more detailed palpation of the frontal bone and its membranous attachments is indicated in a variety of conditions. This is especially true when there is a history of a blow to the forehead, headaches (especially sinus and following lumbar puncture), and post-traumatic alteration of smell, including smelling scents that are not present. In the supine patient, with the physician seated at the patient's head, a *frontal lift* can be either a scanning examination or can be modified into a treatment modality (discussed in

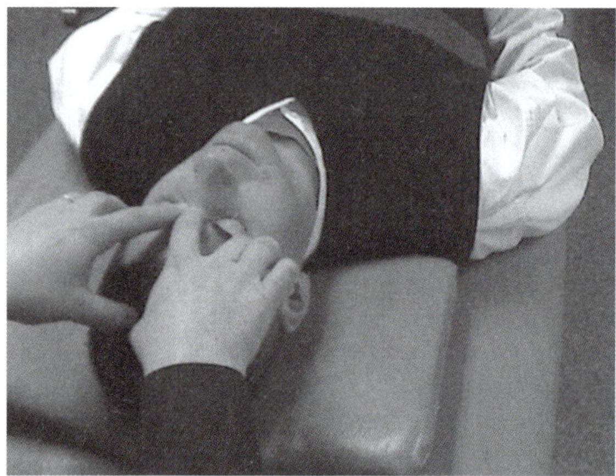

Figure 27.19 Frontal lift.

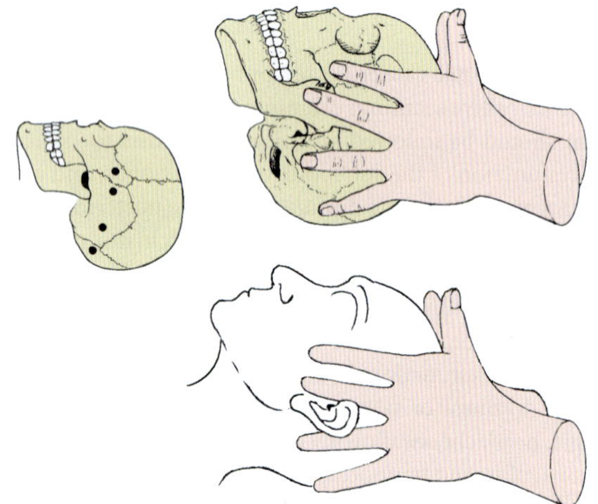

Figure 27.20 Vault hold.

Chapter 50). For this lift, the frontal bone is gently grasped with the index fingers approximated over the glabella and the ring fingers at the lateral aspect of the brow on the orbital portions of the frontal bone. Thumbs are crossed in such a fashion as to provide a controlled lifting pivot (Figure 27.19). The manoeuvre begins with ring fingers slightly compressing toward the centre of the patient's head. The physician then applies a gentle anterior lift (toward the ceiling for a supine patient) of the frontal bone by elevating both ring fingers and pivoting around both thumbs and index fingers. Like the temporal lift, any restriction in joint play constitutes a positive screen for frontal bone somatic dysfunction. Furthermore, when this lift is held at a point of balanced membranous tension, if the patient experiences relief of headache and/or has a sensation of opening of the sinuses, then further palpatory diagnosis of the cranial bones or reciprocal tension membranes is warranted.

The *vault hold* of the cranium provides an extremely useful scanning examination of the cranial base and vault, and many neuromusculoskeletal physicians use it as a general screening examination. The physician sits comfortably and relaxed at the patient's head with forearms resting on the table and fingers relaxed. Hand placement in the supine patient is specific, with index fingers monitoring the sphenoid, fifth digits monitoring the occiput, and the middle two fingers on either side of the ear monitoring the temporal bones (Figure 27.20). The palpable motion sensation, termed the *cranial rhythmic impulse* (CRI), normally has an amplitude of 40 μm to 1.5 mm and a rate of 10–14/minute (Kappler and Ramey 1997, p. 515–40). Altered CRI amplitude, rate, and/or asymmetrical motion indicate a positive scan warranting further palpatory diagnosis. Amplitude has traditionally been believed to be a general indicator of a patient's vitality, but has been the focus of less study than rate or symmetry pattern.

Specific palpatory diagnosis of sphenobasilar somatic dysfunction can be accomplished with the same vault hold previously described. Both passive palpatory monitoring and active motion test assessments of the position as well as inherent motion of midline bones are possible with this hold. Normal palpatory findings include symmetrical movement into flexion and extension while paired bones move into external and internal rotation respectively. Static and dynamic asymmetry or generalized, severely restricted motion indicates somatic dysfunction of the sphenobasilar synchondrosis; dysfunction patterns are illustrated in Figure 27.21.

More detail in diagnosing myofascial somatic dysfunction and TrPs of the head, scanning of facial bone articular dysfunction, or even the specific diagnosis of other cranial bones is beyond the scope of this chapter. Trigger points are covered more completely in Chapter 57. For detailed information about the Sutherland approach to diagnosis and treatment in this region, refer to other standard texts such as *Osteopathy in the cranial field* (Magoun 1976). For a clinical, integrated neuromusculoskeletal approach, the reader is referred to *Osteopathic considerations in HEENT disorders: head, eye, ear, nose, throat* (Kuchera and Kuchera 2012).

Craniocervical junction area

The craniocervical junction includes the occipital condyles and squama, the atlas, the axis, and all of the muscular, ligamentous, and other connective tissues governing the function of these bony structures. Even though each of its component joints is atypical when compared to other cervical vertebral units or even to each other, this superior cervical complex behaves synergistically as a functional unit. Dysfunction here is common, and even 80% of asymptomatic individuals will demonstrate a fascial preference for side-bending and rotating the entire craniocervical complex to the left (Zink and Lawson 1979). Nonetheless, because each of the articulations in this transition area is different in its motion characteristics, a positive palpatory scan of the suboccipital region requires local individual testing of each of these joints (Kappler 1997).

Scanning of this region is best accomplished by palpating the suboccipital region for S.T.A.R. abnormalities. A positive scan here may indicate somatic dysfunction affecting the occipitoatlantal (C0) vertebral unit, the atlantoaxial (C1) vertebral unit, and/or the C2 on C3 (C2) vertebral unit. Articular and myofascial dysfunction within the suboccipital region typically coexist. Travell and Simons cite TrPs in the splenii capitis muscles, commonly found in conjunction with C0 and/or C2 dysfunction, as an example of this close interrelationship (Simons et al. 1999, pp. 432–44). Thus, suboccipital joints should not be examined in isolation. It should also be noted that secondary tension and tissue change present in the suboccipital region and initiated by ipsilateral upper thoracic and rib problems will improve significantly after manipulative treatment of the primary problem (Kapper and Ramey 1997, pp. 515–40).

After screening and/or scanning the area, the examination order for skeletal, arthrodial, and myofascial components of somatic dysfunction becomes an individual decision. Different approaches

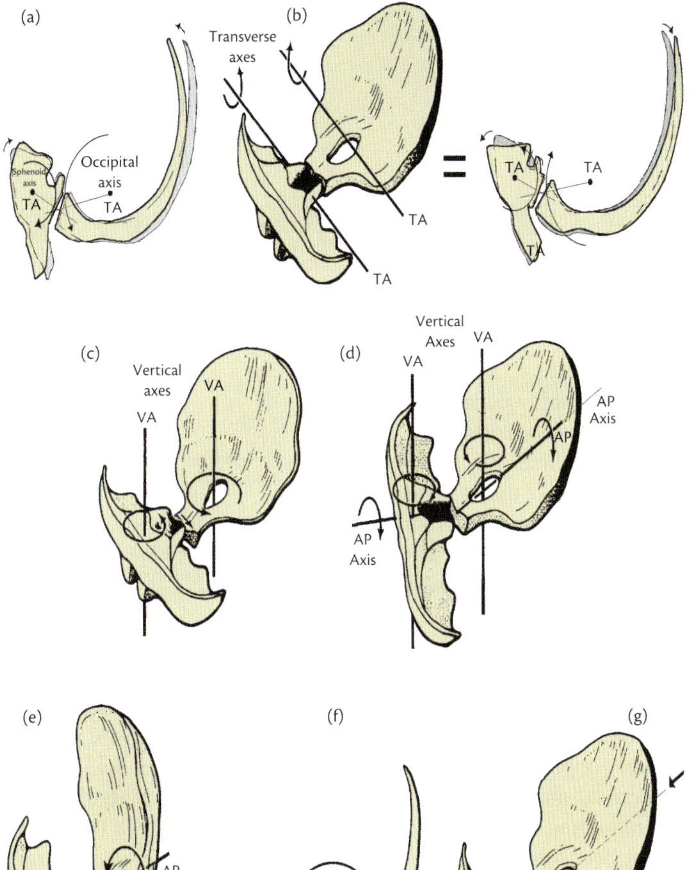

Figure 27.21 SBS strain patterns: (a) extension; (b) flexion; (c) right lateral strain; (d) left side-bending/rotation; (e) right torsion; (f) superior vertical strain; (g) compression.

by different expert practitioners appear to have similar outcomes. For example, because soft tissue dysfunction often alters articular motion characteristics in the craniocervical junction, I prefer to diagnose and address any soft tissue dysfunction before attempting a definitive articular diagnosis through specific segmental examination. Others find that treatment of somatic dysfunction associated with the combined motion characteristics addresses both articular and myofascial components at the same time.

Recent attempts to document the interrelationship between articular and myofascial components and to link them to relevant historical and physical findings have expanded our understanding of the diagnosis and treatment of the suboccipital region. For example, *Travell and Simons' myofascial pain and dysfunction* points out the common combination of C0, C1, and/or C2 articular somatic dysfunctions found in patients with semispinalis capitis TrPs (myofascial somatic dysfunction) (Simons et al. 1999, pp. 445–71). This combination was very likely in a population of patients with cervicogenic headaches, where 91% of patients had C0 or C1 articular somatic dysfunction and 56% had TrPs in the semispinalis capitis muscle predominantly ipsilateral to the symptomatic side (Jaeger 1989). Likewise, Kappler reports that a referred retro-orbital pain pattern, consistent with Travell's upper semispinalis capitis (location 2) trigger point (Figure 27.22), is often found on the palpably anterior portion of a rotated C1 somatic dysfunction (Kappler 1997).

Our understanding has also been expanded through documentation of patterns of dysfunction found within functional units. With respect to the superior cervical complex and headache, for example, Greenman (1996, pp. 550–1) reports a pattern found in most patients presenting with cervical spine stiffness and associated hemicephalgia running from the occiput to the retro-orbital area. The most common palpable structural diagnostic findings including this combination were:

- left occipitomastoid suture restriction
- C0 SRRL
- C1 rotated right
- C2–3 E RLSL

Restriction of motion segmental scanning for C0 dysfunction is often accomplished passively using a *lateral translation test.* Palpating digits placed in the suboccipital triangle sense the end-feel (freedom or resistance) of translation of the skull to the right and to the left with respect to the atlas. Another active scan at this same level is to ask patients who do not have temporomandibular joint dysfunction to actively open their jaw or to tuck in their chin while the physician observes. This active scan is positive for C0 dysfunction if the chin deviates from the midline to either side. Cradling the head with fingertips of the middle digits contacting the tissues

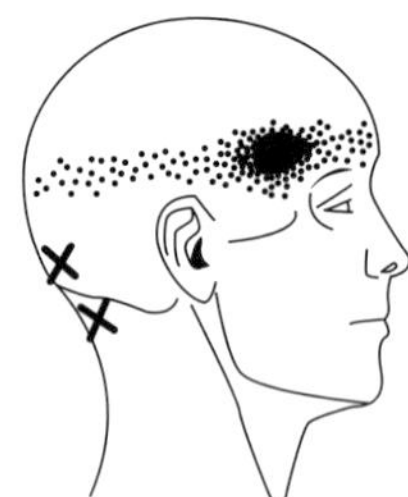

Figure 27.22 Retro-orbital pain pattern seen in both upper semispinalis capitis TrP and in C1 somatic dysfunction. (From Simons et al. 1999)

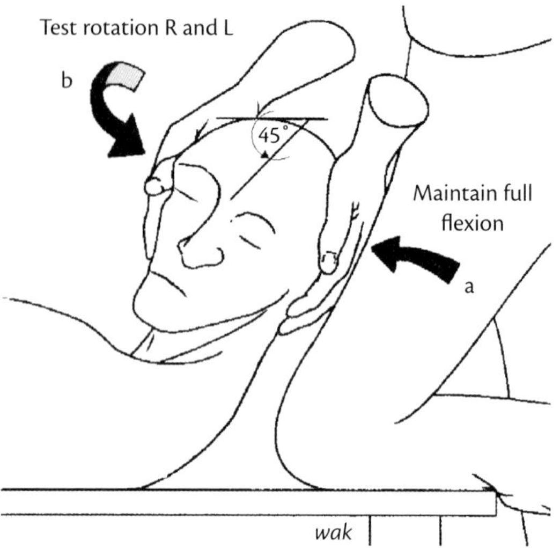

Figure 27.24 Easy atlantoaxial motion test. Locking out other cervicals permits testing of the upper cervical unit. A number of cervical conditions preclude this test however.

in the suboccipital region permits a supine scan for regional motion restriction. Pulling the physician's own forearms and wrists together while hands and fingers traction cephalically automatically pulls the fascia posteriorly and cephalically along the plane of the occipitoatlantal condylar facets. Enough pressure to reach the point where the suboccipital fascia first begins to resist the drag allows evaluation of resiliency (ease) or resistance (drag) to side-bending the region right or left. Scanning tests for C0 dysfunction are shown in Figure 27.23.

Scanning for C1 somatic dysfunction may be accomplished by fully forward bending the entire cervical spine (if tolerated) to physiologically lock out motion below the atlas, followed by rotating the head and atlas on the axis. As rotation is the primary motion allowed between the atlas and the axis, and occipitoatlantal rotation is limited to approximately 3°, asymmetrical motion indicates a positive test. A positive test, or factors prohibiting the performance of this scanning examination, suggests the need for segmental evaluation of C1 (Figure 27.24). C2 will be discussed with the lower cervical complex in the next section.

Related to the extensive neurological interconnections in this region, scanning tests need not be limited to palpation in the suboccipital region. Maigne describes an effective scanning examination for headache patients with the *eyebrow pinch-roll test* (Figure 27.25) (Maigne 1985, pp. 71–134). This scan is positive when the supraorbital skin fold on the symptomatic side is painful to pinch and feels palpably thickened. According to Maigne, a positive eyebrow pinch-roll test, in conjunction with tenderness in the suboccipital triangle over C2, suggests a headache of cervical origin involving the upper cervical complex.

As in all regional scanning examinations, a positive finding should alert the clinician to the need for local or segmental examination. Classification of acute or chronic somatic dysfunction in

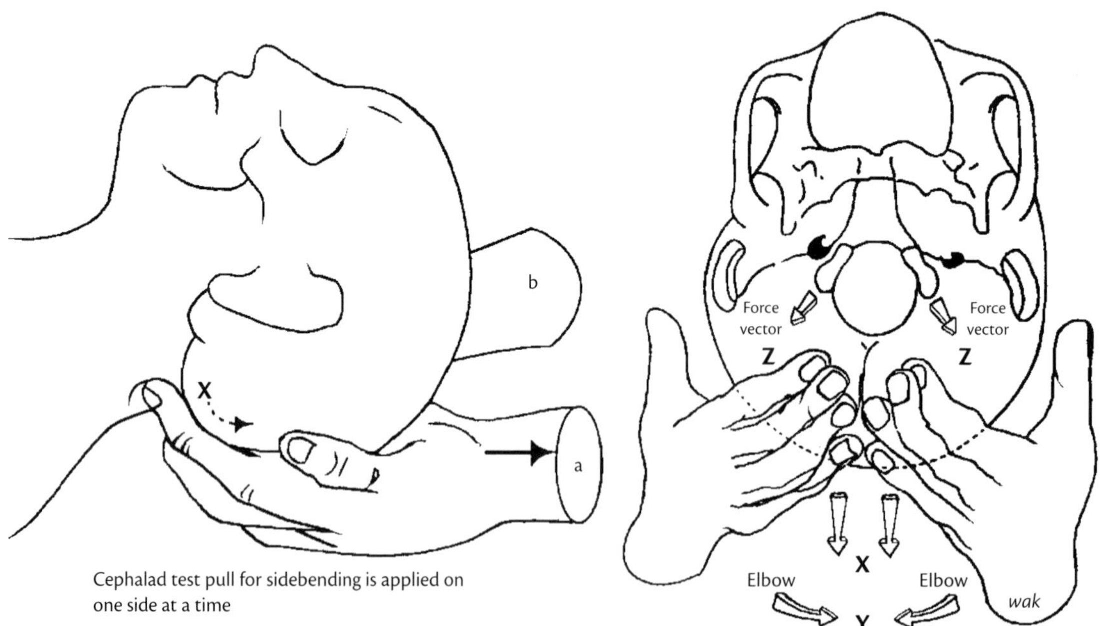

Figure 27.23 Easy occipitoatlantal motion test. Unilateral pull along the facet tests side-bending (which is coupled with rotation in the opposite direction); bilateral traction along both facets tests flexion and is sometimes held to relax suboccipital muscles, thereby allowing more accurate articular diagnosis.

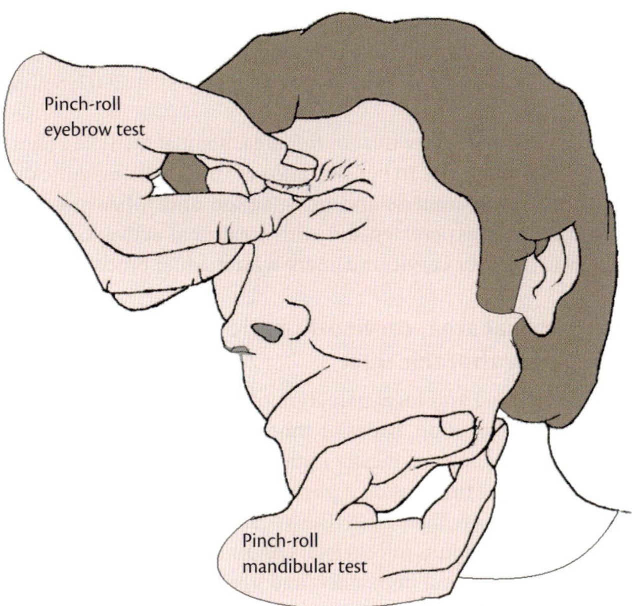

Figure 27.25 Eyebrow pinch test.

this region is largely based on the tissue texture characteristics discussed in Chapter 10.

Segmental examination for occipitoatlantal somatic dysfunction requires recognition that there are two occipitoatlantal joints, one on each side. Anatomically, these joints converge anteriorly (Figure 27.26). In sagittal plane (forward or backward bent) somatic dysfunction of C0, both occipitoatlantal joints are tender, both demonstrate equal tissue texture changes, and together, they typically limit the ability for the joint to fully side-bend or rotate in either direction. In forward-bent C0 dysfunction, the occiput will allow forward bending but is restricted when backward bending is attempted; the opposite is true for a backward-bent C0 dysfunction. In coupled plane somatic dysfunction at this level, side-bending and rotation occur to opposite sides (Kapandji 1970). In a C0 side-bent left, rotated right somatic dysfunction, the occiput is restricted when side-bending to the right and rotation to the left are attempted. Because of the two condylar joints, motion characteristics of C0 somatic dysfunction can be localized further to the right and/or the left occipitoatlantal articulation according to the dominant sensitivity, tissue texture abnormality, and restriction of motion. Thus, in the example of coupled motion above (C0 SLRR), there may be an anterior left occiput, a posterior right occiput, or both. By changing the focus of attention when specifically testing C0, the anterior occiput exhibits restriction of flexion and there is a sense that the occiput cannot glide posterolaterally on that side; the posterior occiput exhibits restriction of extension and cannot glide anteromedially on that side.

Segmental motion examination of C1 (atlantoaxial joint) is best accomplished by stabilizing the axis with one hand. This is accomplished by grasping the posterior spine of C2 (the axis) between the thumb and index finger of one hand; the occiput is cupped in the other hand with the fingers in the suboccipital groove and resting over the posterior arch of the atlas (Figure 27.27). Right and left rotation of the occipitoatlantal unit on C2 is then assessed. Somatic dysfunction in this joint is uniplanar.

The nerve root of C2 has direct anatomical attachments to the vagus and C2 is a common palpatory site of secondary somatic dysfunction. This results from vagal visceral afferent stimuli arising from dysfunction of certain upper respiratory, cardiac, and/or upper gastrointestinal structures. Its own innervation of the posterior scalp and dura of the posterior cranial fossa makes this vertebral segment important when considering diagnosis and treatment of patients with a wide range of problems. Nonetheless, the segmental examination of C2 is conducted in the same manner as all typical cervical vertebral units in the lower cervical area and is discussed in the next section. In interpreting palpatory findings in this region, a wealth of clinical evidence, including a 5-year double-blind study of 5000 hospitalized patients (Kelso 1971), suggests that the differential diagnosis of palpatory findings in this region should include secondary somatic dysfunction from sinus, respiratory, cardiac, and gastrointestinal disorders (D'Alonzo and Krachman 1997; Kuchera and Kuchera 1994). Paterson provides a synopsis of 'bizarre ENT symptoms' resulting from cervical dysfunction and notes that, in the absence of contraindications, manipulation is the treatment of choice (Patterson and Burn 1985, p. 77). Maigne indicates that when cervical somatic dysfunction is eliminated with manipulation, precipitating visceral factors that are still present will no longer trigger the referred headaches (Maigne 1985, p. 99).

Such a variety of symptoms arising from somatic dysfunction in this region should not be unexpected given the connections of C1–3 roots to the cervicotrigeminal nucleus, C2's relationship to the vagus, and the location of the superior cervical sympathetic

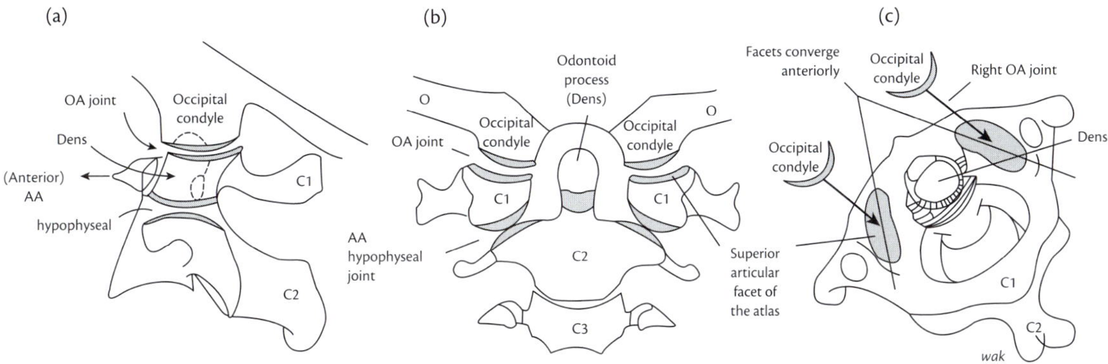

Figure 27.26 Occipitoatlantal and atlantoaxial joints illustrated with direction of superior facets of the atlas: (a) sagittal view; (b) coronal view; (c) superior oblique view.

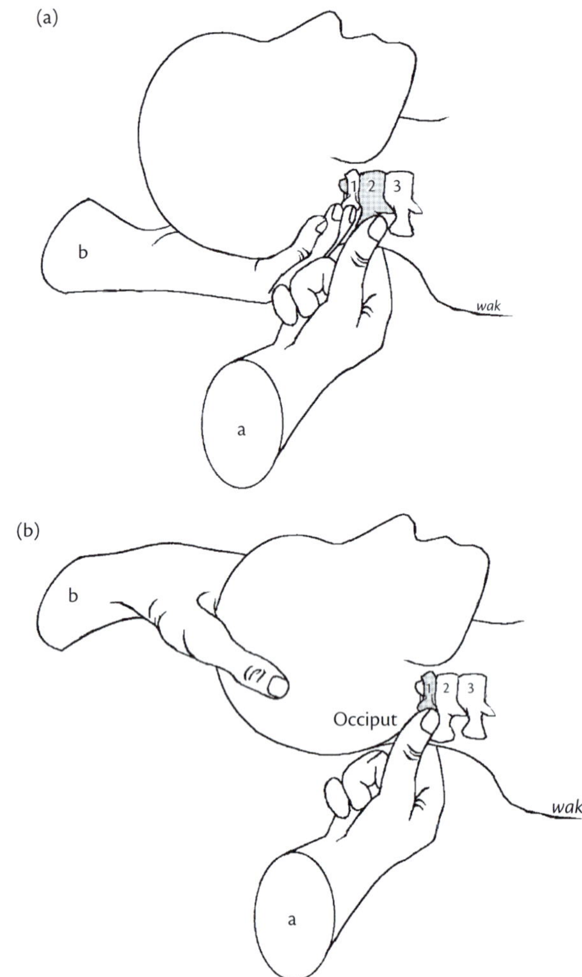

Figure 27.27 Two-hand motion tests: (a) for atlantoaxial joint; (b) for occipitoatlantal joint.

ganglion in the tissues adjacent to C2–3. In isolation, neither cervical screening nor suboccipital scanning provides enough diagnostic information to initiate an individualized neuromusculoskeletal prescription. Thus, local cervical diagnosis for specific somatic dysfunction and a physician's diagnostic capability to investigate and/or co-manage those other conditions are required for formulation of a complete differential diagnosis.

In a final comment about examining this region, it should be noted that previously, some clinicians advocated for a provocative test of the vertebral artery by positioning the upper cervical complex into hyperextension and rotation for up to 1 minute. This position, referred to as a *postural test* (Maigne 1985, p. 186) or a *DeKleyns test* (Kuchera et al. 2002), places the artery in its most precarious position and the clinician carefully observes for any posterior headache, vertigo, or eye nystagmus that might alert him or her to vertebral artery dissection or compromise. In the past, some mandated that this position was prerequisite to any cervical manipulation. Today, many authorities feel that such provocative tests are more likely to cause arterial problems in a susceptible patients than the treatments currently advocated for the area. Therefore currently, the peer consensus of manual medicine physicians regarding this region includes avoiding routine use of provocative postural tests while maintaining a strong awareness that cervical artery dissections are rare but potentially serious events in some patients (Biller et al. 2014; FIMM 2014; Kuchera et al. 2002; Seffinger and Hruby 2007).

To safely and effectively treat in this area, manual medicine physicians should weigh risk to benefit ratios of various therapeutic options after their anamnesis and examination and, when possible, should minimize hyperextension with rotational activation when treating the superior cervical segment with manual procedures.

Lower cervical area, cervicothoracic junction, and superior thoracic inlet

Regional scanning and local palpation of the lower cervical spine, cervicothoracic junction, superior thoracic inlet, and/or any of its component parts are specifically indicated for a patient who has a history and/or the findings on a physical or screening examination that are identified in Table 27.2. This region is particularly important in patients with musculoskeletal conditions that are associated with headache, postural imbalance, and upper extremity problems. Because the thoracic lymphatic duct passes through Sibson's fascia of the thoracic inlet twice before emptying into the brachiocephalic vein, dysfunction of this region of anatomy can be a significant obstruction to lymph flow, resulting in congestive phenomena that manifest almost anywhere in the body. Furthermore, cervical chain ganglia locations, as well as the upper thoracic and rib sympathetic anatomical connections, link palpatory findings of somatic dysfunction in this region to a host of eye, ear, nose, and throat (EENT) and cardiopulmonary disturbances (Figure 27.28).

In this section, some of the considerations discussed previously in relation to the superior cervical functional segment will be relevant to the discussion of the lower cervical segment. Furthermore, somatic dysfunction in this region also reflects compensation for, or causes compensation in, somatic regions above and below. Therapeutic decision making in this region also includes patients with:

- history of cervical trauma, especially whiplash (inertial) injury
- response to prior manual techniques in the region, especially historical presence or absence of vertigo, ataxia, or severe posterior headache afterwards or referral to either upper extremity
- evidence or absence of physical findings suggestive of conditions such as osteoporosis, cervical stenosis, cervical ligamentous laxity or spondylolisthesis, severe rheumatoid arthritis, cervical ribs, or mediastinal tumours.

Lower cervical area

The typical cervical spine extends from C2 through C6 or C7. Together with the cervicothoracic junction, this region is responsible for a wide range of functional disorders affecting the head, neck, and upper extremities and contains sympathetic ganglia whose cell bodies originate in the upper thoracic region.

Some clinicians inappropriately suggest that consideration of the cervical spine in the diagnosis and treatment of patients with headaches is 'controversial'. Seasoned neuromusculoskeletal clinicians, however, have experience in differentiating those patients for whom the cervical spine plays a central rather than a secondary or non-contributory role. The International Headache Society (IHS) agrees with the latter group in recognizing that the cervical spine must be included in classification schema (Olesen 1988).

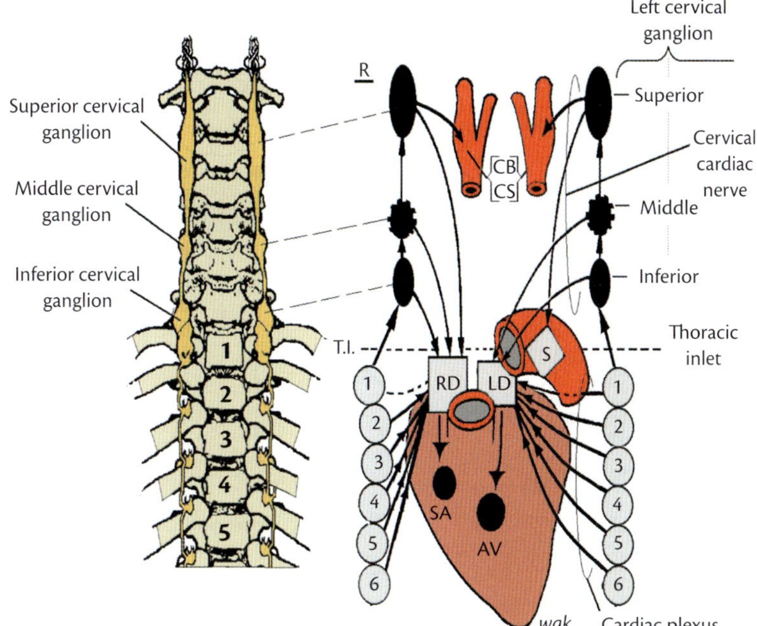

Figure 27.28 (a) Cervical chain ganglia; (b) sympathetic innervation of the heart showing predominance of right side to the sinoatrial node (SA) via the right deep (RD) cardiac plexus and the left side predominance to the atrioventricular node (AV) via the left deep (LD) cardiac plexus.

According to the IHS, inclusion criteria for the cervical spine includes several of the S.T.A.R. characteristics used to diagnosis cervical somatic dysfunction, including:

- local neck or occipital pain projecting to forehead, orbital region, temples, vertex, or ears
- *either* diminished cervical motion, abnormal cervical contour, texture, tone or response to active and passive stretching and contraction *or* abnormal tenderness of neck muscles
- radiographic evidence of pathology, abnormal posture, *or* reduced range of motion.

Lower cervical region dysfunction has also been implicated in symptoms referred to the upper extremities, upper thoracic region and ribs, diaphragm, and cardiorespiratory systems. Regional dysfunction plays a significant role in acute torticollis, cervical radiculopathies, post-whiplash syndromes, cervical vertigo, carpal tunnel syndrome, and superior thoracic outlet syndrome. From a pathophysiological perspective, cervical somatic dysfunction has been implicated in reducing the transport of centrally produced trophic substances to the tissues of the upper extremities (Gilliar et al. 1996; Upton and McComas 1973). This in turn, like the more extreme double crush syndrome, may predispose the upper extremities to increased risk of developing symptomatic entrapment neuropathies and other regional disorders. The area is also subject to secondary somatic dysfunction from disorders of the EENT, cardiopulmonary, and upper gastrointestinal systems.

Both Maigne (1985, pp. 82–4) and Jones (Jones et al. 1995) advocated for use of pressure posteriorly over the cervical spinous processes as a scanning process to identify segmental cervical dysfunction. In their local cervical diagnosis, both of these physicians looked for posterior tender points located approximately one finger's breadth from the median line. Jones' nomenclature for these and other body tender points is standardized and used by practitioners of counterstrain manipulative technique (Figure 27.29).

Each of these neuromusculoskeletal physicians recognizes the importance of additionally examining the anterior cervical region. Jones recorded a large number of anterior cervical tender points after applying pressure to locations from just under the ear on the posterior ascending ramus of the mandible, down the anterolateral aspect (lateral masses) of the cervical spine, to the medial superior end of the sternum. Jones correlated these findings with segmental cervical somatic dysfunction. Maigne described a very similar location for his cervical *pointe sonnette* (doorbell) sign, elicited by applying a few seconds of moderate thumb pressure in the anterolateral region of the cervical spine. Tenderness and replication of the patient's complaints using Maigne's anterior cervical doorbell (push-button or bell-push) sign is said to indicate the involved or irritated cervical root level. Clinically, he interpreted these findings as 'very useful at the level of the middle or lower cervical spine' and noted that this is especially relevant when dealing with atypical upper extremity pain that seems to originate in the cervical region. Both clinical authors noted an anterior palpatory finding at the angle of the jaw (whose cutaneous innervation is supplied by anterior branches of C2 and C3). Jones designated two tender points, one just under the ear on the posterior ascending ramus of the mandible and one 2 cm anterior to the angle of the mandible on the medial side of that bone. Maigne used the skin-rolling method on the mandible to identify dysfunction or pathology associated with either the C2 or C3 level. Note that the differential between cervical region somatic dysfunction and cervical root pathophysiology cannot be made by palpation alone. As pointed out consistently in the work of Simons and Travell, each is capable of creating palpatory change, each is capable of creating neural, vascular, and lymphatic dysfunction, and coexistence is common.

More specific tissue texture scanning for myofascial tender points and TrPs in the lower cervical region is productive if the historical, physical, or screening examinations indicate the need for more definitive information about somatic dysfunction. Simons et al. pointed out that it is common for patients with myofascial points in

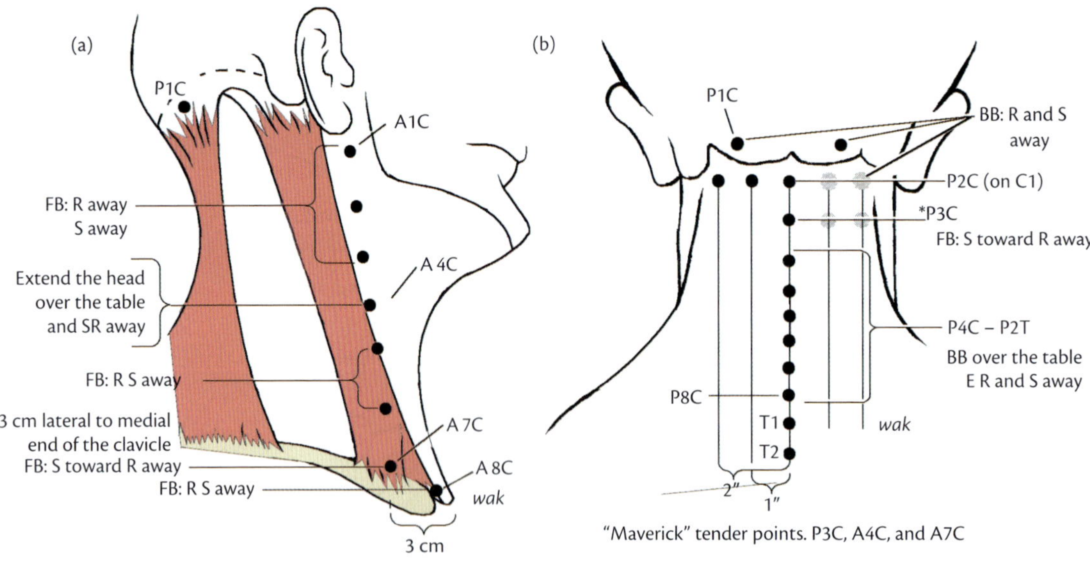

Figure 27.29 Jones' tender points of the cervical region: (a) anterior—occipitoatlantal point posterior to the mastoid process, occipitoatlantal also between mastoid and angle of jaw, C1–7 along anterior margin of the sternocleidomastoid muscle; (b) posterior—occipitoatlantal point on the occiput; A, C1–7 spinous processes; B, C1–7, also 2.5 cm lateral to the spinous processes; C, C1–7, also 5 cm lateral to the spinous processes.

the trapezii muscles to have somatic dysfunction of C2, C3, and/or C4 as well as hypermobility of C4 (Simons et al. 1999, pp. 278–307). They also recorded that TrPs in the splenii cervicis were commonly found in conjunction with C4 and/or C5 dysfunction (Simons et al. 1999, pp. 432–44) and noted that articular somatic dysfunction anywhere between C3 and C6 was frequently associated with TrPs in the levator scapulae (Simons et al. 1999, pp. 491–503).

At the segmental level, palpation of C2–7 motion is most easily accomplished by using the passive segmental rotation and lateral translation tests described previously. Because of the anatomical structure of typical cervical vertebrae and orientation of their articulations, side-bending and rotation are coupled to allow side-bending and rotation to the same side. To test rotation, support the supine patient's head with fingers contacting the posterior surfaces of the articular pillars (Figure 27.30). In the neutral position, rotate each vertebral unit along the plane of its posterior cervical facets (roughly toward the patient's opposite eye) to the right and to the left, assessing the quality of the end-feel in each direction. Additional palpatory information is gained if this is repeated with the cervical spine in both forward-bent and backward-bent positions. In the lateral translation test, the physician contacts the lateral portion of the cervical articular pillars with fingertips while supporting the supine patient's head in his or her hands. Localizing the force to one level, translation is checked in each direction. The test can also be performed with the neck held in flexion and then repeated in extension. The rotation and/or the lateral translation tests may be performed at each level as a scan or used for specific segmental diagnosis of individual levels identified in a scan of the region.

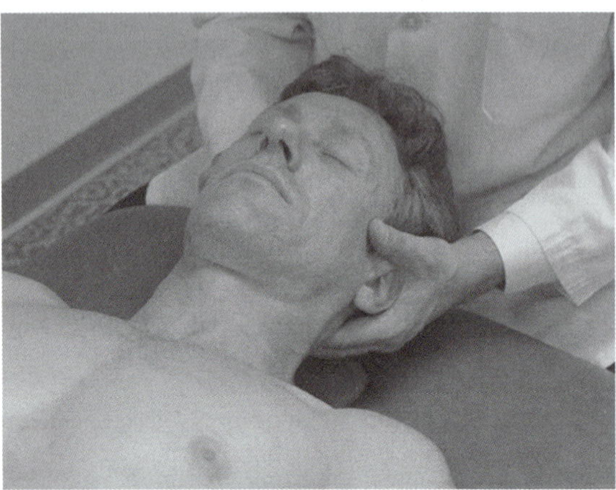

Figure 27.30 Rotational testing of cervical spine respects facet facings. Fingers are on the posterior articular pillars.

Cervicothoracic junction and superior thoracic inlet areas

While the cervicothoracic junction of the spine literally occurs between C7 and T1, the functional superior thoracic inlet region is made up of:

- the first four thoracic vertebrae
- the first two ribs
- the manubrium of the sternum
- all of the attached connecting and restricting tissues.

This region is extremely important from an autonomic and circulatory perspective. The superior thoracic inlet is in close relationship with the superior thoracic outlet, and dysfunction of one affects the other (Figure 27.31). The thoracic duct provides a drainage pathway for lymph from most of the body into the brachiocephalic vein and must pass through this region from the chest into the neck and then back through this region from the neck into the chest. Additionally, the lymphaticovenous valve and peristaltic motions of this terminal portion of the thoracic duct are under sympathetic control governed by lateral horn cell bodies in the spinal cord of this region. These same cell bodies regulate circulation to all the

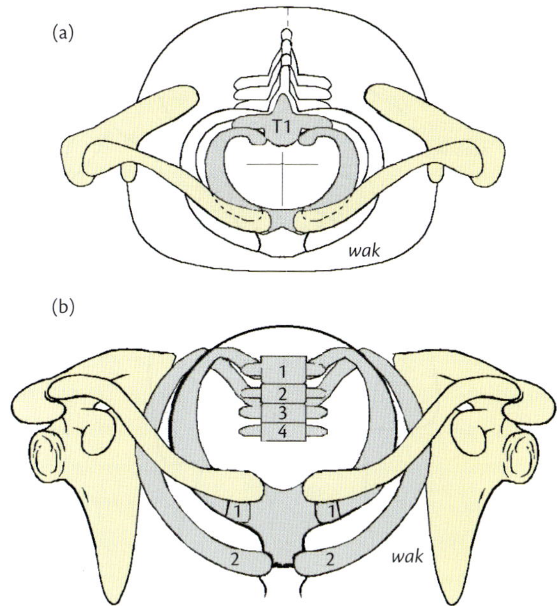

Figure 27.31 Thoracic inlet: (a) anatomical = T1, rib, manubrium; (b) functional = T1–4, rib 1–2, manubrium.

structures of the head and neck, the heart and lungs, and portions of the upper extremities.

Recall that differential diagnostic considerations in this region include viscerosomatic and somatovisceral reflexes. Part of the differential is assisted through palpation of each of the S.T.A.R. characteristics. In primary visceral involvement, the tissue texture abnormalities will often far outweigh the degree of motion restriction and the quality of the restrictive barrier is 'rubbery'. The pattern of the somatic dysfunction sites often is helpful as well. Note that in patients with primary coronary artery/cardiac involvement, somatic patterns include palpable changes, most frequently from T2–4 on the left, as well as left-sided second rib and pectoralis major TrPs (Kuchera 1997a). Upper chest muscle TrPs were reported in 61% of patients with cardiac disease, and treatment of this somatic dysfunction is an important factor in reducing reflex coronary artery spasm (Simons et al. 1999, pp. 833–838). Reduction of chest pain in this particular situation, however, does not eliminate the need to clinically assess and treat the underlying cardiac condition.

Regional motion restriction of the entire functional superior thoracic inlet can be scanned on a supine patient by placing hands over the upper trapezius, with thumbs placed posteriorly to contact the upper thoracic transverse processes and the fingers anteriorly curled into the infraclavicular region and upper ribs. Use enough pressure to move these tissues to a point where the fascia first begins to resist. Then sense their resiliency (ease) or resistance (drag) to side-bend the region right or left and to rotate the region right or left. Few individuals are perfectly symmetrical and 80% of asymptomatic individuals will demonstrate a fascial preference for side-bending and rotating the superior thoracic inlet complex to the right. This, alternating with the directional fascial preference pattern of left side-bending and rotation most commonly palpated for the craniocervical region above and thoracolumbar region below, is part of the common compensatory pattern of Zink (Zink and Lawson 1979).

More specific tissue texture scanning for myofascial tender points and TrPs in the cervicothoracic region is warranted if historical, physical, or screening examinations indicate the need for more definitive information about somatic dysfunction. For example, myofascial points in the middle trapezii muscle fibres are commonly accompanied by a palpatory finding of C6, C7, and/or T1 and first rib somatic dysfunction (Maigne 1985, pp. 82–4). Another reported association is the presence of any two or more dysfunctional vertebral units between C7 and T5 with rhomboid TrPs (Simons et al. 1999, pp. 613–22). Travell and Simons report that this latter combination often appears as a flattened upper thoracic area centred around T3 with motion characteristics which are extended, side-bent, and rotated to the same side as the involved rhomboid muscle. Interestingly, these authors note that the rhomboid TrP resolves with manipulation of the T3 articular somatic dysfunction. Simple extension somatic dysfunctions of T1, T2, T3, and/or T4 vertebral units are found with bilateral posterior cervical TrPs (Simons et al. 1999, pp. 445–71). Likewise, extended somatic dysfunction at T1, with inability to flex forward and an exquisitely tender T1 spinous process, are findings commonly associated with serratus posterior superior TrPs (Simons et al. 1999, pp. 900–7). In yet another example, ipsilateral upper thoracic and rib problems cause secondary suboccipital tension and tissue change that improves significantly after manipulative treatment of the primary problem (Kappler and Ramey 1997, p. 545).

The interrelationship between myofascial dysfunction and articular dysfunction extends to the ribs and adjacent myofascial structures. In this region, Travell and Simons report that rib 1 articular somatic dysfunction often accompanies scalene muscle TrPs (Simons et al. 1999, pp. 504–37) and that both resolve with treatment of the TrP. Conversely, Lewit reports that rib 1 'blockage' (somatic dysfunction) is accompanied by reflex scalene muscle spasm that is abolished by manipulative treatment of that rib (Lewit 1991).

Motion restriction for the first four thoracic vertebrae and the first two ribs may be diagnosed with the patient in a number of positions. In the seated position, screening typically consists of observing and palpating the side-bending curves created by applying vectors of force as shown in the modified acromion drop test (Figure 27.32). Asymmetric flattening of the thoracic side-bending curve or palpable resistance indicates the need for further scanning or local palpation.

Scanning and segmental examinations in any position can be accomplished by alternating pressures over upper thoracic transverse processes or through translation at successive levels of the thoracic spine. A sufficient amount of passive head–neck flexion and extension can also be easily introduced, allowing the physician to feel alternating upper thoracic interspinous gapping and approximation, respectively. Palpatory identification of end-barrier restriction to passive motion in any one plane warrants segmental diagnosis of the remaining planes. When placing fingertips to monitor motion characteristics at the same vertebral (segmental) level, the physician should remember that the transverse processes in the region of the upper thoracic spine (T1–3) are anatomically located at approximately the same horizontal level as their spinous processes. An alternative method for both scanning and segmental diagnosis in this region involves palpating the upper thoracic region with fingertips placed 2–3 cm on either side of the spinous process. The patient is directed to nod their head forwards and then backwards until motion is induced at the palpated site. The aggravation or

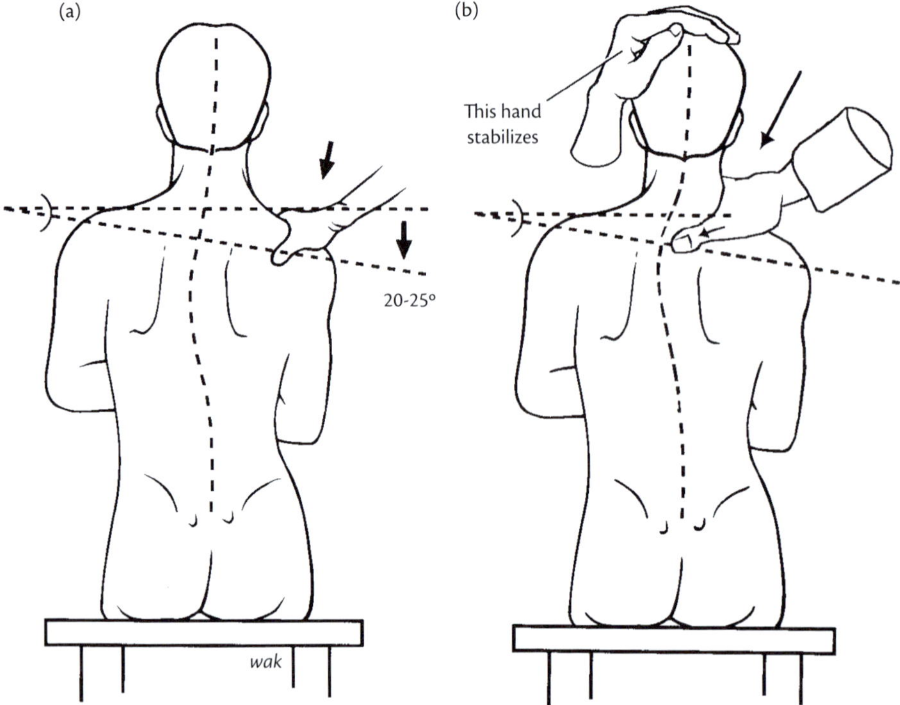

Figure 27.32 (a) Acromion drop test; (b) testing side-bending of the upper thoracic spine, with patient seated, adding a translation component.

reduction of any palpated asymmetry indicates somatic dysfunction that can then be segmentally named. Inter-examiner reliability studies demonstrate that different positions and different tests may result in different palpatory responses. Therefore designation of somatic dysfunction by its motion characteristics should include a description of both the patient's position and the test used.

The first two ribs are atypical compared to other ribs. The relatively immobile anterior synchondrosis of the first rib (R1) means that somatic dysfunction is more commonly palpated over the posterior aspect of the rib (dysfunction occurring at the rib head). Gently grasping just anterior to the superior trapezius border and retracting the tissues slightly posteriorly allows direct fingertip pressure over the posterolateral R1 shaft. Ipsilateral tenderness, superior unlevelling, and resistance to inferior compression are apparent in the more commonly found elevated first rib. The scalene muscles, attaching to the first two ribs, play a significant role in the diagnosis and treatment of the superior thoracic inlet region and somatic dysfunction of the first two ribs. Scalene muscle hypertonicity elevates the rib(s) attached to it, but an elevated first rib can cause a reflex contraction of the anterior scalene muscle.

Although much less common, scalene muscle fatigue or prolonged heavy direct pressure on the first rib may result in inferior subluxation of the first rib's posterior aspect. Clinically, this occurs in the respiratory accessory muscle fatigue found in patients with severe chronic obstructive pulmonary disease or in those carrying a heavy purse or backpack over one shoulder. With this condition, restriction is indicated when the inferior rib fails to rise with a deep inhalation.

Diagnosis of R1 somatic dysfunction is complicated by the fact that the superior thoracic inlet also manifests first rib asymmetry; however, in the superior thoracic inlet dysfunction, the R1–T1 articulations function normally. Thus, coordinating the diagnostic and treatment sequences (discussed in Chapter 50) becomes very important.

The first and second ribs are both subject to acquiring inhalation and exhalation somatic dysfunction. These dysfunctions can also be initiated by the position of their respective thoracic vertebrae. Each of these can also affect the typical ribs and will be more completely discussed in the thoracic cage section that follows. Finally, segmental diagnosis of the manubrium, another important component of the functional superior thoracic inlet, is discussed in relationship to the body of the sternum and is presented in the following thoracic cage section.

Thoracic spine and thoracic cage

Specific regional scanning and local palpation for somatic dysfunction in the T5–12 thoracic region, chest cage, and/or any of its component parts (including the ribs and sternum) are indicated if the patient's history, physical, or screening examinations reveal the findings identified in Table 27.2. The anatomical relationship of the sympathetic chain ganglia to the heads of each rib and the wide distribution of sympathetic fibres from cell bodies in the lateral horn of the thoracic region closely link somatic dysfunction of the thoracic cage to visceral and somatic problems throughout the body (Figure 27.33). With every respiratory cycle, numerous muscle groups and approximately 146 articulations in the thoracic cage are called upon to move. Thus, somatic dysfunction of component parts of the thoracic cage will have wide-ranging systemic, autonomic, and congestive implications. Therefore, the differential diagnosis must include common somatic problems such as costochondritis, other chest wall syndromes, and a wide range of pathological and infectious processes.

In addition to thoracic, costal, and sternal somatic dysfunction, the preceding (cervicothoracic junction) and succeeding (thoracolumbar junction) sections present and direct functional connections

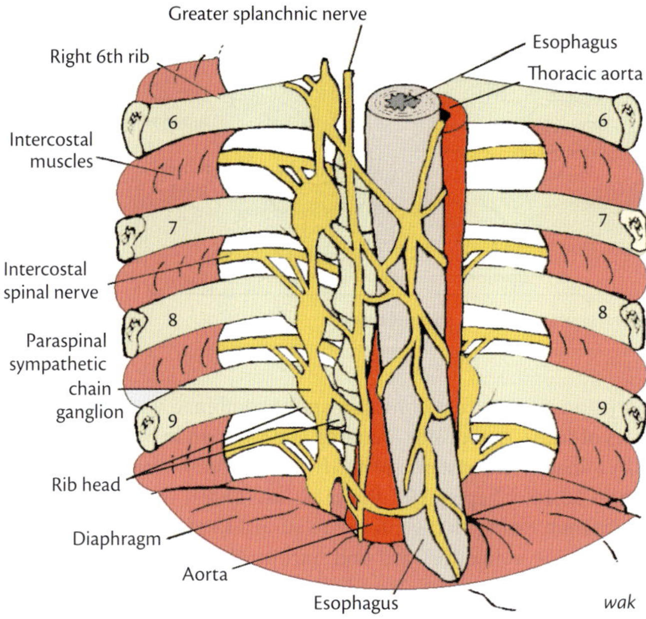

Figure 27.33 Location of thoracic sympathetic chain ganglia in relation to the rib heads.

relevant to this chapter. Likewise, dysfunction in the thoracic cage discussed in this section can be expected to influence function in the cervicothoracic and thoracolumbar junctional areas.

Pathological change in the thoracic cage or of the viscera referring to the region affects the interpretation of somatic diagnostic clues as well as the choice of a treatment plan. Additional evaluation of the thoracic cage region should therefore include appropriate history and physical examination to rule out these processes.

- Any time diagnosis and treatment of somatic dysfunction in this region might be considered, a trauma and fracture history should be explored. Some forms of osteoporosis affect the anterior portion of the thoracic spine early in the process, increasing the importance of uncovering nutritional, metabolic, pharmacological, and/or surgical risk factors associated with this pathophysiological process. Likewise, both osteoporosis and bone metastases can result in spontaneous vertebral or rib fractures when minimal stress is applied to the bone. Thus, these conditions contraindicate most manipulative procedures over the involved site and constitute relative contraindications to certain types of manipulation applied generally.
- Evidence or absence of physical findings suggesting osteoporosis, thoracic kyphosis, or rotoscoliosis should be noted in the neuromusculoskeletal physician's examination, as these conditions affect treatment considerations.
- Visceral disorders stimulate afferents that, in turn, result in progressive and distinctive findings of secondary somatic dysfunction according to the autonomic innervations and sidedness of the involved viscus (Figure 27.34). Progression in the early visceral phase tends to be vague, poorly localized, and midline over the appropriate collateral ganglion. As the visceral condition progresses, somatic clues are added in the form of paraspinal tissue texture changes (more so than restricted motion), Chapman's intercostal reflexes, and rib somatic dysfunction. By the time the visceral problem ruptures or irritates adjacent visceral pleura/peritoneum, the peritoneocutaneous reflex localizes over viscus-specific sites (as in the appendix and its McBurney's point). These somatic findings in visceral disturbances have been extensively documented by osteopathic physicians in the USA (Chila 2011; Kuchera and Kuchera 1994), by surgeons at the Mayo Clinic Foundation (Smith et al. 1961), and by pain management specialists (Melzack and Wall 1989) worldwide.

Thoracic spinal areas

Segmental diagnosis of thoracic somatic dysfunction is quickly and easily accomplished in those areas identified through historical, physical, and/or screening processes. Segmental motion evaluation requires assessment of the end-feel quality of the barriers to rotation, side-bending, and flexion–extension. Finger placement in making these assessments must be precise and the motion characteristics coordinated for each segment. The 'thoracic rule of threes' is useful in guiding hand placement to corresponding thoracic

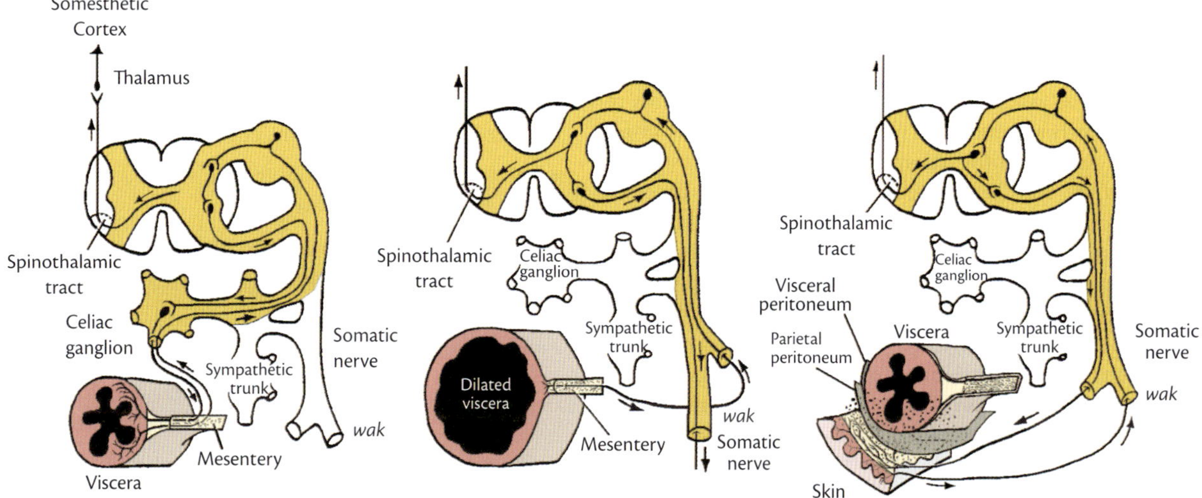

Figure 27.34 Pain pathways from a typical upper GI visceral structure: (a) visceral reflex; (b) viscerosomatic reflex; (c) peritoneocutaneous reflex of Morley. Progression of somatic findings assists in diagnosing visceral disorders and their severity. (Adapted from Kuchera and Kuchera 1994.)

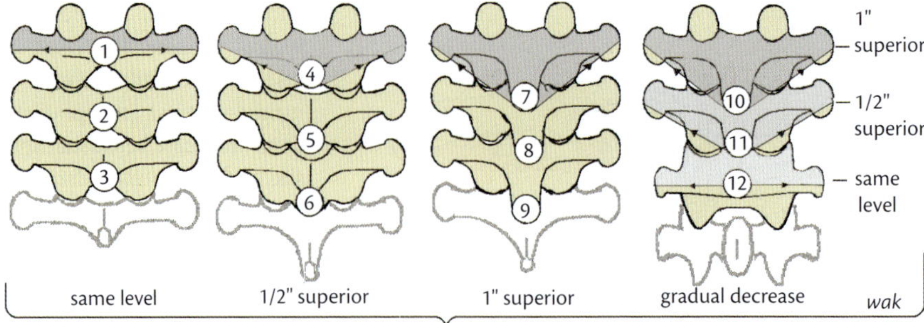

Figure 27.35 Location of transverse processes in relation to their spinous processes: 'rule of threes' for the thoracic region. (Kuchera and Kuchera 2012).

spinous and transverse processes that progressively change their anatomical relationship from the upper to the lower portion of the thoracic vertebral column. Each group of three thoracic vertebral units demonstrates a different positional relationship (Figure 27.35). Once finger placement is assured, segmental motion can be assessed using passive or dynamic methods.

One test unique to the thoracic region is the so-called *shingle test of Kuchera* (Kuchera and Kuchera 1994). It involves placing medial pressure with one thumb on the lateral side of a spinous process at one thoracic level with a counterforce imposed by the other thumb on the spinous process of the thoracic vertebra below. The clinician's thumbs and the pressures are then reversed. Unopposed, pressure on a single spinous process in this manner would typically induce rotation, but in the thoracic region, where the facets lie relatively in a coronal plane, opposite rotations induced at adjacent segments cancel one another. In this manner, only side-bending in the vertebral unit is allowed. Because thoracic spinous processes are situated below the AP axis of lateral flexion, the vertebral unit will attempt to side-bend to the side of the superior thumb (Figure 27.36a). In the shingle test of Kuchera, the quality of the end-feel determines the direction of side-bending; named for the freer motion. Similar thumb placement is employed in a *pre-manipulative test* described by Maigne (1972, pp. 97, 144). In this test, Maigne first checked side-bending at a single thoracic level, seeking pain. When pain was identified, he then assessed for increased pain by adding a counter-force to the spinous process above and below the initial segment. Rather than specifically using this test to determine motion characteristics, Maigne used the test to reinforce his 'rule of no pain and free motion' as shown in Figure 27.36b.

Specific passive motion testing of each of three planes in the thoracic region can be assessed in any position, although for this region it is most easily accomplished with the patient seated or prone. Alternating pressure over the transverse processes of each segment is applied and the end-feel of the barrier to rotation is assessed. Taking into consideration the thoracic rule of threes, translation or passively induced side-bending is applied to assess the quality of that barrier at each thoracic vertebral unit. The third plane of motion is assessed by passively testing interspinous approximation and separation. If there is vertebral unit somatic dysfunction, the quality of each barrier is restrictive in one direction and physiological in the opposing direction. The combination of restrictive barriers determines whether type I or type II dysfunction is present. Pathological change affecting spinal motion is the most prominent consideration in the differential diagnosis of somatic dysfunction. Pathological change in the thoracic region most commonly presents with a capsular pattern of barrier restrictions in which limitation of extension exceeds that of flexion and is combined with varying degrees of restriction of side-bending and rotation in both directions.

In a diagnostic system called *dynamic motion examination* (see Figure 10.10, Chapter 10), the most useful test in this region involves monitoring change in the relationship of transverse process pairs during active forward and backward bending motion from a neutral starting point. Two different *type II somatic dysfunction diagnoses* are possible in this region, using this method:

- The *extended, rotated, and side-bent* (ERS) somatic dysfunction is diagnosed when the transverse process on one side becomes more prominent with forward bending and more symmetric with backward bending.
- The opposite findings are palpated in a *flexed, rotated, and side-bent* (FRS) somatic dysfunction.

Both diagnoses typically involve a single vertebral unit and, in both, the side-bending and rotational restrictions are to the same side. The diagnosis of a *type I somatic dysfunction* typically involves three or more adjacent vertebral units. Dynamic motion testing in type I somatic dysfunction may change the asymmetry of transverse processes slightly, but symmetry is not achieved with either forward or with backward bending.

Specific tissue texture scanning for myofascial tender points and TrPs in the thoracic region is recommended when historical, physical, or screening examinations indicate the need for more definitive information about somatic dysfunction. These points are themselves a specific diagnosis of somatic dysfunction and they commonly coexist with both thoracic articular and costal somatic dysfunction. As their functional anatomy suggests, the interrelationship between thoracic segmental somatic dysfunction and TrPs in the thoracic paraspinal muscles results in the following clinically observed generalities (Simons et al. 1999, pp. 278–307, 913–39):

- rotatores TrPs commonly induce single-segment articular dysfunction at the same level
- multifidi TrPs are commonly seen with dysfunction of two or three adjacent segments
- semispinalis TrPs are often found with group thoracic somatic dysfunction extending over 4–6 vertebral units
- TrPs in the iliocostalis and longissimus muscles are also likely to be associated with group articular thoracic somatic dysfunction.

Greenman went as far as to state that 'palpable muscle hypertonicity of the deepest muscle layers (of the erector spinae mass), including the multifidi and levator costales, is pathognomonic of vertebral motion segment dysfunction at that level'. (1996, p. 206)

(a)

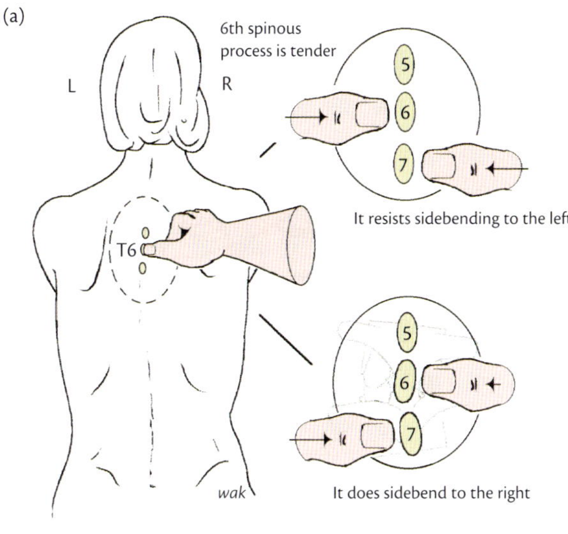

(b)

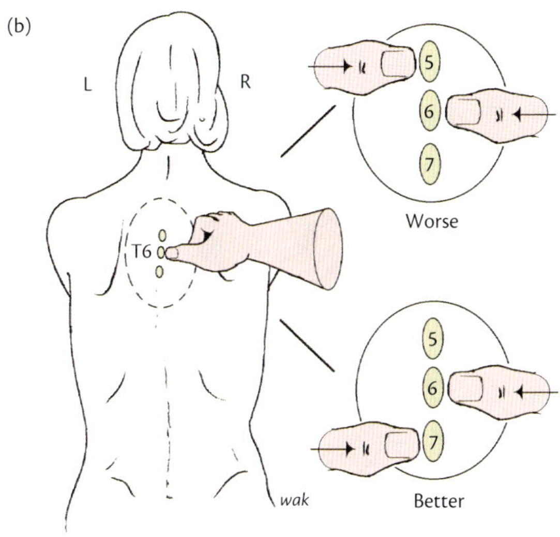

Figure 27.36 (a) 'Shingle test' of Kuchera for the thoracic spine. For example, the sixth spinous process is tender to palpation. Simultaneously, medial and opposite pressure is applied to the spinous processes of the sixth vertebral unit (T6 on T7) in one direction and then the other. Ease or resistance to movement is determined. Ease or resistance to rotations is then independently determined by using knowledge of the 'rule of threes' for the thoracic region. A direct method manipulative treatment is then set up to reverse the restriction in side-bending and rotation. The sagittal plane is used to localize the activating force at the dysfunctional vertebral unit. If rotation was also found to be restricted right, set-up would be to take side-bending left to its barrier, apply a fulcrum that will rotate T6 left, localize at T6 in the sagittal plane, and apply the activating force. (From Kuchera, W.A., Kuchera, M.L. *Osteopathic principles in practice*. Columbus, Ohio: Greyden Press; 1994; 532–533.) (b) 'Shingle test' of Maigne. Medial pressure on a spinous process in the cervical, thoracic, or lumbar spine is found to be tender to the patient. Simultaneous and opposite pressure to the spinous process above and then to the spinous process below determines the direction for direct manipulation. Direct manipulation is given to the joint that is less tender when the test is applied. In this illustration, direct manipulation would be given to the T6 thoracic segment. (From Maigne, R. *Orthopedic Medicine*. Charles C. Thomas: Springfield, IL; 1972; 97.)

Chest cage and typical costal areas

Diagnosis of this region includes evaluation of both costal and sternal elements of the thoracic cage. Specific diagnosis of ribs is usually delayed until thoracic vertebral somatic dysfunction is removed. Likewise, specific sternal diagnosis is delayed until rib somatic dysfunction is treated. These generalities exist because of the tremendous impact thoracic somatic dysfunction plays on rib function and that rib function plays on sternal function.

Ribs identified in the screening or scanning processes can be individually named according to their structural and respiratory characteristics. (Rib 1 subluxation was fully discussed in the previous section.)

Structural, traumatically induced rib dysfunction diagnoses include:

- **Anterior or posterior subluxation:** These ribs exhibit hypermobility and are palpably displaced anteriorly or posteriorly along the axis of motion between the costovertebral and costotransverse articulations. Palpatory findings include a less prominent rib angle with anterior subluxation and a more prominent rib angle with posterior subluxation.
- **Torsion:** This characteristic often occurs in conjunction with thoracic rotation (affecting ribs on both sides) and, unless remodelling of the rib shaft takes place over time, should return to normal bilateral symmetry when the thoracic spine returns to a symmetrical position. With T4 rotation to the right on T5, for example, rib 5 on the right would demonstrate external torsion along its long axis resulting in palpable prominence at the superior border of the rib angle and the inferior border of the sternal end. Internal torsion of the left fifth rib would be present with a sharper inferior border palpated posteriorly and a sharper superior border palpated anteriorly.
- **Anteroposterior or lateral compression:** Trauma from an anteroposterior or a lateral direction may result in sustained deformation. In anteroposterior compression, there is a palpably increased rib shaft prominence in the mid-axillary line and decreased prominence anteriorly and posteriorly. In lateral compression of a rib, the palpable prominence is found anteriorly and posteriorly with less prominence in the mid-axillary line.

Respiratory characteristics and the location of restricted motion also permit useful diagnostic nomenclature for rib dysfunction. These respiratory dysfunction diagnoses include:

- **Pump-handle or bucket-handle costal somatic dysfunction:** The axis of respiratory motion of ribs 2–10 is influenced by a number of factors including the angle between the body of the thoracic vertebra and the transverse processes (Figure 27.37) and the motion of the sternum. In the absence of a true anteroposterior or lateral axis, each of these ribs has a mixture of 'pump-handle' motion (maximally assessed on the anterior chest wall) and 'bucket-handle' motion (maximally assessed on the lateral aspects of the chest wall). By their anatomy, the upper ribs typically have a higher percentage of pump-handle to bucket-handle motion, whereas the lower typical ribs have a higher percentage of bucket-handle type motion. In springing the rib cage for restriction, both the anterior and the lateral aspects of the chest cage should be scanned for dysfunction. Likewise in assessing respiratory motion, both anterior and lateral aspects of suspicious ribs should be assessed. Motion loss to either springing or to a portion of the respiratory cycle that is noted anteriorly is described as pump-handle dysfunction; motion loss noted laterally is consistent with bucket-handle dysfunction.

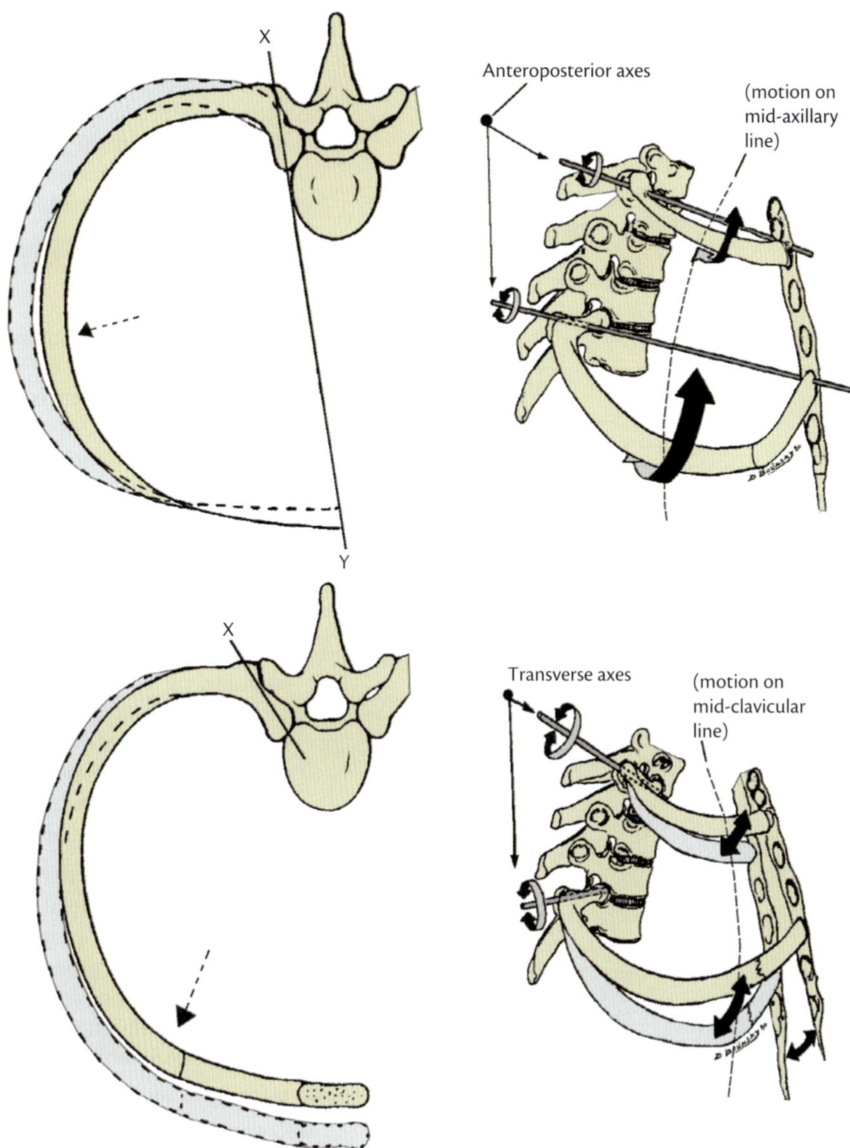

Figure 27.37 (a) Bucket-handle rib motion; (b) pump-handle rib motion.

- **Inhalation or exhalation costal somatic dysfunction:** Costal motion with respiration should be assessed both parasternally (pump-handle component of respiration) and along the lateral chest wall (bucket-handle respiratory component). Rib motion of each rib failing the screening or scanning process is compared to its corresponding rib on the other side of the body. Palpating digits straddle each pair of ribs being tested and the patient is instructed to take a full breath in and to let their breath out. During one phase of the respiratory cycle, the rib with restricted motion will stop moving prior to the normal side. The costal dysfunction is named for the respiratory component that is permitted. An inhalation right fifth rib dysfunction, for example, will have palpatory findings in which both fifth ribs rise in inhalation but, during continued exhalation, the right fifth rib stops moving while the left continues inferiorly. Note that the eleventh and twelfth ribs, without an anterior sternal attachment, have more of a pincer or caliper motion, exhibiting a posterolateral motion during inhalation and an anteromedial motion during exhalation. In general, inhalation rib dysfunction often involves several ribs. Conversely, exhalation rib dysfunction often arises in patients with a persistent cough wherein localized spasm of an intercostal muscle typically results in an exhalation dysfunction of a single rib.

The thoracic cage is host to a number of myofascial points which, by their location and clinical correlations, can be subdivided into Jones' tender points, Travell's/Simons' TrPs, and Chapman's reflex points (Figures 27.9 and 27.38). The system described by Lawrence Jones in his strain–counterstrain system (Jones 1981) is associated with locally tender myofascial points that do not refer pain. The Travell's/Simons' somatic points trigger empirically mapped musculoskeletal pain or visceral dysfunction. Chapman's points (Patriquin 1992, 1997) appear coincident with visceral problems and are interpreted as secondary viscerosomatic findings.

Jones' system recognizes the coexistence of costal dysfunction and related tender points on the anterior and/or posterior chest wall at specific sites. Simons and Travell also record the common coexistence of TrPs with rib somatic dysfunction:

- pectoralis minor TrPs with inhalation R3, R4, and/or R5 costal somatic dysfunction (Simons et al. 1999, pp. 844–56)
- serratus anterior TrPs with pain and palpatory findings anywhere between R2–9, difficult to differentiate from inhalation costal dysfunction (Simons et al. 1999, pp. 887–99)
- abdominal TrPs with exhalation somatic dysfunction in the ipsilateral lower half of the rib cage (Simons et al. 1999, pp. 940–70).

Exhalation costal somatic dysfunction at one or two rib levels also responds well to inactivation of the commonly associated TrPs in intercostal muscles attaching to these ribs (Simons et al. 1999, pp. 862–86).

Sternal area

The sternum is also subject to somatic dysfunction. This is especially true after a motor vehicle accident in which asymmetrical forces from the shoulder harness portion of the seatbelt are transmitted into the sternum, or in the case of cardiac surgery in which the sternum is wired back together. The manubrium and the sternal body are independently assessed for their preference to forward or backward bending, side-bending, and rotation. As in other forms

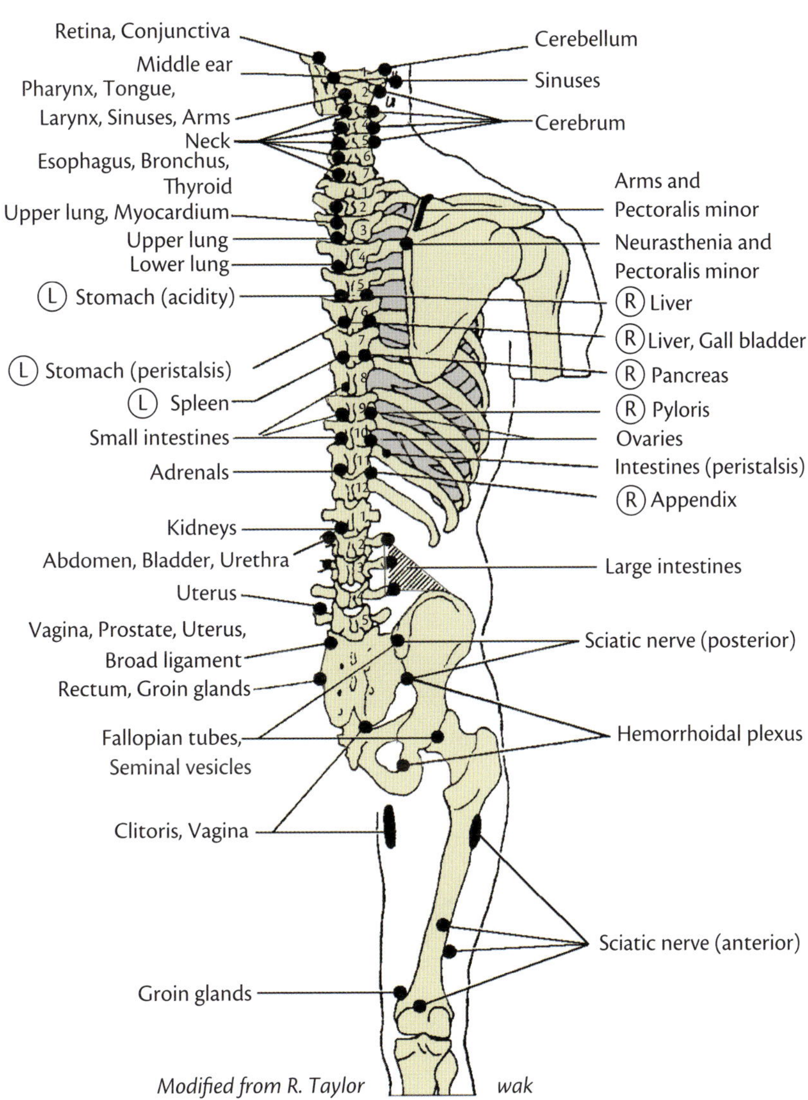

Figure 27.38 Posterior Chapman's tender points. All are bilateral except where indicated as R for right and L for left. See also anterior Chapman's diagnostic points in Figure 27.9.

of somatic dysfunction, restriction in one direction is accompanied by freedom in the opposite direction. Diagnostic testing of various somatic dysfunction combinations of the manubrium, sternal body, and sternal unit is shown in Figures 27.39, 27.40, and 27.41 respectively.

Diagnosis of the sternum is often delayed until other components of the thoracic cage are treated as sternal motion is significantly affected by dysfunction of the ribs that are, in turn, significantly influenced by their thoracic vertebral attachments.

Thoracolumbar junction/inferior thoracic outlet and lumbar spine

While the anatomical thoracolumbar junction of the spine occurs between T12 and L1, the functional inferior thoracic outlet includes the lower rib cage as well as several vertebral segments above and below T12–L1. Regional scanning and local palpation for somatic dysfunction in the thoracolumbar junction, the inferior thoracic outlet, and/or any of their component parts are most likely

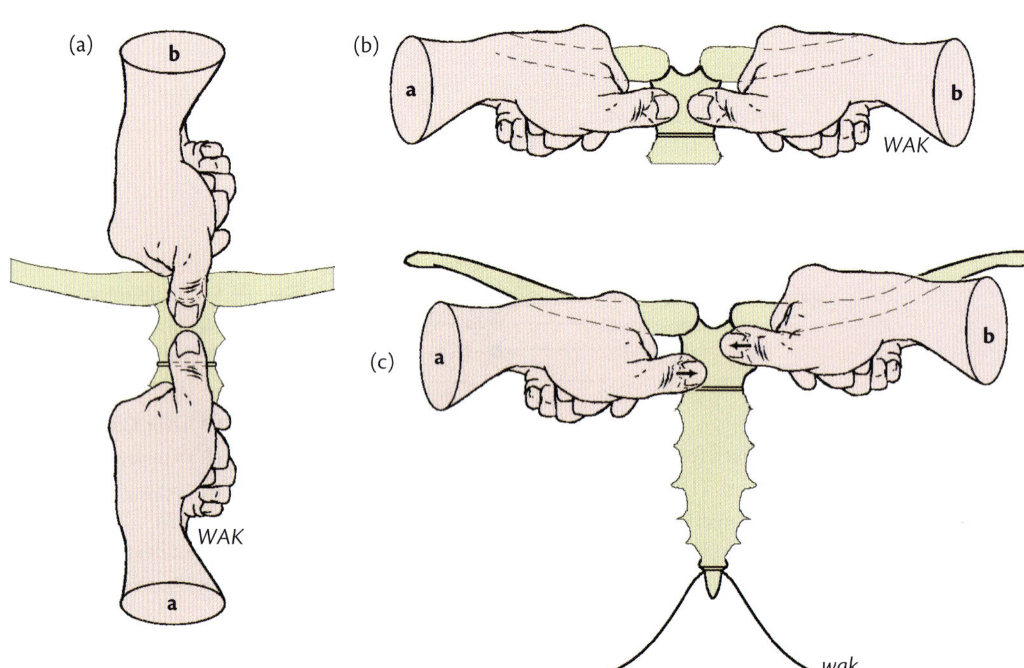

Figure 27.39 Diagnosis of manubrium: (a) flexion or extension; (b) rotation; (c) side-bending.

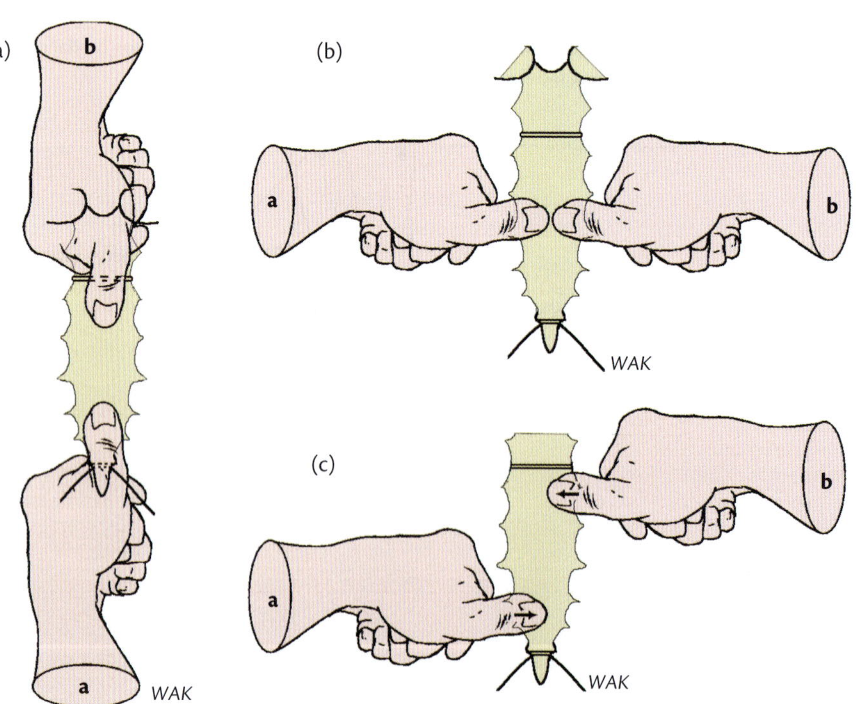

Figure 27.40 Diagnosis of gladiolus: (a) flexion or extension; (b) rotation; (c) side-bending.

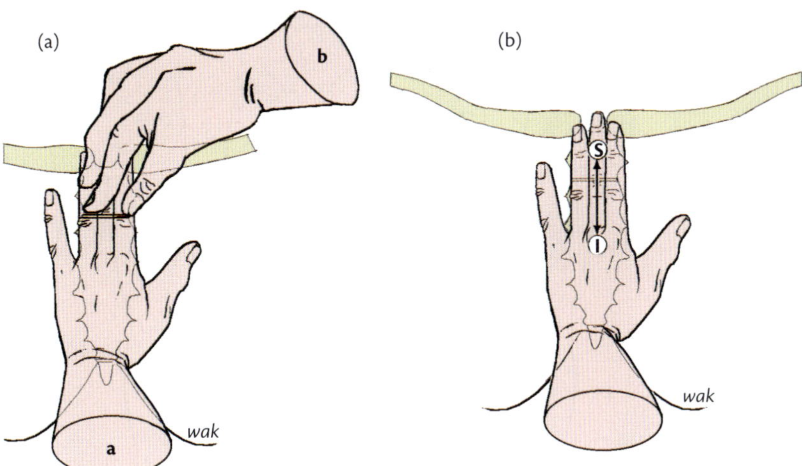

Figure 27.41 Diagnosis of the sternum as a whole: (a) 'plastic hand' method; (b) single hand for F/E, superior or inferior glide, rotation, side-bending.

to be indicated if a patient manifests any of the history, physical, or screening examination findings identified in Table 27.1. Furthermore, dysfunction or compensation occurring in regions above and below affects this transitional region.

As with the rest of the thoracic cage, pathological processes including metastasis significantly affect the interpretation of somatic findings and their treatment. Metastasis in this region is a contraindication to several types of manipulation. Batson's valveless venous plexus of veins in the lumbar spinal region drains the pelvic organs and provides a low-pressure area, predisposing the region to metastasis of regional cancers, such as those arising in the prostate (Scott 1997). Patients with low back pain, especially if it awakens them at night or is accompanied by weight loss or other systemic symptomatology, should therefore have a careful and thorough history and examination of those systems from which metastasis to bone is likely. These additional local and systemic historical and physical examinations are warranted, regardless of the presence or absence of regional somatic dysfunction.

Lumbosacral radiculopathies are not absolute contraindications to any manual technique in this region, but both palpatory and neurological examination are warranted in patients with significant low back pain with or without radiation to one or both lower extremities. Delineation between dermatomal, myotomal, and sclerotomal referral patterns helps the neuromusculoskeletal clinician differentiate between the many causes of low back pain with or without such referral. *Dermatomal* pain is widely recognized, both in distribution and quality. Conversely, *sclerotomal* pain is less well-known and is characteristically described as a deep, dull toothache or arthritic in quality. *Myotomal* involvement can lead to muscle cramps and/or TrPs; individual muscles may test weak or they may be hypertonic from overuse. Ligamentous pain tends to be sclerotomal; severe myofascial TrPs often demonstrate characteristics of both myotomal and sclerotomal patterns.

Recognize that pain and/or dysesthesia can be caused or referred by either neurological or somatic structures in patients with lumbar disk disease, spondylolistheses, and severe lumbar degenerative change. To better illustrate the importance of assessing each of the possible somatic structures involved in the differential diagnosis of this region, see Figure 27.42. Note the similarity in the distribution of an S1 radiculopathy due to a herniated disk, a gluteus minimus myofascial TrP due to hip dysfunction, and posterior sacroiliac ligament strain due to sacroiliac shear somatic dysfunction.

Thoracolumbar junction area

Common musculoskeletal and visceral disorders found to have significant somatic dysfunction in this area are:

- quadratus lumborum TrPs and/or iliolumbar ligament strain
- psoas syndrome
- viscerosomatic referral from the kidneys, gonads, intestines, bladder, or uterus
- signs and/or symptoms of hypertension, dysmenorrhoea, or constipation.

Additionally, the importance of this area through its attachments to the thoracic diaphragm make it a major consideration for somatic dysfunction in the presence of reduced diaphragm motion and in generalized congestive phenomena.

In supine patients, regional thoracolumbar motion is evaluated by exerting rotational and translational pressures over the lower rib cage (Figure 27.43) to the point where the fasciae first begin to resist. The physician evaluates for asymmetrical motion characteristics of resiliency (ease) and resistance (drag) in side-bending and rotation, bearing in mind that 80% of asymptomatic individuals will demonstrate a fascial preference for side-bending and rotating this inferior thoracic outlet region to the left (Zink and Lawson 1979).

A number of regional screening and scanning examinations identify the need for specific segmental diagnosis of thoracolumbar and lumbar somatic dysfunction. The most commonly used screening tests (Figure 27.44) include the hip drop test, trunk side-bending and trunk rotation tests, Schober's test, and the prone lumbar

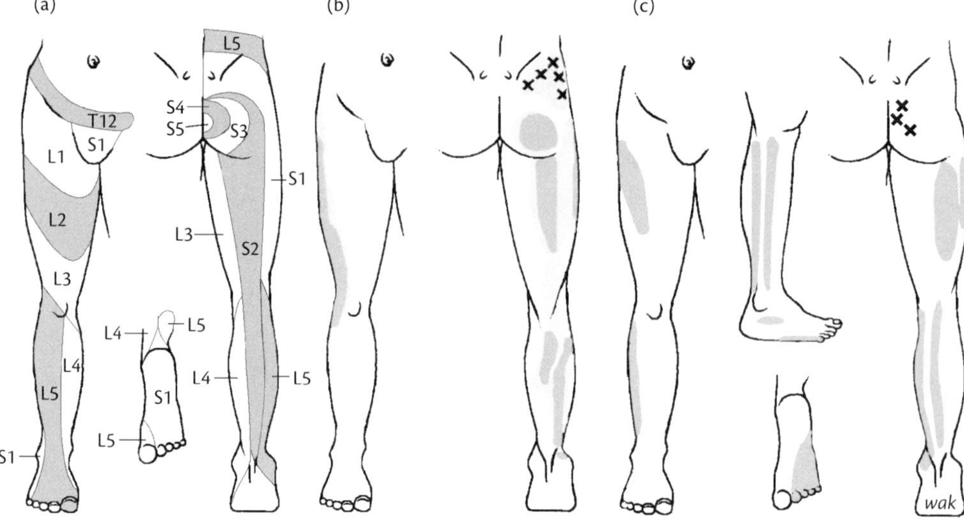

Figure 27.42 Pain pattern distributions: (a) lower extremity nerve root—dermatomal pain quality; (b) gluteus minimus trigger point (Travell)—myotomal pain quality; (c) posterior sacroiliac ligament (Hackett)—sclerotomal pain quality.

springing test. Infrequently performed tests extend to the observation that a positive skin-rolling test over the buttocks may indicate thoracolumbar dysfunction (Patterson and Burn 1985, p. 105).

Should historical, physical, or screening examinations indicate the need for more definitive information about the myofascial component of somatic dysfunction, specific tissue texture scanning for posterior myofascial tender points and TrPs in the thoracolumbar junction region would provide significant information. Travell and Simons point out that it is common to find articular somatic dysfunction spanning several segments from T7 to L4 in patients with myofascial points in the latissimus dorsi muscles (Simons et al. 1999, pp. 572–86). With these dysfunctions, typically, vertebral side-bending occurs toward and rotation occurs away from the involved muscles. Lumbar segmental somatic dysfunction is also commonly seen in patients with myofascial points in the lumbar paraspinal muscles (Simons et al. 1999, pp. 278–307). Here, single-segment articular dysfunction is more likely to be induced by rotatores at the same level, while multifidi TrPs involve two or three adjacent, and semispinalis TrPs involve group lumbar somatic dysfunction extending over 4–6 vertebral units (Simons et al. 1999, pp. 913–39). The authors also note group articular lumbar somatic dysfunction is found with iliocostalis TrPs. The most common articular somatic dysfunctions associated with serratus posterior inferior muscle TrPs are simple T10–L2 dysfunctions that side-bend in one direction and rotate the other. Occasionally, TrPs in this muscle will be linked with exhalation somatic dysfunction involving the ipsilateral lower four ribs (Simons et al. 1999, pp. 908–12).

Another extremely common combination of somatic dysfunction findings consists of psoas and quadratus lumborum TrPs in patients with articular somatic dysfunction at the thoracolumbar junction (Lewit 1986) as well as shortened rectus abdominis muscles with palpable TrPs (Lewit 1986). This is a portion of the total pattern described for gravitational strain pathophysiology (Kuchera 1995b) and postural decompensation. TrPs in the quadratus lumborum are reportedly the most common and most commonly overlooked cause of myogenic low back pain (Simons and Travell 1983).

Lumbar area

In those patients identified through historical, physical, and/or screening processes to benefit from a 'low back' examination,

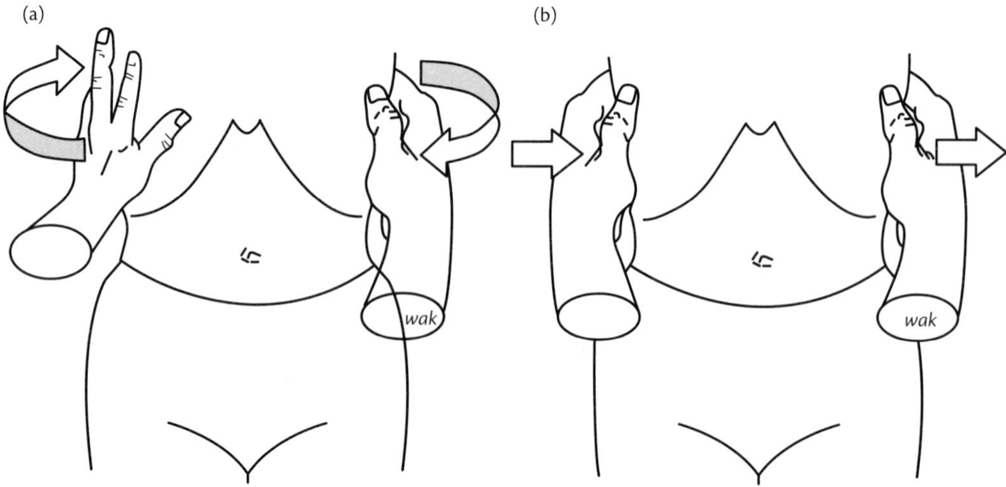

Figure 27.43 Inferior thoracic outlet regional motion: (a) right rotational screen; (b) left translation screen (side-bending right). In each case, reverse test and compare end-feel.

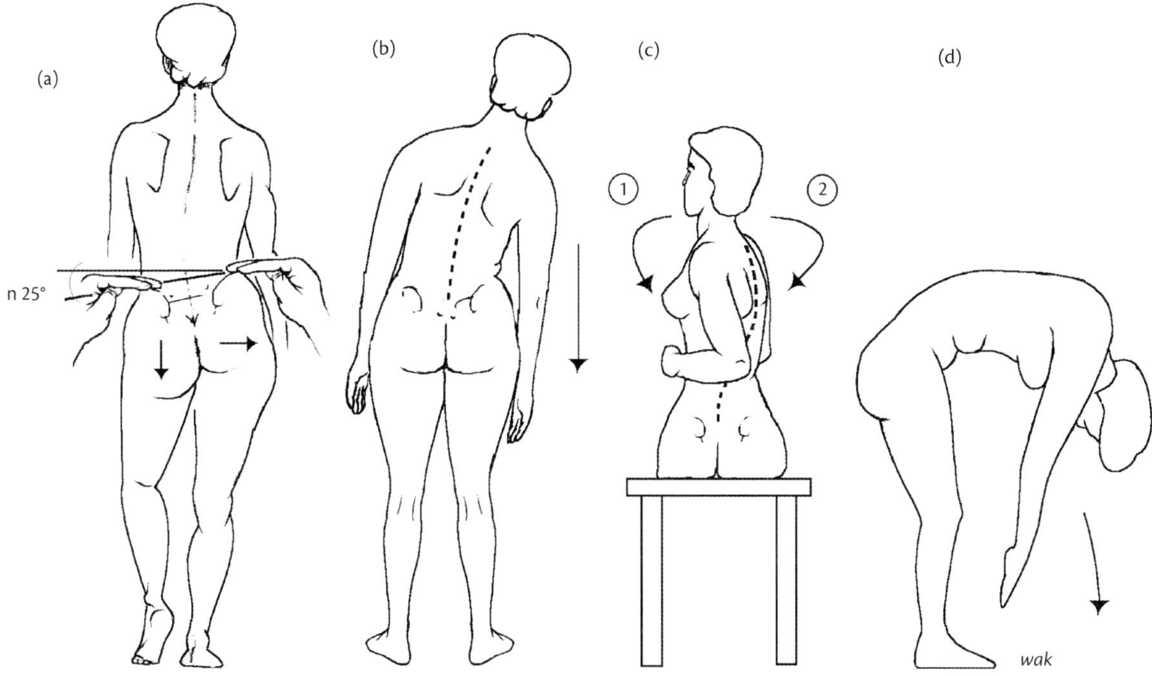

Figure 27.44 (a) Hip drop test; (b) side-bending of spine; (c) thoracolunmbar rotation; (d) spinal flexion (including Schober's test).

segmental lumbar somatic dysfunction is quickly and easily diagnosed. Screening may involve the previously mentioned hip drop test (Figure 27.44a) or lumbar spring test.

In lumbar somatic dysfunction, the quality of each barrier is restrictive in one direction and physiological in the opposing direction. The combination of restrictive barriers determines whether type I or type II dysfunction is present. Pathological change affecting spinal motion is the most prominent consideration in the differential diagnosis of somatic dysfunction. Pathological change, such as occurs in degenerative joint disease, most commonly presents with a capsular pattern of barrier restrictions which, in the lumbar region, involves marked but symmetrical limitation of side-bending accompanied by lesser limitation of both flexion and extension. The sagittal plane capsular barriers arising from degenerative and inflammatory processes (such as ankylosing spondylitis) also create a positive Schober's test (Figure 27.44d).

A number of structural changes predispose to dysfunction in this region. These may be suspected, for example, with palpation of a drop-off sign between lumbar spinous processes as is common in spondylolisthesis (Figure 27.45) or with an isolated midline lumbar tuft of hair as is seen in spina bifida occulta. Spina bifida occulta and isthmic spondylolisthesis have their highest incidence at L5 and S1. Although spina bifida occulta itself is not painful, it is commonly associated with other posterior lumbosacral congenital defects, a higher incidence of acquired isthmic spondylolisthesis, and potential alteration of muscular attachments and function. L5–S1 isthmic spondylolisthesis, affecting 3% of the American population, is associated with extremely high biomechanical risk factors for pathophysiological stress and strain of posterior lumbosacral support structures (Kuchera 1995b, 1997b). Furthermore, patients with the dysplastic form of spondylolisthesis have lumbopelvic articular facets that are nearly horizontal and, as such, they are poorly designed to support upright postural gravitational stress.

For segmental motion evaluation in somatic dysfunction, the quality of the end-feel of barriers to rotation, sidebending, and flexion—extension is assessed. Finger placement must be precise and the motion characteristics coordinated for each segment. Specific passive triplanar motion testing can be individually assessed in any position, although for this region it is most easily accomplished in the lumbar region, with the patient seated or prone. Alternating pressure over the transverse processes of a segment assesses the end-feel of the barrier to rotation at that level. Note that the transverse processes in this region are located essentially in the same horizontal plane as the spinous process of the same vertebra. (In the case of L5, where the anatomy precludes actually palpating transverse processes, the clinician should palpate as far laterally as possible on symmetric portions of the L5 posterior arch.) Translation or passively induced side-bending is applied to assess the quality of that barrier at the same vertebral level. Passively testing interspinous approximation or separation permits assessment of the sagittal plane of motion.

In applying the dynamic motion testing method, patients capable of doing so can change position to permit the clinician to monitor change in the relationship of pairs of lumbar transverse processes. The transverse processes (or lateral posterior arches of L5) are palpated in neutral, extended (sphinx position), and forward bent positions (Figure 27.46). As in the thoracic region, two different type II somatic dysfunction diagnoses are possible in this region, ERS or FRS. The ERS somatic dysfunction is diagnosed when the transverse process on one side will become more prominent with

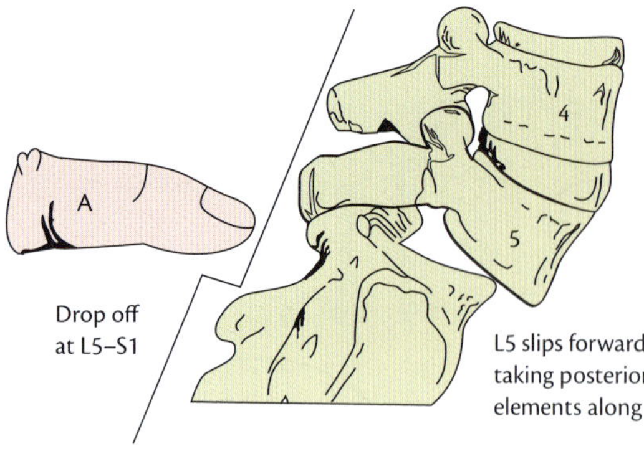

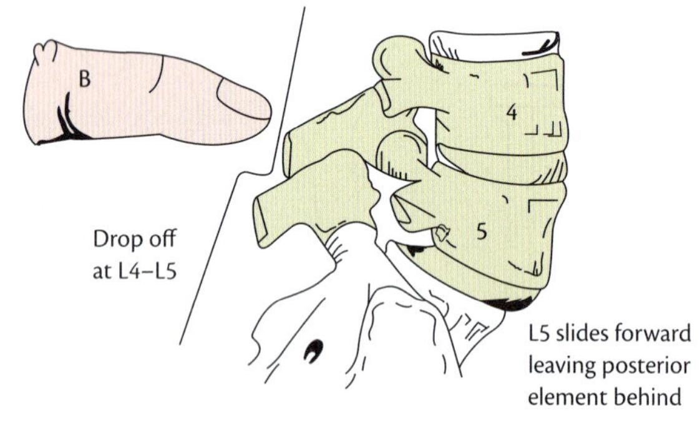

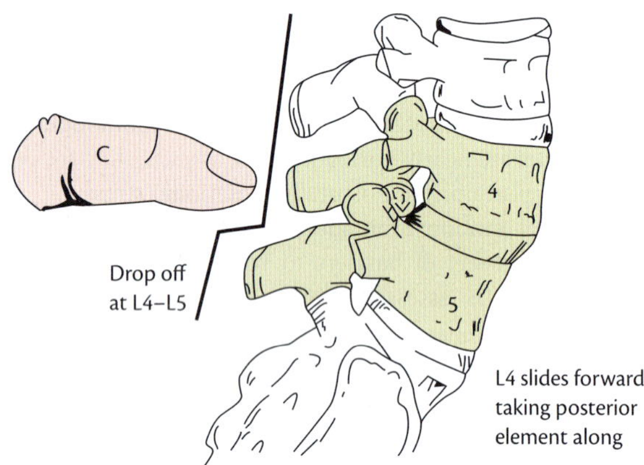

Figure 27.45 Spondylolithesis drop-off sign variations. (A) L5 dysplastic; (B) L5 isthmic; (C) L4 degenerative.

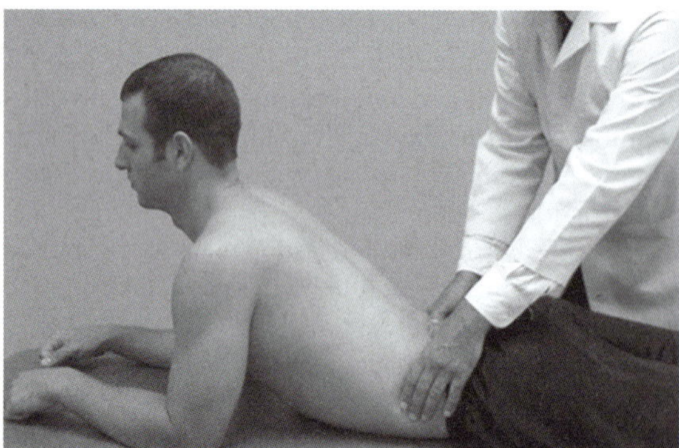

Figure 27.46 Prone to sphinx position creates extension in the lumbar spine and sacral nutation (forward bending). Dynamic motion testing may be performed from multiple start positions.

forward bending and more symmetric with backward bending. The opposite findings are palpated in an FRS somatic dysfunction. Both diagnoses typically involve a single vertebral unit and, in both, the side-bending and rotational restrictions are to the same side. The diagnosis of a type I somatic dysfunction typically involves three or more adjacent vertebral units. Dynamic motion testing in type I somatic dysfunction may change the asymmetry of transverse processes slightly, but symmetry is not achieved with either forward or backward bending.

Pelvis (innominates, pubic symphysis, sacrum, and coccyx) and lumbopelvic junction

This area is strategically located for significant impact on gait, low back function, and postural balance. Therefore, numerous lumbopelvic pain generators have been identified, pain patterns have been mapped, and models have been described to categorize the role of various somatic structures in patient complaints. At the same time, regionally, the pelvis and lumbopelvic junction contain more musculoskeletal congenital anomalies than any other body region. Asymmetry of the lumbar facets (tropism) and sacroiliac joints, important in assessing motion characteristics and the direction of manipulation treatment activation, are ubiquitous. As a consequence of these factors, more variation in lumbopelvic biomechanical models exists amongst different manual medicine schools than perhaps in any other region.

Key differential diagnostic considerations for somatic dysfunction in this region include recognition of hypermobility, structural change due to rheumatological or degenerative disorders, as well as pain and pathology associated with a malignancy or other severe pathological condition.

Because certain arthritic, degenerative, or inflammatory processes first become symptomatic in this region (in young men, for instance, ankylosing spondylitis may begin insidiously, resulting in progressive regional motion loss), additional evaluation should therefore include a number of screening palpatory and neurological tests, including tests for stability and mobility as well as screening for possible significant pathological processes.

- In cases of low back pain of unknown origin, documentation of the presence or absence of pertinent 'red flag' signs and symptoms should appear in the patient record. These include a progressive history of the chief complaint and its response to lying down, movement, or coughing, as well as a detailed description of any neurological radiation of pain, dysesthesia, or muscle weakness. Record any associated weight loss or disturbance of bowel or bladder function, or functional disturbance such as pain waking the patient at night or limiting the ability to walk more than a short distance. A complete neurological examination of the low back and lower extremities should also be recorded. Differential diagnostic considerations will often mandate rectal and/or vaginal examinations to rule out primary pathological sources, permitting a simultaneous palpatory examination of coccygeal and pelvic floor S.T.A.R. characteristics.
- Physical findings such as uveitis, urethritis, or pitting of the nails may indicate associated premature sacroiliac fusion or severe rheumatological disorder, and suggest the need for laboratory or radiographic tests.
- It is a serious sign if the patient experiences more pain when the lower extremity is raised with the hip passively flexed on the

trunk and with the knee bent, than when a typical straight leg raising test is performed. This positive 'sign of the buttock' test (Cyriax and Cyriax 1993) could indicate iliac metastasis, chronic septic sacroiliac arthritis, ischiorectal abscess, sacral fracture, gluteal bursitis, or involvement of the upper femur with neoplasm, bursitis, or osteomyelitis.

Different somatic structures within this region have a significant effect on the function and dysfunction of adjacent structures. For example, sacroiliac articular somatic dysfunction coexists in patients with myofascial points in the quadratus lumborum muscles, while both latissimus dorsi and quadratus lumborum TrPs are accompanied by innominate dysfunction (Simons et al. 1999, pp. 572–86). Pubic and innominate dysfunctions are commonly associated with abdominal TrPs (Simons et al. 1999, pp. 940–70). TrPs in the iliocostalis lumborum are associated with pelvic obliquity secondary to the muscle's insertional aponeurosis onto the sacral base that leads to sacroiliac dysfunction (Simons et al. 1999, pp. 913–39). In this latter case, the positive seated flexion test will be worse than the standing flexion test (Greenman 1996, p. 316).

Somatic structures in adjacent regions also have a significant effect on lumbopelvic function and dysfunction. This is clearly the synopsis of clinical experts in the interdisciplinary text, *Movement, stability and low back pain: the essential role of the pelvis* (Vleeming et al. 1997), in interpreting the lumbopelvic region. One conclusion is that the ultimate balance between regional stability and mobility (Figure 27.47) rests, in part, on form closure contributed by the shape of the sacrum and its angle of nutation/counternutation and, in part, on the proper function of the myofascial *unterkreuz* (Kuchera 1995a) in contributing force closure (Kuchera 1997c).

Finally, it should be noted, upon careful review of Table 27.2, that the importance of the sacral base as the foundation upon which the spine sits extends the impact of dysfunction here far beyond the lumbopelvic area. Thus, regional examination of all areas of the musculoskeletal system is warranted in the presence of an unlevel sacral base. Unlevelling of the sacral base is well documented to be a precipitating and perpetuating cause of muscle imbalance and myofascial TrPs throughout the entire body (Simons et al. 1999; Travell and Simons 1992) as well as a cause of recurrent patterns of somatic dysfunction (Kuchera 2011; Peterson 1983). In addition, segmental facilitated spinal dysfunction arising in compensation for an unlevel sacral base is capable of creating a wide range of visceral and systemic symptomatology.

Lumbopelvic and sacroiliac (sacrum and/or iliac origin) areas

Patients present to neuromusculoskeletal medicine physicians with low back (lumbopelvic) more so than any other area of the body, with the possible exception of headache. Neuromusculoskeletal physicians have moved significantly beyond the historically unifocal preoccupation with discogenic back pain (Mixter and Barr 1934). Farfan, for example, described the cause of low back pain as mechanical (1980) and numerous pain generators are influenced by biomechanical stress and strain. In somatic dysfunction, the lumbar zygopophyseal joints (Fairbank et al. 1981; Mooney and Robertson 1976), the muscular elements associated with lumbopelvic function and dysfunction (Travell and Simons 1992), and the sacroiliac joint itself (Steinbrocker et al. 1953; Travell and Travell 1946) are key pain generators. Although the latter component is perhaps the most 'controversial' (Greenman 1996, pp. 305–11), sacroiliac joint dysfunction is acknowledged to play an 'incontrovertible' (Mooney 1997) role in a number of locally painful spinal disorders. Furthermore, Travell and Simons (1992) and others (Kuchera 1995b) noted the major role of postural imbalance and sacroiliac dysfunction in the perpetuation and precipitation of pain and dysfunction in this region.

Regional scanning and local palpation of the lumbopelvic junction, the pelvic girdle, and its component parts for somatic dysfunction are most likely to be indicated for patients with the presence of the historical, physical, or screening examination findings identified previously in Table 27.2. Here, the different relative symmetry of key structures and their palpatory motion characteristics provide clues to naming the dysfunction but, here, diagnosis also depends largely upon the model used for interpretation.

Lumbopelvic regional restriction of motion may be scanned in the supine patient by first gently placing one hand over one anterior superior iliac spine (ASIS) and reaching across to the opposite side to gently grasp the pelvis posterior to the gluteus medius muscle to lift in a manner to rotate the pelvis on the lumbar spine. Alternating palpation of left and right rotation of the region evaluates for resiliency (ease) or resistance (drag). Gently grasping both sides of the pelvis laterally, just below the iliac crests, and translating the pelvis right and left with respect to the lumbar region, assesses the point where the fasciae first begin to resist side-bending. Few individuals are perfectly symmetrical and 80% of asymptomatic individuals will demonstrate a fascial preference for side-bending and rotating of the pelvic complex at the lumbopelvic junction to the right (Zink and Lawson 1979).

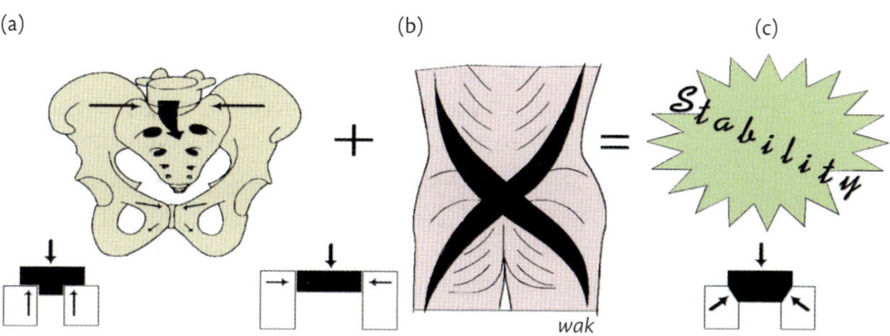

Figure 27.47 (a) Form closure; (b) force closure; and (c) sacroiliac static-dynamic mechanics. (From *Spine: state of the art review*, 1995, 9, 463–90)

Commonly overlooked pain-generating skeletal, arthrodial, and myofascial structures include the quadratus lumborum (Travell and Simons 1992), iliolumbar ligament (Kuchera 1995b), and somatic dysfunction originating in this region as a consequence of a number of diagnoses (Greenman 1996b) including:

- short leg and pelvic tilt syndrome
- type II lumbar somatic dysfunction
- pubic shear somatic dysfunction
- innominate shear somatic dysfunction
- sacral somatic dysfunction restricting nutation (anterior rotation)
- muscle imbalance and dysfunction.

TrPs in the quadratus lumborum (Figure 27.48) are noted to be 'one of the most commonly overlooked muscular sources of low back pain' and are often responsible, through satellite gluteus minimus TrPs (Figure 27.42b), for the 'pseudo-disc' syndrome and the 'failed surgical back' syndrome (Travell and Simons 1992, pp. 28–88). It was also the most commonly involved muscle (32%) in soldiers with musculoskeletal complaints (Good 1942). TrPs in this muscle responded to a variety of manual techniques directed to the muscle itself including massage, tapotement, and post-isometric muscle energy manipulative treatment (Kimberly and Funk 2000; Lewit 1986) (see Chapter 50). This diagnosis also frequently required correction of underlying muscle imbalance, short leg and pelvic tilt syndrome, sacroiliac somatic dysfunction, and twelfth rib somatic dysfunction to prevent recurrence.

The iliolumbar ligament is positioned to provide stability between the lumbar spine and the pelvis. It is consequently one of the first structures to indicate biomechanical dysfunction in the region. Iliolumbar ligament stress arises from the same biomechanical factors already listed for the quadratus lumborum and has a very similar pain pattern (Hackett 1958).

The value of diagnosing lumbar and pelvic (sacral, innominate, pression test, and pubic) somatic dysfunction is well established in the literature. In a study by Greenman of 183 consecutive patients presenting with disabling low back pain (average duration 30.7 months), three or more of the so-called 'dirty half dozen' (Greenman 1992) somatic dysfunction diagnoses already listed were found in 50% of the population. Correction of the dysfunction through integrated rehabilitative means, including manual medicine, resulted in restoration of normal activities of daily living (including return to work) in 75% of these patients.

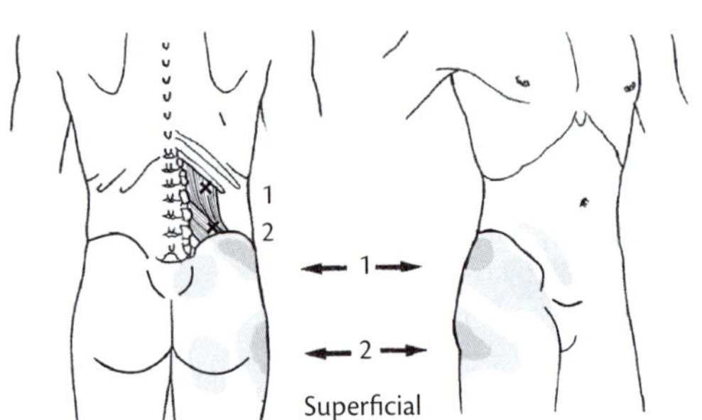

Figure 27.48 Quadratus lumborum trigger point pattern. (From Travell and Simons 1992)

Unfortunately, structure–function interrelationships become especially difficult to evaluate and interpret properly in the presence of anomalies such as sacralization of L5, lumbarization of S1, batwing transverse processes that may or may not have their own articulations with the ilium, and combinations of these and other structural variations at the same spinal level. For these reasons, a significant number of additional screening and scanning examinations have been described to assist the clinician in focusing his or her examination. The most commonly used screening and scanning tests have already been described and include:

- Direct *dynamic tests* for general restriction of sacroiliac motion including the one-legged stork test (also called the spine test by Dvorak, Gillet's test, and march/stork test) as a variation of the Trendelenburg test, or indirect passive examination using long sitting tests (yo-yo sign) and hip rotation tests, and/or the sacroiliac gapping test.
- A variety of *pelvic ligamentous stress tests* (Figure 27.49) including the cranial shear test, pelvic distraction and compression tests, sacroiliac gapping test (also known under many other names including the as the thigh-thrust sacroiliac stress test, the posterior pelvic pain provocation test, and the posterior shear test), sacral thrust test, Gaenslen's test, Yeoman's test, and/or variations of Patrick's FABERE (or figure 4) test.
- Generic identification of sacroiliac dysfunction has been shown to be significant if the patient *using a single finger* (Fortin and Falco 1997) twice localizes a site (within 1 cm) inferomedial to the posterior superior iliac spine (PSIS), with or without stressing the joint with a Patrick's test—noting that five other structures attach or are located within 1.5 cm of the PSIS (the L5/S1 facet joint, sacrospinalis, L5/S1 intervertebral disc, gluteus maximus, and sacroiliac joint).
- *Local motion screening tests* through springing of various areas of the pelvic girdle or through positional changes.

Each of the aforementioned tests may be used in screening or scanning the pelvic region for dysfunction. (In this section, dysfunction at the L5–S1 junction will be discussed as part of pelvic somatic dysfunction. Further insights for the lumbopelvic area can also be obtained in the lumbar section in this chapter.)

Sacroiliac joint

In the widely adopted osteopathic models, three major systems have had significant impact on the nomenclature now commonly employed. Each of these historic systems examined sacral motion as it related to a different anatomical relationship (Strachan 1938; Walton 1966).

- In the *Strachan (high-velocity, low-amplitude, HVLA) model*, diagnosis of the sacrum is named largely with respect to its motion, or restriction, relative to the innominates.
- In the *Mitchell (muscle energy) model* (Mitchell 1958), a series of postulated sacral axes is coupled with diagnoses of sacral torsions to reflect sacral motion, or restriction, relative to the lumbar spine and the mechanics of gait.
- In the *Sutherland (craniosacral) model* (Magoun 1976), motion, or restriction, of the sacrum is described relative to the cranium.

Regardless of the model selected, each diagnosis of somatic dysfunction implies freedom in one direction of motion around an axis with restriction in the opposite direction.

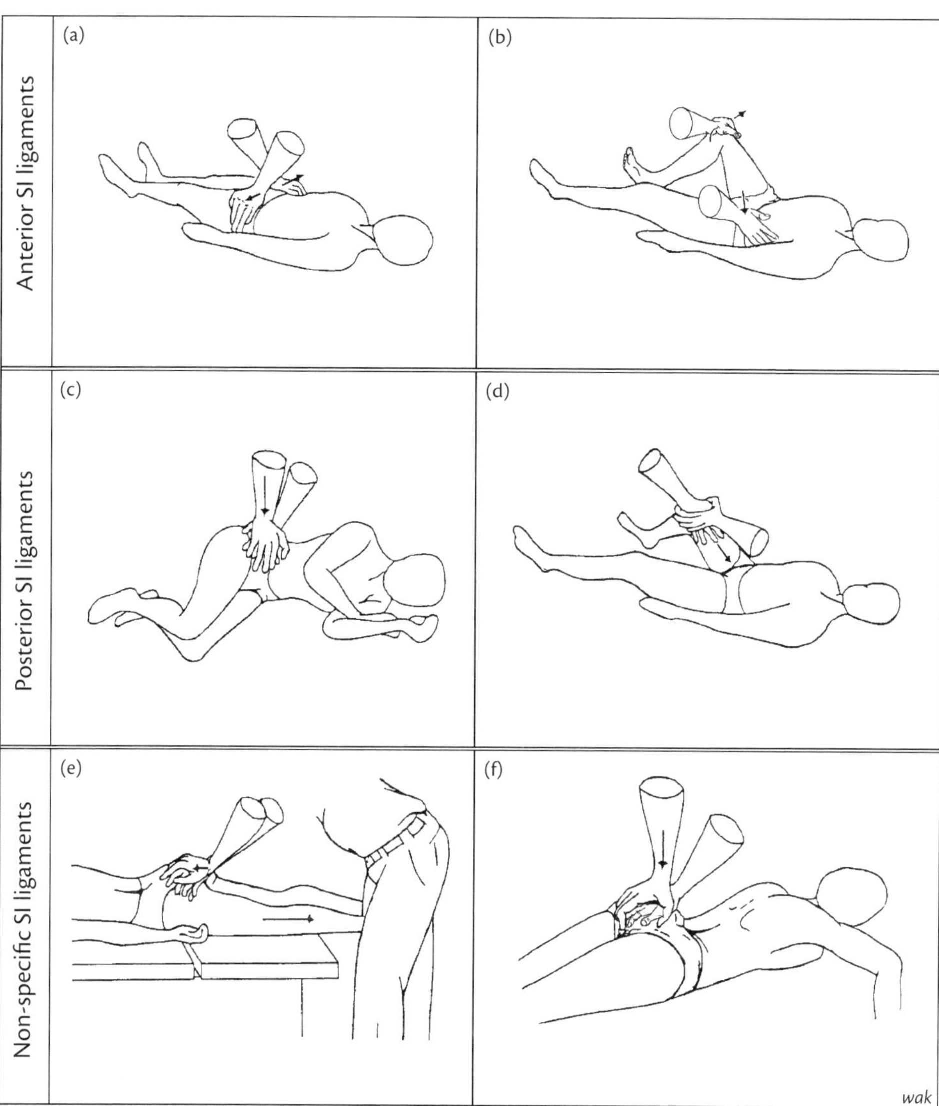

Figure 27.49 Pelvic ligament stress tests.

Each model has relative benefits depending on the clinical situation, the degree of training of the physician, and the type of manual treatment that will be used to treat the dysfunction. Recognition that differing models exist and that nomenclature is model-specific helps manual medicine physicians greatly in sorting through the literature that would otherwise seem contradictory. For a more complete discussion, refer to the chapter on sacrum and pelvis in the standard text, *Foundations for osteopathic medicine* (Heinking and Kappler 2002).

This portion of the chapter limits nomenclature and diagnostic tests to be consistent with the treatment examples presented in Chapter 50. It considers somatic dysfunction of the sacrum relative to motions around postulated transverse, oblique, and vertical axes, as well as one traumatically induced dysfunction (inferior sacral shear) not associated with an axis of motion. A suggested series of local palpatory tests for ascertaining the symmetry of sacral landmarks and the quality of motion available is depicted in Figure 27.50. Their interpretation is described more fully in Tables 27.3 and 27.4.

The goal of local palpatory examination is to compile enough specific information about key landmark asymmetry, sites, and characteristics of restricted motion, and evidence of tissue texture change to extrapolate a tentative diagnosis. The patterns depicted in Table 27.3 help with this interpretation.

Consensus on nomenclature used for descriptive findings and their interpretation permits neuromusculoskeletal physicians to communicate their combinations of objective findings in concise, meaningful ways. Because several different models are used in diagnosing and treating this region, exact agreement between all representative schools of thought is difficult. Nonetheless, while various schools may differ on their interpretation, clinical observation and research, consistent nomenclature, and careful consensus permit certain generalizations.

On the basis of lateralization tests and the resulting tentative diagnosis of dysfunction, the manual medicine physician can then initiate treatment designed to re-establish properties needed for motion, stability (Vleeming et al. 1997), and shock absorption (Wilder et al. 1980). The final goal is to improve function within the

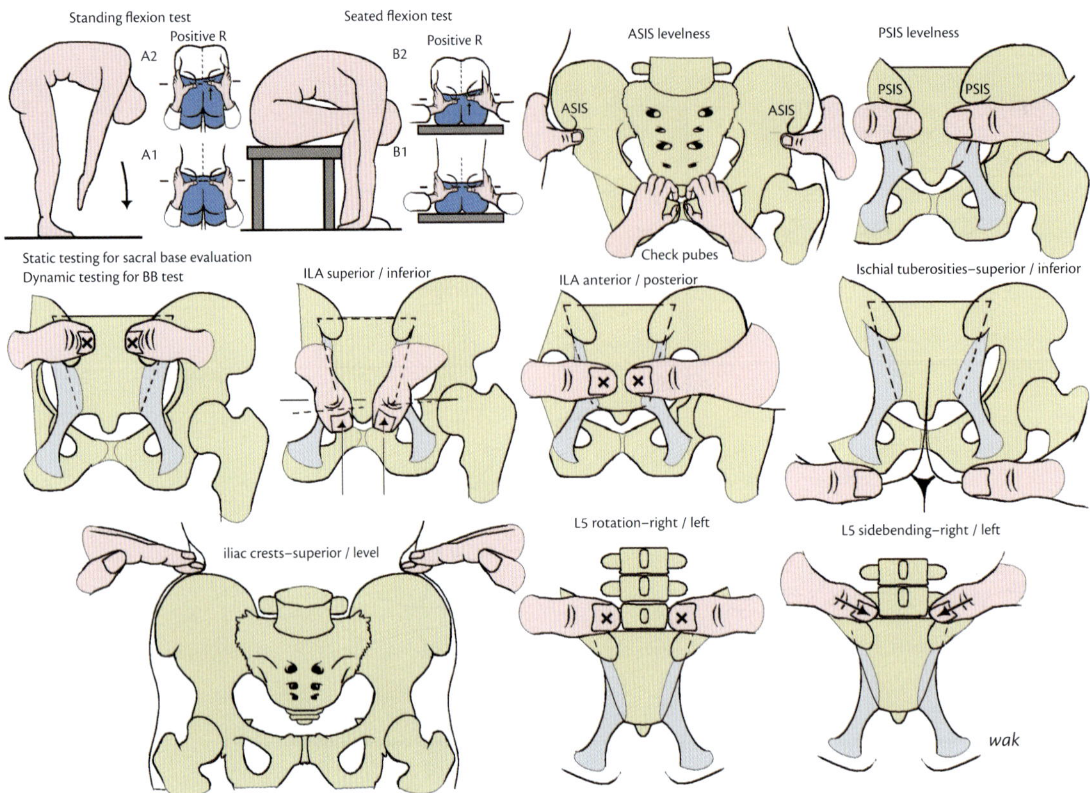

Figure 27.50 Palpation series for gathering pelvic somatic dysfunction data.

Table 27.3 Examination for somatic dysfunction of the sacroiliac articulation

Step	Patient's position	Examination	Results and postulated interpretation
1	Standing	Evaluate anatomical landmarks, standing flexion test	A positive standing flexion test means dysfunction in the lower extremity and/or pelvis on that side
2	Seated	Perform seated flexion test	Will specifically determine whether there is a sacroiliac dysfunction, and if so, which side (but not which arm) of the sacroiliac joint is dysfunctional
3	Supine	Perform ASIS compression test; positional assessment of ASISs, pubic tubercles, and medial malleoli	Helps determine the aetiology of the problem and whether it is purely sacral or a mixed problem, incorporating iliac and pubic dysfunction
4	Prone	Palpate for tissue texture changes, motion testing of the sacrum, motion testing of L5, ligamentous tension testing	Helps the physician discover which axis is involved, find what portion of the SI joint is restricted, determine L5 motion and position, and evaluate pelvic ligamentous tensions

Adapted from Heinking, Jones, and Kappler. Pelvis and sacrum. In: Ward, R.C., *Foundations for osteopathic medicine*, Williams and Wilkins, Baltimore, 1997.

pelvis to permit such vital activities of daily living as required for gait or for providing a level foundation for spinal posture.

Sacral somatic dysfunction diagnoses covered in this portion of the chapter (and treatment presented in Chapter 50) are summarized in Table 27.4. They include the following postulated axes and associated somatic dysfunctions:

- *middle transverse axis (S2 level):* sacral base anterior (bilateral sacral flexion) or sacral base posterior (bilateral sacral extension) somatic dysfunctions
- *left oblique axis (upper left S1 to lower right S3):* left or right rotation on a left oblique axis somatic dysfunctions
- *right oblique axis (upper right S1 to lower left S3):* right or left rotation on a right oblique axis somatic dysfunctions
- *sagittal or parasagittal axis:* left or right sacral margin posterior somatic dysfunctions
- *traumatically induced with no axis:* left or right sacral shear (unilateral sacral flexion or extension) somatic dysfunctions.

The following diagnoses are seen in the literature less frequently and are not fully covered in this chapter: anterior sacrum left or right, superior sacral shear left or right, and posterior sacrum left or right.

Table 27.5 summarizes an example of the importance of moving beyond static landmark assessment and integration of functional

Table 27.4 Sacral somatic dysfunction exemplars

Constellation of static and dynamic findings for common diagnoses of sacral somatic dysfunction	Sacral base anterior (bilateral sacral flexion)	Left rotation on a left oblique axis	Right rotation on left oblique axis	Sacral margin posterior on the left	Left sacral shear (left lateral "unilateral" sacral flexion)
Static findigs palpated over sacrum	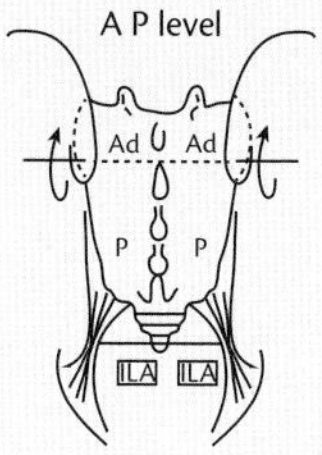 A P level; Ad Ad; P P; ILA ILA	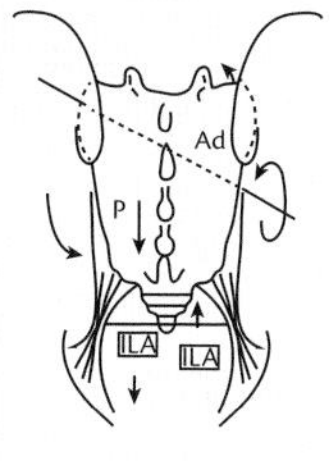 Ad; P; ILA ILA	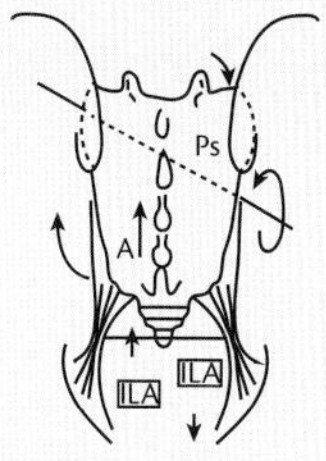 Ps; A; ILA ILA	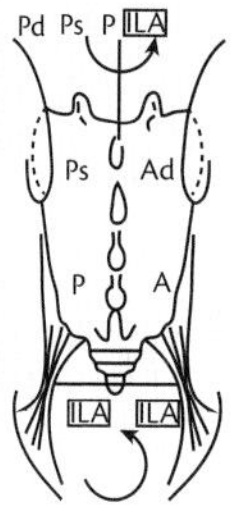 Pd Ps P ILA; Ps Ad; P A; ILA ILA	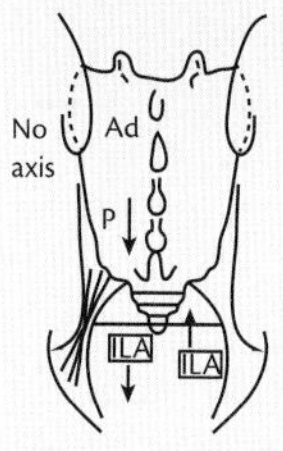 No axis; Ad; P; ILA ILA
Lateralization tests (e.g. restricted side to ASIS springing; longest-last motion in seated flexion test)	N/A	Right commonly reported –theoretically either left upper or right lower pole (or both) could be restricted	Right commonly reported –theoretically either left upper or right lower pole (or both) could be restricted	Left	Left
Sphinx test (backward bending test)	N/A Remains symmetrical	More symmetrical than previously	Less symmetrical than previously	Less symmetrical than previously	More symmetrical than previously
Motion testing or "rattle" of the four poles	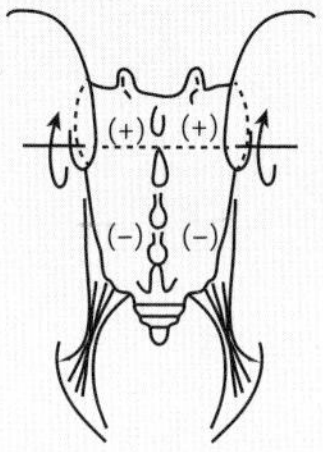 (+) (+); (–) (–)	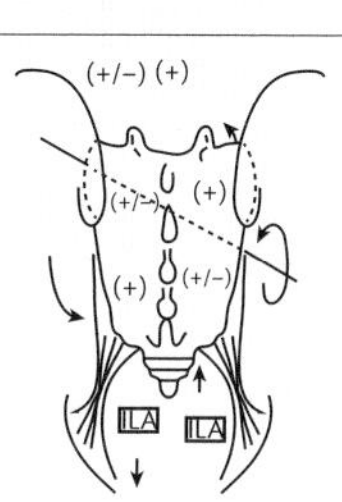 (+/–) (+); (+/–) (+); (+) (+/–); ILA ILA	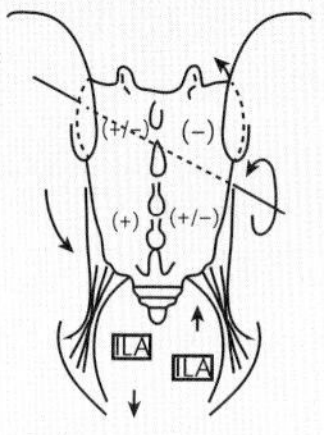 (+/–) (–); (+) (+/–); ILA ILA	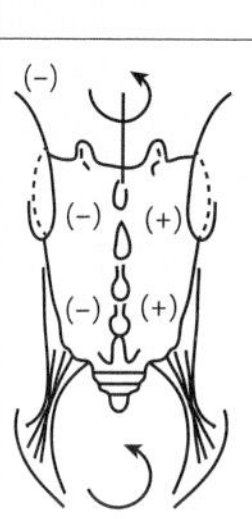 (–); (–) (+); (–) (+)	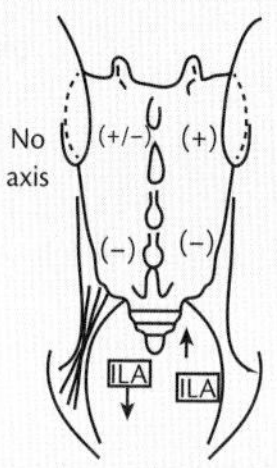 No axis; (+/–) (+); (–) (–); ILA ILA
Restriction of gapping	N/A	Left upper and lower; right lower	Left upper, right upper and lower	Left upper and lower	Left upper and lower

d, deep; s, shallow; A, anterior; P, posterior; I, inferior.

+, moves; –, restricted; ±, some motion.

,normal ligament, , tight ligament, , loose ligament.

tests of motion in making a diagnosis. While each of the five sacral diagnoses has the same static sacral landmarks, variations in the motion characteristics provide different diagnoses and, therefore, different treatment approaches.

With so much individual host variability and so many models of diagnosis in the pelvic region, it is not surprising that this area, more than many others, evokes disagreement concerning biomechanics and clinical approach to diagnosis and treatment. What is generally agreed upon, however, is the importance of the region as a base of function for many important activities of daily living, ranging from sitting and standing postures to ambulation.

With this is mind, greater overall importance might be assigned to screening and lateralization tests that indicate 'if dysfunction exists or not' and, if so, which sites might be monitored to assess return of functional motion and/or reduction of pain. Local tests leading to a diagnosis specific for a particular model will continue to retain their importance for the individual practitioner in selecting a therapeutic technique but should probably bow to reassessment of the big question concerning treatment—namely, do screening and lateralization tests now indicate stability, mobility, and pain-free function in the region?

Coccyx and pelvic floor

The pelvic girdle is important in congestive phenomena and the respiratory–circulatory model of health described by Zink (Zink and Lawson 1979), in part because of its relationship to the pelvic diaphragm. Specific diagnosis of the pelvic floor is usually undertaken after correction of the bony framework to which the muscles attach.

General assessment of the pelvic floor and related muscles often includes observation of the lower extremities (e.g. external rotation of the lower extremity on the side of increased piriformis tension and direct palpation of the ischiorectal fossa using an external approach (see Figure 50.62, Chapter 50) with fingers directed along the ischial tuberosity).

Specific diagnosis of the coccyx or of certain pelvic floor muscles is often done with a gloved finger inserted in the vagina or rectum. This is most commonly performed as part of the pelvic or rectal

Table 27.5 Motion testing importance in differential diagnosis of sacral dysfunction (osteopathic model)

'Diagnoses' listed to the right have the same static findings	Left rotation on left oblique axis	Anterior sacrum right	Posterior sacrum left (only in Strachan model)	Left on left forward torsion	Left rotation on right oblique axis
Static findings palpated over sacrum	(Same)		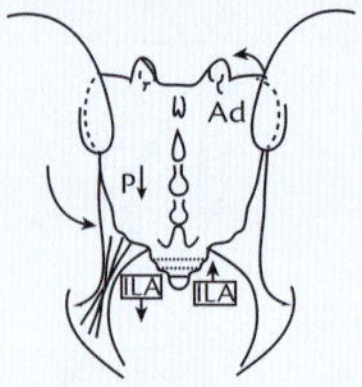 P Ad ILA ILA	(Same)	
Lateralization tests (e.g. restricted side to ASIS springing; longest-last motion in seated flexion test)	+ Right	+ Right with tissue texture change over right upper pole	+ Left with tissue texture change over left lower pole	+ Right	+ Left
Sphinx test (backward bending test)	More symmetrical	More symmetrical		More symmetrical	Less symmetrical
Motion testing or 'rattle' of the 4 poles	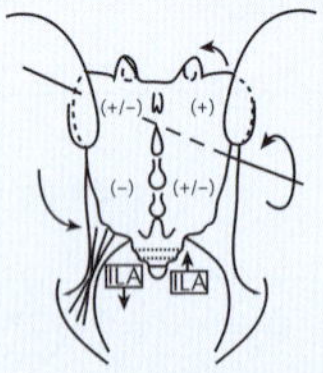 (+/-) (+) (-) (+/-) ILA ILA	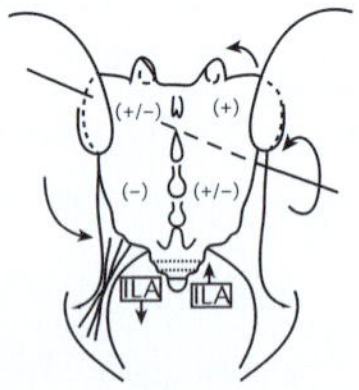 (+/-) (+) (-) (+/-) ILA ILA	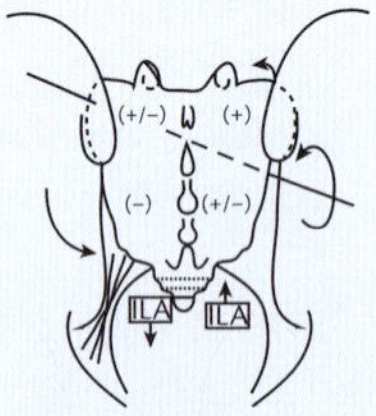 (+/-) (+) (-) (+/-) ILA ILA	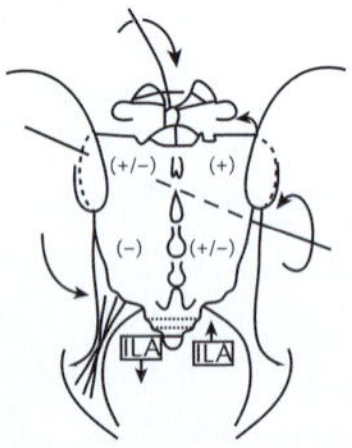 (+/-) (+) (-) (+/-) ILA ILA	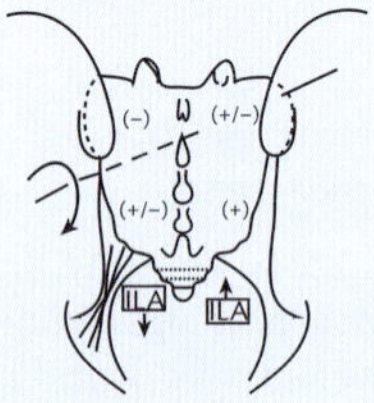 (-) (+/-) (+/-) (+) ILA ILA
L5	N/A	N/A	N/A	$L5S_LR_R$	N/A

d, deep; s, shallow; A, anterior; P, posterior; I, inferior. +, moves; –, restricted; ±, some motion. ,normal ligament, , tight ligament, , loose ligament.

examination during a general physical examination or a detailed examination focusing on constructing the complete differential diagnosis of coccygodynia, pelvic floor spasm, incontinence, prostatodynia, and low back pain of unknown origin.

Innominate (iliosacral) and pubic somatic dysfunction

Somatic dysfunction of the innominate bone is often discussed with respect to the lower extremities, but this chapter includes a few relative diagnostic tests related to their impact on regional function of associated joints, myofascial and ligamentous structures, and of the pelvic ring as a whole.

Much of the iliosacral dysfunction transmitted by way of the innominates can be linked with biomechanical imbalance occurring during gait or from the impact of trauma during different components of the gait cycle. Commonly, function and dysfunction in this context is associated with the physiological motions of anterior and posterior rotation of each half of these pelvic bones around a so-called inferior transverse sacroiliac axis.

Trauma transferred up through a lower extremity (or by landing on one ischial tuberosity during a fall) may create non-physiological dysfunction (Figure 27.51) through forceful gliding of the iliosacral joint (as in a superior innominate shear) or the pubic symphysis (as in a superior pubic shear). Here, there is no postulated axis, rather shearing forces following the joint surface(s) are responsible.

The lateralization test most frequently denoting the side of iliosacral or pubic dysfunction is the standing flexion test; however, shifting the direction of force vectors while performing the ASIS compression test is also very helpful in following outcomes return of function here. Local static landmarks used in deriving somatic dysfunction for the innominate are the ASIS, PSIS, and iliac crests. Static local findings used in pubic shear diagnosis include discovery of a 'step' sign rising up or dropping down a few millimetres as the palpating fingers are drawn across the superior and anterior surfaces of the pubic rami on either side of the pubic symphysis.

Summary: patient-centred approach to somatic dysfunction and diagnosis

Without doubt, somatic dysfunction can be identified in a wide range of patient complaints ranging from local pain and alteration of function to more systemic disturbances. For physicians practicing manual/neuromusculoskeletal medicine, it plays a significant role in the differential diagnosis of a broad spectrum of patient complaints. This is the case for each of the many schools of manual medicine: in spite of their many differences in language, emphases on differing tests, and variety of proposed mechanisms, each recognizes the presence of 'somatic dysfunction', the implications of such altered function on local and distant function, and the patient response to removing that dysfunction.

The experience of physicians in various neuromusculoskeletal fields thereby establishes a definitive role for evaluation and treatment of somatic dysfunction. Nonetheless, much additional work

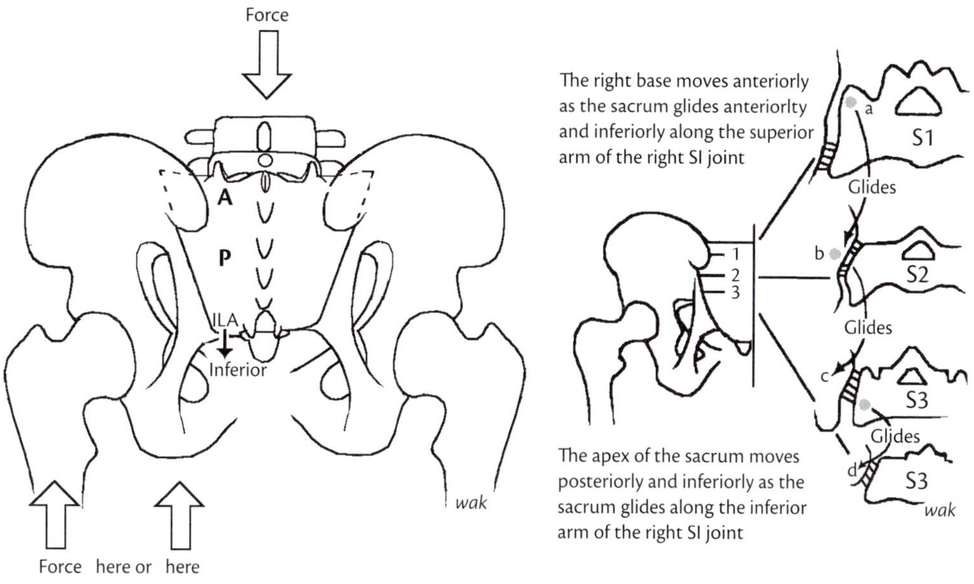

Figure 27.51 Left sacral shear.

needs to be done in standardizing nomenclature, assessing reproducibility and validity of various empirically or theoretically derived clinical–biomechanical models, and expanding the evidence base for the field of manual medicine.

That said, unfortunately the reductionist approach in identifying and studying an isolated somatic dysfunction in a clinical setting may be ineffective. Radin's experience in this regard led to his remark, 'Functional analysis, be it biological, mechanical or both, of a single tissue will fail to give a realistic functional analysis as, in all complex constructs, the interaction between the various components is a critical part of their behavior' (Vleeming et al. 1997). With these factors in mind (and while researchers continue to explore), physicians engaged in manual medicine will most likely continue to practice a multidimensional, patient-centred, total-body approach when assessing somatic dysfunction and the neuromusculoskeletal system. The value of integrating patient-centred and biopsychosocial approaches with diagnosis and treatment of specific anatomical pathophysiology has become the standard of care; for example, its current use in predicting orthopaedic surgical intervention outcomes in back pain patients (SCORE 1996; Waddell et al. 1989).

In summary then, the complete neuromusculoskeletal examination begins with looking at function and dysfunction of the whole patient, examining down to smaller and smaller somatic units, and then reassembling the role of these smaller units back into the total body function.

Acknowledgements

The author gratefully thanks his father, William A. Kuchera, DO (professor emeritus), for the design and clarity of all of the line drawings in this chapter.

References

Amoronso, P.J., et al. *Tobacco and injuries: an annotated bibliography*. US Army Research Laboratory Technical Report, ARTR-1333; 1997.

Biller, J., Sacco, R.L., Albuquerque, F.C., et al. (on behalf of the American Heart Association Stroke Council). Cervical arterial dissections and association with cervical manipulative therapy: a statement for healthcare professionals from the American Heart Association/American Stroke Association. *Stroke*, 2014, 45, 3155–74.

Chaitow, L. *Soft tissue manipulation*. Thorsons: Wellington, UK; 1987.

Chila, A.G. (ed.) *Foundations for osteopathic medicine* (3rd edn). Lippincott, Williams & Wilkins: Baltimore, MD; 2011.

Cyriax, J.H., Cyriax, P.J. *Cyriax's illustrated manual of orthopaedic medicine* (2nd edn). Butterworth-Heinemann: Oxford; 1993.

Cyriax, J. *Textbook of orthopaedic medicine, volume two: treatment by manipulation, massage and injection* (10th edn). Bailliére Tindall: London; 1980.

D'Alonzo, G.E., Krachman, S.L. Respiratory system. Chapter 37 in: Ward, R.C. (ed.) *Foundations for osteopathic medicine*. Williams and Wilkins: Baltimore, MD; 1997; pp. 441–58.

Dananberg, H.J. Lower back pain as a gait-related repetitive motion injury. Chapter 21 in: Vleeming, A., Mooney, V., Snijders, C.J., Dorman, T.A., Stoeckart, R. (eds) *Movement, stability and low back pain: the essential role of the pelvis*. Churchill-Livingstone: New York; 1997; pp. 253–67.

Degenhardt, B.F., Snider, K.T., Johnson, J.C., Snider, E.J. Interexaminer reliability of osteopathic palpatory evaluation of the lumbar spine. *J Am Osteopath Assoc*, 2002, 102(8), 442.

Degenhardt, B.F., Snider, K.T., Johnson, J.C., Snider, E.J. Retention of interexaminer reliability in palpatory evaluation of the lumbar spine. *J Am Osteopath Assoc*, 2002, 102(8), 439.

Dinnar, U. Classification of diagnostic tests used with osteopathic manipulation. *J Am Osteopath Assoc*, 1980, 79, 451–5.

Dinnar, U. Description of fifty diagnostic tests used with osteopathic manipulation. *J Am Osteopath Assoc*, 1982, 81, 314–21.

Education Council on Osteopathic Principles (ECOP). Glossary of osteopathic terminology. In: Chila, A.G. (ed.) *Foundations for osteopathic medicine* (3rd edn). Lippincott, Williams & Wilkins: Baltimore, MD; 2011; pp. 1087–110.

Elkiss, M.L., Rentz, L.E. Neurology. Chapter 34 in: Ward, R.C. (ed.) *Foundations for osteopathic medicine*. Williams and Wilkins: Baltimore, MD; 1997; pp. 401–16.

Fairbank, J.C., Park, T., McCall, W.M. Apophyseal injection of local anesthetic as a diagnostic aid in primary low-back pain syndromes. *Spine*, 1981, 6, 598–605.

Farfan, H.F. The scientific basis of manipulative procedures. *Clin Rheumatol Dis*, 1980, 6, 159.

FCER/Tillinghast. *Data compiled by labor and industry computers in Florida* (FCER: Arlington, VA; 1988) *and Colorado* (Tillinghast: Denver, CO; 1993).

Fédération Internationale de Médecine Manuelle (FIMM) Health Policy Board. *Guidelines on basic training and safety in manual medicine.* FIMM: Belgium; 2014.

Fortin, J.D., Falco, F.J.E. The Fortin finger test: an indicator of sacroiliac pain. *Am J Orthop*, 1997, 24(7), 477–80.

Gerwin, R., Shannon, S., Hong, C., Hubbard, D., Gervirtz, R. Interrater reliability in myofascial trigger point examination. *Pain*, 1997, 69, 65–73.

Gilliar, W.G., Kuchera, M.L., Giulianetti, D.A. Neurologic basis of manual medicine. *Phys Med Rehab Clin N Am*, 1996, 7(4), 693–714.

Glover, J.C., Yates, H.A. Strain and counterstrain techniques. Chapter 58 in: Ward, R.C. (ed.) *Foundations for osteopathic medicine.* Williams and Wilkins: Baltimore, MD; 1997; pp. 809–18.

Good, M.G. Diagnosis and treatment of sciatic pain. *Lancet*, 1942, ii, 597–8.

Greenman, P.E. Sacroiliac dysfunction in the failed low back pain syndrome. *First interdisciplinary world congress on low back pain and its relation to the sacroiliac joint.* San Diego; 1992; pp. 329–52.

Greenman, P.E. Syndromes of the lumbar spine, pelvis, and sacrum. *Phys Med Rehab Clin N Am*, 1996, 7(4), 773–85.

Greenman, P.E. *Principles of manual medicine.* Williams and Wilkins: Baltimore, MD; 1996.

Hackett, G.S. *Ligament and tendon relaxation treated by prolotherapy* (3rd edn). C.C. Thomas: Springfield, IL; 1958.

Heinking, K.P., Kappler, R.E. Pelvis and sacrum. Chapter 52 in: Ward, R.C. (ed.) *Foundations for osteopathic medicine* (2nd edn). Lippincott, Williams and Wilkins: Baltimore, MD; 2002; pp. 762–83.

Jaeger, B. Are 'cervicogenic' headaches due to myofascial pain and cervical spine dysfunction? *Cephalgia*, 1989, 9(suppl 3), 157–64.

Jones, L.H. *Strain and counterstrain.* American Academy of Osteopathy: Newark, OH; 1981.

Jones, L., Kusunose, R., Goering, E. *Jones' strain-counterstrain.* Jones Strain-Counterstrain, Inc.; Boise, ID; 1995.

Kapandji I.A. *The physiology of joints.* Churchill-Livingstone: New York; 1970.

Kappler, R.E. Cervical spine. Chapter 45 in: Ward, R.C. (ed.) *Foundations for osteopathic medicine.* Williams and Wilkins: Baltimore, MD; 1997; pp. 541–6.

Kappler, R.E., Ramey, K.A. Head, diagnosis and treatment. Chapter 44 in: Ward, R.C. (ed.) *Foundations for osteopathic medicine.* Williams and Wilkins: Baltimore, MD; 1997.

Kelso, A.F. A double-blind clinical study of osteopathic findings in hospital patients—progress report. *J Am Osteopath Assoc*, 1971, 70, 570–92.

Kimberly, P. Forming a prescription for osteopathic manipulative treatment. *J Am Osteopath Assoc*, 1980, 79, 512.

Kimberly, P., Funk, S.F. (eds). *Outline of osteopathic manipulative procedures: the Kimberly manual* (millennium edn). Walsworth: Marceline, MO; 2000.

Kuchera, M.L. Gravitational strain pathophysiology and 'Unterkreuz' syndrome. *Manuelle Medizin*, 1995a, 33(2), 56.

Kuchera, M. L. Gravitational stress, musculoligamentous strain, and postural alignment. *Spine*, 1995b, 9(2), 463–90.

Kuchera, M.L. Diagnosis and treatment of gravitational strain pathophysiology: research and clinical correlates (part I and II). In: Vleeming, A. (ed.) *Low back pain: the integrated function of the lumbar spine and sacroiliac joints. Proceedings of the 2nd Interdisciplinary World Congress, 9–11 November 1995.* University of California, San Diego; 1995c; pp. 659–93.

Kuchera, M.L. Travell and Simons' myofascial trigger points. Chapter 66 in: Ward, R.C. (ed.) *Foundations for osteopathic medicine.* Williams and Wilkins: Baltimore, MD; 1997a; pp. 919–33.

Kuchera, M.L. Postural considerations in the sagittal plane. Chapter 72 in: Ward, R.C. (ed.) *Foundations for osteopathic medicine.* Williams and Wilkins: Baltimore, MD; 1997b; pp. 999–1014.

Kuchera, M.L. Treatment of gravitational strain pathophysiology. In: Vleeming, A., Mooney, V., Dorman, T., Snijders, C., Stoeckart R (eds). *Movement, stability and low back pain: the essential role of the pelvis.* Churchill-Livingstone: New York; 1997c; pp.477–99.

Kuchera, M.L. Osteopathic principles and practice/osteopathic manipulative treatment considerations for cephalgia. *J Am Osteopath Assoc*, 1998, 98(Supp 4), S14–9.

Kuchera, M.L. Examination and diagnosis: an introduction. Chapter 39 in: Ward, R.C. (ed.) *Foundations for osteopathic medicine* (2nd edn). Lippincott, Williams and Wilkins: Baltimore, MD; 2002; pp. 566–73.

Kuchera, M.L. Postural considerations in osteopathic diagnosis and treatment. In: Chila, A.G. (ed.) *Foundations of osteopathic medicine* (3rd edn). Lippincott, Williams & Wilkins: Baltimore, MD; 2011; 437–83.

Kuchera, M.L. An integrated perspective on the differential diagnosis of myofascial points. In: Myers, H.L. (ed.) *Clinical application of counterstrain (compendium edition).* Tucson Osteopathic Medical Association: Tucson AZ; 2012; pp. 15–27.

Kuchera, M.L., Kuchera, W.A. *Osteopathic considerations in systemic dysfunction* (2nd edn, revised). Greyden Press: Columbus, OH; 1994.

Kuchera, M.L., Kuchera, W.A. General postural considerations. Chapter 69 in: Ward, R.C. (ed.) *Foundations for osteopathic medicine.* Williams and Wilkins: Baltimore, MD; 1997; pp. 969–77.

Kuchera, M.L., Kuchera, W.A. *Osteopathic considerations in HEENT disorders: head, eye, ear, nose, throat.* Greyden Press; Dayton OH; 2012.

Kuchera, M. L., DiGiovanna, E. L., Greenman, P. E. Efficacy and complications. Chapter 72 in: Ward, R. C. (ed). *Foundations for osteopathic medicine*, 2nd edn (2002). Lippincott, Williams and Wilkins, Baltimore, MD, pp. 1143–61.

Kuchera, W.A., Jones, J.M. III, Kappler, R.E., Goodridge, J.P. Musculoskeletal examination for somatic dysfunction. In: Ward, R.C. (ed.) *Foundations for osteopathic medicine.* Williams and Wilkins: Baltimore, MD; 1997; pp. 489–509.

Levin, S.M. A different approach to the mechanics of the human pelvis: tensegrity. In: Vleeming, A., Mooney, V., et al. (eds). *Movement stability and low back pain: the essential role of the pelvis.* Churchill-Livingstone: New York; 1997.

Lewit, K. *Manipulative therapy in rehabilitation of the motor system.* Butterworth: London; 1985.

Lewit, K. Muscular pattern in thoraco-lumbar lesions. *Manual Med*, 1986, 2, 105–7.

Lewit, K. *Manipulative therapy in rehabilitation of the locomotor system* (2nd edn). Butterworth-Heinemann: Oxford; 1991; pp. 24, 196–7, 244–5.

Magoun, H.I. *Osteopathy in the cranial field.* The Cranial Academy: Indianapolis, IN; 1976.

Magoun, H.I. Temporal bone: trouble-maker in the head. *J Am Osteopath Assoc*, 1974, 73, 825–35.

Maigne, R. Manipulation of the spine. Chapter 4 in: Basmajian, J.V. (ed.) *Manipulation, traction and massage*, (3rd edn). Williams and Wilkins: Baltimore, MD; 1985.

Maigne, R. *Orthopedic medicine: a new approach to vertebral manipulations.* C.C. Thomas: Springfield, IL; 1972.

Melzack, R., Wall, P.D. *The challenge of pain: a modern medical classic.* Penguin: London; 1989.

Mennell, J. *Back pain: diagnosis and treatment using manipulative technique.* Brown and Co: Boston; 1960.

Mense, S., Simons, D. *Muscle pain, understanding its nature, diagnosis, and treatment.* Lippincott Williams and Wilkins: Philadelphia, PA; 2001.

Mitchell, F.L. Structural pelvic function. In: *American Academy of Osteopathy yearbook (1967).* American Academy of Osteopathy: Indianapolis, IN; article date 1958.

Mitchell, F.L., Moran, P.S., Pruzzo, N.A. *An evaluation and treatment manual of osteopathic muscle energy procedures.* Private Publishing Firm: Valley Park, MO; 1979.

Mixter, W.J., Barr, J.S. Rupture of the intervertebral disc with involvement of the spinal canal. *N Engl J Med*, 1934, 211, 210–5.

Mooney, V. Sacroiliac joint dysfunction. In: Vleeming, A., Mooney, V., Dorman, T., Snijders, C., Stoeckart, R. (eds). *Movement, stability and low back pain: the essential role of the pelvis.* Churchill-Livingstone: New York; 1997; pp. 37–52.

Mooney, V., Robertson, J. The facet syndrome. *Clin Orthop*, 1976, 115, 149–56.

Naus, A., et al. Work injuries and smoking. *Industrial Med Surg*, 1966, 35, 880–1.

Headache Classification Committee of the International Headache Society. Classification and diagnostic criteria for headache disorders, cranial neuralgias and facial pain. *Cephalgia*, 1988, 8(suppl 7): 1–96.

Owens, C. *An endocrine interpretation of Chapman's reflexes* (1963 reprint). American Academy of Osteopathy: Indianapolis, IN; 1963.

Paterson, J.K., Burn, L. *An introduction to medical manipulation*. MTP Press: Lancaster, UK; 1985.

Patriquin, D.A. Chapman's reflexes. Chapter 67 in: Ward, R.C. (ed.) *Foundations for osteopathic medicine*. Williams and Wilkins: Baltimore, MD; 1997; pp. 935–40.

Patriquin, D.A. Viscerosomatic reflexes. In: Patterson, M.M., Howell, J.N. (eds). *The central connection: somatovisceral–viscerosomatic interactions, 1989 international symposium*. University Classics: Athens, OH; 1992; pp. 4–18.

Peterson, B. (ed.) *Postural balance and imbalance. 1983 yearbook of the American Academy of Osteopathy*. AAO Press: Newark, OH; 1983.

Reynolds, K.L., et al. Cigarette smoking, physical fitness, and injuries in infantry soldiers. *Am J Preventive Med*, 1994, 19, 145–50.

Rubin, B.R. Rheumatology. Chapter 38 in: Ward, R.C. (ed.) *Foundations for osteopathic medicine*. Williams and Wilkins: Baltimore, MD; 1997; pp. 459–66.

Sciotti, V.M., Mittak, V.L., DiMarco, L. Clinical precision of myofascial trigger point location in the trapezius muscle. *Pain*, 2001, 93, 259–66.

Scott, R.A. Orthopaedics. Chapter 28 in: Ward, R.C. (ed.) *Foundations for osteopathic medicine*. Williams and Wilkins: Baltimore, MD; 1997; pp. 329–47.

Seffinger, M.A., Hruby, R. *Evidence-based manual medicine: problem oriented approach*. Saunders: Philadelphia PA; 2007; pp. 184–7.

Simons, D.G. Muscle pain syndromes. *J Man Med*, 1991, 6, 3–23.

Simons, D.G., Travell, J.G. Low back pain, part 2: torso muscles. *Postgrad Med*, 1983, 73(2), 81–92.

Simons, D.G., Travell, J.G., Simons, L.S. *Travell and Simons' myofascial pain and dysfunction: the trigger point manual, volume 1. Upper half of body*. Williams and Wilkins: Baltimore, MD; 1999.

Smith, L.A., et al. *An atlas of pain patterns: sites and behavior of pain in certain common disease of the upper abdomen*. C.C. Thomas: Springfield, IL; 1961.

Deyo RA. Measuring treatment outcomes for spinal disorders. In Frymoyer JW, Wiesel SW (eds). The Adult and Pediatric Spine, Vol.1. Lippincott Williams & Wilkins: Baltimore; 2004; 1–13.

Steinbrocker, O., Isenberg, S.A., Silver, M., et al. Observations on pain produced by injection of hypertonic saline into muscles and other supportive tissues. *J Clin Invest*, 1953, 32, 1045–51.

Strachan, W.F., et al. A study of the mechanics of the sacroiliac joint. *J Am Osteopath Assoc*, 1938, 43(12), 576–8.

Travell, J.G., Simons, D.G. *Myofascial pain and dysfunction: the trigger point manual. Vol. II*. Williams and Wilkins: Baltimore, MD; 1992.

Travell, J., Travell, W. Therapy of low back pain by manipulation and of referred pain in the lower extremity by procaine infiltration. *Arch Phys Ther*, 1946, 27, 537–47.

Upton, A.R., McComas, A.J. The double crush in nerve entrapment syndromes. *Lancet*, 1973, ii, 359–62.

Vleeming, A., Mooney, V., Dorman, T., Snijders, C., Stoeckart, R. (eds). *Movement, stability and low back pain: the essential role of the pelvis*. Churchill Livingstone: New York; 1997.

Vleeming, A., Snijders, C.J., Stoeckart, R., Mens, J.M.A. The role of the sacroiliac joints in coupling between spine, pelvis, legs and arms. Chapter 3 in: Vleeming, A., Mooney, V., Snijders, C.J., Dorman, T.A., Stoeckart, R. (eds). *Movement, stability and low back pain: the essential role of the pelvis*. Churchill-Livingstone: New York; 1997; pp. 53–71.

Waddell, G., Morris, E.W., et al. A concept of illness tested as an improved basis for surgical decisions in low-back disorders. *Spine*, 1989, 14, 838–43.

Walton, W.J. Osteopathic diagnosis and technique, *Sacroiliac diagnosis*. Matthews Book Co: St. Louis, MO; 1966; pp. 187–97. (Reprinted 1970 and distributed by the American Academy of Osteopathy; Indianapolis IN.)

Ward, R.C. (ed.) *Foundations for osteopathic medicine* (2nd edn). Lippincott, Williams and Wilkins: Baltimore, MD; 2002.

Washington, K., Mosiello, R., Venditto, M., et al. Presence of Chapman reflex points in hospitalized patients with pneumonia. (2003) *J Am Osteopath Assoc*, 103, 479–83.

Wilder, D.G., Pope, M.H., Frymoyer, J.W. The functional topography of the sacroiliac joint. *Spine*, 1980, 5, 575–9.

World Health Organization (WHO). *The international classification of diseases, 9th revision, clinical modification (ICD-9-CM)* (3rd edn). World Health Organization: Geneva; 1979.

Zink, J.G., Lawson, W.B. An osteopathic structural examination and functional interpretation of the soma. *Osteopathic Annals*, 1979, 7, 433–40.

Chapter 28

Thoracic outlet syndrome

John Tanner

The thoracic outlet syndrome (TOS) comprises a number of syndromes involving the upper quarter and hand that are thought to be caused by compression of the subclavian artery, vein, and/or brachial plexus. It is believed that at least one of these structures must be compressed somewhere between the superior opening of the thorax and the axilla to meet this diagnosis.

Anatomy of the thoracic outlet

The thoracic outlet contains many structures in a confined space. The floor of the thoracic outlet is formed by the first rib and fascia of Sibson. This fascia attaches to the transverse process of C7, the pleura, and the first rib. Superiorly lies the subclavius muscle and clavicle; anteriorly, the anterior scalene; and posteriorly, the middle scalene. The brachial plexus and subclavian artery pass over the first rib between the aforementioned muscles (Figures 28.2 and 28.3). The lowest part of the nerve plexus lies behind the subclavian artery. According to Pollack (1980), neurovascular compression occurs at any or all of the three levels:

- in the *superior thoracic outlet* bordered posteriorly by the spine, anteriorly by the manubrium, and laterally by the first rib
- more laterally, in the *costoscalene hiatus* bordered anteriorly by the anterior scalene muscle, posteriorly by the middle scalene muscle, and caudally by the first rib (Figure 28.1)
- most laterally of the three, in the *costoclavicular passage*, bordered laterally by the clavicle, posteriorly by the scapula, and medially by the first rib (Figure 28.1).

Anatomy of the first rib

The anatomy and function of the first rib, and of a cervical rib if present, are critical to the understanding and therapy of the thoracic outlet syndromes.

The orientation of the first rib is different from the other ribs in that its long axis forms a 45° angle with the horizontal. It articulates with the facet on the first thoracic vertebra (the *costovertebral joint*) and the transverse process of the vertebra (the *costotransverse joint*). This latter joint lacks a superior supporting ligament, making it relatively weaker than those of the other ribs. Furthermore, the muscle attachments to this rib, which function during inspiration and to flex and rotate the cervical part of the spine, impose more stress on the rib and its joints than on any of the other ribs. These stresses are probably greatest at the costotransverse joint. Osteoarthritic changes are found in both these joints, but more frequently in the costotransverse joint. Since the axis of its two articulations lie closer to the coronal plane, elevation of the first rib during respiration increases the anteroposterior diameter, often described as a 'pump-handle' movement.

The posterior segment of the first rib relates to the stellate ganglion, the first thoracic spinal root, and the eighth cervical spinal root. The middle segment of the rib extends from the posterior costal angle to the retroscalenic tubercle, providing insertions for the middle scalene, the first digitation of the serratus anterior, and the intercostal muscles of the first intercostal space. The insertion of the pleura on the periosteum of the first rib is very firm. The anterior segment of the first rib relates to the first thoracic nerve, the subclavian artery and vein, the pleura, and the lung apex. The anterior scalene muscle inserts into the pre-arterial tubercle of the first rib between the artery, posteriorly, and the vein, anteriorly. The costoclavicular ligaments and the subclavius muscle insert into this portion of the rib (Figures 28.1 and 28.4).

Developmental anomalies

A *cervical rib* is present in 0.5% of the population, but most remain non-symptomatic. Many anomalous *fibrous bands* (Figures 28.5 and 28.6) attaching to the first rib have been described (Roos 1984). A band from the transverse process of C7 will act as a cervical rib (but not appear on a radiograph). In addition, the first rib receives attachments from any cervical rib. The neurovascular bundle slides up on the first rib as on a pulley. Various *congenital anomalies of the first and second ribs* may occur, with anomalous joints of the first rib and asymmetry due to *cervicothoracic scoliosis*. Pathological positions of the first rib have been shown to cause TOS, such as a high first rib and an upward dislocation of the first rib. (Lindgren 1992)

Neurology

The first thoracic nerve is at greatest risk of tension as it curves over the first rib, and this will be increased by shoulder girdle depression. The C8 root is similarly embarrassed by a cervical rib or fibrous band. This accounts for the limb symptoms being most prominent on the medial aspect of the upper arm, forearm, and hand.

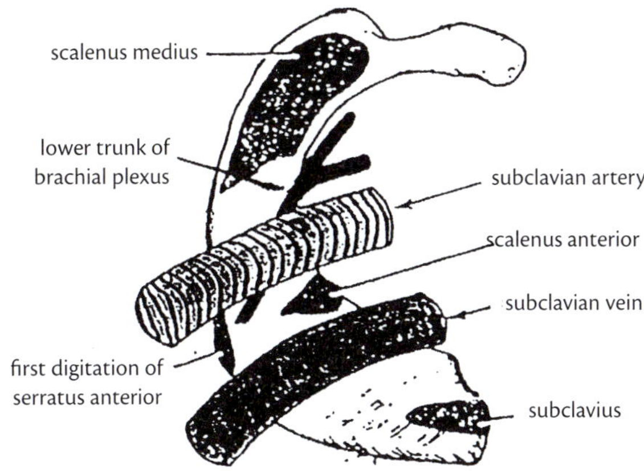

Figure 28.1 Structures related to the superior surface of the first rib. (From Mahran et al., Osteology, 1971, University Book Centre Cairo.)

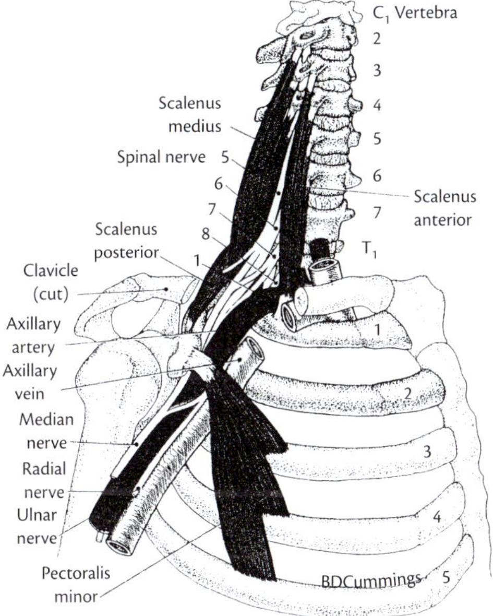

Figure 28.2 Thoracic outlet entrapment by the scalene muscles. The neurovascular bundle is spread out to show the relations of its component parts. A portion of the clavicle has been removed. The brachial plexus and axillary artery emerge above the first rib and behind the clavicle, between the scalenus anterior and scalenus medius muscles. The primal nerves are numbered on the left, the vertebrae on the right. The T1 nerve lies dorsal to and beneath the subclavian artery.

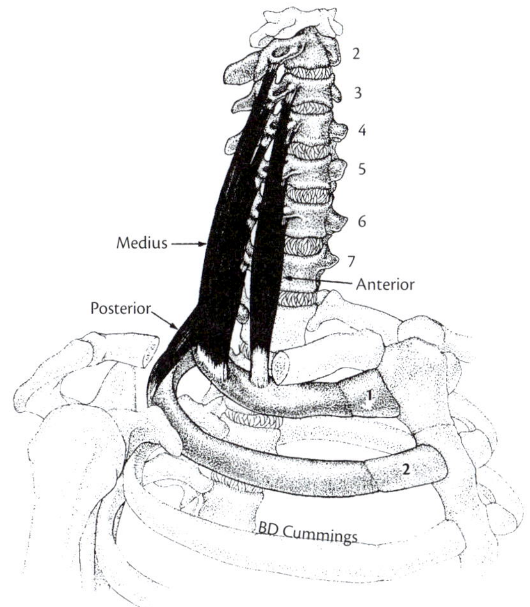

Figure 28.3 Oblique view of the attachments of the three major scalene muscles to the cervical vertebrae and to the first and second ribs. The clavicle has been cut and the section that overlies the scalene muscles removed.

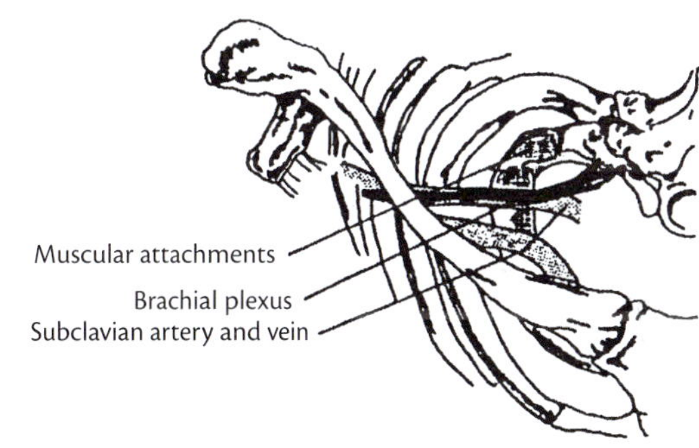

Figure 28.4 The costo-clavicular passage.

Aetiology of thoracic outlet syndrome

The causes most commonly implicated in TOS are cervical ribs, structure or function of the first rib, the anterior scalene muscle, and anomalous fibromuscular bands (see Table 28.1).

Of the 0.5% of the population who possess cervical ribs, only 5–10% ever develop symptoms (Adson and Coffey 1927). The literature cites a cervical rib to be the cause of TOS in 10–100% of cases: American authors favour a higher percentage to be due to fibromuscular bands or scalene muscle abnormalities (see Fig 28.5). A single traumatic episode is reported in 21–91% of the patients in several American studies (e.g. Ellison and Wood 1994; Sanders et al. 1979) or 10% of cases in UK series (e.g. Sharan et al. 1999). Occupational predisposition occurs in over 50% of patients and in these cases, musculoskeletal dysfunction is the major factor, aggravated by structural abnormalities when present.

Structural factors are usually present in the vascular types of TOS; they may be present in cases showing neurological features, but the function of the thoracic outlet is of special importance in occupational cases.

Studies of the normal function of the thoracic outlet are scarce, and the prevalence of neurogenic TOS in the general population is not known. Neurological TOS with objective deficit is a rare lesion with an annual incidence of about 1/1,000,000 (Gilliat 1984): most of the patients are female (9:1) and bony anomalies are usually found.

The most elegant studies of first rib function have been performed by Lindgren et al. (1990) using a cineradiographic technique. Mobility of the first rib during inspiration and expiration was visualized with the patient lying supine, with a fluoroscopic beam at 30°

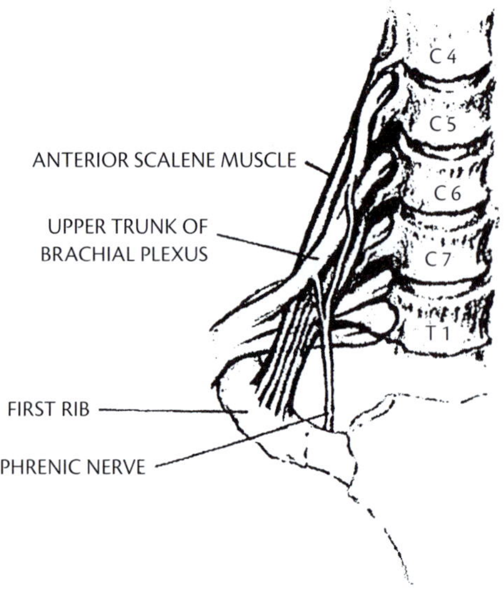

Figure 28.5 Anatomical variant of upper trunk passing through scalenus anterior.

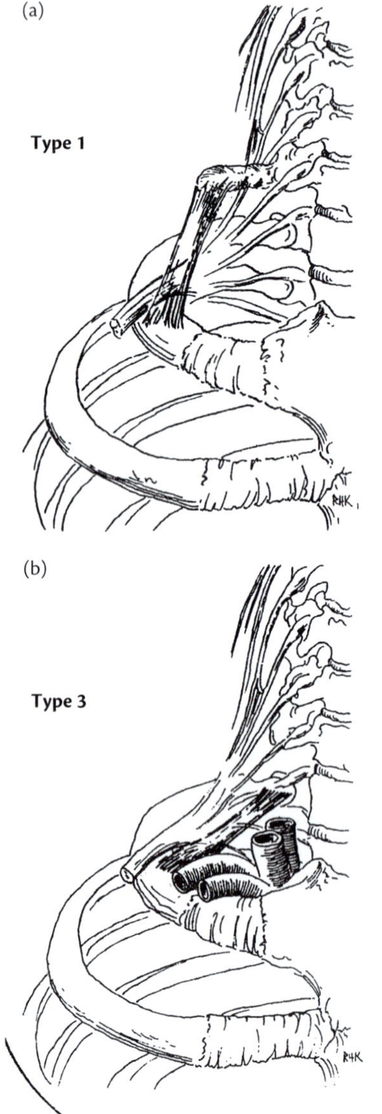

Figure 28.6 Fibrous bands: (a) type 1; (b) type 2. (After Roos).

Table 28.1 Aetiological factors in thoracic outlet syndromes

Anatomical factors		Provocative factors
Structural abnormality	Cervical rib	Trauma
	Clavicle malunion	Occupational stresses
	Fibromuscular bands	Shoulder girdle
		descent
	Pancoast tumour	Overweight conditions
Soft tissue components	Anterior scalene	Pendulous breasts
	Middle scalene	First rib dysfunction
	Pectoralis minor	
	Subclavius	
	Costocoracoid fascia	

of caudal angulation. Movement was considered to be restricted if there was no movement along the axis through the costotransverse joint during expiration and inspiration. The function of the first rib and its stump was studied both clinically and radiologically in unoperated patients with brachialgia and in those whose first rib had been resected. Having visualized abnormal function in a proportion of both conservatively treated and surgically treated cases who continued to have symptoms, Lindgren related these findings to new clinical tests based on the kinesiology of the first rib. These include the expiration–inspiration test and the combined rotation and lateral flexion test (CRLF, Lindgren et al. 1992) (Box 28.1). The inter-examiner reliability of the CLRF test was found to be excellent (kappa reliability coefficient (κ) = 1). The inter-reliability between the clinical and radiological tests was also excellent (κ = 0.84). The sensitivity and specificity of the CRLF test was found to be 92% and 90% respectively as compared with a cineradiographic study.

Asymmetries of the respiratory movements of the first rib have been shown in association with structural asymmetries of the cervicothoracic spine (Girout 1983), when an upward dislocation of the first rib has been suggested to be a cause of brachialgia (McGormick et al. 1981). As a result of these findings, Lindgren proposes a proper trial of conservative treatment including assessment for impaired first rib mobility and appropriate therapy which may include joint mobilization/manipulation but, in particular, long-term self-treatment and maintenance. This aims to restore movements to the first rib by isometric activation of the scalene muscle combined with shoulder girdle exercises. He maintains that if the function is not restored, the symptoms continue despite a transaxillary first rib resection.

Box 28.1 The CRLF test for first rib function

- Start in neutral position of cervical spine
- Passive rotation away from side to be tested, to maximum
- Gentle passive flexion, moving ear towards chest

Test negative: 70° flexion with soft end-feel

Test positive: No movement or half asymptomatic side range with hard end-feel

The diagnosis of arterial TOS is usually made after a severe embolic event involving the arm. Venous TOSs are seen in perhaps 1.5% of all patients, manifest as axillary or subclavian thrombosis, and are more frequent than those of arterial insufficiency (Roos 1976). Thomson (2011) has detailed elegantly the clinical presentation of 'effort thrombosis' in the younger person aged 15–35 involved in strenuous upper limb sport, music, or manual work. This is called the Paget-Schroetter syndrome and results from the 'costoclavicular shearing' of the subclavian vein rather than a cervical rib or fibrous anomaly. The patient describes a 'bursting' feeling on exercise, amongst other vascular symptoms described in the following section. Early recognition and intervention is important since up to 10% can develop pulmonary embolus and in order to prevent post-phlebitic limb.

Clinical presentation of thoracic outlet syndrome

TOS occurs three times more commonly in women, usually around the middle decades. It can present in three ways: neurological, vascular, or combined vascular and neurological.

Symptoms suggesting vascular compression include oedema, heaviness or weakness of the upper extremity and cyanosis, blanching, and erythema similar to Raynaud's phenomenon. Patients may notice that the skin appears blotchy, discoloured, and more often cold. The onset is usually insidious but may follow trauma. The most common complaint is inability to raise or maintain the arm in a static posture for more than short periods without provoking symptoms. The symptoms may also occur with everyday activities, such as cleaning windows, painting a ceiling, or carrying heavy shopping or a briefcase. The symptoms include pain from the neck through the supraclavicular region into the arm and hand, accompanied by a subjective feeling of easy fatiguability and sometimes swelling. Typical of neurological TOS are paraesthesiae experienced in the inner arm and forearm and the ulnar side of the hand. In a series of 27 cases with cervical ribs, Sharan et al. (1999) found symptoms of arm pain, paraesthesia of the lower plexus distribution, pain at the root of the neck, and undue fatigue.

Physical examination for thoracic outlet syndrome

The patient's description of symptoms and their variation with time and activity are often crucial to the diagnosis, particularly in the common case who has few objective signs on examination. Whether symptoms come on with physical activities, or with a sleeping posture (releasing the stretched neural elements over the rib) needs enquiry.

General examination and differential diagnosis

The provocative tests (see following section) are carried out in the context of standard examination of the cervical spine, arm, and upper thoracic spine. This examination should exclude cervical disc and nerve root compression, shoulder dysfunction, and peripheral neuropathies. Particular examination for motor deficit in thenar muscles, intrinsic muscles of hand, and triceps should be made, together with provocative manoeuvres for carpal tunnel and ulnar neuritis (see Box 28.2). Palpation of the supraclavicular fossa may reveal a hard lump (cervical rib), lymphadenopathy, or tumour. Pressure for up to 30 seconds with the thumb over the plexus and first rib may be very tender and elicit familiar symptoms (Spurling's sign). Posture and respiratory pattern should be observed, while soft tissue restriction and accessory joint motion of all the joints of the shoulder girdle and the rib articulations should be examined.

Box 28.2 Differential diagnosis in thoracic outlet syndrome

- Cervical nerve root pressure, e.g. disc
- Cervical joint dysfunction
- Apical lung tumour, other nerve sheath/cell tumours
- Brachial plexitis
- Ulnar neuritis
- Carpal tunnel syndrome
- Peripheral neuropathy
- Chronic regional pain syndromes
- Vasculitis
- Vasospastic disorder, e.g. Raynaud's disease
- Syringomyelia, multiple sclerosis

Examination for vascular features

Auscultation for a bruit above or below the clavicle can be performed (at rest and in the provocative positions) when vascular compromise is suspected. The limb is examined for swelling, discolouration, and temperature change, and for evidence of emboli, e.g. splinter haemorrhages in the nail beds. If arterial compromise is suspected, compare blood pressure with the unaffected side—a drop of more than 20 mm Hg may be significant.

Postural examination

Observe the patient from all views, both at rest and, if possible, when performing tasks which provoke or relieve symptoms.

Poor tone and protraction of the shoulder girdle is often present, while a protracted head position will occur with increased tone in scalenes and sternocleidomastoids. Breathing pattern should be noticed, in particular paradoxical respiration with use of the accessory muscles at rest.

Provocative manoeuvre tests

Anterior scalene or Adson's test (Adson and Coffey 1927)

This evaluates the role of anterior and middle scalene muscles in compressing the subclavian artery which passes between them on its way to the axilla.

The patient hyperextends the neck and rotates the head toward the affected side and takes a deep breath. The examiner monitors the radial pulse which will decrease or become obliterated if the test is positive.

Costoclavicular compression

This is an exaggerated military position designed to narrow the space between the first rib and clavicle, thereby compressing the plexus and/or vessels.

The patient sits with arms relaxed at his/her sides. He/she retracts and depresses the shoulder girdle while the examiner monitors for a change in the radial pulse.

Wright's hyperabduction manoeuvre (Wright 1945)

This involves passive circumduction of the arm overheard while the examiner monitors the radial pulse. This test is positive if the pulse strength changes and/or symptoms are elicited.

Roos' abduction and external rotation (AER) test or the hands-up test (Roos 1976)

This test is performed with the patient sitting, arms abducted 90° and the elbows flexed 90°, with the shoulders braced slightly.

The patient is asked to open and close the fingers slowly and steadily for a full 3 minutes. The examiner observes for drooping of the arms, decreased rate of finger flexion, or the onset of typical symptoms. However, this has been shown to be more accurate in the diagnosis of carpal tunnel syndrome than TOS.

Cervical rotation lateral flexion test (Lindgren et al. 1992)

The neutrally positioned cervical spine is first passively and maximally rotated away from the side being examined and then, in this position, gently flexed as far as possible, moving the ear towards the chest. This is done in both directions. Bony restriction blocking the lateral flexion part of the movement partially or totally indicates a positive test; a free movement indicates a negative test. This test is thought to identify a subluxed first rib.

Expiration–inspiration test (Lindgren et al. 1992)

The movement of the first rib in relation to the clavicle is palpated in the supine position during expiration and inspiration by lightly pressing a finger between the two bones. The right and left sides are compared. In this test, the disturbance of the movement of the first rib can be felt as a restriction of the movement during breathing. This test cannot be done on patients who have previously had rib resections, for obvious reasons.

None of the aforementioned tests unequivocally establishes the presence or absence of TOS, and the first three tests described, using radial pulse obliteration, are so often present in asymptomatic patients (60–70%) that their clinical utility is dubious. Ribbe et al. (1986) used a TOS index requiring at least three of four symptoms or signs for the diagnosis (see Box 28.3). Although the upper limb tension test is not commonly quoted in any of the relevant literature, it is a useful screening test which adds weight to the clinical index of suspicion for nerve mobility restriction (Butler 2000).

Table 28.2 lists the findings in Sharan et al.'s (1999) series of cervical rib cases.

Box 28.3 The thoracic outlet syndrome index

- A history of aggravation of symptoms with the arm in the elevated position
- A history of paraesthesiae in the segments of C8–T1
- Tenderness over the brachial plexus, supraclavicularly
- A positive hands-up (AER) test (see text)

Table 28.2 Findings in a series of cervical rib cases

Atrophy and weakness of the hand muscles	67%
Positive Roos test (AER)	60%
Palpable lump in the posterior triangle	53%
Supraclavicular tenderness	43%
Supraclavicular bruit	8%

Sharan et al 1999- Sharan, D.et al. (1999) Two surgeon approach to thoracic outlet syndrome: Long term outcome. J.Roy. Soc. Med., 92, 239–43.

Investigations for thoracic outlet syndrome

Diagnostic imaging

Diagnosis of TOS is largely based on history and physical examination, but investigation to identify bony abnormality is appropriate where suspicion of the diagnosis is strong. Cervical spine radiographs will show cervical ribs, abnormally long C7 transverse processes, and the apices of the lungs. If vascular compromise is suggested by the examination, then such imaging as magnetic resonance and/or angiography and brachiocephalic venography are the gold standard. The use of Duplex ultrasonography is common but can lead to up to 20% false positive rates. The use of dynamic musculoskeletal ultrasound for neurogenic type may prove to be useful in the future as techniques and technology improve (Fried 2013; Lindgren—personal communication).

Neurophysiology

Claims have been made for the usefulness of ulnar nerve conduction velocity (Urschel and Razzuk 1972), F-wave reflexes (Nishida et al. 1993), and somatosensory evoked potentials (Chodoroff et al. 1985; Machleder et al. 1987), but false positives occur with all tests described and none can be recommended as reliable (Roos 1976; Wilbourne 1990). When the neural type of TOS is suspected clinically, normal practice is to proceed with conservative treatment and to avoid surgery in most cases.

Treatment of thoracic outlet syndrome

Cases with arterial or venous components to the syndrome must be considered for surgical treatment. In the neurological syndromes, conservative treatment by physical methods is the norm.

Role of physical treatment in conservative management of TOS

There are three phases of treatment:

- demonstration of the ability to control the intensity of the symptoms
- exercises to change the symptom-producing faults
- postural maintenance.

Various regimes have been utilized incorporating shoulder girdle elevation and stabilization exercises, flexibility exercises, exercises for the chest and cervical musculature, and controlled breathing routines. McGough et al. (1979) have extended medical management for as long as 2 years before surgical intervention: 90% of their 1200 patients were successfully relieved without surgery. Most practitioners blame faulty posture of the cervicothoracic spine and shoulder girdle in the aetiology of TOS, on the basis of the observation that the symptoms of TOS correspond to a loss of muscular support and/or increased muscular tautness in these regions. The question remains whether abnormalities in bony structure, such as a cervical rib, should determine treatment. Peet et al. (1956) included patients with normal and abnormal cervical radiographs in their treatment regime. After an intensive programme of strengthening and flexibility exercises, they concluded that 70% of all patients, regardless of radiographical findings, had the same chance of achieving relief from their symptoms.

Lindgren (1997), with his self-treatment programme to restore function of the first rib, enabled 88% of 119 patients to achieve a satisfactory outcome, including 73% returning to work. Radiological screening was found to have normalized in 8 of 10 patients. Lindgren's protocol requires intensive training for an exercise routine to be continued at home:

- shoulder girdle active exercises for restoration of mobility
- craniocervical junction nutation for joint mobility and stretching the upper part of the posterior cervical musculature
- scalene muscle activation with active exercise to restore upper rib function
- passive stretching of shoulder girdle muscles, especially upper trapezius, sternocleidomastoids, levator scapulae, and pectoralis minor, using the techniques of Evjenth and Hamberg (1990)

Together with specific exercises customized to the patient's particular requirements should be added a general exercise routine, with attention paid to:

- *Posture*: To counteract protracted head position and protraction of the shoulder girdle. Thoracic kyphosis should be minimized.
- *Breathing pattern.*
- *Muscle imbalance and trigger points*: Abnormality with increased tone, trigger points, and shortening may be found in the muscles previously itemized (and breathing pattern generally: additional treatment techniques such as post-isometric relaxation and trigger point therapy are useful).
- *Joint dysfunction:* Cervical or upper thoracic segmental dysfunction should be corrected, as should first or second rib dysfunction.
- *Ergonomics at home and work:* A change in job or increased workload are common provoking factors for symptoms. Counselling on hours at work, rest periods, posture, and design of workstation is often helpful.

Evaluation of soft tissue restrictions

Recognition of shortened anterior scalene muscle is verified by finding the head position in slight lateral flexion towards the affected side and rotation towards the contralateral side. From the lateral perspective, shortening of this muscle is noted by an increase in lordosis. Spasm of the sternocleidomastoid muscle can be seen from the anterior view and shortening of the upper trapezius will affect the slope of the shoulders seen from the posterior view. Breathing pattern should be noticed, in particular paradoxical respiration with use of the accessory muscles at rest. Observation of shoulder girdle posture may reveal protraction of the shoulder girdle with shortening of the pectoralis muscles, exaggeration of thoracic kyphosis, and abducted shoulder position.

Side-bending to the contralateral side may be limited by up to 30° if scalene muscles are shortened. Furthermore, aggravation or provocation of symptoms can occur with overpressure at the extreme of this range. Assessment of shortened pectoralis minor is achieved by lying the patient supine and observing whether the posterior aspect of the shoulder lies in contact with the surface of the table. If the muscle is shortened, the shoulder will be in a forward position, as a result of the downward pull on the coracoid process. Passive stretching of the pectoralis minor by pushing the posterior aspect of the shoulder down against the surface of the table may elicit the patient's symptoms. Palpation of the upper trapezius, sternocleidomastoid, and scalene muscles is vital to locate trigger points which may refer symptoms to the upper chest, suprascapular area, and arm. Trigger points may extend to the levator scapulae, pectoralis major, and even subclavius muscle (Howell Wright 1991). Botulinus toxin injected into the anterior and middle scalenes has been shown, in uncontrolled series of patients, to significantly prolong the relief of symptoms (Jordan 2000) but controlled studies performed since have failed to support this observation (Finlayson et al. 2011).

Surgical treatment

The outcome of surgical decompression has been difficult to assess in the absence of satisfactory objective tests for comparing preoperative and post-operative states, in the absence of controlled series, and with most series including those with and without structural abnormalities. Furthermore, some patients who were reported by their surgeons to have benefited have subsequently been described by others, on long-term follow-up, as not having been helped by surgery (Carroll and Hurst 1982). Sanders et al. (1979) reported recurrence of symptoms in 17% of 239 scalenectomy patients and in 17% of the 214 patients who had excision of the first rib.

The importance of long-term follow-up is essential although approximately 60% of recurrences occur within 6 months after surgery. Sharan et al. (1999), in a series of 27 cases with cervical ribs (three with bilateral symptomatology), classified the syndromes thus: neurogenic type, 24; arterial, five; venous, one. In the neurogenic group, three patients had upper plexus involvement. The mean duration of symptoms was 24 months. Only three patients gave a history of injury to the neck, and two of the three patients with upper plexus symptoms were found to have a double crush syndrome requiring bilateral carpal tunnel decompression subsequently. The structural lesions detected were as follows: 27 cervical ribs (15 complete, seven incomplete), five C7 exostoses, eight fibromuscular bands, two thickened fibrosed anterior scalenes, one rudimentary first rib and exostosis of second rib. One patient had an axillary subclavian aneurysm in association with a complete cervical rib which required resection and prosthetic grafting. He chose to resect only the middle third of the cervical rib subperiosteally. A two-surgeon approach was used (an orthopaedic surgeon and a vascular surgeon) with prior assessment by a consultant neurologist. They did not resect the first rib, but division of the omohyoid and anterior scalene was done in all cases, while the middle scalene was excised only if the muscle was judged to be abnormal and compressing the neurovascular bundle. Almost all patients were followed up for more than one year and some up to nine years later.

In the long term, excellent or good results were noted in 87%, with 89% returning to their previous lifestyle or occupation. The only complications reported were hypertrophic scarring in one case and five patients with infraclavicular anaesthesia.

An earlier series which discusses surgical treatment is that of Sanders et al. (1979) who found a recurrence rate of over 15% following first rib resections for TOS. On supraclavicular re-exploration, he found the anterior scalene muscle had re-attached to the bed of the first rib. Scalenectomy was successful in each of these cases. This led to the study of anterior scalenectomy as the first operation for all cases of TOS, refractory to conservative therapy. Apart from the usual clinical diagnostic tests, Sanders found a scalene muscle block with local anaesthetic was extremely useful. When comparing the results of scalenectomy and rib resection in a prospective study, results were almost identical, producing 70% good to excellent long-term outcome. He concluded that in patients with a history of neck trauma followed by headache, neck pain, and arm symptoms, scalenectomy should be considered. On the other hand, first rib resection is recommended for patients with no history of neck trauma and symptoms limited to the arm and hand, particularly those with signs of vascular insufficiency.

Roos (1976), writing from his personal experience in evaluating more than 2300 patients for TOS and operating on 776 cases of the most severe category who failed to respond to physical therapy and other conservative measures, finds that the most common anomaly is the presence of the fibromuscular band. He maintained that the most effective means of relieving symptoms is a transaxillary approach, resecting the entire first thoracic rib from sternum to transverse process, cervical rib if present, and complete excision of all anomalous fibromuscular tissue. The important point about his experience is that resection of the first rib alone cannot be considered adequate decompression. A careful search for the presence of congenital bands must also be made, and these bands must be totally excised for complete neurovascular decompression. He claims a 90% success rate if the correct operation is performed with meticulous technique.

In the present climate of controversy, it is right to exercise caution and maintain a relatively high threshold for surgical invasion for 'disputed' neurological TOS in the absence of objective tests such as positive electrodiagnosis, particularly with the improved techniques in manual medicine for treating first rib subluxation, mobilizing the first rib, neuromuscular techniques to relax scalene muscle spasm, and a muscle balance approach for the entire shoulder girdle complex. It is wise to exclude other sites of nerve root compression such as the carpal tunnel (double crush phenomenon) and consider gaining expertise in dynamic ultrasonography of the brachial plexus which may demonstrate reduced gliding of neural structures during the upper limb tension test.

References

Adson, A.W., Coffey, J.R. (1927) Cervical rib. *Ann Surg*, 85, 839.

Butler, D. *The sensitive nervous system*. Noigroup Publications: Adelaide, Australia; 2000, pp. 315–7.

Carroll, R.E. Hurst, L.E. (1982) The relationship of thoracic outlet syndrome and carpal tunnel syndrome. *Clin Orthop*, 164, 149–53.

Chodoroff, G., et al. (1985) Dynamic approach in the diagnosis of thoracic outlet syndrome using somatosensory evoked responses. *Arch Phys Med Rehabil*, 66, 3–6.

Ellison, D.W., Wood V.C. (1994) Trauma-related thoracic outlet syndrome. *J Hand Surg*, 19B, 424–6.

Evjent, O., Hamberg J. (1990) *Autostretching. The complete manual of specific stretching*. Alfta Rehab Forlag: Sweden.

Finlayson, H.C., O'Connor, R.J., Brasher, P.M., Travlos, A. (2011) Botulinum toxin injection for management of thoracic outlet syndrome: a double-blind, randomized, controlled trial. *Pain*, 152(9), 2023–8.

Fried, S.M. (2013) Nazarian Ln dynamic neuromusculoskeletal ultrasound documentation of brachial plexus. Thoracic outlet compression during elevated arm stress. Hand NY, (3), 358–65.

Gilliat, R.W. (1984) Thoracic outlet syndromes. In: Dyck, P.J., Thomas, P.K., Lambert, E.H., et al. (eds.) *Peripheral neurology* (2nd edn). pp. 1402–24.

Girout, J. (1983) Rontgenstudien der dynamik der ersten rippe. *Manuelle Medizine*, 21, 20–2.

Howell Wright, J. (1991) *Physical therapy of the shoulder* (ed. Donatelli, R.A.). Churchill Livingstone: Edinburgh.

Jordan, S.E. (2000) Selective botulinum chemodenervation of the scalene muscle for treatment of neurogenic thoracic outlet syndrome. *Annals Vasc Surg* 14(4), 365–9.

Lindgren, K.A. (1997) Conservative treatment for thoracic outlet syndrome: a 2-year follow-up. *Arch Phys Med Rehab*, 87, 373–8.

Lindgren, K.A., Leino, E., Hakola, M., et al. (1990) Cervical spine rotation and lateral flexion combined motion in the examination of the thoracic outlet. *Arch Phys Med Rehab*, 71, 343–4.

Lindgren, K.A., Leino, E., Manninen, H. (1992) Cervical rotation lateral flexion test in brachialgia. *Arch Phys Med Rehab*, 73, 735–7.

McGormick, C.C., et al. (1981) Upward dislocation of the first rib: a rare cause of nerve entrapment producing brachialgia. *Br J Radiol*, 54, 140–2.

McGough, E.C., et al. (1979) Management of thoracic outlet syndrome. *J Thorac Cardiovasc Surg*, 77, 169.

Nishida, T., et al. (1993) Medial antebrachial cutaneous nerve conduction in true neurogenic thoracic outlet syndrome. *Electromyogr Clin Neurophysiol*, 33, 285–8.

Peet, R.M., et al. (1956) Thoracic outlet syndrome: evaluation of a therapeutic exercise programme. *Staff Meetings, Mayo Clinic*, 31, 281.

Pollak, E. (1980) Surgical anatomy of the thoracic outlet syndrome. *Surg Gynecol Obstet*, 150, 97–103.

Ribbe, E., et al. (1986) Clinical diagnosis of thoracic outlet syndrome—evaluation of patients with cervicobrachial symptoms. *Manual Med*, 2, 82–5.

Roos, D.B. (1976) Congenital anomalies associated with thoracic outlet syndrome. *Am J Surg*, 132, 771–7.

Roos, D.B. (1984) Thoracic outlet and carpal tunnel syndromes. In: Rutherford, R.B. (ed.) *Vascular surgery*. W.B. Saunders: Philadelphia; pp. 708–24.

Sanders, R.J., Monsour, J.W., Gerber, W.F., et al. (1979) Scalenectomy versus first rib resection for the treatment of the thoracic outlet syndrome. *Surgery*, 85, 109–19.

Sharan, D., et al. (1999) Two surgeon approach to thoracic outlet syndrome: long term outcome. *J Roy Soc Med*, 92, 239–43.

Thompson, J.F., Winterborn, R.J., Bays, S., White, H., Kinsella, D.C., Watkinson, A.F. (2011) Venous thoracic outlet compression and the Paget-Schroetter syndrome: a review and recommendations for management. *Cardiovasc Intervent Radiol*, 34, 903–10.

Urschel, H.C., Razzuk, M.A. (1972) Management of thoracic outlet syndrome. *N Engl J Med*, 285, 1140.

Wilbourne, A.J. (1990) The thoracic outlet syndrome is over-diagnosed. *Arch Neurol*, 47, 328–30.

Wright, I.S. (1945) The neurovascular syndrome produced by hyperabduction of the arms. *Am Heart J*, 29, 1.

Chapter 29

Chest wall pain

John Tanner

Background to anterior chest pain

Anterior chest pain is a frequent cause of attendance at emergency departments and of admission to hospital, but it has been estimated that about 25–30% of patients admitted with acute anterior chest wall pain remain undiagnosed despite intensive investigation including chest radiograph, electrocardiography (ECG), coronary angiography, and laboratory tests. Ockene et al.(1980) found that 10–30% of cases of chest pain referred for coronary artery imaging had normal investigations. After some time in hospital and these expensive investigations, the patient is told 'we can't find anything wrong with you, it must be musculoskeletal'. Some of these patients are then referred on to a specialist physician or therapist; others are not. In Ockene's series, 45% still had pain one year later, and over half remained unemployed. In some cases, there appears to be dual pathology: Levine and Mascette (1990) evaluated 62 adults referred for coronary arteriography using a systematic physical examination. In seven patients, the chest pain was reproduced on physical examination: six of these ultimately received a diagnosis of non-anginal chest pain and five had normal coronary arteriograms, although all these patients described their pain in terms often associated with true angina.

Acute chest pain

Obviously, the patient in acute distress from chest pain needs careful screening to rule out serious and possibly life-threatening disorders such as angina pectoris, dissecting aneurysm, pneumonia, pleurisy, or pulmonary embolus. Other viscerogenic sources of pain include oesophagitis and reflux symptoms from hiatus hernia. Less common but equally painful may be Bornholm viral myalgia and pancreatitis. Additionally, some conditions refer pain to the posterior chest, such as pleurisy and pneumonia, angina pectoris, cholecystitis, dissection of an aneurysm, and eroding peptic ulcers.

Chronic chest pain

Chronic insidious onset of chest wall pain requires careful screening for primary tumours of the lung and breast, metastatic deposits in the rib cage, or metabolic bone diseases such as osteomalacia, rickets, and hyperparathyroidism.

Examination

The clinician should include basic screening of the thoracic spine in the initial examination for chest pain unless the diagnosis is very clearly visceral in origin. This may simply involve asking the patient to perform active trunk movements, particularly observing pain or restriction with thoracic rotation in either direction. This can be followed by springing the thoracic spinal joints and rib joints in sequence. If the pain is in the upper pectoral area or posterior chest wall more closely related to the scapula region, then examination of active and passive cervical spine movements may indicate a cervical source.

When no posterior abnormality is identified as a cause of the pain, possibly referred anteriorly, the anterior structures are individually examined, especially the costochondral and sternal joints, and the muscles and their attachments.

Musculoskeletal chest wall pain

Causes of chest wall pain are summarized in Table 29.1.

- *Direct trauma:* Fractures of the sternum or ribs are readily detected clinically and/or by radiography after direct trauma.
- *Indirect trauma* can cause stress fractures of ribs, e.g. in sportsmen such as rowers, and cough fractures are seen in the osteoporotic non-athlete.
- *Cervical spondylosis/strain* may cause pain in the pharynx or upper sternal area. Examination of the cervical spine should reveal the cause: and sometimes imaging, including magnetic resonance imaging (MRI), is useful, or can be used where a more sinister cause is feared.
- *Thoracic spinal joints:* Anterior chest pain can be referred from dysfunction in the joints of the thoracic spine and ribs. Commonly, the patient has developed a pain (possibly also in the posterior chest, but not always) on performing a trivial twisting or bending movement, but it may also follow more vigorous activities from sport or manual work. The patient may describe pain only on deep inspiration. Sometimes paraesthesiae develop, following the course of an intercostal nerve. These pains can also be

Table 29.1 Musculoskeletal causes of chest wall pain

Posterior origin	Anterior origin
Systemic disorders	
Ankylosing spondylitis	Spondylitis or other chronic inflammatory arthritis
	Fibromyalgia
	Hyperventilation syndrome
Local disorders	
Spinal joint dysfunction	Trauma
Disc lesions	Infection
Other spinal pathology	Costochondritis
	Tietze's syndrome

referred from costovertebral joint dysfunction as well as from the zygapophyseal joints, and from thoracic disc lesions.

- Thoracic disc syndromes are rare, but with the advent of new imaging techniques such as MRI, asymptomatic disc bulges or protrusions are found in as many as 30% of individuals. The symptomatic thoracic disc herniation may produce back pain which radiates either in a girdle-like distribution around one side or directly through the chest towards the sternum or upper abdomen. Careful examination for restricted trunk movements, dural signs, and neurological examination of the lower limbs will allow correlation with any imaging findings.

Bruckner et al. (1987) reported on 73 patients with mid dorsal and/or unilateral chest pain seen consecutively in a rheumatology clinic over a three-year period. Visceral disease was excluded. The majority of sufferers were young women with a continuous, dull pain aggravated by coughing and sneezing and relieved by rest. Frequently, tenderness over the thoracic spine and adjacent rib was found, with pain at extremes of thoracic spinal movement. In 16%, cutaneous hyperaesthesia in a radicular distribution was found, but without other neurological abnormalities. Bruckner initially ascribed this clinical picture to a thoracic disc prolapse, but 10 cases were submitted to MRI and no prolapse was seen. However, thoracic intervertebral disc dehydration without associated prolapse was seen in 90% of a later series of patients (and 13% of the controls) and the disc abnormalities corresponded to the symptomatic levels and the clinical examination findings (Bruckner et al. 1989). The condition settled in most of the patients following manipulative therapy and advice on back care. Bruckner concludes that this is a common benign condition which deserves wider recognition. He called it the 'benign thoracic pain syndrome': it fits a syndrome of somatic dysfunction in association with disc change. In cases with disc features but no neural compromise, it is our practice to recommend manual treatment with or without manipulation.

Ankylosing spondylitis

Symmetrical aching in the chest wall, in association with discomfort and possible restriction of movement on examination (in a symmetrical pattern also) should raise a suspicion of inflammatory arthritis of the spine. If the classical features of sleep interruption, morning stiffness, and easing with exercise are added, a trial of anti-inflammatory medication should be made, and further investigation arranged (see Chapter 24). The same pathology can cause synovitis of individual joints in the chest wall, most commonly, the manubriosternal joint. Dawes et al. (1988) studied 45 patients with ankylosing spondylitis together with an age- and sex-matched group of normals for the incidence, nature, and frequency of chest pain. They found 25 of the spondylitic group had experienced recurrent chest pain compared to three normals, and had a significantly reduced chest expansion. The pain was anterior or posterior, sometimes sharp and intermittent, rather than continuous. They concluded that the presence of chest pain in ankylosing spondylitis can be an early presenting feature of the disease (eight patients had chest pain before spinal symptoms) and is associated with more severe disease. Spondyloarthropathy can now be detected relatively early with MRI on both T2 weighted and STIR sequences. High signal at costovertebral joints and the vertebral corners, either anterior or posterior, called Romanus lesions, are diagnostic.

Fibromyalgia

One of the nine pairs of classical tender points of fibromyalgia is adjacent to the second costochondral junction. However, these earlier criteria have since been superceded. It is sufficient to recognize clinically that there is widespread pain and tenderness including the posterior or anterior chest wall, and refer to the new criteria. The examination should then be extended to test the other points, to settle the differential diagnosis between local and more widespread pathology (see Chapter 13).

Hyperventilation syndrome

Patients in acute emotional distress may present with difficulty in breathing, a feeling of suffocation, and a variety of chest pains with paraesthesiae in the upper body including face and head. These patients may be observed to sigh frequently and/or breathe rapidly with predominantly upper chest movement, which characterizes the hyperventilation syndrome. Instruction in correct diaphragmatic breathing to eliminate the paradoxical respiration, or the paper bag rebreathing technique, will help normalize blood gases and reduce symptoms within minutes.

Costochondral joints and chest wall pain

Specific conditions

The costochondral joints are sometimes subject to the inflammatory changes of ankylosing spondylitis and other spondylarthropathies (see previous section); as also are the manubriosternal and sternoclavicular joints. Local tenderness occurs with fibromyalgia (see previous section). Infection of a costochondral or sternal joint has been reported rarely, usually in intravenous drug abusers. The rare autoimmune condition, relapsing polychondritis, can give a more extensive inflammation and softening of the costal cartilages: inflammatory markers such as the erythrocyte sedimentation rate (ESR) will be raised.

Costochondritis and Tietze's syndrome

There is no evidence that these two conditions of unknown cause, giving pain at one or more of the costochondral joints, do not share the same pathology. The conditions are most common in women aged between 20 and 40 (Calabro 1977). Possible precipitating factors include trauma such as a blow to the chest, undue physical exertion, and upper respiratory tract infection, but many cases appear to have a spontaneous onset. Symptoms from particularly tender or painful joints such as the sternoclavicular or other costochondral joints may be treated by local corticosteroid infiltration. This may have to be repeated more than once, since the relief may not last more than 2–3 months. A novel treatment reported by Ricevuti (1985) in a small series of patients with Tietze's showed rapid resolution with human calcitonin.

In *costochondritis* there is localized pain at the costochondral joints, which are tender on examination, but not swollen. It may affect any of the costochondral junctions and more than one site is affected in 90% of cases. The second to fifth costochondral junctions are most commonly involved. The prognosis is excellent. After one year, about one half may continue with some discomfort, but only one third report tenderness with palpation.

In *Tietze's syndrome*, which is less common, there is swelling as well as local tenderness of the joints of the chest wall: 80% of cases involve a single joint. It is rarely bilateral, tending to affect neighbouring articulations on the same side of the sternum.

Unless the swelling presents quite obvious deformity, it may only be possible to distinguish between Tietze's syndrome and costochondritis by performing a computed tomography (CT) or MRI scan to reveal the enlargement of the chondral junction. A recent study of 12 patients diagnosed clinically with Tietze's showed high signal in enlarged costochondral cartilages and subchondral adjacent bone (Volterrani 2008).

References

Bruckner, F.E., et al. (1987) Benign thoracic pain. *J Roy Soc Med*, 80, 286–9.

Bruckner, F.E., et al. (1989) Benign thoracic pain syndrome: role of magnetic resonance imaging in the detection and localisation of thoracic disc disease. *J Roy Soc Med*, 82, 81–3.

Calabro, J.J. (1977) Costochondritis. *N Engl J Med*, 296, 946–7.

Dawes, P.T., et al. (1988) Chest pain a common feature of ankylosing spondylitis. *Postgrad Med J*, 64, 27–9.

Levine, B.R., Mascette, A.M. (1990) Musculoskeletal chest pain in patients with angina: a prospective study. *South Med J*, 83(2), 262–3.

Ockene, I.S., Shay, M.J., Weiner, B.J., Daler, J.E. (1980) Unexplained chest pain in patients with normal arteriograms: a follow-up study. *N Engl J Med*, 303, 1249–52.

Ricevuti, G. (1985) Effects of human calcitonin on pain in the treatment of Tietze's syndrome. *Clin Ther*, 7(6), 669–73.

Volterrani, L., Mazzei, M.A., Giordano, N., Nuti, R., Galeazzi, M., Fioravanti, A. (2008) Magnetic resonance imaging in Tietze's syndrome. *Clin Experim Rheum*, 26(5).

Chapter 30

The joints of the shoulder girdle

John Tanner

Acromioclavicular joint dysfunction and injury

The acromioclavicular joint is as prone to develop degenerative changes as other weightbearing joints. In most patients, osteoarthrosis does not cause symptoms, but an injury such as a fall on the outstretched hand, or repetitive trauma such as is involved in sports as weightlifting, may cause the joint to become symptomatic. People who report a high exposure to physical workload and/or intense sporting activity are more prone to develop osteoarthritis of this joint.

The patient will usually point to the top of the shoulder joint, almost directly over the acromioclavicular joint, as a source of their pain. On examination, passive adduction of the arm in 90° flexion across the chest (Scarf sign) will provoke the pain, which does not radiate down the arm. Direct pressure applied digitally over the joint will also locate tenderness.

If the symptoms are mild, reduction of workload and/or aggravating sporting activity together with the use of topical non-steroidal anti-inflammatory (NSAID) gels or oral NSAIDs may settle the problem. If the symptoms are more severe, restricting everyday activity, then a local joint injection with a small dose of corticosteroid settles the pain very effectively.

Occasionally, inferior osteophytes on the joint will encroach on the subacromial space, resulting in signs of impingement of the rotator cuff and subacromial bursa. If refractory, these osteophytes can be treated by surgical excision. If the osteoarthritis is advanced with gross osteophytosis, removal of the joint by resection of the distal segment of the clavicle is usually curative. Only 5 mm of the distal clavicle needs to be resected to ensure that there is no bone-to-bone abutment.

Osteolysis of the distal clavicle

This is an uncommon condition which tends to occur following trauma or repetitive strain, as in weightlifters and sportsman performing overhead activities. Patients typically present in the second to fourth decade of life with pain localized to the acromioclavicular joint with overhead lifting activity. Radiographs demonstrate osteoporosis, cystic changes, and loss of subchondral bony detail in the distal clavicle. Occasional cystic changes in the acromion may also be found. Radioisotope scan typically shows increased uptake in the distal clavicle and occasionally in the acromion. This can be managed by conservative treatment which includes maintaining range of motion in the shoulder, strengthening, and avoidance of activities inducing pain. If patients do not respond to this regime or are unwilling or unable to modify their activities, surgical excision of the distal end of the clavicle is warranted. Cahill (1982) reviewed 46 patients, all male athletes and, all but one, weightlifters. The surgically treated cases (19) obtained relief, whereas the others only improved by cessation or change of sporting activity and avoidance of weight training.

The cause of osteolysis of the distal clavicle remains obscure. Various proposals for aetiology include autonomic nervous system dysfunction with secondary alterations in blood supply, synovial pathogenesis with invasion of local bone tissue, and subchondral stress fractures due to repetitive trauma. There is a high rate of bilateral involvement of the shoulders.

Acromioclavicular joint injury

The function of the acromioclavicular joint and surrounding ligaments includes suspending the scapula from the clavicle and supporting the weight of the upper extremity. Once the ligaments are destroyed, the stability of the joint must be maintained by the muscles. The loss of suspension can lead to muscle fatigue, encroachment of the acromion on the supraspinatus tendon, and neurological symptoms secondary to traction on the brachial plexus. Strain or dislocation of the acromioclavicular joint is a common injury seen in athletes and in non-athletes who have fallen heavily on the outstretched arm or on the side of the shoulder. The injury can be classified into three grades:

- **Grade I:** Sprain of the acromioclavicular joint without ligament injury or instability; treated conservatively.
- **Grade II:** Disruption of the acromioclavicular joint with tear of the acromioclavicular ligament and upward displacement of the clavicle of up to half the thickness of the shaft; also usually treated conservatively.
- **Grade III:** Complete disruption of the acromioclavicular joint with tear of the acromioclavicular and coracoclavicular ligaments and dislocation of the clavicle by more than half of the shaft thickness (Figure 30.1); in the older non-athletic patient, these injuries can be managed conservatively but throwing power may be

reduced. It is difficult to predict which patients will not do well; however, they can undergo late repair and reconstruction with good results. The younger athlete or manual worker is best managed surgically.

A variety of surgical procedures have been described, and can be divided into three kinds:

- **direct procedure** with sole repair of the acromioclavicular joint and its ligaments
- **indirect procedure** with sole repair of the coracoclavicular ligaments
- **combined procedures**.

In patients whose injury appears to be intermediate between grades II and III, radiological stress views and an axillary view should be obtained. This involves a standard anteroposterior view (usually with a 25° shoot-up angle) followed by asking the subject to hold a 10-kg weight in the affected arm by his/her side for 5 minutes before repeating the radiograph. This should be compared to similar views of the normal side. In some cases, patients who appear to have a grade II injury are shown, in fact, to have a grade III injury under weightbearing stress.

Opinion is divided as to the need for surgical fixation in all cases of complete acromioclavicular separation. Some clinicians recommend conservative management in patients over 45 years of age because of a higher rate of poor results following surgery. However, other authors (Krueger and Frank 1993) obtained good results in older adults who were athletically active. Glick (1987) found that an anatomical reduction was not necessary to obtain a good functional result, although the risk of post-traumatic arthritis in non-surgically treated individuals is somewhat higher. This does not influence clinical symptoms.

There is little information in the literature as to whether better functional results can be obtained with early rather than late operative repair. Weinstein et al. (1995) note a trend towards better results in the group of patients undergoing earlier repair: 96% satisfactory results being obtained with a modified Weaver-Dunn technique with only 77% satisfactory results in those undergoing late repair. They advocate surgery for athletes and manual labourers requiring use of a strong arm, and that operative repair should ideally be made within 3 months of injury. I find that symptomatic grade I and grade II strains usually respond to ligament sclerosant injections (prolotherapy) directed to the acromioclavicular joint, ligament, and capsule, and the coracoclavicular ligaments. The efficacy of this form of injection therapy has been shown in treating chronic ligamentous insufficiency in the lumbar and sacroiliac region but has not been studied in any form of controlled trial in peripheral joints (see Chapter 53). The effectiveness of this treatment obviously depends on at least partial integrity of the involved ligaments.

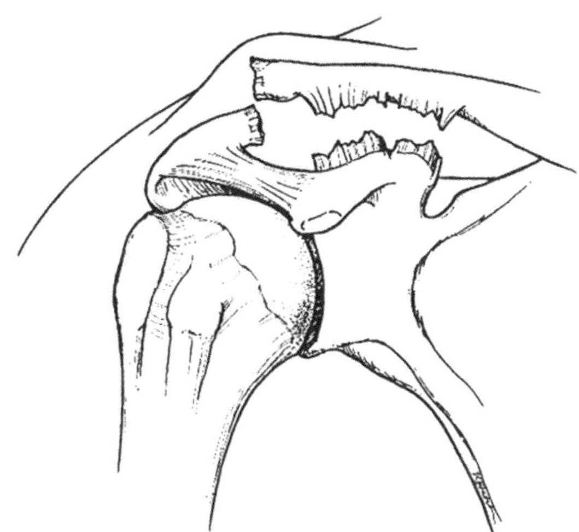

Figure 30.1 Complete acromioclavicular dislocation: there is a complete rupture of the acromioclavicular and coracoclavicular ligaments, damage to the trapezius and deltoid muscle attachments, and tenting of the skin.

Sternoclavicular dysfunction and injury

The sternoclavicular joint may undergo primary osteoarthrotic change which produces some mild tenderness, crepitus, and bony deformity. The symptoms are rarely severe enough to require any local treatment. However, trauma such as a fall on the outstretched arm or a heavy fall on the side of the shoulder, as in a rugby tackle, may strain the capsuloligamentous structures in this joint, producing some degree of synovial swelling and laxity of the anterior joint structures. The patient reports local pain and swelling, often radiating along the length of the clavicle, and this is usually associated with symptoms arising from the acromioclavicular joint, upper trapezius, and cervical spine. The patient reports pain on abduction and elevation of the shoulder together with the presence of swelling, deformity, and tenderness over the joint. Mild symptoms respond to conservative therapy including physiotherapy and anti-inflammatory drugs, topical or oral. More severe symptoms may require local joint injection. Injection of this joint should be performed with great caution using a 25-gauge needle perpendicular to the plane of the joint, taking care to penetrate no further than the anterior joint capsule to avoid puncture of mediastinal structures.

Rarely, the sternoclavicular joint can be dislocated either anteriorly or posteriorly. The posterior dislocation is less common than anterior dislocation because the anterior ligamentous structures are relatively weak. Most of the reported cases occur in young people, mainly men, who have experienced trauma to the shoulder girdle. The patient may present with the neck flexed towards the injured side, supporting the flexed elbow with the opposite hand and complaining of local pain. With an anterior dislocation, the obvious swelling and deformity can be seen and in most cases can be managed conservatively since it rarely causes any long-term dysfunction. With posterior dislocation, the depression may be seen and palpated if swelling has not yet obscured the picture. To confirm the diagnosis in either case, oblique radiographs are recommended since a routine anteroposterior view often does not show the condition. Because of the close relation of the posteriorly displaced medial clavicle to several vital structures, serious complications have been reported which include pneumothorax, haemothorax, and even compression or laceration of the great vessels or trachea. Where the condition has gone unrecognized, the thoracic outlet syndrome (see Chapter 28) has been described. In posterior dislocation, further investigations are therefore important: chest radiograph, computed tomography (CT), and angiography if any vascular involvement is suspected.

In posterior dislocation, closed reduction can be obtained by posterolateral traction of the upper arm and digital traction of the medial clavicle forwards. However, open reduction is sometimes necessary. In late diagnosis, which remains symptomatic, resection of the medial part of the clavicle may be the best option. Conservative management consists of a figure-of-eight bandage for 6 weeks followed by maintenance of active shoulder movement and muscle strength.

Adhesive capsulitis (frozen shoulder) pathology

Historically, Duplay in 1872 first described this condition of a painful, stiff shoulder, referring to it as humeroscapular periarthritis. In 1934, Codman coined the term 'frozen shoulder', attributing the symptoms to a short rotator tendinitis. In 1945, Neviaser surgically explored 10 cases of frozen shoulder, finding absence of the glenohumeral synovial fluid and the redundant axillary fold of the capsule as well as thickening and contraction of the capsule which had become adherent to the humeral head. Thus, he used the term 'adhesive capsulitis'. In the 10 cases he explored, microscopic examinations revealed reparative inflammatory changes in the capsule. However, McLoughlin (1958) reported no evidence of inflammation histologically in the frozen shoulders that he explored. He consistently found that the rotator cuff tendon was contracted and shrunken, which he postulated was due to collagen stiffening.

Simmonds (1949) and McNab (1973) proposed that the diffuse capsulitis was caused by a degenerative inflammatory process in the supraspinatus tendon. Lippmann (1943) confirmed both Schrager and Pasteur's theory that bicipital tenosynovitis preceded frozen shoulder. In examining 12 surgical cases of frozen shoulder, he found tenosynovitis of the long head of the biceps tendon. DePalma (1983) stated that the pathological process of frozen shoulder primarily involves the fibrous capsule. He noted that the normally flexible capsule becomes inelastic and shrunken. The mechanism responsible for these changes is unknown. He also observed involvement of the periarticular structures in the various stages of frozen shoulder. In the early stages, the capsule contracts with loss of the inferior capsular fold. In later phases, increased capsular fibrosis occurs. The synovial membrane becomes thickened and hypervascular. The coracohumeral ligament becomes a thick, contracted cord and the subscapularis tendon also becomes fibrotic. More recent arthroscopic findings include fibrous contracture of the middle glenohumeral ligament and villonodular synovitis at the rotator interval.

Cyriax (1978) documented the clinical examination findings of restriction of active and passive movements in characteristic proportions—which he called the *capsular pattern*. This has most limitation in external rotation, followed by abduction, and then by internal rotation. Both Neviaser (1945) and Kozin (1983) confirmed these findings. Reeves (1975) and McLoughlin (1961) substantiated the capsular pattern in arthrograms of 17 patients with frozen shoulder. He noticed more contrast dye deposited posteriorly than in any other areas of the joint capsule (implying that adhesions, if present, were anterior), reduction of intracapsular volume, and loss of the inferior capsular fold with obliteration of the subscapularis bursa and biceps sheath. Since then, most research and clinical observation has pointed to capsular adhesions as the cause of glenohumeral stiffness in frozen shoulder.

Aetiology

The pathogenesis of capsulitis or true frozen shoulder remains unknown. Cyriax proposed that a history of trauma, such as a fall on the shoulder or on the outstretched hand, may precede the onset of capsulitis by as much as 6 months, but many patients cannot recall such injuries if they appear relatively minor at the time. Most authors consider the onset to be insidious. It usually occurs in people over 40 years old, affecting both sexes but women rather more commonly. Adhesive capsulitis occurs more commonly in association with hemiparesis, ischaemic heart disease, thyroid disease, pulmonary tuberculosis, chronic bronchitis, and diabetes. Capsulitis is five times more common in diabetics, usually involving the non-dominant side, but occurring bilaterally in up to 50%.

Course and clinical features

The natural history of adhesive capsulitis is self-limiting, with an average length of time to recovery of approximately 2 years, but varying from 1 to 4 years. Most patients recover full function, but a minority remain with some functional deficit and up to half do not regain full shoulder motion (Binder et al. 1984). Patients are most likely to require intervention during the painful phase, which may last 2–9 months. Reeves noted that the length of the painful period corresponded to the length of the recovery period in that a shorter period of pain was associated with a shorter recovery period.

Reeves (1975) emphasizes three features which assist in describing phases of the condition: pain, stiffness, and recovery. However, stiffness develops while pain is present, as shown in Figure 30.2.

- *Pain* remains from the onset for 2–6 months, during which the capsule contracts. Arthrography, although not necessary for diagnosis, when performed at this stage will show decreased joint volume, usually less than 10 ml, sometimes as little as 2 ml, with obliteration of the subscapularis bursa and biceps sheath.
- *Stiffness* remains unchanged for 4–12 months.
- The final stage of spontaneous *recovery* lasts from 5 months to 26 months, during which there is a gradual return of external rotation coinciding with the arthrographic reappearance of the subscapular bursa. During this phase, there is a gradual return of abduction and internal rotation.

Symptoms

The typical patient presents with some pain of weeks' or months' duration and insidious onset, and stiffness in the shoulder. They will usually point to the upper arm around the deltoid. The patient will complain of pain produced by attempted movements overhead or behind their back, such as reaching to put on a coat or for the seatbelt in their car. They may complain of spontaneous aching even at rest, but most commonly, patients will describe pain when lying on the affected side at night which may radiate to a varying

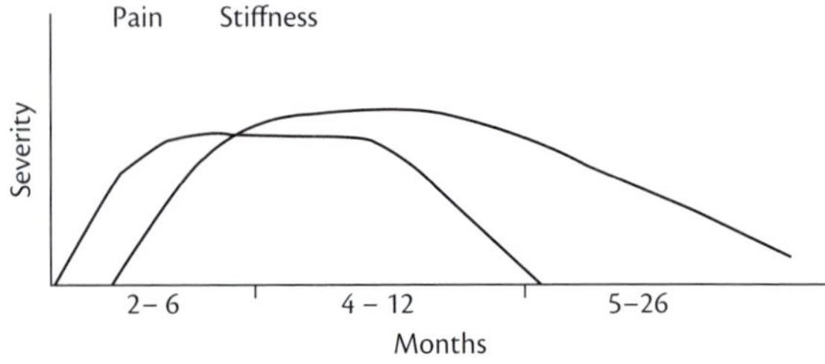

Figure 30.2 Resolution of pain and stiffness: adhesive capsulitis.

degree down the arm to the elbow and sometimes to the forearm, wrist, and hand.

Physical examination

In the painful phase, the patient will present with signs of anxiety due to pain and loss of sleep. Arm swing during gait may be reduced and the patient will be restricted while undressing. Sometimes, the affected side is elevated because of shortening of the trapezius and levator scapulae. As a consequence, there may be referred pain towards the neck and scapular region. Diagnosis is usually clear-cut, using the routine described in Chapter 23.

The cervical spine may show a pattern of strain with features of segmental dysfunction. At the shoulder, active elevation is reduced in all but the earliest cases: the striking findings are of pain and restriction of passive glenohumeral movement; i.e. most marked for external rotation, less so for abduction, and less still for internal rotation. There may be pain on resisted movements, suggestive of concurrent rotator cuff strain, but in typical cases (1) the resisted movements are less painful than the passive ones, and (2) all the resisted movements are painful, not giving the differential pattern typical of trauma to part of the rotator cuff. Specific examination of accessory movements of the glenohumeral joint shows loss of joint play.

In cases that follow trauma, there may be coexistent rotator cuff tendonitis and/or subacromial bursitis which will require treating independently. Urinalysis is useful to detect diabetic cases, who do not have such a good prognosis for early relief.

Investigations

Plain radiographs are usually normal apart from occasionally showing some osteoporosis, and arthrography shows reduced joint volume with obliteration of the subscapularis bursa, bicipital tendon sheath, and inferior capsular fold. Diagnostic ultrasound may show changes in the bicipital tendon sheath and magnetic resonance imaging (MRI) is unhelpful. Therefore, unless there is joint crepitus on passive glenohumeral movements suggesting osteoarthritis in the older patient, imaging investigations are not required to make what is essentially a clinical diagnosis.

Differential diagnosis

Any patient presenting with an acute onset of pain and stiffness in the shoulder, with a capsular pattern on examination, should be adequately screened to exclude other diseases that may present with monoarthritis (Table 30.1). The presence of swelling and warmth to the touch should alert one to the possibility of an inflammatory synovitis or septic arthritis. A brief review of the hands and other joints, looking for evidence of nodules, tenosynovitis, or, in the case of seronegative arthritis, rashes and asymmetric articular involvement, should lead to appropriate investigation and the correct diagnosis. Patients on oral steroids can develop avascular necrosis which, if suspected, is confirmed by plain radiographs and MRI. Bilateral shoulder pain with painful loss of passive external rotation in the 60-year-old patient is more likely to suggest polymyalgia rheumatica.

Table 30.1 Other diseases that may present with monoarthritis

Acute onset	Subacute or chronic onset
Septic arthritis	Crystal deposition, e.g. hydroxyapatite
Gout	Rheumatoid arthritis and variants
Pseudogout	Avascular necrosis

Treatment

The aims of treatment are pain relief and restoration of normal shoulder movement. Treatment should consist of one or more of the following:

- education and reassurance of the patient about the natural history of the condition and support with the use of analgesics or anti-inflammatories
- physiotherapy with the use of mobilization techniques or other modalities
- the use of injection techniques with corticosteroid
- manipulation under anaesthesia.

The choice of treatment depends on the severity and stage of the condition. In terms of severity, a mild case will not merit corticosteroid injection. In terms of stage, we use the criteria developed by Cyriax for gauging whether the case will be sensitive to a steroid injection. We ask the following questions:

- Does pain extend below the elbow?
- Is pain felt at rest?
- Is the patient unable to sleep on that shoulder?

When these questions are answered yes, manual treatment other than accessory movements is likely to increase pain, and not to achieve better range: if active treatment is required, injection is the treatment of choice.

Injection therapy

The trials of Bulgen et al. (1984), Jacobs et al. (1991), and Rizk et al. (1991) all found conclusive benefit for the use of steroids given intra-articularly to the glenohumeral joint, with the best results found in those patients injected early in the course of the illness. Pain relief was the main benefit, although Jacobs also showed an improvement in long-term outcome.

Multiple-injection techniques

A further trial by Winters et al. (1997) was conducted in a primary care setting and this trial reported significant differences between the treatments. In this study, treatment was considered successful after 5 weeks for 35 out of 47 patients (75%) treated with injections and for 7 out of 35 (20%) treated with physiotherapy. The corticosteroid treatment consisted of multiple injections administered by the general practitioners. For the purposes of the research study, passive mobilization was not permitted for patients allocated to the physiotherapy group.

Steinbrocker and Argyros (1974) used a triple injection technique into the joint, bursa, and long head of biceps tendon and found that 95% of patients were dramatically better or cured after 1–3 treatment sessions. Another similar study (Roy 1976) used the same entry criteria and a paired injection technique, joint and bursa, with similarly spectacular results. The authors of this latter study comment that an injection into the subacromial bursa or joint cavity alone carries a very low rate of success compared to a paired approach. It is interesting to compare this comment with Hazleman's findings of combined intracapsular and intrabursal inflammatory change during early arthroscopy (Hazleman 1990).

Accuracy of injection technique

The use of two or three different injection techniques in one treatment may have advantages when one considers a rather uncertain 'hit rate' when performing the technique blind, i.e. without the benefit of radiographic control. Inaccurate placement of intra-articular injections is reported to occur often, even among trained rheumatologists (Eustace et al. 1997; Jones et al. 1993; White et al. 1996): there is a better response to accurately placed injections. The subacromial bursa is known to be in continuity with the joint space in as much as 25% of the individuals and, therefore, a paired injection technique may allow more drug to reach the intended target. Most radiologists, when performing shoulder arthrograms in adhesive capsulitis, prefer the posterior approach since so often the anterior capsular structures are retracted. The anatomy of the posterior approach to shoulder joint injection is shown in Figure 30.3.

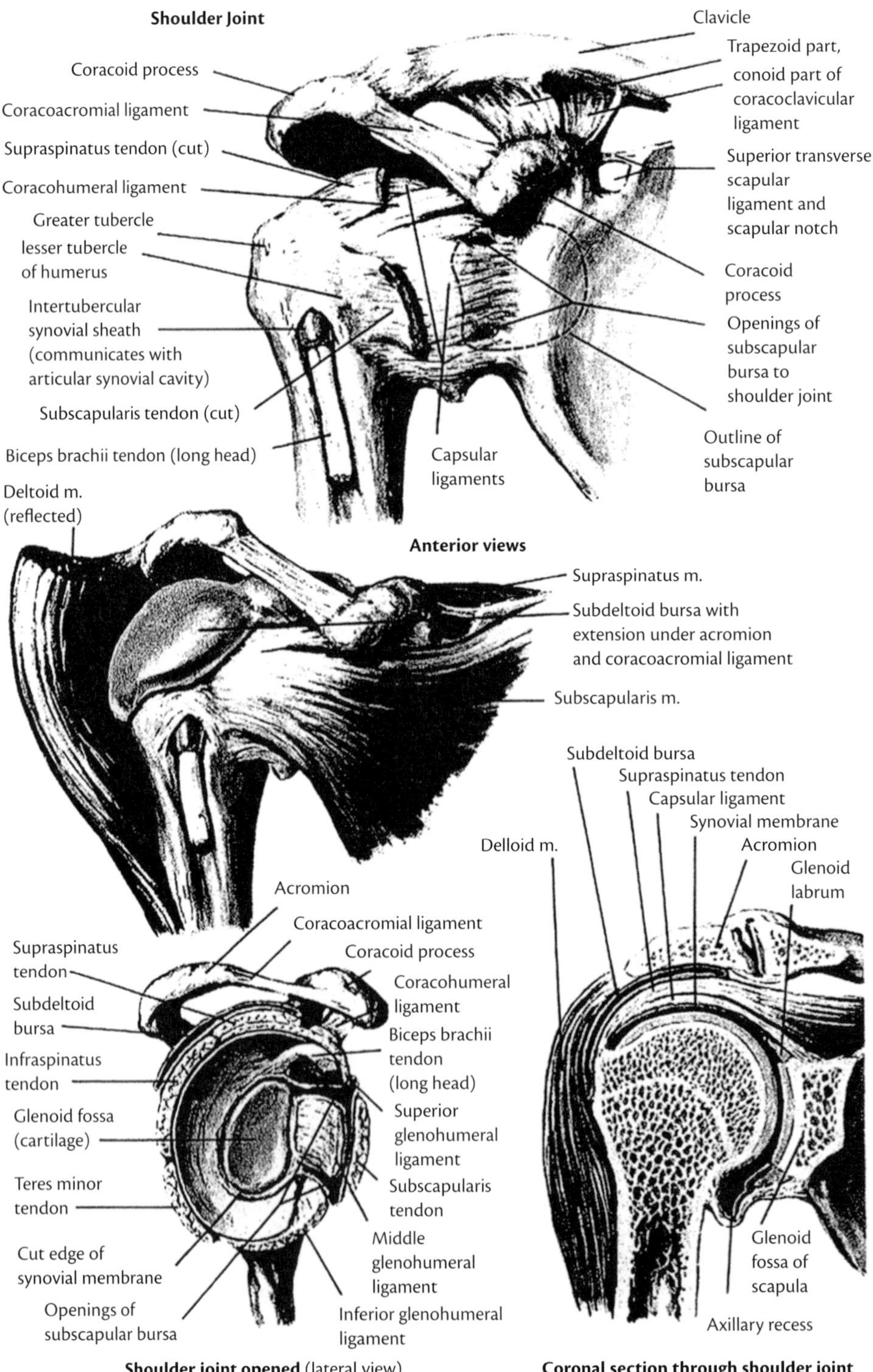

Figure 30.3 Anatomical relations of bursae, biceps tendon, and subacromial space to the joint capsule and associated ligaments.

Jacobs' study used capsular distension with volumes exceeding 25 ml in his study and this could explain the enhanced therapeutic effect in his trial. This may reduce the need for a series of two or three injections, which I find in clinical practice is often required to cover the most painful period of the acute phase.

Injection routine

Appropriate treatment by steroid injection for capsulitis would be initial unguided injection using a single or combined technique as already discussed, followed by review in approximately 3 weeks. The dose I recommend is 20 mg of triamcinolone. Some studies have used up to 40 mg and injected this as many as three times in 6 weeks. This increases the risk of systemic side-effects and, therefore, the minimum dose necessary to achieve the therapeutic result is recommended. Very few patients complain of soreness after the injection. By following up the patient at 3–4-week intervals, the acute phase can be managed by a further booster steroid injection until the most painful phase of the condition has settled. If there is an inadequate response to the first unguided injection, the second injection should be performed with ultrasound or fluoroscopic guidance to assure intra-articular placement. The posterior approach is optimal and, with the use of contrast medium, the abnormal arthrogram can be visualized. Placement of 5–10 ml of local anaesthetic with 20 mg of triamcinolone intra-articularly will very often produce the desired response.

The patient can be reassured that the range of movement will gradually recover with time, although this may take up to 12–18 months. Active and passive exercises can be recommended at this stage, with the caution that over-vigorous mobilization may result in a flare-up of symptoms and therefore require further injection treatment. In my experience, most patients find this approach to management satisfactory. The more refractory and adherent cases may require the hydroinflation/dilatation technique as described by Jacobs (1991) which should be done with image guidance. This can be accompanied by manipulation under interscalene block at the same time to achieve optimal results. Occasionally, the shoulder will remain stiff and restricted in the absence of pain beyond the average 2-year period, and then referral for either arthroscopic capsular release or manipulation under anaesthesia might be indicated. Modern shoulder surgeons prefer the former either at an early or late phase, since they claim best results are obtained without the complications of forceful manipulation of the shoulder joint (see the section 'Manipulation under anaesthesia').

In hospital practice, if two consecutive shoulder joint injections have failed to obtain therapeutic relief, we recommend a third attempt under radiographic control. The posterior approach is optimal and, with the use of contrast medium, the abnormal arthrogram can be visualized. Placement of 5–10 ml of local anaesthetic with 20 mg of triamcinolone intra-articularly will very often produce the desired response.

Physiotherapy

A variety of modalities including heat, ice, diathermy, ultrasound, and infrared have traditionally been used in physiotherapy departments. There is no evidence that any of this is effective except for very short-term relief of symptoms, or perhaps warming of the joint structures before stretching. Mueller et al. (1954) studied the benefit of ultrasound in a placebo control study for periarthritis. Using a power of 2 W/cm^2, he found that this modality was of no value in treating subacute frozen shoulder. Quinn in 1967 found no difference in groups receiving ultrasound at 0.5 W/cm^2 and exercises and those receiving diathermy and exercises.

Active mobilization

In the early, steroid-sensitive phase as already described, all active treatment is contraindicated and treatment should be directed at pain relief, i.e. joint injection. If this is not available, however, the use of ice, analgesics, NSAIDs, and transcutaneous electrical nerve stimulation (TENS) may help. In the later stages, exercise may be cautiously initiated, with close attention to the patient's response. The timing and degree of exercise can be based on the end-feel and point at which pain develops during passive movement. If pain develops before the therapist reaches the end of range, the joint is too irritable to initiate active or passive mobilization. If, however, pain is only experienced at the end of range, exercises may be attempted but if there is undue exacerbation, such as increased pain lasting more than 2 hours after exercise, they should be delayed. Some investigators have concluded that of all the treatments available, active exercise is the most useful (Lee et al. 1974). This study showed that both groups receiving exercises did significantly better than patients receiving analgesics alone.

Active mobilization with the use of mechanical exercise aids such as shoulder wheels, pulleys, and wands has been the traditional mainstay of treatment in the past. Unfortunately, it has a major drawback because there is no stabilization of the scapula, no force to depress the humeral head, and the patient tends to extend the spine to decrease demands on glenohumeral motion. Exactly the same criticisms can be levelled at the use of the shoulder wheel and the finger ladder. These techniques should probably be used only when normal gliding is present, since they involve movement only in the cardinal planes of the joint and do not increase joint play. Similarly, Codman or pendulum exercises, performed with gravity, are pain-free but exercise the joint only in the cardinal planes of movement. These and other exercises may be useful in maintaining flexibility in the joint once it has been obtained through other means.

Passive mobilization

There are a variety of forms of passive mobilization, based on the methods of Maitland (1977), Kaltenborn (1980), and Mennell (1964), but few controlled studies of this method have been undertaken. Bulgen et al. (1984) found no superiority of Maitland mobilization over treatment with ice, steroid injections, or no treatment in patients with more than 1 month's symptoms of frozen shoulder. In fact, after 6 weeks of treatment, he found the group receiving mobilization had greater loss of motion than the other groups. We therefore avoid mobilization when the joint is 'irritable'. After the inflammatory phase, a variety of manual techniques can be tried, if the patient is sufficiently handicapped, using the principles of capsular distraction and improvement of joint play (accessory movements).

Manipulation under anaesthesia

The literature on this subject is controversial, and various manipulative procedures are described. Some authors state that manipulation under anaesthesia only works by rupturing the capsule, usually the adherent inferior fold of the capsule; and indeed, contrast medium can be seen to escape from the capsule during this manoeuvre. Furthermore, long-lever techniques may run the risk of fracturing the humerus, particularly in osteoporotic individuals, and some investigators report tears of the rotator cuff. Despite claims of greatly increasing the range of motion, many physical therapists providing post-operative care find it is common for a patient to have less motion following manipulation, presumably as a result of an acute inflammatory action with muscle spasm. Pain is certainly likely to increase for several days, and modalities such as ice or TENS may be useful.

Thomas et al. (1980) performed a randomized controlled trial on 30 cases with a frozen shoulder of more than 2 months' duration. Both groups received 20 mg of intravenous valium and an injection of 50 mg of hydrocortisone into the shoulder via the posterior approach. One group was manipulated using forced abduction to 90° accompanied by full internal and external rotation. At 1-month follow-up, only two patients had completely recovered, both in the manipulation group. At 3 months, seven patients in the manipulated group (47%) and only two patients in the injected group (13%) had completely recovered. Several authors confirm that capsular rupture is an invariable recurrence during manipulation, although Samilson et al. (1961) suggest that rupture of the rotator cuff is also a frequent complication. This did not occur in any case of 103 manipulations performed with simultaneous arthrography reported by Lundberg (1969).

A promising study by Placzek et al. (1998), using short-lever translational manipulation on 31 patients under interscalene brachial plexus block, has shown significant increases in range of motion both immediately following manipulation and at long-term follow-up (up to 14 months). The average duration of symptoms was over 7 months and all patients were significantly disabled before treatment. Unfortunately, however, all patients also received a 6-day course of 4 mg of prednisolone daily, starting the day before manipulation, and no control group was used. Furthermore, after the manipulation, all patients received a fairly intensive programme of physical therapy. However, the immediate increases in passive range of motion following manipulation obtained in all cases are impressive and there was no tendency to relapse throughout the follow-up period.

Arthroscopic capsular release has been described (Warner et al. 1996) as an alternative for the management of patients who have failed to respond to physical therapy or closed manipulation under anaesthesia, but a recent controlled study (Grant et al. 2013), which was included as part of a systematic review of 22 studies including 989 patients (DARE, University of York), did not find any evidence of improved outcomes over manipulation under anaesthesia.

References

Binder, A.I., et al. (1984) Frozen shoulder: a long term prospective study. *Annals of the Rheumatic Diseases*, 43, 361.

Bulgen, D.Y., et al. (1984) Frozen shoulder. A prospective clinical study with an evaluation of three treatment regimes. *Annals of the Rheumatic Diseases*, 43, 353–60.

Cahill, B.R. (1982) Osteolysis of the distal part of the clavicle male athletes. *Journal of Bone and Joint Surgery*, 64A, 1053–8.

Codman, E.A. (1934) *The shoulder*. Robert E. Kreiger Publishing Company: Malibar, FL.

Cyriax, J. (1978) *Textbook of orthopaedic medicine, Vol. 1* (7th edn). Baillière Tindall: London.

DePalma, A.F. (1983) *Surgery of the shoulder*. J. B. Lippincott: Philadelphia.

Eustace, J.A., et al. (1997) Comparison of the accuracy of steroid placement with clinical outcome in patients with shoulder symptoms. *Annals of the Rheumatic Diseases*, 56, 59–63.

Glick, J.M. (1987) Dislocated acromioclavicular joint: follow up study of 35 unreduced acromioclavicular dislocations. *American Journal of Sports Medicine*, 5, 264–72.

Grant, J.A., Schroeder, N., Miller, B.S., Carpenter, J.E. (2013) Comparison of manipulation and arthroscopic capsular release for adhesive capsulitis: a systematic review. *Journal of Shoulder and Elbow Surgery*, 22(8), 1135–45.

Hazleman, B.L. (1990) Why is a frozen shoulder frozen? *British Journal of Rheumatology*, 29(2), 130.

Jacobs, L.G.H., et al. (1991) Intra-articular distension and steroids in the management of capsulitis of the shoulder. *BMJ*, 302, 1494–501.

Jones, A., et al. (1993) Importance of placement of intra-articular steroid injection. *BMJ*, 307, 1329–30.

Kaltenborn, F.M. (1980) *Mobilization of the extremity joints. Examination and basic treatment techniques*. Olaf Bokhandel: Oslo.

Kozin, F. (1983) Two unique shoulder disorders. Adhesive capsulitis and reflex sympathetic dystrophy syndrome. *Postgraduate Medicine*, 73, 207.

Krueger, M., Frank, E. (1993) Surgical treatment of dislocations of the acromioclavicular joint in the athlete. *British Journal of Sports Medicine*, 27, 2.

Lee, P.N., et al. (1974) Periarthritis of the shoulder. Trial of treatments investigated by multivariant analysis. *Annals of the Rheumatic Diseases*, 33, 116–9.

Lippmann, R.K. (1943) Frozen shoulder peri-arthritis bicipital tenosynovitis. *Archives of Surgery*, 47, 283.

Lundberg, B.J. (1969). The frozen shoulder. *Acta Orthopaedica Scandinavica Supplement*, 119, 55–91.

Maitland, G.D. (1977) *Peripheral manipulation* (2nd edn). Butterworths: Boston.

McLoughlin, H.L. (1961) The frozen shoulder. *Clinical Orthopedics*, 20, 126.

McLoughlin, H.L., Bull N Y. (1958) Management of the painful shoulder. Acad Med. Aug; 34(8); 525–546.

McNab, I. (1973) Rotator cuff tendonitis. *Annals of the Royal College of Surgeons of England*, 53, 271.

Mennell, J. (1964) *Joint pain. Diagnosis, treatment using manipulative techniques*. Little Brown: Boston.

Mueller, E.E., et al. (1954) A placebo-controlled study of ultrasound treatment for periarthritis. *American Journal of Physical Medicine*, 33, 31.

Neviaser, J.S. (1945) Adhesive capsulitis of the shoulder: study of pathological findings in peri-arthritis of the shoulder. *Journal of Bone and Joint Surgery*, 27, 211.

Placzek, J.D., et al. (1998) Long term effectiveness of translational manipulation for adhesive capsulitis. *Clinical Orthopedics and Related Research*, 356, 181–91.

Quinn, C.E. (1967) Humeroscapular periarthritis. Observation on effects of x-ray therapy and ultrasonic therapy in cases of frozen shoulder. *Annals of Physical Medicine*, 10, 64.

Reeves, B. (1975) The natural history of the frozen shoulder syndrome. *Scandinavian Journal of Rheumatology*, 4, 193.

Rizk, T.E., et al. (1991) Corticosteroid injections in adhesive capsulitis, an investigation into their value and site. *Archives of Physical Medicine and Rehabilitation*, 72, 20–2.

Roy, S., Oldham R. (1976) Management of painful shoulder. Lancet, 1:1322.

Roy, S., et al. (1982) Frozen shoulder. *British Medical Journal*, 284, 117–8.

Samilson, R.L., et al. (1961) Arthrography of the shoulder joint. *Clinical Orthopedics*, 20, 21–3.

Shaffer, B., Tibone, J.E., Kerlan, R.K. (1992) Frozen shoulder—a long-term follow-up. *Journal of Bone and Joint Surgery*, 74A, 738–46.

Simmonds, F.A. (1949) Shoulder pain with particular reference to the frozen shoulder. *Journal of Bone and Joint Surgery*, 31B, 426.

Steinbrocker, O., Argyros, T.G.A. (1974) Study on adhesive capsulitis of the shoulder *Archives of Physical Medicine and Rehabilitation*, 55, 209.

Thomas, D., et al. (1980) The frozen shoulder: a review of manipulative treatment. *Rheumatology and Rehabilitation*, 19, 173–9.

Warner, J.J., et al. (1996) Arthroscopic release for chronic refractory adhesive capsulitis of the shoulder. *Journal of Bone and Joint Surgery*, 78A(12), 1808–16.

Weinstein, D.M., et al. (1995) Surgical treatment of complete acromioclavicular dislocations. *American Journal of Sports Medicine*, 23, 3.

White, A., et al. (1996) The accuracy and efficacy of shoulder injections in restrictive capsulitis. J Orthop Rheum, 9:37–40.

Winters, J.C., et al. (1997) Comparison of physiotherapy, manipulation and corticosteroid injection for treating shoulder complaints in general practice: randomized single blind study. *British Medical Journal*, 314, 1320–5.

Chapter 31

Structural disorders of the shoulder

Lennard Funk, Puneet Monga, and Michael Walton

Structural anatomy of the shoulder complex

Bone and joints

Three bones—the clavicle, the scapula, and the proximal humerus—form the shoulder complex (Figure 31.1). These in turn form three synovial joints—the glenohumeral, acromioclavicular, and sternoclavicular—in addition to the scapulothoracic articulation (Figure 31.1.).

The clavicle is an S-shaped bone, which acts as a strut between the sternum and the acromial process of the scapula. The medial half is rounded and convex forward, whereas the lateral end is more flattened and curves posteriorly towards the scapula. The bone is subcutaneous throughout its length and is crossed by the supraclavicular nerves. Anteriorly, the medial half provides the origin of the clavicular head of the pectoralis major and the lateral half, the origin of the anterior deltoid. The clavicle is formed by intramembranous ossification and is the first bone to form in the fetus at around the fifth week of gestation. It is also the last bone to complete ossification in the mid-twenties. The lengthening of the clavicle, leading to a more dorsally placed scapula, is one of the key stages in human evolution as it facilitates the throwing action.

The sternoclavicular joint is the only bony attachment of the shoulder complex to the axial skeleton. The medial end of the clavicle is much larger than the corresponding articular portion of the manubrium and a small part of the articulation occurs with the first costal cartilage. An intra-articular fibrocartilage disc separates the bones into two cavities. Anterior and posterior sternoclavicular ligaments are the primary stabilizers of the joint.

The acromioclavicular joint is a diarthrodial joint and it also has an intra-articular mensical disc. There is a variable degree of articular cartilage cover. The joint is stabilized by condensations of the capsule called acromiclavicular ligaments and also attached to the coracoid by the coracoclavicular ligaments.

The scapula is a flat triangular-shaped bone. It has four important processes; the glenoid, the acromion, the coracoid, and the scapula spine. It lies over the thoracic cage between the second and seventh ribs. It serves as the attachment for 17 muscles. The concave costal surface is the origin of the subscapularis. From inferiorly, the medial border serves as attachment of the serratus anterior, rhomboid major, rhomboid minor, and levator scapulae. The dorsal surface is divided into the supra and infraspinatus fossae by the scapula spine which serves as the origin of the posterior deltoid. The supraspinatus and the infraspinatus arise from their respective fossae. From inferiorly, latissimus dorsi, teres major, and teres minor attach to the medial border.

The junction of the spine and coracoid process anteriorly forms the suprascapular notch and the junction of the free lateral edge and the glenoid, the spinoglenoid notch. A transverse ligament borders the superior outlet of the suprascapular notch. The suprascapular nerve runs under the ligament and the suprascapular artery, above it. The neurovascular bundle then runs along the supraspinatus fossa giving innervation to the muscle before curving round the spinoglenoid notch to supply the infraspinatus.

The lateral border of the scapula is thickened and wedge-shaped to form the glenoid. At the superior apex of the glenoid is the supraglenoid tubercle into which attaches the superior labrum and long head of the biceps; at the inferior margin, the infraglenoid tubercle, which forms the origin of the long head of the triceps. The coracoid process arises from the superior aspect of the base of the glenoid and projects anteriorly and curves laterally. The conjoint tendon of the short head of the biceps and the coracobrachilais originates from the tip, and the pectoralis minor, from the medial border. The coracoacromial and coracoclavicular ligaments arise from the lateral and superior aspects respectively.

The proximal humerus and the scapula glenoid form the glenohumeral joint. This is a large synovial ball and socket joint. The humeral head, however, is approximately four times larger than the shallow glenoid fossa, resulting in the joint being inherently unstable.

Muscles and soft tissue

The glenoid is deepened by the fibrocartilagenous labrum, which encircles the bone and also acts as the insertion of the joint capsule. The capsule is thickened into discrete bands to form the glenohumeral ligaments (Figure 31.2), which are static stabilizers of the joint. Anteriorly are the superior and middle glenohumeral

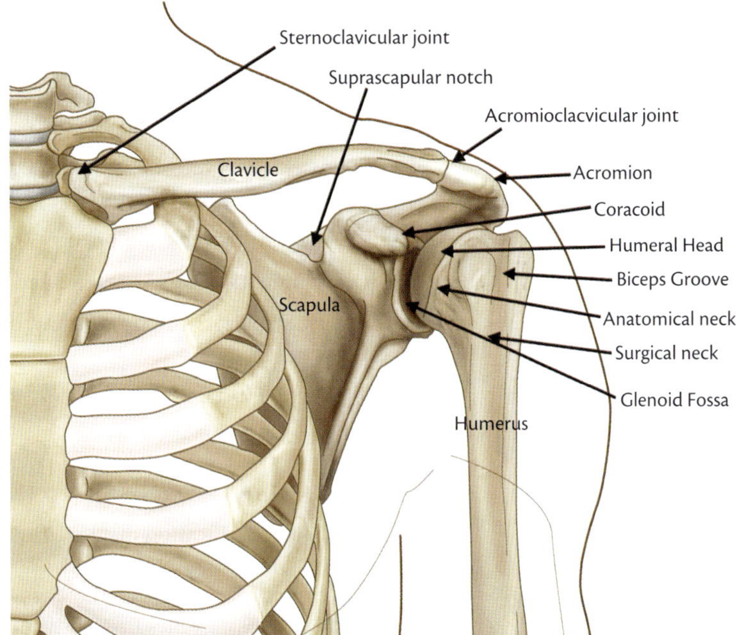

Figure 31.1 Bones and joints of the shoulder. (With permission of shoulderdoc.co.uk)

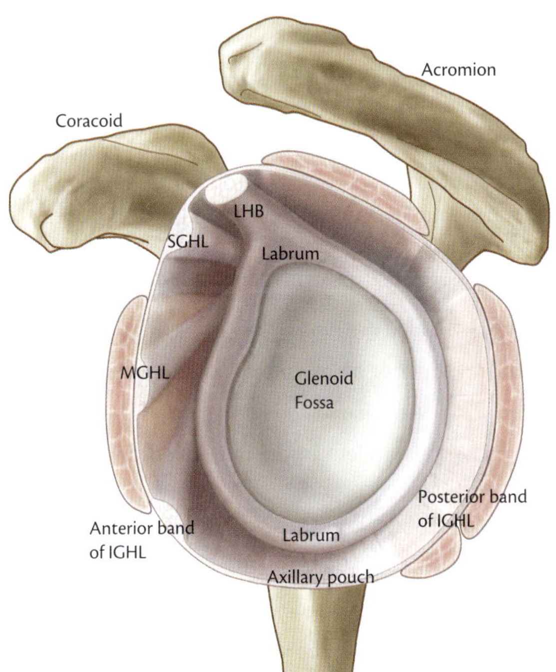

Figure 31.2 Glenoid labrum and the glenohumeral ligaments. (SGHL—superior glenohumeral ligament; MGHL—middle glenohumeral ligament; IGHL—inferior glenohumeral ligament.) (With permission of shoulderdoc.co.uk)

ligaments. Inferiorly is the inferior glenohumeral ligament, which is divided into anterior and posterior bands with an axillary pouch between them. The anterior band of the inferior glenohumeral ligament is the primary restraint to anterior translation of the humeral head in the abducted, externally rotated position. Avulsion of this ligament and its labral attachment leads to the classic 'Bankhart' lesion.

The muscles of the rotator cuff provide dynamic stability of the glenohumeral joint. This group of muscles originates from the scapula and attaches to the proximal humerus. The muscles are best thought of as the anterior and posterior rotator cuff. The anterior cuff (Figure 31.3a) is formed by the subscapularis. This inserts on the lesser tuberosity. The posterior cuff (Figure 31.3b) is formed by the supraspinatus, the infraspinatus, and the teres minor, which insert on the greater tuberosity. The long head of the biceps runs between the two tuberosities in the biciptal groove.

Scapula movement is controlled by the interaction of the force couples of the trapezius and the serratus anterior (Figure 31.4). The trapezius is a large triangular muscle which originates from the nuchal line and ligamentus nuchae of the cervical spine and the spinous processes and supraspinous ligaments of all of the thoracic vertebare. The upper fibres insert into the lateral third of the clavicle, the acromion, and the upper boarder of the scapula spine. The

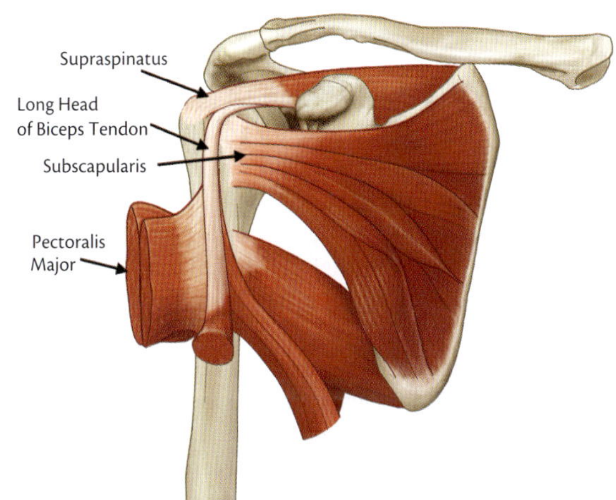

Figure 31.3a Anterior rotator cuff. (With permission of shoulderdoc.co.uk)

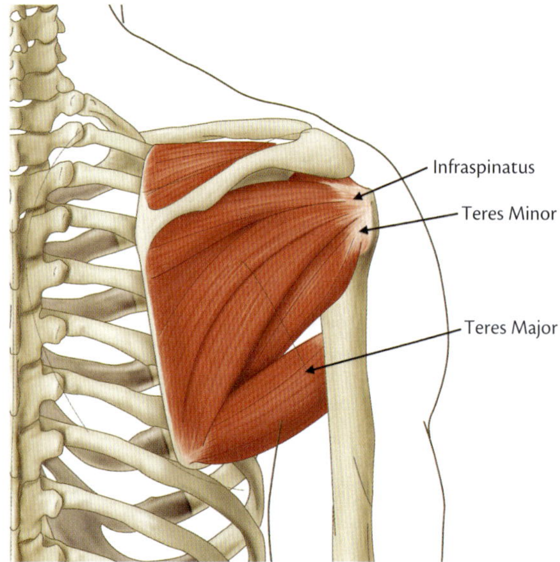

Figure 31.3b Posterior rotator cuff. (With permission of shoulderdoc.co.uk)

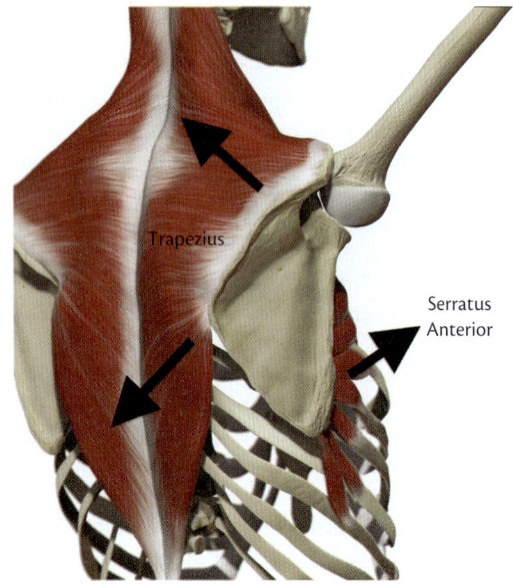

Figure 31.4 Scapula force couples. (With permission of shoulderdoc.co.uk)

lower fibres insert into the medial aspect of the lower boarder of the scapula spine. The serratus anterior arises from the upper eight ribs on the anterior chest wall. The muscle inserts into the medial boarder of the scapula with the upper four digitations at the superior angle and the lower four at the inferior angle.

The pectoralis major is formed by sternal and clavicular components. The sternal component arises from the lateral half of the manubrium and the sternum and from the aponeurosis of the external oblique muscle. The clavicular head arises from the medial half of the clavicle. The muscles insert into the biciptal sulcus on the humerus as a flat tendon with two laminae. The clavicular head and uppermost sternal fibres form the anterior laminae, whereas the remaining majority of the sternal fibres form the posterior laminae. The most inferior muscle fibres insert higher on the humerus giving the tendon an apparent twist.

Glenohumeral joint instability

It is best to think about shoulder instability based on the following aspects, as each of these will affect the management and approach to the patient:

1 The mechanism of original injury or onset (traumatic or atraumatic mechanisms)

2 The affected/injured components:
   - Dynamic stabilizers—muscles and kinetic chain
   - Static stabilizers—bony anatomy, capsule, labrum, and rotator cuff

3 Direction of instability

4 Generalized laxity

Classification

A very good classification that takes into consideration most of the aforementioned components and also acknowledges the change in symptoms over time is the Stanmore Classification (Lewis et al. 2004). This classifies instability into:

- *Polar Type 1*—traumatic dislocation with large structural injuries (e.g. rugby player)
- *Polar Type 2*—minimal trauma, with minor structural injuries (e.g. gymnast)
- *Polar Type 3*—motor control instability with no structural abnormalities or injury

Pathology

The structural injuries in shoulder instability are, in order of decreasing frequency and increasing severity:

1 Soft tissue labral tears
   - Anterior = Bankart lesion
   - Superior = superior labral anterior posterior (SLAP) lesion
   - Posterior = reverse Bankart lesion

2 Hill-Sachs Lesion—indent of the humerus from impact against the glenoid rim

3 Bony Bankart lesion

4 Capsular tears = HAGL (humeral avulsion glenohumeral ligament)

5 Rotator cuff tears

The more severe the lesion, the greater the risk of recurrence and complications; thus the need for earlier surgical intervention.

Clinical assessment

Examination of the unstable shoulder includes evaluation of both laxity and instability, in addition to the standard shoulder assessment.

Laxity

Laxity can be normal. It is simply how loose the ligaments of the joint are. However, differential laxity compared to the opposite, normal shoulder can be pathological. It is also essential to assess the generalized laxity of the patient, using the nine-point Beighton score (Beighton et al.1973).

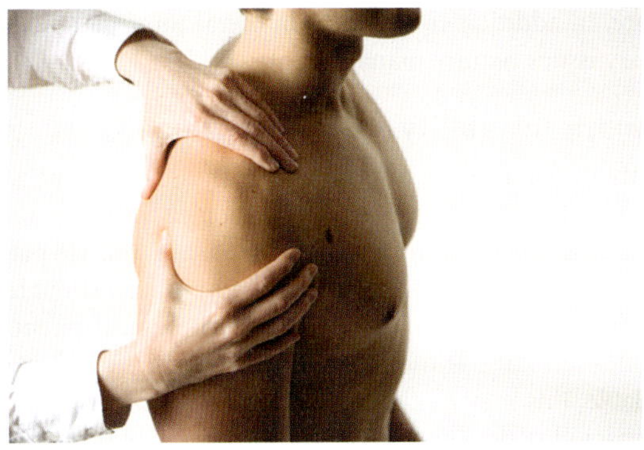

Figure 31.5 Drawer tests for laxity. (With permission of shoulderdoc.co.uk)

Shoulder laxity is assessed by the Drawer tests (Gerber 1984), where the humeral head is translated over the glenoid while stabilizing the scapula (Figure 31.5). It is assessed in the anterior, posterior, and inferior directions. Laxity is graded according to the amount of translation in each direction:

- Grade 0 = no movement
- Grade 1 = translation to the glenoid rim
- Grade 2 = translation beyond the glenoid rim, and relocates spontaneously
- Grade 3 = translation beyond the glenoid rim, and does not relocate spontaneously

Instability

Instability is pathological and includes both symptoms and signs. Instability is never normal. From the history, patients will complain of either true dislocations or subluxations (feelings of the shoulder slipping in and out of joint, feeling loose, or clicking and popping). They may be apprehensive in certain positions—overhead or towards extremes of motion. Pain may be associated, but not always.

Clinically, the 'apprehension tests' demonstrate instability. However, in a muscular athlete these may not always be positive. Our preferred tests are:

- Anterior instability:
  1. Anterior apprehension test (Figure 31.6a)—the arm is brought gently into abduction and external rotation until the patient feels apprehensive. Gradually, more force can be added as the movement progresses. This can be performed with the patient sitting or supine.
  2. Anteroinferior sulcus apprehension (Figure 31.6b)—with the patient leaning forward and the arm dangling down, the examiner gently applies traction to the arm. If the patient feels apprehensive with this, it is positive.
- Posterior instability:
  1. Posterior apprehension test (Figure 31.6c)—the arm is taken into adduction, flexion, and internal rotation. A posterior load is applied gradually until apprehension or pain. This can be performed seated or supine.
  2. Modified O'Brien's test (subtle instability or large athlete) (Figure 31.6d)—with the patient seated and the arm in a fully adducted, internally rotated position in flexion, the patient is asked to resist a downward force on the wrist. If they are unable to maintain resistance, it is suggestive of posterior instability.

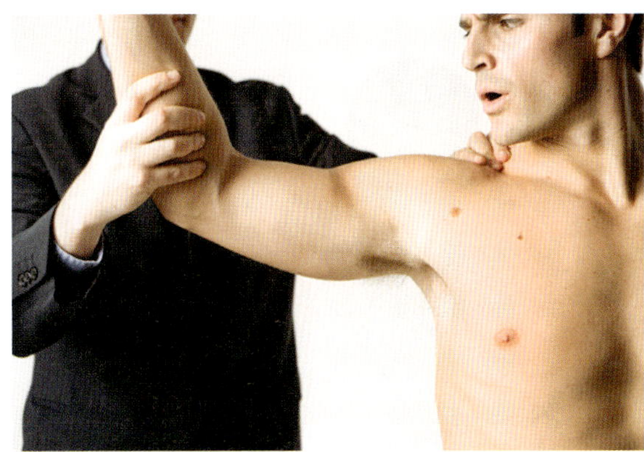

Figure 31.6a Anterior apprehension test. (With permission of shoulderdoc.co.uk)

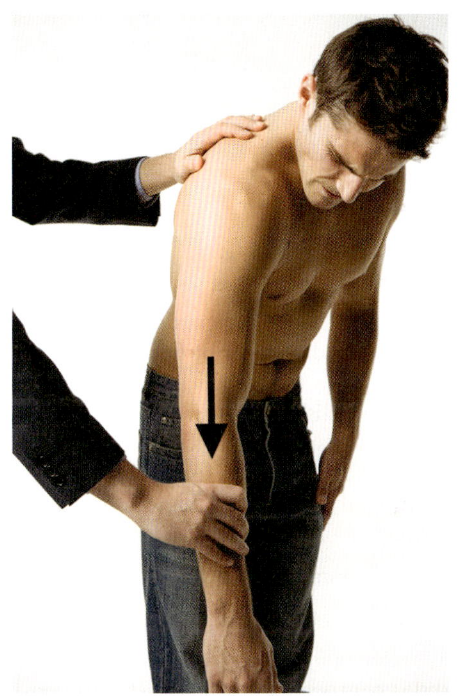

Figure 31.6b Anteroinferior apprehension test. (With permission of shoulderdoc.co.uk)

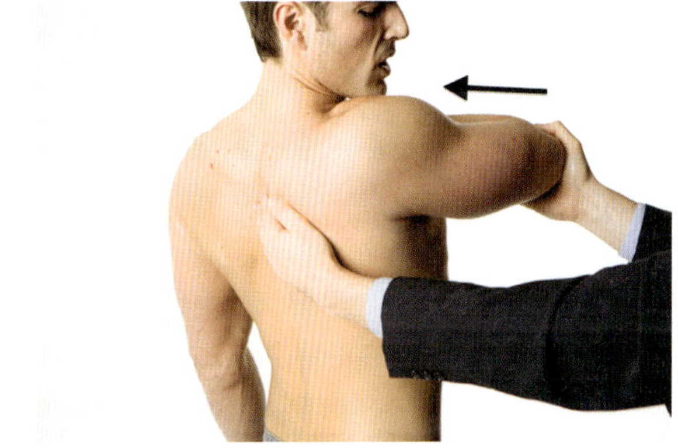

Figure 31.6c Posterior apprehension test. (With permission of shoulderdoc.co.uk)

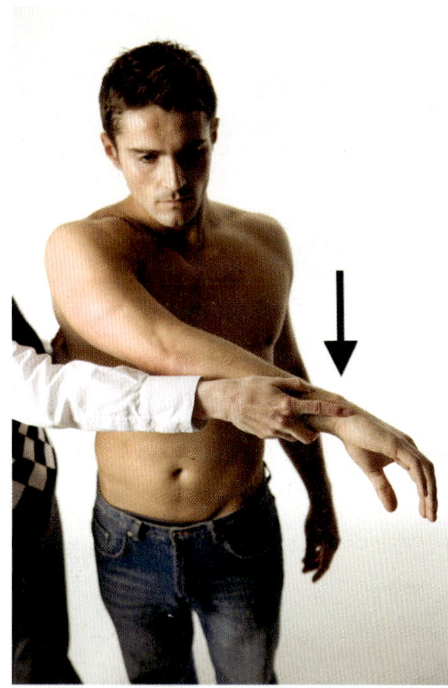

Figure 31.6d Modified O'Brien's test. (With permission of shoulderdoc.co.uk)

Acute traumatic dislocations

Traumatic dislocations may be anterior or posterior. The mechanism of injury usually indicates the direction. Anterior dislocations are usually caused by a force abduction and external rotational force, while posterior dislocations are caused by a posterior force with the arm in flexion and internal rotation (e.g. landing on flexed elbow). In sport, subluxations are generally more common than true dislocations, so the history is essential.

Acute management of a shoulder dislocation involves:

1 Neurovascular assessment before and after reduction
2 Immobilization and pain control
3 Ideally, a radiograph prior to manipulation (to exclude a fracture-dislocation, which would negate a closed reduction)
4 Closed reduction under adequate sedation and muscle relaxation by an experienced clinician
5 Repeat radiographs to confirm the reduction
6 Immobilization in a supportive sling and early, gentle rehabilitation

The recurrence rates after a first-time acute shoulder dislocation depend on the age of the patient, sport, gender, and the structural injuries sustained. High risk of recurrences of over 80% are reported for males, under 20 years of age, playing high-level contact sports, with generalized ligamentous laxity and significant structural injuries (Kralinger et al. 2002). In these high-risk groups, early surgical stabilization is recommended.

Recurrent traumatic instability (Polar Type 1 or 2)

Recurrent instability can be very disabling and requires investigations and treatment. These patients often develop secondary muscular problems with scapula winging and a poor kinetic chain. Therefore, in addition to the glenohumeral joint pathology, these secondary issues require management.

Atraumatic instability (Polar Type 2 or 3)

Instability in the absence of no inciting, traumatic event is rare. It tends to occur in hyper-mobile, young people. The common causes are muscle patterning disorders with abnormal muscle patterning in movement causing subluxation of the hyper lax shoulder joint. Previously, this was thought to be a psychological phenomenon or attention seeking. If the subluxations are purely voluntary and controllable, this may be the case. However, uncontrollable, involuntary instability does require investigation and management. This involves a specialist multidisciplinary shoulder service. Surgery is rarely indicated.

Investigations

Either magnetic resonance imaging (MRI) arthrogram or computed tomography (CT) arthrogram are the preferred investigations for instability. They have the highest sensitivity and specificity in detecting the pathological lesions of instability. However, this is not 100% and is dependent on the equipment, technique, and the radiologist's skill and experience.

Management

Treatment depends on the severity of the symptoms, patient requirements, and the pathological lesions found. All patients should receive specific shoulder physiotherapy. This involves correction of the kinetic chain, muscle patterning problems, scapula correction, lifestyle modifications (if possible), and shoulder stability exercises. Surgery is indicated for significant pathologies, unresponsiveness to good rehabilitation, and high-demand athletes. The surgical procedure depends on the pathology, patient, and surgeon's expertise. Direct repair of the lesions is usually performed, but in revisions, significant bony glenoid erosion, or high-level contact athletes, the coracoid-transfer Latarjet procedure is popular (Burkhart et al. 2007).

Disorders of the proximal biceps

The long head of the biceps (LHB) initially has an intra-articular course from its attachment onto the supraglenoid tubercle of the glenoid via the superior labrum. It then runs within the intertubercular groove, bound by the transverse humeral ligament, and is flanked by the pectoralis major and teres major distally (Buck et al. 2011). This tortuous route is related to the evolutionary development of the upper limb. The function of the LHB is the subject of great interest due to its controversial role as a flexor, depressor, and dynamic stabilizer and its involvement in the throwing action. The three common pathologies affecting the LHB—in the form of tendonitis, instability, and rupture—are described in Table 31.1.

Biceps tendonitis

Tendonitis of the LHB can occur in isolation or as part of rotator cuff disease. Tendonitis usually presents as anterior shoulder pain along the intertubercular groove, localized tenderness in this region, along with a positive Speed's test. The diagnosis is best made by ultrasound scan which reveals fluid in the tendon sheath. Pain relief following a guided local anaesthetic injection into the tendon sheath is confirmatory. A trial of non-operative treatment is usually successful and involves activity modification, pain relief, and

Table 31.1 Common pathologies affecting the long head of the biceps

	Tendonitis	Instability	Rupture
Presentation	Anterior shoulder pain	Clicking	'Popeye' sign
Diagnosis	Localized tenderness, ultrasound	Examination, dynamic ultrasound	Clinical examination
Management	Injection, physiotherapy, tenotomy/tenodesis	Repair stabilizers, tenodesis	Predominantly non-operative

postural and humeral head corrective exercises. Pain relief can best be obtained with a guided injection. Although the risk of tendon rupture associated with corticosteroid injection is small (Karpman et al. 1980), injection of hyaluronan may be preferred in younger patients. Failure of non-operative management is an indication for surgical management in the form of biceps tenotomy or tenodesis (Longo et al. 2011).

Biceps instability

The position of the LHB within its groove is reliant on the anatomical integrity of the biceps pulley. The inferior wall of the biceps pulley is formed by the subscapularis tendon, the anterior wall by the superior glenohumeral ligament, and the superior wall by the coracohumeral ligament (Nakata et al. 2011). Traumatic lesions of this pulley can lead to subluxation of the LHB, with reproducible painful clicking during shoulder rotations. Instability of the biceps tendon can also be associated with tears of the subscapularis tendon. A dynamic ultrasound scan is invaluable for diagnosis of LHB instability. Management of LHB instability depends on the associated lesions. Biceps pulley lesions (Figure 31.7) are most commonly associated with rotator cuff tears and management of such associated pathology is key to the management of biceps instability associated with pulley lesions (Braun et al. 2011).

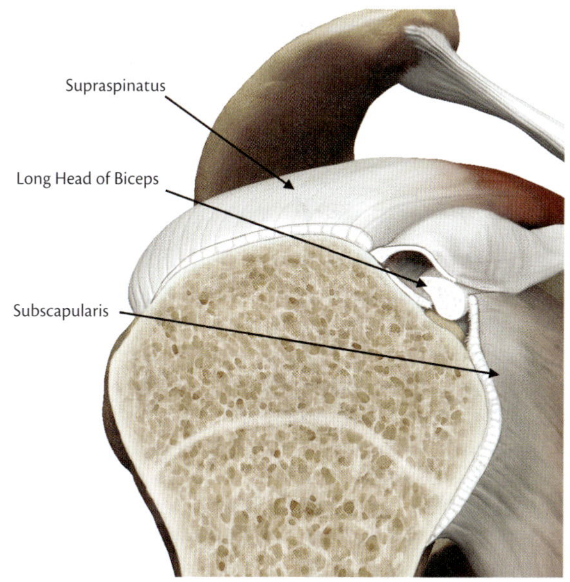

Figure 31.7 Biceps pulley rupture with subscapularis tear leading to medial subluxation of the long head of the biceps tendon from its groove. (With permission of shoulderdoc.co.uk)

Biceps rupture

Spontaneous rupture of the LHB is often associated with rotator cuff tears. Such ruptures may display a 'Popeye' sign, which is a distal bunching of the biceps. Complete distal migration is halted by the short head of the biceps and, in a vast majority of subjects, it is asymptomatic. Clinical and radiological assessment of the rotator cuff is recommended following acute presentation of a 'Popeye' sign.

Traumatic rupture of the LHB is infrequently seen in contact sports or overhead athletes. Although the diagnosis is frequently evident with the presence of a 'Popeye' sign (Figure 31.8), an ultrasound scan is invaluable when diagnosis is in doubt. Tendon to tendon repair of such acute ruptures is not recommended as it usually occurs on a background of tendinopathy. However, acute tenodesis may be selectively offered to preserve acceleration during throwing and supination strength in a high- demand athlete. Surgery should not be offered for cosmetic reasons (Ng et al. 2012).

Tenotomy or tenodesis

Management of a majority of LHB pathologies is in the form of either biceps tenotomy or tenodesis. Tenotomy is division of the LHB near its insertion into the glenoid and is a simple and reliable method of pain relief. There is a high risk of a 'Popeye' sign which may be poorly perceived by the patient. On the other hand, tenodesis of the biceps tendon involves reattachment of the LHB to bone or neighbouring tendons. Tenodesis prevents development of a 'Popeye' sign but can lead to persistent pain at the tenodesis site in a small proportion of patients. There is neither consensus nor quality evidence regarding the choice between tenotomy versus tenotomy (Frost et al. 2009). Popular current practice leans towards tenodesis for young, lean, and athletic individuals and tenotomy for older, less active individuals.

Superior labrum anterior posterior tears

The anatomy of the superior labrum is unique as it is loosely attached (as compared to the inferior labrum) and provides attachment to the long head of the biceps. The superior labrum normally has a recess, which can be mistaken for a labral tear. The blood supply of the labrum is derived from the periphery towards the joint

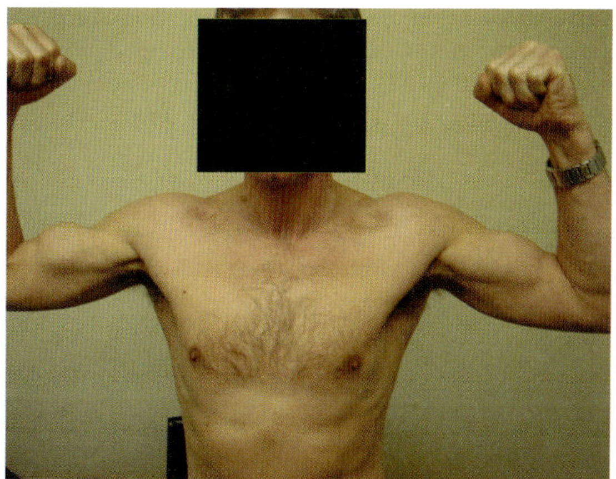

Figure 31.8 'Popeye' sign of long head of the biceps rupture. (With permission of shoulderdoc.co.uk)

and hence predisposing the labrum to degenerative tears (Cooper et al. 1992).

Aetiology

Superior labrum anterior posterior (SLAP) lesions were initially classified by Snyder in 1990 (Snyder et al. 1990). There are three mechanisms of injury that have been proposed:

1 Superior compression—usually due to a fall onto an outstretched arm with the shoulder positioned in an abducted and slightly forward-flexed position, pushing the superior labrum off the glenoid.

2 Traction—a sudden, traumatic pull on the arm with avulsion of the biceps origin (superior labrum) off the glenoid.

3 Repetitive microtrauma from overhead sports activity with associated instability (D'Alessandro et al. 2000). Repetitive overhead external rotation and abduction activity can lead to 'peel back' of the postero-superior labrum. Such overuse injuries are commonly associated with partial articular surface rotator cuff tears. Overhead throwing athletes are particularly predisposed to such injuries and large forces on the biceps tendon during the deceleration phase of the throwing motion may create SLAP lesions (Andrews et al. 1985).

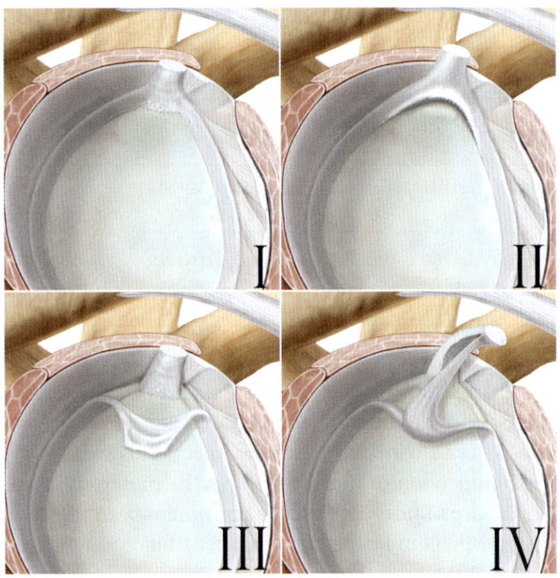

Figure 31.9 SLAP tear classification. (Reprinted from *Arthroscopy*, Vol 6, Issue 4, Snyder, Stephen J. et al., SLAP lesions of the shoulder, p. 274–279, with permission from Elsevier.)

Classification

Based on the arthroscopic appearance, SLAP tears are classified into four main categories with type II being the commonest pathological type seen (55%) (Snyder et al. 1990) (Box 31.1; Figure 31.9). Although there are many further uncommon variants described, it is crucial to recognize the coexistence of SLAP lesions with other labral injuries.

Clinical

Patients with SLAP tears present with a deep pain between the acromioclavicular (AC) joint and the coracoid (D'Alessandro et al. 2000). This pain is typically recreated during the throwing manoeuvre. Painful clicking and popping may also be a feature.

Although a multitude of special tests, including the compression rotation, Kibler's anterior slide, Mayo shear test, and the O'Brien's test, are all described for clinical diagnosis, only the combination of the anterior slide test with a history of popping, clicking, or catching has a moderate diagnostic utility for confirming Type II to IV SLAP lesions (Michener et al. 2011). Differential test injections into the AC joint or subacromial space may be needed to rule out other sources of pain and an MR arthrogram is the preferred investigation to confirm diagnosis (D'Alessandro et al. 2000).

Box 31.1 SLAP tear classification

Type I	Degenerative fraying of the superior edge, which remains firmly attached to the glenoid.
Type II	The superior labrum and the attached biceps tendon are stripped off the superior glenoid, destabilizing the biceps anchor.
Type III	Bucket-handle tear of the superior labrum. The peripheral edge of the labrum and biceps anchor intact.
Type IV	Bucket-handle tear as in Type III, but with extension into the biceps tendon itself.

Treatment

SLAP tears following direct or indirect trauma, with significant inability to return to sports or activities requires surgical repair. Other presentations of SLAP tears can be mostly managed initially with a non-operative trial in a vast majority of patients. Surgical treatment of Type I SLAP involves arthroscopic debridement. Type II and III SLAP tears are usually repaired arthroscopically with suture anchors.

A biceps tenodesis is recommended for Type IV SLAP tears, revision surgery, and in older age groups (usually over 40 years). A biceps tenotomy is preferred over a tenodesis in patients with a low level of physical activity and demand.

Return to play at the same level after surgical treatment of SLAP lesions in overhead athletes range from 22% to 94%, with a lower return to sports in repetitive overhead athletes. Sports-specific rehabilitation is key to achieving optimal outcomes.

Rotator cuff disease

Subacromial impingement

Subacromial impingement is the second most common condition after neck and back pain and accounts for 44–65% of all shoulder complaints (Michener 2011). As such, it represents a significant economic burden on healthcare resources.

The diagnosis of 'impingement' broadly encompasses pain generated from any pathology within the rotator cuff and subacromial space. It gained significant popularity in the 1970s, after Neer published his initial series of successful open anterior acromioplasties, based upon the theory that the pathology was caused by extrinsic compression of the rotator cuff by the acromion or subacromial spur (Neer 1972). However, this theory did not account for the clinical finding, as early as Codman in the 1930s, that much of the tendon disease began on the articular surface.

The current theory of rotator cuff pathology is that it has three contributing mechanisms.

1 *Intrinsic*, age-related tendon degeneration or tendinopathy. This is a non-inflammatory process which, results in decreased tendon integrity and function and may be influenced by tendon vascularity, systemic disease, and injury.

2 *Biomechanical* abnormalities of the scapula and rotator cuff, which may be as a result of tendon damage, pain, or poor posture. Poor cuff function results in abnormal shoulder kinematics frequently with superior humeral translation which, leads to increased pressures within the subacromial space.

3 *Extrinsic* factors limiting the subacromial space can contribute to the mechanical impingement, such as the presence of a subacromial spur formed as an enthesophyte of the coracoacromial ligament, or inferior osteophytes from the AC joint. This increase in subacromial pressure promotes an inflammatory process within the subacromial bursa which, may be a significant pain generator.

Intrinsic tendinopathy may progress to tendon tearing. MRI studies have shown that over 50% of the over-60s population have asymptomatic rotator cuff tears (Sher et al. 1995). The reasons why many rotator cuff tears remain silent and the generator of pain in rotator cuff disorders is very poorly understood.

Diagnosis

The diagnosis of impingement is clinical, not radiographic. Patients usually present with an insidious onset of shoulder pain predominately in the lateral border of the arm, which is exacerbated by overhead activities in internal rotation. Numerous 'special tests' have been described but most have poor specificity. The most common are Neer's sign (pain on elevation in the scapular plane with the shoulder in internal rotation), 'empty can' (pain relief on forward elevation in external rotation), and Hawkins-Kennedy (pain on passive internal rotation with the arm abducted to 90°). Each of the rotator cuff muscles should be tested in turn for power and lag signs.

Investigations

Patients should be investigated with plain radiographs which, may identify the presence of a subacromial spur, calcific tendinitis, or end-stage superior migration of the humeral head. In rare cases, primary or secondary bone tumours may be identified. The rotator cuff itself can be imaged either by ultrasound or MRI. Both modalities have been shown to be highly sensitive and specific for diagnosing rotator cuff tears. Ultrasonography is a more dynamic investigation and is financially less expensive but is highly user-dependent.

Management

The majority of cases of subacromial pain can be treated conservatively. Physiotherapy aims to address the biomechanical changes that predispose to impingement and strengthen the rotator cuff. Rotator cuff function is inhibited in the presence of pain so the judicious use of analgesia is essential. Subacromial injections can be very effective in providing a 'pain-free window' in which to rehabilitate.

If conservative measures fail, then surgical intervention may be indicated. If the rotator cuff is intact, then arthroscopic subacromial decompression may be performed. This procedure is known to be effective in reducing symptoms of impingement, in appropriately selected patients, but it is unclear which element of the operation or rehabilitation is responsible, and debate in the literature continues.

Rotator cuff tears

The presence of a full-thickness rotator cuff tear (or impending in a deep partial thickness tendon tear) in a symptomatic shoulder frequently indicates tendon repair. However, the evidence for this is inconclusive. There is a general consensus that acute traumatic tears, particularly in the younger, active patient should be repaired. The management of degenerate tears is more debatable. Many surgeons would advocate that tendon repair surgery allows a greater reduction in symptoms, better return to function, and a potential reduction in the long-term sequelae of cuff deficiency. However, we also know that many tendon repairs fail, but these patients frequently have a significant improvement in symptoms following surgery despite this.

The technique of tendon repair has advanced greatly in recent years. Arthoscopic surgery has flourished with the advancement in suture and bone anchor technology. These techniques, however, are technically challenging and require sub-specialist training in order to become proficient. Despite this, there remain some tears which, are irreparable, due to tendon retraction and quality. Tendon transfers may be suitable in some instances, while in the elderly, the reverse shoulder replacement has shown good results in those with sufficient pain and disability.

Calcific tendonitis

Deposition of calcium in the tendon of the rotator cuff, usually supraspinatus, is a common disorder. While the calcium is deposited, the patient may complain of mild discomfort. Severe pain occurs in acute calcific tendonitis, when the calcium undergoes resorption. The pain can be so severe that patients often present to casualty departments.

The aetiology of calcific tendinitis is unknown. The deposition of calcium, the calcific stage, is not usually symptomatic. The resting period of the process ends with a resorptive phase that involves granulation tissue and scar formation with removal of the calcium deposits. By this time, the calcium has the consistency of toothpaste. The natural progression of the condition is for spontaneous resolution, with 85% of fluffy deposits and 33% of dense deposits disappearing in 3 years. The calcific deposits can be seen on plain radiographs, as well as ultrasound scan. They often cannot be seen on standard MRI scans.

Management is similar to subacromial impingement, although in the acute calcific phase, more aggressive interventions are usually beneficial for patients in severe pain, in the form of either a subacromial corticosteroid injection or arthroscopic washout and release of the calcific deposit.

Ultrasound-guided barbotage involves release of a deposit under tension (Figure 31.10), allowing the material, which is the consistency of cream cheese, to spurt out under tension in acute cases. Needling the deposit can give short- and long-term relief. It has been shown to be safe, minimally invasive, and better than non-intervention at one month and one year (Serafini et al. 2009). Extracoroporeal shock-wave therapy is popular in some parts of continental Europe, but less so in the UK. The aim is to focus acoustic energy to induce fragmentation of the calcific deposit and induce resorption. In a randomized control trial with sham treatment,

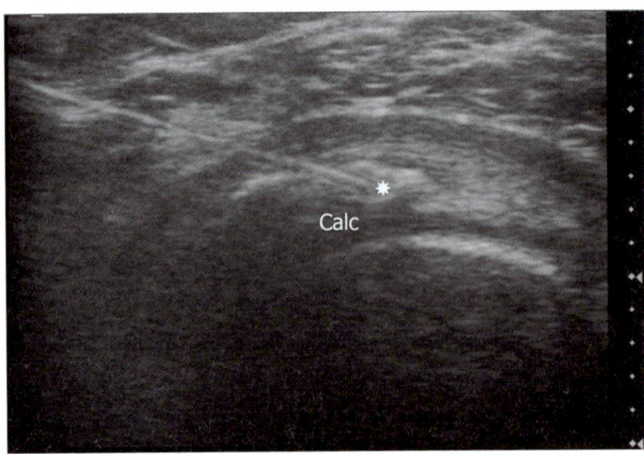

Figure 31.10 Ultrasound-guided barbotage of a calcific deposit. (With permission of shoulderdoc.co.uk)

Gerdesmeyer et al. (2003) demonstrated significantly better results at 3, 6, and 12 months.

Chronic pain in the presence of calcific deposits that has failed to respond to conservative measures may be treated surgically. The majority of surgeons focus on the calcific deposit, which can be identified with arthroscopy. The deposit can be decompressed and, to a variable extent, removed. Surgeons vary in their enthusiasm for the addition of a subacromial decompression. Success rates for surgical decompression are in the region of 92% by 6 months (Seil et al. 2006).

Frozen shoulder

Frozen shoulder, also known as adhesive capsulitis, is a painful restriction of active and passive shoulder movements (Nevaiser and Nevaiser 2011). Although a majority of patients presenting with frozen shoulder do not have an underlying cause (primary frozen shoulder), there is an increased incidence of this condition in patients with diabetes, Dupuytren's contracture, cardiac disease, and stroke. Secondary frozen shoulder can occur after trauma, surgery, or immobilization of the shoulder (Table 31.2).

Aetiology

The key patho-anatomical lesion seen in frozen shoulder is decreased joint volume. Various theories regarding the development of frozen shoulder have been proposed including muscular overactivity, autoimmune disease, abnormal glycosylation, scarring, low-grade infection, and tenosynovitis. The aetiology, pathophysiology, and management of this condition remain controversial (Hand et al. 2008; Nevaiser and Nevaiser 2011).

Table 31.2 Types of frozen shoulder

Primary: associations	Diabetes
	Dupuytren's contractures
	Pulmonary pathologies
	Thyroid pathologies
	Breast cancer
Secondary: associations	Post-traumatic
	Post-operative
	Post-immobilization

Diagnosis

The onset of primary frozen shoulder is typically spontaneous, although some patients may relate the onset of symptoms to a minor injury. Sudden onset, severe pain, particularly at night and aggravated by any movement of the shoulder, is a common presentation. Septic arthritis, acute calcific tendonitis, and neuralgic amyotrophy are the main differential diagnoses in the early stages (Table 31.3). Frozen shoulder is a diagnosis of exclusion. Along with suggestive clinical signs and symptoms, a normal radiograph is essential.

Natural history

Three classic phases of frozen shoulder have been described. In the first 'freezing' phase, the patient typically presents with pain and stiffness. This is gradually replaced by stiffness in the second 'frozen' phase. The third 'thawing' phase is characterized by a gradual improvement in the range of movements. Although frozen shoulder was traditionally thought to resolve spontaneously within 18 to 24 months (Miller et al. 1996), some patients experience continued symptoms for up to 7 years from the onset (Hand et al. 2007).

Treatment

Treatment is proportionate to the severity and duration of symptoms. The first-line treatment includes a combination of oral analgesia, physiotherapy, and glenohumeral joint corticosteroid injection (Nevaiser and Nevaiser 2011; Shin and Lee 2013).

Failure of the primary treatment requires more intervention in sufficiently symptomatic patients. The options are manipulation under anaesthetic (MUA), arthroscopic capsular release, and arthrographic distension (hydrodilatation).

Table 31.3 Differential diagnosis of non-traumatic acute onset shoulder pain

	Frozen shoulder	Septic arthritis	Calcific tendonitis	Neuralgic amyotrophy
X-rays	Normal	Soft tissue swelling	Calcium deposit in rotator cuff	Normal
Features	May have associations like diabetes	Fever, generally unwell, raised local temperature	Deltoid region pain	Neuropathic pain, weakness, and wasting of muscles
(b) Diagnosis	After exclusion	Joint aspirate	X-ray	EMG, NCV

1 MUA involves closed manipulation of the shoulder through a range of motion (Nevaiser and Nevaiser 2011). Although the risks are low, care needs to be exercised in osteoporotic bones.

2 Arthroscopic capsular release involves division of the contracted capsule, rotator interval, and glenohumeral ligaments under direct vision and has become very popular in modern shoulder practice due to the low risk of iatrogenic injury, with improved pain relief and function (Ogilvie-Harris et al. 1995).

3 Arthrographic distension of the glenohumeral joint involves injection of a large volume of saline and long-acting corticosteroid under radiographic guidance. This procedure is particularly appealing as it can be performed as an out-patient procedure, with low risk (Bell et al. 2003). It also has been shown to lead to a rapid improvement in pain and function within one week (Watson et al. 2007).

Treatment choice is usually based on severity of disease, patient's expectation, and surgeon preference.

Glenohumeral arthritis

Cartilage is annueral, alymphatic, and avascular. It forms a shock-absorbing and friction-free surface to joints, which enables smooth, pain-free motion. Arthritis of the glenohumeral joint occurs with progressive loss of articular cartilage. Arthritis is most commonly idiopathic but can be as a result of previous trauma or instability or as a result of altered biomechanics in the absence of a functioning rotator cuff.

The cause of idiopathic arthritis remains poorly understood but is related to fundamental changes in the fluid and biomechanical structure of the cartilage, which results in reduced structural properties. As the thickness of the cartilage reduces, the highly innervated and vascular subchondral bone becomes more exposed to the joint forces, which generates significant pain. The loss of joint lubrication leads to stiffness and crepitus. In response to the increased forces on the subchondral bone, the body produces increased bone surface area in the form of osteophytes.

Non-operative management

The goal of non-operative management is to control pain and maintain movement. Regular oral analgesia is the first-line treatment and should include paracetamol and progress to non-steroidal anti-inflammatory drugs. Physiotherapy may be useful to maintain muscle activity and rotator cuff strength while maximizing pain-free range of motion. If these measures fail, then injections may be beneficial. The two injection modalities are corticosteroids and hyaluronans. Hyaluronans have been shown to be safe and as effective as corticosteroids with potentially less side-effects, although they are significantly more expensive.

Surgical management

The role of surgical intervention should be based upon the patient's health, their symptoms, and their goals. In the physiologically young patient, the aim is to avoid arthroplasty for as long as practically possible. In these young patients, arthroscopic joint debridement accompanied with cartilage-stimulating procedures such as microfracture may provide short- to medium-term symptom relief. However, if symptoms persist, then joint replacement surgery may become inevitable.

Joint replacement or 'arthroplasty' involves replacing the affected joint surfaces, usually with a combination of metal and ultra-high molecular weight polyethylene. Hemiarthroplasty involves replacement of the humeral head only, while total shoulder replacement replaces both the humerus and the glenoid.

It is generally accepted that total shoulder replacement provides better short- to medium-term pain relief and function than hemiarthroplasty. However, loosening of the glenoid component is the leading cause of failure. Hemiarthroplasty, on the other hand, has no glenoid component to fail but may lead to ongoing glenoid pain and bony erosion. The balance of these features should be made on an individual patient basis. In the young patient, who has had no success with non-operative means, the failure rate of a glenoid component may be deemed too high and hemiarthroplasty, a better option.

Rotator cuff arthropathy

The specific form of arthritis that occurs in the presence of a massive rotator cuff tear is called rotator cuff arthropathy. The failure of the rotator cuff to control the pull of the deltoid causes the humeral head to translate superiorly and eventually articulate with the acromion.

Reverse geometry shoulder replacement (Figure 31.11) is often used to treat patients with significant pain and disability. In a reverse geometry shoulder replacement, the ball and the socket of the shoulder are reversed so that the ball is placed on the glenoid and the socket on the humeral side. This has the effect of preventing upward translation of the humerus so that the centre of rotation is maintained but also medialized. Thus, the lever arm of the deltoid is increased and therefore functions better. The results of reverse arthroplasty have been very encouraging and more predictable than hemiarthroplasty. However, the surgery is more challenging, the complication rates higher, and the long-term outcomes are not yet known.

Disorders of the acromioclavicular joint

The S-shaped nature of the clavicle converts large rotational movements at the sternoclavicular joint (SCJ) to smaller movements at the acromioclavicular joint (ACJ) in a similar manner to a 'crank-shaft'.

The stability of the ACJ is governed by both dynamic and static factors. The static restraint is formed by two principal sets of ligaments—the acromioclavicular (AC) and coracoclavicular (CC). During physiological movements (i.e. small displacements), the primary restraint of the ACJ is provided by the AC ligaments. With increasing displacement and force, the AC ligaments continue to provide the primary restraint to posterior translation but the CC ligaments, in particular the conoid, become the primary restraint to superior translation. The trapezoid is the primary restraint to compression. Dynamic stabilization of the ACJ joint is by the muscular insertions of the trapezius and the deltoid and the intervening deltopectoral fascia.

ACJ dislocations

Injuries to the ACJ represent approximately 40% of shoulder girdle injuries in sports. The most common mechanism is a fall onto the point of the shoulder.

The most commonly used classification system was described by Rockwood (Rockwood et al. 1998). This divides the injuries based

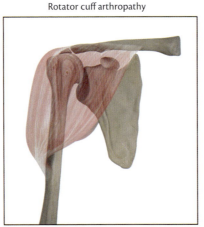

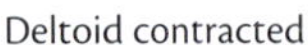

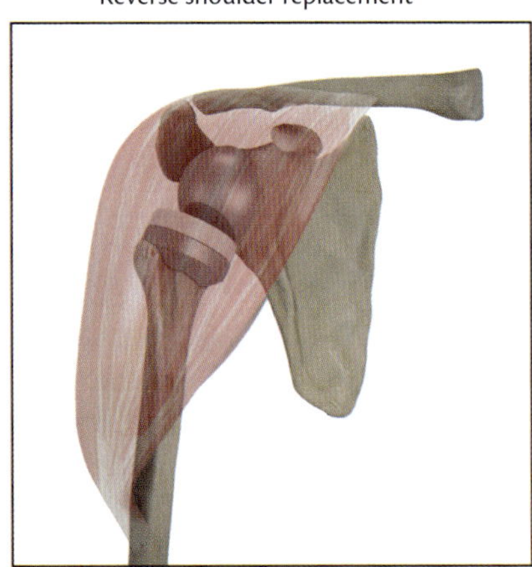

Figure 31.11 The effect of the reverse shoulder replacement in retensioning the deltoid and optimizing shoulder function in the absence of a rotator cuff. (With permission of shoulderdoc.co.uk)

upon the theoretical anatomical lesions and radiographic appearances (Figure 31.12). Types 1 and 2 are stable injuries; types 3–5 are unstable with a spectrum of ligamentous injury; type 6 is extremely rare. The intra and inter-observer reliability of the classification system is poor (Ng and Funk 2012).

Management of ACJ dislocations is very controversial. There is general agreement in the literature that types 1 and 2 injuries should be treated conservatively, and types 4 and 5 treated with surgical stabilization. The management of type 3 injuries remains a source of debate. Most management protocols are based upon the Rockwood classification but most scientific studies are fundamentally flawed due to its poor reliability.

In stable injuries (type 1 and 2), an initial period of rest in a sling may be required. This is then followed by a gradual return to sport as pain allows. Up to 25% of patients may have continual localized ACJ symptoms after 2 years and up to 50% may develop later osteoarthritis.

The literature has been unable to demonstrate the superiority of early surgical intervention over an initial trial of conservative measures for unstable injuries, especially the grade 3 injury. A metanalysis by Phillips et al. (1998) found that those patients treated non-operatively actually returned to pre-injury activities and sports earlier than the surgically treated group, although there was no standardization of surgical technique or non-surgical management

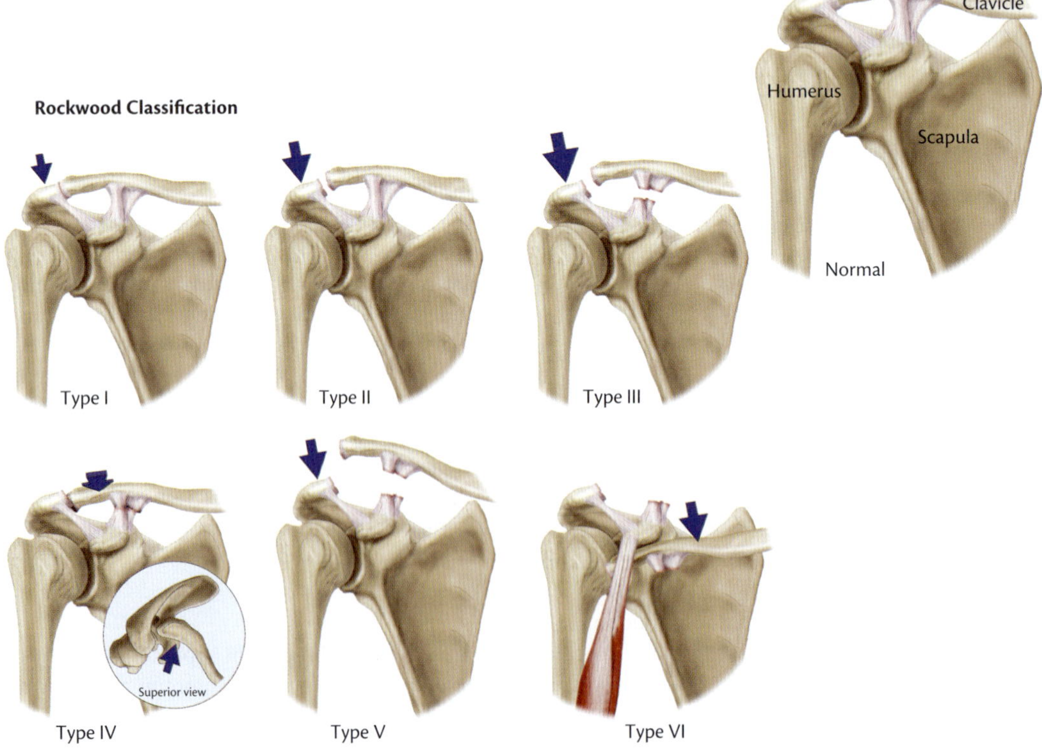

Figure 31.12 Rockwood classification. (With permission of shoulderdoc.co.uk)

regimes. Non-surgical management should incorporate a period of rehabilitation focusing on scapular stabilization exercises and rotator cuff control.

A proportion of patients will have persistent symptoms of instability and require late reconstruction. The symptoms range from mild fatigue discomfort to neurological compromise from brachial plexus traction. The impact of the cosmetic appearance should not be overlooked, particularly in young females.

Acute stabilization can be considered in overhead athletes with unstable injuries either with suture-button techniques or ligament reconstruction (in contact athletes). Late reconstruction is reserved for those patients who fail with conservative strategies and should be performed with a ligament reconstruction.

Distal clavicle osteolysis

Distal clavicle osteolysis (DCO) is a condition most commonly seen in weightlifters or similar heavy training regimes. Patients present with an insidious onset of pain well localized to the ACJ. It is exacerbated by training. There may be accompanying night pain, particularly when sleeping on the affected side.

The pathogenesis is believed to be as a result of repeated microfractures to the subchondral bone and subsequent attempts at repair. There is a osteoblastic reaction with associated synovial proliferation and inflammation. Radiographs will show subchondral reabsorption of the distal clavicle with cyst formation and joint widening. MRI will demonstrate peri-articular oedema.

Initial management is with rest followed by activity modification and a gradual return to sport. A local anaesthetic and steroid joint space injection can be considered both for diagnostic and therapeutic purposes. If non-operative measures fail, then surgery, in the form of distal clavicle excision, either open or arthroscopically, is indicated.

AC joint arthritis

Radiographic osteoarthritis of the ACJ is extremely common over 40 years of age. In most patients, it will remain asymptomatic. In a proportion of patients, the joint will become painful. Patients will present with an insidious onset of pain well localized to the ACJ. There will be tenderness over the joint. Provocative tests, such as cross-body adduction ('scarf' test) will be positive. Radiographs should include an anteroposterior (AP) and oblique at 15–30° cephalad which will enable visualization of the ACJ without the overlap of the scapula spine.

Management is very similar to DCO, with initial conservative treatment followed by ACJ excision in resistant cases.

Clavicle fractures

Fractures of the clavicle are common and represent 2–5% of all adult fractures. These usually result from falls onto the shoulder or onto the outstretched hand (Postacchini et al. 2002).

Clavicle fractures are divided into thirds, depending on the location of the fracture. Fractures of the middle third of the clavicle are most common. The degree of displacement commonly reflects the energy of injury causing the fracture with comminuted and widely displaced fractures representing high energy and significant soft tissue damage associated with these injuries.

AP radiographs are usually sufficient to diagnose clavicle fractures, although a 30° cephalad view is superior in demonstrating displacement of fracture fragments.

The majority of middle third clavicle fractures can be managed non-operatively. Non- operative treatment involves rest in a sling and analgesia. Early operative fixation should be considered in the following circumstances (Martetschlager et al. 2013):

1. Clavicle shortening >15–20 mm
2. Female gender
3. Fracture communion
4. Significant fracture displacement
5. Older age
6. Severe initial trauma
7. Unstable lateral fractures
8. Bony spikes jeopardizing the overlying skin
9. Open fractures

Operative stabilization of clavicle fractures aids early return to sports and work and is a relative indication for early operative fixation in athletes, professional riders, and manual workers. Operative fixation of clavicle fractures is performed either using plating devices applied on the surface of the clavicle (Martetschlager et al. 2013) or intramedullary devices. Choice of implant is primarily driven by fracture configuration and surgeon preference. Although uncommon, patients need to be warned about a tender scar, prominent metalwork requiring removal following fracture healing, metalwork breakage, non-union, and delayed union.

Proximal humeral fractures

The majority of proximal humeral fractures are low-energy and associated with osteoporosis. The frequency therefore increases significantly with age and females are affected approximately three times more frequently than men. Fractures in the younger age group are associated with higher- energy mechanisms of injury.

All fractures can be associated with dislocations of the humeral head. All of the parts become progressively comminuted with increasing energy. Of particular importance is intra-articular extension, which is referred to as a 'head-splitting' fracture.

Treatment

Over 80% can be managed non-operatively. A collar and cuff sling provides a longitudinal traction to the shoulder, which utilizes the principle of ligamentotaxis to help reduce the fracture. Surgery is indicated in the presence of a dislocation or intra-articular extension and relatively indicated with increasing displacement of the fracture parts.

The aim of intervention is to improve the alignment of the fracture, in particular the orientation of the head fragment and the position of the tuberosities such that the sequelae of malunion are avoided. However, surgery has complications and decisions are made on an individual basis determined by the fracture configuration, the patient's comorbidities, and functional expectations.

Surgical options are either open reduction and internal fixation with plate and screws, minimally invasive and percutaneous fixation, or intramedullary fixation. The most common technique for fracture fixation over recent years is with the fixed angle, anatomical locking plates. These implants are more stable in osteoporotic bone and have improved the management of proximal humeral fractures. However, complication rates as high as 36% have been reported, particularly in elderly patients. This has led some surgeons to favour more minimally invasive techniques which, may have less iatrogenic soft tissue disturbance, such as percutaneous pin fixation or intramedullary fixation. However, these techniques can be more challenging and provide less stability. The current scientific base is unable to support one technique at present.

If the bone quality is deemed too poor for fixation or the risk of avascular necrosis (AVN) is high, then arthroplasty should be considered instead of fixation. The principle of arthroplasty is to replace the humeral head as a hemiarthroplasty and fix the tuberosities around the prosthesis. The results of the procedure are directly related to the rates of healing of the tuberosity fragments and, hence, the function of the rotator cuff, which is unpredicatable. A recent development is to use the reverse geometry shoulder replacement. This has the theoretical advantage of leading to a more predictable level of function in the absence of a rotator cuff but is more technically challenging and has a higher complication rate. Early studies are encouraging but are not sufficient, as yet, to fully endorse the technique as the medium- and long-term results are unknown.

Scapula fractures

Fractures of the scapula are uncommon and are usually a result of a relatively high-energy injury. Motor vehicle traffic accidents, along with a fall from height, are the most frequent causes. Scapula fractures are hence associated with other injuries in 85–90% of cases (Table 31.4). Management of such patients is initially based on the Advanced Trauma Life Support® (ATLS®) guidelines, with priority given to life-threatening associated injuries. It is hence not uncommon that there is a delay in diagnosis and definitive management of scapular fractures.

The standard trauma series for shoulder injury includes an AP, lateral, and axillary view of the shoulder. A CT scan is the preferred definitive investigation, which provides delineation of three-dimensional anatomy and aids decision making.

Management of scapula fractures is mostly non-operative, although operative fixation is recommended for the following fracture patterns:

- Displaced fractures of the glenoid articular surface
- Glenoid neck fractures with medial displacement of the glenoid of more than 1cm or angulation of more than 40° (Ada and Miller 1991)

Principles of operative fixation are anatomical reduction of articular fragments, early mobilization, stable fixation, and optimal soft tissue care. Good to excellent functional results can be expected in approximately 85% of cases following surgery, at an average follow-up of over 4 years (Lantry et al. 2008).

Table 31.4 Injuries associated with scapula fractures

1.	Rib fractures
2.	Pulmonary injuries
3.	Humeral fractures
4.	Brachial plexus injuries
5.	Head injury
6.	Vascular injuries
7.	Splenic injuries

References

Ada JR, Miller ME. Scapular fractures. Analysis of 113 cases. *Clin Orthop Relat Res* 1991; 269:174–80.

Andrews JR, Carson WG Jr, McLeod WD. Glenoid labrum tears related to the long head of the biceps. *Am J Sports Med* 1985; 13:337–41.

Beighton PH, Solomon L, Soskolne CL. Articular mobility in an African population. *Ann Rheum Dis* 1973; 32(5):413.

Bell S, Coghlan J, Richardson M. Hydro dilatation in the management of shoulder capsulitis. *Australas Radiol* 2003; 47:247–51.

Braun S, Horan MP, Elser F, Millett PJ. Lesions of the biceps pulley. *Am J Sports Med* 2011; 39:790–5.

Buck FM, Dietrich TJ, Resnick D, Jost B, Pfirrmann CW. Long biceps tendon: normal position, shape, and orientation in its groove on neutral position and external and internal rotation. *Radiology* 2011; 261:872–81.

Burkhart SS, et al. Results of modified Latarjet reconstruction in patients with anteroinferior instability and significant bone loss. *Arthroscopy* 2007; 23(10):1033–41.

Cooper DE, Arnoczky SP, O'Brien SJ, Warren RF, DiCarlo E, Allen AA. Anatomy, histology, and vascularity of the glenoid labrum: an anatomical study. *J Bone Joint Surg Am* 1992; 74:46–52.

D'Alessandro DF, Fleischli JE, Connor PM. Superior labral lesions: diagnosis and management. *J Athlet Train* 2000; 35 (3):286–92.

Frost A, Zafar MS, Mafulli N. Tenotomy versus tenodesis in the management of pathologic lesions of the tendon of the long head of the biceps brachii. *Am J Sports Med* 2009; 37:828–33.

Gerber, C and Ganz, R. Clinical assessment of instability of the shoulder. With special reference to anterior and posterior drawer tests. Journal of Bone & Joint Surgery, British Volume 66.4 (1984); 551–556.

Gerdesmeyer L, et al. Extracorporeal shock wave therapy for the treatment of chronic calcifying tendonitis of the rotator cuff. *JAMA* 2003; 290(19):2573–80.

Hand GC, Athanasou NA, Matthews T, Carr AJ. The pathology of frozen shoulder. *J Bone J Surg* 2007; 89:928–32.

Hand C, Clipsham K, Rees JL, Carr AJ. Long term outcome of frozen shoulder. *J Shoulder Elbow Surg* 2008; 17:231–6.

Karpman RR, McComb JE, Volz RG. Tendon rupture following local steroid injection: report of four cases. *Postgrad Med* 1980; 68:169–74.

Kralinger FS, et al. Predicting recurrence after primary anterior shoulder dislocation. *Am J Sports Med* 2002; 30(1):116–20.

Lantry JM, Roberts CS, Giannoudis PV. Operative treatment of scapular fractures: a systematic review. *Injury* 2008; 39:271–83.

Lewis A, Kitamura T, Bayley J. The classification of shoulder instability: new light through old windows! *Curr Orthop* 2004; 18(2):97–108.

Longo UG, Loppini M, Marineo G, Khan WS, Maffulli N, Denaro V. Tendinopathy of the tendon of the long head of the biceps. *Sports Med Arthrosc* 2011; 19:321–2.

Martetschlager F, Gaskill TR, Millett PJ. Management of clavicle nonunion and malunion. *J Shoulder Elbow Surg* 2013; 22:862–8.

Michener LA, Doukas WC, Murphy KP, Walsworth MK. Diagnostic accuracy of history and physical examination of superior labrum anterior-posterior lesions. *J Athlet Train* 2011; 46:343–8.

Miller MD, Wirth MA, Rockwood CA Jr. Thawing the frozen shoulder: the 'patient' patient. *Orthopaedics* 1996; 19:849–53.

Nakata W, Katou S, Fujita A, Nakata M, Lefor AT, Sugimoto H. Biceps pulley: normal anatomy and associated lesions at MR arthrography. *Radiographics* 2011; 31:791–810.

Neer II CS. Anterior acromioplasty for the chronic impingement syndrome in the shoulder. A preliminary report. *J Bone J Surg (Am vol)* 1972; 54(1):41–50.

Nevaiser AS, Nevaiser RJ. Adhesive capsulitis of the shoulder. *J Am Acad Orthop Surg* 2011; 19:536–42.

Ng CY, Funk L. Symptomatic chronic long head of biceps rupture: surgical results. *Int J Shoulder Surg* 2012; 6:108–11.

Ng CY, Smith EK, Funk L. Reliability of the traditional classification systems for acromioclavicular joint injuries by radiography. *Shoulder & Elbow* 2012; 4(4):266–9.

Ogilvie-Harris DJ, Biggs DJ, Fitsialos DP, MacKay M. The resistant frozen shoulder. Manipulation versus arthroscopic release. *Clin Orthop Relat Res* 1995; 315:238–48.

Phillips AM, Smart C, Groom AF. Acromioclavicular dislocation. Conservative or surgical therapy. *Clin Orthop Relat Res* 1998; 353:10–17.

Postacchini F, Gumina S, De Santis P, Albo F. Epidemiology of clavicle fractures. *J Shoulder Elbow Surg* 2002; 11:452–6.

Rockwood CA, Williams GR, Young DC. Disorders of the acromioclavicular joint. *Shoulder* 1998; 1:413–76.

Seil R, et al. Arthroscopic treatment of chronically painful calcifying tendinitis of the supraspinatus tendon. *Arthroscopy* 2006; 22(5):521–7.

Serafini G, et al. Rotator cuff calcific tendonitis: short-term and 10-year outcomes after two-needle US-guided percutaneous treatment—nonrandomized controlled trial. *Radiology* 2009; 252(1):157–64.

Sher JS, et al. 1995. Abnormal findings on magnetic resonance images of asymptomatic shoulders. *J Bone J Surg (Am vol)* 1995; 77(1):10–15.

Shin SJ, Lee SY. Efficacies of corticosteroid injection at different sites of the shoulder for the treatment of adhesive capsulitis. *J Shoulder Elbow Surg* 2013; 22:521–7.

Snyder SJ, Karzel RP, Del Pizzo W, Ferkel RD, Friedman MJ. SLAP lesions of the shoulder. *Arthroscopy* 1990; 6:274–9.

Watson I, Bialocerkowski A, Dalziel R, Balster S, Burke F, Finch C. Hydrodilatation (distension arthrography): a long-term clinical outcome series. *Br J Sports Med* 2007; 41:167–73.

Chapter 32

Rehabilitation strategies—shoulder disorders

Jo Gibson, Anju Jaggi, and Julia Walton

Introduction to rehabilitation strategies for shoulder disorders

Rehabilitation is commonly the first line of management for shoulder pain and is consistently shown to be superior to placebo interventions. Current evidence supports the use of exercise prescription in the management of many common shoulder conditions. However, there continues to be a lack of consensus as to the specific content and emphasis of exercise interventions. In addition, there is continued controversy as to whether or not the addition of manual therapy techniques to exercise results in superior outcomes. An increased appreciation of the effect of pathology on motor control and dynamic stability of the shoulder complex has been instrumental in guiding popular exercise approaches. However, advances in our understanding of the pathophysiology of common shoulder conditions suggest that strategies to modify pain and address movement restriction should be addressed in conjunction with motor control retraining.

Principles of shoulder rehabilitation

Restriction

While much of the emphasis of current interventions is on exercise prescription, it is important to consider the role of restrictive processes when designing rehabilitation programmes. Restriction within the capsuloligamentous complex potentially impairs the ability of the dynamic stabilizers to perform their role efficiently. Similarly, attempts at rehabilitating function in the dynamic stabilizers without regaining adequate capsuloligamentous flexibility have been shown to result in exacerbation or production of pain. Currently, there is a lack of evidence to suggest which mobilization strategies are most effective. While some authors report no additional benefit of glenohumeral joint mobilization techniques to exercise alone in the management of common shoulder pathologies, their studies commonly include patient populations with minimal movement restriction.

Segmental restrictions in both the thoracic and cervical spine have been shown to negatively impact recruitment patterns in the upper quadrant musculature. Similarly, cervical spine segmental stiffness has been shown to result in reduced pain pressure thresholds and increased muscle stiffness in the shoulder musculature (Mintken et al. 2010). Manual therapy mobilization techniques aimed at the thoracic spine have been shown to optimize recruitment patterns of the scapulothoracic musculature and enhance rehabilitation outcomes (Walser et al. 2009). In addition, specific mobilization techniques (lateral glides, Figure 32.1) addressed to C5, 6 in the cervical spine result in short-term strength gains of the rotator cuff and have a neuro-modulatory effect which leads to reduced pain sensitivity. Authors consistently demonstrate that mobilization techniques aimed at the thoracic and cervical spine (in patients without cervical or thoracic symptomology) augment the outcome of exercise interventions in shoulder rehabilitation (Mintken et al. 2010; Walser et al. 2009).

Scapula

The scapula has been a focus of rehabilitation strategies and exercise interventions in shoulder pathology. Clearly, it is an essential link between the trunk and the arm and is purported to provide a stable base for upper limb function. There continues to be a lack of consensus as to how best to classify scapula kinematics, however; alterations in activation patterns and muscle performance of the scapula muscles are a consistent feature of shoulder pathology (Kibler et al. 2013). This 'scapula dyskinesis' creates an unstable base for upper limb movement and therefore potentially increases loads across the glenohumeral joint during upper-limb activities. It is of note that overload and associated fatigue have been identified as key factors in rotator cuff tendinopathy and impingement-related pathologies. However, increasingly, evidence would suggest that scapula dyskinesis is commonly a secondary rather than a primary feature. Scapula dysfunction can result from a multitude of factors such as postural alignment, capsular restriction, muscle weakness and fatigue, alterations in anatomy/biomechanics, and motor control deficits.

Consequently, clinicians must consider and thoroughly assess potential contributing factors. While there is continued debate as to whether scapula dyskinesis is a primary or secondary feature of pathology, its improvement as a result of exercise interventions has been shown to correlate with symptom resolution (Timmons et al. 2012).

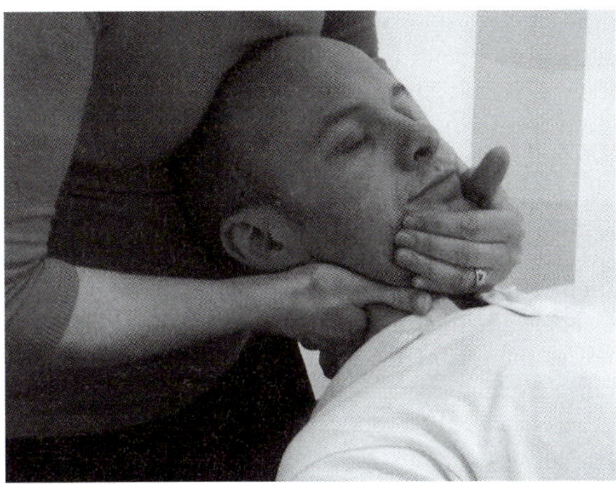

Figure 32.1 Lateral glide mobilization technique.

Rotator cuff

The rotator cuff muscles play a central role in the dynamic stability of the glenohumeral joint and have two key aspects. Firstly, a pre-setting action where they co-activate to stabilize the humeral head prior to movement. Secondly, they control the axis of rotation during movement with a direction-specific activation bias dependent on the plane and direction of movement. The rotator cuff muscles therefore control translation of the humeral head, keeping it relatively centred on the glenoid. This coordinated action counteracts the torque-producing forces of prime mover muscles such as the latissimus dorsi and pectoralis major.

Current evidence would suggest that the pre-setting function is essentially deficient in common shoulder pathologies (David et al. 2000). Similarly, a loss of translational control has been well described in patients with rotator cuff tears, impingement, and instability. This potentially results in increased tensile and shear forces across the glenohumeral joint. The consequential loss of dynamic control is manifested in common compensatory patterns where inhibition of the rotator cuff results in increased activation of the prime movers of the shoulder complex. Rehabilitation strategies should therefore consider these key functions of the rotator cuff and incorporate exercises to re-educate them.

Kinetic chain

The consequence of motor control deficits impacting the shoulder complex should also be considered in terms of the kinetic chain. The kinetic chain depicts the body as a linked system of interdependent segments, working in a proximal to distal sequence, imparting a desired action at the distal segment. Researchers have demonstrated that there is a coordinated pattern of muscle activation and force development from the legs to the arms as unilateral arm movements are initiated. This illustrates the contribution of the whole body during upper limb activity (McMullen 2000). Essentially, the shoulder is a funnel for force transmission from the lower limbs and trunk to the arm. Authors propose that deficits in the kinetic chain resulting in deficient proximal activation can increase the loads at the shoulder and, as a result, create acute or chronic stresses that may cause injury or decreased performance.

Increasingly, the effects of the kinetic chain and poor movement patterns are recognized as key factors in shoulder pathology. Kinetic chain rehabilitation approaches the shoulder as part of a kinetic link system in which proximal segments will impact movement and muscle recruitment. The dynamic nature of such exercises triggers sequential activation through the kinetic chain and allows patients to perform corrective movement strategies more easily (McMullen 2000). In addition, by increasing the functional specificity of kinetic chain exercises for an individual patient, their motor learning potential is enhanced. Assessment and rehabilitation of the patient with shoulder pathology should therefore include evaluation and inclusion of the shoulder, trunk, and lower quadrant.

Rehabilitation for subacromial pain and the rotator cuff

Disorders of the rotator cuff account for up to 70% of all shoulder pain presenting in primary care. Our increased understanding of both the multifactorial nature and pathophysiology of tendon pathology illustrates the challenges of both diagnosis and intervention. Rotator cuff tendon pathology has been attributed to both extrinsic and intrinsic mechanisms (Seitz et al. 2011). Extrinsic factors, including postural abnormalities, rotator cuff and scapular muscle performance deficits, and decreased extensibility of soft tissues around the shoulder girdle, have been postulated to compromise the subacromial space and its contents. Similarly, intrinsic factors relating to alterations in tendon biology, mechanical properties, morphology, and vascularity have been purported to contribute to rotator cuff tendon degradation (Seitz et al. 2011).

Subacromial impingement syndrome (SAIS) is a popular clinical diagnosis that encompasses several patho-anatomical processes and is used to describe a broad spectrum of symptomology. Authors argue that the adoption of a clinical diagnosis of 'subacromial pain syndrome' would better reflect the multifactorial nature of this condition. Clearly then, rotator cuff tendon pathology is not a homogenous entity and rehabilitation interventions attempting to employ a rigid standardized exercise programme fail to reflect this. However, in higher-level trials reporting successful rehabilitation of subacromial pain, rotator cuff tendinopathy, and chronic cuff tears, there are clear commonalities in the principles of rehabilitation interventions; postural correction and motor control retraining, stretching, strengthening of the rotator cuff and scapula muscles, and manual therapy (Kuhn 2009). In addition, there is a general consensus that, other than in the case of an acute rotator cuff tear in a physiologically young patient (who will get the best outcome from early surgical intervention), all patients with rotator cuff pathology should have a period of conservative management as their first-line treatment for a minimum of 6 weeks (Kuhn 2009). Indeed, studies comparing different exercise programmes with surgery in patients with subacromial impingement syndrome have concluded that the two have equivalent outcomes at one year (Lewis 2012).

Rehabilitation priorities for subacromial impingement syndrome

Pain

Pain and functional limitation are commonly the predominant features that cause patients to seek treatment. The complexity of pain-generating mechanisms can provide a challenge for the clinician and it is important to differentiate between peripheral and central sensitization when considering treatment options (Dean et al. 2013).

In SAIS patients with constant background pain, difficulty sleeping, and worsening pain on movement, subacromial injection can be very successful in addressing pain in the short term and facilitating rehabilitation input (Lewis 2010). The outcome of injection in patients not fulfilling these criteria is less predictable. Manual therapy techniques directed to the cervical spine (see Figure 32.1) have been shown to increase pain pressure thresholds and increase pain-free range of shoulder movement in patients with shoulder pain. They can be an extremely useful adjunct to treatment and have been shown to accelerate responsiveness to exercise (Mintken et al. 2010). While electrophysical agents such as interferential, transcutaneous electrical nerve stimulation (TENS), and shockwave therapy are purported to offer a solution for pain relief, currently there is a lack of high-level evidence to support their use specifically for pain relief in patients with rotator cuff pathology.

Restriction

A thorough assessment of the patient should precede any rehabilitation intervention incorporating all the key areas discussed. Before commencing exercises that address motor control and muscle performance, it is essential to identify any restrictive process that may impact the ability of the dynamic stabilizers to perform their role. Evaluation of rotational range of the glenohumeral joint throughout available elevation will enable the clinician to target the specific region of the capsular complex, which is tight. Generic stretches such as the sleeper stretch and cross-body adduction are common inclusions in treatment regimens (Ellenbecker and Cools 2010). However, it is important to ensure that stretches reflect the area of the capsuloligamentous complex that is actually tight, to ensure their efficacy.

Segmental restriction in the cervical and thoracic spine will potentially impact the ability of the dynamic stabilizers to be optimally recruited. Therefore, assessment should include evaluation of these areas. The addition of mobilization of the cervical spine to an exercise intervention in patients with SAIS results in quicker resolution of symptoms. Similarly, mobilization of the thoracic spine enhances recruitment of the scapula stabilizers. Techniques targeted to the cervical and thoracic spine potentially set the system up for success in terms of muscle performance and increased pain pressure thresholds.

Postural correction and motor control retraining

Postural alterations associated with a forward head posture alter scapular kinematics and muscle activity during upper limb activity (Timmons et al. 2012). Similarly, thoracic kyphosis negatively impacts recruitment of the scapula stabilizers and orientation of the scapula. Consequently, any rehabilitation programme should commence with education of the patient regarding the impact of movement and posture on the structures of the shoulder joint and basic cues regarding more efficient postural alignment and movement strategies.

Patients with SAIS and rotator cuff pathology demonstrate common alterations in scapular kinematics characterized by changes in muscle activation patterns. This lack of optimal muscle control is believed to contribute to a reduction of posterior tilt and upward rotation of the scapula during arm elevation (Ellenbecker and Cools 2010). In addition, inhibition of the infraspinatus and inadequate co-activation of the scapulohumeral muscles result in a lack of translation control of the humeral head on the glenoid (Ellenbecker and Cools 2010). Exercise selection should therefore aim to address these deficits. Closed kinetic chain exercises are a very effective tool to facilitate the co-activation role of the rotator cuff (Figure 32.2). However, exercises such as the wall slide, that both encourage weightbearing and active supported movement, achieve both co-activation of the rotator cuff and improvement in muscle activation patterns through range (Figure 32.3).

The simple addition of a low-resistance elastic band or tubing emphasizes the role of the posterior rotator cuff through elevation range. Weightbearing on a surface and the use of an elastic band also enhance the proprioceptive value of these exercises. It is important to emphasize short to long lever elevation in the first instance. The inability of the rotator cuff to cope with load is a feature of cuff-related pathology and clearly by reducing the lever arm during elevation, the rotator cuff is put in a position where it is

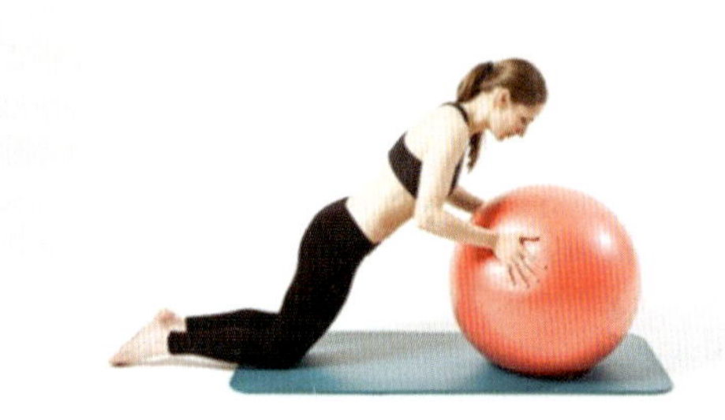

Figure 32.2 Closed kinetic chain exercise. (With permission of shoulderdoc.co.uk)

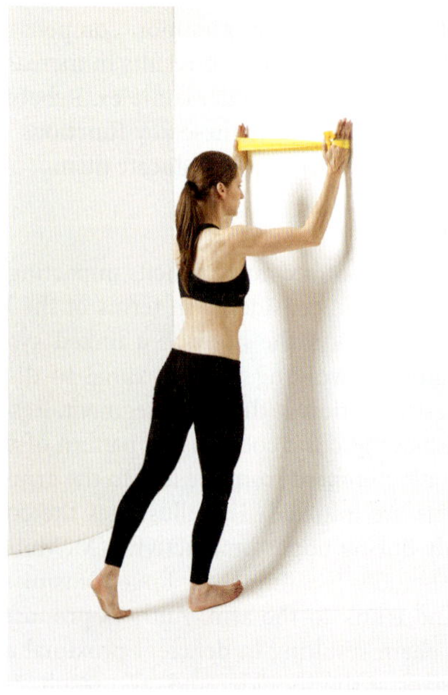

Figure 32.3a Initiation of the wall slide exercise. (With permission of shoulderdoc.co.uk)

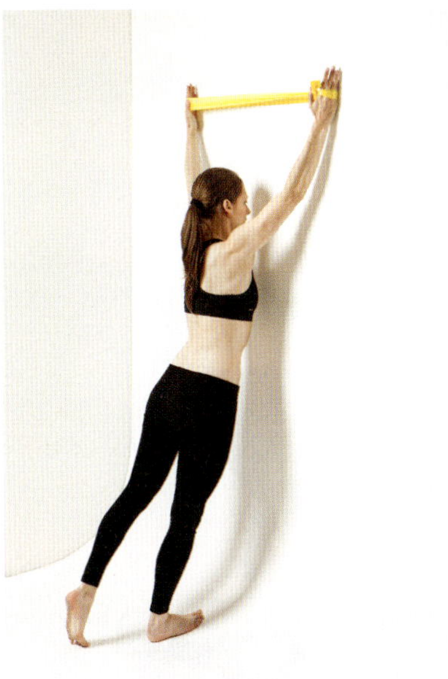

Figure 32.3b Wall slide exercise. (With permission of shoulderdoc.co.uk)

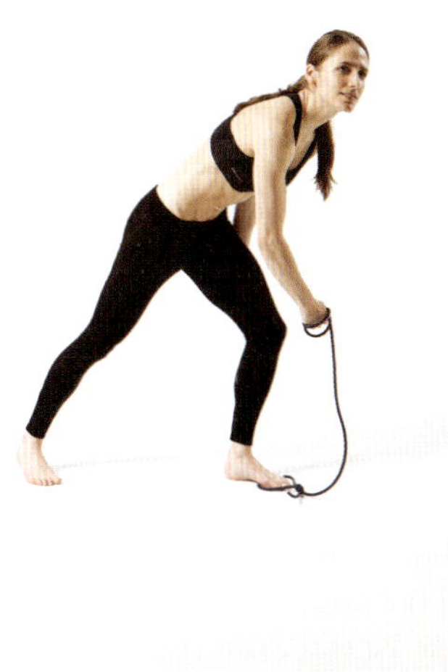

Figure 32.4b 'Robbery' exercise activates key scapular stability muscles. (With permission of shoulderdoc.co.uk)

more able to perform its stability role. Addition of the kinetic chain, using a simple step forward to initiate the wall slide, reinforces the contribution of the rest of the body in function and often makes it easier for the patient to perform the exercise. Exercises such as the 'lawnmower' and 'robbery' exercises (Kibler and Sciascia 2010) also activate the key scapular stability muscles without creating high demands on the glenohumeral joint, making them a useful adjunct in the early stages of rehabilitation. These types of exercises utilize the principles of proprioceptive neuromuscular facilitation in an effort to increase their motor learning potential (Figure 32.4.)

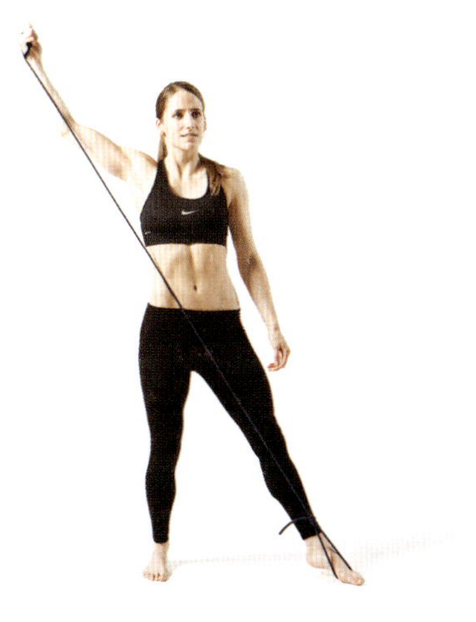

Figure 32.4a 'Lawnmover' exercise activates key scapular stability muscles. (With permission of shoulderdoc.co.uk)

Simple exercises where the patient is encouraged to consciously correct the scapula while performing arm elevation will also impact muscle activation patterns. Patients can be taught to reproduce movements of the scapula into posterior tilt and upward rotation and reliably perform this as a home exercise. It is of note that motor control retraining exercises in isolation have been shown to reduce pain, improve function, and improve posterior tilt/upward rotation of the scapula (Kibler et al. 2013). Furthermore, it is the change in activation patterns of the dynamic stabilizers that most convincingly correlates with pain reduction and functional improvement (Ellenbecker and Cools 2010; Kibler et al. 2013). As a result, there is much debate as to whether rehabilitation should just target motor control retraining or emphasize strengthening of the rotator cuff and scapula musculature. However, in view of what is understood regarding the pathophysiology of rotator cuff pathology, it is important to rehabilitate the dynamic system to cope with the functional load specific to the individual patient. While it is true that motor control retraining alone is effective in symptom reduction, there is a lack of long-term follow-up data to indicate how this may impact recurrence when patients return to full function.

Strengthening

Strengthening exercises are a feature of many rotator cuff rehabilitation regimens. Certainly, current literature consistently reports weakness in the infraspinatus and supraspinatus and the scapula stabilizers in patients with rotator cuff pathology (Lewis 2010, 2012; Seitz et al. 2011). However, it is important to recognize that 'weakness' can result from the lack of dynamic stability inherent to this patient group rather than a true muscle weakness. Undoubtedly, once motor control retraining has been instigated, pain reduced, and muscle activation patterns optimized, there is a significant increase in strength. The key consideration is the functional demands of the individual patient and whether the dynamic system has the functional strength to cope in these situations.

When introducing strengthening exercises, it is important that the patient is able to maintain good control as inappropriate loading that exceeds the stability capability of the upper quadrant is likely to result in overload and the risk of pain recurrence. There is some controversy as to whether pain should be allowed during the performance of strengthening exercises. However, given that we understand that pain inhibits the stability function of the rotator cuff and that comparable outcomes are achieved irrespective of pain production, we would suggest that those exercises that do not provoke pain are preferable. It is of note that, currently, the addition of eccentric exercises to traditional interventions does not result in superior outcomes in pain and function.

There is continued controversy as to whether local muscle-specific exercises or those that incorporate the rotator cuff, scapula, and kinetic chain together are preferable. In reality, it is a question of which exercise works best for an individual patient, as currently there is no robust evidence to suggest which option is superior. However, commonly employed exercises for isolating the posterior rotator cuff and the scapula upward rotators can easily be incorporated within the kinetic chain (Figure 32.5). The theoretical advantage of this approach is that by effectively engaging the kinetic chain, the sensorimotor and motor learning value of the exercises is enhanced (Farina and Falla 2010). The key aim is to achieve functional strength of the rotator cuff and scapula muscles through the full range of shoulder movement.

It is of note that the optimal parameters of exercise have yet to be determined and there is a wide variation of recommendations in the literature (Kuhn 2009). Clinicians should be clear about what they are trying to achieve for an individual patient; range of movement, motor control, fatigue resistance, and strength require very different advice in terms of repetition numbers and frequency of performance. Range of movement exercises will benefit from being performed on a daily basis and motor control exercises require frequent repetition, ideally several times a day (Kuhn 2009). However, strength and endurance training are most effectively achieved with regimes that advocate three sessions per week (Ellenbecker and Cools 2010; Kuhn 2009). Prescription dosage must also reflect the individual abilities of the patient.

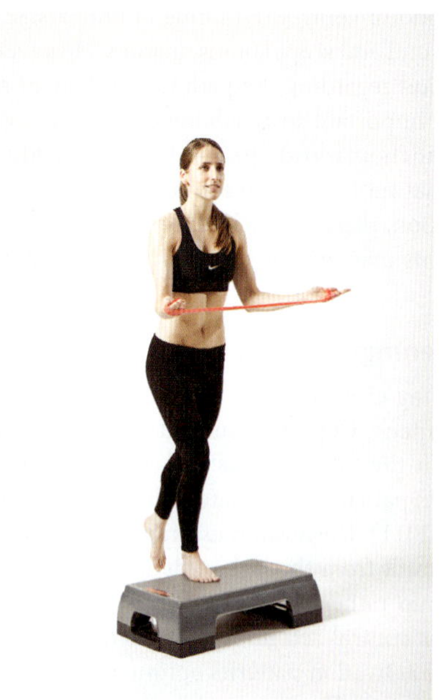

Figure 32.5a Exercise for isolating the posterior rotator cuff and the scapula upward rotation. (With permission of shoulderdoc.co.uk)

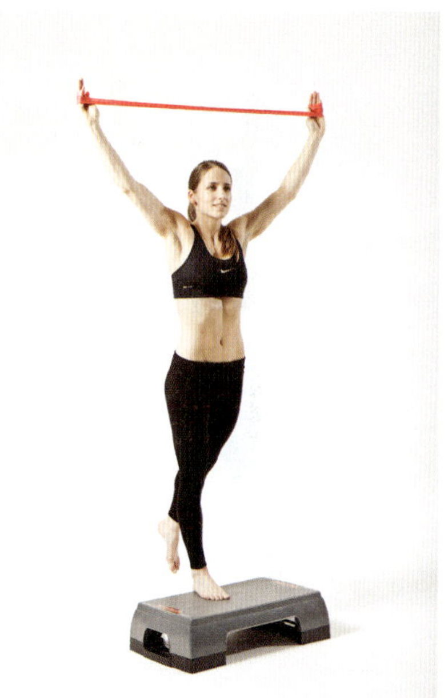

Figure 32.5b Exercise for isolating the posterior rotator cuff and the scapula upward rotation. (With permission of shoulderdoc.co.uk)

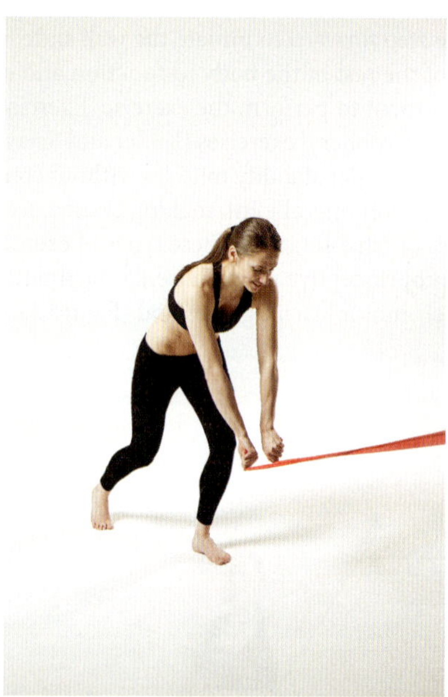

Figure 32.5c Exercise for isolating the posterior rotator cuff and the scapula upward rotation. (With permission of shoulderdoc.co.uk)

Successful rehabilitation interventions report effectiveness at reducing pain and improving function in 6 to 12 weeks. Crucially, if patients with rotator cuff pathology (without stiffness) have failed to show any improvement within 6 weeks, they are unlikely to respond.

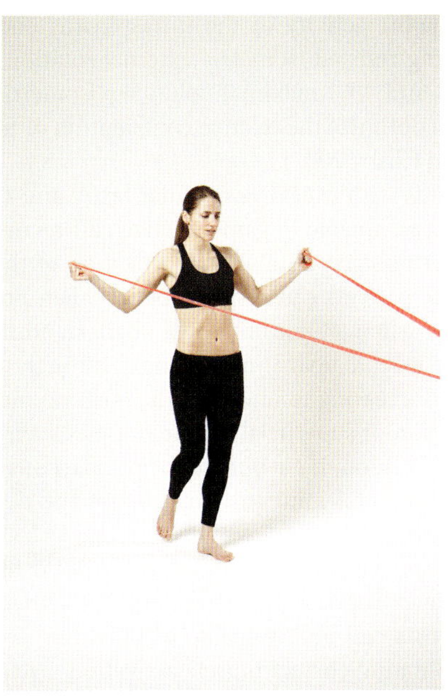

Figure 32.5d Exercise for isolating the posterior rotator cuff and the scapula upward rotation. (With permission of shoulderdoc.co.uk)

Summary

Rotator cuff pathology is multifactorial and dictates a thorough assessment of range of movement, motor control, and individual muscle performance deficits.

There is clear evidence that exercise has a significant effect on pain reduction and improving function in patients with rotator cuff pathology. In the presence of glenohumeral stiffness or stiffness in the cervical or thoracic spine, appropriately directed manual therapy augments the outcome of rehabilitation interventions. Glenohumeral and scapula motor control abnormalities and strength deficits in the scapulohumeral and scapulothoracic muscles are common features of shoulder disability in patients with rotator cuff pathology. Consequently, rehabilitation programmes should incorporate supervised motor control exercise movements and functionally relevant strengthening exercises specific to the rotator cuff and scapula stabilizers.

Rehabilitation for shoulder instability

The shoulder is inherently the most mobile joint in the body, hence why it is the most commonly dislocated. 96% of dislocations are related to a traumatic injury, with anterior dislocation accounting for 97% of these (Kroner et al. 1989); 2–10% of dislocations are posterior, and are often atraumatic; bi-directional (postero-inferior) and multi-directional (posterior, anterior, and inferior) instability are far more common than unidirectional in this cohort (Tannenbaum and Sekiya 2011). There is a fine balance between the structural stability provided by the capsule-labral skeletal complex and the dynamic stability provided through muscular tone and notably the rotator cuff. Disruption or abnormal function of either of these components will result in instability.

Management should therefore be based on the degree of trauma, ease at which symptoms of instability occur, degree of structural damage, and abnormal muscle recruitment.

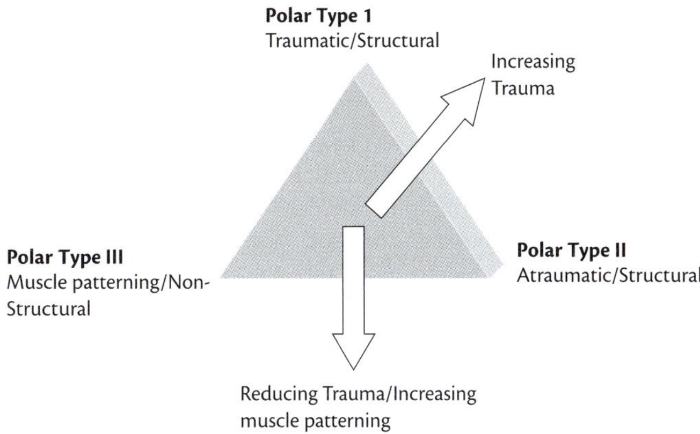

Figure 32.6 Stanmore classification system for shoulder instability. (From Lewis et al. 2004)

The Stanmore classification system recognizes a continuum and coexistence of pathologies which can occur. This can be graphically displayed as a triangle (Jaggi and Lambert 2010) (Figure 32.6). The polar pathologies are labelled Type I (traumatic instability), Type II (atraumatic instability), and Type III (neurological dysfunctional or muscle patterning). The groups are distinguished by an accurate history and clinical examination. Increased trauma and evidence of structural damage indicates a Type I instability and is most likely to require surgical repair for structural insufficiency. Minor damage and muscular weakness (Type II) requires attention to improving function within the rotator cuff and/or repair of minor damage. No structural damage and obvious clinical signs of abnormal muscle activation (Type III) is unlikely to benefit from surgery and there should be a focus on physiotherapy aimed at improving global control of the trunk, scapula, and glenohumeral muscles.

The role of motor control in shoulder instability

The rotator cuff muscles play a relevant role in the dynamic stability of the glenohumeral joint. These muscles are ideally placed to draw the humeral head onto the glenoid and maintain its axis of rotation: the pre-setting action of the rotator cuff provides the concavity compression required for stability prior to movement. Recent electromyographic studies have demonstrated that while the rotator cuff muscles do act synergistically to prevent translation of the humeral head onto the glenoid, the muscles also work independently, dependent on the plane and direction of movement, to prevent translation from the torque action of surrounding muscles (Boettcher et al. 2010). In addition, aberrant activation in superficial torque muscles such as the latissimus dorsi and pectoralis major may have a direct influence on the shoulder girdle and could contribute to ongoing instability, particularly when associated with suppression of the rotator cuff (Jaggi et al. 2012).

The control of the rotator cuff may be further affected by the rhythm and stability of the scapula thoracic muscles which are required to hold the scapula in an optimum position to allow the rotator cuff to function. Scapula dyskinesia is commonly seen in patients with instability and recognized as a sign of abnormal muscular control, either as a primary cause of pathology or a secondary adaptation. General posture and core strength within the trunk can affect scapula position; therefore, attention is often given to the entire kinetic chain when gaining stability at the glenohumeral joint.

Rehabilitation strategies are essentially developed from assessment of dynamic rotator cuff function and observation of faulty movement patterns. Symptom modification tests are often used to guide the therapist to specific muscular regions; these may include postural correction, manual assistance to the scapula, and facilitation to the rotator cuff (Timmons et al. 2012). Improvement to these tests can then help formulate targeted rehabilitation within the kinetic chain.

Testing the rotation control of the rotator cuff in a supine position will help to indicate which parts of the rotator cuff may be eccentrically or concentrically deficient. Most commonly, the external rotators are deficient in anterior instability compared to more dominating, internal-rotating muscles. Exercises encouraging recruitment of the posterior rotator cuff are often prescribed (Figure 32.7), although there is a lack of evidence on which specific exercises are most beneficial for the management of shoulder instability (Ganderton and Pizzari 2013).

Principles of instability rehabilitation

The ultimate aim is to restore a normal functioning rotator cuff; this may be achieved by simply targeting these muscles directly or restoring motor control within the entire kinetic chain. This, to some degree, is dependent on how many compensatory adaptations have occurred with the patient's posture, scapula control, and reliance on other more superficial torque muscles.

Initial phase

Rotator cuff exercises should be performed on a stable scapula. This can either be achieved by supporting the weight of the arm on a table or with the use of closed chain exercises that are suspected to facilitate the pre-setting function of the rotator cuff, enhancing joint stability and stimulating muscle co-activation and proprioception. Early sub-maximal isometric exercises for the rotator cuff should be performed to the exclusion of inappropriate muscle activity. Isotonic exercises of the rotator cuff should focus on repetitions rather than increased load: a yellow cliniband is often sufficient for rotator cuff strengthening. In a study where the electromyographic activity of the infraspinatus and deltoid was analysed during resisted isometric external rotation, low loads of between 10% and 40% maximal voluntary isometric contraction were found to optimize the relative contribution of the infraspinatus (Bitter and Clisby 2007).

Some patients with excessive capsular laxity and/or generalized hypermobility are unable to gain selective cuff recruitment on the background of poor core stability and fixation of the global large muscles. These patients can respond better when postural tone is increased (e.g. when sitting on a Swiss ball, standing on one leg, standing on a wobble board) or enhanced through focus on their core stability. Increasing tone within the postural muscle can help reduce the action of superficial torque muscles such as the latissimus dorsi. In addition, it encourages better placement of the scapula and glenohumeral joint to then prompt the deep stabilizing muscles to work.

Early feedback of posture and shoulder girdle position is important to avoid inappropriate patterning and strengthening. Postural tape and mirrors can be invaluable in providing correct sensory feedback, facilitating correct muscle activation. Facilitation of the scapula via tactile feedback through protraction/retraction/elevation/depression enables the patient to dissociate the scapula from the trunk and appreciate where their scapula is in space (Jaggi and Lambert 2010).

End-stage instability rehabilitation

Closed chain exercises can now also be progressed to weight-bearing on unstable surfaces such as a Swiss ball, thus enhancing neuromuscular control at a reflex level. Placing the unstable base directly under the upper limbs may enhance neuromuscular control; the altering perturbation will challenge proprioception and improve joint position sense. It should be noted that studies have found little difference in upper-extremity muscle activity when using an unstable base (Lehman et al. 2008). Placing the ball under the lower limbs, rather than the upper limbs, may help to enhance core stability and function within the entire kinetic chain (Figure 32.8).

End-stage rehabilitation focuses on continued strength and endurance, and must be about retraining patterns of movement biased towards functional tasks. Repetition, speed, and load may be varied in relation to the desired task, facilitating feed-forward processing.

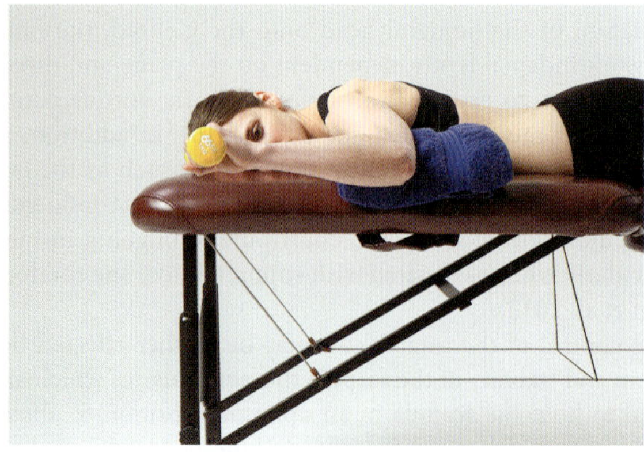

Figure 32.7 Example of exercise to encourage recruitment of the posterior rotator cuff. (With permission of shoulderdoc.co.uk)

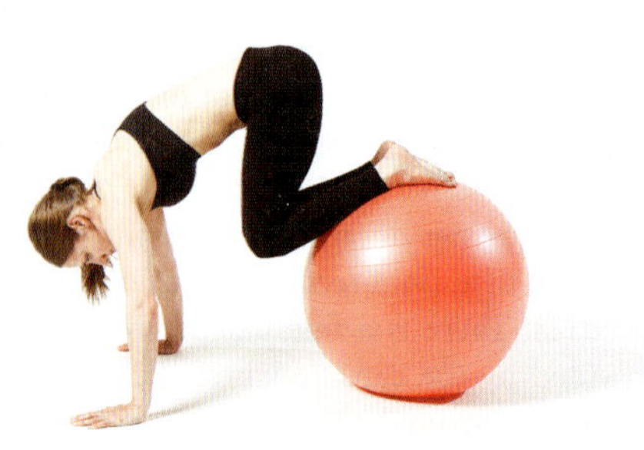

Figure 32.8 Placing the ball under the lower limbs, rather than the upper limbs, may enhance core stability and function within the entire kinetic chain. (With permission of shoulderdoc.co.uk)

Light-weight Swiss balls or bouncing balls off a trampet can be used to increase speed and endurance, and medicine balls can be used for strength training. Proprioceptive neuromuscular facilitation is useful to gain stability and control in functional patterns, strengthening through range. Global upper-limb strengthening can be incorporated with kinetic chain exercises such as step-ups and single leg squats to train patterns of movement rather than isolated muscles (Jaggi and Lambert 2010).

Once recruitment patterns, range of motion, and strength balance have been achieved, rehabilitation principles should incorporate functional training and sport- specific tasks. Cognitive motor learning is enhanced with a goal-specific task (van Vliet and Heneghan 2006). Tasks such as throwing, hitting a specific target, and shooting into a basketball hoop are examples. It is vital an athlete returns to their sport, confident; if this is lacking, they are at risk of compensating with their motor control, increasing their risk of re-injury and instability.

Patients are encouraged to practise exercises on a regular basis and should expect improvement in symptoms within 6–12 weeks of training. More established motor control problems can require treatment regimens of up to 6–9 months. Decisions around the return to sport should be reached collaboratively by surgeons, therapists, coaches, and the patient, as appropriate. Fitness levels must be maintained during the period of rehabilitation.

Summary

Both structural and dynamic components contribute to shoulder instability. The rotator cuff plays a key role in providing this dynamic stability. Therapy should be aimed to optimize its function, taking global posture and scapula stability into account. Abnormal movement patterns and inappropriate muscle activation can be a cause for ongoing shoulder instability.

Rehabilitation for shoulder stiffness

Stiffness at the glenohumeral joint can occur as a result of either pathology of the bony anatomy or adaptation of the soft tissues or a combination of both.

Stiffness as a result of bony abnormalities

The predominant cause of bony stiffness is osteoarthritis (OA). In OA, there is a progressive loss of cartilage leading to increased friction of movement. There may be osteophyte formation which can result in a mechanical block to movement. Through the process, there is a progressive contraction of the periarticular soft tissues—in particular, the capsule.

The literature has very little information on the benefits of physiotherapy for OA of the shoulder. Mobilization techniques should be used to maintain pain-free range of motion. In the early stages of OA, there may also be additional symptoms arising from the rotator cuff, and 'impingement' rehabilitation strategies may also be very beneficial.

Stiffness can also occur following fractures to the shoulder. Malunions of the articular surface can lead to bony impingement and secondary arthritis. Rotational malunions can result in changes to the rotational profile of the joint, leading to changes in the arc of movement and perceived stiffness. The scope of rehabilitation techniques to improve these conditions is limited due to this structural pathology.

Stiffness as a result of soft-tissue contracture

Shoulder stiffness secondary to soft tissue adaptation can be thought of in three types of conditions: idiopathic frozen shoulder, adhesions secondary to trauma (including post-operative) resulting in contracture formation, and poor muscle control. There are many treatment techniques to address shoulder stiffness and the choice of these will be dependent on the diagnosis.

Passive joint mobilization (PJM) techniques, as described by Maitland (1991), are frequently used but, inherently, are not structure-specific. The periarticular constraining structures, including ligaments, capsule, tendons, and muscles, as well as other local structures such as neural tissue and other local joints, may be affected. Theoretically, mobilization will affect the joint articular cartilage and synovial fluid. The agitation of the passive motion is believed to enhance circulation and lubrication of the joint. It is proposed that PJM techniques also transfer kinetic energy which affects the mechanical properties of the connective tissues around the joint. In the remodelling phase of healing, PJM techniques reduce oedema and promote the healing process through circulatory effects encouraging protein synthesis (Frank et al. 1984). The joint movement also influences the orientation of collagen fibres and therefore achieves appropriate tissue compliance and joint range of movement (McConigle and Matley 1994).

The same mobilization theory can be applied to the benefits of active range of motion (ROM) exercises which are, therefore, frequently used in combination with passive mobilization treatments. The advantage of a ROM exercise programme is that it can be performed independently by the patient.

Idiopathic frozen shoulder is a capsular contracture, principally of the coracohumeral ligament, which is a condensation of the capsule within the rotator interval. This leads to shoulder stiffness, especially in external rotation. While individual rehabilitation strategies can be beneficial, there is evidence that in patients with frozen shoulder, group ROM exercise programmes may have additional benefit. The reasons for this remain unclear but group sessions may help to address the psychological element of chronic pain and introduce an element of support or competition to the rehabilitation programme (Russell et al. 2014).

Stiffness as a result of muscle overactivity

Soft tissue adaptation can occur with habitual poor posture and use. However, muscle tightness, as a result of overactivity, rather than adaptive shortening, can also result in a perceived contracture. A common adaptation at the shoulder is overactivity and/or tightness in the pectoralis minor in a protracted shoulder girdle posture. This will adversely affect an individual's ability to improve their scapulothoracic posture and, therefore, improve their shoulder biomechanics. Soft tissue mobilization techniques can be useful to address a patient's symptoms of tightness and the resistance often felt by the clinician when assessing joint range of movement. There are various techniques that can be used to improve circulation and encourage muscle relaxation, thereby lengthening tissue, increasing tissue drainage, and inducing pain relief.

It is important to also assess specific muscle lengths of the shoulder girdle motor control units through the active range of motion.

A poor relationship, resulting in inappropriate co-contraction between agonist and antagonist muscle force couples, may present as a reduction in range of movement, often displaying characteristics of joint restriction and muscle length shortening (Moore and Marteniuk 1986). Poor proprioception and an inability to control movement into these ranges will restrict glenohumeral joint range of movement. This myofascial stiffness can also be a protective response to pain or apprehension, presenting as spasm or muscle guarding (Petty 2011). Proprioceptive neuromuscular facilitation (PNF) techniques encourage normal co-contraction relationships between agonist and antagonists around the shoulder girdle, resulting in a controlled range of movement. PNF involves the stimulation of the proprioceptive system as a basis for muscle re-education and is based on the original work of Herman Kabat (1965). These techniques are a useful treatment to re-establish an increased, controlled range of movement.

In young patients with atraumatic shoulder instability, a restriction in active range at the shoulder may be observed. This type of restriction is a compensatory state caused by inappropriate muscle recruitment patterns and tone as a maladaptive strategy to control shoulder movement in the presence of glenohumeral joint laxity. This overactivity is observed, characteristically, in either the latissimus dorsi or pectoralis major. This type of pathology is rare and, if identified, usually requires a more specialist approach with a detailed movement analysis (Jaggi and Lambert 2010). If a faulty movement pattern is a contributory factor in the reduction of shoulder movement, this should be addressed. The motor relearning theory (Schmidt and Wrisberg 2000) involves the conscious repetition of optimal movement patterns which leads to automatic and subconscious improved motor recruitment. This theory, while essential in these complex cases, is also an important tool in shoulder rehabilitation practice, re-educating movement, and improving muscle function and biomechanics.

Considerations for post-surgical rehabilitation

The key to successful surgical rehabilitation is communication between the surgeon, the therapist, and the patient. It is vital that the surgeon communicates to the therapist and patient, the quality of the tissue repair, any associated procedures, and the peri-operative findings. This allows the therapist to make appropriate decisions during the rehabilitation process.

There is evidence that immobilizing tendons may be detrimental to the healing process. Strict immobilization can result in the formation of irregular and uneven collagen fibres leading to fibrotic adhesions and stiffness. Controlled movement and exercise provides the necessary strain to the tendon, which has been shown to stimulate improvement in cellular activity and collagen deposition at the repair site (Killian et al. 2012). Strict post-operative immobilization of the shoulder can also result in functional instability as a result of rotator cuff inhibition, atrophy, and poor neuromuscular control (Uhl et al. 2003). However, there is a careful balance, as too much activity can lead to repair failure.

Perioperatively, a surgeon is able to assess the quality of a repair and determine a safe range of movement which does not place a strain on the repair site. Post-operatively, this 'safe zone' allows the therapist and patient to determine an active, assisted range of movement, which can be safely performed. In addition, fine needle electromyography (EMG) studies on the rotator cuff muscles have provided evidence of the intensity of muscle activity during specific shoulder exercises (Wilk 1993). This information facilitates the selection of specific exercises with very low levels of rotator cuff activation, allowing safe and controlled post-operative exercise, within this safe zone, without threatening the integrity of surgical repair. Less invasive surface EMG can be used in certain specialist cases to facilitate biofeedback and motor relearning. However, EMG is predominately a research tool and rarely utilized in general physiotherapy practice.

The goal of the therapist is, therefore, to optimize the patient's recovery by safely addressing and maintaining the range of movement, motor control, and proprioception, while respecting tissue-healing physiology.

References

Bitter NL, Clisby EF, Jones MA, et al. (2007) Relative contributions of infraspinatus and deltoid during external rotation in healthy shoulders. *J Shoulder Elbow Surg* 16:563–8.

Boettcher CE, Cathers I, Ginn KA. (2010) The role of shoulder muscles is task specific. *J Sci Med Sport* 13:651–6.

David G, Magarey ME, Jones MA, Dvir Z, Türker KS, Sharpe M. (2000) EMG and strength correlates of selected shoulder muscles during rotations of the glenohumeral joint. *Clin Biomech (Bristol, Avon)* 15(2):95–102.

Dean BJF, Gwilym S, Carr AJ. (2013) Why does my shoulder hurt? A review of the neuroanatomical and biochemical basis of shoulder pain. *British journal of sports medicine* 47:1095–104.

Ellenbecker TS, Cools A. (2010) Rehabilitation of shoulder impingement syndrome and rotator cuff injuries: an evidence-based review. *Br J Sports Med* 44:319–27.

Farina D, Falla D. (2010) The role of motor learning and neuroplasticity in designing rehabilitation approaches for musculoskeletal pain disorders. *Man Ther* 15(5):410–4.

Frank C, Akeson WH, Woo SL-Y, et al. (1984) Physiology and therapeutic value of passive joint motion. *Clin Orthop Relat Res* 185:113–25.

Ganderton C, Pizzari T. (2013) A systematic literature review of the resistance exercises that promote maximal muscle activity of the rotator cuff in normal shoulders. *Shoulder & Elbow* 5:120–35.

Jaggi A, Lambert S. (2010) Rehabilitation for shoulder instability. *Br J Sports Med* 44:333–40.

Jaggi A, Noorani A, Malone A, Cowan J, Lambert S, Bayley I. (2012) Muscle activation patterns in patients with recurrent shoulder instability. *Int J Shoulder Surg* 6:101–7.

Kabat H. (1965) *Proprioceptive facilitation in therapeutic exercise*. New Haven: Waverly Press.

Kibler WB, Sciascia A. (2010) Current concepts: scapular dyskinesis. *Br J Sports Med* 44(5):300–5.

Kibler WB, Ludewig PM, McClure PW, Michener LA, Bak K, Sciascia AD. (2013) Clinical implications of scapular dyskinesis in shoulder injury: the 2013 consensus statement from the 'Scapular Summit'. *Br J Sports Med* 47(14):877–85.

Killian ML, Cavinatto L, Galatz L, Thomopoulos S (2012) The role of mechanobiology in tendon healing. *J Shoulder Elbow Surg* 21(2):228–37.

Kroner K, Lind T, Jensen J. (1989) The epidemiology of shoulder dislocations. *Arch Orthop Trauma Surg* 108:288–90.

Kuhn JE. (2009) Exercise in the treatment of rotator cuff impingement: a systematic review and a synthesized evidence-based rehabilitation programme. *J Shoulder Elbow Surg* 18:138–60.

Lehman GJ, Gilas D, Patel U. (2008) An unstable support surface does not increase scapulothoracic stabilizing muscle activity during push up and push up plus exercises. *Man Ther* 13:500–6.

Lewis JS. (2010) Rotator cuff tendinopathy: a model for the continuum of pathology and related management. *Br J Sports Med* 44(13): 918–23.

Lewis JS. (2012) A specific exercise programme for patients with subacromial impingement syndrome can improve function and reduce the need for surgery. *J Physiotherapy* 58(2):127.

Maitland GD. (1991) *Peripheral manipulation*. London: Butterworth Heinemann.

McConigle T, Matley KW. (1994) Soft tissue treatment and muscle stretching. *J Man Manip Ther* 2(2):55–62.

McMullen J, Uhl TL. (2000) A kinetic chain approach for shoulder rehabilitation. *J Athl Train* 35(3):329–37.

Mintken PE, ClelandJA, Carpenter KJ, Bieniek ML, Keirns M, Whitman JM. (2010) Some factors predict successful short-term outcomes in individuals with shoulder pain receiving cervicothoracic manipulation: a single-arm trial. *Phys Ther* 90(1):26–42.

Moore SP, Marteniuk RG. (1986) Kinematic and electromyographic changes that occur as a function of learning a time-constrained aiming task. *J Mot Behav* 18(4):397–426.

Petty NJ. (2011) *Principles of neuromusculoskeletal treatment and management* (2nd edn). London: Churchill Livingstone.

Russell S, Jariwala A, Conlon R, Selfe J, Richards J, Walton M. (2014) A blinded, randomized, controlled trial assessing conservative management strategies for frozen shoulder. *J Shoulder Elbow Surg* 23(4): 500–7.

Schmidt RA, Wrisberg CA. (2000) Motor learning and performance, a problem-based learning approach (2nd edn). Illinois, Champaign: Human Kinematics.

Seitz AL, McClure PW, Finucane S, Boardman ND III, Michener LA. (2011) Mechanisms of rotator cuff tendinopathy: intrinsic, extrinsic, or both? *Clin Biomech (Bristol, Avon)* 26(1):1–12.

Tannenbaum E, Sekiya JK. (2011) Evaluation and management of posterior shoulder instability. *Sports Health* 3:253–263.

Timmons MK, Thigpen CA, Seitz AL, Karduna AR, Arnold BL, Michener LA. (2012) Scapular kinematics and subacromial impingement syndrome: a meta-analysis. *J Sport Rehabil* 21(4):354–70.

Uhl T, et al. (2003) Shoulder musculature activation during upper extremity weightbearing exercise. *J Ortho Sports Phys Ther* 33(3);109–11.

Van Vliet PM, Heneghan NR. (2006) Motor control and the management of musculoskeletal dysfunction. *Man Ther* 11:208–13.

Walser RF, Meserve BB, Boucher TR. (2009) The effectiveness of thoracic spine manipulation for the management of musculoskeletal conditions: a systematic review and meta-analysis of randomized clinical trials. *J Man Manip Ther* 17(4):237–46.

Wilk KE. (1993) Current concepts in rehabilitation of the athletic shoulder. *J Orthop Sports Physio* 18(1):365–78.

Chapter 33

Upper limb disorders

Michael Hutson, Michael Yelland, and David Rabago

Michael Hutson has written the bulk of this chapter. However, the editors are delighted that Michael Yelland and David Rabago have responded to a request to contribute a substantive section on lateral epicondylalgia.

Introduction to upper limb disorders

The upper limb is a veritable treasure trove for neuromusculoskeletal pathology. Additionally, in terms of body posture and 'posturing', the upper limb acts as a barometer for the stresses and strains that are endemic in the twenty-first century in both the developed and underprivileged worlds.

The recognition that the hand acts as a diagnostic window for many systemic medical conditions and illnesses is an essential component of medical school training. The nails, in particular, are a flag for many types of pathology. Rheumatological and neurovascular conditions may be detected by inspection of the hand. Swellings, deformities, and contractures are often obvious to casual inspection. Both distress and impairment of function may be manifest in patients by observing resting posture and the expressive use (or otherwise) of the hand and upper limb at interview, when undressing and dressing, and during formal examination.

Neuromusculoskeletal disorders in the upper limb are a frequent cause of discomfort and disability, reflecting our use of the hand and upper limb for virtually all domestic, recreational, and workplace tasks. They may be viewed according to a number of models: for instance, pathomorphological ('structural'), biomechanical, pathoneurophysiological ('dysfunctional'), and biopsychosocial. Dysfunction, the common theme throughout this textbook, is sometimes associated with pathomorphology, but not inevitably so. In the upper limb, dysfunction may have devastating consequences.

The disease–illness model, a central pillar of modernist medical thinking over several decades, is as inappropriate in many upper limb disorders as it is in the generality of neuromusculoskeletal disorders. The *biopsychosocial model*, on the other hand, takes account of the behavioural response to illness, injury, and dysfunction. It has a core holistic component and is the preferred model for clinical assessment of neck, shoulder, and arm symptoms, and the construction of appropriate management strategies.

The pathogenesis of neuromuscular disorders in the upper limb is often multifactorial. The time-honoured subdivision of structural pathology into degenerative, traumatic, neoplastic, infective, inflammatory—as taught in medical school—may be standard practice for the orthopaedic surgeon, but this categorization does not adapt easily to the study of neuromusculoskeletal dysfunction. Several of the following aetiological factors may coexist:

- **Overuse:** Repetitive microtrauma, whether associated with domestic activities, sport, leisure, or work, is the principal cause of tendinopathies, which are frequently encountered at the shoulder, elbow, and wrist. Muscle hypertrophy is a consequence of repetitive forceful activities, and may give rise to nerve entrapment (Kopell and Thompson 1963).
- **Degeneration:** Tendinopathies and enthesopathies usually have a substantive degenerative component. Fibroproliferative diseases (found predominantly in the hand) are also basically degenerative in type. Arthropathies may of course be degenerative.
- **Posture:** Adverse body posture at work, rest, or play, particularly at the proximal thoracic spine and shoulder girdle, should always be considered as a possible aetiological factor. Hence the need for a thorough examination of the cervicodorsal spine and shoulder region in patients presenting with upper limb symptoms. The close anatomical relationship between neurovascular, myofascial, and osseous structures at the thoracic inlet, proximal thoracic cage, and pectoral girdle should raise clinical awareness at initial assessment of the potential for neuromuscular and/or vascular dysfunction. Postural vigilance by the patient and medical attendant is required during rehabilitation from many upper limb problems to prevent recurrence of dysfunction.
- **Biomechanics/ergonomics:** A study of the technical aspects of gripping, lifting, and the use of the hand and arm during all manual activities is often revealing. A basic knowledge of ergonomics in the factory and at the keyboard is essential. Ergonomists may be recruited to assist in evaluation and management of upper limb disorders that are associated with work.
- **Comorbidity—systemic and psychiatric illness:** Systemic conditions that include diabetes, nutritional deficiencies, hormonal disturbances, alcohol abuse, and inflammatory joint disease contribute to increased vulnerability to neuromusculoskeletal dysfunction. Diabetes in particular, affecting a significant proportion

of the population, is associated with an increased incidence of fibroproliferative conditions (such as trigger finger and Dupuytren's contracture), and also with carpal tunnel syndrome. Psychosocial factors are the principal cause of chronicity in many somatic syndromes, particularly back pain, whiplash, and upper limb disorders. Prognosis is substantively adversely affected by the coexistence of frank psychiatric illness.

- **Neural dysfunction:** Neural disturbances, whether playing a primary, secondary, or contributory role, are particularly common in the upper limb. Hence the need to evaluate function at the cervical and proximal thoracic spines when presented with a symptomatic upper limb. The so-called *double crush phenomenon* (Upton and McComas 1973), although a somewhat crude label with regard to increased neural tension and neural plasticity, is a helpful concept to some clinicians. The possibility of the additive effect of nerve compression at diverse sites such as the intervertebral foramen, the brachial plexus, and the periphery needs to be considered in the aetiology of many conditions, particularly work-related. It is a reminder of the continuum of this delicate but vital structure throughout the upper limb. To others, the pathogenesis of non-specific upper limb pain is more easily understood when predicated on the hypothesis of abnormal sensory neural processing—in other words, a reduced threshold for pain perception (Mitchell et al. 2000)—a feature of central neurosensitization. The cause of central sensitization in patients with 'non-specific' arm pain is disputed. Indeed, it may vary from one patient to another. Cervical spinal nerve entrapment has to be considered. Reduced median nerve mobility in the carpal tunnel is mooted as another possibility in some patients (Greening et al. 1999). In yet another vulnerable group, neural compression between neck and shoulder, often associated with poor upper body posture and adverse biomechanics, is a possibility.
- **Iatrogenesis:** Causation and/or aggravation of symptoms as a result of clinical processes is common throughout medical practice, and may be a major factor in the development, severity, and chronicity of upper limb disorders. The devastating potential of iatrogenesis may only be reduced by improved post-graduate tuition, leading to a better understanding by clinicians of the principles of neuromusculoskeletal medicine.
- **Beware: Neuropathic pain and iatrogenesisis are common** in patients with upper limb disorders.

The emphasis in this chapter is on those soft tissue and neural conditions of the upper limb that occur relatively frequently in family medical practice and also in secondary medical care. Conditions that primarily affect the joints of the elbow, wrist, and hand are excluded. (In general, these are associated with pathomorphology such as inflammatory joint disease, degenerative joint disease, and post-traumatic capsulitis, and are dealt with adequately elsewhere.) Shoulder joint dysfunction is discussed in Chapters 30, 31, and 32. Epicondylalgia is sufficiently common in the population generally, and such a useful musculoskeletal condition for teaching purposes, that Yelland and Rabago, to whom the editors are much indebted, have written on lateral epicondylalgia in this chapter.

Examination of the elbow, wrist, and hand

The examiner observes demeanour, posture, and the use of the hand and arm at interview and during examination. In general, behaviour at interview and during examination is often as important as more formal functional assessment. By way of illustration: a weak, limp handshake is typical of neuropathic pain syndromes. The use of a wrist support could have similar connotations, or could indicate soft tissue pathology. The systemic manifestations of diseases such as rheumatoid arthritis, nodal osteoarthritis (of the hands), and endocrine disorders may be detected.

Elbow and forearm

Soft tissue swellings include olecranon bursitis, sometimes referred to as 'beat elbow'. A more modest degree of soft tissue swelling may be present over the common extensor origin in lateral epicondylitis. The range of active/passive movements at the elbow is –10/150°. More than 10° of extension is referred to as *hyperextension*. Sometimes this is a component of the hypermobility syndrome. The end-feel in flexion is soft, whereas the end-feel to extension should be hard. A springy block to extension is indicative of synovitis/capsulitis or an intra-articular loose body. The capsular pattern of joint dysfunction is a greater loss of flexion compared to extension.

Resisted elbow flexion and extension (testing biceps and triceps primarily) are undertaken routinely. Weakness may be caused by biceps/triceps muscle lesions or by nerve dysfunction (for a variety of reasons). Resisted supination and pronation are undertaken primarily to assist with the diagnosis of muscle lesions in the proximal forearm. Palpation of the lateral epicondyle, medial epicondyle, and distal biceps tendon should be routine. Biceps tendonitis and distal biceps rupture are relatively uncommon but may cause long-term loss of function if not diagnosed. 'Tennis elbow' may give rise to tenderness of the extensor muscle mass as well as the lateral epicondyle. Tenderness at the head of the radius may be present in an atypical tennis elbow. Tenderness in golfer's elbow is usually maximal 0.5–1 cm distal to the point of the medial epicondyle. The presence of more widespread tenderness should alert the examiner to the possibility of neurogenic conditions. Palpation at the medial epicondyle may reveal a hypermobile ulnar nerve in the cubital tunnel.

Resisted dorsiflexion of the wrist and extension of the fingers is undertaken routinely in lateral epicondylalgia. The examination should always include resisted forearm rotation (supination and pronation), resisted palmar flexion of the wrist, and resisted flexion of the fingers. The examiner may occasionally be caught out by neuropathic arm pain (in which all these manoeuvres are painful as a consequence of regional mechanical hyperalgesia) manifesting as 'apparent' epicondylalgia. In medial epicondylalgia, resisted pronation is very commonly more painful than resisted palmar flexion of the wrist or resisted flexion of the fingers, reflecting its origination, in many cases, in the pronator teres part of the common flexor origin.

Joint play (accessory) movements should be undertaken at the inferior radioulnar joint. The techniques described by John Mennell are to be commended (Mennell and Zohn 1976).

Wrist

Bony deformities may be the result of a previous fracture. Soft tissue swellings over the dorsum of the wrist are more common than swellings over the volar aspect. Diffuse synovial proliferation suggests an inflammatory disorder. The dorsum of the wrist is the most common site for a ganglion. The active movements of dorsiflexion, palmar flexion, radial deviation, and ulnar deviation are tested sequentially. Passive movements provide the examiner with a test of end-feel. Radial and ulnar deviation should be assessed with the wrist held in zero flexion. Comparison with the other limb is recorded, as there is a considerable variation in the normal ranges of movement. Phalen's test demands full palmar flexion of the wrist for 1 minute. This should be undertaken with the arms held in a dependent position. The *reversed Phalen's test* is undertaken by combining wrist dorsiflexion with extension of the fingers and forearm, commonly uncomfortable with finger flexor tendonitis. *Finkelstein's test* is undertaken with the wrist passively ulnar-deviated and the thumb passively opposed across the palm (held in position by active flexion of the fingers): discomfort (a positive test) is experienced in de Quervain's syndrome.

The joint play movements described by Mennell are again commended. Loss of anteroposterior glide is a useful indicator of dysfunction at the wrist. Palpation at the wrist should be undertaken gently but methodically. A heavy-handed approach will reveal spurious tenderness (for instance, in the anatomical snuff box) (Hutson 1997). A careful progression by palpation along the bony and tendon landmarks is essential for confirmation of the provisional diagnoses that may have been made by history, movement assessment, and resisted muscle contraction. Careful palpation is required to detect localized tenderness and thickening of tendons, particularly when tendinopathy is at a subacute or chronic stage. A comparison should always be made with the asymptomatic contralateral wrist.

Hand

Neurological contractures are not described here. Thenar or hypothenar wasting are commonly observed, and should stimulate a search for the primary cause in the neurological system or an adjacent joint. Swellings of the finger joints are examined for the bony hardness of osteoarthritis, including Heberden's nodes, or the soft synovial swelling and squeeze tenderness of inflammatory arthritis. The squaring at the base of the thumb indicative of osteoarthritis of the first carpometacarpal joint is noted. Vasomotor changes and palmar fascia thickening should also be recorded. Asking the patient to 'make a fist' is useful for demonstration of the movements at the carpometacarpal, metacarpophalangeal, and interphalangeal joints of the thumb and fingers, but flexion can also be limited by the swelling of tenosynovitis in the palm and fingers. At the carpometacarpal joint of the thumb, the capsular pattern is more loss of abduction than extension. As at the hip joint, axial compression combined with rotation is often uncomfortable in osteoarthritis. Ulnar laxity at the first metacarpophalangeal joint may result from 'skier's thumb' when traumatic or from 'gamekeeper's thumb' as a consequence of repetitive stress.

Joint play movements at all the interphalangeal and metacarpal joints may be undertaken. Although such techniques are useful during workshop-type training, in practice, they are often discarded because of their failure to contribute much to diagnosis.

Conventionally, neurological examination includes assessment of motor and sensory function. Motor function is routinely tested by resisted contraction during the examination of the joints and soft tissues. Whether formal sensory examination, for instance by the two-point discrimination test, yields much information is somewhat contentious. It is my opinion that the symptoms of sensory blunting reported by a patient are probably the most reliable guide to reduced sensation. Tinel's test for the median or ulnar nerves is notoriously unreliable. The concept of neural 'tension' in the upper limb is also a contentious issue; neural 'sensitivity' is a more appropriate concept. The test commonly referred to as *adverse neural tension* should be considered to reflect such upper limb neural sensitivity; when positive, it should stimulate the examiner to search for the cause of the sensitivity. For further information on neural tension tests and neural sensitivity, the reader is referred to Hall and Robinson (Chapter 15).

Tendinopathies in the upper limbs

At the hand, wrist, and forearm, a frequently applied diagnostic label in family practice is tenosynovitis, tendinitis, or 'teno'. Indeed, many patients suffering from unexplained wrist and forearm pain, particularly when they are engaged in repetitive stereotyped activities (most often in the workplace), are prescribed non-steroidal anti-inflammatory drugs (NSAIDs) and frequently wrist supports on the basis of a presumed inflammatory tendinitis. There is in fact little evidence of a significant inflammatory reaction in tendinopathies in the upper limb other than for the inflammatory disorders such as rheumatoid arthritis. Should florid signs of inflammation be present, rheumatoid arthritis or an associated inflammatory condition is the most likely cause.

This book concentrates on non-inflammatory disorders, but it is always necessary for the musculoskeletal physician to exclude inflammatory arthritis, particularly with any degree of soft tissue swelling. The conventional view of tendinitis (more appropriately labelled 'tendinopathy') is that cumulative stress or overload, often in the form of repetitive vigorous manual activities, gives rise to viscoelastic deformation of collagen. Compensatory mechanisms may be overwhelmed, causing collagen fibril microfailure. Light microscopy in surgical cases reveals frayed fibrils with disrupted architecture (Khan et al. 2002). Histopathological changes include collagen and mucoid degeneration (see the section 'Lateral epicondylagia' by Yelland and Rabago, in this chapter). Should a tendon be covered by a paratendon, a secondary inflammatory reaction may then occur, giving rise to paratendonitis, as in Achilles' paratendonitis in the lower limb.

When tendons run through fibro-osseous channels, they have a lining synovium in addition to a fibrous sheath. Although 'tenosynovitis' is an appropriate term for tendon pathology associated with inflammatory disorders such as rheumatoid arthritis, tendon degeneration (with no significant inflammation) is more accurately labelled 'tendinopathy'. Conditions such as de Quervain's disease, in which there is thickening of the tendon sheath, should be labelled 'tenovaginitis'.

In the hand, thickening of the fibrous sheath may give rise to tenovaginitis stenosans; for instance, trigger thumb or trigger finger. The association between repetitive manual activities and tenovaginitis is unclear. Many conditions that give rise to thickened collagenized fibrous structures, such as trigger finger and Dupuytren's contracture, are more common in diabetics. Biopsy findings in de Quervain's tenovaginitis reveal increased fibroblastic activity and vascular proliferation, but the more obvious features are an increase in glycosaminoglycan content (hyaluronic acid, condroitin sulphate, and dermatin sulphate), synovial thickening, and fibrocartilaginous transformation.

Overuse leads to degradative changes (tendinosis). These should be interpreted as the response to stress and not merely the inevitable age-related changes of degeneration (Hutson 1997). In view of the morphology, it should come as no surprise to find that NSAIDs have little effect on symptoms or on chronicity. They are, however, associated with risk of significant morbidity.

De Quervain's disease

Fritz de Quervain described this condition in 1895. He called it 'fibrose, stenosierende tenovaginitis'. It is likely, however, that Tillaux (1892) described the same condition a few years previously.

De Quervain's disease is relatively common. Although it is seen most frequently in middle age, mothers of young children are at risk (Harvey et al. 1990). Symptomatic de Quervain's disease is seen in workers whose tasks include repetitive use of the thumb and hand, particularly repetitive use of the pinch grip and radioulnar deviations at the wrist. Although Leao (1958) stated that de Quervain's disease could be considered an occupational condition in many cases, it is unclear whether repetitive manual activities cause the condition or simply convert a previously asymptomatic condition to a symptomatic one.

In de Quervain's disease, discomfort at the radial wrist is predominantly activity- related. Although crepitus is sometimes associated with the acute phase of the condition (and indeed Tillaux, in his initial description of the condition, labelled it as 'tenosynovitis crépitante'), the more commonly encountered chronic condition rarely exhibits crepitation on examination. Patients are nearly always aware of, and certainly complain of, 'swelling' of the distal forearm. Because the condition is work-related, discomfort is maximal at work, lessening with rest. Manual activities in the kitchen are particularly stressful. Although pain may radiate proximally and distally, it is experienced maximally over the radial styloid and slightly distal to this.

The most reliable clinical features are thickening ('swelling') of the combined tendons of the extensor pollicis brevis and abductor pollicis longus at the level of the radial styloid, and a positive Finkelstein's test. To experienced examiners, the thickened tendinous structures are not often a diagnostic challenge. Finkelstein's test, however, should always be undertaken with considerable care. A false positive test (when the patient complains of pain due to other conditions) may be the result of a poor examination technique. A comparison should always be made with the other (presumably painless) side. The examiner should be careful to apply pressure to the radial margin of the second metacarpal to create ulnar deviation at the wrist once the thumb has been passively flexed across the palm and held there by the patient's fingers. My advice is to apply passive radial deviation in the first instance, and then ulnar deviation to distinguish between those conditions at the wrist that have an articular component and de Quervain's tenovaginitis.

The most common differential diagnosis is degenerative change (osteoarthritis) at the first carpometacarpal joint. Other degenerative changes within the carpus, such as scaphotrapezoid osteoarthritis, may also cause radial wrist pain. In these conditions, tenderness is expected over the affected joint. However, in patients who are difficult to assess because of abnormal hyperalgesia, for instance when neurosensitized, tenderness may be somewhat diffuse. Under these circumstances, the clinical features of neurosensitization may be augmented by articular hyperalgesia (in which all passive movements and indeed virtually all examination procedures at the wrist, however gentle, evoke discomfort).

Management strategies include the use of NSAIDs, physiotherapy (usually disappointing), wrist support, steroid injections, and surgery. A trained musculoskeletal physician would usually treat by localized low-dose steroid (combined with local anaesthetic) infiltration around and along the line of the affected tendons, to which most patients respond. The injection may be given proximal to distal, or the other way around, at the level of the radial styloid or just proximal to the base of the first metacarpal. No more than 5–10 mg of triamcinolone is necessary. Harvey et al. (1990) quote an 80% success rate for resolution of de Quervain's disease with steroid injections. However, more than one injection may be necessary. A reasonable treatment protocol is to review the patient one month after the initial injection, and to repeat the low-dose steroid injection if symptoms persist. Should symptoms recur, surgical decompression is nearly always effective if the correct diagnosis is made.

A common clinical error is to confuse de Quervain's disease with intersection syndrome. The conditions are at different anatomical sites, and it is in intersection syndrome that crepitus is a marked diagnostic feature. De Quervain's disease affects the extensor pollicis brevis and abductor pollicis longus in the first dorsal compartment of the wrist (see Figure 33.1). An understanding of the dorsal compartments facilitates the assessment of wrist pain.

Intersection syndrome

This condition affects the tendons of the second dorsal compartment at the wrist, more accurately described as the distal forearm as this condition is situated more proximally than other tendinopathies at the wrist. The condition arises at the intersection between the extensor carpi radialis longus and brevis tendons (by definition, the tendons of the second dorsal compartment) and the tendons of the extensor pollicis brevis and abductor pollicis longus. It is a crossover point, thus explaining the histopathological features of a sticky fibrinous deposit between these tendons. In a seminal article, Thompson et al. (1951) considered that unaccustomed work, or a return to work after a period of absence, was the stressor in a significant proportion of cases.

Intersection syndrome is otherwise known as peritendinitis crepitans, reflecting the clinical feature of crepitus secondary to an inflammatory reaction at the site of the musculotendinous junction of the affected tendons. Although first described by Velpeau (1841), it was probably Troell (1918) who used the term 'peritendinitis crepitans'. Troell compared the condition to similar tendinopathies of the lower leg, including of the Achilles' tendon.

Intersection syndrome is an overuse condition. Patients complain of pain, swelling, tenderness, and 'creaking' (crepitus). As is common to other tendinopathies, not only in the upper limb but also throughout the body, patients usually complain of 'weakness', probably because of pain inhibition.

Manual workers constitute a high-risk group, though rowers and canoeists are frequently affected, as are weightlifters and dog handlers (Hutson 2001). In Thompson's series (Thompson et al. 1951), most of the 544 patients with forearm tendinitis (of which 419 cases were due to peritendinitis crepitans) worked in the Vauxhall motor factory.

Intersection syndrome is found approximately 6 cm proximal to Lister's tubercle at the wrist. Crepitus is a constant feature in the acute state. Tenderness and swelling are present, and Finkelstein's test may be positive.

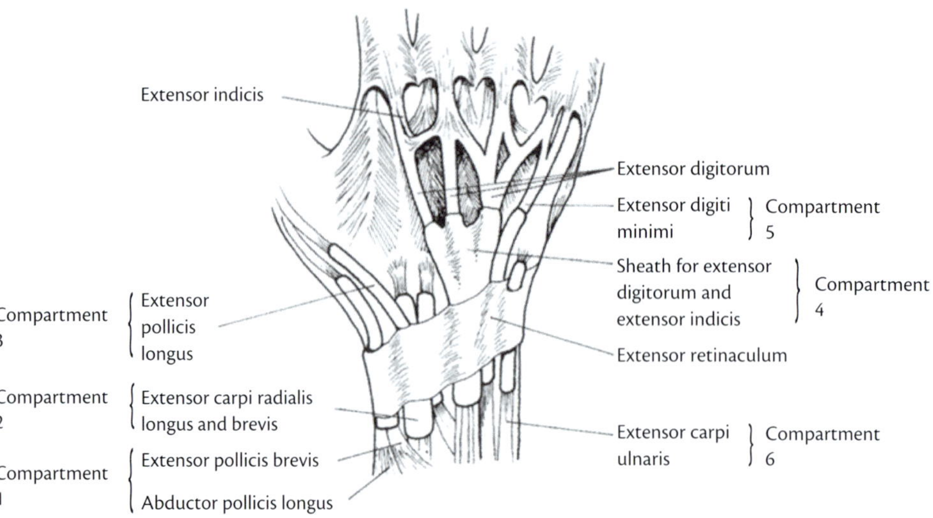

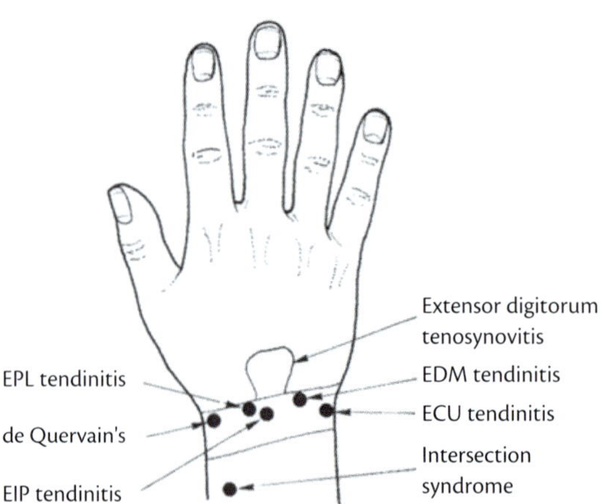

Figure 33.1 De Quervain's disease.

Very slow progress is to be expected with splinting or physiotherapy. This is one of the few crepitating inflammatory conditions found in clinical practice that resolves within a few days of administering a steroid injection. Nevertheless, a full assessment of the aetiological factors is necessary to prevent recurrence. As with all tendinopathies, an appropriate period of rest or at least reduction of biomechanical stresses is necessary to prevent recurrence. It is my experience that increased vulnerability to recurrence persists for months, possibly years.

Extensor pollicis longus tendinopathy

The extensor pollicis longus lies in the third dorsal compartment. Extensor pollicis longus tendinopathy was described by Dums (1896) in Prussian drummer boys in whom rupture occurred as a result of attrition at Lister's tubercle. Extensor pollicis longus rupture may also be a consequence of a fracture of the radial styloid, more commonly, a minimally displaced Colles' fracture than a fracture requiring manipulative reduction. Gross weakness of active extension at the interphalangeal joint of the thumb is found in extensor pollicis longus rupture. The clinical findings are pain on passive flexion of the thumb and on resisted thumb extension.

Extensor digitorum tenosynovitis

The labelling of this fourth dorsal compartment condition reflects its aetiology. It is appropriately labelled tenosynovitis, as it is most commonly due to rheumatoid arthritis. The presentation, in the form of swelling, tenderness, and deformity, is often relatively florid. The swelling distal to the extensor retinaculum is often in the form of a 'goose foot' when marked.

It may be an isolated lesion in the hand, but a high index of suspicion with respect to an inflammatory disorder should be present when there is swelling. Impairment of function is often severe in well-established rheumatoid arthritis.

Extensor digiti minimi tendinopathy

This condition is rare, although it has been reported as a consequence of trauma or overuse (Hooper and McMaster 1979). Attempts to flex the wrist after making a fist are described as painful.

Extensor carpi ulnaris tendinopathy

After de Quervain's tenovaginitis and intersection syndrome, extensor carpi ulnaris tendinopathy is the next most common tendinopathy at the wrist that is not due to inflammatory disease. It occurs in the sixth dorsal compartment of the wrist, giving rise to ulnar wrist pain. It is an overuse condition, occurring in work or recreational activity in which there are repetitive radioulnar wrist deviations, particularly when combined with rotation. It occurs in professional golfers who may need to revise grip and swing to offload the extensor carpi ulnaris as part of the management of this condition.

A reliable clinical finding is discomfort on passive radial deviation of the wrist with a fully pronated forearm/wrist. Full passive supination may also be painful. As with many tendinopathies at the wrist, resisted contraction of the affected tendon is not painful, other than in the acute phase. Care needs to be taken to localize tenderness over the ulnar styloid. Clicking raises the possibility of recurrent subluxation of the extensor carpi ulnaris.

The most common differential diagnosis is a lesion of the inferior radioulnar joint. This condition also gives rise to discomfort on passive rotations of the forearm and to localized tenderness. Occasionally, a sprain of the ulnar collateral ligament at the wrist is found, although a ligamentous injury tends to be overdiagnosed by the inexperienced physician.

Flexor carpi ulnaris tendinopathy

This condition may result from repetitive flexion movements of the wrist (as an overload phenomenon) or from repetitive direct trauma to the volar–ulnar aspect of the wrist (as in racquet players, golfers, or cricketers). In practice, the at-risk group appears to be industrial workers, particularly those involved in the building and demolition industries. The use of a heavy hammer combines a high degree of force with repetition.

The flexor carpi ulnaris tendon is tender, maximally just proximal to the pisiform bone. In those activities in which compression of a tool or sporting implement is an aetiological factor, compression of the pisiform against the underlying triquetral may evoke discomfort. Stretching of the flexor carpi ulnaris tendon by combined extension and radial deviation of the wrist usually evokes discomfort.

As a consequence of the topographical relationship between the flexor carpi ulnaris tendon (and pisiform) and the ulnar nerve at the wrist, entrapment neuropathy of the deep branch of the ulnar nerve in Guyon's canal, during its course around the pisiform, is an occasional associated finding. A change in working or sporting technique is often necessary to reduce overload. Localized steroid/local anaesthetic injections are effective.

Flexor carpi radialis tendinopathy

This is relatively uncommon. Figure 33.2 demonstrates a case of calcific flexor carpi radialis tendinitis at the volar aspect of the wrist that gave rise to acute pain and loss of function of the hand. This example reveals the usefulness of plain radiology in acute pain and swelling of the hand.

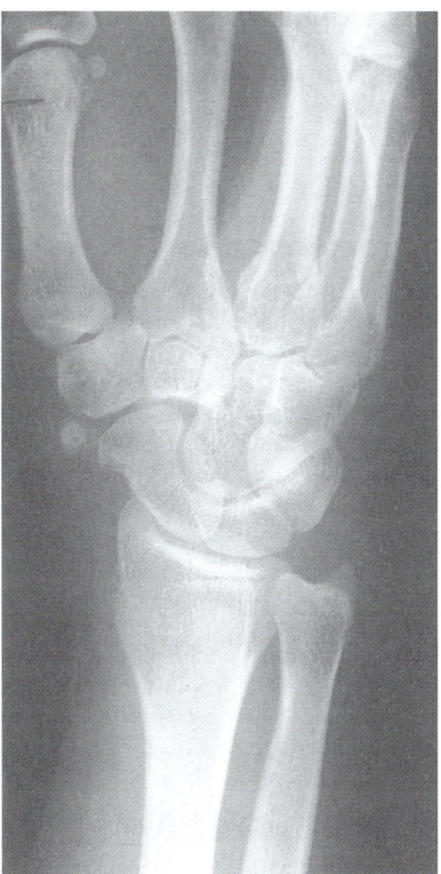

Figure 33.2 Calcific flexor carpi radialis tendinitis at the volar aspect of the wrist.

Flexor digitorum tendinopathy

Although not often described as a discrete tendinopathy, flexor digitorum tendinopathy is commonly found as a mild chronic condition in workers whose job tasks include repetitive grasping. Chronic tendinopathy gives rise to a minor flexion contracture and a positive 'prayer' sign. This stenosing form of tendinopathy is found in a subgroup of patients with carpal tunnel syndrome. In the acute form, swelling may be observed proximal to the wrist creases (Kiefhaber and Stern 1992).

Power of finger flexion is retained. Attempts by the examiner to passively extend the fingers evoke discomfort. If detected early, a programme of graded stretching exercises is a logical management strategy, but it is apparent that patients appear to accept symptoms at a relatively minimal or nuisance level and rarely seek advice.

Stenosing tenovaginitis of the digital flexors (trigger finger; trigger thumb)

This condition is characterized by thickening of the first annular (A1) pulley of the fibrous flexor tendon sheath at the level of the metacarpophalangeal joint. Patients complain of triggering and clicking. The thumb, middle, or ring fingers are most commonly affected.

Repetitive compression during strong grasping is a logical, but unproven, aetiological factor. Bonnici and Spencer (1988) established an increased incidence in women and an association with occupations that require repetitive hand movements. There appears to be a subgroup of the population, particularly but not exclusively people with diabetes, who are vulnerable to fibroproliferative conditions of the hand such as trigger finger and Dupuytren's contracture. Low-dose steroid injections are effective. Early relief of discomfort and triggering is the expected outcome (Marks and Gunther 1989) although, as with de Quervain's tenovaginitis, cases that are refractory or recurrent may be treated by surgical decompression.

The most effective injection technique, using a 23-gauge needle, is to advance the tip of the needle at a more or less 90° angle to the palm, through the tendon, withdraw slightly from the bone, and then inject 10 mg triamcinolone (or equivalent). Some practitioners prefer an angled technique or an approach through the web between the digits.

Dupuytren's contracture

Repetitive manual activities were considered by Baron Dupuytren (1834) to be the cause of this condition, which he described in a coachman and in a wine merchant. This association is now much more uncertain, although alcohol may be a causative factor (Noble et al. 1992). It is rarely seen in non-white people, and often has a familial distribution. The palmar condition is usually described, although the plantar fascia is also affected in many patients.

It is more common in men than women, and is usually found to be bilateral over time. The earliest feature, usually unnoticed initially by the patient, is thickening of the palmar fascia, often with a nodular component. Puckering soon becomes evident, and subsequently the characteristic flexion deformity of the right and little fingers. Massage and stretching in the early stages may prevent or delay flexion contracture. There appears to be no inflammatory element, and steroid injections are ineffective. Pronounced contractures can only be effectively treated by surgery.

Ganglion (synovial cyst) in an upper limb

A ganglion is a tense cystic swelling, containing thick viscous fluid, associated with a joint or tendon sheath. Probably the most common site, certainly the most frequently described, is the dorsum of the wrist. Often there is tethering to the carpal joints. However, ganglia are also seen elsewhere, and are more common in women than men (Nelson et al. 1972).

Ganglia are not manifestations of rheumatoid arthritis or associated conditions. Distinguishing between a ganglion and a rheumatoid swelling is usually not difficult as the former is tense and yields a sticky fluid when aspirated; rheumatoid swelling is typically soft, warm, and more diffuse. Ganglia are often painless, but their presence is often disturbing and cosmetically unsightly. They are also unpredictable with respect to their natural history. For the majority, spontaneous resolution is to be expected. However, many recur, and treatment is often sought.

Discomfort, particularly on manual activities, may develop and be associated with impairment of function at the wrist. In a subgroup of patients, dorsal wrist discomfort may precede the development of swelling. Localized tenderness may be present; also discomfort on dorsiflexion and palmar flexion at the wrist, but there are no features of tendinitis or of synovitis. Aspiration with a 20-gauge needle, with or without a steroid injection, is often effective (Varley et al. 1997). The more traditional management strategy of 'bashing' with a heavy object (commonly a family bible in Victorian times) is outdated.

Although the majority of patients recover satisfactorily after surgical excision, dissection may be tedious, and recurrence is not unusual. In Nelson's series of 222 patients (in whom 50% of ganglia occurred over the dorsal aspect of the wrist), the cure rate of 94% with surgery under general anaesthesia was significantly better than other groups treated by digital pressure or by aspiration.

Peripheral nerve entrapment in the upper limb

The neural system in the upper limb should be viewed as a continuum, both anatomical and physiological, extending from the cervical spine to the fingertips. Nerve compression occurs at well-recognized sites at which constrictions and compressions result from a variety of osseous, muscle, and fascial structures. Increased susceptibility to abnormal neural dynamics may be caused by the double crush phenomenon (in which there are multiple sites of neural compression or irritation). The entrapment neuropathies are the most common, and will be dealt with in some detail, either in this chapter or elsewhere:

- **Intervertebral foramina of the cervical spine:** Nerve root compression is most commonly caused by degenerate bulging discs combined with fibro-osseous hypertrophy of the apophyseal joints. Cervical spinal extension and ipsilateral rotation reduce the dimensions of the foramina. Thus, compressive (axial) injuries, particularly when associated with extension of the neck, often cause nerve root compression. Activities that are associated with prolonged flexion of the neck often provoke radicular symptoms, probably because of increased tautness of the spinal cord and the emerging roots. Unpleasant symptoms that radiate to the upper limb from the neck, whether radicular (dermatomal) or pseudoradicular (sclerotomal) in type, do not always conform to recognized pathways (Slipman et al. 1998). It is often difficult, on clinical grounds, to state categorically whether such symptoms are arising in the neck, as it has been established that many tissues other than nerve roots may refer pain (Feinstein et al. 1954; Kellgren 1939), giving the clinician good cause to rely on an appropriate neuromusculoskeletal examination and not just on the presence of neurological signs. Symptoms in the arm that seem to be consistent with a radicular or pseudoradicular syndrome, based on the clinical features of somatic dysfunction at the cervicodorsal spine, may have their origins elsewhere in the upper limb; a local cause of neural irritation in the arm must be excluded—an important theme of this text.
- **Brachial plexus/thoracic outlet syndrome:** The components of the brachial plexus may be compressed between the anterior and middle scalene muscles (the 'scalenous gap'), or under the pectoralis minor muscle, or between the clavicle and the first rib, or by compression from a cervical rib or fibrous band. See Tanner (Chapter 28) for further information.
- **Median nerve entrapment:** The median nerve may be compressed just above the elbow by an accessory ligament from the tip of a supracondylar bony spur (the ligament of Struthers). At the elbow, compression may occur as the median nerve passes between the two heads of the pronator teres muscle, by a sharp lacertus fibrosus (the broad aponeurotic expansion of the distal biceps brachii), or under the edge of the flexor digitorum superficialis (Howard 1986). Occasionally, the anterior interosseous nerve—a branch of the median nerve, arising in the proximal forearm—is traumatized, giving rise to weakness of pinch grip. The most common site of median nerve compression is at the wrist, beneath the flexor retinaculum (transverse carpal ligament), where it is universally referred to as *carpal tunnel syndrome* (CTS).

- **Ulnar nerve entrapment:** Because of its relatively exposed position, the ulnar nerve is vulnerable to compression or trauma at the elbow, either in the condylar groove (cubital tunnel) behind the medial epicondyle, or as it pierces the flexor carpi ulnaris muscle. A less common site is at the canal of Guyon at the wrist.
- **Radial nerve entrapment:** Most commonly, radial nerve compression occurs following injury, such as humeral fracture, in the upper arm. Compression injuries to the radial nerve, as it winds around the humerus, are sometimes referred to as 'Saturday night palsy'. At the elbow, compression occurs in the radial tunnel (giving rise to both motor and sensory components) at the arcade of Fröhse (the thickened superior edge of the supinator muscle) or by tightening of the fibrous edge of the extensor carpi radialis brevis (Kopell and Thompson 1963), when a motor deficit only is the consequence. Occasionally, compression of the superficial radial nerve occurs in the distal forearm, giving rise to paraesthesiae over the dorsal aspect of the base of the thumb.

As a general comment, frequent, repetitive and forceful movements of the hand, wrist, forearm, and elbow may give rise to muscle hypertrophy that has the capacity for constricting an adjacent nerve. This is the more likely with coexistent constitutional anatomical variants such as tight tunnels or fascial envelopes, resulting in a vulnerability to dynamic (in the first instance) and, subsequently, chronic (or fixed) nerve entrapment. These conditions are seen most frequently in sportsmen and in assembly workers, construction engineers, and the like.

Carpal tunnel syndrome (CTS)

CTS is the most common peripheral nerve entrapment in the upper limb, affecting the middle-aged predominantly (but with a large overlap from the 30s to over 60). It affects women more commonly than men. It is not uncommonly bilateral. The essential characteristic is compression of the median nerve at the wrist in the carpal tunnel. At one end of the spectrum of severity, in the younger age groups, it may be dynamic (and reversible). At the other end, it is refractory to management other than surgical decompression. Most cases of somewhat moderate severity are often helped by non-surgical management strategies.

The carpal tunnel is bounded to the radial side by the tuberosity of the navicular (scaphoid) bone and the trapezoid, and to the ulnar side by the pisiform bone and the hook of hamate. All but the trapezium are palpable. The musculoskeletal physician is recommended to become familiar with the surface anatomy. This is helpful when undertaking steroid injections.

At the wrist, the median nerve has both sensory and motor components, supplying the muscles of thumb opposition. The manifestations of median nerve compression in the carpal tunnel include:

- Paraesthesiae and numbness in the distribution of the median nerve in the hand (usually the thumb and adjacent 2½ fingers, although it is well recognized that this is variable, and should not be relied upon for diagnosis).
- Discomfort in the wrist and hand, often with radiation proximally to the forearm, and sometimes to the shoulder and the neck.
- More intense nocturnal symptoms. Patients commonly wake and hang their hand out of bed for relief.
- Worsening of symptoms on elevation of the hand for everyday tasks.
- Clumsiness (as a consequence of altered superficial sensation distally) for intricate finger/manual activities.
- A usually insidious onset, although it may sometimes follow trauma.

Although CTS is commonly labelled as idiopathic, there are a number of clinical conditions that reduce the space for the median nerve in the carpal tunnel and with which CTS is associated:

- rheumatoid arthritis
- non-specific tenosynovitis of the finger flexors
- pregnancy
- acromegaly
- hypothyroidism
- diabetes
- amyloidosis
- occasionally, other space-occupying lesions within the carpal tunnel, such as a ganglion.

Of these conditions, the most contentious, principally because of its (even casual) work-related connotations, is 'non-specific' flexor tendonitis. I have no doubt that this is responsible for reversible CTS, usually seen in relatively young factory workers and referred to by Braun et al. (1989) as 'dynamic' CTS. These cases, incidentally, are not necessarily seen or recognized in hand clinics that are associated with long waiting lists. It also occurs in a subgroup of the more typical, middle-aged CTS sufferers in whom chronic flexor tenosynovitis gives rise to fixed flexion contractures of the fingers (as demonstrated, on examination, by the 'prayer' sign).

Additionally, the so-called double crush syndrome (Upton and McComas 1973) may also play a role. This is not difficult to understand once the basic concepts of abnormal neurodynamics are appreciated. CTS is one cause of neural irritation in the upper limb. However, it does not take much imagination to appreciate that neural irritation in the upper limb may develop from compression at more than one site, such as at the neck or the thoracic outlet. It follows that in some patients with demonstrable CTS, symptoms are also experienced in the neck and in the upper limb. A full evaluation of the possible additional sites for neural compression in the upper limb, to identify a double crush phenomenon, should be undertaken before patients are subjected to carpal tunnel decompression.

In view of the possible dual pathology, the clinician should examine the cervicodorsal spine as well as the upper limb in patients with symptoms, however vague or diffuse, in the arm and hand. The 'specific' tests for CTS are:

- *Reproduction of symptoms* (burning, paraesthesiae, numbness in the thumb and fingers) by pressure over the volar aspect of the wrist. This is based on the same principle as the Tinel test (or sign), but I recommend that firm pressure over the volar aspect of the wrist for 30 seconds is preferable to tapping.
- *Positive Phalen's test* (Phalen 1966) undertaken bilaterally and simultaneously by holding the dorsum of the palmar-flexed wrists against each other during forward flexion at the shoulders and elbow flexion. However, this test may also be positive in the presence of neural compression proximally, and it is advisable to undertake the modified Phalen's test one arm at a time, by active

or passive palmar flexion of the wrist, with the arm in the dependent position.

- Wasting of the thenar eminence.
- Weakness of opposition of the thumb and/or abduction of the thumb.
- Blunted sensation in the distribution of the median nerve.

None of these tests offers a better than 75% sensitivity or specificity (Katz et al. 1990). Muscle wasting and muscle weakness are late signs, and it is poor medical practice to await positive clinical findings in the form of sensory blunting or muscle weakness for the diagnosis of CTS.

The 'gold standard' is often considered to be positive neurophysiological studies. Beware, however, the possibility of minor neurophysiological abnormalities without symptoms (false positive test), and negative neurophysiological findings with characteristic symptoms (particularly in the younger, dynamic, reversible case). Be aware, too, of the not uncommon association with other conditions in the upper limb, particularly at the cervical and proximal dorsal spines, that contribute to neural tension (see relevant sections). Patients who unexpectedly do not improve following carpal tunnel decompression are often considered by their medical attendants to have alternative agendas (for instance, compensation), but in fact the issue of adverse neural tension in the upper limb, and the possible contributory sites, may not have been explored.

Traditionally, allopathic medical management has been predicated on the use of night splints and decompression surgery. Patients often find that the maintenance of a flexed position of the wrist, or repetitive wrist flexion, is provocative (by further compression of the median nerve in the carpal tunnel), hence the usefulness of cock-up splints (to provide slight dorsiflexion at the wrist) at night.

I recommend the use of low-dose steroid injections (for instance 5 mg triamcinolone) to the carpal tunnel. When combined with a small amount of local anaesthetic, this management strategy has both diagnostic and therapeutic usefulness in the majority of patients. With practice, correct needle placement is not difficult. Imagine a vertical line dividing the carpal tunnel midway between the pisiform bone and the tuberosity of the navicular (more or less in the position of the palmaris longus tendon, if present); then place the needle just to the ulnar side of this line between the proximal and distal wrist creases, angulating distally and dorsally at approximately 45°. The preferred technique of injecting the ulnar aspect of this vertical dividing line avoids impinging the needle on the median nerve.

Improvement or abolition of symptoms (even if only for a few days or a few weeks) is confirmatory diagnosis of CTS. In a significant proportion of patients, approximately 50% overall, one injection successfully abolishes symptoms or reduces them to a level that is compatible with normal day-to-day activities (Dammers and Veering 1999). A minority of patients in whom the symptoms recur within a few months are helped on a long-term basis by further injections, but the law of diminishing returns usually applies, in which case surgical decompression is a reliable fall-back procedure.

The disadvantages and/or side-effects of the described management strategies are few, but they are more frequent after surgery than after non-surgical techniques. Median nerve damage has been reported after impingement by a needle, but the precaution of 'backing off' if electric shock feelings are experienced at the time of needle penetration should prevent this. CRPS (chronic regional pain syndrome) type 1 may follow carpal tunnel decompression, and it is not unusual for patients to express dissatisfaction, either because of persistence or recurrence of symptoms, tenderness of the scar, or an unsatisfactory cosmetic result. Surgery is never without the occasional hazard. Traditional osteopathic approaches include neural mobilization of the median nerve in the carpal tunnel.

Upper limb symptoms due to neural irritation are often associated with cervical spinal dysfunction and/or proximal thoracic spinal dysfunction (but without substantive loss of spinal mobility, which is sometimes referred to as a 'hard' clinical sign by many orthopaedists).

Successful treatment often requires the combination of cervical spinal mobilization, thoracic spinal mobilization, paravertebral block injections in both the neck and upper thoracic spine, advice regarding postural awareness and ergonomic improvements, neural release and stretching, and carpal tunnel injections. The clinician should not be afraid to address a complex case in this manner. A satisfactory conclusion may be obtained by spinal mobilization alone, but it is my experience that in the entrenched case, usually in factory workers, a battery of treatments is necessary, combined with ergonomic advice and (often) liaison with employers or supervisors regarding work practices.

When assessing the relationship of CTS to work, both intrinsic factors ('constitutional' narrowing of the carpal tunnel or swelling of its contents) and external factors (repetitive flexion and extension of the wrist, long periods of wrist flexion, or repetitive grasping/finger flexion as in the pinch grip) should be considered. The studies by Silverstein et al. (1987) and Wieslander et al. (1989) are often cited. Silverstein identified a significant association between forceful use of the hand and repetitive wrist motion and symptoms in the wrist and hand, but a specific diagnosis of CTS was not made in the study population. Wieslander noted that CTS is most common in workers using hand-held vibrating tools, those undertaking repetitive and/or forceful hand/wrist movements such as assembly workers, grinders, keypunch operators, musicians, and bricklayers. Feldman et al. (1987) noted an increased incidence of symptoms and signs suggestive of CTS in workers with high-risk jobs.

The increased association with exposure to vibration is generally accepted (Koskimies et al. 1990; Rosenbaum and Ochoa 1993). There are numerous (anecdotal) accounts of a sudden painful flush of paraesthesiae in the hand from the unaccustomed use of vibrating equipment, such as electric shears, with the wrist flexed. For those exposed to the use of vibrating tools on a regular basis as part of their work, CTS is accepted as an industrial injury (PD A12) in the UK. Nevertheless, it has to be distinguished from the condition of hand–arm vibration syndrome (HAVS) that may also give rise to discomfort and paraesthesiae in the hand but, critically, also has a substantive component of circulatory disruption.

Pronator syndrome

Hypertrophy of the pronator teres muscle arises from repeated forceful pronation of the forearm, often accompanied by prolonged firm finger flexion, as in assembly workers, sports such as tennis, and also in musicians (Bejjani et al. 1996). Direct trauma or compression by fibrous bands is occasionally found. Both motor and sensory deficits may result, as in CTS, but in addition, painful weakness of pronation is usually present. Most cases respond to local infiltration of steroid and local anaesthetic, failing which, surgical exploration may be necessary.

Ulnar nerve entrapment

Ulnar nerve entrapment at the elbow is the second most common peripheral nerve entrapment in the upper limb. However, at least two other possibilities should always be considered for neuritic symptoms along the ulnar border of the hand: thoracic outlet syndrome and ulnar nerve entrapment in the canal of Guyon at the wrist.

The ulnar nerve enters the forearm via the fibro-osseous cubital tunnel in the groove behind the medial epicondyle. The boundaries are the elbow joint, a fascial arcade intimately associated with the heads of the flexor carpi ulnaris, and the flexor carpi ulnaris muscles themselves. Compression by the fascial band, by muscle hypertrophy, and by osteophytic spurs in osteoarthritis are possibilities. Additionally, in evaluating the possible cause of ulnar nerve compression at the elbow, direct compression (usually repetitive in nature and work- related) should be distinguished from the more occasional and unpredictable trauma to a hypermobile ulnar nerve. (Treatment of the two conditions may be radically different.)

Paraesthesiae and numbness of the little finger and the ulnar margin of the ring finger are virtually always present. An early presentation may be a manual worker's inability to undertake intricate or repetitive tasks as competently as previously. Symptoms from ulnar nerve compression at the elbow are always experienced distally, but also sometimes proximally (when additional or alternative causes of neural dysfunction have to be considered). Progressively, hypothenar wasting becomes apparent, and in the late stages, clawing of the fingers due to weakness of the intrinsic hand muscles. Symptoms are often worse at night as the elbow is often held in the flexed position in which the ulnar nerve at the elbow is relatively taut.

Workers at risk are those who rest their elbows on a work surface to stabilize their arms for manual activities. Baseball pitchers, tennis players, and field athletes are susceptible as a consequence of valgus forces at the elbow, causing fibrosis and, in some cases, osteophytosis. Symptoms may be caused or aggravated when driving a car by resting the elbow on an inner ledge of the adjacent door. Repetitive flexion and extension of the elbow are cited as provocative activities. This is based on the fact that the ulnar nerve moves in the cubital tunnel during sagittal plane movements, becoming relatively taut in flexion.

A standard neurological examination is necessary. An early feature is weakness of the abductor digiti minimi. Sensory assessment usually reveals sensory blunting (although this part of the examination is often forgotten or deliberately ignored by many clinicians who feel that the subjective awareness of altered sensation is evidence enough of a sensory component to a neural problem). At the elbow, the ulnar nerve should be palpated for hypermobility, first in elbow flexion and then in extension, and also during the movement from flexion to extension. Tapping the ulnar nerve (a Tinel test) or compressing it digitally at the elbow may give rise to discomfort and/or paraesthesiae distally as a normal finding, but patients with ulnar nerve entrapment experience increased discomfort when compared with the normal side. Nerve conduction studies are commonly undertaken but, in many cases, this confirmatory examination is unnecessary.

A conservative approach is reasonable in early cases, particularly when there is no (or no substantive) sensorimotor deficit. This is particularly important in those patients in whom compression of the nerve during daily activities, usually working at a bench, is considered to be an aetiological factor. Liaison with employers or with an ergonomist may need to be considered in order to reduce the stresses at the elbow.

The ulnar nerve may be compressed at the wrist as it passes through the canal of Guyon, possibly by the pisohamate ligament. Trauma, as a single event or repetitively, to the region of the hamate (for instance, in golfers or cricketers) or repetitive compression at work (for instance, when using a hammer or similar tool) may be the cause. In cyclists, 'handlebar palsy' may result from prolonged compression against dropped handlebars. The deep branch of the ulnar nerve as it traverses the palm may be compressed in those workers who hold an implement or tool in or across the palm; Jones (1988) described pizza-cutter's palsy.

Entrapment of the radial nerve and posterior interosseous nerve

The radial nerve curves round the humerus in the spiral groove, piercing the lateral intermuscular septum to lie in front of the elbow. It then enters the radial tunnel, bounded medially by the brachialis muscle and anterolaterally by the brachioradialis muscle and extensor carpi radialis longus. At the distal aspect of the tunnel, it divides into a superficial branch and the deep branch—the posterior interosseous nerve.

In the radial tunnel, first described by Roles and Maudsley (1972), subsequently by Lister et al. (1979), compression may occur as a consequence of fibrous bands or arches, including the arcade of Fröhse, and by a sharp margin to the extensor carpi radialis. Compression of the radial nerve may result in mixed sensory and motor manifestations. However, when the posterior interosseous nerve is compressed (giving rise to the 'posterior interosseous nerve syndrome'), the consequences are motor only. The posterior interosseous nerve is vulnerable to compression between the two heads of the supinator muscle in those athletes and workers whose supinator is hypertrophied. In my experience, this problem occurs most commonly in workers who use relatively heavy tools such as industrial hammers and who supinate their forearms repetitively (for instance, in the tightening movement with a screwdriver), and occasionally in athletes.

Roles and Maudsley reported cases of resistant tennis elbow that were helped by surgical decompression of the radial nerve. The diagnosis of tennis elbow is far more complex than might appear to the novice clinician; the possibility of nerve compression masquerading as tennis elbow should always be considered. In my experience, when muscle hyperalgesia is found around the elbow (particularly when accompanied by more extensive regional muscle hyperalgesia), this is most likely to be the consequence of proximal nerve compression or irritation. However, an index of suspicion with respect to the radial nerve and posterior interosseous nerve at and just below the elbow should always be maintained.

Neurological examination of the upper limb, particularly a search for motor defects, is paramount. Assessment of supination and dorsiflexion of the wrist is particularly important. Lesions of the radial nerve or posterior interosseous nerve commonly give rise to weakness of supination (often a reflection of pain inhibition, when it is accompanied by discomfort on resisted contraction) and weakness of dorsiflexion of the wrist and sometimes of the finger extensors. The presence of paraesthesiae in the forearm or back of the hand suggests that the compression is occurring relatively proximally in the radial tunnel, affecting the radial nerve rather than the posterior interosseous nerve.

In the established case, ergonomic adjustments at work or technical adjustments during sporting activity (for instance, the backhand at tennis) are of prime importance. Partial relief of symptoms may be gained by intramuscular stimulation (dry needling) or injections (for instance of local anaesthetic) as the extensor muscle mass in the proximal forearm, including both the extensor carpi radialis muscles and the supinator muscle, are commonly hyperalgesic and hypertonic. Nerve conduction studies may be helpful. Surgical decompression should be considered in the established case that is refractory to conservative management.

The superficial radial nerve may be traumatized or compressed distally in the forearm. The condition is sometimes referred to as Wartenberg's syndrome. Paraesthesiae are experienced over the dorsiradial aspect of the hand; frequently in occupations that require repetitive supination and pronation and/or hyperpronation (Dellon and Mackinnon 1986), and occasionally as a consequence of over-tight splints or even handcuffs.

Neuropathic arm pain

The regional pain syndrome, commonly referred to as neuropathic arm pain (NAP), 'RSI', or type II work-related upper limb disorder (WRULD) (Hutson 1997) to distinguish it from those upper limb disorders in which there is demonstrable pathomorphology (type I WRULD), is characterized by persistent pain and dysaesthesiae. Initially experienced peripherally, often in the hand(s) or forearm(s), discomfort often extends diffusely to the shoulder, neck, and upper back. In a minority of patients it is experienced in the contralateral upper limb. Usually, the pain has a deep, burning, 'toothache' quality, sometimes accompanied by a subjective sensation of swelling and by a variable degree of numbness and tingling in the hand and/or fingers. It is commonly associated with repetitive stereotyped activities of the hands and digits, but perhaps more relevant in causation is the upper body posture that is maintained for long periods in office workers. The symptoms are often related to a particular task, for instance, the use of a keyboard or mouse or (commonly) to an intensive spell of keyboard activities.

Initially, the symptoms resolve with rest. Gradually, the symptoms become more persistent, intense, and refractory to either rest or conventional treatment. Sleep pattern is often disturbed. The discomfort becomes increasingly intrusive with respect to work and home activities. Psychological symptoms are commonly found at this stage—for instance, depression, headaches, chronic fatigue, and frustration. Not infrequently, there is a history of unsuccessful surgery for suspected tennis elbow or CTS.

The pathogenesis is evident from the acronym NAP. It has long been established that pain and altered sensation following peripheral nerve damage results from pathophysiological changes within the nervous system. The hypothesis with respect to the pathogenesis of NAP is that these pathophysiological changes within the central nervous system, and possibly in the peripheral nervous system too, are precipitated by repetitive or prolonged stresses applied to the soft tissues of the upper limb. Afferent stimulation at a consistently intense level may arise in the hands and fingers, but may also arise proximally at the shoulder girdle or at the cervicodorsal spine. The overloaded sensorineural mechanisms for pain production and perception are augmented by sensitization of the wide dynamic range (WDR) neurones situated in the dorsal horns of the spinal cord. Pain amplification develops, resulting in allodynia (reduced threshold to painful stimuli), hyperalgesia (increased response to stimuli), wind-up (increased response to repeated stimulation), hyperpathia (prolonged response to stimuli), and the expansion of receptive fields (giving rise to relatively widespread symptoms).

It may be noted from the seminal work of Cohen and associates (1992) that the clinical features are remarkably consistent. Secondary hyperalgesia, manifesting as 'regional' muscle tenderness and sometimes terminal discomfort on joint movements, is present in the majority of patients. The proximal forearm muscles, extensor and flexor, are usually tender. The proximal scapular fixator muscles are also hyperalgesic. There are usually signs of segmental dysfunction in the cervical spine or proximal thoracic spine or both. Adverse neural tension is commonly present. It is noteworthy that although it is generally recognized that adverse neural tension may be associated with cervical spinal dysfunction, it is extremely common in this group of patients for proximal thoracic spinal dysfunction (between D3 and D5) to be present. It is hypothesized that in many patients, poor work postures, associated with a proximal thoracic kyphosis and protracted shoulders, cause proximal thoracic spinal and cervical spinal dysfunction, and altered neurodynamics. The addition of repetitive stereotyped activity of the hands and fingers to the long periods of static muscle activity at the shoulder girdle overwhelm the already compromised peripheral nervous system, giving rise in vulnerable patients to neurosensitization.

Conventional investigations such as cervicodorsal spinal radiographs, nerve conduction studies, and magnetic resonance imaging (MRI) are negative with respect to nerve root or peripheral nerve compression. Occasionally, nerve conduction studies may be equivocal for CTS, leading the unsuspecting orthopaedic surgeon to undertake carpal tunnel release. Neuropathic pain, however, remains refractory to such operative intervention.

Other aetiological factors often play a role. These include psychosocial factors (such as premorbid psychological profile, environmental stresses, misattributions and beliefs, adverse posture and ergonomics, iatrogenesis, and litigation). Of these factors, iatrogenesis is often a powerful aggravating factor. Just when a patient sorely needs a knowledgeable medical practitioner in the early stages to deal with the described factors appropriately, help is not always to hand. Regrettably, the failure of the medical profession in general to recognize the early presence of neuropathic pain leads to misdiagnosis, inappropriate management, and an increasingly frustrated and despondent patient. It is not surprising that reactive depression often develops, sometimes compounded by the prescription for amitriptyline, useful in low dosages for pain relief, without an appropriate explanation of the use of a tricyclic antidepressant, thereby inculcating in the patient's mind the impression that the medical attendant believes 'it's all in the mind'.

The most appropriate management strategy is an explanation to the patient of the nature of the complaint. Attention to ergonomics and work environment in general is required, if this has not already been undertaken. My preferred tricyclic is amitriptyline, commencing at 10–20 mg at night, gradually increasing in dose by titrating against tolerance and efficacy. Manual treatment includes neural stretching and treatment for spinal dysfunction. In my experience, spinal mobilization alone is insufficient. Localized paravertebral block injections of low-dose steroid and local anaesthetic to the appropriate cervical spinal or proximal thoracic spinal segments are often helpful. If necessary, follow-up treatment by prolotherapy (see Chapters 24 and 25) is helpful. A pragmatic approach incorporating most if not all of these modalities, combined with reduction of provocative physical stresses, yields the best results. For patients with established neuropathic arm pain, I have found that the most effective interventional therapy is the combination of neural blocks and neural mobilization (Hutson 1997).

Medial epicondylalgia (epicondylitis)

Medial epicondylalgia ('golfer's elbow') is a tendinopathy (or 'enthesopathy') that affects the common flexor origin at the medial epicondyle of the humerus. It gives rise to medial elbow discomfort, sometimes radiating to the volar and ulnar aspects of the forearm. It is less common than lateral epicondylalgia. It affects primarily the middle-aged and, in particular, those engaged in work or sport that involves repetitive forceful grasping and pronation of the forearm. Hence, it occurs in right-handed golfers with a 'strong' right hand: uncocking the wrist before ball contact is associated with greater pronation than is the case with a 'weak' grip on the club. (Right-handed golfers tend to experience medial epicondylalgia of the right elbow or lateral epicondylalgia of the left elbow.)

As the name of the condition (medial epicondylalgia) suggests, pathological changes may occur at the tendons attached to the medial epicondyle. These changes have been confirmed by the work of Nirschl (1986). The pronator teres muscle and the flexor carpi radialis are the principal muscles involved. Of these, it would appear to be the pronator teres that is the more important aetiologically. This is borne out by the clinical observation that resisted pronation is painful and weak, more so than resisted wrist or finger flexion, in these patients. Patients usually complain of medial elbow tenderness in addition to discomfort on manual activities.

Examination reveals a full range of movements at the elbow. There is rarely any significant swelling. Tenderness is localized to the teno-osseous junction, maximal 1 cm distal to the tip of the medial epicondyle. Resisted pronation is painful and associated with variable degrees of weakness on resisted contraction. There is rarely weakness of other muscle groups. Should weakness be apparent of the muscles used in the pinch grip (the muscles of flexion and opposition of the thumb, and flexion of the index finger), the *pronator syndrome* should be suspected. In this condition, the median nerve is compressed during its passage through the pronator teres muscle. (According to Bejjani et al. 1996, musicians are a particularly vulnerable group as a consequence of frequent repetitive pronation of the forearm.) In a relatively straightforward case of medial epicondylalgia, there are no neuritic symptoms. Movements at the elbow and wrist are normal, although stretching the common flexor/pronator origin by the combination of passive extension of the elbow, supination of the forearm, and dorsiflexion of the wrist evokes medial elbow discomfort.

Management is much the same as for lateral epicondylalgia (see the following section). Although a low-dose steroid injection is expected to be symptomatically beneficial, a relapse of the condition is frequently found unless appropriate advice is given with respect to reduction of biomechanical loading of the common flexor origin. Tennis players with a 'wristy' (heavy top-spin) forehand usually benefit from an adjustment to their technique. Similarly, golfers often need to weaken their grip on the club. Factory workers, for instance those on assembly lines, often benefit from an ergonomic assessment, particularly with respect to the use of tools. Physiotherapy gives modest returns. Medial elbow pain that is refractory to conventional treatment may be a manifestation of secondary hyperalgesia. A neurogenic aetiology is always a possibility in patients with elbow and forearm pain; hence the need for a comprehensive cervicodorsal spinal evaluation and an assessment of upper limb neurodynamics in all patients. Indications that abnormal neurodynamics are playing a significant role are:

- the coexistence of medial and lateral elbow pain
- bilaterality of symptoms
- relatively widespread upper limb symptoms and hyperalgesia, particularly the presence of hyperalgesia of the proximal scapular fixator muscles and adverse neural tension
- an adverse upper body posture, particularly protracted shoulders.

Lateral epicondylalgia (by Michael Yelland and David Rabago)

Epidemiology

Lateral epicondylalgia (LE), also known as tennis elbow, is a common overuse tendinopathy primarily of the extensor carpi radialis brevis at its proximal insertion, with pain experienced over the lateral epicondyle (Allander 1974; Hamilton 1986). It is characterized by muscle weakness, decreased upper extremity function, and decreased quality of life (Macdermid 2005; Newcomer et al. 2005; Smidt et al. 2003) resulting in compromised daily living, sport, and work activities. The prevalence of LE is approximately 3% in the general population, (Allander 1974; Bot et al. 2005; Walker-Bone et al. 2004), 7% among 40–50 year-olds (Linaker et al. 1999), and as high as 30% in some occupational groups (Bernard 1997). Age is a risk factor (Werner et al. 2005). The condition has a natural time course of 6 to 48 months, but up to 10% of patients develop chronic symptoms that are recalcitrant to conservative management and undergo surgical intervention (Coonrad and Hooper 1973; Nirschl and Pettrone 1979). Due to its high prevalence in the workplace, the overall economic impact of LE is high (Silverstein et al. 2002).

Pathology

LE is an overuse tendinopathy characterized by local tendon pathology and pain and motor system dysfunction (Riley 2007). Such local tendon pathology includes failure of normal tissue healing and loss of normal homeostasis of collagen remodelling in response to repeated injury (Kraushaar and Nirschl 1999; Riley 2007). Histopathological changes include collagen and mucoid degeneration. Ultrasound studies indicate a strong association between LE and neovascularity and several structural changes, including thickening of the common extensor tendon, focal hypoechoic tendon regions, linear intrasubstance tears, intratendinous calcification, diffuse heterogeneity, and peritendinous fluid (Levin et al. 2005). Changes in biomechanical characteristics, including pain-free grip strength, rate of force development, and electromechanical delay, are associated with the diagnosis of LE but not with the self- reported clinical severity of disease.

Historically, the term most commonly used for lateral elbow pain is 'lateral epicondylitis', reflecting the deeply ingrained belief that LE is an inflammatory condition. This view extends to most other chronic tendinopathies, but the pathophysiological model for tendinopathy has evolved over time (Rees et al. 2013). 'Tendinitis' was the common term used before the 1990s, as it was purported that inflammation was responsible for the pain and disability, leading to treatments for tendinopathy being predominantly anti-inflammatory in nature.

In the 1990s, this view was challenged by the results of several studies that noted the absence of inflammatory cell infiltrates and the presence of the degenerative changes of collagen separation, thinning, and disruption, consistent with degeneration. There was a gradual shift in thinking towards tissue degeneration as the prime pathology. By the 2000s, the paradigm had shifted to tendinosis, as signalled by a landmark 2002 editorial by tendinopathy content leaders in the *British Medical Journal* entitled 'Time to abandon the "tendinitis" myth' (Khan et al. 2002). These 'degenerative' models have led to attempts to improve treatment and rehabilitation of the failing tendon with physical exercise regimes that load the tendon and injection treatments that stimulate healing through inflammation and growth factors or simply try to reduce the pain associated with tendinopathy.

The 'tendinosis' paradigm may have become as deeply ingrained in the recent medical literature as the original 'tendinitis' concept was in older literature. However, subsequent research based on advances in immunohistochemistry and gene expression analysis suggests that the degenerative/tendinosis model may be oversimplified. Tenocyte hyperplasia and hypertrophy provide indirect evidence of up-regulated inflammatory mediators. It is likely that elements of the inflammatory response play a role in the progression or continuation of tendon disrepair. The neovascularization that is commonly associated with tendinosis involves elements of the inflammatory response, including stimulation by substance P, COX-1, and COX-2. Other biochemical mediators of the development and progression of chronic tendinopathy include the matrix metalloprotineases and calcitonin gene-related peptide (CGRP).

Clinical features

The pain of lateral epicondylalgia, as the name suggests, is experienced at the lateral elbow in the region of the lateral epicondyle. Often there is an associated ache in the muscle bellies of the wrist extensors distal to this. Although the patient may recall a particular incident, such as a blow to the lateral elbow, as the inciting cause, most commonly, the pain is of insidious onset and may be associated with recent increases in occupational or sporting activities. Typically, patients report increased pain with gripping and with lifting light or heavy objects with the forearm pronated or in the neutral position (Tosti et al. 2013). Symptoms are generally worse with the elbow extended and better with the elbow flexed and the forearm supinated.

LE remains a clinical diagnosis. The cardinal features on examination include reproduction of the pain with gripping and an associated reduction in grip strength (Boyer and Hastings 1999; Tosti 2013). There is pain with resisted extension of the wrist with the elbow extended. This test is best done by resisting extension of the middle finger or third metacarpal as the extensor carpi radialis brevis tendon inserts into the base of the third metacarpal. Resisted supination of the elbow may also be painful. There may be some terminal resistance with passive extension of the elbow, but normal elbow flexion. Passive stretching of the common extensor origin may be painful. Tenderness should be elicited just distal and anterior to the lateral epicondyle. Other potential sites of tenderness include the lateral supracondylar ridge, over the annular and radial collateral ligaments related to the radial head, and the muscle bellies of the wrist extensors just distal to these ligaments. Few data speak of the reliability and validity of these clinical features (Cleland et al. 2010).

Differential diagnosis

Other elbow pathologies in the differential diagnosis of elbow pain include chondral lesions and intra-articular loose bodies, both suggested by clicking or limitation of range of motion of the elbow. The presence of a joint effusion suggests consideration of avascular necrosis and osteochondritis dissecans or an inflammatory arthropathy (Tosti et al. 2013).

Examination of the shoulder should be performed for conditions that may refer pain to the elbow. Likewise, neck examination is indicated for sources of somatic referred pain or radicular pain that may compound the assessment. Allodynia or marked hyperalgesia over the lateral elbow should invite consideration of neuropathic pain from a cervical nerve root or the radial nerve (Hutson 2006). Pain and tenderness well distal to the lateral epicondyle over the common extensor bellies, rather than near the lateral epicondlyle, suggests compression of the posterior interosseous nerve in the radial tunnel (Boyer and Hastings 1999).

The baseline association between LE and regional pain syndromes has been reported. However, potential mechanistic relationships between the two, and potential treatment that addresses both conditions, have not been studied.

Investigations

If the clinical features are typical of LE, radiological investigations are not required. They may be obtained when atypical features of the examination suggest an alternative diagnosis (Tosti et al. 2013). Nonetheless, if performed, X-rays may show soft tissue calcification in the common extensor origin. Magnetic and ultrasound imaging of tendinopathic tissue may show tendon thickening and collagen disruption, mucoid degeneration, partial and full thickness tendon tears and neovascularization, and assessment of biomechanical markers have all been associated with baseline LE. However, definitive correlation between the severity of these changes and the clinical severity measured by the Patient-Rated Tennis Elbow Evaluation (Chourasia et al. 2013) has not been reported, and clinical improvement in response to treatment has not been clearly associated with improvement in radiological abnormalities (Chourasia et al. 2013; Rabago et al. 2009, 2010).

Nerve conduction studies may have a role when cervical radicular pain and the radial tunnel syndrome are suspected. An assessment of the pain pressure threshold of the lateral elbow and of pain-free grip strength, often used as outcomes in research studies, may have a role in monitoring the progress of treatment.

Management

Management of LE begins with education about the pathology and natural history of the condition. A discussion about aggravating and relieving movements and postures may be helpful in planning modification of activities while the condition gradually resolves;

simple suggestions to limit LE pain can include picking up objects with the palm facing upwards, workstation modifications to reduce wrist extension, and preferential use of the unaffected arm (see Box 33.1).

The results of numerous negative or equivocal studies of treatment for LE may lead the clinician to wonder if any are effective; active therapies have generally been found to be no better in the long term than watchful waiting. The data is often of limited quality, as existing studies frequently suffer from inadequate sample size; inconsistency of diagnostic criteria, treatment protocols, and outcome measures; and short (less than 6 months) follow-up. Key issues, such as quality of life, the cost and benefit of various therapies, and work-related impacts are relatively unstudied. Very few studies compare a given intervention with either watchful waiting or physical therapy designed specifically for epicondylosis. While better research is sorely needed, recommendations based on clinical experience, clinical trial data, and meta-analyses (Bisset et al. 2005; Buchbinder et al. 2011; Coombes et al. 2010) provide some guidance.

Elbow bracing, taping, and relative rest are commonly used and have intuitive appeal; their use addresses the current understanding of LE as an overuse injury by resting the damaged tissue. Among physical interventions, eccentric exercise may improve pain but not maximum grip strength (Pienimaki et al. 1996). Positive initial effects for elbow manipulative therapy techniques have been reported but there are no long-term studies showing the durability of this effect. These modalities may have short-term benefits on pain and grip strength, but there are no long-term studies that support their use, particularly in severe cases.

Non-steroidal anti-inflammatory drugs (NSAIDs) are often used and target the potential inflammatory process thought to play a role in the early stage of LE; though as noted, the role of inflammation is not clear. While oral NSAIDS have not been found to be better than either placebo or comparison treatment (Bissett et al. 2011), a systematic review of the use of topical NSAIDs (diclofenac and benzydamine) reported that pain was significantly improved after 4 weeks' use compared with placebo (Green et al. 2001).

Acupuncture offers significant short-term benefits over placebo, which wane after 2 months (Trinh et al. 2004). Low-level laser therapy at the optimal doses of 904 nm and possibly 632 nm wavelengths gives short-term pain relief and reduced disability, both alone and together with an exercise regimen (Bjordal et al. 2008).

There seems to be no benefit from extracorporeal shockwave therapy, which may even confer a higher rate of short-term adverse events (Buchbinder et al. 2005). Electromagnetic field therapy is not supported by strong evidence supporting its efficacy, and iontophorsesis has shown positive long-term results in only one trial and so needs further research. There are some early indications that therapeutic ultrasound is better than placebo for pain but not for grip strength or global improvement at 3 months; adding transverse friction massage or hydrocortisone coupling gel has not been shown to add benefit (Bisset et al. 2005).

There are early suggestions that combination therapies may be better than monotherapies. A combined programme of massage, ultrasound, and exercises is somewhat better than control therapy at 6 weeks and 12 months, and better than steroid injections at 12 months (Smidt et al. 2003). There were similar findings in a later study showing that physiotherapy combining elbow manipulation and exercise was superior to 'wait and see' in the first 6 weeks and to corticosteroid injections after 6 weeks. Corticosteroid injections were superior to both other approaches at 6 weeks but, paradoxically, had higher recurrence rates at 12 months (Bisset et al. 2006). Combining the physiotherapy/exercise programme with the corticosteroid injections does not seem to alter the effect of the corticosteroids (Coombes et al. 2013).

These findings have been reflected more broadly in a meta-analysis of trials using corticosteroid injections showing a superior reduction in pain scores in the short term (0–12 weeks) compared with other interventions but an overall negative effect in the intermediate (13–26 weeks) and long term (≥52 weeks) (Coombes et al. 2010). In contrast, injections of sodium hyaluronate show both good short-, intermediate-, and long-term results. Injections of botulinum toxin have evidence for good short-term results. Placebo-controlled trials on arteparon injections and on aprotinin injections have been negative.

Two injection therapies directly address the hypothesis that tendinopathic pain and functional loss result from degenerative effects (Rabago et al. 2009). Several recent trials have assessed the use of platelet-rich plasma injections for LE, but high-quality research on this treatment is still emerging. The strongest published randomized controlled trial (RCT) compares it with corticosteroid injections and, similar to trials of other treatments, shows it to be inferior to corticosteroids in the short term and superior in the intermediate and long term (Peerbooms et al. 2010). A similar trial with an additional arm with saline control injections is under way (Buchbinder et al. 2013).

Two RCTs assessing prolotherapy injections of hypertonic d-glucose (dextrose) and combined d-glucose/morrhuate sodium report good intermediate-term results compared to control or watchful waiting. However, these were pilot-level efforts with small sample sizes (Rabago et al. 2013; Scarpone et al. 2008). D-glucose remains the most commonly used prolotherapy solution as morrhuate sodium is difficult to procure and no longer in active production; a larger, more rigorous clinical trial on d-glucose injections is still in progress.

Due to the relatively small amount and poor quality of research on surgical interventions for lateral elbow pain, there is insufficient evidence to support or refute its effectiveness (Buchbinder et al. 2011).

Appropriate and comprehensive treatment of patients with risk factors for LE and with early and refractory LE involves an appreciation and application of a broad range of prevention and treatment strategies (Box 33.1).

Upon making the diagnosis, we begin with education about the condition and its prognosis. We establish a time course for healing; most patients recover in weeks to months, but up to 20% may take up to a year or longer. Patients are advised on the symptom prevention strategies. We avoid steroid injections in almost all circumstances; in the recent past, we have injected musicians with LE who have upcoming concert dates, and have advised them on the potential for long-term worsening compared to waiting or other strategies. If possible, patients are advised on relative and complete avoidance of exacerbating activity and use of a simple wrist splint. We will write limited work-release excuses for this. Topical NSAIDS can be used if early (less than 4–6 weeks) in the time course.

Patients who are refractory to such conservative care are then referred for mobilization with movement and a concentric/eccentric exercise programme. Acupuncture can be used at this treatment

Box 33.1 Preferred management strategy for lateral epicondylalgia

Patients present to our primary care clinic with a variety of predisposing risk factors for LE and a varied degree of disease severity. The ideal management involves never getting LE to begin with; therefore, risk assessment is appropriate and the following guidelines apply.

Prevention

Physicians can make the following patient-specific general recommendations for a healthy lifestyle and LE risk reduction among patients with professions or sporting activities associated with increased risk of LE or in patients who have recovered from prior LE. These steps, individually or in concert, may also reduce symptoms of active LE but have not been rigorously assessed:

General

- Smoking cessation
- Stress reduction

Avoidance of exacerbating activities

- Reduce or avoid the lifting of objects with the arm extended
- Reduce repetitive gripping
- Decrease overall tension of gripping
- Avoid extremes of bending and full extension
- Work or train with the elbow in a partially flexed position
- Use wrist supports when weight-training
- Enlarge the gripping surface of tools or rackets with gloves or padding, use a hammer with extra padding to reduce tensions and impact, and hold heavy tools with two hands

Ergonomic evaluation

Evaluate repetitive motion activity, duties, equipment, and techniques, especially in work situations. Information on ergonomic evaluation of computer, laboratory, and industrial settings is available through the Centers of Disease Control at: <http://www.cdc.gov/ od/ohs/Ergonomics/ergohome>.

Exercise

Stretching and strengthening exercises once daily, along with frequent periods of short rest.

Treatment

Many of the techniques described under 'Prevention' also offload affected tendons and may assist tissue healing.

stage but has only been found effective for relatively short-term pain relief (Bissett et al. 2011).

Patients in our medical system who fail active use of the described treatment may be candidates for injection therapy, including prolotherapy and PRP injection, intended to directly affect degenerative tissue. Decision making is often influenced by financial issues since neither is typically covered by third-party payers. Both are supported by some high- quality RCTs that they may safely improve the symptoms and functional loss associated with LE in carefully selected patients with refractory LE.

Rarely, referral for surgical evaluation is made for the very small number of patients refractory to these more conservative modalities.

References

Allander, E. (1974) Prevalence, incidence and remission rates of some common rheumatic diseases or syndromes. *Scand J Rheum* 3, 145–53.

Bejjani, F. J., Kaye, G. M., Benham, M. (1996) Musculoskeletal and neuromuscular conditions of instrumental musicians. *Arch Phys Med Rehabil* 77, 406–13.

Bernard, B.P. (1997) *Musculoskeletal disorders and workplace fractures: a critical review of the epidemiological evidence for work-related musculoskeletal disorders of the neck, upper extremity and low back. NIOSH Publication 97-141.* Washington D.C.: National Institute for Occupational Safety and Health.

Bisset, L., Beller, E., Jull, G., Brooks, P., Darnell, R., Vicenzino, B. (2006) Mobilisation with movement and exercise, corticosteroid injection, or wait and see for tennis elbow: randomised trial. *BMJ* 333(7575), 939.

Bisset, L., Coombes, B., Vicenzino, B. (2011) Tennis elbow. *Clin Evid (Online).* 27 Jun 2011, pii, 1117.

Bisset, L., Paungmali, A., Vicenzino, B., Beller, E. (2005) A systematic review and meta-analysis of clinical trials on physical interventions for lateral epicondylalgia. *Br J Sports Med* 39(7), 411–22, discussion-22.

Bjordal, J. M., Lopes-Martins, R. A., Joensen, J., et al. (2008) A systematic review with procedural assessments and meta-analysis of low level laser therapy in lateral elbow tendinopathy (tennis elbow). *BMC Musculoskelet Disord*, 9, 75, doi: 10.1186/1471-2474-9-75.

Bonnici, A. V., Spencer, J. D. (1988) A survey of trigger finger in adults. *J. Hand Surg*, 13B, 202–3.

Bot, S. D. M., et al. (2005) Incidence and prevalence of complaints of the neck and upper extremity in general practice. *Ann Rheum Dis*, 64, 118–23.

Boyer, M. I., Hastings, H. II. (1999) Lateral tennis elbow: 'Is there any science out there?'. *J Shoulder Elbow Surg*, 8(5), 481–91.

Braun, R. M., Davidson, K., Doehr, S. (1989) Provocative testing in the diagnosis of dynamic carpal tunnel syndrome. *J Hand Surg*, 14A, 195–7.

Buchbinder, R., et al. (2013) *Comparative effectiveness of ultrasound-guided injection with either autologous platelet rich plasma or glucocorticoid for ultrasound-proven lateral epicondylitis: a three-arm randomised placebo-controlled trial. ACTRN12613000616774.* Available at: <http://www.anzctr.org.au/TrialSearch.aspx> (Accessed 29/11/13)

Buchbinder, R., Green, S., Youd, J. M., Assendelft, W. J. J., Barnsley, L., Smidt, N. (2005) Shock wave therapy for lateral elbow pain. *Cochrane Database Sys Rev*, 4, CD003524, doi: 10.1002/14651858.CD003524.pub2.

Buchbinder, R., Johnston, R. V., Barnsley, L., Assendelft, W. J. J., Bell, S. N., Smidt, N. (2011) Surgery for lateral elbow pain. *Cochrane Database Sys Rev*, 3, CD003525, doi: 10.1002/14651858.CD003525.pub2.

Chourasia, A. O., Buhr, K. A., Rabago, D. P., et al. (2013) Relationships between biomechanics, tendon pathology, and function in individuals with lateral epicondylosis. *J Orthop Sports Phys Ther* 43(6),368–78.

Cleland, J., Koppenhauer, S. (2010) Netter's orthopaedic clinical examination: an evidence-based approach. Saunders, Elsevier.

Cohen, M. L., Arroyo, J. F., Champion, G. D., Browne, C. D. (1992) In search of the pathogenesis of refractory cervicobrachial pain syndrome. *Med J Aust* 156, 432–6.

Coombes, B. K., Bisset, L., Brooks, P., Khan, A., Vicenzino, B. (2013) Effect of corticosteroid injection, physiotherapy, or both on clinical outcomes in patients with unilateral lateral epicondylalgia: a randomized controlled trial. *JAMA* 309(5), 461–9.

Coombes, B. K., Bisset, L., Vicenzino, B. (2010) Efficacy and safety of corticosteroid injections and other injections for management of tendinopathy: a systematic review of randomised controlled trials. *Lancet* 376(9754), 1751–67.

Coonrad, R., Hooper, W. (1973) Tennis elbow: its course, natural history, conservative and surgical management. *J Bone Joint Surg Am* 55, 1177–82.

Dammers, J. W. H. H., Veering, M. (1999) Injection with methylprednisolone proximal to the carpal tunnel. *BMJ* 319, 884–6.

Dellon, A. L., Mackinnon, S. E. (1986) Radial sensory nerve entrapment in the forearm. *J Hand Surg* 11A, 199–205.

Dums, F. (1896) Uber trommlerlahmungen. *Deutsch Militarztliche Zeitschr* 25, 144–55.

Dupuytren, Baron G. (1834) Permanent retraction of the fingers, produced by an affection of the palmar fascia. *Lancet* ii, 222–5.

Feinstein, B., Langton, J. N. K., Jameson, R. M., et al. (1954) Experiments on pain referred from deep somatic tissues. *J Bone Joint Surg* 36A, 981–97.

Feldman, R. G., Travers, P. H., Chirico-Post, J., et al. (1987) Risk assessment in electronic assembly workers: carpal tunnel syndrome. *J Hand Surg* 12A, 849–55.

Green, S., Buchbinder, R., Barnsley, L., et al. (2001) Non-steroidal anti-inflammatory drugs (NSAIDS) for treating lateral elbow pain in adults. *Cochrane Database Syst Rev* 4, CD003686.

Greening, J., Smart, S., Leary, R., Hall-Craggs, M., O'Higgins, P., Lynn, B. (1999) Reduced movement of median nerve in carpal tunnel during wrist flexion in patients with non-specific arm pain. *Lancet* 354, 217–8.

Hamilton, P. G. (1986) The prevalence of humeral epicondylitis: a survey in general practice. *J Roy Coll Gen Pract* 36(291), 464–5.

Harvey, F. J., Harvey, P. M., Horsley, M. W. (1990) de Quervain's disease: surgical or non-surgical treatment. *J Hand Surg* 15A, 83–7.

Hooper, G., McMaster, M. J. (1979) Stenosing tenovaginitis affecting the tendon of extensor digiti minimi at the wrist. *Hand* 11, 29–301.

Howard, F. M. (1986) Controversies in nerve entrapment syndromes in the forearm and wrist. *Orthop Clin North Am* 17(3), 375–81.

Hutson, M. A. (1997) *Work-related upper limb disorders: recognition and management*. Oxford: Butterworth-Heinemann.

Hutson, M. A. (2001) *Sports injuries: recognition and management* (3rd edn). Oxford: Oxford University Press.

Hutson, M. A. (2006) Upper limb disorders. In: Hutson, M. A., Ellis, R. (eds). Textbook of musculoskeletal medicine. Oxford: Oxford University Press.

Jones, H. R. (1988) Pizza-cutters's palsy (letter). *N Engl J Med* 319, 410.

Katz, J. N., Larson, M. G., Sabra, A., et al. (1990) The carpal tunnel syndrome: diagnostic utility of the history and physical examination findings. *Ann Intern Med* 112, 321–7.

Kellgren, J. H. (1939) On the description of pain arising from deep somatic structures with charts of segmental pain areas. *Clin Sci* 4, 35–46.

Khan, K. M., Cook, J. L., Kannus, P., Maffulli, N., Bonar, S. F. (2002) Time to abandon the 'tendinitis' myth. *BMJ* 324(7338), 626–7.

Kiefhaber, T. R., Stern, P. J. (1992) Upper extremity tendinitis and overuse syndromes in the athlete. *Clin Sports Med* 11(1), 39–55.

Kopell, H. P., Thompson, W. A. L. (1963) *Peripheral entrapment neuropathies*. Baltimore, MD: Williams & Wilkins.

Koskimies, K., Farkkila, M., Pyykko, J., et al. (1990) Carpal tunnel syndrome in vibration disease. *Br J Industr Med* 47, 411–6.

Kraushaar, B. S., Nirschl, R. P. (1999) Tendinitis of the elbow (tennis elbow). Clinical features of histological, immunohistological, and electron microscopy studies. *J Bone Joint Surg* 81-A, 269–78.

Leao, L. (1958) de Quervain's disease: a clinical and anatomical study. *J. Bone Joint Surg.*, 40A(5), 1063–70.

Levin, D., Nazarian, L. N., Miller, T. T., et al. (2005) Lateral epicondlyitis of the elbow: US findings. *Radiology* 237, 230–4.

Linaker, C. H., et al. (1999) Frequency and impact of regional musculoskeletal disorders. *Best Pract Res Clin Rheumatol* 13(2), 197–215.

Lister, G. D., Belsole, R. B., Kleinert, H. E. (1979) The radial tunnel syndrome. *J Hand J* 4A, 52–9.

Macdermid, J. (2005) Update: the Patient-rated Forearm Evaluation Questionnaire is now the Patient-rated Tennis Elbow Evaluation. *J Hand Ther* 18(4), 407–10.

Marks, M. R., Gunther, S. F. (1989) Efficacy of cortisone treatment in treatment of trigger fingers and thumbs. *J. Hand Surg* 14A, 722–7.

Mennell, J. McM., Zohn, D. A. (1976) *Diagnosis and physical treatment: musculoskeletal pain*. Boston, MA: Little, Brown.

Mitchell, S., Cooper, C., Martyn, C., Coggon, D. (2000) Sensory neural processing in work-related upper limb disorders. *Occup Med* 50(1), 30–2.

Nelson, C. L., Sawmiller, S., Phalen, G. S. (1972) Ganglions of the wrist and hand. *J Bone J Surg* 54A, 1459–64.

Newcomer, K. L., et al. (2005) Sensitivity of the Patient-rated Forearm Evaluation Questionnaire in lateral epicondylitis. *J Hand Ther* 18(4), 400–6.

Nirschl, R. P. (1986) Soft-tissue injuries about the elbow. *Clin Sports Med* 5(4), 637–52.

Nirschl, R., Pettrone, F. (1979) Tennis elbow: the surgical treatment of lateral epicondylitis. *J Bone Joint Surg Am* 61-A(6), 832–9.

Noble, J., Arafa, M., Royle, S. G., McGeorge, G., Crank, S. (1992) The association between alcohol, hepatic pathology and Dupuytren's disease. *J Hand Surg* 17B, 71–4.

Peerbooms, J. C., Sluimer, J., Bruijn, D. J., Gosens, T. (2010) Positive effect of an autologous platelet concentrate in lateral epicondylitis in a double-blind randomized controlled trial: platelet-rich plasma versus corticosteroid injection with a 1-year follow-up. *Am J Sports Med* 38(2), 255.

Phalen, G. S. (1966) The carpal-tunnel syndrome—seventeen year's experience in diagnosis and treatment of six hundred and fifty-four hands. *J Bone Joint Surg* 48A, 211–28.

Pienimaki, T., Tarvainen, T., Siira, P., et al. (1996) Progressive strengthening and stretching exercises and ultrasound for chronic lateral epicondylitis. *Physiotherapy* 82, 522.

Rabago, D., Best, T. M., Zgierska, A., Zeisig, E., Ryan, M., Crane, D. (2009) A systematic review of four injection therapies for lateral epicondylosis: prolotherapy, polidocanol, whole blood and platelet rich plasma. *BJSM* 43, 471–81.

Rabago, D., Kijowski, R. X., Zgierska, A., Yelland, M., Scarpone, M. A. (2010) Magnetic resonance imaging outcomes in a randomized controlled trial of prolotherapy for lateral epicondylosis. *Int Musculo Med* 32(3), 117–23(7).

Rabago, D., Lee, K. S., Ryan, M., et al. (2013) Hypertonic dextrose and morrhuate sodium injections (prolotherapy) for lateral epicondylosis (tennis elbow): results of a single-blind, pilot-level randomized controlled trial. *Am J Phys Med Rehab* 92(7), 587–96.

Rees, J. D., Stride, M., Scott, A. (2013) 47,9 e2 Tendons—time to revisit inflammation. *Br J Sports Med.*

Riley, G. (2007) Tendinopathy—from basic science to treatment. *Nat Clin Pract Rheum* 4(2), 82–9.

Roles, N. C., Maudsley, R. H. (1972) Radial tunnel syndrome: resistant tennis elbow as a nerve entrapment. *J Bone Joint Surg* 54B(3), 499–508.

Rosenbaum, R. B., Ochoa, J. L. (1993) *Carpal tunnel syndrome and other disorders of the median nerve*. Stoneham, MA: Butterworth-Heinemann, pp. 233–49.

Scarpone, M., Rabago, D., Arbogest, J., Snell, E., Zgierska, A. (2008) The efficacy of prolotherapy for lateral epicondylosis: a pilot study. *Clin J Sports Med* 18, 248–54.

Silverstein, B. A., Fine, L. J., Armstrong, T. J. (1987) Occupational factors and carpal tunnel syndrome. *Am J Ind Med* 11, 343–58.

Silverstein, B., ViikariJuntura, E., Kalat, J. (2002) Use of a prevention index to identify industries at high risk for work-related musculoskeletal disorders of the neck, back and upper extremity. *Am J Ind Med* 41, 149–69.

Slipman, C. W., Plastaras, C. T., Palmitier, R. A., Huston, C. W., Sterenfeld, E. B. (1998) Symptom provocation of fluoroscopically guided cervical nerve root stimulation: are dynatomal maps identical to dermatomal maps? *Spine* 23(20), 2235–42.

Smidt, N., et al. (2003) Effectiveness of physiotherapy for lateral epicondylitis: a systematic review. *Ann Med* 35(1), 51–62.

Thompson, A. R., Plewes, L. W., Shaw, E. G. (1951) Peritendinitis crepitans and simple tenosynovitis: a clinical study of 544 cases in industry. *Br J Ind Med* 8, 150–8.

Tillaux, P. (1892) *Traité d'anatomie topographique. Avec applications à la chirugie* (7th edn). Paris: Asselin et Houzeau.

Tosti, R., Jennings, J., Sewards, J. M. (2013) Lateral epicondylitis of the elbow. *Am J Med* 126(4), 357 e1–6.

Troell, A. (1918) Uber die sogenannte tendovaginitis crepitans. *Dtsch Z Chir* 143, 125–62.

Upton, A. R. M., McComas, A. J. (1973) The double crush in nerve-entrapment syndromes. *Lancet* ii, 359–62.

Varley, G. W., Needoff, M., Davis, T. R. C., Clay, N. R. (1997) Conservative management of wrist ganglia. *J Hand Surg* 22B(5), 636–7.

Velpeau, A. (1841) Crepitation douloureuse des tendons. Article 2, *Leçons orales de clinique chirurgicale a l'Hôpital de la Charité, vol. 3*. Paris: Gernser-Baillière; p. 94.

Walker-Bone, K., et al. (2004) Prevalence and impact of musculoskeletal disorders of the upper limb in the general population. *Arth Care Res* 51(4), 642–51.

Werner, R. A., Franzblau, A., Gell, N., Hartigan, A., Ebersole, M., Armstrong, T. J. (2005) Predictors of persistent elbow tendonitis among auto assembly workers. *J Occup Rehab* 15, 393–400.

Wieslander, G., Norback, D., Gothe, C-J., Juhlin, L. (1989) Carpal tunnel syndrome and exposure to vibration, repetitive wrist movements, and heavy manual work: a case referent study. *Br J Ind Med* 46, 43–7.

Chapter 34

The pelvis

Michael Hutson and Bryan English

This chapter, written by Michael Hutson and Bryan English, is based on a chapter written by Malcolm Read for the first edition of the *Textbook of Musculoskeletal Medicine*. We are very grateful to Malcolm, who is now retired, for being able to update the chapter.

Introduction to the pelvis

The pelvis is formed from the sacrum and two innominate bones, the innominate being a composite of the ilium, ischium, and pubis, which fuse in the region of the acetabulum. Apart from protecting the viscera and providing attachment for muscles, the pelvis transmits the weight of the body from the vertebrae through the sacrum and onto the femora when standing, or the ischia when sitting. The sacrum forms an auricular L-shaped joint with the two iliac bones (Figure 34.1). This sacroiliac joint is a diarthrodial joint because it contains synovial fluid and has matching articular surfaces. However, it is different from all other joints in the body because the ilial surface has fibrocartilage that articulates with the hyaline cartilage of the sacrum. The joint is synovial on its anterior aspect and fibrous on its posterior aspect.

The sacroiliac joints (SIJs) are capable of a nutational or nodding movement in the anteroposterior plane, but this movement is small and is limited by the ridges and depressions which produce a rough surface that locks the joint into a stable position that will allow the transmission of impact forces from the leg to the body, and support the body weight. The anterior, posterior, and interosseous ligaments are associated functionally with the sacrotuberous and sacrospinous ligaments (Figure 34.2) and the fascia of the gluteals and hamstrings, producing a linked stabilizing system. The anterior aspect of the pelvic ring is formed from the pubic bones on both sides meeting at the pubic symphysis. This joint is an ovoid synovial joint with strong ligaments forming the arcuate ligament inferiorly. The fascia over the adductors is contiguous with the abdominal fascia and it is this anatomical continuity, and the continuity of the gluteals and hamstrings with the sacrotuberous and sacrospinous ligaments and gluteal fascia, that produce diagnostically challenging disorders from the spine and hamstrings, and anteriorly, the groin strain and adductor tear.

This diagnostic conundrum is further complicated by referred pain from the discs, facet joints, and SIJs. The whole pelvis may be looked on as a ring, one feature of which is that it cannot be disturbed in only one place at a time, so that a disturbance in one area produces an associated disturbance in another part of the ring. An illustration of the ring mechanism in musculoskeletal practice is the condition of pelvic dysfunction, often referred to as SPD (symphyseal-pelvic dysfunction), that may be experienced in the later stages of pregnancy. These features of interdependency involving the fascial connections, and referred pain from disc, facet, and dura, makes the management of pelvic injuries a problem, for it sometimes appears as though one injury improves only for another injury to appear in its stead. The apparent stability of the SIJ belies the fact that it can move, and the stresses across the joint are manifest by osteophytes on its anterior surface (Figure 34.3). The joint can ankylose from ageing or from the effect of inflammatory arthropathies.

Pain may be referred from proximal structures to the pelvis. Accordingly, any examination of the pelvis must include an examination of the spine and, particularly, the thoracolumbar junction where the ilioinguinal nerve (T12) originates to supply the groin. Pain may be referred to the buttock and the groin from lumbar segmental disturbances such as discal pathology and facetal dysfunction, as well as the connecting ligaments. Sometimes, invasive diagnostic interventions, for instance, infiltrating the facet joints under direct vision or even a provocative probe when the disc, facet joint, and SIJ are stimulated under narcoleptic anaesthesia, may be required to establish the cause of pelvic pain. Those practitioners whose training conditions them to search for referred pain must be aware of local conditions that can also be a cause of pelvic pain.

Sacroiliac joint

Vleeming et al. (1997) and Bowen and Cassidy (1981) have demonstrated, by injecting the SIJ with contrast and steroid, that the SIJ is a source of pain. However, it is not quite so easy clinically to differentiate a sacroiliac lesion from facetal or discal pathology.

History

The patient's history can range from a diffuse sacroiliac or buttock pain, to pain referred down the leg as far as the ankle. However, the referred sacroiliac pain is not accompanied by pins and needles or numbness. The young age of a patient (especially if he is a man in his 20s), will raise the suspicion of ankylosing spondylitis, which

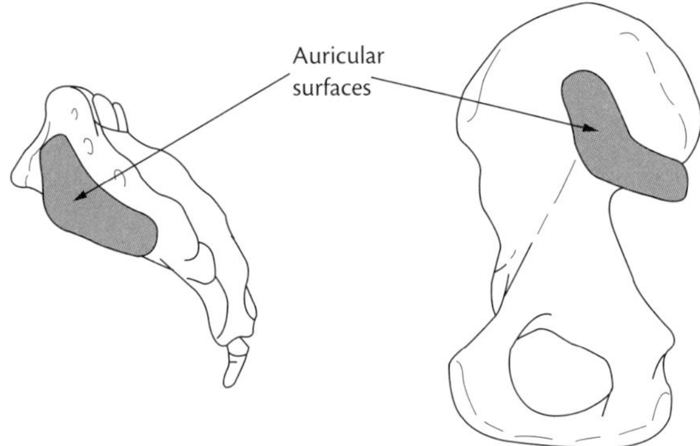

Figure 34.1 The auricular L-shaped sacroiliac joint. (Reproduced with permission of Malcolm Read.)

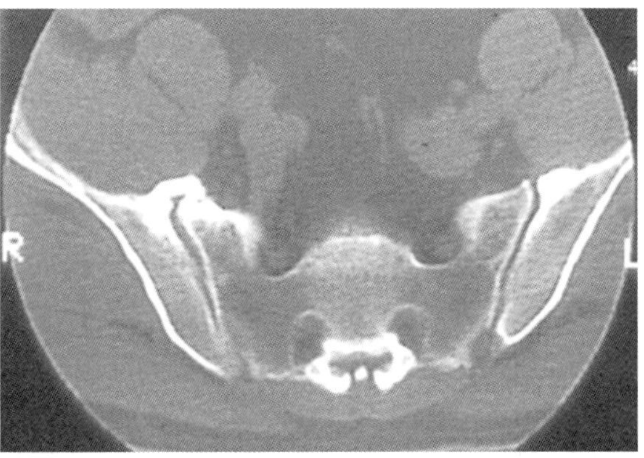

Figure 34.3 CT scan with large right and developing left osteophytes. (Reproduced with permission of Malcolm Read.)

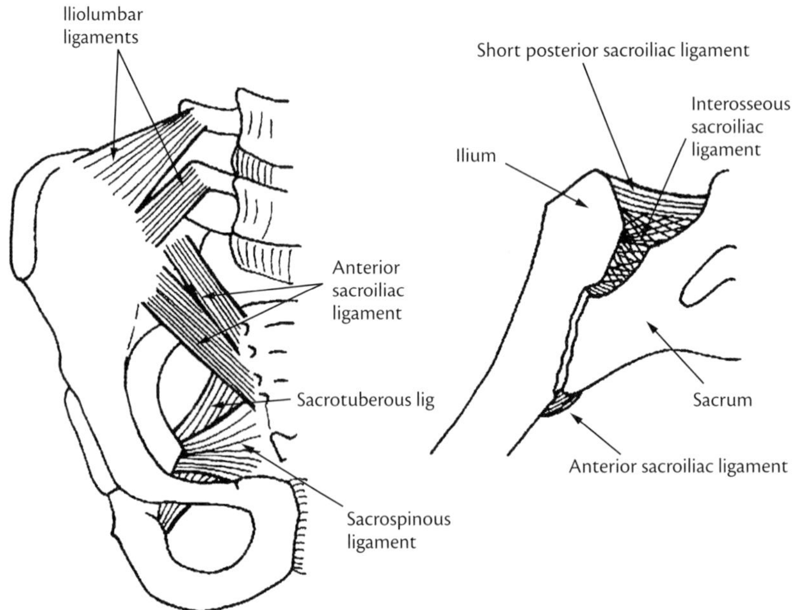

Figure 34.2 Ligaments of the sacroiliac joint. (Reproduced with permission of Malcolm Read.)

has a male/female ratio of 8:1, but this condition can present in the 30s and 40s as undiagnosed back pain. Ankylosing spondylitis may be so severe that the patient is carried into the consulting room on a stretcher, exhibiting all the signs of an acute prolapsed disc with severe limitation of straight leg raise. Specifically, a young patient or a patient with undiagnosed back pain should be asked about any family history of ankylosis and whether there has been any history of iritis, urethritis, or bowel disease. Recurrent enthesitis affecting multiple sites and/or a groin strain also may be presenting features of ankylosing spondylitis. Schober's test (Box 34.1) and a reduced chest expansion (below 4 cm) are indicative.

Investigations include blood tests for ESR (erythrocyte sedimentation rate), CRP (C-reactive protein), and HLA (human leukocyte antigen) B27, radiographs, and possibly computed tomography (CT) scanning of the SIJ. The radiographs will show sclerosis on the ilial side of the SIJ and may also show irregularity and lytic areas within the joint (Figure 34.4). CT scanning may display these areas of erosion and sclerosis even in the presence of normal radiographs (Figure 34.5). Magnetic resonance imaging (MRI) may not be quite so effective for displaying problems with cortical bone, but the inflammatory nature of ankylosing spondylitis can be seen on T2-weighted or STIR (Short T1 Inversion Recovery) -related sequences of the SIJ (Figure 34.6).

A history of direct trauma to the SIJ may indicate an apparent springing or crushing of the pelvis. On the other hand, falling off a horse but catching the foot in the stirrup, so that the limb is pulled out from the pelvis, will produce a distraction or shearing of the SIJ. Running downhill or driving the foot into the ground with the back in extension, as in the pole vault take-off, produces a compressive shearing force. Compression and some shearing force to the right SIJ is probably applied by the right-handed golfer who is concentrating on coiling the pelvis at the top of the backswing. Here, the hip is prevented from full internal rotation by the muscle tension, and the twisting force is transferred to the SIJ. The hormone relaxin, which is secreted both perimenstrually and in the later stages of pregnancy, relaxes the pelvic ligaments. This may be reflected

Box 34.1 Schober's test

Schober's test for the lumbar spine may be carried out by taking a lower mark in the standing position at the level of the posterior inferior iliac spines, measuring 15 cm up from this mark, and making another mark on the skin in the midline. The patient is then asked to flex their spine forwards towards their toes while the tape measure is held on the upper mark. The distance between the two marks should lengthen by at least 5 cm. Failure to lengthen suggests some degree of spinal ankylosis.

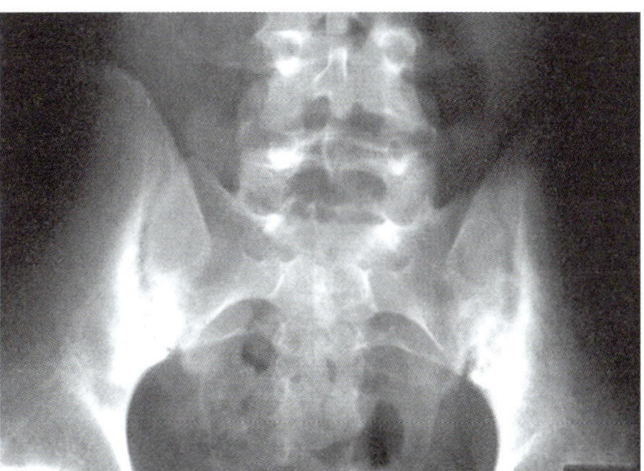

Figure 34.4 X-ray of the SIJs showing ileal sclerosis typical of ankylosingspondylitis. (Reproduced with permission of Malcolm Read.)

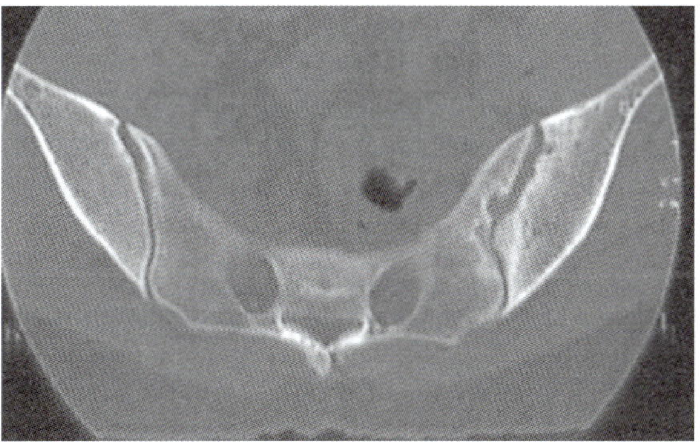

Figure 34.5 A CT scan showing ankylosing spondylitis. This 30-year-old female had normal X-rays and MRI scan. (Reproduced with permission of Malcolm Read.)

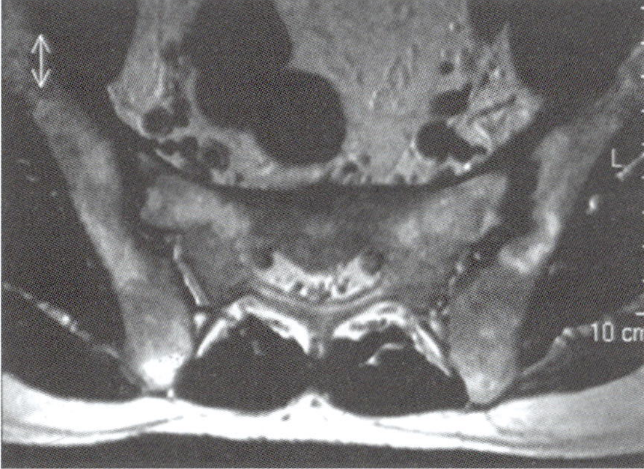

Figure 34.6 Increased signal can be seen in the left ileum in this seronegative sacroiliitis. (Reproduced with permission of Malcolm Read.)

by perimenstrual backache and the backache of pregnancy experienced by some women. Though the lithotomy position may be used during delivery, especially with forceps, there is an increased incidence of SIJ pain following this procedure. Care should be taken not to force the hips too far into abduction, so that the loads are transferred to the SIJ where they cause problems. This is particularly important when the patient is under general anaesthetic and has no ability to resist the abduction forces on the hips and, subsequently, the SIJ.

Examination

Assessment should always include examination of the spine to exclude segmental instability. However, weightbearing extension of the spine can produce pain from the SIJs and, therefore, the *one-legged extension test* (Figure 34.7) and the *Fitch catch test* (Figure 34.8), which require increased extension and rotation and are a test for a pars interarticularis defect, may also prove positive in SIJ problems. Both of these manoeuvres increase the extension of the spine with weightbearing (Box 34.2); the Fitch catch adds rotation.

The *Piedallu sign* (Box 34.2) is perhaps more difficult to interpret. It is thought to be a consequence of SIJ fixation, but lumbar segmental disorders can produce the same response. Equally, a stance with one hemipelvis held forward of the other or one anterior superior iliac spine being rotated anteriorly or posteriorly, may be produced by SIJ dysfunction, a genuine short leg, segmental dysfunction, or muscular imbalance. Unfortunately, this finding is often described as a short leg, which leads to confusion. A true short leg can only be accurately assessed on a standing radiograph or light-ray grid screen. Without a true short leg, this sign only represents a *functional short leg*, which is what it should more appropriately be called.

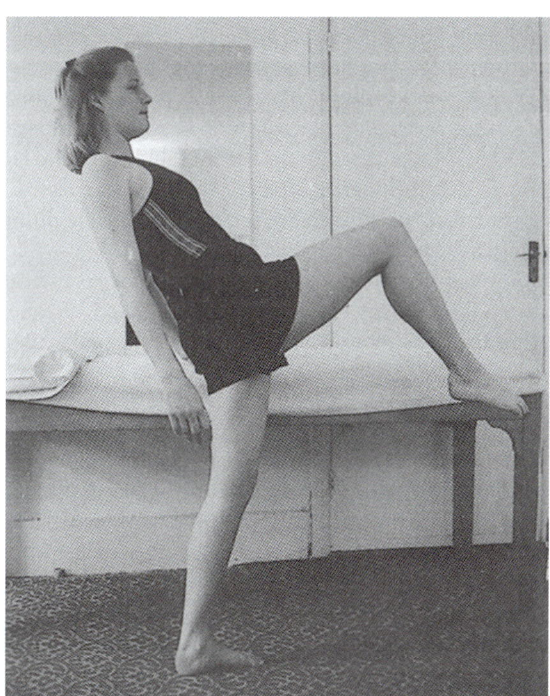

Figure 34.7 The one-legged hyperextension test. (Reproduced with permission of Malcolm Read.)

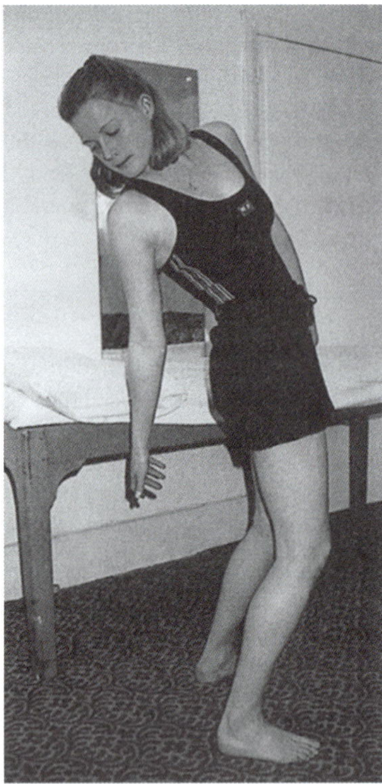

Figure 34.8 The Fitch catch. (Reproduced with permission of Malcolm Read.)

Box 34.2 Tests for SIJ dysfunction

- The *one-legged hyperextension test* (Figure 34.7) is performed with the patient standing on one leg while the other leg is raised with the knee flexed to about 90°, and at this stage the patient extends the back.
- The *Fitch catch* (Figure 34.8) is performed with the patient standing with legs apart and leaning the back into extension, but at the same time, the hand stretches backwards to reach for the contralateral Achilles. This is then repeated on the other side.
- The *Piedallu sign* test is performed with the patient standing, and the thumb of one hand is placed over the spinous process of the fifth, fourth, and third segment consecutively, while the thumb of the other hand is placed over the posterior inferior iliac spine (PIIS). The patient is asked to raise the ipsilateral knee towards the chest. The ischium will move outwards and the PIIS should swing downwards, but will rise cranially in the presence of a dysfunctional SIJ.
- For the *Downing sign* test, the patient is laid supine with ankles together. The hip is flexed, externally rotated, and then abducted, before being returned to its position on the couch. An increase in the apparent leg length, as noted from the position of the medial malleoli as they lie together, is said to indicate a mobile joint, whereas a fixed SIJ will produce shortening of the affected leg. With a reversal of this movement, the apparent lengthening should return to its pre-test state.
- *Pelvic spring* is a provocative stress test that produces SIJ pain when the iliac crests are compressed or distracted in the supine patient. The patient should then be asked to lie on their hand, which supports the fifth segment, and the compression or distraction force reapplied. Pain that disappears on supporting the fifth segment is suggestive of segmental dysfunction.
- For *Ongley's test*, the hip on the side to be tested is flexed to 90° and then axial compression with some adduction is applied through the femur. It is thought that 90° of hip flexion stresses the sacroiliac ligaments; greater than 90°, the sacrotuberous ligament; and less than 90°, the iliolumbar ligaments.

None of these tests for a short leg is accurate, and before the results are given credence, at least three of the tests should indicate the same leg is short. Indeed, as many individuals have a leg length discrepancy that causes them no functional disability, leg length correction, as a therapeutic measure, should be approached with caution. Perhaps the quickest way to make a clinical assessment is to ask the patient to stand and supinate their feet, in case any tendency to pronation has dropped one side lower than the other, and check iliac crest levels either by palpation or with a spirit level (see Box 34.3). For greater certainty, the patient should turn and face the other way in case the floor is not level, and the test repeated. Only if this gives a significant difference is it worth following through to further tests of true leg length difference.

The *Downing sign* (Box 34.2) is used by some to indicate SIJ fixation, but the accuracy of this sign has been called into question, suggesting that it is more related to the thoracolumbar junction (Sweetman 1998).

Pelvic spring (Box 34.2) is indicative of quite severe SIJ dysfunction, but the fifth lumbar segment disc or facet joint will also produce a positive pain response if inflamed. Pain that disappears on supporting the fifth segment is suggestive of segmental dysfunction. Sacroiliac stress tests also load the sacrotuberous, sacroiliac, and iliolumbar ligaments. These may be a cause of pain when stressed.

Ongley's test (Box 34.2) is performed with the patient supine. Direct pressure over the posterior aspect of the SIJ with the patient lying prone may also be painful, as may be compression of the ilial wing with the patient side-lying.

Dural stress tests such as straight leg raising, Lasegue, and slump test are negative, but facet rocking tests can be equivocal. The dura is capable of sliding within the spinal canal, lateral canal, and fascia to accommodate movement, but if it is tethered, then a pull is exerted on the nerve linings producing pain. Stretching of the dura and neural complex is the rationale behind dural stress tests. In the lower limb, this can be performed by raising the straight leg of the supine-lying patient to stretch the sciatic nerve. The patient's pain is felt in the back and/or leg. Dorsiflexing the foot and/or internally rotating the leg at the same time will stretch the sciatic nerve further, which is the *Lasegue test* (Figure 34.9). The dural assessment may be added to this test by sitting the patient on the couch with their back straight or in slight extension, and then raising the straight leg. This manoeuvre is then repeated with the patient's back curled into flexion and their chin on their chest (Figure 34.10). This position will be more painful if the dura is involved and will be relieved, to some degree, by raising the chin from the chest, while returning the chin to the chest reproduces the increased pain. This is the *slump test*.

Box 34.3 Assessment of a short leg

Clinically, a short leg may be assessed somewhat inaccurately by comparing the measurements on each side from the umbilicus to the tip of each medial malleolus; from the anterior superior iliac spines to the tip of the medial malleolus; from the greater trochanter to the tip of the lateral malleolus and by placing the thumbs on the tips of the medial malleoli, while making certain they are level and then asking the patient to sit up. The malleoli should remain level and an alteration in their position, with one rising cranially, suggests a short leg on that side. Similarly, if the buttocks are actively raised off the couch and dropped back on the couch, a malleolus may move cranially to indicate the short leg.

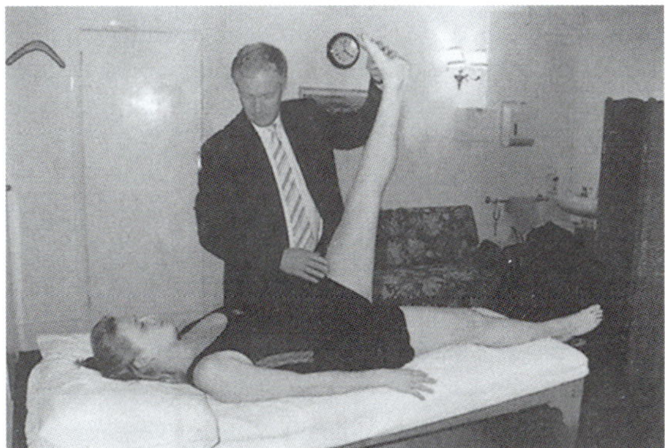

Figure 34.9 The Lasegue test. Straight leg raising tensions the sciatic nerve. This pull is increased by adding ankle dorsiflexion. (Reproduced with permission of Malcolm Read.)

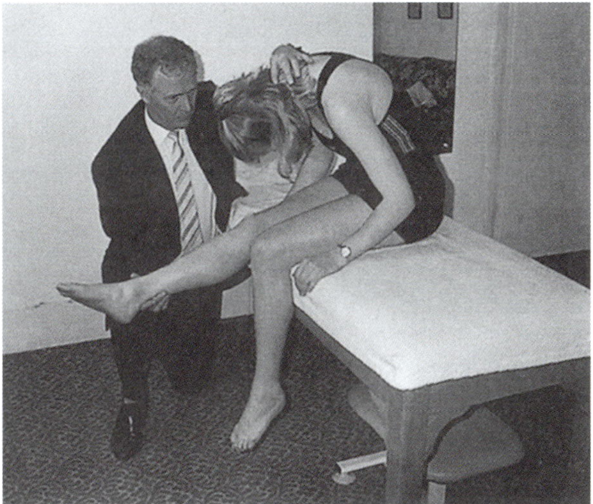

Figure 34.10 Slump test. A positive test eases the pain with neck extension and increases pain with neck flexion. (Reproduced with permission of Malcolm Read.)

Inestigations

Plain radiographs may display the sclerosis on the ilial aspect of the SIJ that is associated with ankylosing spondylitis (Figure 34.4) and, in severe cases, irregular lytic areas may be visualized, until the joint reaches a state of ankylosis visible by radiography. Look also for vertebral signs of ankylosis plus any erosion of the gracilis margin of the pubic symphysis (Figure 34.11). Degenerative or adaptive changes may be demonstrated as inferior osteophytes which may not be reported upon by the radiologist as they are interpreted as normal changes, but presumably are representative of stress forces across the joint (Macdonald and Hunt 1951; Solonen 1957).

Technetium-99 bone scanning excludes any bone injury or disease such as Paget's disease, tumours, or stress fractures, but local areas of increased signal may still be visualized within the SIJ. Nowadays, it is rarely undertaken for SIJ problems; MRI is the more usual investigative test.

CT and MRI through the SIJ can display areas of sclerosis, lysis (Figure 34.5), and sacroiliitis (Figure 34.6) that may be missed on standard radiographs and MR scans of the spine. These areas of altered bone architecture presumably reflect the weightbearing stresses transferred from the legs through the pelvis and on to the spine. CT examination of an area that has a 'hot' bone scan can differentiate the lesion further, such as an underlying stress fracture of the SIJ or ilial wing. MRI must be directed specifically at the SIJ as the standard lumbar views do not display this area well (Read 1998). They can demonstrate an increased T2-weighted signal with an inflammatory iliitis (Figure 34.6), but MRI is not as effective for cortical bone and may miss the areas of sclerosis and anterior osteophytosis.

Bone densitometry will be required when pelvic or sacral stress fractures have been diagnosed (see section 'Stress fractures' in this chapter), and this must be accompanied by a dietary and hormonal profile and advice, as oligo- and amenorrhoeic athletes are susceptible to unusual stress fractures. Blood tests may reveal a raised ESR or CRP, RBC (red blood count), and WBC (white blood count) in leukaemia which may present as bone pain, and markers of bone activity such as alkaline phosphatase, myeloma fractions, and prostate specific antigen (PSA).

Treatment

Inflammatory sacroiliitis should be treated as appropriate for the underlying systemic disease, with non-steroidal anti-inflammatories (NSAIDs) as required for pain control. Exercise should in preference be non-impact and swimmers should avoid the breast stroke, though the reduced abduction and external rotation of the wedge kick, as opposed to the frog kick, may be tolerated. Spinal mobilization and muscle-stretching exercises should be undertaken and maintained.

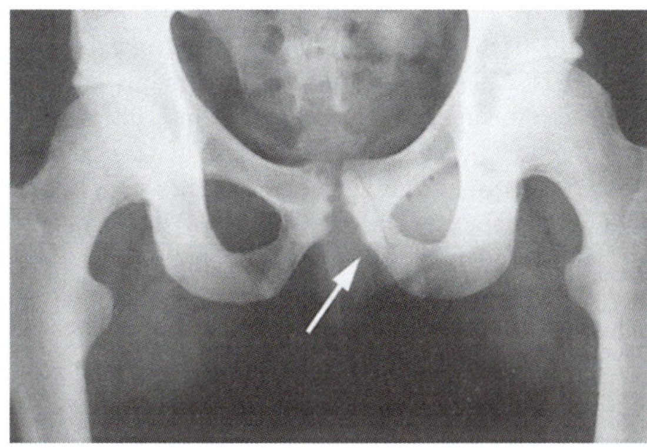

Figure 34.11 X-rays show cysts and sclerosis with erosion of the gracilis margin (arrow) in a 19-year-old footballer with ankylosing spondylitis. (Reproduced with permission of Malcolm Read.)

Dysfunctional SIJ pain may respond to manipulation both of the ileum and the sacrum itself, but excessive manipulation may well maintain an unstable and inflamed joint.

An acute flare of the joint can be treated with steroids injected into the posterior sacroiliac ligaments and the joint from the posterior superior aspect. These ligaments can be strengthened by sclerosant injections ('prolotherapy') to the sacroiliac and iliolumbar ligaments. They are particularly useful for women who have perimenstrual or postpartum ligamentous insufficiency and SIJ instability (Cyriax and Cyriax 1983).

Posterior lumbar ligament strain

Posterior lumbosacral ligament strain occurs in the interspinous and supraspinous ligaments, but particularly in the iliolumbar, lumbosacral, and sacroiliac ligaments (Figure 34.2). The diagnosis may be one of exclusion, as these ligaments can produce radiation of pain to the buttock, leg, or groin, and the nature of the pain may mimic other mechanical disorders; indeed, strain of these ligaments can accompany and be part of the pain complex from the intervertebral disc or facet joint.

History

Primarily, the history may be the persistence of symptoms following the resolution of a disc, facet joint, or SIJ lesion. In its pure form, if that exists, it is rest pain relieved by movement. Accordingly, the history of morning pain, and sitting pain that are relieved by movement, can be considered typical. Indeed, this ligamentous pain is sometimes referred to as the 'cocktail party' or 'theatre-goer's' back, as the individual is not able to sit or stand for long without having to alter position. A less frequent presentation is a history of pain in the popliteal fossa that appears after a back lesion has settled, and this seems to respond to appropriate treatment to the posterior lumbar ligaments.

Examination

A principal requirement is the exclusion of disc, facet, or SIJ disorders, bony disease or neural referrals of pain, or their detection alongside features that could be associated with ligamentous dysfunction. The absence of mechanical signs apart from outer range discomfort on spinal flexion and extension in the presence of pain that has no other cause is suggestive of ligamentous strain.

Treatment

Correction of the primary underlying cause such as a disc lesion will enable the ligamentous pain to settle over time, but this may be aided by NSAIDs or a local intraligamentous cortisone injection. Electrotherapeutic physiotherapy modalities to reduce inflammation can be effective. Persistence of the pain suggests stress of the posterior lumbar ligaments, and these may be strengthened by prolotherapy (see Chapters 54 and 55). Following this, the patient should be advised on how to adopt a spinal neutral position whenever possible and institute muscle balance work/core stability to stabilize the pelvic posture.

Side-lying external hip rotation

The patient lies on their side with the knees slightly bent, and the back is taken into lumbar neutral, and splinted into this position by tightening the abdominal muscles. The upper knee is then raised but the ankles are kept in contact, so that the external rotators of the hip are active but the lumbar spine is fixed in neutral. This should be repeated 30–40 times on each side.

One leg half-squat balancing

The patient stands evenly balanced on both legs and then tightens the gluteals, at which stage they balance on one leg and lower themselves into a half squat (Figure 34.12). This exercise is to strengthen the external rotators of the hips, so the pelvis must not be allowed to slide out sideways nor the ipsilateral anterior superior iliac spine to rotate forwards and medially. This should be held for 20 seconds. Repeat on the other side.

'Super woman'

Kneel on all fours and hold the lumbar spine in neutral. Splint this position by tightening the abdominal muscles, and then raise one leg backwards followed by the contralateral arm forwards (Figure 34.13). Care must be taken not to lose the horizontal plane of the pelvis or to lose spinal neutral. This balance should be held for 30–40 seconds.

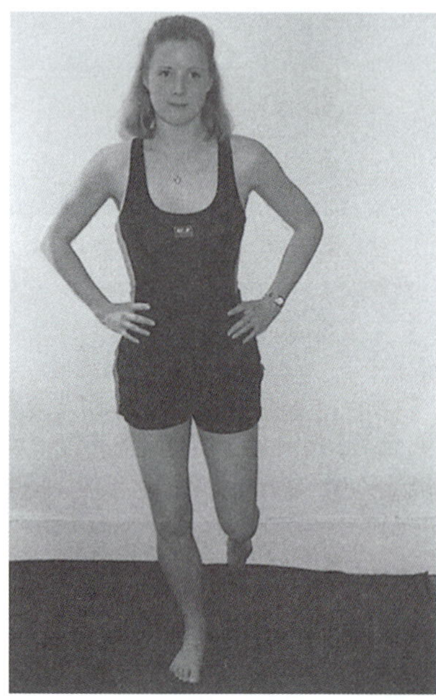

Figure 34.12 The half squat. The pelvis is straight and the knee in line with the foot. This works the hip stabilizers. (Reproduced with permission of Malcolm Read.)

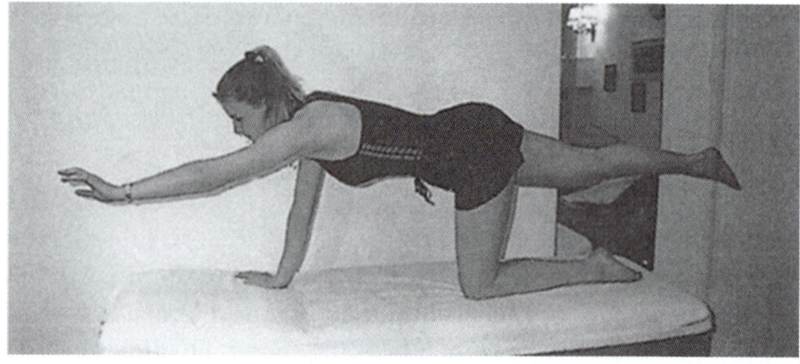

Figure 34.13 'Super (wo)man' exercises the pelvic and back stabilizer muscles. (Reproduced with permission of Malcolm Read.)

Entrapment of the long cutaneous nerve of the thigh

The long cutaneous nerve to the thigh supplies an area over the posterolateral pelvis and the thigh. The area of pain referral overlies the tensor fascia lata and the iliotibial band.

History

The pain can radiate to the lateral aspect of the knee and is difficult to distinguish from the tensor fascia lata and the iliotibial tract syndrome. There may be some subjective awareness of numbness in this area. It is possible that continual pressure from clothing and local trauma may be causative.

Examination

The diagnosis is made by the absence of resisted abduction pain from the tensor fascia lata and absence of resisted hip external rotator pain. Palpation reveals a non-tender trochanteric bursa and piriformis insertion. Hip pathology and referred pain from other sources such as the spine must be excluded. Palpation over the crest of the ilium shows a local tender area that may also refer pain down the outside of the thigh.

Treatment

A local cortisone injection may be effective. Sometimes a neuroma exists, when the nerve must be decompressed in its fascia.

Meralgia paraesthetica (compression of the lateral cutaneous nerve of the thigh)

The presenting symptoms are usually altered sensation and pain over the anterior thigh. The lateral cutaneous nerve to the thigh is commonly compressed as it emerges through the superficial fascia, but it may emerge near the anterior superior iliac spine or close to the groin crease. In sportspeople, the tight elastic from clothing around the top of the leg can cause compression of the nerve, in which case it is cured by releasing such elastic tension. It has also been noted in female gymnasts who compress the front of their thighs on the asymmetric bars during many of their gymnastic routines.

Examination

There is a delineated area of altered sensation over the anterior aspect of the thigh, commensurate with the lateral cutaneous nerve distribution. A small area of increased discomfort may be palpated somewhere from the anterior superior spine to the upper mid-thigh, and this area of nerve entrapment can be further delineated by pressure from a blunt probe such as a retracted ballpoint pen.

Investigations

Electromyography (EMG is of little value).

Treatment

Alteration of clothing will be effective if that is the cause. Local infiltration with corticosteroid around the fascial entrapment can help, but infrequently, and surgery to release the fascia may be required in patients in whom the symptoms are distressing. Patients may find that the symptoms resolve spontaneously, usually over the course of some years.

Gluteal bursitis

History

Occasionally, after a lot of running or leg extension exercises, the gluteal bursa may become inflamed, producing pain over the upper buttock that is worse on these movements and on local pressure.

Examination

Care must be taken to exclude spinal and SIJ pathology, but the diagnostic features are pain on both passive hip flexion and supine straight leg raise, with localized palpable tenderness over the upper outer quadrant of the buttock. With respect to differential diagnosis, it is worthy of note that myofascial pain from the glutei is common in the population at large, often associated with low lumbar or sacroiliac dysfunction.

Treatment

A reduction in gluteal exercises is required, especially in martial arts and circuit training exponents, who specifically exercise the glutei. Electrotherapeutic modalities to reduce inflammation and a steroid injection into the upper, outer quadrant with the needle reaching the bone, when allied to a diminution of gluteal-specific exercises, can be curative. Care must be taken to avoid the sciatic nerve during any massage or injection techniques.

Tensor fascia lata dysfunction

History

An uncommon source of lateral pelvic, hip, and thigh pain, it occurs primarily with gymnasium activities when abduction of the leg is overworked and is often accompanied by trochanteric bursitis, and sometimes iliotibial band syndrome. It occurs in running when the tensor fascia lata is overworking to stabilize the pelvis. Camber running, with the painful side lower than the pain-free side, is contributory. Theoretically, a grossly supinated foot with weak external rotators may also overload the tensor fascia lata.

Examination

Both active movement of the hip and resisted abduction are painful. Maximum tenderness is under the lip of the ilium, though a more general tenderness may be present over the whole muscle. Palpation of the iliotibial band will reveal a degree of tightness/hypertonia comparing one side to the other. *Ober's test* (Box 34.4) can reveal a lack of passive adduction of the thigh due to tightness within the iliotobial band. The *modified Thomas test* (Box 34.4; see also Box 34.6 and Figure 34.20) may reveal abnormal abduction of the thigh.

Treatment

The most effective treatment is massage and stretching by a physiotherapist of the straight leg into adduction behind the other leg; also by the patient standing with the affected leg crossed behind the other. The body is swung out and over the affected hip but the actual weight is still supported by the normal leg. Electrotherapeutic modalities to settle inflammation help. NSAIDs and a steroid injection under the ilial rim ease the discomfort. Rehabilitation includes relaxing the hip during running and reduction of active exercises that abduct the leg. However, tightness within the ilitobial

Box 34.4 Tests for trochanteric bursitis

- *Ober's test* is performed with the patient lying on their side. The lower leg is flexed at the knee and then at the hip. The upper femur is then taken into abduction and extended, and following this is then adducted behind the lower leg. A normal band should allow adduction beyond the upper aspect of the other leg. A tight iliotibial band either produces pain or does not adduct beyond the upper aspect of the other leg.
- The *modified Thomas test* can demonstrate a tight iliotibial band (Figure 34.14). The patient lies supine with their buttocks on the end of the couch but one leg bent at the hip and held into full flexion. The other hip is extended. The normal iliotibial band allows the extended leg to lie straight in line, whereas the tight iliotibial band pulls the thigh into abduction.

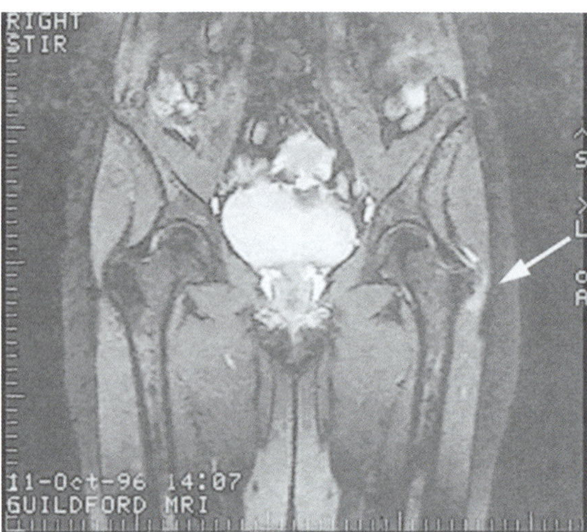

Figure 34.14 STIR-sequence MRI displays left trochanteric bursitis (arrow). (Reproduced with permission of Malcolm Read.)

band can be multifactorial with primary issues being related to lack of strength in muscle groups in and around the pelvis. Lack of strength, lack of stability in and around the pelvis, decreased range of movement within a hip joint, dysfunction in the lower lumbar spine, abnormal cadence due to structural or functional problems in either or both lower limbs can all have a role to play in assessing the cause of this pathology.

Trochanteric bursitis

Three trochanteric bursae are described by name, situated deep to and facilitating the action of the distal gluteus minimus, medius, and maximus tendons. The bursae lie over the greater trochanter, into which the tendons of gluteus medius and minimus are inserted. Gluteus maximus is inserted largely into the iliotibial band (ITB), which originates from the tensor fascia lata and inserts at Gurney's tubercle at the knee. The ITB is a strong ligamentous band that also provides attachment to the lateral quadriceps and hamstrings, and its function is to stabilize the hip and leg against abduction forces. During hip movement, particularly walking and running, the iliotibial band moves across the greater trochanter from which it is separated by the trochanteric bursa complex. Inflammation of the bursa usually arises from increased friction, and occasionally from direct trauma, when it may produce a haembursitis.

History

The history may include trauma from a fall, or hitting a wall or another individual with the outer hip. Far more commonly, trochanteric bursitis comes on insidiously, though sometimes after increased unaccustomed activity. It is worse on walking and running, but is also painful to lie on or to cross the painful leg over the non-painful leg.

Examination

Examination should exclude referral of pain from the back and the hip joint, though the hip is less easy to exclude because internal rotation and flexion may produce pain from the bursa. Local tenderness to palpation directly over the greater trochanter is very suggestive of bursitis, though gluteal enthesopathy (see following section) has to be excluded. Sometimes, resisted abduction of the hip may be painful.

Investigations

Investigations are undertaken to exclude underlying bony or hip pathology, but specific views of the bursa are best obtained with diagnostic ultrasound, especially with a haembursitis which may be aspirated at the same time. Like all haembursae, they tend to recur and require further draining on a few occasions. Steroids into the haembursa may reduce the recurrence. Complications such as accompanying bony trauma or even an enthesitis from the external rotators of the hip may lead to a bone scan or MRI investigation being required; the inflamed bursa being best seen on T2 or STIR-related sequences (Figure 34.14).

Treatment

Treatment of the bursitis may be with electrotherapeutic modalities to reduce inflammation, NSAIDs, or intrabursal cortisone. If the iliotibial band is tight and Ober's test positive, as is often the case, stretching of the iliotibial band, as described for the tensor fascia lata, is required. Frequently, the external rotators of the hip and, in particular, the piriformis are weak, allowing the pelvis to slide outwards over an adducted and internally rotated hip. Thus, strengthening exercises to the hip stabilizers are essential. Paradoxically, race walkers, who particularly slide past their hip in this fashion, do not seem to produce this injury even in their early days of training. Surgical Z-plasty may be effective in recalcitrant cases.

Gluteal enthesopathy

Over recent years, and particularly with the increased use and sophistication of MRI and USS (ultrasound scanning), gluteal enthesopathy, equivalent to insertional tendinopathy, has become increasingly recognized. It is assumed to be intimately associated with trochanteric bursitis as the gluteus medius and minimus tendons are, in part, separated from the greater trochanter by bursae, and gluteus maximus is in close anatomical relationship.

Evidence of (degenerative) pathology at tendon insertions does not equate necessarily to localized tenderness and pain, though other clinical findings in the buttock such as weakness of the glutei, tender muscle, and trigger points in the bellies of the relevant muscles, as is often the case, are strongly supportive of a contribution to trochanteric pain being made by the musculotendinous unit. It would appear to be a reasonably safe assumption that in a significant percentage of patients with 'trochanteric bursitis', there are both underlying stress changes at the gluteal bony attachments to the proximal femur and an inflammatory bursitis.

Clinically, it is difficult to be certain of the exact diagnosis in many patients, though a low-dose steroid injection followed by rehabilitation of the hip abductors and internal rotators is a pragmatic treatment strategy.

Box 34.5 Hip pointer

According to American literature, baseball players who are likely to slide into the bases on their sides will often produce a haematoma over the iliac crest. Direct trauma following contact in sports such as football and rugby can also induce this disabling condition that can take several weeks to resolve. The bleed into the bowl of the pelvis and pelvic floor produces a space-occupying lesion that causes notable pain and the contraction associated with general ambulation. Though this may be aspirated, surgical release of the haematoma may occasionally be required.

Dysfunction of the external rotators of the hip

This group of deep pelvic muscles is probably as important to the hip as the rotator cuff is to the shoulder. The external rotators probably function in a similar way to fix and stabilize the hip.

History

Patients may present with pain over the buttock, trochanter, and the line of the gluteal insertion along the lateral aspect of the femur, which may radiate down towards the ankle and foot. Painful external rotators are often seen in golfers who hit into a 'closed' left side, and this problem can be relieved by opening out the left foot at the stance, allowing the left side to swing through and out of the way. Unfortunately, established pain in the external rotators is difficult to handle and indeed to establish as a correct diagnosis. The patient may have pain at rest, lying in bed, and on walking. This pain is flared on climbing stairs when the painful hip leads on to the next stair and begins to raise the weight of the body.

Examination

External hip rotator dysfunction is a common finding that accompanies tracking problems at the knee. The weakness of the external rotators of the hip, rather than pain, may be the prime cause of the malfunction at the knee. During foot strike, the external rotators should hold the hip firmly, but if they are weak, the hip will be allowed to roll into internal rotation and the pelvis on that side moves anteriorly. This movement increases the functional anteversion of the femur, which becomes translated into a valgus movement at the knee with increased Q angle. Examination of the hip reveals an unclear pattern of painful movement that is suggestive of hip pathology but is not quite a capsular pattern, and hip flexion is often sore, consistent with Cyriax's sign of the buttock (Cyriax and Cyriax 1983).

Palpation demonstrates tenderness over the insertion of the piriformis at the posterolateral aspect of the greater trochanter, but there may also be tenderness over the gluteal insertions. Variably, there is tenderness over the origin of the piriformis at the inferior medial margin of the ilium and SIJ, and often there is tenderness over the ischial aspect of the sacrotuberous ligament. *Per rectum,* the obturator internus may be tender. Resisted external rotation of the hip is usually painful. The complex situation may be complicated by a trochanteric bursitis and a tight iliotibial tract with a positive Obers' sign. Finally, as if there was not enough to confuse the diagnosis, the rare piriformis and hamstring syndromes must be excluded (see following relevant section). Here, straight leg raise and Lasegue tests should be positive but the slump test negative. Pelvic instability at the SIJ and pubic symphysis will often cause dysfunction in the external rotators.

A tear of the external rotators of the hip may occur in activities that involve a forced degree of rotatory movement and control (Box 34.5). Tears of the gemelli, obtutator externus, quadratus femoris, and piriformis can occur. The discomfort may persist for up to 3 weeks, though activity can remain at a relatively optimal level depending on discomfort, due to the supporting network of the bulk of the adjacent muscles.

Investigations

MRI is the investigation of choice in musculotendinous lesions, but usually shows no clinical evidence of inflammation or dysfunction in this condition (though abnormalities have been demonstrated in the quadratus femoris tendon) (Klinkert et al. 1997).

Treatment

Correction of the muscular weakness at the hip is required rather than exercises for the knee. Orthotics that prevent or limit valgus movement at the knee will, therefore, be of value in the short term to the hip as well, but rehabilitation must be directed to retraining the strength of the external rotators of the hip. Techniques of side lying, maintaining pelvic stability, and then externally rotating the hip, or of balancing on one leg in a half squat, can aid strengthening of the hip rotators, as may step-ups on the affected side while taking care to maintain hip and pelvic stability (see the previous section 'Posterior lumbar ligament strain'). During the half squat, the ipsilateral anterior superior iliac spine must not be allowed to rotate forwards, the hip must not slide outwards, and the contralateral leg must not be permitted to swing behind the balancing leg, as all of these manoeuvres prevent the external rotators from working properly (Figures 34.12 and 34.15). Sitting with the affected leg crossed over the other leg, and the foot placed on the couch alongside the knee, permits an increased internal rotation to stretch the muscles, which may also be strengthened by external rotation isometrics. The history of buttock pain and sometimes referral down the leg is similar to that produced by dural or SIJ irritation, and an injection of the piriformis insertion at the posterior lateral aspect of the greater trochanter can cause referred pain to the foot. Discomfort from these muscles can produce a painful straight leg raise, but Lasegue and slump tests are negative.

Treatment is difficult and lengthy for the painful syndromes, and involves stretching of the external rotators and iliotibial tract. The external rotators are stretched by sitting with the affected leg

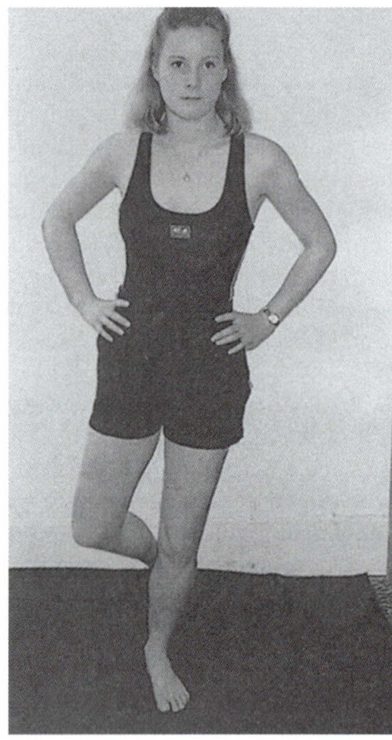

Figure 34.15 The left pelvis has swung forwards. (Figure 34.12 shows the right external rotators stabilizing the hip.) (Reproduced with permission of Malcolm Read.)

crossed over the straight extended contralateral leg. The ipsilateral foot is placed as proximal as possible on the couch, alongside the lateral aspect of the contralateral leg. The knee is then pulled, by the hands, towards the midline to achieve a passive stretch. In the figure-of-four stretch, the patient lies supine with the foot of the hip to be stretched crossed over and resting just above the contralateral knee (Figure 34.16). The affected hip is externally rotated as far as possible and then the contralateral knee is pulled, by the hands, towards the chest, thus flexing the spine. As the pelvis becomes lifted off the couch by this manoeuvre, so the external rotators come under stretch. This must be accompanied by isometric exercises to the piriformis and isotonic exercises with external rotation in side-lying position to the piriformis and obturator. However, pelvic stability is a functional problem and the balancing exercises, with a half squat and 'running tall', are essential. Running tall concentrates the running style on maintaining pelvic stability and moving over the hips, rather than sliding the hips outwards and 'rolling through' the gait.

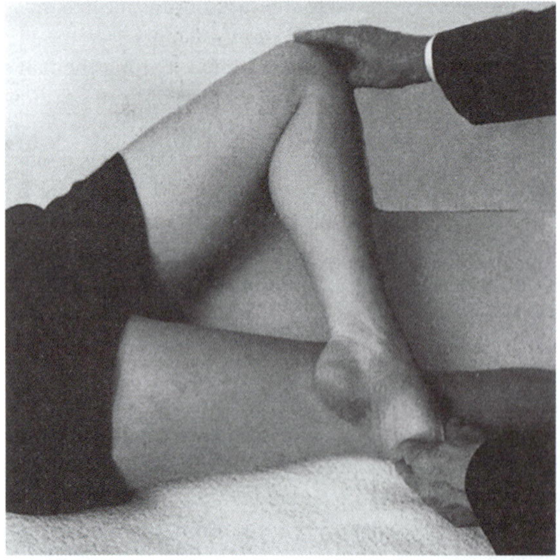

Figure 34.16 Figure-of-four test. (Reproduced with permission of Malcolm Read.)

Like all inflammatory lesions, rehabilitation sometimes cannot continue until the inflammation has resolved. Accordingly, massage, electrotherapeutic modalities, and cortisone to the piriformis origin and insertion or the sacrotuberous ligament and trochanteric bursa may be of value.

Sacrotuberous ligament sprain

The sacrotuberous ligament is a strong ligament running from the sacrum to the ischial tuberosity and is not frequently disrupted.

History

When this ligament is injured, there is usually a history of an external rotation strain of the pelvis on a fixed, flexed, weightbearing hip. An example is digging out a trench with a spade and throwing the soil out sideways and backwards towards the affected side, without fully straightening up.

Examination

Referred pain from the back must be excluded and any accompanying external hip rotator dysfunction must be dealt with, but the sacrotuberous ligament is locally tender to palpation over the superior surface of the ischial tuberosity. This can sometimes be palpated more easily with the patient kneeling on all fours, but lying the patient prone on the couch with the knee on the affected side dropped on to a chair placed alongside the couch will flex the hip to allow easy palpation of the sacrotuberous ligament and prove less threatening to the patient.

Treatment

The inflammation settles over time with appropriate anti-inflammatory physiotherapy, but if resistant, it can respond to a carefully placed steroid injection into the sacrotuberous insertion on the ischial tuberosity, being aware of the sciatic nerve approaching the lateral aspect of the tuberosity. Stretching as for external rotators of the hip is of benefit.

Piriformis and hamstring syndromes

The sciatic nerve may be trapped by the piriformis or gemelli as it passes between these muscles; this being an anatomical variant. It may also be bowed or tethered by the biceps femoris insertion onto the lateral aspect of the ischial tuberosity in athletes who have trained the hamstring.

History

The history is of sciatica with pain and perhaps pins and needles and numbness in the sciatic distribution, but there is no history of back pain. The piriformis syndrome may have some greater trochanteric element to the pain distribution.

Examination

Initially, this is a diagnosis of exclusion, when the common causes of sciatic nerve entrapment are ruled out by normal back movements. The indicative findings are of positive straight leg raise and Lasegue tests because the sciatic nerve is tethered, but the slump test is negative because there is no dural tethering. It is unusual to have signs of motor nerve involvement, but altered sensation may be detected. Sometimes, resisted piriformis contraction tested with the ipsilateral hip flexed and the foot crossed over the contralateral thigh may reproduce the referred pain.

Investigation

Investigations are undertaken to exclude other causes of sciatica. EMG may differentiate between an intraspinal lesion and this extraspinal cause.

Treatment

Stretching of the type used for adverse neural tension may benefit both conditions, but takes time. An injection close to the biceps femoris insertion can be curative, but the sciatic nerve must be avoided. Surgery may be required to release the nerve entrapment.

Stress fractures

History

Stress fractures of the pelvis seem to be confined to runners. They may occur in either sex but are predominant in oligo- or amenorrhoeic women, in whom atypical pelvic pain should immediately raise the possibility of a stress fracture. The pain is located over the site of the lesion and is worse with foot impact to the ground. Look particularly for sacral (Figure 34.17) and ilial stress fractures (Bottomley 1990), but, more commonly, fractures of the inferior pubic ramus (Figure 34.18). Stress fractures of the superior pubic ramus are reported less commonly.

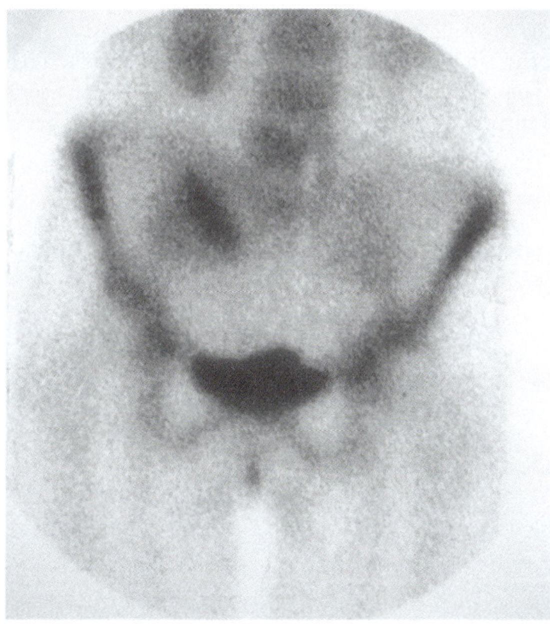

Figure 34.17 Bone scan shows the stress lesion across the right sacroiliac joint. (Reproduced with permission of Malcolm Read.)

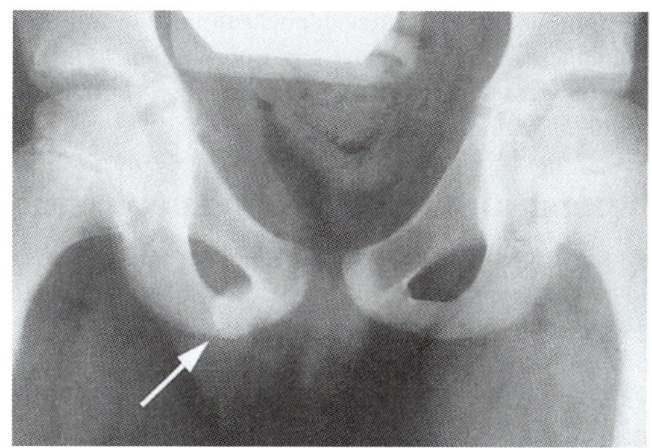

Figure 34.18 Callus in the inferior pubic ramus from a healing stress fracture (arrow). (Reproduced with permission of Malcolm Read.)

Examination

Clinical assessment may be confusing, with both hip and lumbar spinal movements producing pain, as may pelvic compression tests. The lack of a clear diagnosis in the presence of pain on weightbearing or foot impaction in a runner should lead to a bone scan or MRI to exclude any underlying bony problems. Indeed, the lack of a clear diagnosis in a sportsperson should generally lead to investigations for bony stress injuries.

Investigation

A decade ago, the watershed diagnostic aid was a bone scan, in which increased radiation from the active bone technetium-99 appears more intense (hot) on the scan. In the current decade, it is deemed more appropriate to scan the lesion further with CT or MRI to attempt to differentiate it from a tumour, bone cyst, or osteoid osteoma. Particular scrutiny should be made of the sacrum, the ilial wing, and the inferior pubic ramus, though stress fractures of the superior pubic rami do occasionally occur.

Investigation of bone density and a dietary profile should be undertaken, especially looking at the calcium intake. Many runners are confused about power/weight ratio, as they believe that by losing weight they will have less bulk to carry around. Unfortunately, for proponents of this theory, all racers have to be able to generate speed up to a sprint level to win high-class races, and the type 2 white fibres, which are required for sprinting, have bulk. Muscle weighs more than fat, but the athlete confuses the benefits of the muscle bulk with the weight of fat. Monitoring of skin thickness, rather than weight, should be advocated for these individuals. Among this group, there will also be some people with genuine anorexia nervosa, whose body image is acceptable to society as long as they run. These individuals respond quite well to a therapeutic approach orientated around their athletic performance, such as 'muscle needs to be provided with energy and this is carbohydrate', and discussions centred upon their running performance, with positive support, as opposed to a dietary approach. However, there are hormonal problems within this group, and gynaecological and endocrinological opinions are of value.

Treatment

Impact training, such as running, should be suspended and the athlete cross-trained on non-impact modalities such as the bike, rowing machine, and swimming or pool running. Running is introduced and increased incrementally against pain, and at this stage, a biomechanical assessment of running style, muscle balance, and leg length should be undertaken.

Enthesopathies and avulsion apophysitides

During the growth phase, children become less supple as the muscle–tendon complex grows more slowly than the bony length. However, the muscle–tendon complex is stronger than the epiphysis, so that the adolescent injury is usually entheseal. Particular problems occur around the pelvis in adolescence, which therefore require a radiograph to exclude an apophyseal avulsion. These same problems occur in adults, but they are more likely to be tendinous or muscle lesions rather than apophyseal.

Therapy, in the adult or child without an avulsion, is directed towards stretching the muscle complex just to pain, and by strengthening the muscle group. The child with an avulsion must be rehabilitated carefully, with due attention to pain, and, in the early stages, transcutaneous electrical nerve stimulation (TENS) or interferential stimulators set to twitch the muscle may be sufficient to maintain muscle loading. As the injury improves, so isometrics within the restraints of pain and then isotonic exercises against resistance may be added. Later, controlled running ladders through to sprinting, and kicking ladders for those who require them, should be introduced (Read 2000).

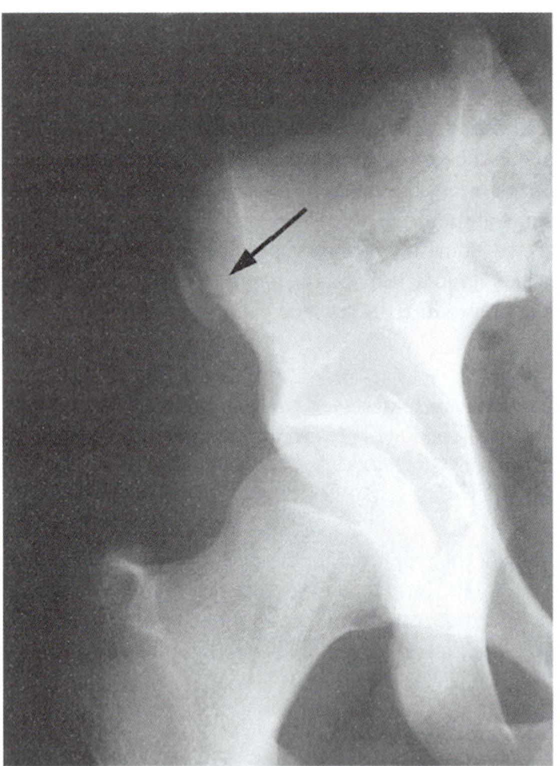

Figure 34.19 Anterior superior iliac spine avulsion in an adolescent following a sprint race. (Reproduced with permission of Malcolm Read.)

Lesions of the rectus femoris origin

History

The acute injury presents as a sudden pain while sprinting or kicking, whereas the chronic problem often presents as weakness or fatigue when running, accompanied by groin pain of a more diffuse nature.

Examination

The pain is centred over the anterior aspect of the hip. Tenderness to palpation is present over the anterior superior iliac spine or the reflected head of the rectus femoris from the acetabular lip (Figure 34.19). Active or resisted supine straight leg raising is painful, whereas a psoas lesion causes pain on resisted testing of the flexed hip as well as, or instead of, an extended hip. The *modified Thomas test* (Box 34.6) is painful and limited for quadriceps stretching.

Investigations

The more persistent chronic presentation with an acute initial onset, especially if getting worse over 5 days or so, should be radiographed, as myositis ossificans is a fairly common complication of this traumatic muscle injury and will delay healing (Figure 34.21). Children must be radiographed for a possible avulsion lesion (Figure 34.19).

Box 34.6 Modified Thomas test

The patient sits on the end of the couch with the opposite knee pulled up to the chest. The patient is then laid down and the opposite leg stretched out with the knee straight. The amount of hip extension is a reflection of psoas tightness. The knee may then be flexed from this position and the degree of knee flexion is a function of quadriceps tightness. The good side should be compared to the bad side (Figure 34.20).

Treatment

The injury is treated as for any enthesopathy, but particular attention should be paid to graded rehabilitation to sprinting and kicking. Any myositis has the added requirement of rest in the initial stages, though indomethacin is reputed to be of benefit; if rehabilitation fails, surgical excision should be considered. The complication of surgery is that the lesion reforms if the surgery is performed too soon.

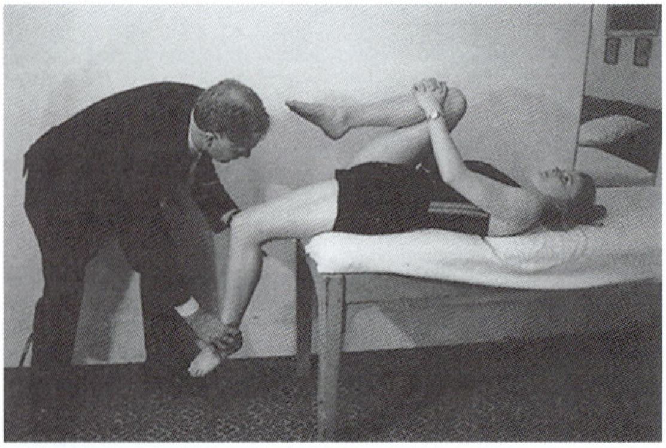

Figure 34.20 Modified Thomas test for quadriceps tightness. (Reproduced with permission of Malcolm Read.)

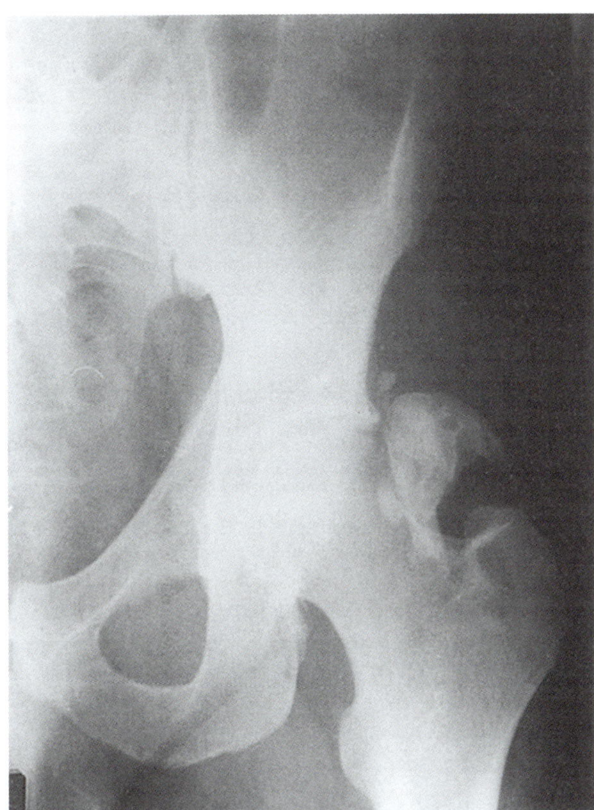

Figure 34.21 Myositis ossificans in the rectus femoris. (Reproduced with permission of Malcolm Read.)

Psoas muscle lesions

History

The psoas is a flexor and external rotator of the hip. It is injured during sprinting and kicking, but particularly in high knee-lift exercises and running in mud, when the foot has to be pulled out of the clinging mud. Lesions arise after hill running and sometimes in running sports such as field hockey in which the trunk is often in a half-bent position. Because the psoas, working on a fixed leg, aids abdominal curls, most sit-up exercises are done with the hips flexed, but sit-up exercises done with straight legs or leg raises may overload the psoas and may encourage extension of the spine, which is a problem for those suffering from extension-orientated spinal dysfunction.

Examination

The pain is located anteriorly and just lateral to the femoral canal in the groin. Passive hip flexion may be painful, which suggests the psoas bursa is inflamed. Resisted testing of the hip flexors at 90° of hip flexion indicates a muscle lesion or an enthesopathy at the psoas attachment at the lesser trochanter. However, this is a strong muscle, and sometimes manual testing just does not produce sufficient tension across the enthesis to produce pain. The modified Thomas test (see Box 34.6) for psoas tightness is restricted and painful.

Investigation

Radiography may show an avulsion at the lesser trochanter, and MRI or diagnostic ultrasound may reveal a psoas bursa or muscle tear on T2-weighted STIR sequences; but often no abnormality is detected.

Treatment

Management is by reduction of the inflammation by electrotherapeutic modalities and then gradual reintroduction of resisted hip flexion as an isometric exercise, followed by repetition of active high knee raises. Rehabilitation should then be graded into running drills that include high knee exercises, and finally, incremental load increases up to sprinting and hill running. Stretching of the psoas and rectus femoris is required to lengthen the musculotendinous junction and to prevent scar tissue contraction. Localized tenderness over the psoas bursa, which lies below Poupart's (inguinal) ligament and approximately two fingerbreadths lateral to the femoral canal, may respond well to a cortisone injection placed on the surface of the muscle, and then followed by appropriate rehabilitation.

The mechanics of the psoas muscle are integral to lumbar and pelvic movement. Prevention of injury in and around the pelvis can be assisted by regularly monitoring the strength and hypertonia of the psoas and its related structures. Contractile tissue lesion with structures such as the hamstring (a hip extensor) can be due to a quiet non-symptomatic dysfunction of the psoas.

Adductor tendinopathy

It is difficult to be certain as to which adductor is involved in individual cases, as the muscles vary in their activity depending upon the degree of hip flexion at the time of testing, but the majority of localized palpable tenderness will centre over the adductor longus at the pubic symphyseal area and, less frequently, the adductor magnus insertion, with tenderness running along the inferior pubic ramus to the ischial tuberosity.

History

Adductor longus tendinopathy is situated at the enthesis, but there is frequently a musculotendinous variant that is locally tender about 6 cm distal to the origin. This can produce a partial rupture with bruising and a palpable gap. The cause may be acute, either from a blocked side-foot tackle or a sudden sideways abduction stretch of the hip during a slip, or it may be caused by chronic overload from repetitive abduction stretches or adduction forces such as side-footing a ball. The fascia encasing the adductors is contiguous with the abdominal fascia, and the patient may also present with suprapubic abdominal pain. This pain can be difficult to distinguish from symphyseal pain and the pain from the conjoined tendon at the inguinal ring and pubic tubercle. Indeed, the myriad of symptoms in this area may have their primary focus in weakness of the posterior abdominal wall (a so-called sports hernia; more common in the male due to anatomical variation from the female). The scrotal invagination test may detect tenderness and patency at the inguinal ring in such cases.

The adductor magnus injury does not seem to refer pain suprapubically; by contrast, it mimics a hamstring lesion. It is seen more frequently during fast acceleration where the adductors often contribute as much power as the hamstrings.

Examination

Adductor tendinopathy is invariably tender to local palpation over the origin, whereas the absence of localized tenderness but the presence of a history of groin pain suggests the adductors are not primarily involved. Examination may reveal hip discomfort, but not in a capsular pattern. Resisted adduction is painful when the supine-lying patient squeezes a fist held between their knees, adducts the neutral hip from about 45° against resistance, and the 90° flexed hip is adducted against resistance. The pain produced by this resisted muscle testing is localized to the adductor areas. Tenderness is found over the adductor origin or about 6 cm from the origin in the case of a musculotendinous lesion. The adductor magnus lesion may also give rise to pain on resisted hamstring contraction as well as adduction, and tenderness is palpated along the inferior pubic ramus.

Treatment

Treatment is by electrotherapeutic modalities to reduce inflammation, frictions to organize scar tissue, and stretching exercises of the adductors to prevent scar tissue contraction. An injection of cortisone at the adductor origin settles inflammation in the acute and chronic case. Although its use is eschewed in the acute lesion, it may be required in spite of extensive physiotherapy to this area. Resisted isometric adduction is then initiated at both inner and outer range to commence therapy for any concomitant tendinopathy. This is followed by cross-leg swinging in front and behind the uninvolved leg, crossover steps in front and behind the other leg, and sideways steps leading to sideways bounds. Running starts with the use of a rehabilitation ladder. When straight-line sprints can be tolerated, side steps, figure-of-eight runs, and cutting runs should be added, as may a kicking ladder (Read 2000). The partial rupture will heal by itself and often leaves a palpable gap. Surgery is infrequently required to close the defect. Rarely, surgical debridement of the adductor origin may be required.

Shearing of the adductor longus tendon from the pelvis may occur. This tendon has a 'design fault' with its very short and bifid nature making it susceptible to this frustrating and chronic pathology that can be monitored with diagnostic ultrasound. The superficial aspect of the tendon tends to be the area that shears away from its insertion and is the cause of the majority of symptoms. The deeper tendon then requires some time to re-establish control and ability to accept load. An intact superficial tendon can be injected; however, the risk in this procedure is in initiating a shearing pathology. Partial shearing causes more long-term problems than a complete shear, which is why surgical tenotomy may be suggested. The long-term results of tenotomy as compared to a conservative approach appear to be no different according to long-term follow-up and, therefore, seem to be somewhat aggressive to a non-surgical referrer (Schlegel et al. 2009).

An appropriate way to manage this condition is to accept that it may be a 3-month process, allowing the creation of a realistic prognosis and a more considered rehabilitation phase. Avoiding such actions as long kicking for a ball player is advised until the very end of the process, despite the obvious temptation as running is possible after about 5 weeks.

Ischial tuberosity lesions

The hamstring origin may suffer from a traction apophysitis. In a child, the apophyseal avulsion may remain unattached (Figure 34.22). The avulsion may be of sufficient force to separate the apophysis at such a distance that surgery to screw the apophysis

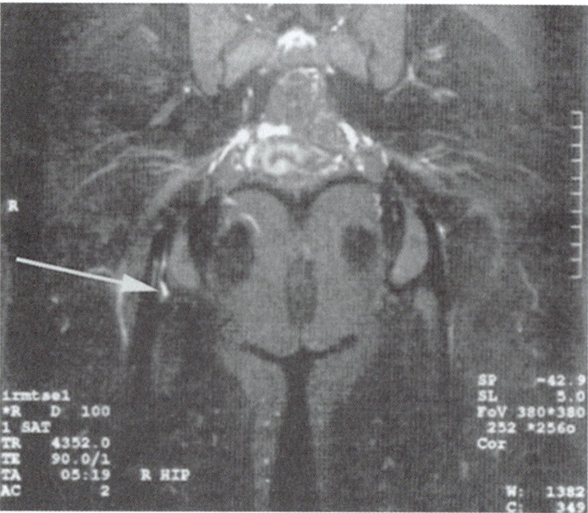

Figure 34.22 This avulsion of the ischeal tuberosity is chronic having remained detached during growth. (Reproduced with permission of Malcolm Read.)

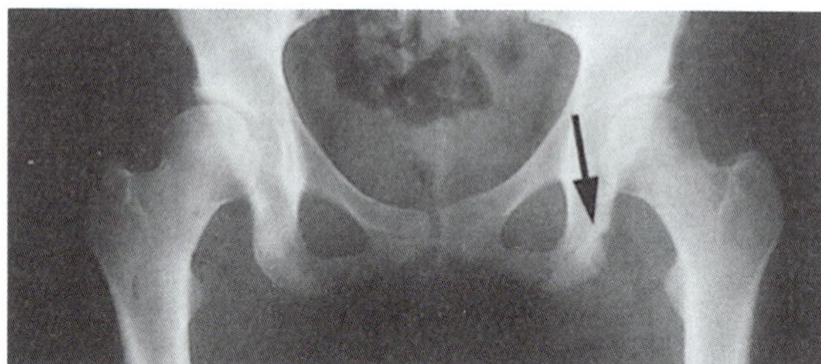

Figure 34.23 MRI shows a degenerative tear in the hamstring tendon and an ischeal bursa. (Reproduced with permission of Malcolm Read.)

back is required (Kurosawa et al. 1996). A localized tendinous tear adjacent to the origin occurs in the adult, and a bursitis between the hamstring tendon and the ischium can form (Figure 34.23).

History

Great forces are applied to the hamstring origin by a fall that whips the hip into full flexion with extended knees, such as a fall onto the back. However, stretching exercises can also avulse the origin in moves such as the front/back splits of dancers (Figure 34.24) and the hurdle stretch, where the leg is raised onto an object and the body is flexed over the straight leg. Osternig et al. (1986) demonstrated coactivation between the ipsilateral hamstrings and quadriceps. Basically, the hamstrings start contracting in the last third of knee extension to decelerate the swing phase and prepare to stabilize the leg for foot impact. Unfortunately, the hurdles stretch, which requires knee extension and hip flexion can, if forced, provoke a coactivation contraction from the hamstring, the very muscle one is trying to stretch and, thus, a powerful eccentric force on the ischial origin.

Lombard's paradox, in which one end of a muscle is contracting while the other is relaxing, is exhibited by any muscle that crosses two joints. The hamstring contraction should produce extension of the hip and flexion of the knee, but some movement patterns, such as dipping for the line at the end of a race, or bending to pick up a ball at speed, require flexion of the knee and flexion of the hip.

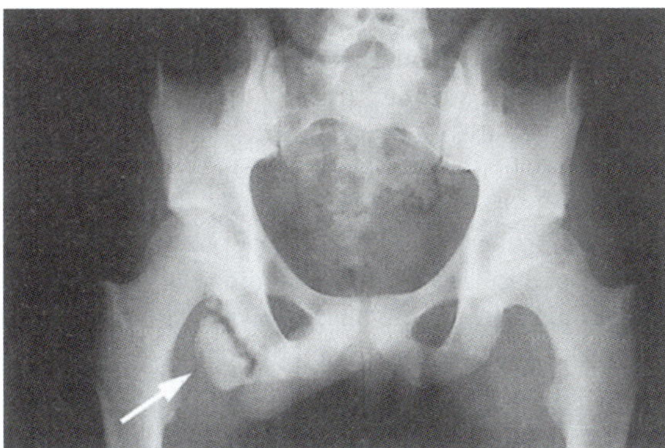

Figure 34.24 X-ray shows a discrete avulsion of the ischeal tuberosity following 'front and back' splits. (Reproduced with permission of Malcolm Read.)

Mistiming of this muscle movement makes for a torn hamstring, and is the reason that rehabilitation drills must build up this paradoxical skill to higher speeds. The aetiology of an ischial lesion includes an acute episode of stretching or exercising the hamstring, though some martial art kicking drills may gradually overload the enthesis.

Examination

Resisted testing of hamstrings in prone lying evokes pain at the tuberosity. Passive supine straight leg raising is painful, but the Lasegue and slump tests do not increase the pain. Primary posterolateral disc prolase, renowned for producing sciatica without lumbar pain, is often mistakenly diagnosed as a hamstring tear, and must be excluded. The use of the *bowstring sign* (Box 34.7) at this stage is perhaps most helpful.

Local palpation of the tuberosity or the tendinous junction is painful. The hamstring can maintain high loads and manual testing may be insufficient to produce pain in minor lesions. If the patient lies on the floor with heels resting on a chair and then raises the hips off the ground as high as possible, the extra power required for this manoeuvre may evoke the pain. It is also an excellent rehabilitation exercise. This test may be performed with one leg taking the load and the other raised clear of the chair.

Investigation

Radiography may demonstrate the avulsion; bone scan, a hot tuberosity; and MRI, the tendon tear and a bursitis. Real-time ultrasound in skilled hands may also be diagnostic. When healing has progressed to a sufficient level, isokinetic dynamometry, tested sitting and prone, registers the muscle balance (or imbalance), both between the ipsilateral and contralateral hamstrings and quadriceps. It is important to assess muscle balance so that appropriate strategies for rehabilitation may be undertaken. It may be preferable

Box 34.7 Bowstring sign

The straight leg raise is undertaken to a point at which pain is felt, and then the knee is flexed, relieving the pain. Pressure on the popliteal fossa and, particularly, the posterior tibial nerve will cause the sciatic pain to recur if the nerve is involved, but not if it is a hamstring lesion.

Box 34.8 Ballistic stretching

Here, the standing patient actively swings the straight leg into a full straight leg raise position, thus encouraging active quadriceps activity and coactive contraction of the hamstrings over as great a swing range as possible.

for the muscle to be exercised with the hip flexed or extended, and either at slow or fast speeds. Experience with hamstring dynamometry in athletes indicates that the damaged leg may be weak or strong, so that a damaged hamstring in the strong leg will require strengthening of the non-damaged weak leg during rehabilitation.

Treatment

Treatment is directed to reducing inflammation with electrotherapy or cortisone injection, organizing scar tissue with isometrics and massage, and preventing scar contraction with stretching exercises. For the non-athlete, a simple eccentric loading exercise for the hamstring is repetitive, slow (controlled) flexion of the spine from the upright position with straight legs. However, *ballistic stretching* (Box 34.8) is required for the hamstring of the dedicated sportsperson so that both the range and control of hamstring coactivation is improved. A hamstring rehabilitation ladder through running drills is required to return the patient to full activities.

Pathologies of the hip joint

The hip is a major loadbearing joint within the body, with ligamentous and bony configurations so strong that instability within the joint is almost unknown, except as a result of major trauma. It is, however, prone to its own peculiar pathologies.

The neonate

The standard assessments of the newborn baby include testing the hip for any clicking or limitation of abduction, in which case the baby is treated by frog splinting and is under the care of the orthopaedic or paediatric department.

The toddler

The young child, up to about 6–8 years old, may present with a painful hip on loadbearing and on passive testing when a capsular pattern of pain is found. This requires radiography to exclude other pathology such as a tumour or infection. If a bone scan and blood test are normal, treatment for the symptomatic hip is non-weightbearing until the joint has settled, at which stage all may have returned to normal without future recurrence of the problem. As the mechanism is not well understood, this is referred to as an *irritable hip*.

From about 5–10 years, children may have hip pain which, in its early stage, is associated with a normal radiograph, but bone scan may show a diminished uptake in the femoral head. This may be associated with an irritable hip. Alternatively, there may be no history of malfunction until examined as an adult who presents with an early degenerate hip with a flattened femoral head. This is the Legg-Calvé-Perthe malformed hip, where the normal rounded contour of the femoral head is replaced by a flattened elongated femoral head caused either by some degree of avascularization or even a mild slipped capital femoral epiphysis that was unrecognized and untreated. The Legg-Perthe hip, in the adult, is in itself not painful, but the joint is prone to early degenerative changes, which are painful.

Growth spurt

The growth spurt is generally thought to occur between the ages of 12 and 16, but as children develop at different rates, so the range of the age spectrum must always be considered. Knee pain in an adolescent that occurs during their growth spurt must always raise an index of suspicion about the hip. Clinical examination of all knee and thigh pain should begin by excluding hip pathology, and this is vital in an adolescent, who may sustain a slipped capital femoral epiphysis. Here, movement of the hip is immediately referred to the knee as pain. Internal rotation of the hip may be impossible, and there may be a fixed external rotation of the hip with shortening. Radiography may show a slipped capital femoral epiphysis. If there is any doubt about the diagnosis, it should be treated as a slipped capital epiphysis and a paediatric orthopaedic opinion sought for possible femoral capital epiphyseal pinning.

Avascular necrosis of the hip

Pain in the hip that presents soon after scuba diving should raise the possibility of avascular necrosis from the 'bends'—a nitrogen gas infarct from depressurizing too rapidly. Avascular necrosis may be a long-term consequence of the use of alcohol, steroids, or barbiturates.

Osteoarthritis of the hip

The most common problem is the degenerate osteoarthritic hip. There appears to be a familial element to degenerative joint disease, but some research suggests that impact exercise may increase its likelihood.

History

The pain usually starts with activity and presents as groin pain, but posterior hip pain is not uncommon. This pain may then become almost continuous, disturbing sleep. There are probably two elements to the pain source; osteochondral damage and the capsular soft tissue inflammation. The capsulitis causes the more continuous pain, and is present without loadbearing. It occurs when getting in or out of a car or crossing the legs one over the other, whereas the osteochondral damage gives rise to loadbearing pain and is often pain-free at rest. This history can govern treatment, in that the capsular pain does respond to anti-inflammatories such as NSAIDs and intra-articular injection of cortisone, or electrotherapy, whereas the osteochondral joint damage may respond to electrotherapeutic measures such as interferential and short-wave diathermy, but does not respond so well to NSAIDs and cortisone.

Examination

Examination is always thought to be easy, but this is often not the case. The patient may enter the consulting room with pain or a limp, or with a Trendelenburg gait. Here, the gluteal muscles are weak on the side of the lesion so that the patient cannot fix the pelvis to raise the leg, and thus leans towards the non-affected side to assist the raising of the painful side. The Trendelenburg gait is probably diagnostic, and the Trendelenburg sign is confirmatory, but the external rotators of the hip can mimic this sign when weak or painful, as can nerve damage to the gluteals. Hip flexion and rotation at its extreme end of range will be enhanced by flexion of the spine, and thus restriction of hip range can load the SIJ and vertebral column. Equally, testing the vertebral column with the patient standing may also place stresses throughout the hip, so the lumbar spine should be tested with the patient sitting, at which stage the pain from lumbar movements will not be influenced by hip movement.

If examination of the hip demonstrates a capsular pattern, then the capsule is inflamed; but a degenerative osteochondral joint may not have a true capsular pattern. The finding of a capsular pattern is diagnostic of hip disease. Pain on flexion of the hip alone is difficult to interpret, as this may be relieved by adding slight external rotation suggesting some local impingement or labrial tear. These lesions are displayed by MRI. Hip flexion pain that is felt in the buttock was described by Cyriax and Cyriax (1983) as 'the sign of the buttock': not diagnostic of a lesion in the buttock, but indicative that the lesion is not in the hip. It is then wise to look elsewhere, such as the lumbar facet joints, external rotators of the hip, sacrotuberous ligament, or possibly a capsular impingement of the hip. Facet joint pain may be felt directly in the groin on hip flexion. The capsular pattern at the hip, with pain in all planes of movement, should be detected with the patient sitting on the edge of the couch, and while lying supine and lying prone. The passive movements include flexion and extension, internal and external rotation, plus abduction and adduction. When the examiner is unable to distinguish between the hip and the back as the cause of symptoms, then, as a general rule of thumb, the back should be treated first.

Investigation

Investigations of the hip are primarily by radiography, preferably undertaken in the standing position, which will reveal narrowing of the joint space and osteophytic lipping in early degenerative disease. Cystic and sclerotic changes in the head of the femur and the acetabulum develop at a later state. Radiography may demonstrate the flattened femoral head of a Perthe's hip which is prone to early degenerative changes. Occasionally, an os acetabulare is seen at the acetabular rim and though this is recognized as a normal variant, it can limit abduction of the hip, with some discomfort, which in high-kicking sports, such as martial arts, presents a long-term problem. The os acetabulare develops as an apophysis and, in some sports that require a large range of hip movements, may produce pain on passive movement and on resisted muscle testing of the rectus femoris, which attaches in this area. The apophysis fuses up to the age of 25, which can produce problems of management in the young professional sportsperson.

Treatment

It must be remembered that degeneration of a joint is a continuum that gets worse with time. Radiography may be normal, but capsular signs are present, in which case, the pain is predominantly from the soft tissues which will respond to conservative therapeutic measures. It is when bony changes occur that conservative measures are less effective, as they only treat the soft tissue elements. The extent of disability and amount of pain caused by osteochondral degeneration will govern the criteria for a possible surgical replacement of the hip. Activities should be encouraged but should be non-weightbearing and involve high repetitions and low-resistance work. This is best done on a cycle or rowing ergometer, though swimming is of value as long as the outer ranges of the hip movement are not stressed. Because movements at the outer range of the joint range are painful, smaller walking paces are advised, as is getting out of the car with both legs together. A bicycle seat may have to be raised to accommodate limited hip flexion and the left foot turned further out at the golf address to permit a follow-through after ball-strike.

Stress fracture of the femoral neck

Stress fractures of the hip occur through the femoral neck. They are divided into compression and tension fractures. The compression fracture lies on the inferior surface of the femoral neck (Figure 34.25) and the tension fracture on the superior surface (Figure 34.26). The tension stress fracture is more likely to convert to a complete fracture (Figure 34.27), with serious consequences, such as avascular necrosis of the femoral head.

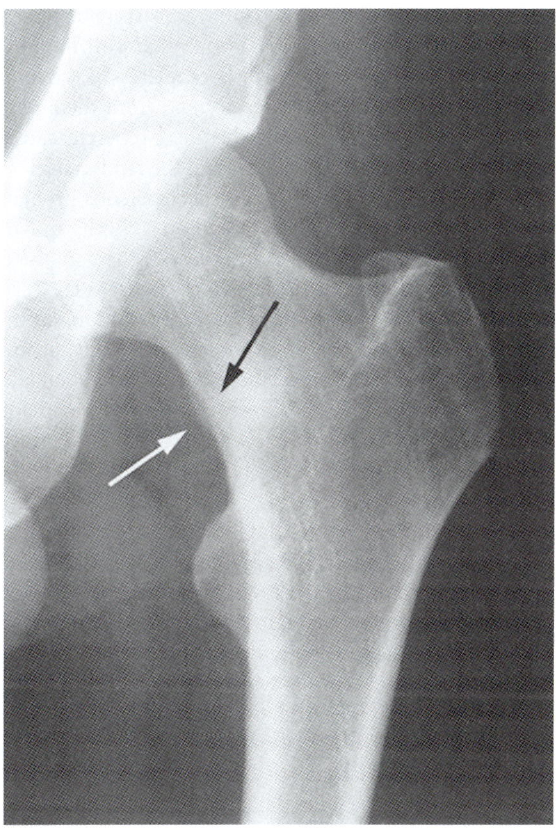

Figure 34.25 X-ray showing a compression stress fracture with callus (arrow). (Reproduced with permission of Malcolm Read.)

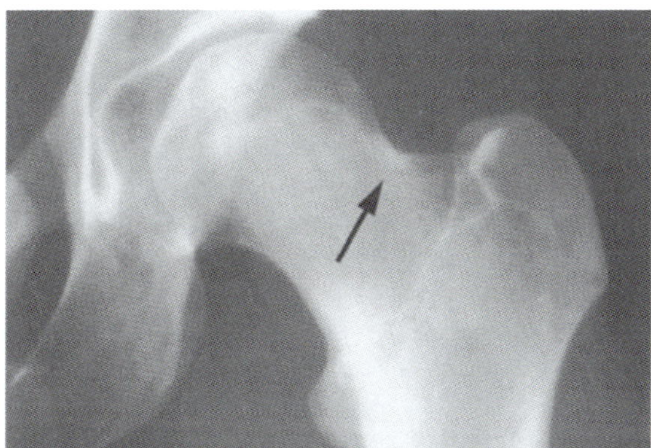

Figure 34.26 The sclerosis of this tension stress fracture suggests healing. A CT scan would exclude or display non-union (arrow). (Reproduced with permission of Malcolm Read.)

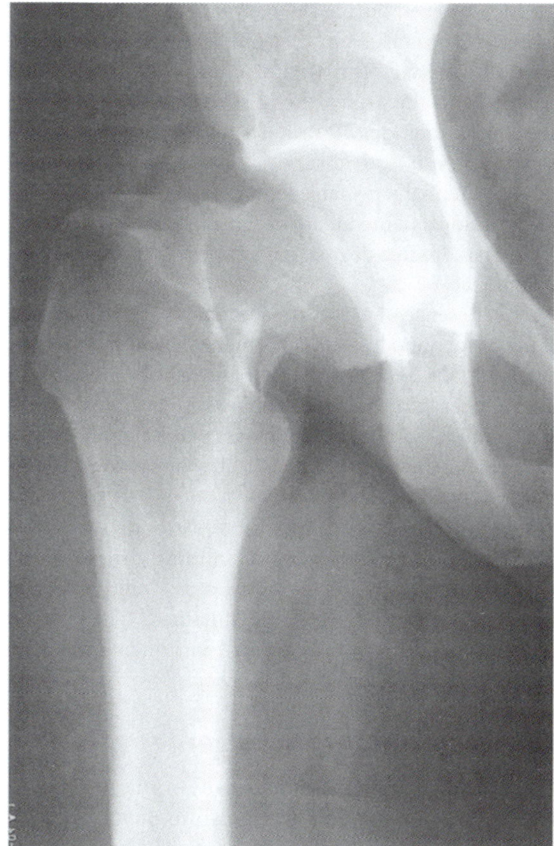

Figure 34.27 A disaster in a young athlete, this tension stress fracture has completed and needs surgery. Avascular necrosis may still occur. (Reproduced with permission of Malcolm Read.)

History

A history of groin pain in an active 18–40-year-old individual, especially a runner or military recruit (Stoneham and Morgan 1991), should raise the possibility of a stress fracture. The pain is relieved at rest and is worse on activities though, when severe, the pain may be present when moving the non-weightbearing hip. Sometimes this pain presents in the buttock as well.

Examination

Clinical findings will differ, depending on the extent of the lesion, but will be provoked by passive hip movements and weightbearing. Resisted hip muscle testing may evoke the pain as it is impossible to prevent some movement at the hip. Most important of all is an awareness of this lesion, and that the possibility of a stress fracture in a sportsperson must be excluded from a presentation of hip pain because the missed diagnosis can lead to bony collapse of the femoral neck, avascular necrosis, and a replacement hip in a 20-year-old. A disaster!

Investigations

Investigations will be initially by radiography. In the subacute lesion, callus or sclerosis at the superior or inferior femoral neck is revealed. However, during the early stages of this lesion, radiographs may be negative, and the clinician should investigate further with a bone scan. This will demonstrate increased uptake of technetium-99 in the presence of a stress lesion. A tension stress fracture should then be CT scanned to assess whether a fracture line is apparent; if it is, then surgical pinning is probably required, for this is a potentially unstable lesion. Though MRI may show the early stress lesion as a medullary oedema, it may not display the extent of the fracture to a degree that a surgical opinion can be given with confidence.

Once the presence of a stress fracture has been established, a full menstrual history and history of hormonal balance, dietary regime, and possible bone density should be instigated. However, this lesion does appear in men, and a training history of too rapid an increase of loads should be sought; biomechanical faults should also be corrected, together with biochemical bone markers.

Treatment

If there is no requirement for surgical pinning, the management is rest from all impact training. However, cross-training on a bicycle or rowing ergometer, or in water, is maintained. When impact pain from walking has settled, then gradual incrementation of impact loads may be considered.

Femoro-acetabular impingement (FAI)

In recent medical practice, supported by medical literature, the diagnosis of hip impingement has grown in popularity. Impingement of the neck of the femur onto the acetabular rim may produce bony bruising or a tear or shear of the hip labrum. Surgical intervention of such lesions may indeed be indicated if there is profound exostosis of the femoral neck causing a 'pincer' lesion. However, the advent of superior techniques of hip arthroscopy suggests that there has been a degree of over-diagnosis and over-treatment of such lesions. Functional pathology within the area, revealed by radiological diagnosis, can be addressed by manual therapy and rehabilitation techniques governing hip range, power, and proprioceptive control, before considering arthoscopic intervention (Gerhardt et al. 2012).

Obturator neuropathy

The obturator nerve arises from the nerve roots L2–4 and exits the pelvis as an anterior and posterior branch, through the obturator foramen. It is thought that the anterior branch may become trapped at the level of the obturator foramen (Brukner et al. 1999).

The history is of exercise-related groin pain in a sportsperson, often of some months' duration, centred on the adductor origin at the pubic bone. This may radiate down the medial aspect of the thigh to the knee. Adductor spasm and weakness is more likely after exercise, and in longstanding cases, there may be some paraesthesia over the medial thigh.

Examination

Obturator neuropathy is suspected when groin pain is reproduced when the patient stands in a partial lunge position with the affected leg backward, externally rotated and abducted. Investigations are undertaken to exclude other causes of groin pain. EMG may be diagnostic of denervation in the adductor longus and brevis muscles in longstanding cases. A nerve block injection, under radiographic control, into the roof of the obturator foramen, confirmed with radio-opaque dye, may block the post-exercise pain and reproduce the weakness.

Treatment

Conservative measures may fail, and surgical release of the nerve is then the treatment of choice, followed by early rehabilitation to jogging and running.

Pubic symphyseal lesions

Historical perspective and terminology

Traumatic osteitis pubis symphysis (TOPS) consists of damage to the ligaments and/or joint of the pubic symphysis, with the potential for destabilization of the pelvic ring, whereas stress to the *conjoined tendon* of the external inguinal ring, formed from the abdominal muscular and fascial insertions into the pubic tubercle, causes microtears and disruption to the enthesis and the tendon itself.

Early papers that describe TOPS in sportspersons probably include cases of conjoined tendon disruption as well, and indeed there may well be a continuum of injury from the conjoined tendon disruption through to the unstable pubic symphysis. Certainly, there seems now to be a plethora of conjoined tendon disruptions that either reflect altered training (perhaps too many sit-ups and crunches) or a failure to diagnose these in the past, when all groin strains were classified as TOPS. However, it must be remembered that many of these lesions get better with rest for 12–18 months.

Harris and Murray (1953) described TOPS in footballers who had associated sacroiliac problems, which would support the hypothesis of a pelvic ring injury. The literature does refer to this as a sporting problem, possibly from one-legged overload as in kicking a ball, but perhaps more pertinent is twisting over a fixed foot such as when tackling an opponent in soccer. Here, the support leg is moved into external rotation and abduction as the tackle leg is stretched out into abduction, and when the outer limits of the range of the hip movements are reached, the load is transferred to the pelvic ring, producing a distraction force across the pubic symphysis. Indeed, MRI scanning has revealed several cases with oedema in the adjacent pubic bone (Figure 34.28).

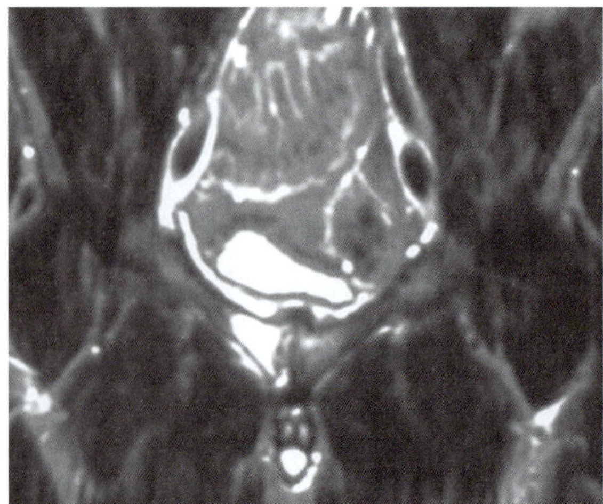

Figure 34.28 Oedema in the pubic bone with underlying adductor entheseal inflammation. (Reproduced with permission of Malcolm Read.)

In females in the later stages of pregnancy or in labour, a similar destabilizing problem at the pelvis may arise and is then often referred to as *symphysis pubis dysfunction* (SPD). Careful examination, that should include SIJ stress tests, reveals SIJ dysfunction in these patients. Indeed, management of this condition by prolotherapy to the SIJs appears to be the most effective management strategy (see Chapter 55).

History

The history of both lesions is of groin/anterior pelvic pain. Adductor muscle enthesopathy may also be present, but the indicator of pelvic ring dysfunction is the accompanying low suprapubic abdominal pain. The apparent connection to the adductors may well come from the fact that the adductors are involved not only in stabilizing the pelvic ring, but also because the adductor fascia passes deep to the symphysis pubis and becomes contiguous with the abdominal fascia. In its mildest form, pain is produced by twisting and turning and by sprinting rather than just running, but as the lesion becomes more severe, so there may be a constant suprapubic ache that is worse turning over in bed, sitting up, and walking. Some will complain of perineal or rectal pain, which suggests TOPS rather than a conjoined tendon lesion. Coughing and especially sneezing are painful.

Examination

The patient indicates the site of pain as over the adductor origin and the pubic tubercle, and this pain is worse on resisted adduction and sitting up. However, with TOPS or a conjoined tendon lesion, the adductor origin is classically not tender to palpation, whereas it is when the adductor origin lesion is present. The external inguinal ring, palpated through the invaginated scrotum, is tender and dilated. Tenderness may not be present if the patient has been resting from sport, and a therapeutic trial of cortisone to the adductor origin, followed by 10–14 days of incremental activities building up to sprints, is a reasonable procedure at this stage. If there is a flare of symptoms, the diagnostic signs of a conjoined tendon lesion may then be found. TOPS is tender to palpation over the pubic symphysis, and the conjoined tendon lesion is tender over the pubic tubercle. There is usually no pathological cough impulse to be palpated through the inguinal canal in either case. The diagnosis is not always easy and, unfortunately, investigations may not be helpful.

In SPD associated with pregnancy, symptoms are also primarily experienced anteriorly, though it is the author's opinion that treating the symphysis pubis, for instance by injection, is ineffective if similar treatment is not given to the SIJs.

Investigations

Investigations in the sportsperson should include the one-legged standing radiograph (the *stork or flamingo test*). If there is symphyseal instability, there is a shift in the level of the contralateral two pubic bones by over 2 mm (Figure 34.29). The radiograph may reveal sclerosis and lysis through the symphysis, indicative of TOPS, rheumatoid arthritis, or ankylosing spondylitis (Figure 34.11). Ankylosis of the pubic symphysis (Figure 34.30) and erosion of the gracilis margin are indicators of ankylosing spondylitis.

A bone scan excludes any other bony injury; in particular, stress fractures of the femur and pelvis. The standard anteroposterior view of the bone scan does not separate the bladder from the symphysis and, therefore, a rather arbitrary assessment is made of a 'hot lesion'. The squat view separates the bladder signal from the pubic symphysis and is, therefore, more reliable, but there are still problems of interpretation. MRI can demonstrate pubic symphyseal shift, particularly in the horizontal plane, and can display bone marrow oedema. An MRI can confirm disruption of the surrounding soft tissues.

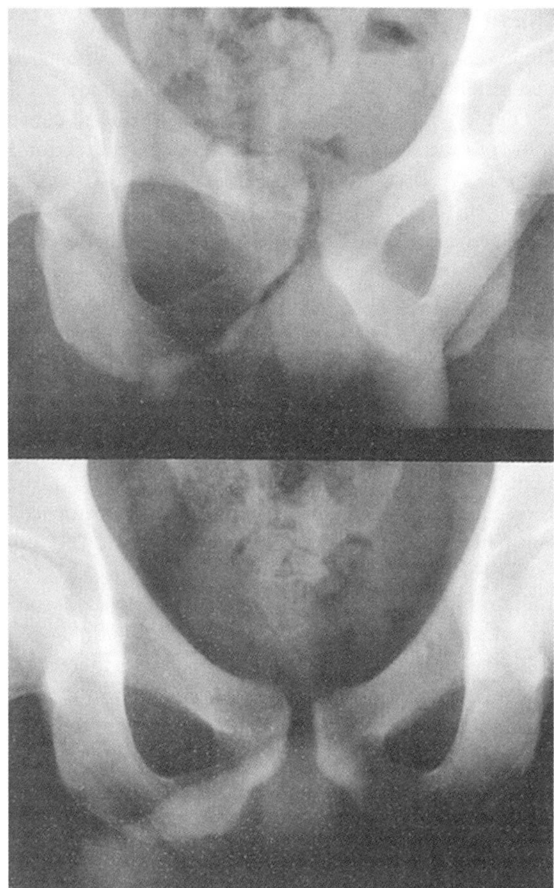

Figure 34.29 Flamingo or Stork views. Standing on one leg and then the other shows movement of the pubic symphysis greater than 2 mm. (Reproduced with permission of Malcolm Read.)

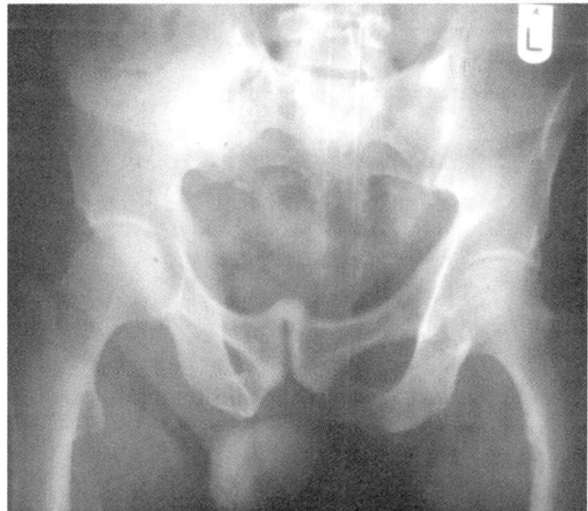

Figure 34.30 Ankylosis of the pubic symphysis. (Reproduced with permission of Malcolm Read.)

Treatment

Sometimes circumstances require short-term treatment of the inflamed lesion. Cortisone and local anaesthetic may be injected into the pubic symphysis, with or without ultrasound control for TOPS, or into the pubic tubercle for the conjoined tendon lesion (Holt et al. 1995). The vogue is for a surgical repair to the conjoined tendon, which returns players rapidly to their sport. However, it should be remembered that this lesion does get better with rest, albeit 12–18 months of controlled non-impact rest. Many sportsmen experience a contralateral injury, or a recurrence, presumably because the causative factors have not been identified and treated or because they have returned too soon to their causative sport. As yet, this is a very uncommon sporting injury in women.

Some surgeons will not repair the conjoined tendon if the pubic symphysis shifts by more than 2 cm on the stork test, and then the treatment of the unstable pelvis becomes a problem. Rest from impact is essential and any training should be by non-impact cross-training methods, although in the severe stages of TOPS, swimming is also painful. It may be possible to stabilize the pelvis by prolotherapy (sclerosing the SIJs with dextrose selerosant solution), on the principle that a ring cannot be disturbed in only one place, and that if the SIJ ligaments are strengthened, then there is a stabilizing effect on the symphysis. Time and reduction in twisting and impaction exercises are essential, as is proper rehabilitation and a graded return to sporting activities. Rarely, the symphysis is surgically fused.

The pelvic pain from SPD in females often resolves very slowly, and prolotherapy in experienced hands is strongly recommended. Failing that, a gradual recovery is to be expected over the course of a year or two. Recurrence of the condition with further pregnancies is to be expected.

References

Bottomley, M. B. (1990) Sacral stress fracture in a runner. *Br J Sports Med*, 24(4), 243–4.

Bowen, V., Cassidy, J. D. (1981) Macroscopic and microscopic anatomy of the SIJ from embryonic life until the eighth decade. *Spine*, 6(6), 620–8.

Brukner, P., Bradshaw, C., McCrory, P. (1999) Obturator neuropathy: a cause of exercise related groin pain. *Phys Sports Med*, 27(5), 62–73.

Cyriax, J. H., Cyriax, P. J. (1983) *Illustrated manual of orthopaedic medicine* (2nd edn). Butterworth-Heinemann, Oxford.

Gerhardt, M. B., Romero, A. A., Silvers, H. J., Harris, D. J., Watanabe, D., Mandelbaum, B. R. (2012) The prevalence of radiographic hip abnormalities in elite soccer players. *Am J Sports Med*, 40(3), 584–8.

Harris, N. H., Murray, R. O. (1953) Osteitis pubis of traumatic etiology. *J Bone Joint Surg*, 35A, 685.

Holt, M. A., Keen, S. J., et al. (1995) Treatment of osteitis pubis in athletes. Results of corticosteroid injections. *Am J Sports Med*, 23(5), 601–6.

Klinkert, P., Porte, R., de Rooje T. P., deVries, A. G. (1997) Quadratus tendinitis as a cause of groin pain. *Br J Sports Med*, 31(4), 348–50.

Kurosawa, H., Nakasita, K., Saski, S., Takeda, S. (1996) Complete avulsion of the hamstring tendons from the ischial tuberosity. A report of two cases sustained in judo. *Br J Sports Med*, 30(1), 72–4.

Macdonald, G. R. Hunt, T. E. (1951) Sacroiliac observations on the gross and histological changes in the various age groups. *Can Med Assoc J*, 66, 157.

Osternig, L. R., Hamill, J., Lander, J. E., Robertson, R. (1986) Co-activation of sprinter and distance runner muscles in isokinetic exercise. *Med Sci Sport Exercise*, 18(4), 431–5.

Read, M. T. F. (1998) Specific computerised tomographic views of the SIJ shows lesions that are undiagnosed with standard investigations of the lumbar spine. *J Orthop Med*, 20(1), 22–4.

Read, M. T. F. (2000) *A practical guide to sports injuries*. Butterworth-Heinemann, Oxford.

Schlegel, T. F. I., Bushnell, B. D., Godfrey, J., Boublik, M. (2009) Success of nonoperative management of adductor longus tendon ruptures in National Football League athletes. *Am J Sports Med*, 37(7), 1394–9.

Solonen, K. A. (1957) The SIJ in the light of anatomical roentgenological and clinical studies. *Acta Orthop Scand*, 27 (suppl. 27), 1–127.

Stoneham, M. D. Morgan, N. V. (1991). Stress fractures of the hip in Royal Marine recruits under training, a retrospective analysis. *Br J Sports Med*, 25(3), 145–8.

Sweetman, B. J. (1998) Low back pain and the leg twist test. *J Orthop Med*, 20(2), 3–9.

Vleeming, A., Mooney, V., Snijders, C., Dorman, T., Stoeckart, R. (eds) (1997) *Movement, stability and low back pain. The essential role of the pelvis.* Churchill Livingstone, Edinburgh.

Further reading

Brukner, P., Khan, K. (1993) *Clinical sports medicine*. McGraw-Hill, New York.

Reid, D. C. (1992) *Sports injury assessment and rehabilitation*. Churchill Livingstone, Edinburgh.

Chapter 35

Sacroiliac joint disorders

Simon Petrides

. . . the pelvic girdle is the crossroads of the body, its architectural center, the meeting place of the locomotive apparatus, the resting place of the torso, the temple of the reproductive organs, the framework within which new life develops, the place of the two main functions of elimination and last but not least a place on which to sit down.

(Fred L. Mitchell D.O.)

Introduction to sacroiliac joint disorders

Hippocrates apparently observed that the female pelvis separates during labour and remains so after birth (Lynch 1920). Goldthwait and Osgood first described the sacroiliac joint (SIJ) as a painful entity in 1905. SIJ dysfunction has been proposed as a cause of low back pain by osteopaths and chiropractors for many years. More recently, physiotherapists, musculoskeletal physicians, sport and exercise medicine specialists, and pain physicians have researched further into the concepts of SIJ pain and dysfunction. History, clinical signs, and radiological investigations individually are inadequate to diagnose SIJ pain. However, as with all musculoskeletal assessment, careful analysis of all the presenting features can direct the physician to the diagnosis with reasonable accuracy.

Prevalence of sacroiliac joint disorders

The prevalence of SIJ pain has not been widely studied but is in the region of 13–30% of patients with low back pain. Schwarzer used diagnostic block injections and pain provocation during injection and computed tomography (CT) arthrography to establish this generally accepted range (1995).

In a larger study of 1293 patients with low back pain, there was 22.5% prevalence, mostly using a range of clinical tests (Bernard and Cassidy 1991; Bernard and Kirkaldy-Willis 1987). Diagnostic block injections remain the gold standard in this respect. Maigne used comparative SIJ local anaesthetic blocks and concluded that the prevalence was 15–25% in unilateral low back pain (Maigne et al. 1996). A systematic review of literature in 2009 estimated the prevalence of SIJ pain to range between 10% and 38% using double blocks in the study population (Ruper et al. 2009).

Anatomy of the sacroiliac joint

The SI joint is the largest axial joint in the body with an average surface area of 17.5 cm^2 (Bernard and Cassidy 1991). It is auricular-shaped, diarthroidal, and a synovial joint with only the anterior third being a true synovial joint. Wide variations in size and shape exist between individuals and within the same individual (Dijkstra et al. 1989). Hyaline cartilage lines the sacral surface and fibrocartilage lines the iliac surface. The adult joint surfaces develop interlocking ridges. The rest of the articulation comprises a complex arrangement of ligamentous connections:

- The *anterior SI ligament* is just a thickening of the anterior capsule.
- The *posterior SI ligament* (Figure 35.1) is made up of the short (upper) and long (lower) posterior SI ligaments.
- The *interosseus SI ligament* is deep to the posterior SI ligament and is made up of shorter fibres.
- The *sacrotuberous ligament* runs between the sacrum and the ischial tuberosity.
- The *sacrospinous ligament* runs between the sacrum and the ischial spine.
- The *iliolumbar ligament* effectively acts as an SI ligament and crosses the joint connecting the transverse process of L5 with the inner posterior iliac crest.

Nerve supply to the sacroiliac joint

The extra-articular ligamentous posterior joint is considered by several authorities to be innervated by the lateral branches of the L4–S3 dorsal rami (Bernard and Cassidy 1991). Other authors state that L3 to S4 may be the full extent of the innervation (Grob et al. 1995). There is physiological evidence that there is dorsal and ventral innervation of the intra-articular portion of the SI joint (Dreyfuss et al. 2009). This extent of sensory supply may account for the wide variation in pain referral patterns (Cohen 2005).

Bone scintigraphy and SPECT (single-photon emission computed tomography)-CT scanning has recently been shown to

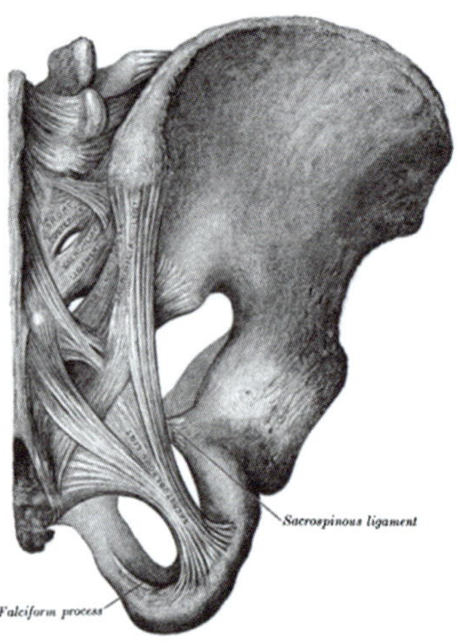

Figure 35.1 Right hemi-pelvis image showing the posterior SI ligaments. (Professional Health Systems with permission.)

demonstrate metabolic alterations in an SI joint with established involvement, and also in the posterior ligaments, thus confirming the importance of the nerve supply to both structures (Cusi et al. 2012).

Sacroiliac joint function

The SIJ primarily functions as a structure with the ability to transfer and dissipate load from the trunk to the lower extremities and vice versa. Motion, although a matter of 2–4° (Vleeming et al. 1992), is available in all three axes (White and Panjabi 1990). Whilst SIJ motion occurs mostly from sitting to standing, there is a maximum of 2° of rotation in extension and 0.5–1.6 mm translatory movement. However, no difference in motion has been found when comparing painful to non-painful joints (Sturesson et al. 1989).

'*Form closure*' is a term which describes how the shape and integrity of the joint and its ligaments help prevent shearing and translation of its surfaces under load (Pool-Goudzwaard et al. 1998). Vertical forces are controlled during walking, sitting, and standing, while antero-posterior forces are controlled during bending activities.

'*Force closure*' is a term coined by the same authors and addresses the compression force required to control the translatory forces across the joint. These forces are primarily supplied by co-activation of the latissimus dorsi and the contralateral superficial gluteus maximus linked by the superficial layer of the thoracolumbar fascia (*the posterior oblique sling*) (Figure 35.2). This system may work well under high load such as pushing, pulling, throwing, and running. Under low load, such as walking, standing, or sitting, 'force closure' is provided by co-activation of the posterior fibres of internal oblique linking with the deep fibres of the contralateral gluteus maximus via the middle layer of the thoracolumbar fascia.

Therefore, it is erroneous to believe that muscles play little part in supporting the SIJs. There are, in fact, several other muscles which directly connect to the SI supporting ligaments. These muscles are directly associated with pain and dysfunction in the SIJ and include the piriformis, biceps femoris, and iliacus.

'*Tensegrity*' is a term describing tension and compression forces through connective tissue (ligaments and fascia), soft tissues, and the pelvic floor which stabilize the sacrum between the iliac bones. Levin described this mechanism as analogous to a bicycle wheel where the hub (sacrum) is suspended by spokes (SI ligaments) within the wheel rim (pelvic ring) (Levin 2006).

'*Motor control*' and co-activation of tonic deep stabilizers such as the transversus abdominis and multifidus have been described by Richardson as affecting 'stiffness' of the SIJ measured by Doppler imaging of vibrations, and this contributes to 'force closure' at the SIJ (Richardson et al. 2002).

Sacroiliac joint dysfunction

SIJ dysfunction refers to aberrant 'function or position' of the SIJ which may or may not cause pain.

Extrinsic causes of SIJ dysfunction

Axial loading, compression, shearing, and sudden rotatory forces centred around the SIJ are primarily responsible for disruption of the joint capsule and surrounding ligaments. Chou assessed the events leading to SI pain, which was confirmed by local anaesthetic injection, and found that trauma was the cause in 44% of patients

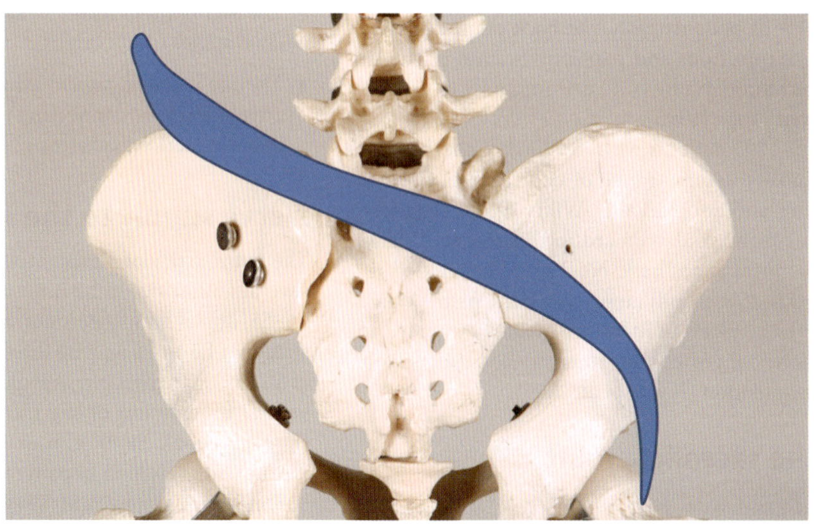

Figure 35.2 Latissimus dorsi and the contralateral superficial gluteus maximus linked by the superficial layer of the thoracolumbar fascia (the posterior oblique sling). (Blackberry Clinic with permission.)

(road traffic accidents were the main cause of trauma, followed by a fall onto the buttock and childbirth) (Chou et al. 2004).

Repetitive asymmetric movements in sports such as the triple jump, the high jump, and hockey are recognized causative factors.

Intrinsic (non-traumatic) causes of SIJ dysfunction

Causes of 'hypermobility' and 'hypomobility' along with 'SIJ malposition' can be subdivided:

- *Myofascial causes:* Tension on ligamentous and connective myofascial tissues may result from lumbar dysfunction, muscle imbalance (lower cross syndrome), leg length discrepancy, over-pronation, poor footwear, scoliosis, gait abnormalities, hip osteoarthritis (OA), post-lumbar fusion, and pregnancy.
- *Arthrogenic causes:* SIJ malpositioning, along with intra and peri-articular SIJ degenerative changes can lead to dysfunction and vice versa. Inflammatory SIJ disorders are also often accompanied by dysfunction.
- *Post-surgical causes:* SIJ pain is often a consequence of lumbar interbody or lumbosacral fusion, but this may *not* be due to a resulting increase in mechanical load borne by the SIJ (Frymoyer et al. 1978a). Onsel demonstrated an increase in SIJ uptake on isotope bone scan after lumbar fusion surgery (Onsel et al. 1992); however, the biomechanical basis for this observation has been refuted by other studies (Frymoyer et al. 1978b). SIJ dysfunction can also be related to alteration in load transmission after total hip replacement.
- *Inflammatory causes:* Inflammatory sacroiliitis is often a presenting feature of sero-negative spondylarthropathies such as ankylosing spondylitis, psoriatic arthropathy, reactive arthropathy (e.g. Reiter's syndrome), enteropathic arthropathy, systemic lupus erythematosus (SLE), and others, suggesting an autoimmune or genetic predisposition or an infective aetiology.
- *Other causes*: Stress fractures of the sacrum are occasionally encountered in runners and can be confirmed by magnetic resonance imaging (MRI) and/or CT scan.

Primary and secondary bony tumours of the sacrum or ilium can present in the same way as more innocent SI dysfunction. Attention should always be paid to the coexistence of any 'red flags' in the history.

History and pain referral patterns of sacroiliac joint disorders

History

There is often a history of a fall, slip, or trip resulting in the patient landing on one buttock. Involvement in a road traffic accident with a rear end collision may injure the SIJ, especially if the ipsilateral foot is on the brake. Various repetitive asymmetrical sports such as golf, the high jump, and skating can be associated with SIJ pain. The characteristic pain can be aggravated by sitting on the ipsilateral buttock and weightbearing on that side while walking or standing (Fortin et al. 1994a,b). Pain may also be aggravated by climbing stairs and turning in bed.

Pain referral patterns

SIJ pain is typically unilateral, located near or just inferior to the posterior superior iliac spine (PSIS), and dull in character. There can also be a history of catching, clunking, or clicking associated with a sharp pain. Patients often report a subjective feeling of the pelvis 'going out' along with an awkwardness of gait.

The pain can radiate down the posterior thigh, into the groin or even anterior thigh. It may even refer as far as the posterolateral calf, foot, and toes.

Evidence

Groin pain has been described as the only referral site to distinguish SIJ from non-SIJ pain (Schwarzer et al. 1995). However, in asymptomatic volunteers, sensory examination immediately after sacroiliac injection of contrast and local anaesthetic reveals an area of buttock hypoaesthesia extending approximately 10 cm caudally and 3 cm laterally from the PSIS. This area of hypoaesthesia corresponded to the area of maximal pain noted upon injection (Fortin et al. 1994a). Slipman demonstrated pain in patients with local anaesthetic confirmed SI pain to radiate to the buttock (94%), lower lumbar area (72%), lower extremity (50%), groin (14%), upper lumbar area (6%), and abdomen (2%). Pain radiated below the knee in 28%, with 12% reporting foot pain (Slipman et al. 2000).

Inflammatory back pain

Criteria in the history pointing to a diagnosis of 'inflammatory back pain' have been proposed when two out of four of the following are present:

(1) morning stiffness lasting more than 30 minutes

(2) improvement of back pain with exercise but not rest

(3) night pain in the second half of the night only

(4) alternating buttock pain.

These criteria yield a sensitivity of 70% and a specificity of 81% (Rudwaleit et al. 2006).

The sacroiliac joint in pregnancy

The SIJ is vulnerable during pregnancy as a result of laxity due to the increased levels of oestrogen and relaxin combined with the biomechanical postural stresses of late pregnancy. The lax ligaments can also become symptomatic as a direct result of parturition when the SIJs and pubic symphysis undergo deformation during the final stages of delivery (Daly et al. 1991).

Pelvic girdle pain (PGP) and symphysis pubis dysfunction (SPD)

These are both a result of the pelvic ring disturbance during pregnancy and delivery. PGP can be non-pregnancy related but has a point prevalence of 20% in pregnancy. Pain is experienced in the vicinity of the lumbosacral, SI, and symphysis pubis joints (Keriakos et al. 2001). It can radiate to the posterior thigh and can coexist with SPD. Characteristic features include:

- Difficulty climbing stairs
- Pain and difficulty turning over in bed
- Having to sit to dress
- Pain getting in and out of the car or bed
- Pain with squatting
- Difficulty swimming breast stroke
- Pain on lifting one leg to step over something

Diagnosis can be made from specific pain provocation and functional tests (as described in a later section in this chapter); for example, Patrick's (Faber) test, thigh thrust, Gaenslen's test, modified Trendelenburg's test, and the active straight leg raise (ASLR) test. Pain on palpation of the posterior SI ligaments and the symphysis can also help with the diagnosis. Exclusion of lumbar causes is another prerequisite (Vleeming et al. 2008).

Treatment of the condition is similar to other forms of SI pain, with adequate reassurance and education regarding the nature of the condition. A study in women with PGP after pregnancy found that specific stabilization training resulted in 50% disability reduction, a 30% pain reduction on a visual analogue scale (VAS), and quality of life improvement compared to a control group. This effect persisted at a 2-year follow-up (Stuge et al. 2004).

Sacroiliac joint imaging

Ankylosing spondylitis

Inflammatory changes in the SIJs are often seen early in ankylosing spondylitis (AS) and are useful in the diagnosis and follow-up of patients with the condition (Van der Heijde and Spoorenberg 1999). Radiographic involvement of the SIJ is a prerequisite for diagnosing AS. Sacroiliitis is bilateral, symmetric, and progressive with bony erosions, sclerosis, and pseudo-widening of the joints, eventually leading to fusion.

Enteropathic sacroiliitis

Enteropathic arthritis develops in 9–20% of people who suffer from inflammatory bowel disease (i.e. Crohn's disease and ulcerative colitis). About 20% of people with enteropathic arthritis have sacroiliitis. It is similar radiographically to AS, with bilateral symmetric sacroiliitis along with the other characteristic features of 'continuous' spondylitis. It flares up in relation to the exacerbations of the inflammatory bowel disease.

Reactive arthritis and psoriatic arthritis

This causes an asymmetric sacroiliitis with 'discontinuous' spondylitis.

MRI scan (STIR – Short Tau Inversion Recovery sequences), CT, SPECT scans, radio-isotope bone scans

These can all show features of inflammatory or degenerative SIJ arthropathy but are not part of the routine work-up unless there is doubt regarding SIJ involvement and in order to rule out other pathology.

Clinical tests for sacroiliac joint disorders

There are at least 50 sacroiliac tests which have been described in the diagnosis of SIJ dysfunction. These include 'positional palpation tests', 'motion palpation tests', and 'pain provocation tests'.

Positional palpation tests

These tests look for asymmetry by palpation of bony landmarks such as the anterior and posterior iliac spines (ASIS/PSIS), the iliac crests, the sacral sulcus, the infero-lateral angle of the sacrum, and the greater trochanters.

Reliability

The tests have insufficient reliability to be able to assess their usefulness in relating asymmetry to SIJ pain. However, osteopaths and chiropractors use the positional assessments as part of the multimodal evaluation of SIJ dysfunction and low back pain. The presence of a leg length discrepancy (LLD) is arguably related to the presence of pelvic or SIJ torsional asymmetries whether as a cause or effect, although pelvic torsion does not appear to be associated with the presence of low back pain (Levangie 1999).

The symphysis pubis (SP) can experience significant loads and helps stabilize the pelvic ring. Motion palpation at the SP includes assessment of vertical shear and slight rotatory motion. This is often associated with SI torsional disturbance.

'Pelvic torsion'

The positional tests are, however, in everyday use by almost all practitioners of manual therapy. They are used in a pragmatic approach to assess pelvic asymmetries and to direct treatment. There are situations in which anterior rotation of one innominate bone and posterior rotation of the contralateral innominate coexist and the asymmetry of the landmarks is easily palpable. These features, along with LLD, can be measured on *standing anteroposterior (AP) pelvic X-ray*, making it difficult to refute. Most pelvic torsions are, however, much less easily palpable, leading to the poor results in reliability studies. Such results do not, in the author's opinion, disprove the existence of the phenomenon, since there is a wide spectrum of types of SI dysfunction and a wide variation in observers' technical ability to detect the asymmetries in movement and position.

Motion palpation tests

These include the Gillet test, Piedallau test, and joint play (Menell) test. Detailed description of these tests can be found in technique manuals. It is important, however, to appreciate the varying approaches used by osteopaths, chiropractors, and physiotherapists and the information deduced from these tests, along with the potential shortcomings of the subjective nature of some of the assessments.

The tests involve palpation of the SIJ sulcus and landmarks on movement of the trunk or lower limb. Tests which have been extensively studied include the standing flexion, sitting flexion, standing hip flexion, sacral springing, supine to sit, and prone knee flexion tests.

Reliability

These tests are regularly used by osteopaths and chiropractors but they seem to have poor inter-observer and intra-observer reliability (Freburger and Riddle 1999, O'Haire and Gibbons 2000); although some studies have shown adequate reliability. The reliability can improve when using groups of tests; however, the 'validity' of these tests is also unproven.

Validity

A reference standard for SIJ dysfunction is not readily available, so validity of the tests for this disorder is unknown. SIJ palpation tests of movement, position, or symmetry have not been studied with any meaningful methodology in view of the lack of a gold standard against which the dysfunction can be measured. The presence of dysfunction in relation to the existence of pain has been studied. In this trial, a group of tests demonstrated a sensitivity of 82% and a specificity of 88%, but the tests themselves were individually unreliable and the study was non-blinded (Cibulka and Koldehoff 1999).

The presence of pregnancy-related pelvic pain (PRPP) during and after pregnancy has been related to asymmetric SIJ laxity by using Doppler imaging of vibrations over the joints, which supports the construct linking SIJ dysfunction to an underlying SIJ instability (Damen et al. 2002).

Pain provocation tests

Reliability

Pain provocation tests have been shown to have acceptable inter-examiner reliability when well standardized (Laslett et al. 2005; Robinson et al. 2007). In a systematic review in 2009, the conclusion was that the evidence for provocative testing to diagnose SIJ pain is Level II-3 or limited (Rupert et al. 2009).

Validity

Although no single test has been demonstrated to be highly specific or sensitive for SIJ pain (Dreyfuss et al. 2009), Laslett concluded that three or more positive pain provocation tests in a diagnostic accuracy study have a sensitivity of 91% and a specificity of 78%, and in patients whose pain cannot be made to centralize using the McKenzie method (1981), the specificity rises to 87% (Laslett et al. 1994, 2003, 2005, 2008; Levin U 2004). The use of three or more tests was corroborated by van der Wurff et al. (2006) who used a similar selection of tests (Figures 35.3–35.7).

Stuber carried out a systematic review of the literature in 2007 to determine the specificity, sensitivity, and predictive values of such clinical tests of the SIJ. He concluded that the distraction test (Figure 35.3), compression test (Figure 35.4), thigh thrust/posterior shear (Figure 35.5), sacral thrust, and resisted hip abduction were the only tests to have specificity and sensitivity greater than 60% in at least one study, and that further investigation is warranted to determine which tests or combinations of these tests are the best for diagnosing SIJ dysfunction (Stuber 2007).

There is also debate as to the ideal force that should be used and the number of repetitions that should be carried out when performing these tests (Levin 2004).

In chronic back pain populations, patients who have three or more positive provocation SIJ tests and whose symptoms cannot be made to centralize have a probability of having SIJ pain of 77%, and in pregnant populations with back pain, a probability of 89%. This combination of test findings could be used to evaluate the efficacy of specific treatments for SIJ pain.

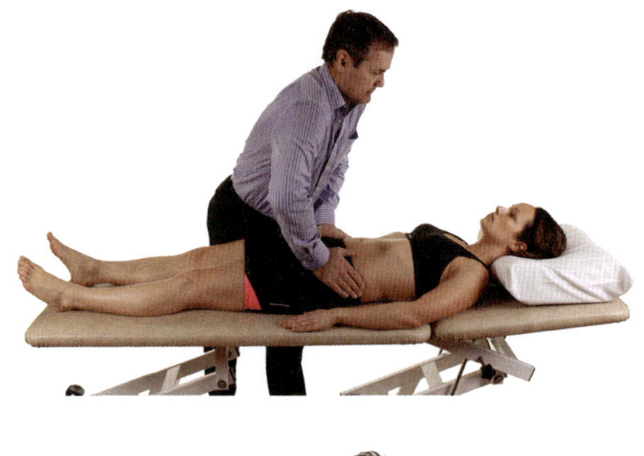

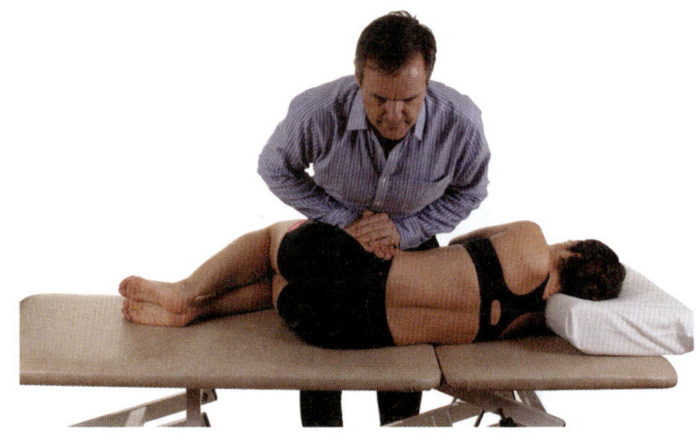

Figure 35.4 ASIS compression test, and alternative technique.

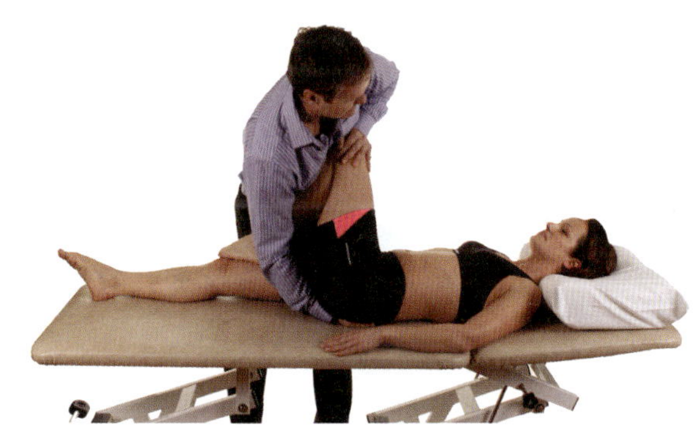

Figure 35.5a Left thigh thrust test. Pain reproduction implies a positive test.

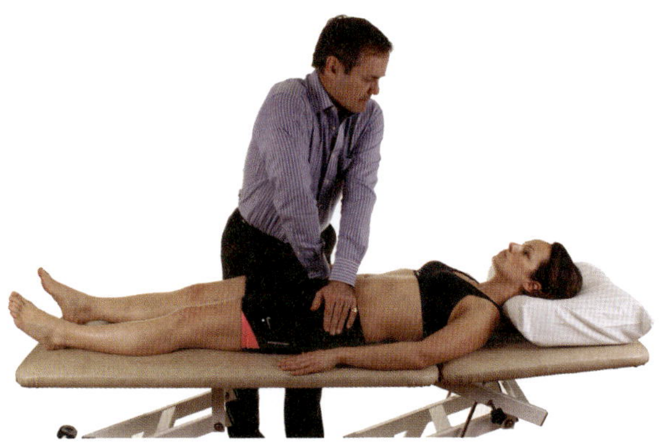

Figure 35.3 ASIS distraction test.

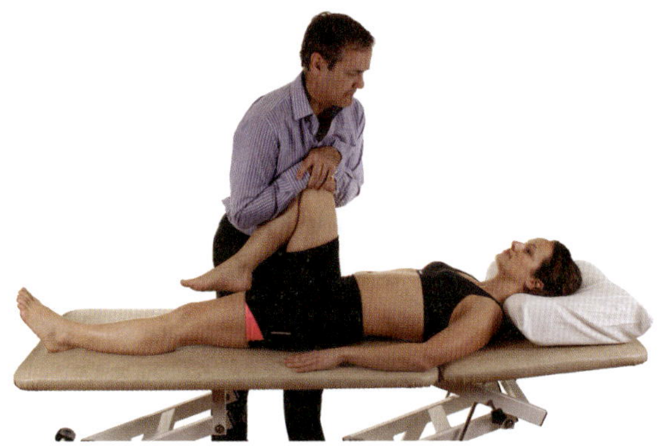

Figure 35.5b Right thigh thrust.

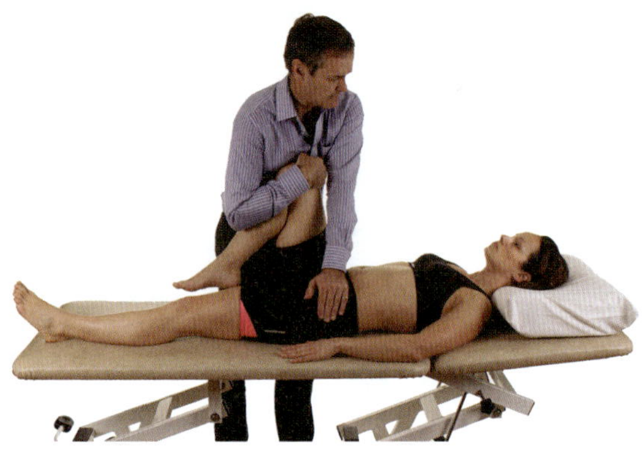

Figure 35.5c Right thigh thrust, alternative techniques.

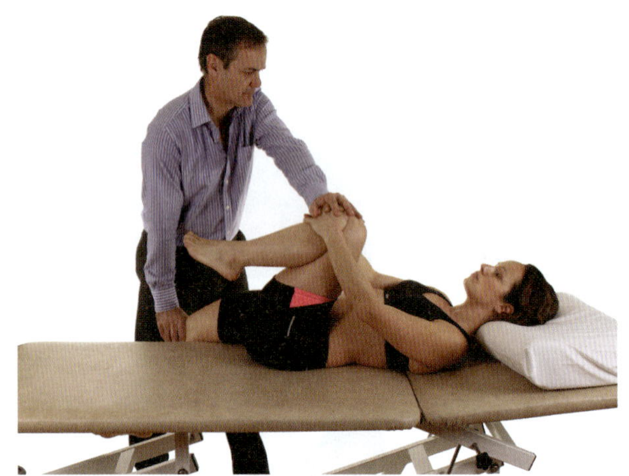

Figure 35.6 Gaenslen's test stressing the right SI joint.

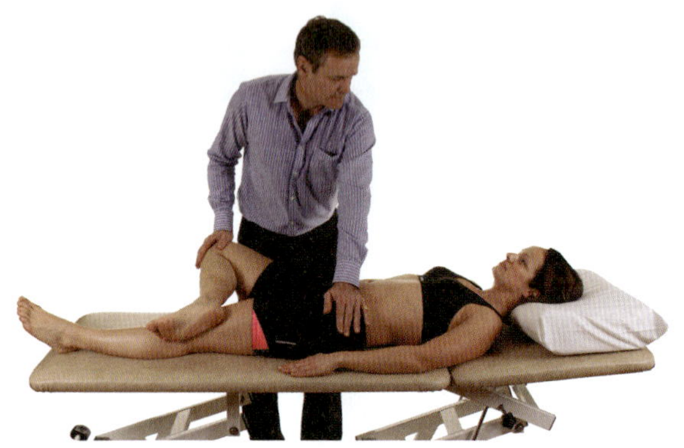

Figure 35.7 Patrick's (FABER) test of right SIJ.

It is not however known if the pain provocation tests can reliably identify extra-articular SIJ sources of pain, although it is the author's opinion that a significant proportion of SI pain seen in most types of practice is extra-articular and ligamentous. A study by Murakami et al. suggests that this may indeed be the case (2007).

Active straight leg raise (ASLR) test

The ASLR test (Figures 35.8 and 35.9) not only assesses pain provocation but also mobility, stability (force closure), and ways to

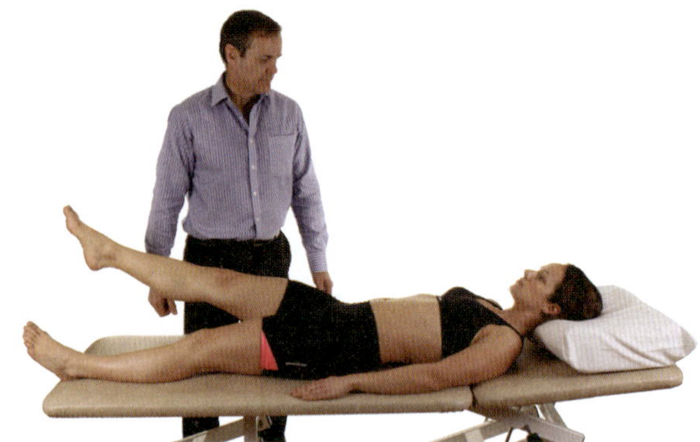

Figure 35.8 Active straight leg raise test (ASLR).

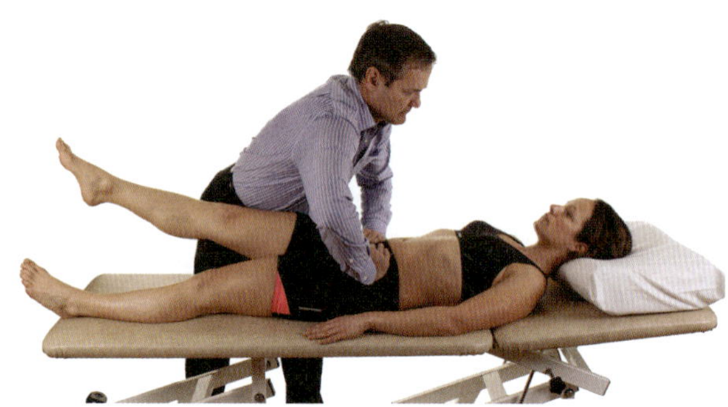

Figure 35.9 Active straight leg raise test (ASLR) with pelvic stabilization.

correct any instability (Mens et al. 2002). It tests the ability of the SIJ to transfer load through the pelvis. A subjective score of difficulty and pain is monitored on ASLR on a 0–5 scale. It has also been shown to have predictive value for post-partum SIJ-related pain (Damen et al. 2002).

Method

The supine patient actively raises the straight leg 20 cm whilst noting pain and difficulty as the clinician assesses trunk rotation (Figure 35.8). Resistance can be added (Turner 2009) (Figure 35.9). If either test is positive, then:

1 the patient braces the lumbar spine

2 manual compression is applied through the ilia

3 a SI belt is tightened around the pelvis.

The test is repeated and any difference, particularly an easing of pain or a subjective feeling that the leg is lighter, is considered a positive test. The ASLR test has been reported as having a sensitivity of 0.87 and a specificity of 0.94 (Mens et al. 2002). A positive test has correlated with excessive mobility of the pelvis on X-ray, severity of pain and disability, overall clinical state, and hip flexor electromyography (EMG) output, and is predictive of outcome (de Groot et al. 2008; Mens et al. 2002; Stuge et al. 2004).

The more recently described '*drop test*' (Figures 35.10a and b) has a high reliability (Kappa score) but has yet to be tested for validity to demonstrate diagnostic accuracy (Robinson et al. 2007).

In all of the pain provocation tests, there is a wide variety of techniques used by practitioners, irrespective of experience. The

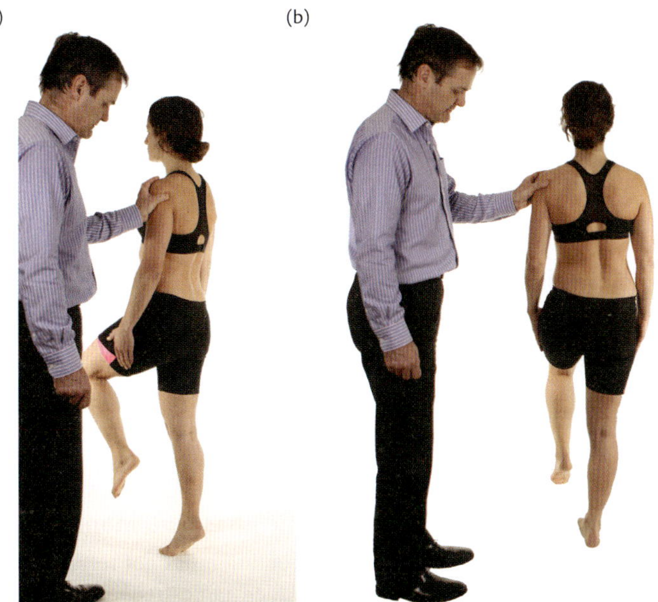

Figure 35.10(a–b) The drop test: the patient drops down from a single leg tip-toe position keeping the knee straight. Reproduction of pain denotes a positive test.

amplitude of force used, the direction of force, the duration of force, and the interval between application of forces all vary widely and can affect the likelihood of a test being negative if inadequate force is used (Levin et al. 2001).

Muscle adaptive shortening tests

These tests are used to evaluate the shortening or lengthening of muscles related to innominate rotation and pelvic torsion. These muscles can become vulnerable to injury as a result of adaptations of this kind.

- *Ober's test* (Figure 35.11): assesses the shortening of the tensor fascia lata and the ilio-tibial band.
- *Passive prone knee flexion test* (Figure 35.12) *and the modified Thomas test* (Figure 35.13): assess the flexibility or shortening of the rectus femoris and other hip flexors.
- *Hamstring tightness test:* commonly tested by a passive straight leg raise with bent or straight knee.

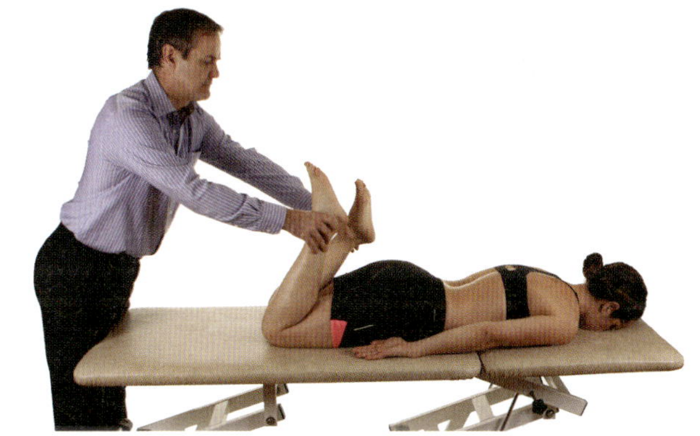

Figure 35.12 Passive prone knee flexion test; end-feel resistance to movement is assessed.

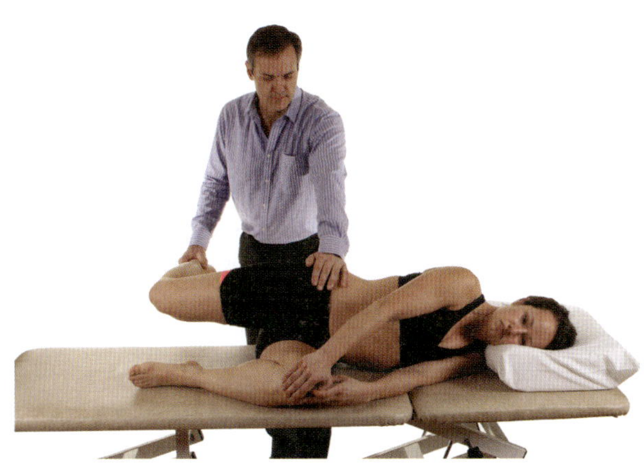

Figure 35.11 Ober's test.

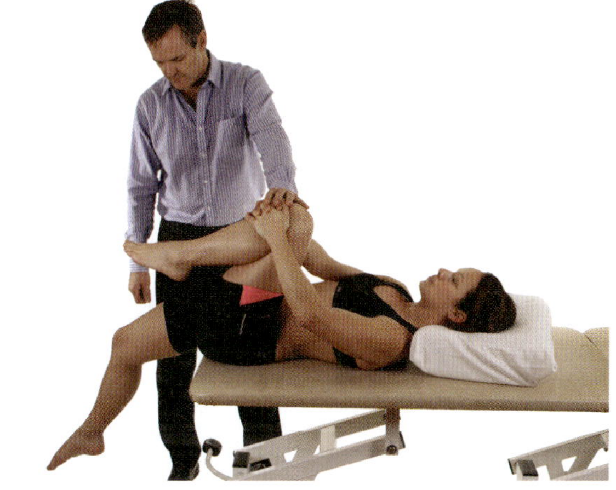

Figure 35.13 The modified Thomas test can be used to assess tightening of rectus femoris in SIJ dysfunction. The angle of ipsilateral knee flexion is noted.

Trigger points in SI dysfunction

The presence of trigger points in gluteal muscles can be associated with SIJ pain (Travell and Simons 1982). Imbalance of tension in muscles and fascia around the SIJ echoes the concepts advocated by A.T Still (osteopathy) and Palmer (chiropractic) by focusing on dynamic aspects of the musculoskeletal system rather than pathological structure.

Diagnosis of sacroiliac joint disorders

The gold standard diagnostic procedure for SI pain is a fluoroscopic or CT-guided local anaesthetic intra-articular injection using comparative or placebo-controlled diagnostic blocks (Bogduk 2004). However, the International Association for the Study of Pain (IASP) criteria for SIJ pain are still appropriate and include:

1 pain in the region of the SIJ

2 positive pain provocation tests

3 response to local anaesthetic injection under fluoroscopic guidance (Merskey and Bogduk 1994).

Diagnostic intra-articular or multi-depth, multi-site lateral branch blocks can help direct treatment (Dreyfuss et al. 2009).

Differential diagnosis

The following differential diagnoses must be kept in mind before concluding that pain originates from the SIJ:

- Ankylosing spondylitis
- Other sero-negative spondylarthropathies
- Hip fracture
- Illiotibial band syndrome
- Discogenic pain
- Piriformis syndrome
- SIJ infection
- Superior cluneal nerve (iliac crest) syndrome
- Trochanteric bursitis
- Gluteal enthesopathy.

Blood tests

When clinically indicated, it may be necessary to exclude sero-positive and sero-negative spondylarthropathies. Consideration should be given to ordering ESR (erythrocyte sedimentation rate), CRP (C-reactive protein), RhF (Rheumatiod Factor), FBP (Full Blood Picture), HLAB27 (Human Lymphocyte Antigen B27). The anti-nuclear antibody (ANA) test can help to exclude a systemic autoimmune connective tissue disorder such as systemic lupus erythematosus or Sjogren's syndrome. If the symptoms exist in the elderly or red flags are present, then the prostate specific antigen (PSA) test may be indicated. Protein electrophoresis for multiple myeloma and other malignancy screening tests may also help.

Treatments for sacroiliac joint disorders

Acute phase: 0–10 days

Use non-steroidal anti-inflammatory drugs (NSAIDS), muscle relaxants if there is a myofascial component (manipulation may be too painful), cryotherapy, ultrasonography, iontophoresis, myofascial release techniques, soft tissue massage, positional release, muscle energy techniques, hold relax, reciprocal inhibition, strain–counterstrain, functional technique, support belt, exercises, trigger point injection (one or two injections may help—relief is often temporary but provides a pain-free window for functional rehabilitation).

Sub-acute phase: 10 days to 6 months

Manipulation has been reported in many studies as beneficial in this phase; also de-rotatory or mobilizing manipulation, contrast bathing, intra-articular or intra-ligamentous steroid injection under fluoroscopic or CT guidance (Luukkainen et al. 1999, 2002). Image-guided prolotherapy may help if the condition is recurrent or recalcitrant (Cusi et al. 2010) (see Chapter 55).

Chronic phase: >6 months

If the condition has not responded to any of the traditional treatments, then radio-frequency neurolysis can be tried. In a meta-analysis of SIJ interventions published in 2012, the evidence in favour of cooled radio-frequency was fair (Hansen et al. 2012).

If there are features of chronic pain, then cognitive behavioural therapy (CBT), antidepressants and TENS (transcutaneous electrical nerve stimulation) units may be indicated. Stress, anxiety, fear, and pain all affect the ability to rehabilitate effectively. Anti-epileptics such as Pregabalin or Gabapentin can be tried, along with a functional restoration programme (FRP).

It is the author's experience that the interventional treatments most likely to be effective are manual therapy, specific lumbo-pelvic stabilization training, prolotherapy, and injections of corticosteroid into the intra-articular space or peri-articular ligaments. Radio-frequency neurolysis may also provide significant relief lasting for up to a year (Cohen et al. 2013).

Manipulation techniques for treating sacroiliac joint disorders

Osteopathy, chiropractic, and physiotherapy

Abnormal loading on the structures in the dysfunctional pelvis may mediate the aberrant patterns of neuromuscular control seen in patients. Manual therapy may normalize the loads on the joint, capsule, and surrounding ligaments (Indahl et al. 1999).Many of the accepted approaches to the SIJs are based on models of pelvic mechanics such as those proposed by Fryette, Mackinnon, and Mitchell (Stone 1999).

Osteopathy, physiotherapy, and chiropractic practitioners have much common ground in the techniques currently taught at training establishments in the UK and used in practice:

For iliac rotatory dysfunction and sacral nutation/counter-nutation restrictions, some of the techniques used include:

- *Myofascial muscle energy techniques* (MET) while supine, side-lying, or prone.
- *High-velocity thrust* (HVT)/*high-velocity low-amplitude* (HVLA) manipulation in a range of positions, such as the 'Chicago' manipulation (Figure 35.14) while supine.
- *Mobilization/articulation* (Figures 35.15 and 35.16) using gapping, shearing (Figure 35.17), and rotatory techniques.

- *'Pelvic blocking'* techniques and the use of an instrument called an *'activator'* are specific to chiropractic approaches to combat nutation or counter-nutation.
- Acupuncture, trigger point therapy, positional release techniques, taping, SIJ stabilization belts, re-education of gluteal, pelvic, and trunk motor control, soft tissue and stretching of associated musculature.

For pubic dysfunction, myofascial muscle energy and HVT techniques can be employed.

A prospective study by Flynn attempted to find a clinical prediction rule for a positive outcome following application of a widely-used SIJ manipulation. Twenty-one SIJ tests were evaluated, including tests for symmetry, pain provocation tests, and motion tests. None of the SIJ tests used were found to be predictive of the outcome of the manipulation, although the authors concluded that SIJ manipulation is thought to be indicated in the presence of hypomobility (Flynn et al. 2003).

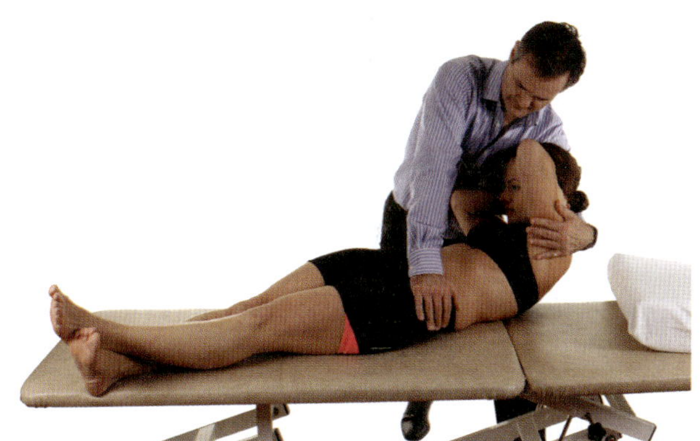

Figure 35.14 'Chicago technique'; left SI manipulation posteriorly.

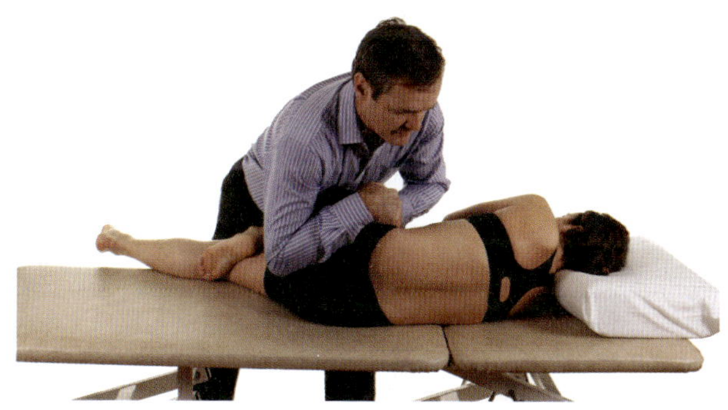

Figure 35.15 Articulatory mobilization of the left SI joint.

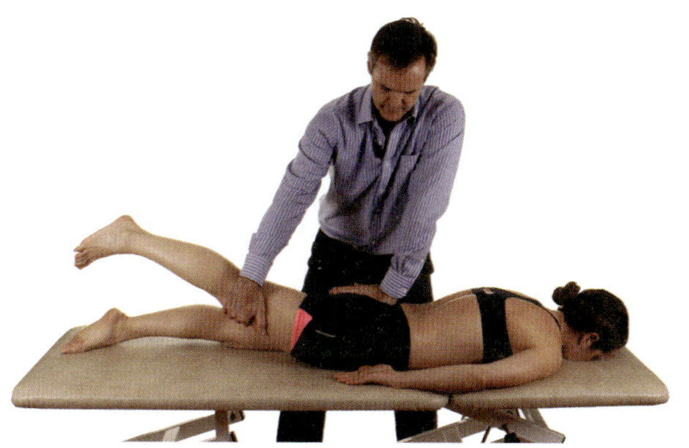

Figure 35.16 Passive long-lever posterior articulatory mobilization of the right ilium anteriorly while holding back the sacrum.

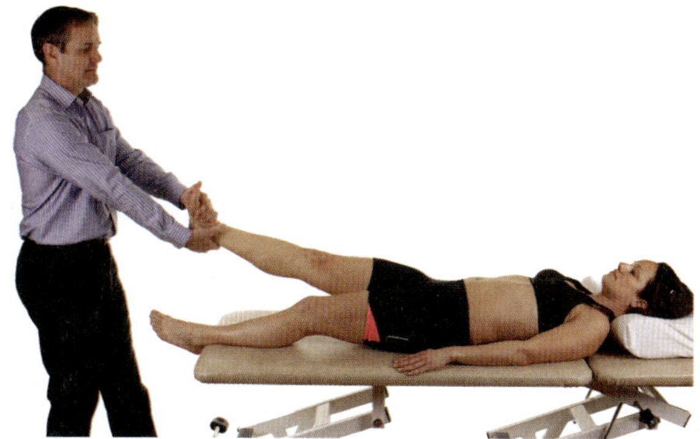

Figure 35.17 The 'leg-tug' shearing technique for right iliac up-slip.

Acupuncture

Acupuncture has been shown to provide additional benefit to stabilization exercises in a study similar to that by Stuge (Elden et al. 2005).

Rehabilitation

It is important to refer for physical therapy in treatment of SIJ disorders as a first line of treatment. This should include a multimodal rehabilitation programme (Vanelderen et al. 2010).

The essential approach to SIJ rehabilitation is to strengthen weak or inhibited muscles such as those of the *posterior oblique sling*, stretch tight/shortened muscles, address muscle imbalances, address subtalar control and foot biomechanics, along with any LLD. Lumbopelvic stability, balance, and proprioceptive programmes are essential and, in athletes, can be enhanced later by sport-specific training before final return to play.

SI belts

An SI belt can serve to stabilize hypermobile SIJs and provide feedback to gluteal muscles, but is not to be relied upon without using other simultaneous approaches to aid stabilization. Data from one study supports the use of SI pelvic compression belts to modify activation patterns of hip extensors among patients with SIJ pain (Jung et al. 2012).

Refractory sacroiliac joint pain

In cases which do not respond permanently to manual therapy, it may be necessary to re-address any unresolved issues and reconsider the diagnosis. It is worth considering further investigations to exclude malignancy and inflammatory spondylarthropathy.

However, it is common to find that manipulation, having initially been successful in treating SIJ dysfunction, can become temporary in its effect, with progressively shorter episodes of pain relief. These patients may be amenable to more advanced techniques such as intra- or extra-articular injections, prolotherapy stabilizing injections, or radio-frequency neurolysis of the SIJ.

Sacroiliac injections

Clinical studies have shown that intra- or extra-articular SIJ injections/interventions can have a significant effect on SIJ pain, suggesting nociception from internal and external structures (Braun et al. 1996; Luukkainen et al. 1999, 2002; Maugars et al. 1996; McKenzie 1981).

Diagnostic intra-articular SIJ blocks

A single intra-articular local anaesthetic injection has diagnostic utility in that it can, if positive, identify the SIJ as the source of pain. There is, however, a risk of a false positive response. A 'control' or 'comparative' block, using a longer-acting anaesthetic can be used to confirm the diagnosis or demonstrate the likelihood of a false positive block (ISIS 2004). Further diagnostic confidence can be gained from a negative response to medial branch blockade of the lower ipsi-lateral facet joints (Schwarzer et al. 1995).

However, Murakami et al. demonstrated that intra-articular SIJ injection does not rule out the SIJ as a cause of symptoms in a significant proportion of patients. Twenty-five consecutive patients with established SIJ pain were injected with intra-articular lidocaine and another 24 were injected with peri-articular lidocaine into the posterior ligaments. Only 9 out of 25 of the intra-articular group reported an improvement, while all 24 patients with peri-articular injection reported a significant outcome. All of the 16 patients who had not responded to intra-articular injection were crossed over and all completely responded to peri-articular injection. This indicates that the posterior SI ligaments have nociceptive innervation and may well be involved in a large proportion of patients with SIJ pain (Murakami et al. 2007). Cheng reported that patients with SIJ pain on extension and axial rotation were less likely to respond to intra-articular injection (Cheng 2012).

Extra-articular corticosteroid injections

Some reports have suggested benefit from the use of extra-articular corticosteroid injection for presumed SIJ pain (Luukkainen et al. 2002).

Intra-articular corticosteroid injections

Intra-articular injections have been shown to be effective, in many studies, in treatment of sacroiliitis due to spondylarthropathy. One retrospective case series has shown promising results with idiopathic SIJ pain (Slipman et al. 2001).

Preparation

The patient should lie in the prone position under a C-arm fluoroscope. The skin should be sterilized using an iodine-, chlorhexidine-, or alcohol-based solution, which should be allowed to dry. Sterile gloves and a no-touch technique should be employed.

Procedure

Under anteroposterior view, the C-arm is rotated to separate the posterior joint margins from those of the anterior joint (Figure 35.18). The posterior joint appears medially and the medial cortical line should be made as distinct as possible. A cephalad tilt may be required to identify the posterior joint lines.

The needle is directed to touch the sacrum 1 cm above the inferior end of the joint. The needle is then re-directed a few millimetres into the joint space. A lateral view can confirm that placement of the needle should not be beyond the anterior margin of the sacrum. Injection of up to 0.3 ml contrast such as Omnipaque should confirm intra-articular placement. Thereafter, a mixture of local anaesthetic (lidocaine 2% or bupivacaine 0.5%) with a suitable corticosteroid is injected to a maximum of 2.5 ml. Any escape of contrast from the joint margins should be noted.

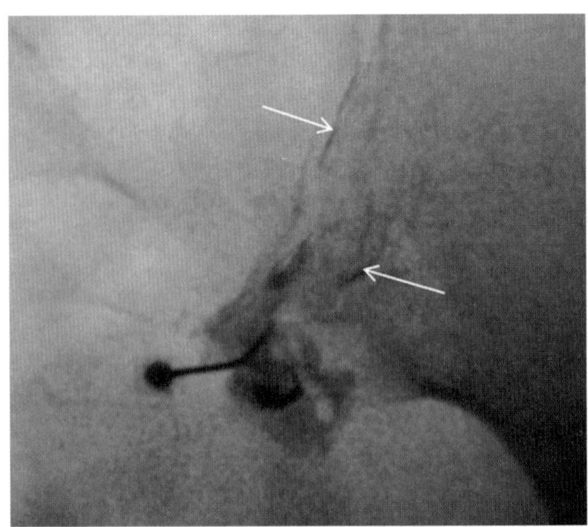

Figure 35.18 Intra-articular injection of contrast; right SIJ. White arrows denote the anterior and posterior SIJ margins. (Blackberry Clinic with permission.)

Post-procedure

A record should be made of the extent and duration of pain relief over the next few hours. More than 75% relief would suggest a positive response. There may be extended relief due to the steroid action (ISIS 2004).

A systematic review of the literature on SIJ interventions in 2009 concluded that the level of evidence for the diagnosis of SIJ pain using comparative, controlled, local anaesthetic blocks is II-2. The false positive rate of single, uncontrolled, SIJ injections is 20% to 54% (Rupert et al. 2009).

Lateral branch blocks

It has recently been shown that multi-site, multi-depth injections under fluoroscopic guidance to anaesthetize the lateral branches of the dorsal rami of S1–3, along with the L5 dorsal ramus, can help diagnose *extra-articular* (posterior ligamentous) SIJ pain. These injections do not effectively block the intra-articular portion of the SIJ since it is innervated from both ventral and dorsal sources. Comparative blocks of this kind may be valuable in identifying patients who could respond to lateral branch radio-frequency neurotomy (Dreyfuss et al. 2009).

Prolotherapy

Multi-site injections of a proliferant solution around the SI ligamento-periosteal junctions can be a useful treatment for persistant SI dysfunction or instability. The hyper-osmolar solution acts as an irritant which results in production of growth factors and a subsequent fibro-proliferative augmentation and thickening of dense connective tissue within the SI ligaments (Dagenais et al. 2005). The technique used is similar to that described in Chapter 55, with more emphasis placed on injections at either end of the iliolumbar ligament, the posterior SI and interosseus ligaments, along with the sacral insertion of the sacrotuberous and sacrospinous ligaments.

Preparation

The patient should lie in the prone position under a C-arm fluoroscope. The skin should be sterilized using an iodine-, chlorhexidine-, or alcohol-based solution, which should be allowed to dry. Sterile gloves and a no-touch technique should be employed.

Procedure

Under anteroposterior view, the needle insertion is from the midline at the L5–S1 interspace (Figure 35.19). Several insertions are made along the iliac and sacral margin of the posterior SIJ. A proliferant solution (P2 G) is mixed 50:50 with lidocaine to result in a solution containing lidocaine 0.5%, dextrose 12.5%, phenol 1%, glycerol 12.5%. Further specific injections can then be made under image guidance to the origin of the iliolumbar ligament on the inferior surface of the tip of the transverse process of L5 and onto the inside of the posterior portion of the iliac crest. In recalcitrant cases, it may be necessary to include the sacral insertions of the sacrotuberous and sacrospinous ligaments.

Post-procedure

The patient is warned regarding the possibility of a post-procedural flare of pain for 1–2 days.

Course of injections

Prolotherapy in the UK is normally carried out as a course of three injections, each at 1-week intervals. Patients are instructed to avoid painful situations as much as possible during the course. A gradual return to normal activity is advised over the following 4 weeks as the ligament strengthens and the joint stabilizes.

A recent study on SI pain diagnosed using clinical signs followed by CT-guided posterior and interosseus SI ligament prolotherapy injections showed significant improvements for those followed up at 3, 12, and 24 months (Cusi et al. 2010).

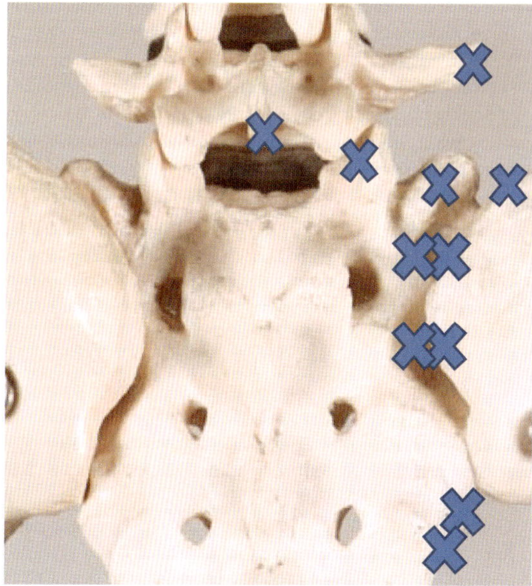

Figure 35.19 Target points for right SI ligament prolotherapy: posterior SI ligament insertions, iliolumbar ligament origin and insertion, interosseus SI ligament, L5–S1 facet capsule, and supraspinous ligament insertion on L5 spinous process. The sacrospinous and sacrotuberous ligament origins on the lateral border of the sacrum can also be included.

Radio-frequency neurolysis

This is a minimally invasive treatment and appears to be effective in a proportion of cases of SIJ pain, especially if there is imaging evidence of sacroiliitis (Burnham and Yasui 2007; Cohen and Abdi 2003; Vallejo et al. 2006; Yin et al. 2003). Radio-frequency denervation may provide relief for up to a year in cases which have failed to experience sustained relief from steroid injections (Cohen et al. 2013).

More recently, a retrospective study by Stelzer showed promising lasting improvement in pain, quality of life, and analgesia usage in a large European study population, with benefits lasting, in some subjects, at 20 months after treatment (Stelzer et al. 2013). In a meta-analysis of SIJ interventions published in 2012, the evidence in favour of cooled radio-frequency was fair (Hansen et al. 2012). In a systematic review of the literature in 2009, the conclusion was that for radio-frequency neurolysis (RFN), the indicated evidence is limited (Level II-3) for short- and long-term relief (Rupert et al. 2009).

The difficulty in SIJ radio-frequency neurolysis lies in the variable site and depth of the lateral branches of the dorsal rami at S1–3 which supply the posterior structures of the SIJ. New types of RFN cannulae and 'cooled' electrodes have been introduced to cater for this variation and to widen the lesion (Vanelderen et al. 2010).

Surgery for sacroiliac joint disorders

Surgical fusion is more invasive and is rarely carried out in the UK. The limited studies available appear to offer a moderate chance of pain reduction and functional improvement in patients with confirmed SIJ pain which has been unresponsive to conservative interventions (Buchowski et al. 2005).
(Hansen H 2007). Laslett (2008).

References

Hansen H.(2007) Sacroiliac joint interventions a systematic review. *Pain Physician* 10:165–84.

Bernard T, Cassidy J. (1991) The sacroiliac syndrome. Pathophysiology, diagnosis and management. In: Frymoyer J. (ed.) *The adult spine: principles and practice*. New York: Raven; pp. 2107–30.

Bernard T, Kirkaldy-Willis W. (1987) Recognising specific characteristics of non-specific low back pain. *Clin Orthop Relat Res* 217:266–80

Bogduk N. (2004) *Practice guidelines: spinal diagnostic and treatment procedures.* San Francisco: International Spine Intervention Society.

Braun J, Bollow M, Seyrekbasan F, et al. (1996) Computed tomography guided corticosteroid injection of the sacroiliac joint in patients with spondyloarthropathy with sacroiliitis: clinical outcome and follow-up by dynamic magnetic resonance imaging. *J Rheumatol* 23:659–64.

Buchowski J, Kebaish K, Sinkov V, Cohen D, Sieber A, Kostuik J. (2005) Functional and radiographic outcome of sacroiliac arthrodesis for the disorders of the sacroiliac joint. *Spine J* 5:520–8.

Burnham R, Yasui Y. (2007) An alternate method of radiofrequency neurotomy of the sacroiliac joint: a pilot study of the effect on pain, function, and satisfaction. *Reg Anesth Pain Med* 32:12–9.

Cheng J. (2012) Sacroiliac steroid injections do not predict ablation relief (abstract 136). *Pain Med* 13:281–349.

Chou L, Slipman C, Bhagia S, et al. (2004) Inciting events initiating injection-proven sacroiliac joint syndrome. *Pain Med* 5:26–32.

Cibulka M, Koldehoff R. (1999) Clinical usefulness of a cluster of sacroiliac joint tests in patients with and without low back pain. *J Orthop Sports Phys Ther* 29:83–99.

Cohen S. (2005) Sacroiliac joint pain:a comprehensive review of anatomy, diagnosis, and treatment. *Anesthes Analges* 101(5):1440–53.

Cohen S, Abdi S. (2003) Lateral branch blocks as a treatment for sacroiliac joint pain: a pilot study. *Reg Anesth Pain Med* 28:113–9.

Cohen S, Chen Y, Neufeld N. (2013) Sacroiliac joint pain: a comprehensive review of epidemiology, diagnosis and treatment. *Expert Rev Neurother* 13(1)99–116.

Cusi M, Saunders J, Hungerford B, Wisbey-Roth T, Lucas P, Wilson S. (2010) The use of prolotherapy in the sacroiliac joint. *Br J Sports Med* 44(2):100–4.

Cusi M, Saunders J, Van der Wall H, Fogelman I. (2013) Metabolic disturbances identified by SPECT-CT in patients with a clinical diagnosis of sacroiliac joint incompetence. *Eur Spine J*. 7:1674–82.

Dagenais S, Haldeman S, Wooley J. (2005) Intraligamentous injection of sclerosing solutions (prolotherapy) for spinal pain: a critical review of the literature. *Spine J* 5:310–28.

Daly J, Frame P, Rapoza P. (1991) Sacroiliac subluxation: a common treatable cause of low-back pain in pregnancy. *Fam Pract Res J* 11:149–59.

Damen L, Buyruk H, Gueler-Ysal F, Lotgering F, Snijders C, Stam H. (2002) The prognostic value of asymmetric laxity of the sacroiliac joints in pregnancy-related pelvic pain. *Spine* 27: 2820–4.

Dijkstra P, Vleeming A, Stoeckart R. (1989) Complex motion tomography of the sacroiliac joint: an anatomical and roentgenological study. *Rofo* 150:635–42.

Dreyfuss P, Henning T, Malladi N, Goldstein B, Bogduk N. (2009) The ability of multi-site, multi-depth sacral lateral branch blocks to anesthetize the sacroiliac joint complex. *Pain Med* 10: 679–88.

Elden H, Ladfors L, Olsen M, Ostgaard H, Hagberg H. (2005) Effects of acupuncture and stabilising exercises as adjunct to standard treatment in pregnant women with pelvic girdle pain: Randomised single blind controlled trial. *BMJ* 330:761.

Flynn T, Fritz J, Whitman J, et al. (2003) A clinical prediction rule for classifying patients with low back pain who demonstrate short-term improvement with spinal manipulation. *Spine* 27:2835–43.

Fortin J, Aprill C, Ponthieux B, et al. (1994b) Sacroiliac joints: pain referral maps upon applying a new injection/arthrography technique. Part II: clinical evaluation. *Spine* 19:1483–9.

Fortin J, Dwyer A, West S, Pier J. (1994a) Sacroiliac joint: pain referral maps upon applying a new injection/arthrography technique. Part I: asymptomatic volunteers. *Spine* 19(13):1475–82.

Freburger J, Riddle D. (1999) Measurement of sacroiliac joint dysfunction: a multicenter intertester reliability study. *Phys Ther* 79:1134–41.

Frymoyer JW, Hanley E, Howe J, et al. (1978b) Disc excision and spine fusion in the management of lumbar disc disease: a minimum ten-year follow-up. *Spine* 3:1–6.

Frymoyer JW, Howe J, Kuhlmann D. (1978a) The long-term effects of spinal fusion on the sacroiliac joint and ilium. *Clin Orthop* 134:196–201.

Goldthwait J, Osgood R. (1905) A consideration of the pelvic articulations from an anatomical, pathological and clinical standpoint. *Boston Med Surg J* 152:593–601.

Grob K, Neuhuber W, Kissling R. (1995) Innervation of the sacroiliac joint in humans. *Z Rheumatol* 54:117–22.

de Groot M, Pool-Goudzwaard A, Spoora C, Snijders C. (2008) The active straight leg raising test (ASLR) in pregnant women: differences in muscle activity and force between patients and healthy subjects. *Man Ther* 13:68–74.

Hansen H, Kenzie-Brown A, Cohen S, Swicegood J, Colson J, Manchikanti L. (2007) Sacroiliac joint interventions: a systematic review. *Pain Physician* 10:165–84.

Hansen H, Manchikanti L, Simopoulos T, et al. (2012) A systematic evaluation of the therapeutic effectiveness of sacroiliac joint interventions. *Pain Physician* 15(3):E247–78.

van der Heijde D, Spoorenberg A. (1999) Plain radiographs as an outcome measure in ankylosing spondylitis. *J Rheumatol* 26(4):985–7.

Indahl A, Kaigle A, Reikerås O, Holm S. (1999) Sacroiliac joint involvement in activation of the porcine spinal and gluteal musculature. *J Spinal Disord* 12(4):325–30.

Bogduk N (ed). Practice Guidelines for Spinal Diagnostic and Treatment Procedures, 2nd edn. International Spine Intervention Society, San Francisco, 2013.

International Spine Intervention Society (ISIS). (2004) *Spinal diagnostic & treatment procedures, practice guidelines.*

Jung H, Jeon H, Oh D, Kwon O. (2013) Effect of the pelvic compression belt on the hip extensor activation patterns of sacroiliac joint pain patients during one-leg standing: a pilot study. *Man Ther*. 18(2): 143–148

Keriakos R, Bhatta S, Morris F, Mason S, Buckley S. (2001) Pelvic girdle pain during pregnancy and puerperium. *J Obstet Gynaecol* 31(7):572–80.

Laslett M. (2008) Evidence-based diagnosis and treatment of the painful sacroiliac joint. *J Man Manip* 16:142–52.

Laslett M, Williams M. (1994) The reliability of selected pain provocation tests for sacro-iliac joint pathology. *Spine* 19:1243–9.

Laslett M, Aprill C, McDonald B, Young S. (2005) Diagnosis of sacroiliac joint pain: validity of individual provocation tests and composites of tests. *Man Ther* 10:207–18.

Laslett M, Young S, Aprill C, McDonald B. (2003) Diagnosing painful sacroiliac joints: a validity study of a McKenzie evaluation and sacroiliac joint provocation tests. *Aust J Physiother* 49:89–97.

Levangie P. (1999) The association between static pelvic asymmetry and low back pain. *Spine* 24:1234–42.

Levin S. (2006) Tensegrity, the new biomechanics. In: Hutson M, Ellis R. (eds) *Textbook of musculoskeletal medicine*. Oxford: Oxford University Press.

Levin U, Nilsson-Wikmar L, Harms-Ringdahl K, Stenstrom CH. (2001) Variability of forces applied by experienced physiotherapists during provocation of the sacroiliac joint. *Clin Biomech* 16:300–6.

Luukkainen R, Nissila M, Asikainen E, et al. (1999) Periarticular corticosteroid treatment of the sacroiliac joint in patients with seronegative spondyloarthropathy. *Clin Exp Rheumatol* 17:88–90.

Luukkainen R, Wennerstrand P, Kautiainen H, et al. (2002) Efficacy of periarticular corticosteroid treatment of the sacroiliac joint in non-spondyloarthropathic patients with chronic low back pain in the region of the sacroiliac joint. *Clin Exp Rheumatol* 20:52–4.

Lynch F. (1920) The pelvic articulations during pregnancy, labor, and the puerperium: an X-ray study. *Surg Gynecol Obstet* 30:575–80.

Maigne J, Aivaliklis A, Pfefer F. (1996) Results of sacroiliac joint double block and value of sacroiliac pain provocation tests in 54 patients with low back pain. *Spine* 21:1889–92.

Maugars Y, Mathis C, Berthelot J, Charlier C, Prost A. (1996) Assessment of the efficacy of sacroiliac corticosteroid injections in spondylarthropathies: a double-blind study. *Br J Rheumatol* 35:767–70.

McKenzie R. (1981) *The lumbar spine: mechanical diagnosis and therapy.* Waikanae, NZ: Spinal Publications Ltd.

Mens J, Vleeming A, Snijders C, Koes B, Stam H. (2002) Validity of the active straight leg raise test for measuring disease severity in patients with posterior pelvic pain after pregnancy. *Spine* 27(2):196–200.

Merskey H, Bogduk N. (1994) *Classification of chronic pain: descriptions of chronic pain syndromes and definitions of pain terms* (2nd edn). Seattle, WA: IASP Press.

Murakami E, Tanaka Y, Aizawa T, Ishizuka M, Kokubun S. (2007) Effect of peri-articular and intra-articular lidocaine injections for sacroiliac joint pain: prospective comparative study. *J Orthop Sci* 12:274–80.

O'Haire C, Gibbons P. (2000) Inter-examiner and intra-examiner agreement for assessing sacroiliac anatomical landmarks using palpation and observation: a pilot study. *Man Ther* 5:13–20.

Onsel C, Collier B, Meting K, et al. (1992) Increased sacroiliac joint uptake after lumbar fusion and/or laminectomy. *Clin Nucl Med* 17:283–7.

Pool-Goudzwaard A, Vleeming A, Stoeckart R, Snijders C, Mens J. (1998) Insufficient lumbopelvic stability: a clinical, anatomical and biomechanical approach to 'a specific low back pain'. *Man Ther* 3(1):12–20.

Richardson C, Snijders C, Hides J, Damen L, Pas M, Storm J. (2002) The relationship between the transversely oriented abdominal muscles, sacroiliac joint mechanics and low back pain. *Spine* 27(4):399–405.

Robinson H, Brox J, Robinson R, Bjelland E, Solem S, Telje T. (2007) The reliability of selected motion and pain provocation tests for the sacroiliac joint. *Man Ther* 12:72–9.

Rudwaleit M, Metter A, Listing J, et al. (2006) Inflammatory back pain in ankylosing spondylitis: a reassessment of the clinical history for application as classification and diagnostic criteria. *Arthritis Rheum* 54(2):569–78.

Rupert M, Lee M, Manchikanti L, Datta S, Cohen S. (2009) Evaluation of sacroiliac joint interventions: a systematic appraisal of the literature. *Pain Physician* 12(2):399–418.

Schwarzer A, Aprill C, Bogduk N. (1995) The sacroiliac joint in chronic low back pain. *Spine* 20:31–7.

Slipman C, Jackson H, Lipetz J, et al. (2000) Sacroiliac joint pain referral zones. *Arch Phys Med Rehabil* 81:334–8.

Slipman C, Lipetz JS, Plastaras C, et al. (2001) Fluoroscopically guided therapeutic sacroiliac joint injections for sacroiliac joint syndrome. *Am J Phys Med Rehabil* 80:425–32.

Stelzer W, Aiglesberger M, Stelzer D, Stelzer V. (2013) Use of cooled radiofrequency lateral branch neurotomy for the treatment of sacroiliac joint-mediated low back pain: a large case series. *Pain Med* 14:29–35.

Stone C. (1999) *Science in the art of osteopathy, osteopathic principles and practice*. Nelson Thornes Ltd; 1st edition.

Stuber K. (2007) Specificity, sensitivity, and predictive values of clinical tests of the sacroiliac joint: a systematic review of the literature. *J Can Chiropr Assoc* 51(1):30–41.

Stuge B, Bragelien V, Laerun E. (2004) The efficacy of a treatment program focusing on specific stabilizing exercises for pelvic girdle pain after pregnancy: a two-year follow-up of a randomized clinical trial. *Spine* 29(10):197–203.

Stuge B, Laerum E, Kirkesola G, Vollestad N. (2004) The efficacy of a treatment program focusing on specific stabilizing exercises for pelvic girdle pain after pregnancy: a randomized controlled trial. *Spine* 29:351–9.

Sturesson B, Selvik G, Uden A. (1989) Movements of the sacroiliac joints: a roentgen stereophotogrammetric analysis. *Spine* 14:162–5.

Travell J, Simons D.(1982) *Myofascial pain and disfunction: the trigger point manual. The lower extremities.* Baltimore, MD: Lippincott, Williams & Wilkins.

Turner H. (2009) The combined approach to the sacroiliac joint. *Health Educ Sem* www.heseminars.com

Levin U. (2004: unpublished) Sacroiliac pain provocation testing in physiotherapy time and force recording.

Vallejo R, Benyamin R, Kramer J, Stanton G, Joseph N. (2006) Pulsed radiofrequency denervation for the treatment of sacroiliac joint syndrome. *Pain Med* 7:429–34.

Vanelderen P, Szadek K, Cohen S, et al. (2010) Sacroiliac joint pain. *Pain Pract* 10(5):470–8.

Vleeming A, Albert HB, Östgaard HC, Sturesson B, Stuge B. (2008) European guidelines for the diagnosis and treatment of pelvic girdle pain. *Eur Spine J* 17(6):794–819.

Vleeming A, van Wingerden J, Dijkstra P, et al. (1992) Mobility in the sacroiliac joints in the elderly: a kinematic and radiological study. *Clin Biomech* 7:170–6.

White A, Panjabi M. (1990) *Clinical biomechanics of the spine* (2nd edn). Philadelphia: JB Lippincott.

van der Wurff P, Buijs E, Groen G. (2006) A multi-test regimen of pain provocation tests as an aid to reduce unnecessary minimally invasive sacroiliac joint procedures. *Arch Phys Med Rehabil* 87:10–4.

Yin W, Willard F, Carreiro J, Dreyfuss P. (2003) Sensory stimulation-guided sacroiliac joint radiofrequency neurotomy: technique based on neuroanatomy of the dorsal sacral plexus. *Spine* 28:2419–25.

Chapter 36

Structural disorders of the knee

Fazal Ali and Derek Bickerstaff

Structural disorders of the knee relate to the articular cartilage that lines the surface of the bones, the menisci, and the ligaments that provide the stability to the knee.

History of a patient presenting with a knee complaint

General questions

All histories begin with the presenting complaint and, in the case of a joint, the site and side affected. This is then followed by the patient's age, occupation, and, specifically in knee-related problems, sporting participation (including type and intensity). The latter three are important in ascertaining the patient's degree of functional disability, which clearly has a bearing on the range of treatments offered. For instance, a 20-year-old professional footballer with an anterior cruciate ligament tear may be offered different advice to a 40-year-old office worker who has no active sporting participation but presents with the same injury.

It is then important to ascertain the duration of symptoms, exact details of the precipitating injury, and the general course of events including response to any treatment already received.

Usually, patients present with a combination of symptoms relating to pain, swelling, locking, and giving way. The diagnostic specificity of each of these symptoms in isolation is poor; rather, they are used in combination to guide the examiner to a differential diagnosis.

Specific questions

Pain

The site of pain within the knee is an indication as to the structure damaged but is by no means diagnostic, particularly with traumatic disorders such as meniscal tears. As an example, lateral joint pain from a patello-femoral disorder is frequently mistaken for a lateral meniscal tear. The site of pain following an episode of injury however, such as a medial collateral ligament strain, is a clear indication of the possible structures involved.

It is then important to relate the pain to the level and type of activity, such as whether the symptom appears after a few steps walking or only after running. In addition, questions about the pain related to specific actions such as twisting and turning may indicate a problem with the main weight-bearing areas of the knee such as a meniscal tear or chondral defect. Bent-knee activities such as kneeling, crouching, or squatting may indicate a patello-femoral problem, though posterior horn tears of the medial meniscus are aggravated by loaded bent-knee activities such as coming up from a squatting position.

The examiner should always be aware of the possibility of referred pain from the hip or lumbar spine, particularly when assessing a patient with degenerative symptoms.

Swelling

Swelling can be localized, such as a lateral meniscal cyst, or generalized, such as a haemarthrosis. Localized swellings such as bursae, meniscal cysts, and ganglia may vary in size, sometimes associated with activity levels, and are common findings. Swellings which are constant and increasing in size should be investigated as a matter or urgency; soft tissue or bony tumours around the knee are rare but well reported.

Generalized swellings are effusions secondary to an inflammatory process. The commonest effusion is related to some mechanical derangement within the knee such as a meniscal tear or chondral damage. There is usually a history of injury with the effusion appearing within 24 hours. Effusions also occur secondary to inflammatory arthropathies and can be massive if chronic. There is usually no record of injury but a careful history should be taken to identify other features of rheumatoid arthritis or sero-negative arthropathies. These generalized swellings are not necessarily pure effusions; at least part of the swelling may be synovial hypertrophy, which will become apparent on examination if suspected from the history.

A haemarthrosis presents as a generalized swelling within 4 hours of an injury. The main differential diagnosis of a haemarthrosis is an anterior cruciate ligament (ACL) rupture, an osteochondral fracture (often associated with a patella dislocation), or a peripheral meniscal tear. Indeed, if an athlete gives a history of a twisting injury on the sports field followed by swelling within 4 hours, they have a 70–80% chance of having sustained an ACL rupture (Maffuli et al. 1993). The commonest misdiagnosis in this setting is to confuse an ACL rupture with a lateral patella dislocation; indeed, rarely, both can occur together (Simonian et al. 1998). Both occur on the slightly flexed weight-bearing knee forced into external rotation.

Not surprisingly, haemarthroses are painful due to the degree of tension within the knee. A relatively painless diffuse swelling as opposed to a true haemarthrosis should alert the examiner to the possibility of a more extensive ligamentous injury with disruption of the capsule. The examiner can be lulled into thinking the injury is less severe than is the case.

Locking

Locking can be subdivided into true locking and pseudo-locking. True locking is relatively rare. It occurs when an intra-articular structure, loose body, or meniscal tear interposes between the femoral condyle and tibial surface. Classically, the patient loses terminal extension but is able to flex the knee (though usually also losing some terminal flexion which is less noticeable). Loose bodies may also be felt by the patient in the supra-patella pouch but, more commonly, in either the medial or lateral gutter. They are classically elusive and, once found, immediately move to another area, hence their eponym of 'joint mouse'.

Pseudo-locking is a far more common presentation, and usually occurs in patients with anterior knee pain secondary to some form of patella maltracking. Classically, it is associated with marked pain and the knee is solidly locked. Over a period of time, the knee movement gradually returns.

Giving way

There are two types of giving way: true giving way, which is usually associated with some form of ligamentous instability, and a buckling type sensation, which is usually associated with anterior knee pain and the symptom of pseudo-locking previously described.

An example of true giving way is seen in ACL instability. The patient has no problem running in a straight line but on planting the foot and twisting with the upper body internally rotating, the knee suddenly collapses, quickly followed by pain and, later, swelling.

Chronic medial instability usually presents with difficulty performing cutting movements rather than rotation. Isolated posterior cruciate ligament (PCL) rupture does not usually present with instability unless there is associated posterolateral or posteromedial instability. In these situations, the knee feels unstable with rotatory movements but also on walking downstairs, due to the unimpeded anterior displacement of the femur on the tibia. Often, patients with these complex problems present with marked instability with active daily living and may constantly need the use of a knee brace.

Buckling of the knee is seen in patients with anterior knee pain and is associated with pain. These patients often report their knee buckling without any rotary movement, usually occurring when walking in a straight line or down stairs. The knee buckling is rarely associated with an effusion.

Orthopaedic examination of the knee

Orthopaedic examination of the knee follows the usual routine of inspection, palpation, movement, ligaments, and special tests. (The musculoskeletal physician may well be trained in the Cyriax routine of inspection, active movements, passive movements, stress tests, muscle contraction tests, and palpation.) One must always remember to use the opposite limb for comparison and leave any possible painful tests to the end. A tense patient will make any assessment of subtle instabilities impossible.

Inspection

Initial inspection should begin with the patient standing, to assess overall limb alignment, any shortening, and any rotational abnormalities which may have a bearing on patello-femoral function (Figure 36.1). In addition, the foot position should be assessed for evidence of any abnormalities such as hyperpronation which again can affect patello-femoral function. It is easier at this stage to assess the posterior aspect of the knee for scars, swellings, or bruising. The anterior aspect can be assessed now or later when the patient is supine.

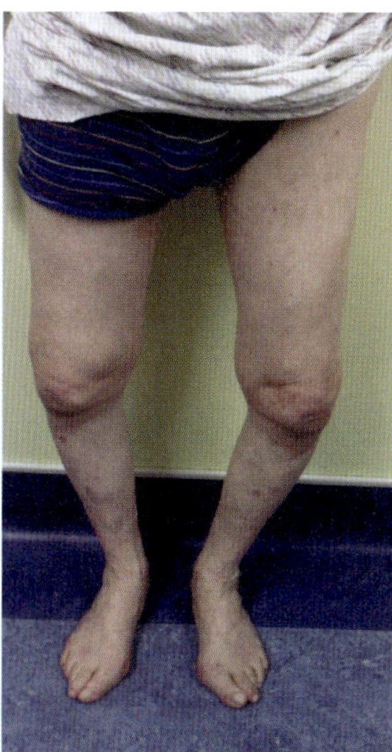

Figure 36.1 A patient with bilateral varus knees from osteoarthritis of his medial compartments. When he walks, he will demonstrate a varus lurch.

Gait pattern is observed when the patient walks both towards and away from the examiner. When observing the gait, look at the foot progression angle (the angle the foot makes with an imaginary straight line—typically 10–15°) and the patella progression angle (the angle the patella makes with an imaginary straight line—typically 0°). Look also for a varus (lateral) lurch or a valgus (medial) lurch. A varus lurch signifies medial compartment osteoarthritis or lateral collateral ligament laxity. A valgus lurch signifies lateral compartment osteoarthritis or medial collateral ligament laxity.

Sitting the patient with the legs hanging over the side of the couch allows the examiner to look for patella height, assess tracking, and feel for crepitus as the knee bends and straightens. Look for a J-sign, which is the lateral movement of the patella as the knee goes into extension, and signifies patella instability.

The patient is now laid supine on the examination couch with their head relaxed. A patient straining to watch an examination may increase muscle tone affecting observations such as knee laxity. As well as inspecting the anterior aspect of the knee for scars, swellings, or bruising, any quadriceps or calf wasting can be observed and measured if thought appropriate.

Palpation

There are three basic tests for the presence of an effusion. The first is the ballotment test for a massive effusion. This is performed in a similar way to a fluid thrill in the abdomen. It involves pushing the swelling on one side and feeling it on the other. The patella tap is for a moderate effusion. The patella is pushed onto the femoral

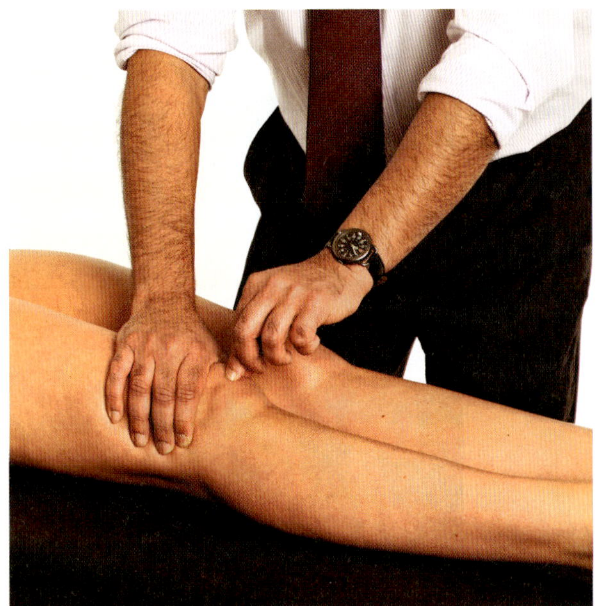

Figure 36.2 Patella tap for a moderate effusion.

trochlea having first obliterated the suprapatella pouch by pressure on it from the other hand (Figure 36.2). The third is the bulge test for very small effusions which involves stroking the lateral gutter to empty the fluid and watching for a fluid wave in the medial gutter. If there is the appearance of swelling in the knee and yet no effusion, one must consider synovial hypertrophy as seen in conditions such as pigmented villo-nodular synovitis (Flandrey et al. 1994).

The knee is largely subcutaneous apart from posteriorly and, as such, many structures can be palpated directly. This is best done with the knee flexed to 90° with the foot firmly planted on the examination couch in a neutral position. The fingers can then be used to palpate along the joint lines starting with the painless side. Tenderness along the joint line, particular posteromedially, may indicate a meniscal tear. The borders of the femoral and tibial condyles, the patella tendon, and medial (MCL) and lateral (LCL) collateral ligaments can also be palpated for tenderness.

The site of tenderness is important in an MCL strain. Most commonly, there is tenderness on the medial epicondyle at the site of the femoral attachment of the MCL. This can be confused with disruption of the medial patello-femoral ligament seen in lateral patella dislocation. Tenderness along the medial joint line in an MCL strain is indicative of disruption of the deeper fibres and suggests a potentially more complicated injury.

The best way to isolate the LCL is to put the patient's leg in a figure-of-four position. This puts the ligament under tension, making it more pronounced and easier to palpate. The patella tendon should be palpated in full extension and when tensed at 90° of flexion. In chronic patella tendinosis, tenderness at the proximal tendon is more noticeable in extension; in flexion, the normal superficial fibres cover the damaged deep fibres resulting in less pain on palpation.

The posterior aspect of the knee should also be palpated to identify soft tissue masses in the popliteal fossa, which may not have been evident on inspection.

Movement

The normal range of passive movement in the sagittal plane is assessed comparing both sides and including hyperextension. The range can be noted as degrees of movement such as –10° to 140°. Alternatively, hyperextension can be measured as the distance the heel can be lifted off the examination couch and flexionby the heel to buttock distance. The patient should be asked to actively perform a straight leg raise to assess the integrity of the extensor mechanism and flex the knee as far as possible.

Ligament instability

This will be split into three subsections, ACL instability, MCL and LCL instability, and PCL instability including posterolateral rotatory instability (PLRI).

Anterior cruciate ligament instability

Prior to assessing ACL or PCL instability, both knees are viewed from the side when flexed to 90° to identify any posterior sag indicating PCL instability. If this is not recognized, anterior movement from an abnormally posterior placed tibia may be misinterpreted as anterior instability. If there is a posterior sag, then the quadriceps active test can be performed. In this position, hold the patient's foot and ask them to try to extend the knee. The quadriceps muscle will contract and pull the tibia forwards.

The anterior and posterior drawer tests are performed with the patient's knee flexed to 90°. A positive anterior drawer test is indicative of an ACL rupture together with the secondary restraints (posterior capsule, collaterals) and signifies a severe injury.

The classic test for ACL instability is the Lachman test (Torg et al. 1976). With a normal-sized knee, the best technique is to grasp the distal thigh with one hand, holding the femur while flexing the knee to 20° (which isolates the ACL by relaxing the secondary restraints), and then the other hand grasps the proximal tibia and displaces the tibia anteriorly (Figure 36.3). The amount

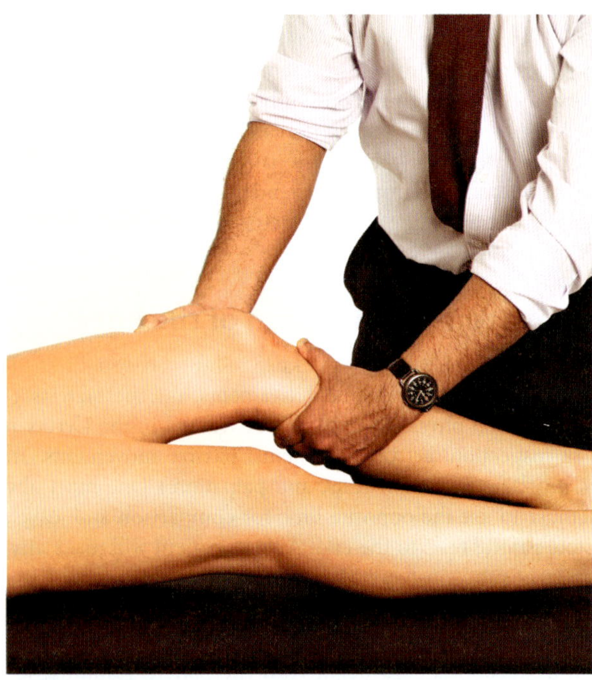

Figure 36.3 Lachman's test for ACL laxity.

of anterior displacement is then estimated and can be graded. One method of grading is: grade 0 = 0–3 mm (normal), grade I = 3–5 mm, grade II = 5–10 mm, grade III = >10 mm with no end- point. These measurements are estimated on comparison with the uninjured knee. The amount of displacement is subjective and, while useful to the same examiner with subsequent examinations, is of less use to another examiner. True measurement of displacement is better undertaken with some form of laxity measurement device, though even these are subject to inter-observer error. Of more importance on examination is whether there is definite anterior displacement and whether there is a soft or hard end point. A soft end point is indicative of a complete rupture. In patients with large thighs or examiners with small hands, it is better to fix the femur over the examiner's flexed knee while displacing the tibia with the other hand (Draper and Schulthies 1995).

The other classic test for ACL instability is the pivot shift test which can be performed a number of different ways, though the basic principle is the same (Galway and MacIntosh 1980). The pivot shift test recreates the anterolateral subluxation of the tibia on the femur which results in the giving way sensation experienced by the patient when twisting on a planted foot. The patient's leg is held in full extension with the hands around the knee and the foot tucked under the arm. The lower leg is then internally rotated by twisting the examiner's body and a valgus strain applied to the knee via the laterally placed hand and the elbow and body. In this position, the tibia is anterolaterally subluxed. The knee is then flexed gently and, at about 20°, the tibia suddenly reduces, which can be seen in obvious cases (usually under anaesthetic) and palpated by the hands around the knee in more subtle cases. The degree of instability is increased if the hip is abducted as this decreases tension in the iliotibial band (Bach et al. 1988). It is not possible to perform this test with medial instability, as the medial pivot is lost. The key to this test is obtaining the patient's confidence as, if performed too forcibly, it can be distressing for the patient.

Collateral ligament instability

MCL injury is the commonest form of knee instability. In the acute situation, the patient guards the knee and although an impression of medial instability may be gained, the extent of the instability is difficult to assess. In the chronic setting, the examination is much easier.

With the leg held as described for the pivot shift, the knee is placed in full extension including hyperextension. A valgus force is then applied to the knee by pushing the lower leg, held by the elbow and body, against the laterally placed hand. The degree of opening can be assessed as described in the Lachman test but the most important point is whether there is a soft or hard end point. If there is no end point with the leg in full extension, this signifies a major disruption of the knee with damage to the cruciate ligaments, which act as secondary stabilizers to valgus strain. Some opening with an end point may represent disruption of the deep fibres of the MCL. The test is then performed in 20° of flexion, which relaxes the secondary restraints and allows an assessment of the superficial fibres of the MCL. Again, an assessment is made as to the degree of movement and the presence of an end point.

Posteromedial rotatory instability is a major instability in which there is damage to the posteromedial structures of the knee, principally the posterior oblique ligament, and occurs with severe ligament disruptions, usually affecting the PCL (Nielsen et al. 1984). As well as medial opening in extension and flexion, the posterior subluxation of the medial tibial plateau off the femur can be demonstrated using a 'dial test' which is described in the section on posterolateral instability.

LCL instability in isolation is unusual and usually associated with posterolateral instability, which will be described in the next section. Essentially however, the test is the same as for the MCL. There is greater normal laxity in the lateral structures and care should be taken to compare movement with the uninjured knee.

Posterior cruciate and posterolateral rotatory instability

These two instabilities are described together as they frequently coexist but also because there are subtle differences in differentiating the two on examination. The examination for these instabilities should take place concurrently (Miller et al. 1999).

As described earlier, before cruciate ligament examination, both knees are flexed to 90° with the patient supine and both feet planted on the examination couch. In this posterior sag test, gravity displaces the tibia relative to the femur, indicating a PCL disruption. Proceed with the posterior draw test with the knees in this position and the feet planted in neutral rotation. The examiner sits on the feet with hands around the knee; the fingers can ensure the hamstrings are relaxed and the thumbs can palpate the joint line. At this angle of flexion the anterior tibial condyles should be anterior to the corresponding femoral condyles. The injured knee is compared with the normal knee and the posterior translation is measured as described earlier in the Lachman test. Another method of grading is grade I if it is 0–5 mm (tibia still anterior to the femur), grade II if 5–10 mm (tibia flush with femur), and grade III if over 10 mm with no end point (tibial condyles sagging behind femoral condyles). In the PCL-deficient knee, the posterior draw test at 20°, or 'posterior Lachman test', is also mildly positive but more strongly positive in the presence of posterolateral rotatory instability.

In the quadriceps active test, the patient is positioned as previously described. Anterior translation of the proximal tibia with quadriceps contraction indicates a PCL injury.

There are many tests described to diagnose posterolateral instability. One has already been described—the 'posterior Lachman test'. This is most positive in combined PCL and PLRI, slightly less in isolated PLRI, and least in PCL instability.

The varus stress test is performed by positioning the patient in exactly the same way as the valgus test described for the MCL, but with a varus force applied to the knee in full extension and 20° of flexion. Increased opening in flexion indicates injury to the LCL, which is usually associated with damage to the posterolateral corner. Increased opening in extension may still be present in an isolated injury to these structures but is more obvious when combined with anterior or posterior cruciate instability. Comparison with the normal side is important.

The 'dial test' is passive external rotation of the tibia (relative to the femur), with the knee at 30° and 90° of flexion. This is best performed with the patient prone, when the feet indicate the degrees of rotation from neutral. In the rare case of isolated PLRI, increased external rotation is noted at 30° but less so at 90°. When combined PCL and PLRI are present, increased external rotation is noted in both positions (Staubli 1994; Veltri and Warren 1994).

Tests such as the external rotation recurvatum test, reversed pivot shift test, and a posterior draw test performed with the foot in external rotation may also be carried out for additional confirmation.

Limb alignment and gait pattern must be observed to ensure there is no lateral thrust on walking which is seen in chronic PLRI, usually associated with PCL injury, but also seen in ACL injury. If this is not recognized, the ligament reconstructions may fail in the absence of a corrective osteotomy.

PCL and posterolateral corner injuries are major events and, in the acute setting, particular care must be taken to ensure there is no neurovascular injury, in particular to the common peroneal nerve.

Special tests

Meniscal pathology

McMurray's test was intended to recreate displacement of a painful meniscal tear, and is probably not in the patient's best interests. A modification of this is a compression test to produce discomfort along the joint line, which may indicate pathology in the medial or lateral compartment. For McMurray's test, the patient is supine with the knee flexed. The examiner places one hand on the top of the knee with the fingers and thumb positioned to palpate the joint line and the other under the heel. The examiner can then compress the joint by pushing down on the top hand while the lower hand controls flexion and can also provide a varus or valgus strain, thereby compressing each compartment in turn in varying degrees of flexion. This test is most specific for a tear of the posterior horn of the medial meniscus. The patient reports discomfort on the posteromedial joint line with the knee compressed in full flexion and external rotation. Similar compression of the joint can be achieved using Apley's compression test with the patient prone (Apley and Solomon 1982). Compression, flexion, and rotation of the knee are controlled by the examiner's hand on the patient's heel.

Another less specific test is to ask the patient to fully squat and, if possible, duck walk. This action compresses the posterior horns of the menisci but can also cause patello-femoral pain. The absence of positive signs does not definitely exclude a meniscal tear but other investigations such as a magnetic resonance imaging (MRI) scan should be undertaken.

Patello-femoral pathology

With the patient supine, an assessment of the patella size, position, and height is made in both extension and flexion. The patella is then observed with the patient flexing and extending the knee to observe patella tracking. This is often easier done with the patient's knee flexed over the end of the couch. Rarely, one can identify a sudden jerk of the patella as it moves from its laterally placed position into the trochlea at the onset of flexion. Medial displacement of the patella is extremely uncommon and usually iatrogenic.

With the patient supine, the borders of the patella and the retinaculae are carefully palpated for tenderness. In acute patella dislocation, there is a boggy feel to the medial retinaculum with tenderness along the medial border of the patella or over the medial epicondyle at the site of insertion of the medial patello-femoral ligament (MPFL). With chronic anterior knee pain from maltracking, there may be tenderness over the superolateral border of the patella.

An assessment should then be made of lateral retinacular tightness which one finds with patella tilting, such as seen in excessive lateral pressure syndrome. To do this, the patella should be just engaged in the femoral trochlea. The knee is flexed slightly by placing one hand balled into a fist under the knee while the other moves the patella maximally, medially, and laterally. The patella should be able to move at least one quadrant medially; any less indicates lateral retinacular tightness. The medial retinaculum is naturally more lax, but movement of greater than two quadrants laterally indicates laxity in the medial retinaculum that one may see in recurrent patella dislocation. With the patella held in this lateral position, the knee is now flexed and the patient's reaction observed. A positive patella apprehension test is seen when the patient resists further flexion for fear of the patella dislocating.

Meniscal lesions

Structure

The medial and lateral menisci lie interposed between the femur and tibia in their respective compartments of the knee. As with articular cartilage, they are specialized connective tissue structures, principally formed by type 1 collagen. They are crescent- shaped structures designed to resist compression forces and, by effectively increasing the surface area of the joint, avoid high point contact and, therefore, spread the load applied across the joint. The majority of collagen fibres are orientated circumferentially around the meniscus in the shape of a hoop (Figure 36.4).

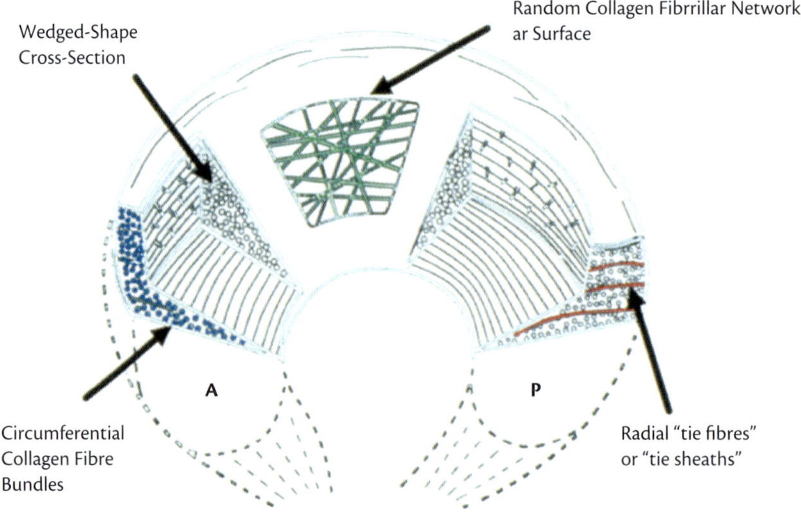

Figure 36.4 Ultrastructure of the meniscus.

These fibres are anchored to bone at the anterior and posterior horns of the meniscus and, therefore, when a compressive load is applied, the hoop fibres effectively resist extrusion of the meniscus, sharing load across the joint. There are also radial tie fibres which tether the meniscus to the peripheral capsule and a mesh of obliquely orientated fibres on the surface of the meniscus that resist shear forces.

The medial and lateral menisci are shaped differently, conforming to the respective joint surfaces. The lateral meniscus is generally more mobile than the medial, which reflects the increased laxity in the lateral compartment when compared to the medial. As such, the peripheral attachments of the medial meniscus are more secure, particularly in the posterior aspect, which may explain the higher incidence of meniscal tears in the posterior horn of the medial meniscus caused by a compressive and rotary force on a fixed structure.

Menisci are largely avascular, except for the peripheral third; hence, it is only in this area that the normal reparative process occurs (Arnoczky and Warren 1982). More central tears, which include the vast majority of meniscal tears, do not heal.

Pathology and presentation

Meniscal tears are common events and usually produced by rotation on the flexed loaded knee. Medial meniscal tears are 5–7 times more common than lateral, and the vast majority occur in the posterior third of the meniscus. The patterns of tear differ from side to side. There have been numerous classifications of tear but most relate to the type of tear rather than aetiology. The basic types are longitudinal split, flap, radial, oblique, and horizontal cleavage (Dandy 1990) (Figure 36.5). Degenerate tears can be a combination of tears occurring with chondral changes of early osteoarthritis. Cystic degeneration is a common finding on MRI scan and is believed to predispose a meniscus to tearing if sufficient load is applied. Cystic degeneration is associated with a meniscal cyst that occurs more commonly in the lateral meniscus in its anterior third and, when symptomatic, is almost always associated with a tear, usually a horizontal tear. Discoid menisci occur in 5% of the population (rising to 20% in Japan) and are 10 times more common in the lateral meniscus. They are usually only symptomatic when torn or, far more rarely, if the posterior horn attachments are deficient (Wrisberg type), with instability and locking.

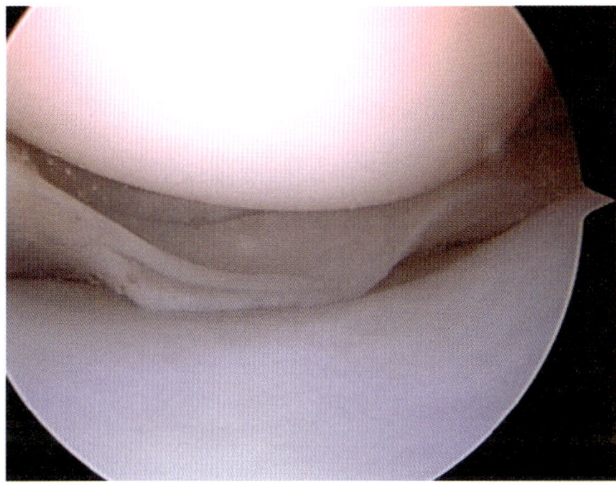

Figure 36.5 A longitudinal split is seen towards the periphery of the meniscus associated with a horizontal cleavage tear.

Meniscal tears are commonly associated with injuries to other structures, notably the chondral surface or ACL. A torn meniscus may present in one of two ways: either as intermittent locking or simply pain with weight-bearing activity, made worse by rotary movements. This becomes a recurrent problem as if the patient rests, the symptoms often resolve, only returning once activity is resumed. There may be an effusion in these acute episodes but this is usually mild unless associated with chondral damage. There is often a 'buckling' sensation—a sensation that the knee may collapse—but in the absence of any ligamentous instability. The clinical signs of a meniscal tear have been dealt with earlier but often the diagnosis is made from the history, as there may be few clinical signs at presentation, especially with lateral meniscal tears. With regards to the medial meniscal tear, if there is tenderness in the posteromedial joint line with a positive compression rotation test as described earlier, then one can be confident of a tear of the posterior horn of the medial meniscus.

MRI has been of great benefit in the diagnosis of knee pathology and has reduced the need for unnecessary arthroscopy. The sensitivity of the clinical diagnosis of meniscal tears is in the order of 75–80% compared with greater than 90% for MRI. This does not mean to say that all knees need an MRI scan. If there is doubt, which is usually with lateral meniscal tears, then an MRI scan is justified.

Management

The initial management of a meniscal tear may be conservative. Immediate treatment is necessary if the patient presents with a locked knee or with a peripheral tear of the meniscus. Attempts to try and manipulate the knee should be avoided as this could potentially cause further damage. The patient should undergo surgery at the earliest opportunity to unlock the knee and treat the tear with excision of the torn segment or suture. With the uncomplicated tear, the initial symptoms often resolve but may recur with increased activity. As meniscal tears do not heal, the patient often returns with further recurrent problems or the tear may extend with an episode of further trauma. If a patient has such recurrent problems, then the next stage in management is arthroscopic removal of the torn fragment.

Menisci were originally thought to be of little function and were removed through an open arthrotomy. Total menisectomy results in a reduction of the contact area of approximately 50% (Ahmed and Buke 1983). Partial menisectomy increases the contact pressure. Resection of as little as 20% of the meniscus increases contact pressures by more than 350% (Seedholm and Hargreaves 1979). Therefore, even partial menisectomies have resulted in less than satisfactory long-term results (Andersson-Molina et al. 2002; Chatain et al. 2003). Despite this, most meniscal tears are treated by partial menisectomies, with many studies in the literature documenting the clinical and radiological outcomes (McDermott and Amis 2006). Hede et al. described the long-term results of patients undergoing partial or total mensiectomy. They found that the function of the knee was inversely related to the amount of tissue resected (1992).

There are clear anatomical differences between the medial and lateral compartments of the knee, and between the medial and lateral menisci. On the lateral side, the meniscus carries 70% of the load in the lateral compartment, whereas the medial meniscus carries only 50% of the load of the medial compartment. Because of this, worse results have been reported after lateral than after medial menisectomy. McNicholas et al. found that after medial menisectomy, 80% of patients had good or excellent results at long-term follow-up, whereas only 47% had such an outcome after lateral menisectomy (2000).

Loss of meniscus means loss of the functions of the meniscus. Functions include load-bearing, shock absorption, joint stability, lubrication, and proprioception. The current trend is to preserve as much meniscus as possible. This includes trying to repair the meniscus in order to save it. The theory of meniscal repair is based on the blood supply to the meniscus, the outer 30% of the medial meniscus being vascular (red zone) with a transition to avascular meniscus in the inner third (white zone). In the lateral meniscus, this vascularized area is slightly less than on the medial side.

The results of repair have been encouraging. Kotsovolos et al. showed that at a mean follow-up of 18 months, just over 90% of 58 meniscal repairs were clinically successful, with absence of joint-line tenderness, locking, or swelling (2006).

The indications for meniscal repair are any peripheral tears in the red zone, any tears in the red–white zone, and any tears in the younger patient. Stable longitudinal tears (<1 cm in length) and partial thickness tears often remain asymptomatic or heal without suturing (Shelbourne and Heinrich 2004). Various techniques have been tried to enhance the healing of a meniscal repair, especially in the red–white zone but also in the white–white zone. These include techniques whereby bleeding is promoted, such as debridement of the meniscal ends, trephination of the peripheral aspect of the meniscal rim, and synovial abrasion (Uchio et al. 2003).

It has been shown that meniscal healing is better following an ACL reconstruction as opposed to following a repair alone. Cannon found that the healing rates improved from 53% to 93% when the repair was performed in conjunction with an ACL reconstruction. The reason for this is thought to be the blood and marrow elements created at the time of the ACL reconstruction may provide a milieu, bathing the healing meniscus (Cannon and Vittori 1992).

The use of a fibrin clot has stemmed from these findings. Clinical studies have suggested improved healing rates in red–white meniscal tears in which a fibrin clot was used (Van Trommel et al. 1998). Another potential way to provide growth factors to the area of an avascular meniscal lesion, but in a higher concentration than a fibrin clot, is the use of platelet-rich plasma (PRP). PRP is created through centrifugation of whole blood into its cellular components (Sanchez et al. 2003).

If a meniscus is unavoidably lost, there is a place, particularly in the younger patient before degenerative changes ensue, to consider replacing the meniscus with an allograft. Meniscus allograft transplantation may be performed in these patients if pain is a major symptom. The results are variable and there is little long-term data on the prevention of degenerative changes. Rath et al. (2001) reported a 64% success rate following meniscal allograft transplantation. Noyes was able to achieve a reduction in pain in 89% of his patients (Noyes et al. 2004).

Another new development is tissue engineering by regeneration of the meniscus with collagen scaffolding. This scaffold is made out of tissue such as bovine Achilles' tendon. It may be used in situations such as previous large partial menisectomies and irreparable meniscal tears. Results show that at 6 years, the average amount of meniscal defect remaining filled was 69% (Steadman and Rodkey 2005).

Over the past 30 years, with the advent of arthroscopic surgery, meniscal preservation has become the norm, with removal of only the torn fragment or suturing of the meniscus if the tear is in the peripheral zone. Theoretically, this should reduce the incidence of late degenerative changes, though in view of the long time frame, there is little data available yet to support this claim.

The availability of meniscal suturing should mean there is no excuse for sacrificing the meniscus, particularly in the young athlete. The patient should be warned of the poor healing capacity of the meniscus. When associated with an ACL rupture, the chance of healing is in the order of 80%, but this drops to 50% with an isolated meniscal tear. In addition, the rehabilitation is far slower, with a return to contact sport at 6 months rather than 6 weeks if the tear is removed. This, and the consequences of a major meniscectomy, should be carefully explained to the patient.

Chondral lesions of the knee

Structure

Articular cartilage is a specialized connective tissue, the matrix of which consists of a gel of proteoglycan and water, which is reinforced by collagen fibres. These fibres are firmly anchored to the subchondral bone, giving stability to the cartilage. Chondrocytes synthesize and maintain the matrix of collagen and proteoglycan within which they lie. The collagen is predominantly of type II. The collagen fibres are arranged in the form of arcades that arise from subchondral bone (**Figure 36.6**). The proteoglycans and cells are embedded within the collagen fibres. The proteoglycans are long chain polysaccharides linked to hyaluronate that are negatively charged and hold water within the cartilage. This proteoglycan–water gel gives the cartilage matrix a high osmotic pressure. The tendency of the proteoglycan to swell is balanced by the elastic resistance of the collagen network. The collagen arcades thus aid in absorption of compressive forces.

Pathology and presentation

Articular cartilage is avascular, aneural, and alymphatic and nutrition must therefore be derived either deeply from blood vessels in the subchondral bone and/or from the synovial fluid bathing the

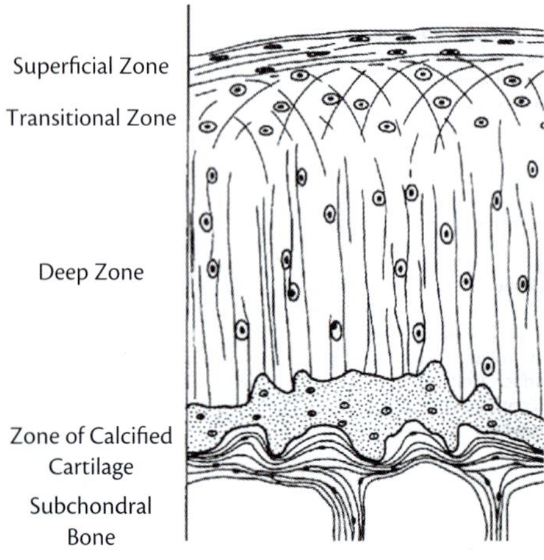

Figure 36.6 Diagrammatic representation of the articular cartilage.

cartilage surface. The chondroblasts in the cartilage tissue are relatively few and their metabolic rate is low. The capacity of chondrocytes to divide and migrate in the articular cartilage is restricted by the matrix fibres. As a consequence, the articular cartilage does not repair significantly after injury.

The proteoglycan structure can be damaged by trauma, or by enzymes from inflammatory disease and infection. If this happens, the proteoglycan structure disintegrates and the water-holding capacity is lost. Progressive breakdown of the collagen meshwork occurs, leading to exposure of bone that is responsible for the symptoms of severe pain and disability. A number of classification systems are in use, but no single system seems to be universally applicable. The spectrum of grades is from softening and fissuring to fragmentation and erosion.

Partial-thickness injuries of the articular cartilage do not heal. They stimulate only a minimal and short-lived reaction in the adjacent chondrocytes in the form of increased cell replication and matrix turnover. Full-thickness injuries penetrating the subchondral bone produce the normal response associated with wound healing, including vascular invasion, cell migration, and inflammatory reaction, filling the defect with fibrocartilage. Fibrocartilage primarily functions as a resistor to tension, in contrast to hyaline cartilage which mainly resists compressive forces. The end product of fibrocartilage is thus inadequate, biomechanically. Articular defects increase surface stresses in the remaining cartilage, increasing wear in the affected compartment.

Damage to articular cartilage is a common problem. In a review of 31,516 knee arthroscopies by Curl et al. (1997), 53,569 hyaline cartilage lesions were documented in 19,827 patients. Grade III lesions of the patella were the most common. Grade IV lesions were predominantly located on the medial femoral condyle. Patients under 40 years of age with grade IV lesions accounted for 5% of all arthroscopies; 74% of these patients had a single chondral lesion (4% of the arthroscopies). No associated ligamentous or meniscal pathology was found in 36.6% of these patients.

Levy et al. (1996) examined 23 isolated chondral defects in 15 soccer players; 33% of the lesions were less than 10 mm in diameter, but all players had knee pain. Their study indicated that even small lesions are significant in producing symptoms. It appears that pain is caused by the stimulation of nerve endings in the subchondral bone due to compromised load-transmitting and energy-absorbing capabilities.

There is increasing clinical evidence that full-thickness articular cartilage defects slowly and progressively advance, leading to premature arthritis. Twyman et al. (1991) prospectively followed 22 knees in which osteochondritis dissecans had been diagnosed before skeletal maturity At an average age of 34 years, 32% had radiographic evidence of moderate or severe osteoarthritis.

These lesions may be encountered incidentally during ligament or meniscal surgery, having been silent or asymptomatic for an unknown period of time, or they may mimic a meniscal tear in their presentation. The usual symptoms and signs include pain with weight-bearing, mechanical catching, clicking, or locking, and effusion. Untreated lesions can lead to debilitating joint pain, dysfunction, and degenerative arthritis.

MRI using cartilage sequencing can provide reliable information on the state of articular cartilage (Potter et al. 1998). Diagnosis is adequate with the standard 1.5 Tesla MRI scanners but is much more accurate with the newer 3T scanners.

Management

Cartilage repair strategies

- Bone marrow stimulation
- Whole tissue transplantation
- Cell-based techniques

Bone marrow stimulation

- Abrasion techniques
- Microfracture

Bone marrow stimulation is the most frequently used technique for treating small symptomatic lesions of the articular cartilage of the knee.

Microfracture involves the perforation of the subchondral plate in order to recruit mesenchymal stem cells (MSC) from the bone marrow space into the lesion (**Figure 36.7**). The MSC are then able to differentiate into fibrochondrocytes, which contribute to fibrocartilage repair of the lesion. This fibrocartilage consists of Type I, II, and III collagen in varying amounts. This is unlike hyaline cartilage which is mainly Type II collagen.

The formation of a stable clot that maximally fills the chondral defect is important. There is a direct correlation with the success of the bone marrow stimulation procedure and the ability of the clot to adhere to the defect (Frisbie et al. 2003).

The advantages of microfracture are that these techniques are technically straightforward and the cost is low compared to other techniques. Disadvantages are that the overall concentration of MSC is quite low. In addition, the results are worse in the older patient and declines with age.

The post-operative regime following microfracture is important in order to maximize the chance of success of this technique. This includes non-weight-bearing with crutches for 6 weeks and CPM (continuous passive movement) for 6–8 hours per day for 6 weeks. CPM has been shown to improve cartilage nutrition and stimulate MSC differentiation (Salter 1989).

Steadman et al. reported the first long-term follow-up of microfracture: 71 knees followed up for 11 years showed a significant improvement in multiple clinical outcome measures (Steadman and Briggs 2003). Mithoefer et al. in 2009 showed 67% good to excellent results, with 25% fair and 8% poor. Microfracture has also been

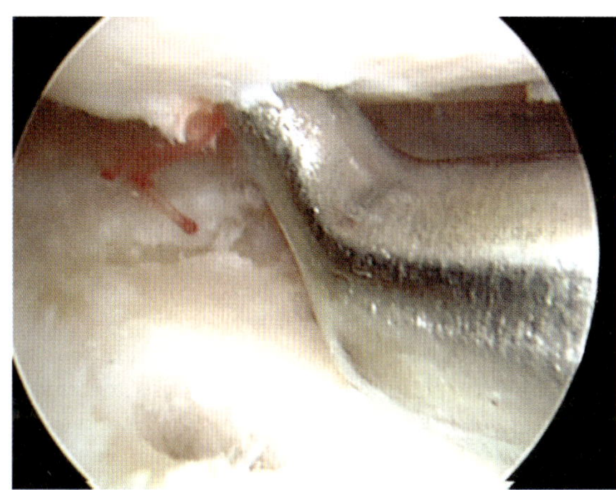

Figure 36.7 An area of chondral loss being treated by microfracture.

compared with other cartilage restoration procedures showing very similar results (Gudas et al. 2005; Knutsen et al. 2004).

The ideal candidate for microfracture, who is most likely to benefit and be able to return to sport, is a patient who is less than 40 years old, has a lesion less than 2 cm^2, has had pre-operative symptoms for less than 12 months, and has had no prior operative intervention (Gobbi et al. 2005; Kreuz et al. 2006).

Whole tissue transplantation

- Autologous osteochondral transplantation (OATS/mosaicplasty)
- Osteochondral allograft transplantation

Autologous osteochondral transplantation involves transplantation of multiple, small, cylindrical autogenous osteochondral plugs harvested from the less weight-bearing periphery of the articular surface of the femoral condyle and transferred to create a congruent and durable resurfaced area in the defect. The donor site heals with cancellous bone and fibrocartilage. The advantages are that transplantation is of viable hyaline cartilage, there is a relatively brief rehabilitation period, and the procedure can be performed in a single operation. Disadvantages include donor site morbidity, graft subsidence with weight-bearing, and the absence of fill and potential dead space between cylindrical grafts.

The majority of outcomes from studies have been encouraging. Ozturk et al. showed 85% good–excellent results in 19 patients (2006). Hangody and Fules reviewed 831 patients showing 92% good–excellent outcomes in the femur, 87% for the tibia, and 79% for patella lesions (2003). Its efficacy has been compared to ACI (autologous chondrocyte implantation) where similar results between the groups were found (Dozin et al. 2005).

Osteochondral allograft transplantation is a cartilage resurfacing procedure that involves transplantation of a cadaver graft, consisting of intact, viable articular cartilage and its underlying subchondral bone, into the defect. Advantages include the ability to achieve precise surface architecture and immediate transplantation of viable hyaline cartilage as a single procedure. Disadvantages are limited graft availability (needs to be fresh), high cost, and risk of immunological rejection and disease transmission.

A number of retrospective studies have demonstrated favourable good–excellent results (Chu et al. 1999; Ghazavi et al. 1997).

Cell-based techniques

Autologous chondrocyte implantation (ACI), originally described in 1994, is a technique to restore hyaline cartilage, rather than fibrocartilage, to a chondral defect.

A biopsy is taken from the non-weight-bearing segment of the medial or lateral femoral condyle. Cells are then cultured over the next 3–4 weeks to about 15–20 million chondro-lineage cells. At a second operation, the bed is prepared and a periosteal patch is sewn onto the defect before the suspension of cells are injected into the defect. This is first generation ACI.

Because of the problems associated with the first generation techniques, further advances have been made. Instead of periosteum, Gooding et al. (2006) demonstrated the superiority of Type I/III porcine collagen membrane as a cover for the graft. Now, in addition to avoiding the periosteal patch and in order to speed up the whole process of chondrocyte implantation, the second generation ACI technique has been developed—MACI (matrix assisted chondrocyte implantation). This uses a scaffold Type I/III collagen or, more recently, hyaluronan. The cells are cultured on the surface of the scaffold which is then implanted into the defect and secured with a fibrin glue.

The ideal candidate for ACI is a younger patient (<40 years) with less than 2 years of symptoms, a single defect, a defect on the trochlea or the lateral femoral condyle, and with less than two previous surgeries.

The original results of ACI were described by Brittberg et al. (1994). Zaslav et al. (2009), in a prospective study in patients with failed prior treatment, demonstrated 76% good to excellent results. Compared with microfracture, Knutsen et al. (2007) showed no difference in macroscopic and clinical results in the two groups at 5 years. Compared with mosaicplasty, Bentley et al. (2003) showed 88% good to excellent results in the ACI group versus 69% in those treated by mosaicplasty. Kon et al. in 2009 compared microfracture with MACI using a hyaluronan scaffold, where both groups had a satisfactory outcome but MACI was better clinically.

The future

Third generation ACI

A 3D scaffold mimicking cartilage structure is now being used to provide an increased surface area:volume ratio for cellular migration, adhesion, and differentiation. This can be made from fibres, sponges, or gels and, after the integration of chondrocytes, can be used as a scaffold for implantation.

Bone marrow derived MSCs

MSCs have been shown to differentiate into bone, cartilage, fat, marrow, muscle, skin, and tendon. Any of these tissues are therefore potential sources of MSCs. Bone marrow however has the highest chondrogenic potential (Nejadnik et al. 2010). It may therefore be used to form chondrocytes then, via a subsequent operation, implanted into the defect.

Replacements

Different devices are now on the market. These are used to fill a defect. Only short-term data is available for these. However, they may offer an option for this difficult treatment group.

Knee instability

The normal stability and kinematics of the knee joint are maintained by the shape of the femoral and tibial condyles and the menisci, in combination with the passive supporting structures consisting of the four major ligaments—the anterior cruciate ligament (ACL), the posterior cruciate ligament (PCL), the medial collateral ligament (MCL), and the lateral collateral ligament (LCL). Significant contributions are also made by the posteromedial and posterolateral capsular components and the iliotibial tract. All the aforementioned structures provide primary static stability. The muscles acting over the joint provide secondary dynamic stability. Instability resulting from ligament injury results from both direct and indirect trauma.

The medial collateral ligament

The MCL is attached proximally to the medial femoral condyle and distally to the tibial metaphysis, 4 to 5 cm distal to the medial joint line beneath the pes anserinus insertion. Posterior to the MCL is the posterior oblique ligament (POL) which is a thickening of the capsule. Immediately deep to the MCL is the medial capsular ligament. These constitute the medial ligament complex. The MCL has a superficial portion (the primary static stabilizer to valgus stress) and the deeper meniscotibial and meniscofemoral portion. In full extension, the POL and the posteromedial capsule resist valgus stresses. These relax at 20–30° of flexion, when the MCL becomes the primary restraint. The MCL, together with the POL, resists abnormal internal tibial rotation. Isolated injuries occur usually as a result of a direct blow to the lateral aspect of the knee in a slightly flexed position. When the deforming force includes a rotational component, associated injuries to the cruciate ligaments can occur.

Assessment of the acute injury includes looking for a localized bruise or swelling, localized tenderness, and application of a gentle valgus force with the patient's knee in 15–20° of flexion. The degree of medial joint opening compared to the normal knee is a measure of damage to the MCL. A difference of only 5–8 mm is indicative of significant structural damage to the MCL because of its parallel collagen arrangement (Indelicato 1995). This is now repeated with the knee in full extension to evaluate the extent of the medial soft tissue damage. Excessive opening in full extension is indicative of combined MCL and POL damage and should alert the examiner to the strong possibility of an associated ACL or PCL injury. If the knee is stable in full extension, there is unlikely to be damage to the POL.

Treatment of acute, isolated MCL injury is conservative (Indelicato 1995: Jacobson and Chi 2006). Incomplete tears (sprains) of the MCL without significant instability are treated with **R**est, **I**ce, **C**ompression, and **E**levation (RICE) during the first 48 hours. This is followed by temporary immobilization, then protected range of movement, and the use of crutches for pain control. Weight-bearing, as tolerated, is encouraged as soon as pain allows, followed by early functional rehabilitation. Very occasionally do isolated acute tears need surgery (Narvani et al. 2010).

Treatment of acute MCL injuries combined with ACL injuries is usually surgery for both ligaments, although bracing for the MCL, followed by ACL reconstruction, is an alternative **(Figure 36.8)**.

Chronic MCL insufficiency is rare in isolation and is usually associated with ACL or PCL injury. Careful examination must differentiate between MCL with or without posteromedial rotary instability. Symptomatic medial instability not improved with conservative treatment may require surgery in the form of proximal advancement of the MCL (Shahane and Bickerstaff 1998). Reconstructive procedures involve the use of autograft (hamstring or patella tendon), allograft, or synthetic ligaments (Borden et al. 2002).

The anterior cruciate ligament

The ACL is intracapsular but extrasynovial. Its femoral attachment is on the lateral wall of the intercondylar notch at its posterior aspect. The tibial attachment is on the anterior aspect of the tibial plateau near the tibial spines. The ACL has been described as having an anteromedial band which is tighter in flexion and a posterolateral band which is tighter in extension (Amis 1991). This arrangement of the fascicles allows different portions to be taut throughout the range of motion, permitting the ligament to be functional in all the degrees of flexion and extension. Its main source of blood supply is the middle genicular artery, a branch of the popliteal artery that approaches by piercing the posterior capsule. It has also been shown to contain proprioceptive nerve endings (Biedert et al. 1992). The ACL is the primary restraint to anterior translation of the tibia onto the femur and to hyperextension (Fu et al. 1993). It functions as a secondary restraint to varus or valgus angulation at full extension. It also resists internal and external rotation, mostly near full extension than in early flexion.

Diagnosis: This is made by a positive Lachman's test and a positive pivot shift test. Plain radiographs may show an avulsion of the insertion of the ACL or a Segond fracture (a lateral capulsar avulsion fracture from the margin of the lateral tibial plateau that is often associated with an ACL injury) **(Figure 36.9)**. MRI has an overall accuracy of greater than 90% in assessing the ACL, although this need not be used routinely (Glashow et al. 1989). MRI is mainly used to detect associated injuries, of which, lateral meniscal tears are the most common. MRI also shows bone abnormalities not seen on conventional radiographs. These include 'bone bruises', seen in approximately 60% of ACL injuries, the significance and long-term sequelae of which have yet to be determined, although the

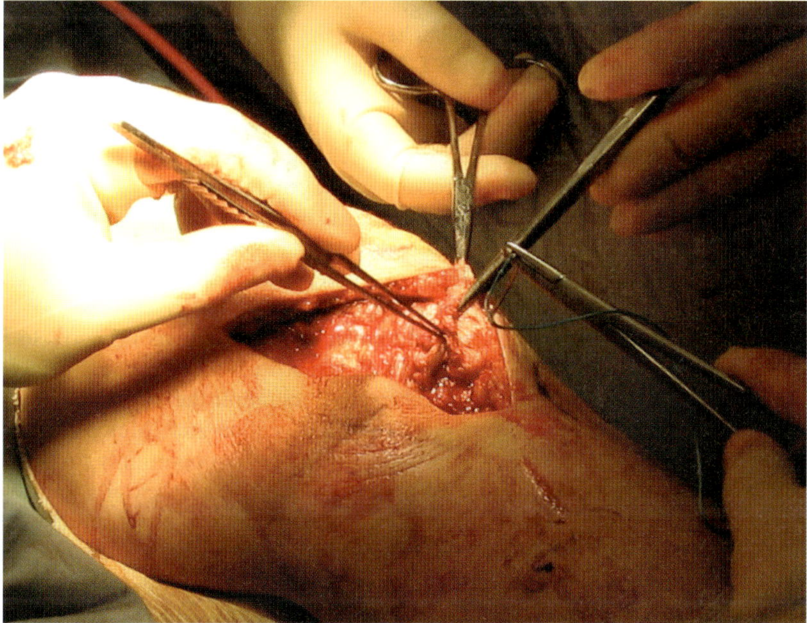

Figure 36.8 Complete rupture of the MCL being repaired surgically.

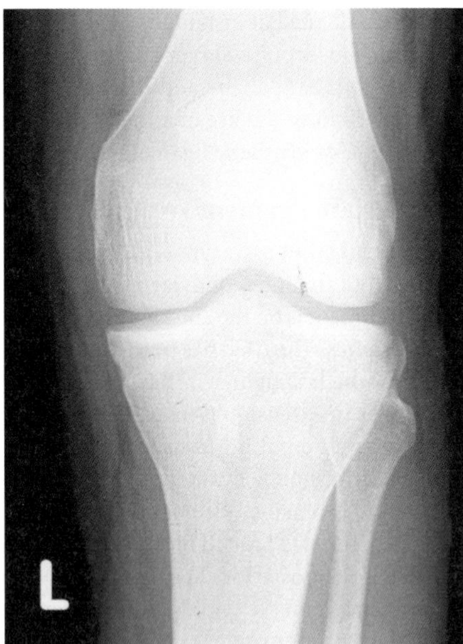

Figure 36.9 Segond fracture. Lateral capsular avulsion indicating an ACL rupture.

evidence is towards no clinical significance (Costa-Paz et al. 2001; Graf et al. 1993).

Management: An acute repair is associated with poor results, including a higher re-rupture rate and arthrofibrosis (Harner et al. 1992). No functional advantage is gained by early reconstruction (Meighan et al. 2003). Hence, the initial treatment is based on the reduction of pain and swelling and early restoration of normal joint movement. For peel-off lesions from the femur, primary repair in conjunction with microfracture has recently been advocated. The treatment of 'partial' ACL tears remains controversial. They are difficult to diagnose on MRI. Non-operative treatment may be sufficient in most cases. However, ACL reconstruction is recommended if there is functional instability or a positive pivot shift test (DeFranco and Bach 2009).

The goal of treatment for ACL deficiency is to prevent re-injury which otherwise may lead to chondral injuries, meniscal injuries, or laxity of secondary restraints. These secondary injuries are thought to lead to arthritis, although progression to radiologically detectable osteoarthritis appears to be variable (Hart et al. 2005).

Once ACL deficiency is diagnosed, the decision between operative and non-operative treatment is based on variables that are unique to each individual. Among the factors considered are the patient's age, activity level (recreational/occupational), the degree of laxity, associated meniscal or ligamentous pathology, ability and willingness to participate in a physiotherapy programme, and future expectations, including the type of sporting activity in which the patient wishes to participate.

Non-operative management of acute ACL tears may be successful in those patients who have no associated injuries and are willing to give up high-demand sports. The rehabilitation programme emphasizes proprioceptive muscle training to maximize the dynamic stability, hamstring strengthening, and avoidance of unbalanced quadriceps strengthening to prevent anterior translation. Non-operative management also includes counselling concerning high-risk activities and measures to prevent recurrent injuries. The role of functional knee bracing remains controversial. Braces were thought to offer protection by improving joint position sense and by providing mechanical constraint of joint motion.

Older individuals are often more willing to modify their activities, but surgery may be required even in these individuals, if the instability is so great that their activities of daily living are impaired or, as is increasingly seen, they are unwilling to stop pivoting sports. In carefully selected patients, similar results to younger patients can be achieved (Dahm et al. 2008).

As patients do not tolerate instability in two major ligaments very well, the presence of associated injuries also influences decision making in the direction of surgery. Also in cases in which meniscal repair is undertaken ACL reconstruction is advisable because the failure rate of meniscal repair is increased in the presence of ACL instability (Hanks et al. 1990).

Surgery: Historically, techniques have been described for intra-articular and extra-articular reconstructions of the ACL using the iliotibial band, the semitendinosus and gracilis tendons, the patella tendon, allograft tissue, and various synthetic materials. Currently, intra-articular open or arthroscopic techniques are used. The arthroscopic technique is used by most surgeons. The surgical technique requires proper placement and tensioning of the graft, avoidance of impingement and stress risers on the implanted tissue, and adequate fixation on both femoral and tibial sides. The available graft materials are broadly divided into autografts, allografts, and synthetic grafts.

Autogenous grafts are most commonly employed in ACL reconstruction. They provide a framework for revascularization and regeneration of the ligament and, with modern fixation techniques, allow rapid rehabilitation. Allografts heal in a similar fashion but at a slower rate. They are therefore more widely used when there are no autograft alternatives. There is however a risk of disease transmission. Synthetic grafts have not proved successful in the long term. Recent meta-analysis showed no difference in short- term clinical outcome between allografts and autografts (Carey et al. 2009).

Surgeons differ in their preference of autogenous tissue. The patella tendon graft (B-PT-B) **(Figure 36.10)** has greater initial tensile strength and allows more secure bone-to-bone fixation. Most surgeons report 80–90% good or excellent results using autogenous B-PT-B. Patellar fracture, tendinitis, anterior knee pain, and increased incidence of infra-patellar contracture syndrome have been described with their use. Patellar fracture can usually be avoided by improved technique. Patellar tendinitis is usually short-lived and after one year is generally not a problem. Anterior knee pain, however, appears to be more significant with this graft source than with hamstring reconstruction.

Use of semitendinosus and gracilis tendon grafts for reconstruction of ACL has now been well established as they have been theorized to offer certain advantages **(Figure 36.11)**. They provide a stronger ACL substitute when both are used together. Their stiffness characteristics mimic the normal ACL more closely than does the stiffer patellar tendon graft. Multiple strands of the hamstring grafts also allow a better opportunity for revascularization. These offer an ideal alternative in skeletally immature patients (where harvesting patellar graft can jeopardize the tibial apophysis), in women (for cosmetic reasons), or when there is extensor mechanism pathology. Hamstring harvest is associated with minimal graft site morbidity. Both direct and indirect clinical comparisons have

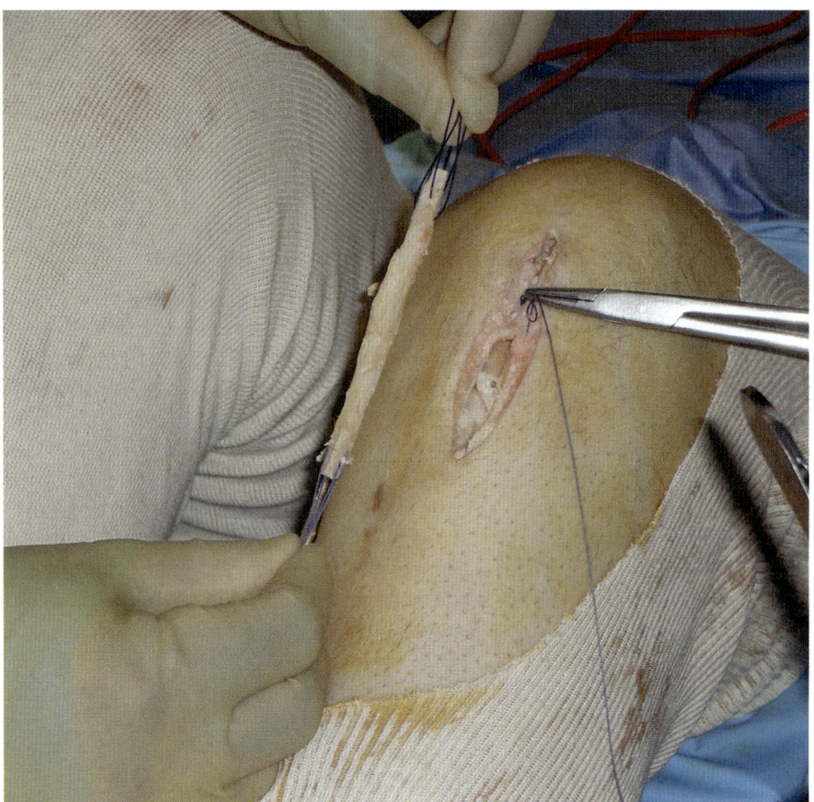

Figure 36.10 Bone–patella tendon–bone ACL reconstruction via the open technique.

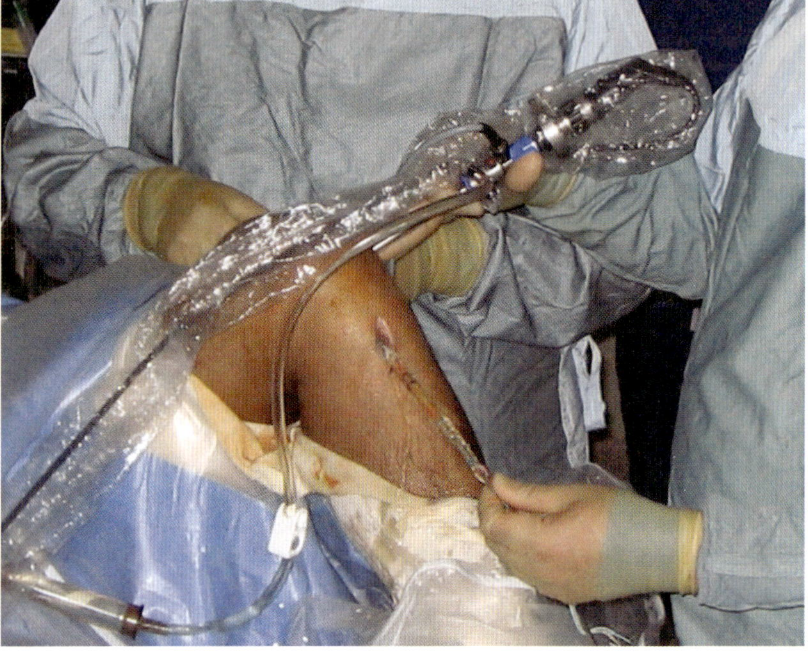

Figure 36.11 Arthroscopic ACL reconstruction using hamstring tendons.

shown that B-PT-B grafts and hamstring grafts have similar rates of effectiveness in adults, with only minimal variations in knee stability and muscle strength at an average of 3 years after implantation (Aglietti et al.2004).

A recent vogue has been double-bundle ACL reconstruction, which proposedly demonstrates biomechanical advantages over single-bundle technique by providing increased rotational stability. Most studies to date have shown no difference in clinical outcome between the two groups (Adachi et al. 2004; Longo et al. 2008).

Rehabilitation: Post-operative rehabilitation is an important aspect of care of ACL deficient patients. Previously, rehabilitation focused on protection of the new ligament with block to full extension and avoidance of active quadriceps contraction to prevent anterior tibial translation stressing the graft. This led to stiffness of the knees and patello-femoral problems. Shelbourne advocated an accelerated rehabilitation protocol, the objective being early and long-term maintenance of full knee extension, improving results. This protocol was based on the use of patellar tendon graft, although the principles are similar with other types of grafts (Shelbourne and Nitz 1990).

Injury prevention programmes have been developed to try to decrease the incidence of ACL injuries, especially in females, who are more likely to have a rupture of their ACL in playing sport. These programmes involve plyometrics and neuromuscular training, especially on landing and cutting (Mandelbaum et al. 2005).

The lateral collateral ligament and the posterolateral corner

The LCL originates on the lateral epicondyle of the femur and is attached distally on the fibular head. The LCL is relatively rarely injured in isolation and is usually injured as part of a complex involving the posterolateral corner (PLC), the PCL, or the ACL. The PLC is a complex anatomical region of the knee consisting of the popliteus tendon, the popliteo-fibular ligament, the arcuate ligament, and the posterolateral joint capsule. The lateral and the PCL complex can be considered as consisting of three layers—the iliotibial tract and the superficial portion of the biceps femoris forming the first layer; the LCL as the second layer; and the joint capsule, the arcuate ligament, the popliteo-fibular ligament, and the popliteal tendon as constituting the third layer. The LCL is the primary static stabilizer to the lateral opening of the joint, supplemented by the popliteo-fibular ligament and the cruciates. The popliteo-fibular ligament is the primary restraint to posterolateral rotation, supplemented by the LCL and the popliteus tendon (Shahane and Bickerstaff 1999).

The most useful tests in differentiating between isolated LCL, PCL, and PLC or combined PCL–PLC injuries are the varus stress test and the dial test (passive external rotation of the tibia, relative to the femur, with the knee at 30° and 90° of flexion (see 'Collateral ligament instability' within the 'Orthopaedic examination of the knee' section). The patient's limb alignment and gait pattern must be observed to ensure there is no lateral thrust on walking. If this is not recognized, the ligament reconstruction may fail in the absence of a corrective osteotomy. MRI is useful in the acute setting to identify associated cruciate injury, the site of injury to the structures in the PLC, which will help plan surgery. Despite clinical examination and imaging, up to 72% of PLC injuries are commonly missed on initial presentation (Pacheco et al. 2011).

The data available on surgical outcomes for posterolateral reconstruction is limited. The wide variety of procedures used to treat patients with posterolateral instability makes it difficult to derive a consensus on the most effective and appropriate approach to this clinical entity. Grade I injuries can be treated in an extension brace. With more significant acute injuries of the PLC, surgical intervention within 2 weeks of the initial injuries is optimal, with the direct repair of all injured structures where possible (Ross et al. 2004). If the LCL or the popliteo-fibular ligament is ruptured mid substance, then consideration should be given to reconstruction of these structures, as direct repair in isolation may be insufficient. In the chronic setting, direct repair is often not possible and a variety of techniques can be used including tissue advancement and augmentation with autograft or allograft tissues. The authors use hamstring autografts to reconstruct the LCL and the popliteo-fibular ligaments, similar to the technique described by Larson (Kumar et al. 1999). If there is a varus thrust, the authors prefer to perform an opening medial wedge osteotomy to avoid any further slackening of the lateral structures one may see with a lateral closing wedge osteotomy.

Posterior cruciate ligament

There is a wide variation in the incidence of PCL injuries. Various studies quote figures that range from 2% to 40%, but probably they average 15% of all knee ligament injuries (Cooper et al. 1991; Fanelli and Edson 1995). They are increasingly recognized as sporting injuries. It is likely that the apparent increase in incidence is due to more frequent recognition. The PCL takes origin from the medial femoral condyle, with its attachment in the shape of a semi-circle. It inserts in a depression between the posterior aspects of the two tibial plateaus, approximately 1 cm below the articular surface. Functionally, it is composed of two bundles, anterolateral and posteromedial. In mid range of flexion (40–120°), the anterolateral bundle is the primary restraint to the posterior drawer. The posteromedial bundle increases its contribution towards full flexion (Race and Amis 1996). Earlier studies have shown the anterolateral bundle to be structurally and biomechanically more significant (Harner and Xerogeanes 1995). Some studies suggest reconstruction of both bundles to restore the normal function of the PCL throughout the range of motion (Race and Amis 1998; Stahelin et al. 2001).

The PCL is the primary static restraint to posterior translation of the tibia. It is a secondary stabilizer to varus angulation and external tibial rotary displacement at 90° (of knee flexion). The mechanism of most sporting PCL injuries is a fall on the flexed knee with the foot in plantar flexion. This imparts the force to the tibial tubercle, pushing the tibia posteriorly and usually resulting in an isolated PCL rupture. Hyperflexion of the knee without a direct blow to the tibia can also cause isolated PCL injury. Forced hyperextension can injure the PCL, but this usually is combined with injury to the ACL. Posteriorly directed force to the anteromedial tibia with the knee in hyperextension may also cause a PLC injury. Significant varus or valgus stress will injure the PCL only after rupture of the appropriate collateral ligament. In isolation, there is often little instability, whereas when associated with posterolateral or posteromedial injuries, stability of the knee is dramatically reduced.

Plain radiographs may show a PCL avulsion fracture. MRI has proved to be sensitive and specific for diagnosis of acute PCL injury. It can be used to confirm meniscal and chondral damage. Instrumented knee testing can also be used to confirm the diagnosis of PCL injury, in combination with the quadriceps active test.

Management of acute isolated PCL injuries is conservative. Reconstruction is usually not required. They have a high likelihood of healing (Shelbourne et al. 1999). If the degree of posterior translation is less than 10 mm, as in the majority of isolated injuries or even in those with small tibial PCL avulsion fractures, a non-operative aggressive rehabilitation programme is arranged. Following an initial period of R I C E, an extension splint is worn for 3–4 weeks. A posterior tibial support (PTS) splint is ideal. Physiotherapy is focused especially on quadriceps strengthening. Close follow-up is necessary in order that combined instability is not missed.

If the avulsed fragment is large, it can be reduced and fixed through a posterior approach. If the posterior translation is greater than 10 mm, without a firm end point, reconstruction is advised, since it is likely that additional secondary restraints have been compromised. Acute surgical treatment of complete PCL tears can include primary repair or reconstruction, depending on the location of injury. PCL reconstruction can be performed with a patellar tendon autograft, semi-tendinosus and gracilis autograft, or a patella or Achilles' tendon allograft. The reconstruction of the PCL can be performed with open or arthroscopically assisted techniques. Arthroscopic procedure is performed under X-ray control using an additional posteromedial portal to assist in tibial tunnel preparation. This procedure is technically demanding. When an acute injury has posterolateral, ACL, or Grade III MCL components (that usually occurs in a spontaneously reduced dislocation of the knee), it appears best to operate early, between 2–3 weeks, to maximize healing potential and minimize stiffness.

Despite the lack of prospective studies, it appears that progressive degenerative changes may occur in some PCL deficient knees, especially to the medial femoral and patello-femoral components.

Post-operative rehabilitation following PCL reconstruction is designed to restore range of motion without stressing the graft. Exercises that produce posterior tibial translation are avoided. For the first 6 weeks, flexion is carried out in a prone position, limited weight-bearing using crutches is necessary, and a PTS brace is worn. Following the early rehabilitation programme, running begins at about 5 months, and sports and physical activity commences at 6–7 months. A full range of sports is allowed when adequate quadriceps and hamstrings strength is demonstrated after about 9 months.

References

Adachi N, Ochi M, Uchio Y, et al. (2004) Reconstruction of the anterior cruciate ligament. Single versus double-bundle multistranded hamstring tendons. *J Bone Joint Surg (Br)* 86B:515–20.

Aglietti P, Giron F, et al. (2004) Anterior cruciate ligament reconstruction: bone-patellar tendon-bone compared with double semitendinosus and gracilis tendon grafts. *J Bone Joint Surg Am* 86A(10):2143–54.

Ahmed AM, Buke DL. (1983) In vitro measurement of static pressure distribution in synovial joints—Part I: Tibial surface of the knee. *J Biomech Eng* 105:216–25.

Amis AA, et al. (1991) Functional anatomy of ACL: fibre bundle action related to ligament replacement and injuries. *J Bone Joint Surg (Br)* 73(2): 260–7.

Andersson-Molina H, Karlsson H, Rockborn P. (2002) Arthroscopic partial and total menisectomy: a long term follow-up study with matched controls. *Arthroscopy* 18:183–9.

Apley AG, Solomon L. (1982) *Apley's system of orthopaedics and fractures* (6th edn). London: Butterworths.

Arnoczky SP, Warren RF. (1982) Microvasculature of the human meniscus. *Am J Sports Med* 10:90.

Bach BR Jr, Warren RF, Wickiewicz TL. (1988) The pivot shift phenomenon: results and a description of a modified clinical test for anterior cruciate ligament instability. *Am J Sports Med* 16(6):571–6.

Bentley G, Biant LC, Carrington RW, et al. (2003) A prospective, randomised comparison of autologous chondrocyte implantation versus mosaicplasty for osteochondral defects in the knee. *J Bone Joint Surg Br* 85:223–30.

Biedert RM, Stauffer E, Friederich NF. (1992) Occurrence of free nerve endings in the soft tissues of the knee joint—a histologic investigation. *Am J Sports Med* 20:1430–3.

Borden PS, Kantaras AT, Caborn DN. (2002) Medial collateral ligament reconstruction with allograft using double-bundle technique. *Arthroscopy* 18(4):E19.

Brittberg M, Lindahl A, Nilsson A, et al. (1994) Treatment of deep cartilage defects in the knee with autologous chondrocyte transplantation. *N Eng J Med* 331:889–95.

Cannon WD Jr,Vittori JM. (1992) The incidence of healing in arthroscopic meniscal repairs in anterior cruciate reconstructed knees versus stable knees. *Am J Sports Med* 20:176–81.

Carey JL, Dunn WR, et al. (2009) A systematic review of anterior cruciate ligament reconstruction with autograft compared with allograft. *J Bone Joint Surg Am* 91:2242–50.

Chatain F, Adeleine P, Chambat P, et al. (2003) A comparative study of medial versus lateral arthroscopic partial menesectomy on stable knees: 10-year minimum follow up. *Arthroscopy* 19:842–9.

Chu CR, Convery FR, Akeson WH, et al. (1999) Articular cartilage transplantation. Clinical results in the knee. *Clin Orthop Relat Res* 360: 159–68.

Cooper DE, Warren RF, et al. (1991) The PCL and the posterolateral structures of the knee: anatomy, function and patterns of injury. *Instr Course Lect* 40:249–70.

Costa-Paz M, Muscolo DL, Ayerza M, et al. (2001) Magnetic resonance imaging follow-up study of bone bruising associated with anterior cruciate ligament ruptures. *Arthroscopy* 17:445–9.

Curl WW, Krome J, Gordon S, Rushing J, Smith BP, Poehling GG. (1997) Cartilage injuries: a review of 31,516 knee arthroscopies. *Arthroscopy* 13:456–60.

Dahm DL, Wulf CA, et al. (2008) Reconstruction of the anterior cruciate ligament in patients over 50 years. *J Bone Joint Surg (Br)* 90–B:1446–50.

Dandy DJ. (1990) The arthroscopic anatomy of the symptomatic meniscal lesion. *J Bone Joint Surg Br* 72(4):628.

DeFranco MJ, Bach BR. (2009) A comprehensive review of partial anterior cruciate ligament tears. *J Bone Joint Surg Am* 91:198–208.

Dozin B, Malpeli M, Cancedda R, et al. (2005) Comparative evaluation of autologous chondrocyte implantation and mosaicplasty: a multicentered randomized clinical trial. *Clin J Sport Med* 15:220–6.

Draper DO, Schulthies SS. (1995) Examiner proficiency in performing the anterior draw and Lachman tests. *J Orthop Sports Phys Ther* 22(6): 263–6.

Fanelli GC, Edson CJ. (1995) Posterior cruciate ligament injuries in trauma patients. *Arthroscopy* 11:526–9.

Flandrey F, Hughston JC, McCann SB, Kurtz DM. (1994) Diagnostic features of diffuse pigmented villonodular synovitis of the knee. *Clin Orthop* 298:212–20.

Frisbie DD, Oxford JT, Steadman JR, et al. (2003) Early events in cartilage repair after subchondral bone microfracture. *Clin Orthop Relat Res* 407:215–27.

Fu FH, Harner CD, et al. (1993) Biomechanics of knee ligaments—basic concepts and clinical applications; ICL *J Bone Joint Surg* 75A(11):1716–27.

Galway HR, MacIntosh DL. (1980) The lateral pivot shift: a symptom and sign of anterior cruciate ligament instability. *Clin Orthop*147:45–50.

Ghazavi MT, Pritzker KP, Davis AM, et al. (1997) Fresh osteochondral allografts for post traumatic osteochondral defects of the knee. *J Bone Joine Surg Br* 79:1008–13.

Glashow JL, et al. (1989) Double blind assessment of the value of MRI in the diagnosis of ACL, meniscal lesions. *J Bone Joint Surg* 71A:113–9.

Gobbi A, Nunag P, Malinowski K. (2005) Treatment of full thickness chondral lesions of the knee with microfracture in a group of athletes. *Knee Surg Sports Traumatol Arthrosc* 13:213–21.

Gooding CR, Bartlett W, Bentley G, et al. (2006) A prospective, randomised study comparing two techniques of autologous chondrocyte implantation for osteochondral defects in the knee: periosteum covered versus type I/III collagen covered. *Knee* 13:203–10

Graf BK, Cook DA, De Smet AA, et al. (1993) Bone bruises on MRI evaluation of ACL injuries. *Am J Sports Med* 22:220–3.

Gudas R, Kalesinskas RJ, et al. (2005) A prospective randomized clinical study of mosaic osteochondral autologous transplantation versus microfracture for the treatment of osteochondral defects in the knee in young athletes. *Arthroscopy* 21:1066–75.

Hangody L, Fules P. (2003) Autologous osteochondral mosaicplasty for the treatment of full-thickness defects of weight bearing joints: ten years of experimental and clinical experience. *J Bone Joint Surg Am* 85(Suppl 2):25–32.

Hanks GA, Gause TM, Handal JA, et al. (1990) Meniscus repair in the ACL deficient knee. *Am J Sports Med* 18:606–13.

Harner CD, Xerogeanes JW. (1995) The human PCL complex: an interdisciplinary study—ligament morphology and biomechanical events. *Am J Sports Med* 23:736–45.

Harner CD, Irrgang JJ, Paul J, et al. (1992) Loss of motion after ACL reconstruction. *Am J Sports Med* 20(5):499–506.

Hart AJ, Buscombe J, Malone A, Dowd GSE. (2005) Assessment of osteoarthritis after reconstruction of the anterior cruciate ligament. *J Bone Joint Surg (Br)* 87–B:1483–7.

Hede A, Larsen E, Sandberg H. (1992) The long term outcome of open total and partial menisectomy related to the quantity and site of the meniscus removed. *Int Orthop* 16:122–5.

Indelicato PA. (1995) Isolated MCL injuries in the knee. *JAAOS* 3:1.

Jacobson KE, Chi FS. (2006) Evaluation and treatment of the medial collateral ligament and medial-sided injuries of the knee. *Sports Med Arthrosc* 14:58–66.

Knutsen G, Drogset JO, Engebretsen L, et al. (2007) A randomised trial comparing autologous chondrocyte implantation with microfracture. Findings at five years. *J Bone Joint Surg Am* 89(2):105–2112

Knutsen G, Engebretsen L, et al. (2004) Autologous chondrocyte implantation compared with microfracture in the knee. A randomized trial. *J Bone Joint Surg Am* 86:455–64.

Kon E, Gobbi A, Filardo G, et al. (2009) Arthroscopic second-generation autologous chondrocyte implantation compared with microfracture for chondral lesions of the knee: prospective non randomized study at 5 years. *Am J Sports Med* 37:33–41.

Kotsovolos ES, Hantes ME, et al. (2006) Results of all-inside meniscal repair with the FasT-Fix meniscal repair system. *Arthroscopy* 22:3–9.

Kreuz PC, Erggelet C, et al. (2006) Is microfracture of chondral defects in the knee associated with different results in patients aged 40 years or younger? *Arthroscopy* 22:1180–6.

Kumar A, Jones S, Bickerstaff DR. (1999) Posterolateral reconstruction of the knee: a tunnel technique for proximal fixation. *The Knee* (6): 257–260

Levy AS, Lohnes J, Sculley S, et al. (1996) Chondral delamination of the knee in soccer players. *Am J Sports Med* 24 (5):634–9.

Longo UG, King JB, et al. (2008) Double bundle arthroscopic reconstruction of the anterior cruciate ligament. Does the evidence add up? *J Bone Joint Surg (Br)* 90–B:995–9.

Maffuli N, Binfield PM, King JB, Good CJ (1993) Acute haemarthrosis of the knee in athletes. A prospective study of 106 cases. *J Bone Joint Surg (B)* 75(6):945–9.

Mandelbaum BR, Silvers HJ, et al. (2005) Effectiveness of neuromuscular and proprioceptive training program in preventing anterior cruciate ligament injuries in female athletes: a 2 year follow up. *Am J Sports Med* 33:1103–10.

McDermott ID, Amis AA. (2006) The consequences of menesectomy. *J Bone Joint Surg Br* 88B:1549–56.

McNicholas MJ, Rowley DI, McGurty D, et al. (2000) Total menisectomy at adolescence: a thirty-year follow up. *J Bone Joint Surg Br* 82B:217–21.

Meighan AAS, Keating JF, Will E. (2003) Outcome after reconstruction of the anterior cruciate ligament in athletic patients. A comparison of early versus delayed surgery. *J Bone Joint Surg (Br)* 85–B:521–4.

Miller MD, Bergfeld JA, Fowler PJ, Harner CD, Noyes FR. (1999) The posterior cruciate ligament injured knee: principles of evaluation and treatment. *Instr Course Lect* 48:199–207.

Mithoefer K, McAdams T, et al. (2009) Clinical efficacy of the microfracture technique for articular cartilage repair in the knee: an evidence based systematic analysis. *Am J Sports Med* 37:2053–63.

Narvani A, Mahmud T, Lavelle J, Williams A. (2010) Injury to the proximal deep medial collateral ligament. *J Bone Joint Surg (Br)* 92–B:949–53.

Nejadnik H, Hui JH, Feng C, et al. (2010) Autologous bone marrow-derived mesenchymal stem cells versus autologous chondrocyte implantation: an observational cohort study. *Am J Sports Med* 38:1110–6.

Nielsen S, Rasmusson O, Oveson J, Andersen K. (1984) Rotatory instability of cadaver knees after transection of collateral ligaments and capsule. *Arch Orthop Trauma Surg* 103(3):165–9.

Noyes FR, Barber-Weston SD, Rankin M. (2004) Meniscal transplantation in symptomatic patients less than fifty years old. *J Bone Joint Surg Am* 86:1392–404.

Ozturk A, Ozdemir MR, Ozkan Y. (2006) Osteochondral autografting(mosaicplasty) in grade IV cartilage defects in the knee joint:2–7 year results. *Int Orthop* 30:200–4.

Pacheco RJ, Ayre CA, Bollen SR. (2011) Posterolateral corner injuries of the knee. A serious injury commonly missed. *J Bone Joint Surg (Br)* 93–B:194–7.

Potter HG, Linklater JM, Allen AA, et al. (1998) Magnetic resonance imaging of articular cartilage in the knee. *J Bone J Surg* 80(A):1276–84.

Race A, Amis AA. (1996) Loading of the two bundles of the PCL—an analysis of bundle function in a posterior drawer. *J Biomech* 29(7):873–9.

Race A, Amis AA, et al. (1998) PCL reconstruction: in vitro biomechanical comparison of 'isometric' versus single and double bundle anatomic grafts. *J Bone Joint Surg (Br)* 80(1):173–9.

Rath E, Richmond JC, Yassir W, et al. (2001) Meniscal allograft transplantation. Two to eight year results. *Am J Sports Med* 29:410–4.

Ross G, DeConciliis GP, et al. (2004). Evaluation and treatment of acute posterolateral corner/anterior cruciate ligament injuries of the knee. *J Bone Joint Surg Am* 86A(Supp2):2–7.

Salter RB. (1989) The biologic concept of continuous passive motion of synovial joints. The first 18 years of basic research and its clinical application. *Clin Orthop Relat Res* 242:12–25.

Sanchez AR, Sheridan PJ, Kupp LI. (2003) Is platelet-rich plasma the perfect enhancement factor? A current review. *Int J Oral Maxillo-fac Implants* 18:93–103.

Seedholm BB, Hargreaves DJ. (1979) Transmission of the load in the knee joint with special reference to the role of the menisci. *Eng Med* 8:220.

Shahane SA, Bickerstaff DR. (1998) Proximal advancement of the medial collateral ligament for chronic medial instability of the knee joint. *The Knee* 5:191–7.

Shahane SA, Bickerstaff DR, et al. (1999) The popliteo-fibular ligament—an anatomic study of the posterolateral corner of the knee. *J Bone Joint Surg (Br)* 81(4):636–42.

Shelbourne KD, Heinrich J. (2004) The long term evaluation of lateral meniscal tears left *in situ* at the time of anterior cruciate ligament reconstruction. *Arthroscopy* 20:346–51.

Shelbourne KD, Nitz P. (1990) Accelerated rehab after ACL reconstruction. *Am J Sports Med* 18:292–9.

Shelbourne KD, Jennings RW, Vahey TN. (1999) Magnetic resonance imaging of posterior cruciate ligament injuries: assessment of healing. *Am J Knee Surg* 12:209–13.

Simonian PT, Fealy S, Hidaka C, O'Brien SJ, Warren RF. (1998) Anterior cruciate ligament injury and patella dislocation: a report of nine cases. *Arthroscopy* 14(1):80–4.

Stahelin AC, Sudkamp NP, Weiler A. (2001) Anatomic double bundle posterior cruciate ligament reconstruction using hamstring tendons. *Arthroscopy* 17:88–97.

Staubli HU. (1994) Posteromedial and posterolateral capsular injuries associated with posterior cruciate ligament insufficiencies. *Sports Med Arth Rev* 2:146–64.

Steadman JR, Rodkey WG. (2005) Tissue engineered collagen meniscus implants: 5 to 6 year feasibility study results. *Arthroscopy* 21:515–25.

Steadman JR, Briggs KK, et al. (2003) Outcomes of microfracture for traumatic chondral defects of the knee: average 11 year follow-up. *Arthroscopy* 19:477–84.

Torg JS, Conrad W, Kalen V. (1976) Clinical diagnosis of anterior cruciate ligament instability in athletes. *Am J Sports Med* 4(2):84–93.

Twyman RS, Desai K, Aichroth PM. (1991) Osteochondritis dissecans of the knee. A long term study. *J Bone J Surg* 73(B), 3:461–4.

Uchio Y, Ochi M, Adachi N, et al. (2003) Results of rasping of meniscal tears with and without anterior cruciate ligament injury as evaluated by second-look arthroscopy. *Arthroscopy* 19:463–9.

Van Trommel MF, Simonian PT, Potter HG, et al. (1998) Arthroscopic meniscal repair with fibrin clot of complete radial tears of the lateral meniscus of the avascular zone. *Arthroscopy* 14:360–5.

Veltri DM, Warren RF. (1994) Posterolateral instability of the knee. *J Bone Joint Surg* 76-A:460–74.

Zaslav K, Cole B, Brewster R et al(2009) A prospective study of autologous chondrocyte implantation in patients with failed prior treatment for articular cartilage defect of the knee; results of the Study of the Treatment of Articular Repair (STAR) clinical trial. Am J Sports Med;37(1):42–55.

Chapter 37

Patellofemoral/extensor mechanism disorders

Nicholas Peirce

It is clear that the patellofemoral joint is a complex articulation, depending on both dynamic and static restraints for stability. Often referred to as anterior knee pain, the large number of attempts to classify patellofemoral pain make the diagnosis and management of these set of conditions both challenging and somewhat confusing. Nevertheless, in order to facilitate appropriate treatment, patellofemoral problems in the skeletally mature patient can be helpfully divided into three broad categories, as shown in Figure 37.1, which can usually be ascertained from the history and examination (Fulkerson and Shea 1990):

- patellofemoral pain with instability, i.e. subluxation or dislocation
- patellofemoral pain with malalignment but no episodes of instability
- patellofemoral pain without malalignment.

Patellofemoral disorders

Anterior knee pain has received extensive attention over the years, both in the clinical and the academic setting. It represents up to 50% of all knee injuries, and is the most common presentation to sports injuries clinics, accounting for 25–33% of all visits (Hahn and Foldspang 1998; Kannus et al. 1987; Mummery et al. 1998). Anterior knee pain customarily follows chronic overload of the extensor mechanism, including the patellofemoral joint, the patellar tendon, and its bony attachments, but can be associated with traumatic episodes. As the name implies, it is very much an umbrella term encompassing a huge variety of disorders of the extensor mechanism, patellofemoral joint, and associated structures outlined in Table 37.1. In this chapter, an attempt will be made to distinguish between the different conditions that predispose to anterior knee pain including patellofemoral pain, patella dislocations, synovial plica, extensor mechanism pains (including patella tendonopathy), and some of the uncommon but important differential diagnoses to consider. After an injury has been defined as traumatic or non-traumatic, the anterior knee pain can be classified using the algorithm in Figure 37.1.

Patellofemoral pain

Aetiology

Patellofemoral pain syndrome (PFPS) has become increasingly accepted as a unifying description of any condition that produces retropatellar pain and possible cartilage changes, excluding acute episodes of dislocation of the patella. Despite the prevalence of PFPS, there is still some controversy over its aetiology and diagnosis. This is highlighted by the huge variety of titles that have been used to describe the spectrum of retropatellar discomfort: chondromalacia patellae, patellar chondropathy, patellofemoral arthralgia, patellalgia, lateral pressure syndrome, runner's knee, retropatellar knee pain. What is certain is that PFPS causes significant morbidity, threatening both routine activities and sporting ambitions, typically in adolescents of both sexes, although with greater severity in young women.

The cause of pain is unknown, although until recently it was thought to relate to the softening of the patella cartilage, chondromalacia patella, originally described by Koenig in 1924 (Owre 1934). Although this clinical condition does exist, cadaveric, imaging, and arthroscopic studies have clearly demonstrated it to be an incidental finding in asymptomatic individuals and have conversely demonstrated normal cartilage in patients with longstanding anterior knee pain (Bentley and Dowd 1984; Casscells 1975; McGinty and McCarthy 1981). Early changes in cartilage (softening, fissuring, and blister-like formations) have sometimes been shown to progress to underlying bone changes, appearing frequently over the areas of increased lateral pressure. Consequently, numerous studies have attempted both to map these changes and correlate them with patient symptoms and sites of established loading, with only partial success. Furthermore, as the cartilage itself has no neural innervation, mechanisms for retropatellar pain are only speculation and may be multifactorial, such as trauma-induced irritation of the retinacular nerves (Fulkerson et al. 1985), osteochondral microfractures, marginal synovitis (Radin et al. 1984), and painful retinacular structures. What is strikingly apparent, however, is the correlation of anterior knee pain with increased activity and hours of participation in sport (Milgrom et al. 1996; Mummery et al. 1998).

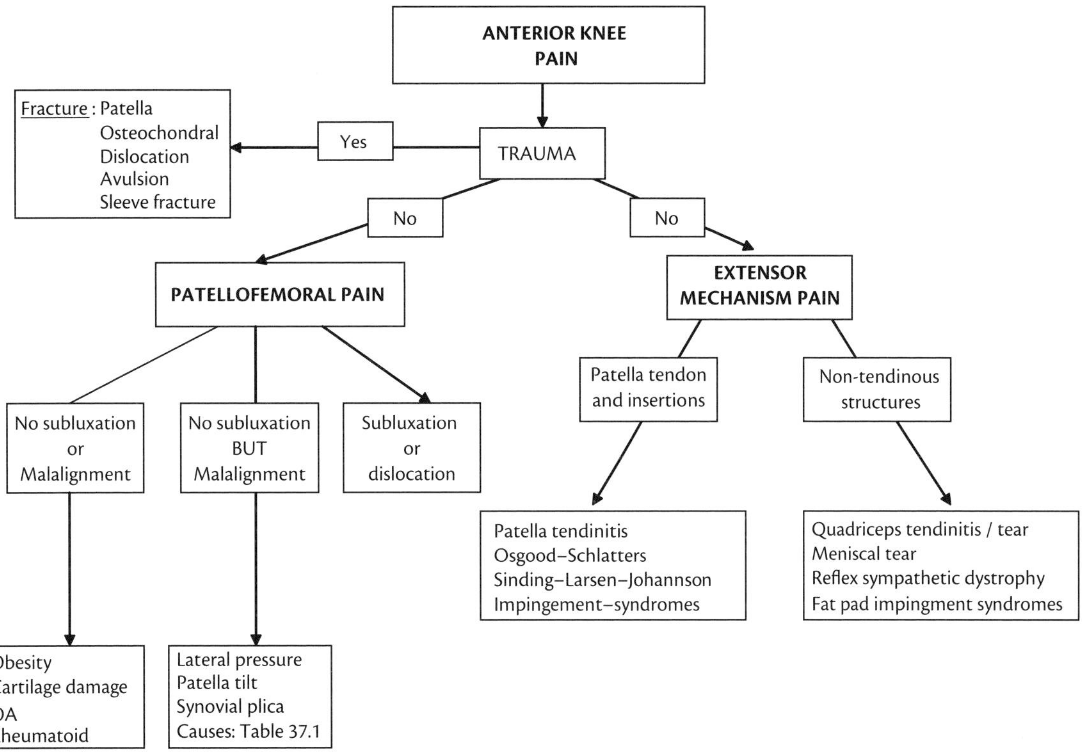

Figure 37.1 Anterior knee pain algorithm.

Table 37.1 Causes of anterior knee pain

Common cause	Moderately common	Rare
Patellofemoral pain syndrome	Bursae: Prepatellar superior/deep infrapatellar	Reflex sympathetic dystrophy
Patella tendonosis (jumper's knee)	Lateral retinacular / medial plicae	Referred pain
Osgood–Schlatters disease	Sinding-Larsen–Johansson syndrome	Malignancy
Patellar subluxation/dislocation	Fat pad syndrome	Anterior impingement
	Quadriceps tendinitis/rupture	Nerve injuries

Anatomy

The patellofemoral joint represents a functionally distinct articulation separate from the tibiofemoral joint, and some authors have considered it to be insufficiently advanced for the loads delivered by erect activity in humans (Dye 1987). The anterior distal femur forms a saddle-shaped trochlear groove in which the patella glides, with the lateral femoral condyle slightly more prominent to ensure midline patella tracking and prevent lateral subluxation (Table 37.2) (Tria et al. 1992). As the femoral sulcus increases beyond 150°, the patella is increasingly likely to subluxate or dislocate laterally (Figure 37.2), referred to as the *glide* of the patella (Figure 37.3).

The patella itself is, in essence, a large sesamoid bone within the extensor mechanism that articulates through the medial (convex) and lateral (concave) facets (Table 37.2). Only distinct parts of these surfaces are in contact with the trochlea during flexion, further increasing the loading across the joint. This can reach up to 7–8 times body weight during jumping and squatting (reflected in the thickness of the articulator cartilage) and is often referred to as the patellofemoral joint reaction force (Figure 37.4). Thus, the joint is exposed to significant stresses that may be exacerbated by uneven load distribution, produced by abnormalities in patella shape, malalignment, obesity, overuse, and subluxation or dislocation of the patella. An enormous continuum of patella shapes has been classified, e.g. by Wiberg (1941). Those that are most likely to produce problems are the dysplastic shapes such as patella magna and parva, and dysplasia of the femoral condyles (Table 37.2) (Ficat and Hungerford 1977).

Maintenance of normal patellar alignment and tracking within the trochlear groove is achieved by the V of the lateral and medial walls of the trochlear groove, the control of the quadriceps muscle groups, in particular the vastus medialis oblique (VMO), and the relative mobility of the medial and lateral retinaculum. Maltracking nevertheless appears to be common and is, in part, dependent on the resultant forces formed by the angle between the quadriceps insertion (anterior superior iliac spine and the mid-patella) and that of the patellar tendon (mid-patella to tibial tubercle)—the *Q angle* (Figure 37.5) (Grabiner et al. 1994; Kaufner and Arbor 1971). An excessive angle (more than 10° in men and 15° in women)

Table 37.2 Summary of radiological views and patellofemoral indices predisposing to patellofemoral disorders. (Adapted from Carson et al, with permission.)

View	Knee flexion	Technique and position	Measurement	Implications
AP	0°	Standing feel straight ahead	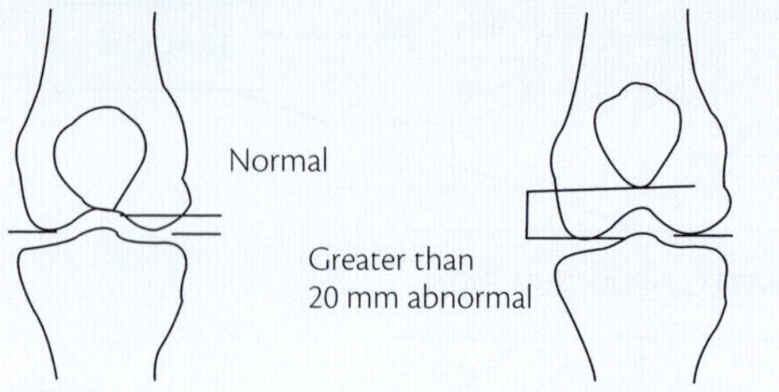 Normal Greater than 20 mm abnormal	- Hypoplastic patella - Lateral subluxation patella - Biparlite patella - Asymmetry of femoral condylar (abnormal femoral anteversion or femoral rotation)
	90°	Supine	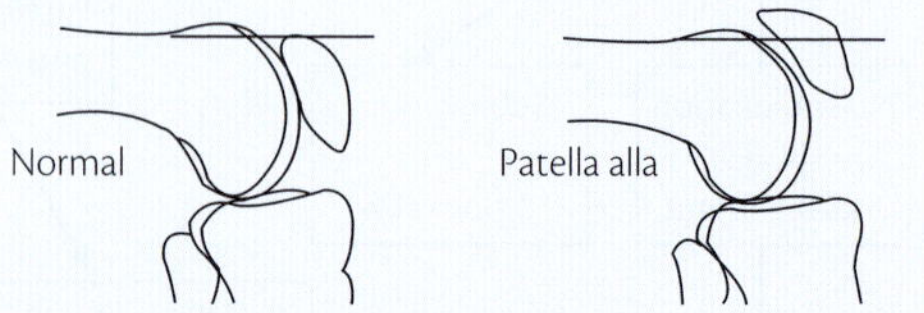 Normal Patella alla	- Patella intera - Patellar tracture
Lateral	Approx 30°	Supine (Insali-Salvati)	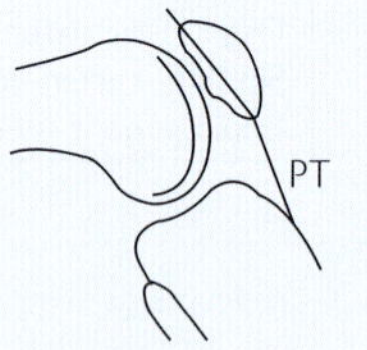 PT Ratio of P PT = 10 More than 20% vanation is abnormal	
	30°	Supine	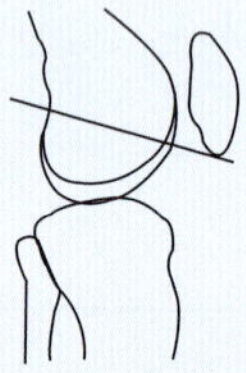 Blumensaat's line (see text)	
(Hughston) Tangenfial	55°	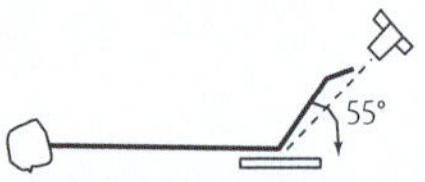 55° Prone position Beam duecled cephalad and intenor. 45 degrees from vertical	1) Sulcus angle: 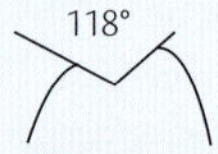 118° 2) Patella index: 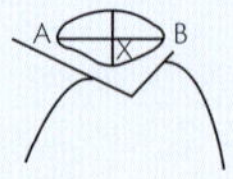 A B X AB / XB - XA NL Male 15 Female 17	- Patellar dislocation - Osteochondral tracture - Soft tissue calciticalion (old dislocated patella or tracture) - Patellar subluxation Patellar lilt Increased medial joint space Apex of patella lateral to apex of femoral sulcus Lateral patella edge lateral to femoral condyle Hypoptastic lateral lemoral condyle (usually proximal) - Patellofemoral osleophyles - Subchondral trabeculae onentation (increase or decrease) - Patellar configuration (Wiberg-Baugarll)
(Merchant) Tangenfial	45°	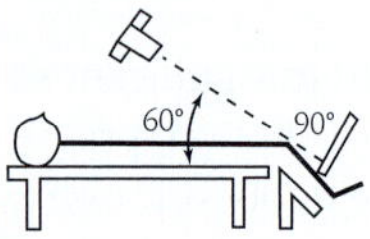 60° 90° Supine position Beam duecled caudal and intenor. 30 degrees from vertical	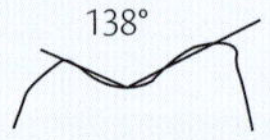 1) Sulcus angle: 138° 2) Congruence angle: − Med -6° Lat + 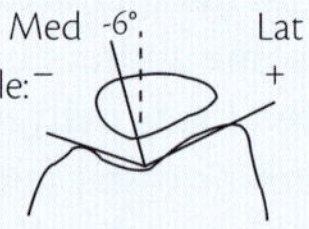	
(Laurin) Tangenfial	20°	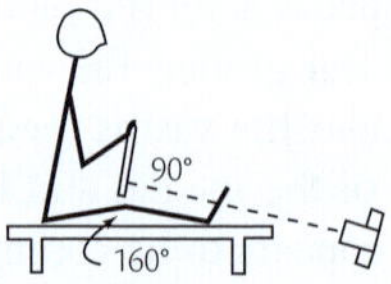 90° 160° Sitting posilion Beam duecled cephaled and supenor. 160 degrees from vertical	1) Lateral patellofemoral angle: 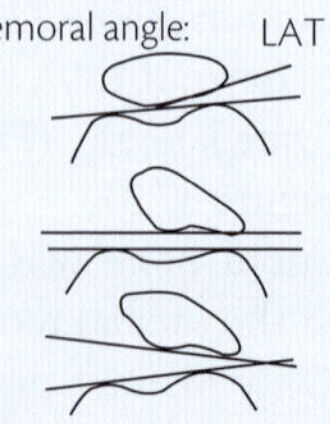 LAT NL ABNL ABNL 2) Patellofemoral index: Ratro A/B Med Lat Normal = 16 or less 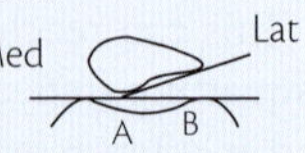 A B	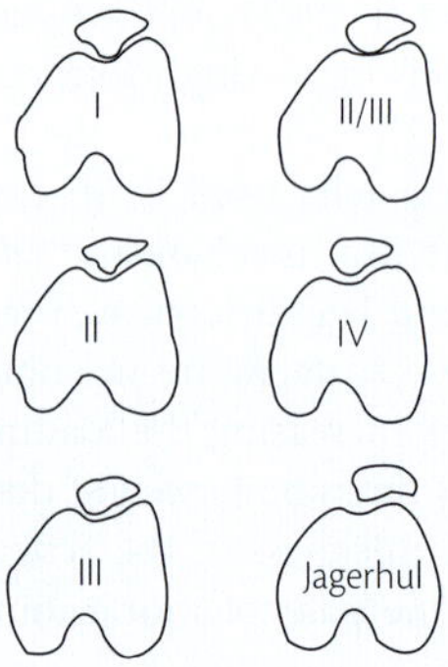 I II/III II IV III Jagerhul

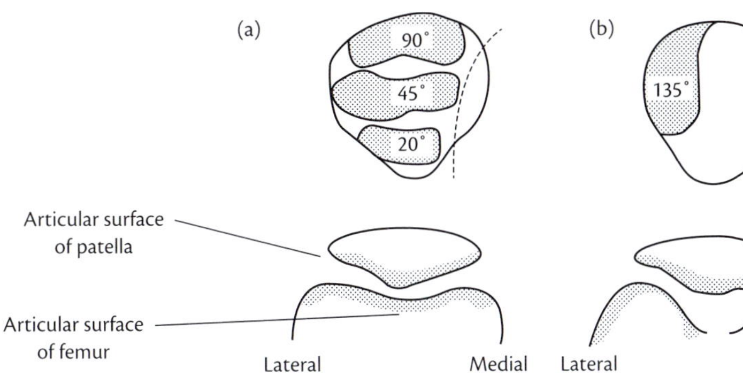

Figure 37.2 Articular surfaces of the patella during flexion: (a) at 80° flexion; (b) at 135° flexion. Contact remains minimal until 10–20° of flexion, when the inferior pole of the patella and the femoral condyle meet. As flexion continues, contact is made between the middle and, finally, superior facets, only making contact with the odd facet after 120°. (Modified from Ficat and Hungerford 1977.)

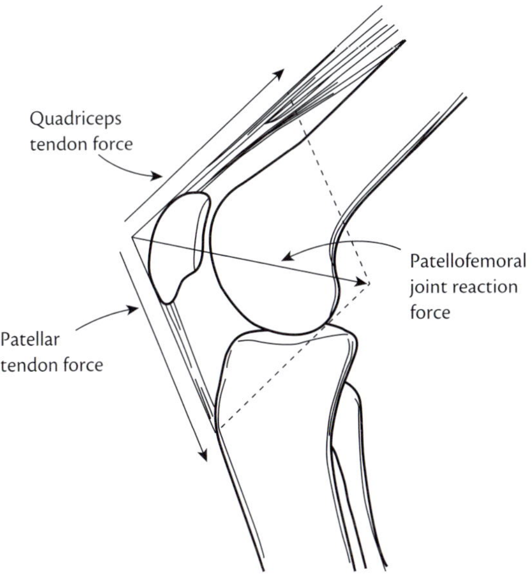

Figure 37.3 Lateral glide of the patella.

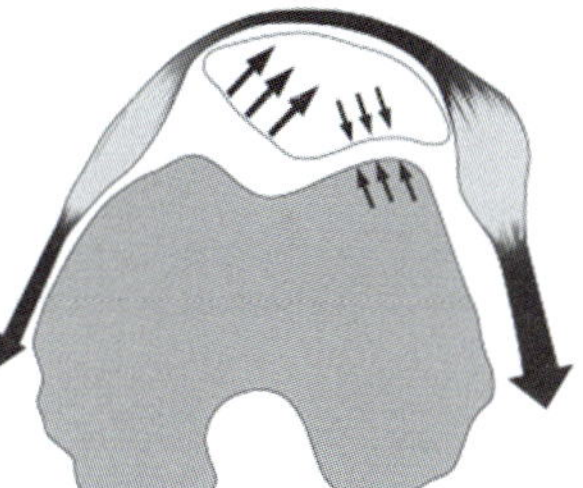

Figure 37.5 Normal alignment. Patellofemoral alignment is maintained by the Q angle—the angle formed between the line of the quadriceps (superior anterior iliac spine to the mid-patella) and the patellar tendon (mid-patella to tibial tuberosity) produces a resultant lateral force. Angles greater than 10° in men and 15° in women are considered abnormal and predispose to malalignment and an increasing displacement of the patella laterally. (Reprinted with permission from Chan et al.)

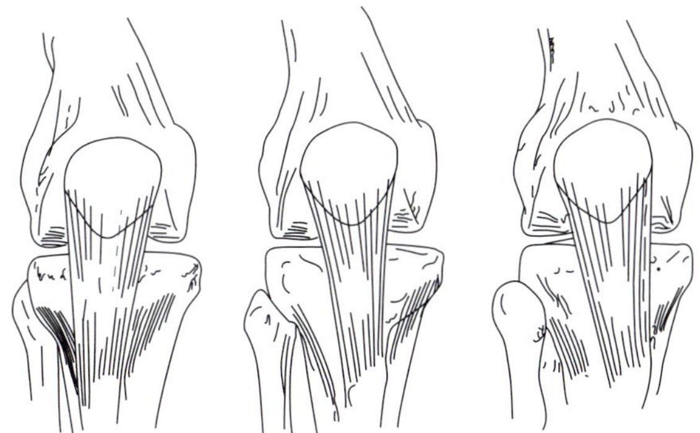

Figure 37.4 Patellofemoral joint reaction force. (Reprinted with permission from Chan et al.)

encourages the patella to subluxate laterally, normally abolished after 30° flexion.

Patella maltracking

There now seems to be a general acceptance of the relationship between maltracking and PFPS, although there is a variety of possible causes for pain (Fulkerson and Shea 1990; Kannus and Nittymaki 1994). Increased patella height has been also shown to correlate with unilateral PFPS as determined by lateral radiographs. Patella height, defined as the ratio of the patellar ligament to the length of the patella, is measured by the Insall–Salvatti index. A value of greater than 1.2 is referred to as *patella alta*. This condition may predispose to subluxation, with a mean index of 1.17 for normal subjects and 1.30 for those with anterior knee pain (Kannus and Nittymaki 1994). The relationship between the patella configuration and the sulcus angle is also referred to as the *patella congruence* and can be represented by a variety of measurements outlined in Figure 37.5. These have been extensively described by Laurin et al. (1979) and Merchant (1988) and also include additional radiographic measures such as the lateral patellofemoral angle and patellofemoral index (Laurin et al. 1979) (Table 37.2). Together, these may be used to try and predict a tendency to subluxate, as well as the degree of patella tilt and glide.

Maltracking and PFPS are also thought to arise from an imbalance of the medial restraints of the patella (53% of the total soft tissue restraining force derived from the medial patellofemoral ligament, with a small contribution from the medial patellomeniscal ligament and retinaculum; Conlan et al. 1993). Additionally, maltracking clearly appears to arise from inaction of the vastus medialis obliquus (VMO) (Lieb and Perry 1968), and it is widely recognized that weakness of the VMO and imbalance of the quadriceps musculature predisposes to maltracking

VMO weakness can occur as a result of disuse atrophy, congenital dystrophy, or reflex pain inhibition and may not be detectable unless end-of-range and variable testing is undertaken

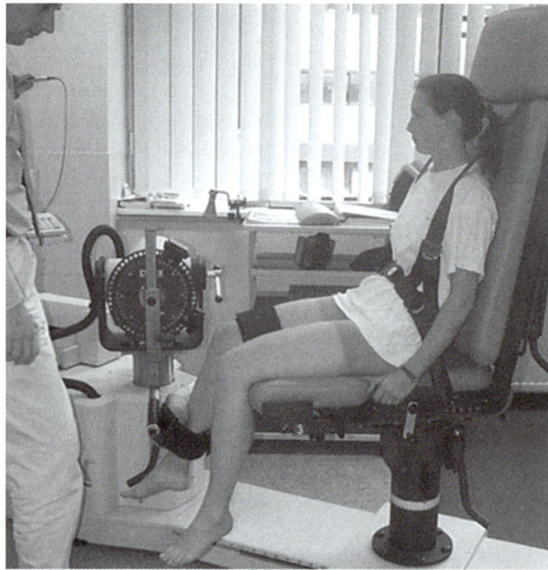

Figure 37.6 Assessment of lateral pressure syndrome and VMO dysplasia. Excessive lateral pressure can result from tight lateral retinacular structures, VMO dysplasia (resulting in lateral glide), maltracking (seen), and lateral facet overload.

with electromyography (EMG) and isokinetic measurements (Figure 37.6). Some of the many causes of malalignment are shown in Table 37.3.

Lateral patellar pressure syndrome

Also referred to as lateral compression syndrome, this condition describes PFPS that may arise from a tight lateral retinaculum, tight iliotibial band, and patella tilt. The distinguishing feature is no history of subluxation or variable maltracking, but instead, constant loading of the lateral facets. This condition, characteristically, is no longer considered separately from PFPS and they are covered together here.

Table 37.3 Causes of patella malalignment

Structure	Condition
Pelvis/hip/lumbar spine	Gynecoid pelvis
Tibia	Genu varus/valgum/recurvatum
	Tibia vara/torsion
	Hyperpronation
Femur	Anteversion/retroversion
	Trochlear dysplasia
	Sulcus angle: widening
	Previous fractures/shortening
Quadriceps	VMO dysplasia/weakness/atrophy
	Vastus lateralis hypertrophy
	Rectus femoris tightness
Patella	Alta/baja/parva
	Dysplasia/odd facet
	Tilt
	Dysplasia/odd facet
Lateral structures	Tight ITB
	Tight lateral retinaculum

History

The patient with PFPS often has a variety of nondescript pains with an insidious onset and present since childhood. Crepitus, clicking, and pseudo-locking may all be associated with the dull aching, which is frequently bilateral. However, a history of trauma may be present, including a direct blow to the patella that may indicate localized articular cartilage changes. Otherwise, patellofemoral pain is associated with eccentric activity, ascending and especially descending stairs, squatting, or prolonged flexion such as with sitting and driving. This has led to the term 'movie-goer's sign', when extension of the knee in an aisle seat may relieve patellofemoral pressure. Many of the symptoms have also been described as, in part, related to inflamed plicae, which can also be associated with clicking and locking. Patella subluxation or dislocation is important to distinguish and is most commonly accompanied by subjective episodes of 'giving way', often not associated with rotation. The patient may feel a popping sensation and often pain, causing the knee to buckle, probably as a result of inhibition of the quadriceps mechanism. Swelling may also be seen occasionally in all forms of patellofemoral pain.

Examination

The assessment of patellofemoral pain is dependent on a careful analysis of the gait and alignment of the lower limb of the individual. As well as routine observation of effusions, deformity, and bruising, the tracking of the patella can be observed in standing, walking, and squatting. Sit the subject over the edge of a couch and palpate the femoral condyles. The lateral should be higher than the medial and, in this position, the knee can be taken through resisted extension with any lateral deviation or glide provoked. Palpate the medial edges for plica and retropatellar articular changes while assessing the glide and mobility of the patella and any apprehension indicative of subluxation (Figure 37.7). Inspection of the quadriceps musculature bulk, strength, flexibility, and activity during contractions is also important, as well as assessing the tilt of the patella that may be associated with tight lateral retinaculum and iliotibial bands (Figure 37.8). The key examination points are outlined in Table 37.4.

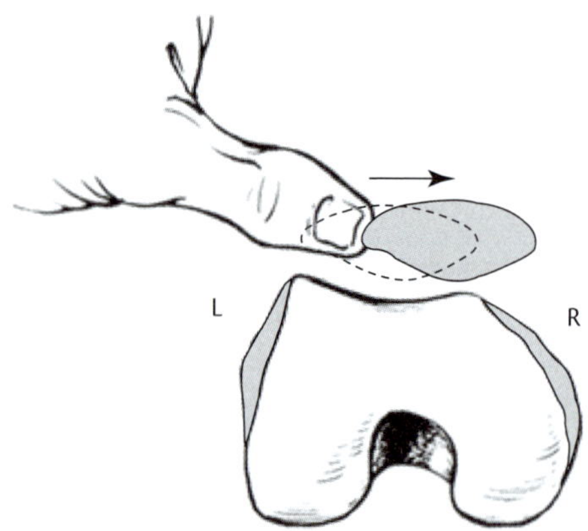

Figure 37.7 Glide/dislocation of the patella. Lateral displacement of the patella demonstrates the glide of the patella and may reproduce apprehension of an impending dislocation.

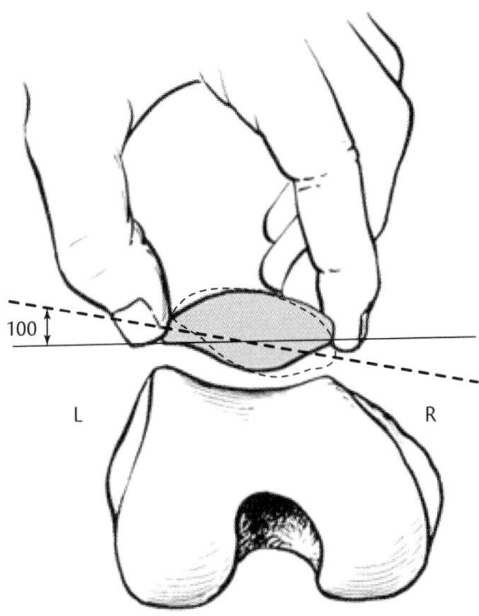

Figure 37.8 Tilt of the patella. Excessive tilt is demonstrated by deviation of more than 100° around the central axis. (Modified from Post et al.)

Investigations

The radiographic imaging of patellofemoral disorders includes standard radiographs taken through the sulcus of the femoral condyle at varying degrees. These include skyline views at 30° and further views at 40° and 60° that may show tilting or displacement of the patella. These are illustrated in Table 37.2 (Hughston and Walsh 1979; Insall and Salvati 1971; Laurin et al. 1979; Merchant 1988). Recently, ultrasound has been tried with varying success (Joshi and Heatley 1998) and most promising may be results from dynamic imaging using magnetic resonance imaging (MRI) (Miller et al. 1998).

Treatment

Non-surgical treatment

Non-surgical management of the PFPS centres on correcting any maltracking, improving tracking, and removing abnormal loads from the lateral facets and retinaculum. Provided gross traumatic changes of the cartilage and significant subluxating or dislocating individuals are identified, conservative measures for the treatment of patellofemoral pain are often successful and in up to 95% of cases produce resolution or significant improvement in symptoms (Natri et al. 1998; Post 1998). This may also reflect the self-limiting nature of PFP. A wide variety of different management strategies is practiced, reflecting the lack of consensus and evidence for consistent benefit from each technique. In a series of recent reviews, no one treatment strategy has been shown to be consistently effective when subject to randomized prospective study (Powers 1998). Treatment regimes include activity modification, exercises, stretches and regional soft tissue mobilization, orthotics, analgesia, and taping and bracing techniques, with only 2–3% requiring surgical intervention. A recent meta-analysis of clinical studies of many of these techniques found only five trials matched strict methodological criteria. Of these, only strengthening exercises and injections with glycosaminoglycan polysulphate produced short-term benefits, with the remainder producing equivocal results (Arroll et al. 1997).

Table 37.4 Key examination points

Palpation	
Patella	Shape? Hypotrophic? Bipartite? Dystrophic Bony tenderness? apophysitis/stress fracture/ avulsion? Trauma
	Inferior and superior poles? apophysitis/enthesopathy? tendonopathy
Medial/Lateral Patella Joint Line	Plica, Retropatella Discomfort, ITB referred pain
Surrounding Structures	Tibio-femoral joint line, condylees, superior tibio-fibular joint, quadriceps muscle
Observation	
Alignment: (Static and Dynamic)	Medialisation/Lateralisation/Q-angle
	Alta/Baja/Tilt/Rotation
	Quadriceps tone and contractile activity
Inflammation	Bursa/Inflammation/Deformity/atrophy/Chronic Pain Syndrome
Gait	Hind-foot, forefoot pronation, hip ante-retroversion, leg length descrepancy, gluteal control, antalgia
Tibia/Ankle/Foot	Tibial torsion, cavoid foot, pes planus
Test	
Neural Tests	Femoral Nerve/Slump/SLR? referred lumbar spine Component
Active Test	Clarks Compression? patello-femoral joint pain, Crepitus
	Apprehension Test? instability
	Plica fold test (lateral stretch of plica)
	Resisted Muscle tone
	Squatting/duck walk
Ultrasound	Routine observation of apophyseal/tendon pathology
Other Tests	Joint Hypermobility, local anaesthetic test, heel wedge/orthotic tests, taping, isokinetic, aspiration, activity provocation

The mainstay of non-surgical treatment remains the correction of maltracking which can arise from VMO dysplasia or disuse atrophy. McConnell reported 96% success rate with an exercise and taping regime that is now extensively incorporated into many rehabilitation protocols (Crichton 1989; Gerrard 1989; McConnell 1986). The purpose of the programme is to improve the timing, strength, and coordination of VMO/vastus lateralis contractions which have a reciprocal action in controlling patellar position. A normal ratio of contractile activity is reported as 1:1, which may be reduced in people with PFPS, although others have questioned this association with PFPS (Herrington 1998). Certainly, the results of taping and VMO strengthening have not always been reproduced (Hilyard et al. 1989; Wood 1998) and taping has been shown to produce no change in EMG activity (Herrington and Payton 1997; Powers 1998). In addition, VMO strengthening is arguably difficult to achieve in isolation. Nevertheless, there is no doubt that both passive stretching and active training, preferably in the last 30° of extension, can provide painless and impressive results in some individuals (Morrish and Woledge 1997; Natri et al. 1998; Voigt and Wieder 1991).

Closed chain programmes incorporating electrical stimulation may also be helpful, although biofeedback techniques have met with variable success, but the use of open chain techniques such as isokinetics remains controversial. Anti-inflammatory modalities such as ice, cryocuffs, interferential, and ultrasound have a limited role in immediate management. Braces are now widely used in the management of PFPS (Figure 37.9), acting as biomechanical restraints and corrective devices, and corrective orthotics have been reported to have positive benefits. A variety of sleeve devices are also used in an attempt to relocate and maintain the patella within the femoral sulcus. The Palumbo lateral buttress brace (Palumbo 1981) is well known, with one study suggesting that muscle activation of the VMO and vastus lateralis was reduced with the use of the brace (Gulling et al. 1996). There are now a variety of different devices including ones to correct tilt, glide, and even rotation. Stretching of the lateral structures, including the iliotibial band, is also part of most physiotherapy protocols. Stretching is centred on quadriceps, hamstrings, calf muscles, and lateral structures that may cause maltracking, rotation of the tibia or femur, and lateral deviation of the patella during contraction (Gose and Schweizer 1989). Hydrotherapy may have a strong place in rehabilitation, but access to it is limited.

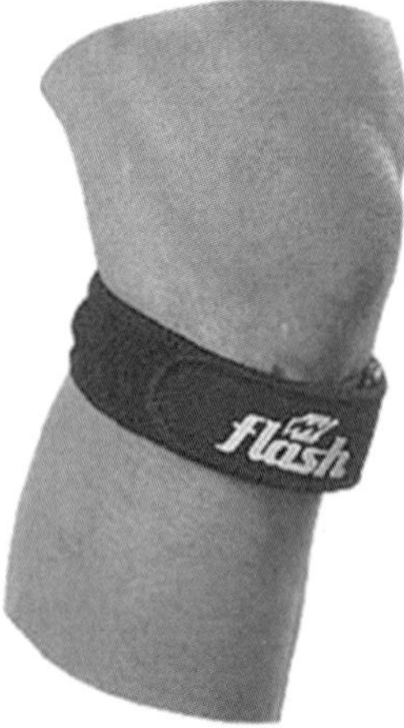

Figure 37.9 Patella control brace. Knee braces can help prevent lateral displacement. This particular brace (Dynev Tilt and Glide Brace, Promedics Ltd) also helps prevent tilt as well as glide. (Reprinted with permission from Promedics Ltd.)

Conservative measures appear to benefit many people. Those with negative findings in the clinical tests of patellar pain and crepitation, non-appearance of bilateral symptoms during the follow-up, low body height, and young age are associated with good long-term outcome (Natri et al. 1998).

The use of supplement injections, such as hyaluronic acid, has increased significantly. A number of meta-analyses have shown some benefit, especially higher molecular weight compounds (Wang 2004). In addition, at 7 years' follow-up, Kannus and colleagues found that glycosaminoglycan polysulphate injection, combined with intensive quadriceps-muscle exercises, compared favourably to injections of a placebo combined with exercises, and to exercises alone. Interestingly, the remaining patients who still had symptoms or objective signs of a patellofemoral disorder had an increased appearance of overt signs of osteoarthritis (Kannus et al. 1999). One should also remember that many patients with patellofemoral pain might have a chronic maladaptive syndrome and an increased likelihood of a variety of underlying psychological problems (Witonski et al. 1999).

Surgical treatment

Surgical treatment may sometimes be necessary. In the chronic and extreme patella subluxer or dislocator, surgical procedures may be clearly indicated. However, surgical treatment for PFPS should be reserved for:

(1) failure of conservative management,

(2) unremitting pain localized to the patella,

(3) pain with activities of daily living,

(4) patellar subluxation/dislocation, or

(5) associated trauma.

Only 2–3% of patellofemoral pain normally requires surgery. For those patients with lateral patellar pressure, odd facet syndrome, and tight lateral retinaculum, a lateral retinacular release can reduce lateral tension and improve tracking. First advocated in 1970, this procedure has now been widely adopted as the technique of choice (Christensen et al. 1988; Fu and Maday 1992; Harwin and Stern 1981; Hughston et al. 1996; Krompinger and Fulkerson 1983; Wilner 1970). It can be performed openly, arthroscopically, or subcutaneously, and is a relatively safe procedure. Nevertheless, it is sometimes used indiscriminately and can produce haemarthrosis, vastus lateralis disruption, medial instability, and post-operative stiffness (Post 1997). The exact mechanism for improvement is unknown, but destruction of pain fibres and restoration of normal alignment in lateral patellar tilt has been suggested.

A large number of other surgical procedures are used, including arthroscopic debridement, tibial transfer procedures such as a Maquet procedure (tibial advancement), Elmslie-Trillat procedure (medialization of the tibial tuberosity), lowering of the patella, vastus medialis plasty, and trochleoplasties. More recently, it has become clear that early identification of potential disruption of the medial patellafemoral ligament is increasingly important in relation not only to the mechanism of injury but also to repair. The huge variety of treatments again reflects the individual nature of each case and underlying malalignment, as well as the variable success of each procedure.

Patellar subluxation/dislocation

This most commonly occurs in a lateral direction accompanying direct trauma to the knee, or with forced external rotation of the tibia. The subject normally experiences extreme pain, may cry out, and will often notice a spontaneous reduction. An immediate effusion usually develops and there may be considerable tenderness along the medial border after disruption of the meniscofemoral ligaments and medial retinaculum. Radiographs are important to exclude osteochondral lesions, and additional damage to ligaments, including cruciates and collaterals, should be considered.

If the patella remains dislocated, gentle medial pressure, with the knee in full extension, followed by a PRICE (Protection, Rest, Ice, Compression, Elevation) regime to help reduce haemarthrosis is valuable. Many dislocations can be managed conservatively with initial immobilization and casting or bracing, followed by an intense mobilization and quadriceps strengthening programme. At long-term follow-up, good to excellent results have been seen in 75% of patients (Hawkins et al. 1986; Henry and Craven 1981). Nevertheless, in the presence of considerable soft tissue disruption, osteochondral fractures, inadequate reduction, or recurrent dislocation, realignment of the extensor mechanism may be necessary and is often successful (Metcalf 1982). Interestingly, recurrent dislocations are not more likely to produce osteoarthritis changes but may require surgical intervention to correct underlying malalignment abnormalities (Maenpaa and Lehto 1997).

The plica (synovial)

During fetal development, three synovial compartments fuse within the knee. Remnants can be left overlying medial retinaculae. Plicae are some of the normal synovial structures of the knee joint cavity. They are remnants of the mesenchymal tissue that occupies the space between the distal femoral and proximal tibial epiphyses in the 8-week-old embryo. The incomplete resorption leaves synovial pleats in most of the knees (Figure 37.10). The superior and the inferior plicae are the most common (50–65%) but have little clinical relevance. There are many morphological types. The lateral plica is rare (1–3%). The medial plica is present at autopsies in one of every three or four knees. It also is of various types; wide and thick in one of every fifteen knees. Arthrography, ultrasonography, computer tomography (CT) scan with arthrography, and MRI can demonstrate their presence and measure their size with good accuracy. Arthroscopy allows a very precise assessment of the plica, including dynamic examination. It may detect medial impingement against the patellofemoral articular surfaces and secondary (localized chondromalacia) as well as other incidentally associated pathological conditions of the knee. Medial plicae rarely become symptomatic, but can follow blunt trauma. Nevertheless, no predisposing factors are necessary.

The plica causes symptoms such as pain, crepitus, snapping, or popping and may be seen with an effusion related to patellofemoral joint motion. The clinical picture mimics a torn medial meniscus or a maltracking patella. Clinical examination is extremely helpful if the snapping plica is palpated at the medial edge of the patella, reproducing the patient's symptoms. If chronic, these symptoms may be treated with non-steroidal anti-inflammatory drugs (NSAIDs), physiotherapy, electrophoresis, or local injection. Surgical treatment is indicated if conservative therapy fails. Arthroscopic complete resection of the plica cures the symptoms in a few days, thereby confirming the correct diagnosis and the effectiveness of the treatment. Histological examination often confirms chronic irritation between the plica and the femoral condyle. The syndrome probably only occurs in one in ten medial plicae, and less than 3% of arthroscopies for patellofemoral pain. In addition, associated lesions are very common, which makes it difficult to evaluate the role of the plica in the production of symptoms.

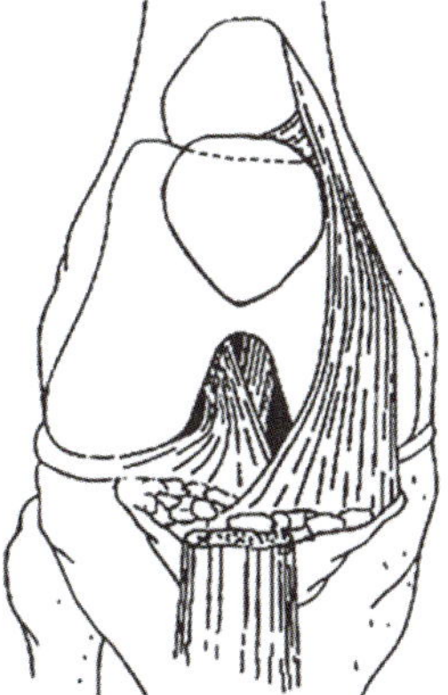
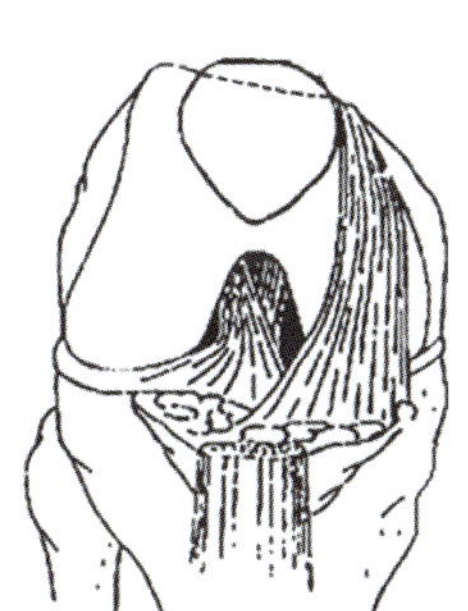

Figure 37.10 Medial plicae. Synovial plicae are vestigial remnants found superolaterally and medially. During flexion, loading of the plicae between the patella and femoral condyle increases and can produce pain, clicking, and even locking sensations.

Patella stress lesions

Patella stress may have probably been previously identified as patella hypertension, which was first voiced as a possible cause of anterior knee pain when Lempberg and Arnoldi (1978) identified a rise in interosseous venous pressure in association with anterior knee pain, and in the absence of articular degeneration. Raised bone marrow pressure has also been identified with hip pathology and several studies have shown changes in interosseous pressure, possibly caused by delayed venous blood flow of the patella during flexion and kneeling. Several studies have demonstrated an association with anterior knee pain and articular changes but, at present, clinical identification of the affected individual, measurements of interosseous pressure, and treatment through drilling or osteotomy remain uncertain.

Bipartite patella

The patella initially ossifies at between 3 and 5 years of age, commencing as multiple foci that rapidly coalesce. As the patellar ossification centre enlarges, the expanding margins may be irregular and associated with accessory ossification centres. These are most common superolaterally and may lead to the development of a bipartite patella, which has cartilaginous continuity despite the appearance of osseous discontinuity. During development, cartilage may not be replaced in the superior two thirds of the articular surface (the lower one third is covered by the fat pad) (Ogden 1984). These are frequent incidental findings on radiography and are unlikely to contribute to symptoms. Occasionally, a fracture must be considered.

Extensor mechanism pain

The extensor mechanism of the knee comprises the quadriceps musculature, the patella, and the patellar tendon. Rectus femoris,

VMO, vastus intermedius, and vastus lateralis unite to form a single tendon (the quadriceps tendon) that inserts into the superior pole of the patella with the superficial fibres forming a sheath over the patella and dispersing as the medial and lateral retinaculum (Figure 37.11). These fibres then align together, at the inferior pole, to become the patellar tendon (patellar ligament) that runs distally, 6–8 cm long and 2.5–3 cm wide, to insert into the tibial tuberosity. The forces transmitted through the patellar tendon can exceed eight times body weight during eccentric activities such as jumping and landing. Inferior fibres of the patellar tendon insert into the posterior surface of the patella apex through a gradual transition from tendon to fibrocartilage and mineralized fibrocartilage to bone, dispersing stress evenly from tendon to bone (Roels et al. 1978). The conditions that affect the extensor mechanism are less common than those of the patellofemoral joint, producing significant morbidity and, occasionally, catastrophic failure. They are often predictable through chronology with the enthesopathies. Osgood-Schlatter's disease and Sinding-Larsen-Johannson syndrome present in the prepubertal child, quadriceps and patellar tendinitis in early adult life, and fractures or rupture usually in the middle decades.

Patellar tendinopathy

Our understanding of tendon pathology has evolved over recent times and the nomenclature used has been adapted to reflect this. Patella tendinopathy, originally described by Blazina et al. in 1973, is the name applied to the clinical syndrome of pain and thickening of the patella tendon, as opposed to the older term 'tendinitis' which is reserved for the more uncommon pathology related to true inflammatory conditions.

Epidemiology

Patella tendinopathy is relatively uncommon in the general population but has an extremely high incidence in a number of sports including basketball (50%), volleyball (40%), football (20%), and dancing (25%) (Cook et al. 1997; Gisslén and Alfredson 2005; Hägglund et al. 2011; Øystein et al. 2005). As one of its previous names, 'jumper's knee', would suggest, it is associated with those sports that require repetitive and explosive eccentric quadriceps activity (Blazina et al. 1973; Stanish and Curwin 1984), but it also linked with those demanding rapid acceleration or deceleration, cutting, and kicking (Cook et al. 1997). Hence, it is therefore seen commonly in basketball, football, athletics, and volleyball. There appears to be a male predominance, with many athletes affected below the age of 20 (Cook et al. 1997; Øystein et al. 2005). Increasingly, it is also seen in sports that have moved from grass to artificial surfaces, such as field hockey.

Pathophysiology

The pathogenesis of tendinopathy is still relatively poorly understood. At a microscopic level, an established tendinopathy appears as collagen degeneration with an increase in ground substance consisting of glycosaminoglycans and proteoglycans; an increase in the number of fibroblasts; and a change in tenocyte morphology (Khan et al. 1998, 1999; Peers and Lysens 2005). Scattered vascular ingrowth, termed 'neovascularity', is also a feature (Sharma and Maffulli 2006).

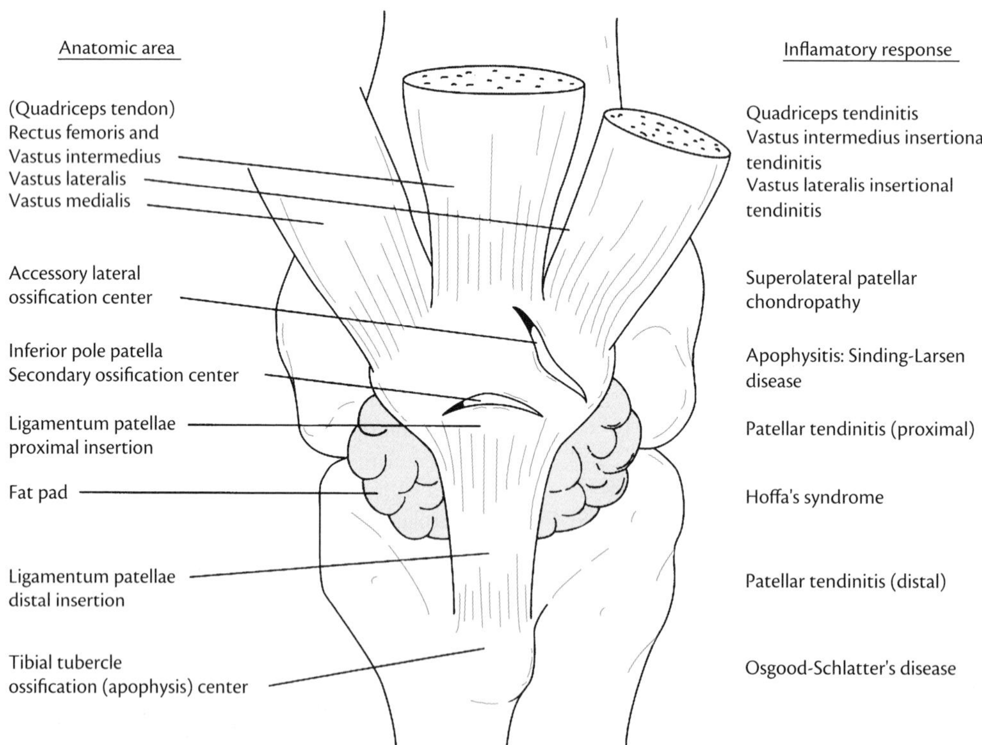

Figure 37.11 Extensor mechanism. Anterior knee pain includes inflammation and trauma to the extensor apparatus. A spectrum of conditions can disrupt the quadriceps musculature, patellar tendon, and secondary ossification centres. The regional areas are highlighted on the left and the corresponding pathological entity on the right. (Modified from Reid 1992.)

Various models have been proposed to account for tendinopathy including failed healing and dysrepair (Peers and Lysens 2005; Sharma and Maffulli 2006). It has been suggested that there is a continuum of pathology beginning with a reactive tendon in response to an acute overload, which may progress to tendon dysrepair and then degeneration with the conditions and load continuing to be detrimental (Cook and Purdam 2009) (Fig 37.12). The reversibility of the pathological process decreases once degeneration is present (Cook and Purdam 2009). Overuse or overload is thought to be the main instigator; however, the slow metabolism of tendons, hypoxia, ischaemic damage, oxidative stress, and matrix metalloproteinase imbalance have all been proposed as potential contributors to the process (Sharma and Maffulli 2006). A genetic susceptibility to tendinopathy is thought to exist (Magra and Maffulli 2007; in particular, polymorphisms in the COL5A1 and tenascin-C genes have been associated with higher rates of tendinopathy. The role of inflammation has attracted much attention. The absence of inflammatory cells on microscopy is well recognized (Rees et al. 2013); however, the presence of other inflammatory mediators such as interleukin-1 and -6, cyclo-oxygenases, and substance P suggests there may be an element of the inflammatory pathway involved (Rees et al. 2013).

The pain associated with tendinopathy is also not fully understood. The lack of inflammation suggests that alternative pain-generating mechanisms exist. A combination of mechanical and biomechanical processes has been implicated (Khan et al. 2000; Peers and Lysens 2005; Rio et al. 2014; Sharma and Maffulli 2006). Dysregulation of peripheral pain receptors and mediators, including substance P and glutamate, is thought to play a role (Peers and Lysens 2005; Sharma and Maffulli 2006). Other suggested mechanisms include activation of nociceptors on the prepatellar fat pad and synovium by biochemical mediators released from the tendon (Khan et al. 2000) and neovascularity within the tendon accompanied by nerve fibres and vessel wall receptors (Cook et al. 2005). However, given that neovascularity is not universal, this would not explain the pain generation is all cases (Cook et al. 2005; Gisslén and Alfredson 2005). There may also be a central component to the pain generation (Rio et al. 2014).

Clinical presentation

The diagnosis of patella tendinopathy is usually a clinical one. It usually presents as anterior knee pain exacerbated by activity (Khan et al. 1998; Peers and Lysens 2005). The pain may be mild with an onset following activity but as the severity increases, pain is experienced at the onset of activity. In its severe form, pain can limit or prevent activity. There may also be pain during periods of sitting (Peers and Lysens 2005). The onset of pain often coincides with a recent increase in either training load, volume, or intensity.

On physical examination there is localized tenderness at the inferior pole of the patella when the knee is fully extended and the quadriceps are relaxed (Khan et al. 1998; Peers and Lysens 2005).

The VISA-P questionnaire is a method of scoring severity in patella tendinopathy based on questions related to symptoms and function (Visentini et al. 1998). It can also be used to monitor progress and response to treatment, but should not be used as a diagnostic aid.

Imaging

Ultrasound and MRI are the main imaging modalities used to confirm the presence of tendinopathy (Scott et al. 2013). Ultrasound has the advantage of greater spatial resolution, demonstration of neovascularity (Scott et al. 2013), and relative cost; it is, however, user-dependent. MRI can be better at demonstrating the exact location and extent of tendinopathy (Khan et al. 1998) (Figure 37.12 and 37.13).

Imaging findings do not correlate with severity or clinical improvement (Khan et al. 1998; Peers and Lysens 2005; Scott et al. 2013). In addition, there may be evidence of tendinopathy on imaging in the absence of symptoms and, vice versa, symptoms may be present with normal findings on imaging (Gisslén and Alfredson 2005; Khan et al. 1998; Peers and Lysens 2005).

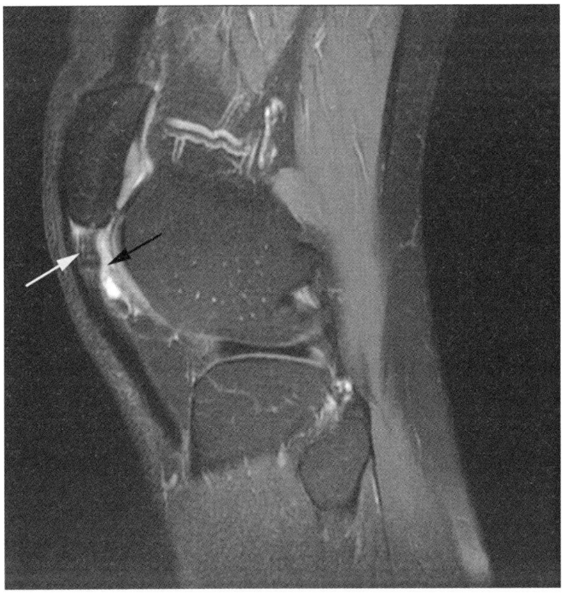

Figure 37.12 Early patellar tendinosis with swelling and abnormal signal of the proximal patellar tendon (white arrow). Note fat pad oedema due to impingement (black arrow).

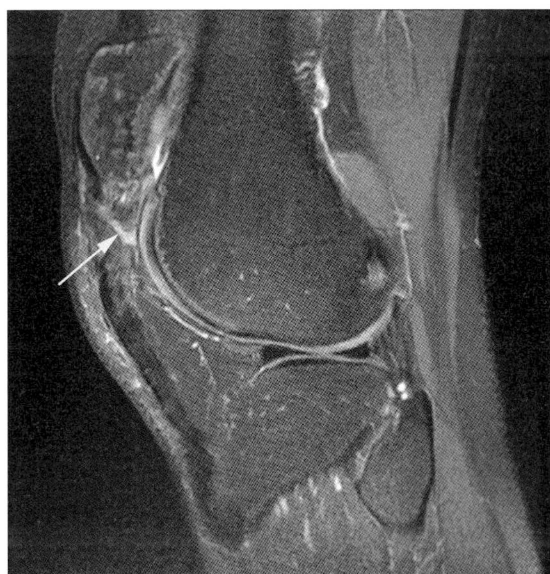

Figure 37.13 Advanced proximal patellar tendinosis with partial fluid-containing tear of the tendon (arrow).

Ultrasound examination reveals diffuse thickening of the tendon either segmentally or over its length, with hypoechoic areas within the tendon and irregular fibre structure (Fritschy and de Gautard 1988; Khan et al. 1996; Lian et al. 1996). There may also be thickening of the paratenon and areas of calcification. New vessels are seen as increased blood flow within the tendon on power and colour Doppler (Gisslén and Alfredson 2005; Khan et al. 1998). The ultrasound appearances can be graded according to greyscale appearance or the degree of neovascularity (Tables 37.5 and 37.6).

Management

There are a variety of types of treatment used in patellar tendinopathy and a lack of evidence to support a unified approach. The treatments applied are similar to those used in other tendinopathies including exercise therapy, injections, extracorporeal shockwave therapy (ESWT), and surgery (Larson et al. 2012). The management approach may also differ according to the chronicity and severity of presentation and may be limited to activity modification or require a more comprehensive rehabilitation programme (Larson et al. 2012). In view of the relationship with activity and overload, reducing or modifying activity is often suggested. This may take the form of avoidance of particular activities such as kicking or jumping, and alternative activities such as stationary cycling or aqua jogging may be performed in preference to the usual sport (Khan et al. 1998; Rutland et al. 2010). Alternatively, technique modifications (e.g. landing with two as opposed to one leg) or complete rest from all sporting activity may be recommended (Khan et al. 1998; Rutland et al. 2010). There is little evidence to guide this; however, it would appear that during a period of eccentric exercise rehabilitation, the outcome is better if all activity is avoided (Visnes and Bahr 2007). Care needs to be taken with the reintroduction of activity, with regard to the load, volume, and intensity, to reduce the risk of symptom recurrence.

Table 37.5 Ultrasound grading of tendinopathy

Grade	Appearance
1	Normal appearing tendon (parallel margins with homogeneous echotexture)
2	Enlarged tendon (bowed margins with homogeneous echotexture)
3	Hypoechoic area, with or without tendon enlargement (dark area, with or without bowed margins)

Archambault, J., Wiley, J., Bray, R., Verhoef, M., Wiseman, D., Elliott, P. (1998) Can sonography predict the outcome in patients with Achillodynia? *Journal of Clinical Ultrasound*, **26**, 335–339. Reprinted with permission of John Wiley & Sons.

Table 37.6 Grading of neovascularity in tendinopathy

Grade	Appearance
0	No visible vessels
1	1 or 2 blood vessels (low blood flow)
2	Some blood vessels (some blood flow)
3	Many blood vessels (strong blood flow)

Hoksrud, A., Öhberg, L., Alfredson, H., Bahr, R. (2008) *American Journal of Sports Medicine*, **36**, 1813–1820. © 2008 by SAGE. Reprinted by permission of SAGE publications.

Exercise-based therapy

The most widely used treatment in patellar tendinopathy is exercise therapy, and the greatest amount of supporting evidence exists for eccentric exercise (Khan et al. 1998; Larson et al. 2012; Peers and Lysens 2005; Visnes and Bahr 2007), which has also been shown to be superior to concentric exercise. The use of eccentric exercise in tendinopathy was originally developed by Curwin and Stanish in 1984 (Curwin et al. 1985), and further developed by Alfredson et al. (1998) in their work on Achilles' tendinopathy. It is suggested that slow movement progressed by increasing load rather than speed is important. There are still many potential variables including the number of repetitions, number of sets, frequency, load, presence of pain, and continuation of sporting activity. It is difficult to compare all of these variables in randomized controlled trials and many protocols have evolved through clinician experience. Examples of eccentric exercise for patellar tendinopathy include drop squats, single leg squats on the flat, and decline single leg squats. The latter is generally preferred and is performed using a decline board at 25°. The use of the decline board increases the load on the patellar tendon while limiting involvement of the hip flexors (Purdam et al. 2003; Visnes and Bahr 2007). The affected leg is trained with the slow eccentric knee flexion and both legs are used in the returning concentric knee extension. The importance of training with or without pain, and the influence of a warm-up or ice application following exercise, is not known. It is suggested that the exercises are performed as a home-based programme with three sets of 15 repetitions, twice daily for 12 weeks. With this programme, improvement levels of 50–70% can be seen (Visnes and Bahr 2007; Woodley et al. 2007).

The mechanism by which eccentric exercises exert their effect is not known. It is thought to be related to the mechanical–biological interaction. It has been shown that they increase the collagen synthesis in tendons (Miller et al. 2005). The halting of blood flow in neovessels during the loading may also contribute (Rees et al. 2009). The improvements seen in patellar tendinopathy following eccentric training might suggest that prophylactic eccentric training would be beneficial. However, this has been associated with the development of other injuries and is therefore not recommended (Larson et al. 2012).

Improving flexibility through stretching develops tendon function and is recommended alongside other treatments, although the specific nature of the stretches and whether static or ballistic is not clear (Rees et al. 2009; Witvrouw et al. 2007; Woodley et al. 2007).

Analgesia

Although NSAIDs have previously been widely advocated in the management of tendinopathy, the realization that there is a degenerative rather than inflammatory process has led to questioning of the role of anti-inflammatories (Khan et al. 1999; Peers and Lysens 2005; Rees et al. 2009). They may additionally have a detrimental effect on healing (Peers and Lysens 2005; Rees et al. 2009). Paracetamol is not known to have such adverse effects.

Ice application is useful for its analgesic properties and may also have a vasoconstrictive effect on neovessels within the tendon (Peers and Lysens 2005). It should not be used before sporting activity as decreased temperature reduces tendon compliance.

Orthotics/braces

Orthotics and offloading the patellar tendon through bracing can be helpful in certain cases, particularly where there is thought to be a significant biomechanical contribution to the tendinopathy (Khan et al. 1998). The chopat strap is one example of a patellar tendon brace in use (Khan et al. 1998; Larson et al. 2012).

A proportion of those with tendinopathy will not make sufficient improvement with exercise therapy alone and a large menu of alternative treatments have been explored and developed (van Ark et al. 2011).

Injections

Tendinous and peri-tendinous injections of a variety of substances are given to promote tendon healing, reduce neovascularity, or reduce pain.

Corticosteroids

Corticosteroids, via injection or iontophoresis, can result in short-term relief of pain (Coombes et al. 2010; Peers and Lysens 2005; Rees et al. 2009) and possibly act by directly reducing pain. However, the long-term results are less favourable. Intra-tendinous injections also carry the risk of weakening tendon structure and increasing the risk of rupture. They are therefore not currently recommended in patellar tendinopathy.

Sclerosants

Sclerosis is the injection of a chemical irritant which targets the neovascularity within the tendon and the associated pain-generating mechanisms (van Ark et al. 2011; Rees et al. 2009). Examples include polidocanol and lauromacroglycol, both of which have been shown to have a positive effect in the treatment of patellar tendinopathy (van Ark et al. 2011; Larson et al. 2012; Rees et al. 2009).

Prolotherapy

Prolotherapy involves injecting an irritant substance to promote a healing response (van Ark et al. 2011; Longo et al. 2012). Hyperosmolar dextrose and morrhuate sodium are used most frequently (Longo et al. 2012). There is limited evidence for its use in patellar tendinopathy, although there are positive results from the data available (van Ark et al. 2011).

Autologous blood injection (ABI), platelet-rich plasma (PRP), and dry needling

PRP is derived from an autologous blood sample. It has a high density of platelets and growth factors which are thought to stimulate healing (van Ark et al. 2011). Studies on its use in patellar tendinopathy are lacking in quantity and quality, but do suggest some promising results. Whole blood can also be injected directly and shows similar promise (van Ark et al. 2011).

Dry needling is the repeated needle penetration of the abnormal tendon (van Ark et al. 2011). It can be used alone or in combination with other injection therapies. The introduction of acute tendon damage is thought to trigger a healing response. It is unclear whether it produces a significant clinical effect either alone or in combination (van Ark et al. 2011).

Apoprotinin

The use of apoprotinin is based on the finding that matrix metalloproteinases (MMPs) are increased in tendinopathic tissue (Rees et al. 2009; van Ark et al. 2011). It is hypothesized that collagenases delay recovery and that injecting a collagenase inhibitor such as apoprotinin may improve recovery. Again, although promising, there is a paucity of experimental data.

High-volume injections

High-volume injections, as the name suggests, involve the injection of a large volume of fluid around the tendon, producing a mechanical stretch on the paratenon and proposed method of action of stripping away neovessels and nerves from the tendon (Loppini and Maffuli 2011). Normal saline is the fluid used, with the possible addition of a corticosteroid to reduce the inflammatory reaction to the injection of a large volume of fluid around the tendon (Loppini and Maffuli 2011). Positive results are reported, including an earlier return to play, although further work is still needed.

Other therapies

Glyceryl trinitrate (GTN) patches have been used in the management of tendinopathy. Their use is counterintuitive as they have a vasodilatory action. However, they may enhance the extracellular matrix and therefore promote healing (Rees et al. 2009).

ESWT is used in other tendinopathies such as the Achilles. Either high-energy or low-energy shockwaves can be used; the latter is painful and requires local or regional anaesthesia (Loppini and Maffuli 2011). The small-scale studies available suggest that its use in patellar tendinopathy is safe and effective (van Leeuwen et al. 2009). However, the type of shockwave and further details are not deducible from data as yet.

Ultrasound, transverse friction, and low-level laser therapy have all been used in tendinopathies, including patellar tendinopathy. However, there is no evidence that their use improves symptoms or function (Rees et al. 2009; Tumilty et al. 2012).

Surgery

The surgical management of tendinopathy is generally reserved for those who have undergone conservative management without an adequate improvement (Khan et al. 1998; Larson et al. 2012; Peers and Lysens 2005; Rees et al. 2009). There are many different surgical techniques available including tenotomy with excision of the macroscopic necrotic area, via either open or arthroscopic technique; drilling or resection of the tibial attachment with realignment; minimally invasive stripping; and radio-frequency microtenotomy (Maffulli et al. 2010; Rees et al. 2009).

Quadriceps tendinopathy

Quadriceps tendinopathy is a relatively uncommon cause of anterior knee pain. The causes of quadriceps tendinopathy are probably similar to those of patella tendinopathy in that they are related to volume and intensity of loading and seen in explosive/jumping sports including basketball, volleyball, fencing, and American football (Almekinders 1998; Giombini et al. 2013). There is little or no published literature but it is sometimes associated with traction changes of the quadriceps enthesis. Clinical features are of pain on or just above the common quadriceps tendon insertion, associated with activity and helped initially by reduced loading. Ultrasound and MRI findings demonstrate a pattern of thickening, loss of fibre definition, and calcification, in keeping with degenerative processes. Management is very much akin to that of patella tendinopathy.

Although the quadriceps tendon is particularly thick (properties that lend it to use in anterior cruciate ligament grafts), interestingly, there are a number of cases of quadriceps rupture associated with possible preceding tendinopathic changes. These have been most commonly reported in American Football but are also associated with males, over 40 years of age, and underlying systemic conditions including inflammatory arthritides, diabetes, and gout (Boublik et al. 2013).

Pre-patella and infra-patella bursitis

Bursae are discrete spaces or sacs of synovial fluid emanating from synovial tissue lining the structure. Pre-patella bursitis ('housemaid's knee') is a subcutaneous lesion found in front of the patella/patella tendon. It is normally a consequence of repetitive or acute trauma but may result from infective or inflammatory conditions. Infra-patella bursae, as the name suggests, are deep to the patella tendon and have also acquired a number of occupation-related names. Although repetitive micro-trauma may cause some, it has become apparent that many fluid collections in this area may also be linked to an underlying tendinopathy. The condition is often diagnosed through palpation but ultrasound and/or MRI both provide clear diagnostic certainty. Management is frequently through a combination of conservative measures, including ice, compression, and anti-inflammatory modalities. Ultrasound-guided aspiration and injection can also be effective, provided infection and underlying tendinopathy are excluded.

Osgood-Schlatter's disease

This is one of the most common apophysitides. It is an exercise-induced growth disorder primarily affecting boys aged 10–15 years and girls aged 8–13, with pain and swelling of the tibial tubercle most commonly reported in the active individual (18%) (Kannus et al. 1988).

The tibial tuberosity begins ossification at 7–9 years of age as a distal focus. This progressively enlarges proximally and anteriorly, while the main tibial ossification centre concomitantly expands downward into the tuberosity (Figure 37.11). A section of epiphyseal cartilage (Henke's disk) usually remains between these two ossification centres until close to physeal maturity (as late as 19 years of age) and, as such, the anterior chondro-osseous region at the site of patellar tendon attachment is a susceptible region. This may be acutely or chronically traumatized to create an Osgood-Schlatter lesion, which can eventually elongate to form an enlarged ossicle. The closure of the tuberosity physis occurs at puberty and usually resolves the problem (Ogden 1984).

The most common presenting symptom is pain. In a survey of 412 young athletes, symptoms first occurred at 13.1 years on average. Several biomechanical associations have been made, including patella alta (Aparicio et al. 1997). Initially, pain is managed by activity modification, NSAIDs, and ice, as well as ultrasound and interferential treatment, while cross-training with avoidance of loading activities. Infrapatellar braces may be used (Levine and Kashyap 1981). Occasionally, there may be severe night pain, and the differential diagnosis of malignancy must be considered. Bone scans are usually unhelpful because of the activity of the apophysis, and plain radiograph and MRI are more appropriate. Successful reduction in symptoms has been reported in one study with cessation of training for an average of 3.2 months, and interference with activity for an average of 7.3 months. Pain is typically found in 21% of those physically active and 4.5% in the inactive. Interestingly, the incidence appears higher in siblings (45%) and those who suffer from Sever's disease (calcaneal apophysitis) (68%) (Kujala et al. 1985), although it is more common in soccer, volleyball, and basketball players. Occasionally, surgical removal of painful ossicles is considered (Fisher 1980; King and Blundell-Jones 1981); however, the treatment is usually delayed until after puberty. Initially, drilling of the tuberosity was largely unsuccessful, but results from surgery are now encouragingly good (Fisher 1980; Glynn and Regan 1983; King and Blundell-Jones 1981).

Sinding-Larsen-Johannson syndrome

This condition, described by Sinding and Larsen in 1920 and Johannson in 1921, occurs as a result of traction enthesopathy of the inferior pole of the patella. The pathological process is similar to Osgood-Schlatter's disease, and is a result of overuse in the prepubertal child. It is similar in presentation to patellar tendinitis and management remains consistent with treatment protocols for patellar tendinitis and Osgood-Schlatter's disease (Traverso et al. 1990). Occasionally, sleeve fractures occur in conjunction with pre-existing Sinding-Larsen-Johannson syndrome (Gardiner et al. 1990).

Failure of the extensor mechanism; rupture/fractures

The patellar tendon, insertions, and quadriceps musculature can all rupture in extreme cases of sudden overload or trauma. Fortunately rare in athletes, these failures can occur in the presence of pre-existing disease states, with quadriceps ruptures most likely in the over-40s and patellar tendon ruptures in younger people. A variety of systemic disease states, as previously described, may predispose to this condition, and the implication that previous steroid injections can induce rupture still remains controversial. Occasionally, the distal pole of the patella or the tibial tubercles can be avulsed, which is usually managed conservatively in the prepubertal child.

Fat pad syndrome (Hoffa's disease)

Hoffa's disease, an obscure cause of anterior knee pain, may result from impingement and inflammation of the infrapatellar fat pad (Figure 37.14). First reported by Albert Hoffa in 1904, the condition remains uncommon, is infrequently reported, and is sometimes seen in association with surgical procedures (Faletti et al. 1998; Jerosch and Schroder 1996; Tsirbas et al. 1991). The exact role of the fat pad is ill-defined, although it may act in helping anterior stability of the soft tissue structures. Inflammation of this structure (Figure 37.12 and 37.14) often follows direct trauma or surgery, producing ill-defined pain. This may be anterolateral or anteromedial and can be accompanied by considerable stiffness. Occasionally, a bulging fat pad can be identified, but often the diagnosis is missed, leading to chronic changes and disability. Regional injections of anaesthetic may help establish the diagnosis, although concomitant pathology such as with patellar tendonitis and adjacent bursa are frequently well established (Duri et al. 1997). A possible relationship between impingement of the infrapatellar fat pad and the development of ossifying chondroma has also been reported (Krebs and Parker 1994). Treatment includes initial rest from provocative activities with quadriceps stretching, patella mobilization, regional anti-inflammatory modalities, steroid injection, and, occasionally, surgical resection. Fat pad entrapment may also mimic anterior meniscal pathology and can produce catching, jumping, and locking sensations as well as a positive McMurray's test.

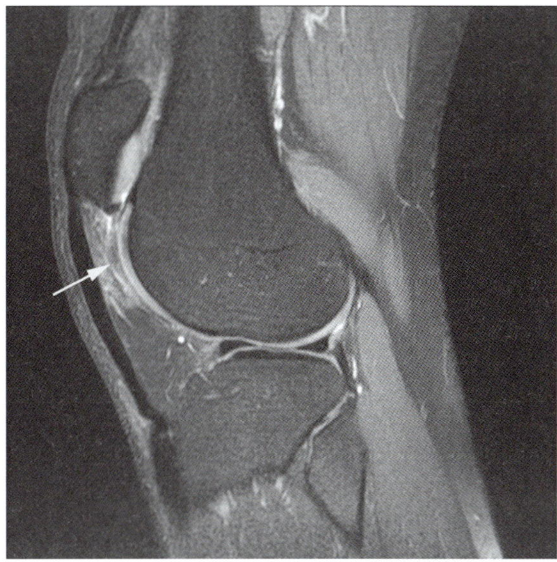

Figure 37.14 Hoffa's fat pad oedema. Sagittal PD FATSAT image of the knee showing oedema of the Hoffa's fat (arrow).

Stress fractures are uncommon but should be considered in all unexplained patella discomfort. These are most commonly seen in endurance athletes. Underlying stress fracture lines may also be difficult to identify in what are perceived to be normal fractures. MRI will initially demonstrate bone stress but CT may be needed to better identify fracture margins.

Differential diagnosis

Anterior knee pain is commonly seen in the adolescent, and a variety of different underlying diagnoses must therefore always be borne in mind (see Table 37.1). Osteochondritis dissecans of the tibiofemoral and, less commonly, the patellofemoral joint (not dealt with in this book) are essential to identify early. Probably more important are tumours of the soft tissue and bone that, although infrequent, occur most commonly in the long bones of the femur and tibia. Thus night pain, pain unrelated to activity, and pain that is failing conservative treatment, with no obvious malalignment, should always flag up possible underlying pathology. Patella fractures, non-ossifying fibromas, necrosing lipomas, infection, and neuritis may all present with anterior knee pain. With surgery and arthroscopy frequently performed, the possible sequel must also be considered including infrapatellar contracture syndrome and infrapatellar neuritis, nerve root entrapment of lumbosacral nerve roots L2–4, and the poorly understood reflex sympathetic dystrophy, now classified as chronic pain syndrome (CPS) type 1 (Youmans 1989).

References

Alfredson, H., Pietila, T., Jonsson, P., and Lorentzon, R. (1998) Heavy-load eccentric calf muscle training for the treatment of chronic Achilles tendinosis. *American Journal of Sports Medicine*, 26(3), 360–6.

Almekinders, L. C. (1998) Tendinitis and other chronic tendinopathies. *Journal of the American Academy of Orthopedic Surgeons*, 6(3), 157–64.

Aparicio, G., Abril, J. C., Calvo, E., and Alvarez, L. (1997) Radiologic study of patellar height in Osgood-Schlatter disease. *Journal of Pediatric Orthopedics*, 17, 63–6.

van Ark, M., Zwerver, J., van den Akker-Scheek, I. (2011) Injection treatments for patellar tendinopathy. *British Journal of Sports Medicine*, 45, 1076.

Arroll, B., Ellis-Pegler, E., Edwards, A., and Sutcliffe, G. (1997) Patellofemoral pain syndrome. A critical review of the clinical trials on nonoperative therapy. *American Journal of Sports Medicine*, 25, 207–12.

Bentley, G. and Dowd, G. (1984) Current concepts of etiology and treatment of chondromalacia patella. *Clinical Orthopaedics*, 189, 209–28.

Blazina, M. E., Kerlan, R. K., Jobe, F. W., Carter, V. S., and Carlson, G. J. (1973) *Orthopedic Clinics of North America*, 4, 665–78.

Boublik, M, Schlegel, T.F., Koonce, R.K., James W. Genuario, J.W., and Kinkartz, J.D. (2013) Quadriceps tendon injuries in National Football League players. *American Journal of Sports Medicine*, 41, 1841–6.

Casscells, W. (1975) *Journal of Bone and Joint Surgery*, 57, 1033.

Christensen, F., Soballe, K., and Snerum, L. (1988) *Clinical Orthopaedics and Related Research Issue*, 234.

Conlan, T., Garth, W. P., and Lemons, J. E. (1993) *Journal of Bone and Joint Surgery*, 75A, 682–93.

Cook, J., Khan, K., Harcourt, P., Grant, M., Young, D., and Bonar, S. (1997) A cross sectional study of 100 athletes with jumper's knee managed conservatively and surgically. *British Journal of Sports Medicine*, 31, 332–6.

Cook, J., Malliaras, P., De Luca, J., Ptasznik, R., Morris, M., and Khan, K. (2005) Vascularity and pain in the patella tendon of adult jumping athletes: a 5 month longitudinal study. *British Journal of Sports Medicine*, 39(7), 458–61,

Cook, J. and Purdam, C. (2009) Is tendon pathology a continuum? A pathology model to explain the clinical presentation of load-induced tendinopathy. *British Journal of Sports Medicine*, 43, 409–16.

Coombes, B., Bisset, L., and Vicenzino, B. (2010) Efficacy and safety of corticosteroid injections and other injections for management of tendinopathy: a systematic review of randomised controlled trials. *The Lancet*, 376, 1751–67.

Crichton, K. (1989) *Australian Journal of Physiotherapy*, 35.

Curwin, S., Rubinovich, R., and Stanish, W. (1985) Tendinitis: its etiology and treatment. *Clinical Orthopaedics and Related Research*, 208, 65–8.

Duri, Z. A. A., Aichroth, P. M., Dowd, G., and Ware, H. (1997) *Knee*, 4, 227–36.

Dye, S. F. (1987) *Journal of Bone and Joint Surgery*, 69A, 976–83.

Faletti, C., De Stefano, N., Giudice, G., and Larciprete, M. (1998) *European Journal of Radiology*, 27, S60–9.

Ficat, R. P. and Hungerford, D. S. (1977) *Disorders of the patellofemoral joint*. Williams and Wilkins, Baltimore.

Fisher, R. L. (1980) *Orthopaedic Review*, 9, 93–6.

Fritschy, D. and de Gautard, R. (1988) Jumper's knee and ultrasonography. *American Journal of Sports Medicine*, 16, 637–40.

Fu, F. H. and Maday, M. G. (1992) *Orthopedic Clinics of North America*, 23, 601–12.

Fulkerson, J. P. and Shea, K. P. (1990) *Journal of Bone and Joint Surgery*, 72A, 1424–9.

Fulkerson, J. P., Tennant, R., Jaivin, J. S., and Grunnet, M. (1985) *Clinical Orthopaedics and Related Research*.

Gardiner, J. S., McInerney, V. K., Avella, D. G., and Valdez, N. A. (1990) *Orthopaedic Review* 19.

Gerrard, B. (1989) *Australian Journal of Physiotherapy*, 35, 71–80.

Giombini, A., Dragoni, A., Di Cesare, M. A. Del Buono, A., and Maffulli, M. (2013) Asymptomatic Achilles, patellar, and quadriceps tendinopathy: a longitudinal clinical and ultrasonographic study in elite fencers. *Scandinavian Journal of Medicine & Science in Sport*, 23(3), 311–6.

Gisslén, K. and Alfredson, H. (2005) Neovascularisation and pain in jumper's knee: a prospective clinical and sonographic study in elite junior volleyball players. *British Journal of Sports Medicine*, 39, 423–8.

Glynn, M. K. and Regan, B. F. (1983) *Journal of Pediatric Orthopedics*, 3, 216–9.

Gose, J. C. and Schweizer, P. (1989) *Journal of Orthopaedic and Sports Physical Therapy*, 10, 10.

Grabiner, M. D., Koh, T. J., and Draganich, L. F. (1994) *Medicine Science Sport and Exercise*, 26, 10–21.

Gulling, L. K., Lephart, S. M., Stone, D. A., Irrgang, J. J., and Pincivero, D. M. (1996) *Isokinetics and Exercise Science*, 6, 133–8.

Hägglund, M., Zwerver, J., and Ekstrand, J. (2011) Epidemiology of patellar tendinopathy in elite male soccer players. *American Journal of Sports Medicine*, 39(9), 1906–11.

Hahn, T. and Foldspang, A. (1998) *Scandinavian Journal of Social Medicine*, 26, 44–52.

Harwin, S. F. and Stern, R. E. (1981) *Clinical Orthopaedics and Related Research*.

Hawkins, R. J., Bell, R. H., and Anisette, G. (1986) *American Journal of Sports Medicine*, 14, 117.

Henry, J. H. and Craven, P. R. (1981) *American Journal of Sports Medicine*, 9, 82.

Herrington, L. (1998) *Critical Reviews in Physical and Rehabilitation Medicine*, 10, 257–63.

Herrington, L. and Payton, C. J. (1997) *Physiotherapy*, 83, 566–72.

Hilyard, A., Moore, C., and Pope, J. (1989) *Australian Journal of Physiotherapy*, 35.

Hughston, J. C., Flandry, F., Brinker, M. R., Terry, G. C., and Mills, I. J. (1996) *American Journal of Sports Medicine*, 24, 486–91.

Hughston, J. C. and Walsh, W. M. (1979) *Clinical Orthopaedics*, 144, 36.

Insall, J. and Salvati, E. (1971) *Radiology*, 101, 101.

Jerosch, J. and Schroder, M. (1996) *Archives of Orthopaedic and Traumatic* Surgery, 115 195–8.

Joshi, R. P. and Heatley, F. W. (1998) *Knee*, 5, 129–35.

Kannus, P., Aho, H., Jarvinen, M., et al. (1987) *American Journal of Sports Medicine*, 15, 79–85.

Kannus, P., Natri, A., Paakkala, T., and Jarvinen, M. (1999) *Journal of Bone and Joint Surgery*, 81A, 355–63.

Kannus, P., Niittymaki, S., and Jarvinen, M. (1988) *Clinical Pediatrics*, 27, 333–7.

Kannus, P. A. and Nittymaki, S. (1994) *Medicine Science Sport and Exercise*, 26, 289–96.

Kaufner, H. and Arbor, A. (1971) *Journal of Bone and Joint Surgery*, 63, 1551–60.

Khan, K. M., Bonar, F., Desmond, P., et al. (1996) Patellar tendinosis (jumper's knee): findings at histopathologic examination, US and MR imaging. *Radiology*, 200, 821–7.

Khan, K., Cook, J., Bonar, F., Harcourt, P., and Astroma, M. (1999) Histopathology of common tendinopathies: update and implications for clinical management. *Sports Medicine*, 27(6), 393–408.

Khan, K., Cook, J., Maffulli, N., and Kannus, P. (2000) Where is the pain coming from in tendinopathy? It may be biochemical, not only structural, in origin. *British Journal of Sports Medicine*, 34, 81–3.

Khan, K., Maffuli, N., Coleman, B., Cook, J., and Taunton, J. (1998) Patellar tendinopathy: some aspects of basic science and clinical management. *British Journal of Sports Medicine*, 32, 346–55.

King, A. G. and Blundell-Jones, G. (1981) *American Journal of Sports Medicine*, 9, 250–3.

Krebs, V. E. and Parker, R. D. (1994) *Arthroscopy*, 10, 301–4.

Krompinger, W. J. and Fulkerson, J. P. (1983) Lateral retinacular release for intractable lateral retinacular pain. *Clinical Orthopaedics and Related Research*, 179, 191–3.

Kujala, U. M., Kvist, M., and Heinonen, O. (1985) *American Journal of Sports Medicine*, 13, 236–41.

Larsson, M.E.H., Kall, I., Nilsson-Helander, K. (2012) Treatment of patellar tendinipathy – a systematic review of randomized controlled trials. Knee Surg. Sports Traumatol. Arthrosc., 20, 1632–46.

Laurin, C. A., Dussault, R., and Levesque, H. P. (1979) *Clinical Orthopaedics*, 144, 16–26.

van Leeuwen, M., Zwerver, J., van den Akker-Scheek, I. (2009) Extracorporeal shockwave therapy for patellar tendinopathy: a review of the literature. *British Journal of Sports Medicine*, 43, 163–8.

Lempberg, R. K. and Arnoldi, C. C. (1978) *Clinical Orthopaedics*, 136, 143–56.

Levine, J. and Kashyap, S. (1981) A new conservative treatment of Osgood-Schlatter disease. *Clinical Orthopaedics and Related Research, N.O.*, 158, 126–8.

Lian, O., Holen, K. J., Engebrestson, L., et al. (1996) Relationship between symptoms of jumper's knee and the ultrasound characteristics of the patellar tendon among high level male volleyball players. *Scandinavian Journal of Medicine & Science in Sports*, 6, 291–6.

Lieb, F. and Perry, J. (1968) *Journal of Bone and Joint Surgery*, 50A, 1535.

Longo, U., Franceschetti, E., Rizzello, G., Petrillo, S., and Denaro, V. (2012) Elbow tendinopathy. *Muscles, Ligaments, and Tendons Journal*, 2(2), 115–20.

Loppini, M. and Maffuli, N. (2011) Conservative management of tendinopathy: an evidence-based approach. *Muscles, Ligaments, and Tendons Journal*, 1(4), 134–7.

Maenpaa, H. and Lehto, M. U. K. (1997) *Clinical Orthopaedics and Related Research Issue*, 339.

Maffulli, N., Longo, U., Loppini, M., Spiezia, F., and Denaro, V. (2010) New options in the management of tendinopathy. *Open Access: Journal of Sports Medicine*, 1, 29–37.

Magra, M. and Maffuli, N. (2007) Genetics: does it play a role in tendinopathy? *Clinical Journal of Sport Medicine*, 17(4), 231–3.

McConnell, J. (1986) *Australian Journal of Physiotherapy*, 32, 215–23.

McGinty, J. B. and McCarthy, J. C. (1981) *Clinical Orthopaedics*, 167, 9–18.

Merchant, A. C. (1988) *Arthroscopy*, 4, 235.

Metcalf, R. (1982) *Clinical Orthopaedics*, 167, 9.

Milgrom, C., Finestone, A., Shlamkovitch, N., Giladi, M., and Radin, E. (1996) *Clinical Orthopaedics and Related Research*, 331, 256–60.

Miller, B.F., Olesen, J.L., Hansen, M., et al. (2005) Coordinated collagen and muscle protein synthesis in human patella tendon and quadriceps muscle after exercise. *Journal of Physiology*, 567, 1021–33.

Miller, T. T., Shapiro, M. A., Schultz, E., Crider, R., and Paley, D. (1998) *American Journal of Roentgenology*, 171, 739–42.

Morrish, G. M. and Woledge, R. C. (1997) *Scandinavian Journal of Rehabilitation Medicine*, 29, 43–8.

Mummery, W. K., Spence, J. C., Vincenten, J. A., and Voaklander (1998) *Canadian Journal of Public Health*, 89, 53–6.

Natri, A., Kannus, P., and Jarvinen, M. (1998) *Medicine and Science in Sports and Exercise*, 30, 1572–7.

Ogden, J. A. (1984) *Skeletal Radiology*, 11, 246–57.

Owre, A. (1934) *Acta Chiolurgica Scandinavica*, 77.

Øystein, L., Engebretsen, L., and Bahr, R. (2005) Prevalence of jumper's knee among elite athletes from different sports: a cross-sectional study. *American Journal of Sports Medicine*, 33(4), 561–7.

Palumbo, P. M. (1981) *American Journal of Sports Medicine*, 9, 1.

Peers, K. and Lysens, R. (2005) Patellar tendinopathy in athletes: current diagnostic and therapeutic recommendations. *Sports Medicine*, 35(1), 71–87.

Post, W. R. (1997) *Techniques in Orthopaedics*, 12, 145–50.

Post, W. R. (1998) *Physician and Sports Medicine*, 26, 68–78.

Powers, C. M. (1998) *Journal of Orthopaedic and Sports Physical Therapy*, 28, 345–54.

Purdam, C., Cook, J., Khan, K., and Hopper, D. (2003) Discriminitive ability of functional loading tests for adolescent jumper's knee. *Physical Therapy in Sport*, 4, 3–9.

Radin, E. L., Pail, I. L., and Lowy, M. (1984) *Journal of Bone and Joint Surgery*, B, 660.

Rees, J., Maffulli, N., and Cook, J. (2009) Management of tendinopathy. *American Journal of Sports Medicine*, 37(9), 1855–67.

Rees, J., Stride, M., and Scott, A. (2013) Tendons—time to revisit inflammation. *British Journal of Sports Medicine*, 0, 1–7.

Rees, J., Wolman, R., and Wilson, A. (2009) Eccentric exercises; why do they work, what are the problems and how can we improve them? *British Journal of Sports Medicine*, 43, 242–6.

Reid, D. C. (1992) *Sport injury assessment and rehabilitation*. Churchill Livingstone, New York.

Rio, E., Moseley, L., Purdam, C., et al. (2014) The pain of tendinopathy: physiological or pathophysiological?

Roels, J., Martens, M., Mulier, J. C., and Burssens, A. (1978) *American Journal of Sports Medicine*, 6, 362–8.

Rutland, M., O'Connell, D., Brismée, J., Sizer, P., Apte, G., and O'Connell, J. (2010) Evidence-supported rehabilitation of patellar tendinopathy. *North American Journal of Sports Physical Therapy*, 5(3), 166–78.

Scott, A., Docking, S., Vicenzino, B., et al. (2013) Sports and exercise-related tendinopathies: a review of selected topical issues by participants of the second International Scientific Tendinopathy Symposium (ISTS), Vancouver, 2012. *British Journal of Sports Medicine*, 47, 536–44.

Sharma, P. and Maffulli, N. (2006) Biology of tendon injury: healing, modeling and remodelling. *Journal of Musculoskeletal and Neuronal Interactions*, 6(2), 181–90.

Stanish, W. D. and Curwin, S. (1984) *Tendonitis: its etiology and treatment*. Collamore Press, Lexington, MA.

Traverso, A., Baldari, A., and Catalani, F. (1990) *Journal of Sports Medicine and Physical Fitness*, 30, 331–3.

Tria, A. J., Palumbo, N. C., and Alicea, J. A. (1992) *Orthopedic Clinics of North America*, 24, 545–53.

Tsirbas, A., Paterson, R. S., and Keene, G. C. R. (1991) *Australian Journal of Science and Medicine in Sport*, 23, 24–6.

Tumilty, S., McDonough, S., Hurley, D., and Baxter, D. (2012) Clinical effectiveness of low-level laser therapy as an adjunct to eccentric exercise for the treatment of Achilles' tendinopathy: a randomized controlled trial. *Archives of Physical Medicine and Rehabilitation*, 93, 733–9.

Visentini, P., Khan, K., Cook, J., Kiss, Z., Harcourt, P., Wark, J. (1998) The VISA score: an index of severity of symptoms in patients with jumper's knee (patellar tendinosis). *Journal of Science and Medicine in Sport*, 1(1), 22–8.

Visnes, H. and Bahr, R. (2007) The evolution of eccentric training as treatment for patellar tendinopathy (jumper's knee): a critical review of exercise programmes. 41, 217–23.

Voigt, M. L. and Wieder, D. L. (1991) *American Journal of Sports Medicine*, 19, 131–7.

Wiberg, G. (1941) *Acta Orthopodica Scandinavica*, XII, 319.

Wilner, P. (1970) *Clinical Orthopaedics*, 669, 213.

Witonski, D., Karlinska, I., and Musial, A. (1999) *Medicine and Science Monitor*, 4, 1019–23.

Witvrouw, E., Mahieu, N., Roosen, P., and McNair, P. (2007) The role of stretching in tendon injuries. *British Journal of Sports Medicine*, 41, 224–6.

Wood, A. (1998) *Journal of Sports Chiropractic and Rehabilitation*, 12, 1–14.

Woodley, B., Newsham-West, J., and Baxter, G. (2007) Chronic tendinopathy: effectiveness of eccentric exercise. *British Journal of Sports Medicine*, 41, 188–99.

Youmans, W. T. (1989) *Clinics in Sports Medicine*, 8, 331–42.

Chapter 38

Soft tissue injuries at the knee

Steve McNally

Overview of soft tissue injuries at the knee

Injuries of the soft tissues of the knee encompass a wide range of aetiological and pathological processes including infective, inflammatory, and biomechanical dysfunction as common causes alongside the traumatic and degenerative. The clinician must also remain aware of soft tissue presentations as manifestations of systemic disease, anatomical variants, malformations, or neoplasms. Conservative management and physical therapy is usually the preferred first line, although surgery may be indicated for some conditions for refractory cases or in the acute phase for severe infections such as bursal abscess. The intracapsular structures and collateral ligaments are excluded from this chapter.

As the knee joint is a key component in the centre of the lower limb kinetic chain, it is implicated in every aspect of locomotor function (including standing still). Also, as the joint is only ever completely stable in the fully extended 'close-packed' position (assuming intact structural anatomy), it follows that there are varying degrees of potential instability in one or more of the movement planes during every type and phase of motion which includes flexion, extension, rotation, varus, valgus, forwards and backwards translation; all occurring in complex combinations and subject to sudden changes of direction while absorbing impact forces and generating propulsive power. The distal tendons of the quadriceps, sartorius, hamstrings, and gracilis muscles, the tendon of popliteus, and the origins of gastrocnemius (that provide both co-ordinated movement and functional stability) are sites of potential injury in the tendon substance and/or bony attachments/entheses or the bursae that are closely related anatomically. Several of these muscles span two joints and have actions affecting both; hence the knee should never be assessed in isolation. The iliotibial band is another structure that falls into this category, having actions on both the hip and knee.

Presentations in the form of symptoms and/or detectable pathology around the knee may be due to primary problems several joints above or below in the kinetic chain. Every medical student is taught to consider the hip joint when faced with a presentation of knee pain but the originating problem may lie in sites as variable as the sacroiliac joint (either by referred pain or alteration of functional limb length) or in the first metatarsophalangeal joint (leading to tension in the plantar fascia transmitted up through the continuum of the posterior myofascial chain). The same is true for virtually the whole musculoskeletal system. Therefore, the clinician should approach a presentation of soft tissue knee pain or dysfunction with a completely open-minded approach and not have their attention focused entirely on the knee alone, even if a glaringly obvious local pathology is present. Injecting steroid around an inflamed iliotibial band will not resolve the condition without concomitant management of the underlying biomechanical, neurodynamic, or anatomical dysfunction.

After careful assessment of the pathophysiological process and confirmation of the tissue/structural diagnosis, the injury must be placed within context of the individual patient and the functional demands required of their knee. One needs to consider factors such as age, gender, occupation, and athletic/leisure pursuits in order to tailor management of their problem in line with their expectations. A small area of patellar tendinosis that may look identical on ultrasound scans will have very differing impacts on a jumping athlete and a patient with a more sedentary occupation, and the management plans will also differ considerably.

Superficial bursitis of the knee

The subcutaneous bursae on the anterior aspect of the knee are exposed to traumatic injury by acute contact or penetrative insult, or repetitive shearing or friction between skin and bone (prepatellar bursitis), or the infrapatellar tendon (superficial infrapatellar bursitis). While predominantly haemorrhagic or inflammatory, micro-organisms entering externally from overlying skin puncture (traumatic or iatrogenic), systemically, or by local internal spread from patellar osteomyelitis (Choi 2007) can lead to infective bursitis and abscess formation. A wide range of micro-organisms have been implicated in infectious bursitis including staphylococci, streptococci, brucella species, and mycobacterium tuberculosis. Inflamed bursae in any location may also be manifestations of systemic, non-infectious disease such as sarcoidosis (Fujimoto et al. 2006), gout (Dawn et al. 1997), or idiopathic arthritis (Aydingoz et al. 2011).

Repetitive external compression and friction is the commonest aetiology and, as the layman's names of housemaid's, parson's, carpet layer's, and beat knee suggest, there is usually an occupational association. 'Beat knee' is a prescribed industrial disease (PD A6) defined as 'manual labour causing severe or prolonged external friction or pressure at or about the knee'; this is not to be confused

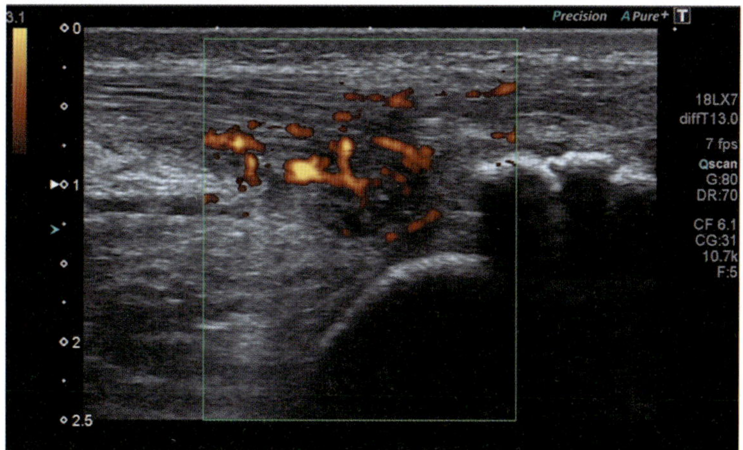

Figure 38.1 Ultrasound scan of an adolescent footballer's knee showing neovascularity around the deep infrapatellar bursa and distal patellar tendon insertion into an immature tibial apophysis, consistent with typical Osgood-Schlatter's disease.

with another prescribed disease, 'miner's knee', which is also related to compression effects from repetitive squatting and kneeling but refers to elevated intra-articular pressure leading to chondral degeneration and premature osteoarthrosis. Certain sporting disciplines, such as wrestling, can predispose to anterior knee bursitis and massive pre-patellar bursitis is occasionally reported in individuals whose ambulation involves frequent crawling through impairment/disability, e.g. cerebral palsy or post-poliomyelitis paralysis.

Morel-Lavallée lesions have been increasingly reported in the literature in recent years as a recognized variant of pre-patellar bursitis with subtle distinguishing diagnostic features on magnetic resonance imaging (MRI), whereby a hyper-intense fluid signal extends beyond the anatomical boundary of the bursa (Borrero et al. 2008; Ciaschini and Sundaram 2008). Rarely, anatomical variants (Karkos et al. 2002) may mimic superficial knee bursitis and must be borne in mind in the differential diagnosis.

Clinical symptoms and signs are usually obvious in the form of localized pain, swelling, heat, and erythema with limitation of knee flexion and function. Additional imaging investigations are rarely needed, although ultrasound scanning can assist with differentiation between semi-solid and cystic collections, and from guided-aspiration procedures, fluid can be sent for culture and microscopy to determine any infective agent, cytology, or crystals. MRI may be required to confirm a diagnosis of a Morel-Lavallée lesion in chronic presentations, although clinical management alters little as a result. Care must be taken not to diagnose a soft tissue sarcoma incorrectly if calcification is noted in a chronically traumatized or haemorrhagic bursa (Stahnke et al. 2004).

Management should be directed at the underlying cause and pathological process, with removal of direct or repetitive pressure and prescription of anti-inflammatory or anti-microbial modalities including physical therapies, electrotherapies, or medication in line with the severity of presentation. Needle aspiration can be therapeutic as well as diagnostic. Surgery is reserved for severe or refractory cases, and endoscopic bursectomy under local anaesthesia may confer advantages in terms of reduced skin morbidity and improved cosmetic results in comparison to open bursectomy (Huang and Yeh 2011; Ogilvie-Harris and Gilbart 2000). Preventive measures, including protective knee pads, are important for certain occupations, athletes, or individuals with unusual mobility issues as described earlier.

Deep anterior bursitis of the knee

Although classified here as 'deep', due to the fact that they are not immediately subcutaneous, the deep infrapatellar bursa and anserine bursa may still be injured as a result of direct contact trauma or repetitive external friction as per the superficial bursae. Infection from external trauma is less likely due to protection from the overlying tendons but these bursae may be implicated in any of the systemic conditions described in the section 'Superficial bursitis of the knee'. More commonly, bursitis in these locations is closely associated with biomechanical factors and kinetic chain dysfunction, leading to excessive tension in the overlying tendons, overloading the cushioning capacity of the bursae to the point of irritation and inflammation. The key to management therefore tends to lie in correction of those abnormalities in addition to anti-inflammatory modalities directed at the bursa itself.

Anserine bursitis, in particular, often coexists with a degree of pes anserinus tendinopathy affecting one or more of the components of the sartorius, gracilis, and semitendinosis. Deep infrapatellar bursitis can be associated with osteophyte formation adjacent to the tibial insertion of the patellar tendon or bony fragmentation of the apophysis in classical Osgood-Schlatter's disease in adolescents (Figure 38.1). Impingement pain during end-range knee extension may be a feature, alongside the usual inflammatory symptoms and signs.

Anterior impingement and Hoffa's fat pad

The extensive extrasynovial collection of fat anterior to the knee joint and deep to the infrapatellar tendon may have functions other than simply filling space and maintaining anatomical relationships during functional movement. Highly vascular and well-innervated, Hoffa's fat pad is implicated as a source of neovessels that penetrate the inferior aspect of the patellar tendon in the advanced stages of tendinosis, and various forms of invasive management are directed at this plane between the fat pad and tendon including prolotherapy, saline injection 'stripping', and surgical debridement (Pascarella et al. 2011). Cytokines produced by adipocytes in this region may also play an important role in cartilage damage associated with knee osteoarthrosis (Distel et al. 2009). Hoffa's fat pad should therefore be regarded as an active organ as opposed to inert connective tissue (Dragoo et al. 2012).

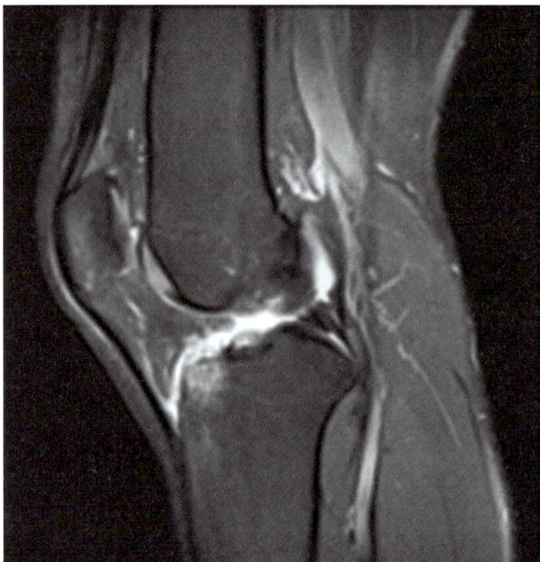

Figure 38.2 Sagittal MRI of a professional footballer's knee following a hyper-extension episode; bony oedema is present in the anterior tibial plateau with high signal in and around the overlying inferior part of Hoffa's fat pad, consistent with contusion.

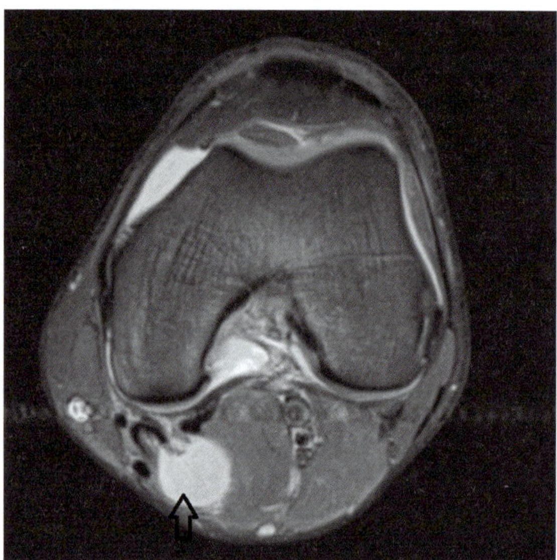

Figure 38.3 Axial MRI showing a popliteal cyst (arrow) communicating with the joint capsule between the tendon of semimembranosus and the medial head of gastrocnemius.

In individuals with anatomical knee recurvatum, hyperextension trauma can cause fat pad contusion and haemorrhage which is often intensely painful due to the high sensory innervation and pressure effects from bleeding in an enclosed space which is compressed further by activities requiring forceful knee extension, such as kicking in sports (Figure 38.2). Less severe conditions may present as areas of focal or diffuse oedema or, more severely, in the form of tearing leading to fibrosis, scarring, and chronic impingement. Knee arthroscopy is a common cause of fat pad trauma at the sites of medial and lateral portal entry. Irritation and oedema can be due to patellofemoral maltracking (Subhawong et al. 2010).

Neoplastic masses have been described in the form of chondromas (Ingabire et al. 2012) and osteochondromas (De Maio et al.2011; Singh et al. 2009) and can be viewed as an end stage of chronic 'Hoffitis' via metaplastic change (Turhan et al. 2008). The differential diagnosis of a swelling arising from Hoffa's fat pad should include ganglion cysts, haemangiomas, vascular malformations, and pigmented villonodular synovitis (Dean et al. 2011; Ghate et al. 2012).

Management of non-neoplastic presentations should focus on correction of biomechanical predisposition where possible and enhancement of functional eccentric quadriceps and hamstring muscle strength to improve control of knee extension during foot strike and deceleration/landing. Surgical removal of solid or cystic masses is usually required to clear the associated impingement and confirm a histological diagnosis.

Popliteal swellings of the knee

The vast majority of swellings situated at the back of the knee are benign in nature and will fall under the spectrum of 'Baker's cysts' (as they are popularly known), although in most cases, this is an incorrect terminology given that most lesions are not true, fully encapsulated cysts in that they communicate with the synovial sac of the joint itself (Figure 38.3). A true popliteal cyst is a distension of the semimembranosus bursa or a direct bulge of the posterior synovial sac between the tendons of the semimembranosus and the medial head of gastrocnemius. In adults, there is virtually always an underlying pathological process within the joint capsule that has led to joint effusion and increased intra-articular hydrostatic pressure. Previously, this was not thought to be the case in children presenting with popliteal cysts (most were assumed to be sporadic) but the presence of such cysts is probably underreported and associations with arthritic conditions and hypermobility syndromes have been demonstrated (Neubauer et al. 2011). Having observed many such lesions in paediatric and young adult athletes with varying structural knee injuries, or as a post-surgical finding, it is possible that these cysts act as a natural 'relief valve' mechanism to reduce intra-articular synovial pressure, which may be beneficial for long-term chondrocyte health, thereby slowing progression to joint degeneration. However, this is not reported in the literature.

Most swellings are noted as a coincidental finding when examining a knee with the patient prone, but some may complain of restricted deep knee flexion, fluctuations in size of the swelling (with or without pain), or, occasionally, local neurovascular compression symptoms may be a feature. These lesions are usually secondary manifestations of the underlying primary pathology, but cysts can rupture and cause severe local irritation and inflammation (Abdelrahman et al. 2012). Treatment is best directed at the underlying cause (e.g. addressing intra-articular structural disorders or inflammatory arthropathy), although local treatment to the cyst itself, in the form of aspiration, steroid injection (Bandinelli et al. 2012; Köroğlu et al. 2012), or prolotherapy may be indicated, with surgical excision reserved for the most troublesome only. Surgery is more likely to be successful if concomitant pathology is dealt with, and a valvular communication may also be detected arthroscopically (Malinowski et al. 2011).

Accuracy of diagnosis is essential prior to any invasive procedure as failure to recognize a cystic or pseudocystic lesion arising from tissues other than synovium may be disastrous. Similarly, solid masses must be differentiated from those with predominantly liquid contents and ultrasound scanning is the simplest way of achieving this. If the source of the lesion cannot be easily identified, MRI may also be required. Septic arthritis (Izumi et al. 2012), cystic adventitial disease of the popliteal artery (Drac et al. 2011), aneurysms, posterior horn meniscal cysts (Sivasubramanian et al. 2012), ganglion cysts (Spinne et al. 2012), and pigmented villonodular synovitis (Tosti and Kelly 2011) have been implicated in mimicking the classical Baker's cyst. A lipoma or (rarely) a schwannoma of the common peroneal nerve (Andrychowski et al. 2012) may present as a solid popliteal mass.

Tendinoses around the knee

Symptoms arising from tendon pathology at the knee are usually a manifestation of abnormal loading of the specific musculotendinous unit involved by dysfunctional biomechanics, excessive extrinsic load (e.g. unaccustomed exercise), or weakness (particularly of eccentric strength) in the muscle to which the tendon is anatomically attached. Tendinosis may also occur intrinsically, secondary to systemic quinolone antibiotic therapy, and there is emerging opinion that certain genotypes may predispose individuals to tendon pathology. Once a tendon generates pain, either by neural or chemical mediation, there is a secondary inhibition of the agonist muscle and a vicious cycle is established leading to further weakness and stress on the tendon, thereby propagating any structural changes that have been established. Hence, tendinosis generally poses significant challenges for the treating clinician.

The location of the pathological process within the tendon also significantly alters the clinical presentation and management; patellar tendinosis is predominantly enthesopathic at its bony origin on the inferior patellar pole, although it can occur mid-substance or at the distal tibial insertion, and while there are some common treatment options, the underlying pathology and aetiology may be very different. Tendinosis can be reactive (with a temporary inflammatory component), degenerative (classical overuse tendinosis without a cellular inflammatory response), traumatic (tears and fissures), or iatrogenic (post-graft harvest for anterior cruciate ligament reconstruction). Moving away from the prime focus of symptoms in the affected tendon, the anatomical and/or biomechanical fault(s) may lie several joints proximal and/or distal to the knee. An holistic approach is therefore essential in the assessment of knee tendinosis in order to arrive at the correct conclusion with respect to causation and then to plan a logical and systematic approach to management to achieve symptom relief, restoration of function, and prevention of recurrence.

Anterior tendinosis (quadriceps and patellar)

Conditions affecting the knee extensor tendon mechanism are among the spectrum of patellofemoral syndromes discussed in detail in Chapter 37. Therefore, this section will be restricted to an outline of the extensive published literature, in conjunction with the author's own experiences and observations of managing such presentations.

Whilst tendinopathic changes do occur in the mid portion of both tendons, the majority of presentations occur at the entheses into the superior and inferior patellar poles, with the deep portion being predominantly affected. Both distractive and compressive load stress has been implicated in the aetiology of these conditions (Cook and Purdam 2012). Anatomical changes on ultrasound and/or MRI ranging from tendon thickening, increases in matrix, through to defects and clefts/micro-tears, with or without varying degrees of neovascularization, may be noted in both symptomatic and asymptomatic tendons (Figure 38.4). Moreover, the extent of neovascularization noted by Doppler ultrasound scanning may differ according to timing of the scan (e.g. before or after athletic activity) and to knee position during scanning (flexed with tendon under tension or extended and relaxed). Conversely, symptomatic tendons may look anatomically normal on imaging. Caution is therefore advised in interpreting such findings when detected during screening examinations or in the assessment of a presentation of anterior knee pain, although research evidence

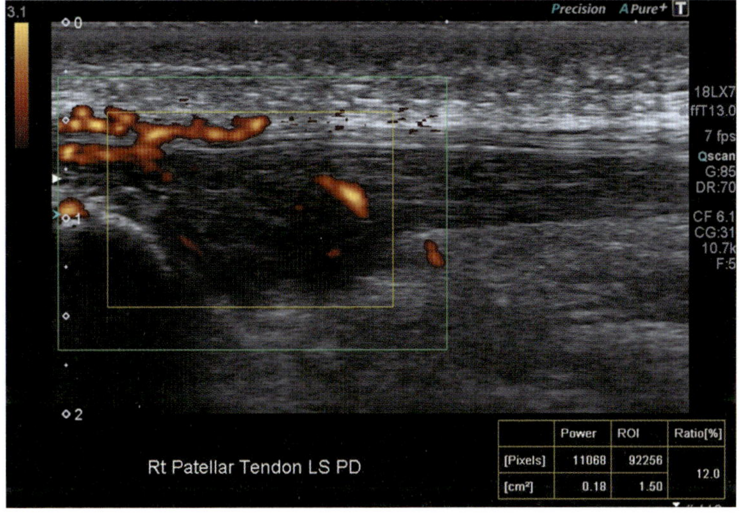

Figure 38.4 Power Doppler ultrasound scan of proximal patellar tendon showing hypoechoic area in deep tendon fibres with neovascularization, consistent with advanced tendinosis.

generally supports the hypothesis that tendons with detectable structural changes are more likely to become symptomatic (Giombini et al. 2011).

Another interesting observation, supported also by case reports and studies, is that the extent of anatomically detectable symptomatic tendinosis (patellar in particular) does not necessarily correspond to the severity of pain and/or functional disability experienced, suggesting that there are several pathways of pain mediation or perception involved in these conditions, including psychological or situational factors (van Wilgen et al. 2011). The holistic management approach referred to earlier is probably more vital to adopt in cases of recalcitrant patellar tendinosis than tendinoses elsewhere, in order to achieve a favourable outcome, and even then, there is a group that remain resistant to all modalities employed. Patellar tendinosis will continue to be a focus for further research for some time until this clinical conundrum is solved.

Extensive progressive tendinosis can lead to rupture of either the quadriceps or patellar tendon components (Arumilli et al. 2009); bilateral cases have been reported, although this should alert the clinician to individual predisposition to tendon mechanical weakness due to systemic illness (alkaptonuria), hormonal imbalance (hyperthyroidism), drug therapy (quinolone antibiotics), or drug misuse (anabolic steroids) affecting collagen synthesis/regeneration.

A myriad of treatments directed at the tendon itself have been proposed (van Ark et al. 2011; Larsson et al. 2012) including shockwave therapy, laser, topical nitrates, sclerosant, prolotherapy, growth factor, and stem cell infiltration; all with the aim of stimulating local collagen synthesis and promoting regeneration of the defective areas within the tendon. Scientific evidence is mixed at best and it is not appropriate to generalize or be too prescriptive in recommending therapeutic interventions. Therefore, each presentation should be assessed in isolation before employing such modalities (especially those that are invasive). Additionally, there is differing expert opinion as to whether such treatments are best directed within or around the tendon, or even targeted towards the interface with Hoffa's fat pad from which neovessels and accompanying sensory nerves arise. A variety of surgical procedures have been employed in resistant cases, again with varying success rates (Marcheggiani Muccioli et al. 2012).

Faced with a vast and confusing array of potential options, there are two constants with good supporting evidence that must form part of any therapeutic plan—namely, load management and quadriceps resistance exercise. The former should employ sufficient load restriction relative to the patient's pre-morbid activity levels (excessive complete rest may be disastrous for an athlete) with respect to volume, intensity, and type. Slow resistance exercises with progressive increases in load, e.g. eccentric decline squat protocols (Visnes and Bahr 2007), are effective in reducing pain and restoring function, even before tendon structure is noted to improve (as illustrated in Figure 38.5).

Primary prevention can be attempted by addressing anatomical, clinical, and imaging findings noted on screening assessments in vulnerable individuals such as jumping athletes, for whom quadriceps and patellar tendinosis is a common occurrence and can be severely debilitating or career-threatening, although predictive power is relatively weak (Mann et al. 2012; van der Worp et al 2011).

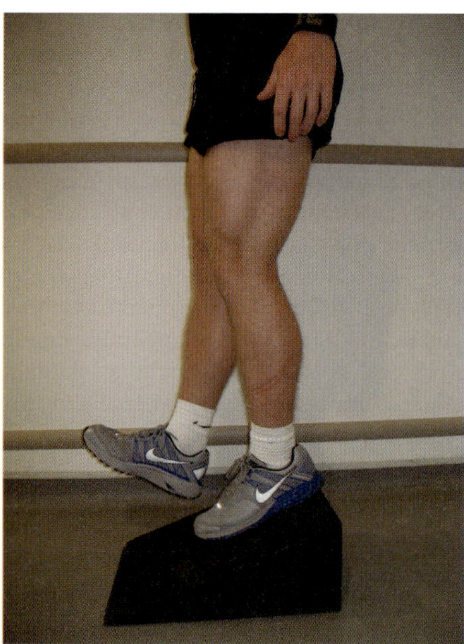

Figure 38.5a Demonstration of the eccentric decline squat exercise for quadriceps/patellar tendinosis: start position.

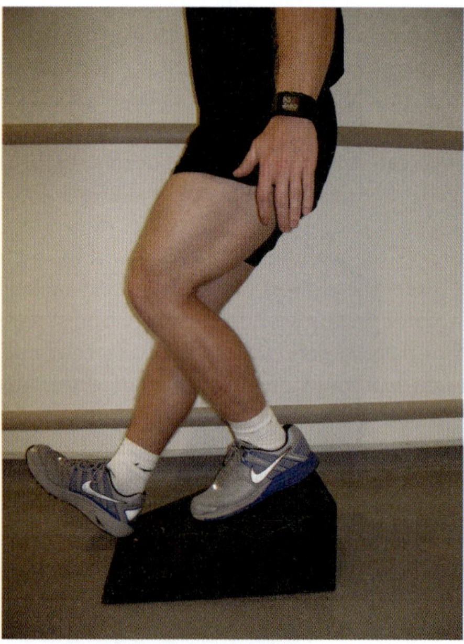

Figure 38.5b Demonstration of the eccentric decline squat exercise for quadriceps/patellar tendinosis: end position.

Anteromedial tendinosis (pes anserinus)

As already discussed in the section 'Deep anterior bursitis of the knee', this condition of a painful insertion of the pes anserine tendons into the anteromedial border of the tibia often coexists with anserine bursitis and is probably best considered as an 'anserine syndrome' or 'tendino-bursitis (Helfenstein and Kuromoto 2010), in contrast to discrete tendinosis that can occur more proximally (and posteriorly) which is described in the following section 'Posteromedial tendinosis'.

Symptoms localized to this region may be misdiagnosed as distal medial collateral ligament injury, although there is usually a clear history of acute trauma in the latter. Chronic valgus strain from obesity or increased Q-angle (females) can predispose to anserine tendino-bursitis and associations have been claimed with diabetes mellitus, osteoarthritis, antero-posterior knee instability, and other lower limb malalignments causing biomechanical stress, but the evidence base is inconclusive (Alvarez-Nemegyei 2007).

Posteromedial tendinosis (semimembranosus, semitendinosus, and gastrocnemius)

As part of the hamstring/calf posterior myofascial chain, these muscle/tendon units (see Figure 38.6) are involved in concentric knee flexion and work eccentrically in controlling knee extension during deceleration and late swing phase, with most hamstring injuries thought to occur during the latter function. In addition, the semimembranosus 'complex' of five tendinous arms is closely related anatomically to the posterior oblique portion of the medial collateral ligament, and hence makes an important contribution to dynamic medial knee stability, acting also synergistically with the popliteus muscle to pull the posterior horn of the medial meniscus backwards during knee flexion (Beltran et al. 2003).

Primary semimembranosus tendinosis is rarely reported but should be considered in a presentation of chronic, aching, posteromedial knee pain in combination with accurate localization of tenderness on palpation over the main body of the tendon or its tibial insertion (Bylund and de Weber 2010). Ultrasound/MRI may assist in confirming the diagnosis by detection of thickening or structural/stromal changes within the tendon substance, associated bursitis, and exclusion of pathology in other structures in the vicinity. More commonly, this condition is seen in middle-aged/elderly individuals (often with concomitant knee pathology such as osteoarthritis) but can present in younger endurance athletes subjected to sudden increases in exercise volume or intensity. Increased valgus stress from foot over-pronation or an increased Q-angle stresses the medial knee tendons and should be looked for and addressed.

The semitendinosus tendon follows a course medial to the semimembranosus and is smaller and more discretely defined on palpation. Again, reports in the scientific literature are few but this tendon seems more prone to irritation from friction or 'snapping' as it passes over the posteromedial tibial condyle in conjunction with the gracilis tendon (Bae and Kwon 1997), as opposed to an

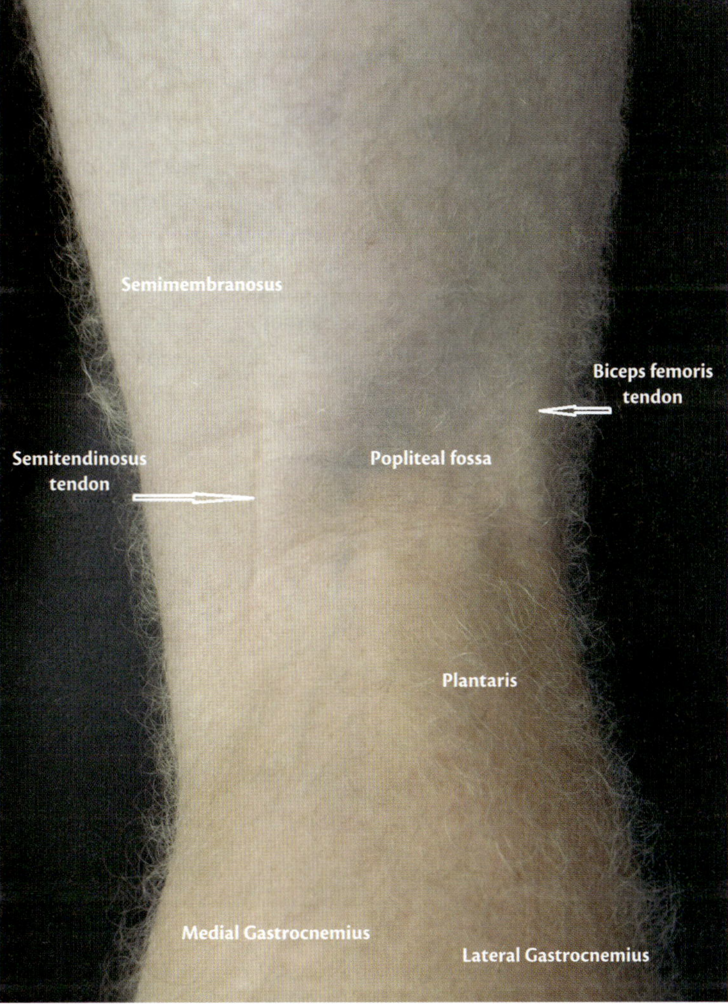

Figure 38.6 An illustration of the anatomical landmarks of the popliteal region; of importance when localizing symptoms and clinical signs.

intrinsic degenerative process. Conservative management is the norm, focusing on release of kinetic chain tension and appropriate adjustment of biomechanics/anatomical predisposition, although surgery has been undertaken, with reported success, in a refractory case (Karataglis et al. 2008).

Calcifying tendinosis of the medial head of gastrocnemius has been reported in a series of three elderly female patients presenting with both acute and chronic posteromedial knee pain, restriction of extension, localized tenderness, and pain on passive stretching, with calcific deposits in the tendon substance on X-ray. Refractory to conservative management, all required steroid infiltration and one needed surgery to decompress and excise calcific deposits, with good symptomatic relief and restored function (Iguchi et al. 2002).

Posterolateral tendinosis (biceps femoris and popliteus)

Symptoms arising from the posterolateral corner of the knee can be very difficult to localize accurately given the close anatomical relationship of several structures within a confined area. It is important to distinguish between conditions of primarily biomechanical origin, such as tendinosis, from those affecting the structural integrity of this area of the knee, as misdiagnosis may result in unnecessary surgery (e.g. arthroscopy for a suspected posterior horn lateral meniscus tear) or failure to recognize posterolateral rotatory or varus instability which can have significant consequences for long-term joint health or athletic performance.

The distal biceps femoris tendon arises from a fusion of the long and short heads of the biceps femoris muscle, although anatomical variants, including bifurcation of the tendon at the level of the fibular head, commonly occur and can be detected sonographically (Smith et al. 2011). Assumed to represent varying separate continuations of the long and short head, the sonographer may initially suspect pathological tendinosis on first inspection due to apparent 'thickening' and anisotropy effects. The biceps tendon can be reliably identified as the cause of pain in this region if noted to be 'snapping' or dyskinetic in motion and associated with true hypoechoic clefts or tendon fibre tearing on sonography. Peritendinous fluid, as opposed to distension of the bursa between the fibular collateral ligament and the biceps femoris tendon, is another diagnostic clue that may require confirmation by MRI. Imaging findings should correlate closely with clinical findings of tenderness on palpation and a suggestive clinical history, features of which may include a sensation of painful snapping or friction or predisposition, such as inappropriate saddle height causing posterolateral knee pain in a cyclist.

As with similar conditions, management should focus on correction of biceps femoris hypertonia, anatomical or functional shortening, and restoration of rotatory knee mechanics in the first instance, followed by local management of the painful tendon as described earlier. Surgical tenolysis, multiple tenotomy, and/or reconstruction has proven successful in managing this condition in athletes following failure of conservative therapy (Longo et al. 2008).

The tendinous portion of the popliteus muscle has a close anatomical relationship to the posterior horn of the lateral meniscus, with varying secondary attachments into it, alongside others to the fibular head and its primary insertion into the lateral femoral condyle. Unlocking the fully extended knee by means of its internal rotatory action on the tibia, the popliteus tendon has complex functional roles in controlling lateral meniscus displacement and retraction during knee flexion, with contributions to varus and valgus stability, and assisting the quadriceps muscle and cruciate ligaments in preventing excessive posterior tibial translation relative to the femur, all occurring dynamically in a co-ordinated fashion. Damage to the popliteus tendon may therefore occur by a variety of means, but the classical presentation is one of insidious onset pain on deceleration, checking movements, or downhill running.

Acute ruptures may be found in conjunction with structural posterolateral complex disruption from trauma, where instability is present, but also, rarely, without significant instability (Guha 2003). A more acute presentation of severe posterolateral knee pain in a less athletic middle-aged/elderly patient may indicate calcific tendinosis of popliteus akin to similar pathology seen commonly in supraspinatus. Locally targeted therapy such as steroid/local anaesthetic infiltration (Tibrewal 2002), dry needling, or shockwave therapy may be helpful, although this condition can be resistant and require surgical debridement of the calcific deposits to relieve pain and restore function (Shenoy et al. 2009; Tennent and Goradia 2003).

Popliteus tendinosis of biomechanical origin is best managed by addressing factors that place excessive strain on the popliteus, predominantly fatigue of the quadriceps during stance phase of gait. While usually presenting with gradual onset of pain, it can occur after a short period of overload and typically gets worse with attempts at continued activity. Tenderness along the course of the tendon can be elicited by palpation in either the prone or 'figure 4' position; provocation of pain by passive external tibial rotation with the knee flexed to 90° or active dynamic assessment using Garrick's test (Figure 38.7) is confirmatory. Physical therapy and reconditioning should focus on enhancing quadriceps recruitment/activation, eccentric strength, and endurance, while maintaining flexibility and normal muscle tone (avoiding both reduced and excessive tone). Confidence in the diagnosis (which may not be readily supported by positive imaging findings), together with patience and commitment to the remedial conditioning programme, while avoiding provoking activities, should prove successful in the majority of cases without resorting to invasive tendon therapy or surgery.

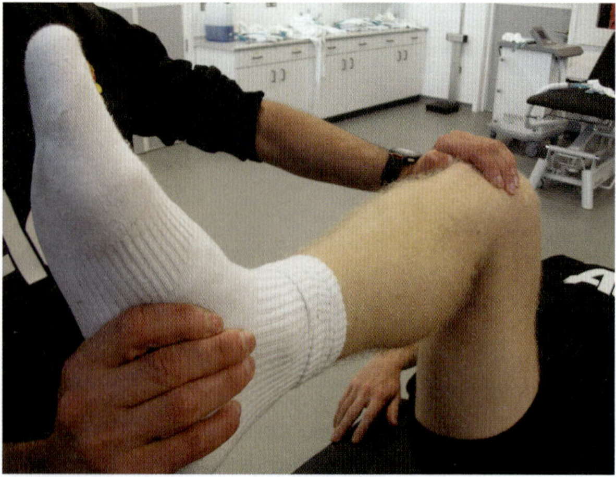

Figure 38.7 Demonstration of Garrick's test; the patient actively resists passive lower leg external rotation by the examiner. Pain provocation indicates a positive test for popliteus injury.

Iliotibial band syndrome

This painful condition over the lateral epicondyle of the femur, precipitated by repetitive knee flexion and extension, is not simply attributable to friction of a discrete anatomical structure over a bony prominence or a 'bursa' that lies between the two. The iliotibial 'band' is more of a thickening of the fascia lata that surrounds the thigh, which distally has multiple insertions into the linea aspera, the lateral epicondyle of the femur, and Gerdy's tibial tubercle. At the focal point of pain (which may radiate proximally and/or distally), there is often no separate bursa but, rather, a recess of the lateral knee joint synovium with surrounding adipose and connective tissue.

By transmitting contractions of tensor fascia lata, the iliotibial band assists with hip flexion, abduction, and medial rotation as an open-chain action. However, in the closed-chain, weight-bearing situation, it has an important stabilizing action on the hip while the contralateral limb goes through the swing phase of ambulation. Distally, it acts as a lateral dynamic stabilizer of the knee together with the biceps femoris and popliteus tendons. There is conflicting opinion on the biomechanical mechanisms by which these effects are exerted; some observers believe that the iliotibial band remains under tension in both a flexed and extended knee position, and others report an elongation under load when running. Similar debate exists as to whether the band glides posteriorly during knee flexion and anteriorly during extension (hence the 'friction' theory) or gives an illusion of doing so due to repetitive tightening under load (creating an 'impingement' effect on the deeper structures) (Fairclough et al. 2006).

Whatever the true mode of action, the majority of presentations are relatively similar, affecting individuals where repetitive knee flexion/extension under load is required, such as in running, cycling, or rowing. This condition is sometimes a complicating factor following total knee arthroplasty. The characteristic history of localized burning pain that begins after a period of exercise and worsens with attempts to continue (eventually causing cessation of the activity) usually clinches the diagnosis without the need for imaging investigations.

Ober's test, or variations thereof (passive knee flexion/extension with the hip extended and adducted), usually reproduces pain in the more severe cases, but the supporting evidence for this test is weak and it may be negative or equivocal in more subtle presentations (Figure 38.8). There may be other clues in the history such as training errors/sudden increases in activity, and clinical assessment may detect weakness of the larger hip abductor muscles, impairment of hamstring/quadriceps activation and strength imbalance, or poor rotatory knee control when hopping/landing. Other findings, such as rear-foot eversion or increases in knee flexion angle in stance phase (as when running downhill or when fatigued), have also been implicated, although research quality is questionable (Lavine 2010). Atypical presentations occur without a history of repetitive flexion/extension overload and symptoms can develop suddenly in individuals who engage in multi-directional sport with frequent cutting, checking, or deceleration movements.

As with patellar tendinosis, there may be features of allodynia or neuropathic pain either as a primary component or secondary to iatrogenic insult such as repeated injections.

Likewise, an individualized approach should be taken when managing this condition, aiming to optimize anatomical and biomechanical predisposition, increasing flexibility in the proximal thigh/hip girdle musculature where excessive 'tension' is a feature (Baker et al. 2011) or, alternatively, increasing hip abductor muscle activation and strength where the opposite predominates. Topical/oral analgesics or anti-inflammatory preparations may afford temporary pain relief but rarely assist with resolution. Sustained relief may be obtained with corticosteroids injected beneath the distal band into the inflamed tissues/synovial bursa/recess and, more recently, hyaluronic acid preparations have been used in a similar fashion with mixed anecdotal success and no supportive scientific studies to date.

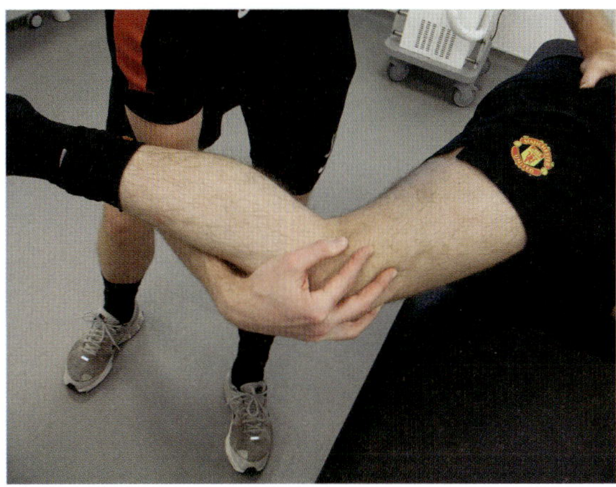

Figure 38.8a A variation of the classical Ober's test utilizing rotational stress in addition to knee flexion and extension while the hip is extended and adducted. A positive test is indicated by pain around the lateral epicondyle of the femur.

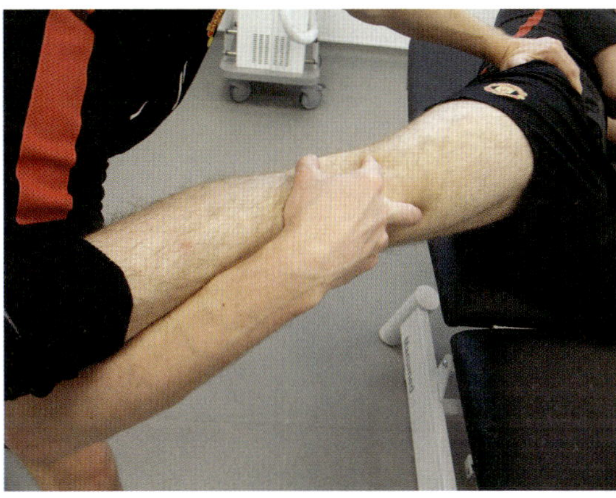

Figure 38.8b A variation of the classical Ober's test utilizing rotational stress in addition to knee flexion and extension while the hip is extended and adducted. A positive test is indicated by pain around the lateral epicondyle of the femur.

If imaging is undertaken (usually to exclude other pathology in recalcitrant cases), this usually shows little or no change in the band/fascial thickening itself, but signs of inflammation and/or disruption may be noted in the underlying connective tissue around the lateral synovial recess (Figure 38.9). Consideration must be given to changes that may be due to previous treatment interventions including injections.

Surgery has historically been reserved for the most resistant cases, with a lengthening procedure (Barber et al. 2007) affording positive outcomes, although not universally, which may be explained by

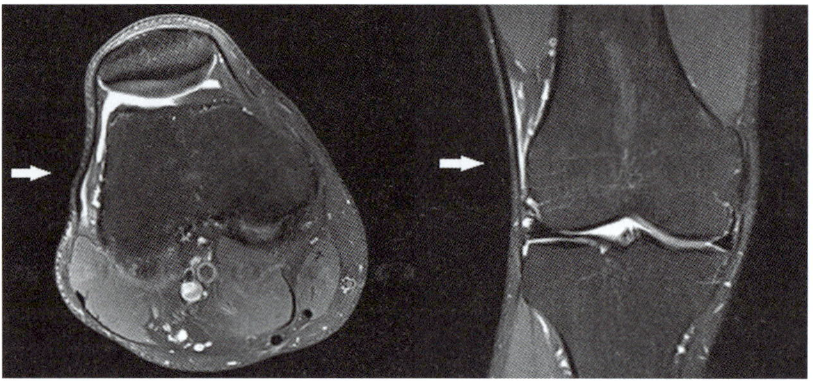

Figure 38.9 MRI appearances of chronic iliotibial band syndrome in a professional footballer; an area of intense high signal is seen deep to a structurally normal iliotibial band extending into the lateral retinaculum and distal fibres of vastus lateralis.

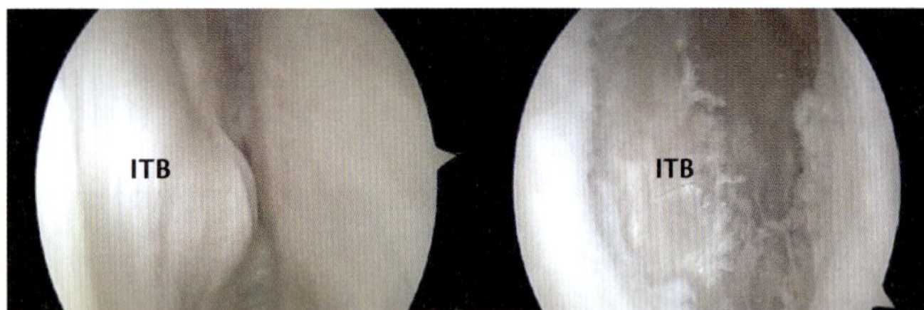

Figure 38.10 Arthroscopic appearances pre- and post-lateral gutter synovectomy procedure performed on the same patient shown in Figure 38.9. A soft tissue mass deep to the iliotibial band is clearly visualized on the left image; on the right image, following excision, the lateral gutter space has been increased thereby reducing impingement.

subsequent theory that the iliotibial band *should* be under a degree of tension in order to perform its knee-stabilizing function. Recent surgical preference has shifted to arthroscopic fenestration procedures whereby accumulation of inflamed tissue around the lateral synovial recess is resected (Figure 38.10), decompressing the area of impingement by the overlying band (Michels et al. 2009). Arthroscopy also allows exclusion of other intra-articular pathology and rarities such as lateral synovial cysts or sarcoma, which may mimic iliotibial band syndrome. There may be justification for considering such surgery earlier when treating an atypical case, in an elite athlete, where biomechanical and neurodynamic factors have been addressed.

Coronary (meniscotibial) ligament sprain

Traditionally thought to be an injury suffered by middle-aged recreational sportspersons undertaking sporadic, high-demand twisting and turning activities with less than ideal general conditioning, it is the experience of the author and others that this presentation is also seen in younger patients undertaking similar sporting pursuits (Hudes 2011), particularly if contact tackling is a feature. Coronary ligament injury often coexists with structural disruption to the collateral ligaments and/or menisci, particularly on the medial side of the knee, due to the close anatomical attachments between the medial capsule, deep portion of the collateral ligament, and the meniscus. Lateral coronary ligament sprains may also be associated with meniscal injury but less so with lateral collateral ligament injury as the structures are not in continuity. It is important to recognize the isolated coronary ligament injury (or those with minimal meniscal and collateral ligament involvement) as the management is almost universally non-surgical and prognosis more favourable.

Although the mechanism of injury is usually identical to that which causes structural derangement (i.e. rotation of a flexed knee against resistance or with the foot planted), the clinical signs differ in that there is usually little or no swelling and minimal loss of movement other than at end-range flexion. Precise, careful palpation may delineate tenderness to the tibial margin of the meniscus on the affected side, with pain on rotational stress or McMurray meniscal tests, but without the 'click' associated with unstable meniscus tears. The onset commonly occurs after an acute episode but may also present from chronic rotational stress, particularly in individuals with knee/foot malalignment.

Sonography is of limited value in assessing the isolated coronary ligament sprain (and also subtle meniscocapsular separation). MRI may be useful in excluding concomitant pathology, thereby raising confidence in a diagnosis of isolated sprain based on history and clinical examination, but is not helpful in detecting the lesion itself. Injection of contrast for MRI arthrography is probably not justifiable as management is not likely to alter as a result and the potential risk of iatrogenic infection from this procedure could be avoided.

Some cases may only be detected at arthroscopy (Lougher et al. 2003), performed following a period of chronic symptoms or in order to exclude internal derangement following inconclusive clinical or imaging assessment. Management, however, is virtually always conservative with full resolution expected within a few months by avoidance of provoking activities with correction of abnormal biomechanics, alongside standard anti-inflammatory modalities. Steroid/local anaesthetic injection around the chronically painful ligament may be useful and friction massage to break up adhesions from scarring will both desensitise pain and restore normal meniscal mobility.

References

Abdelrahman MH, Tubeishat S, Hammoudeh M. Proximal dissection and rupture of a popliteal cyst: a case report. *Case Rep Radiol* 2012; 292414. DOI: 10.1155/2012/292414.

Alvarez-Nemegyei J. Risk factors for pes anserinus tendinitis/bursitis syndrome: a case control study. *J Clin Rheumatol* 2007; 13(2):63–5.

Andrychowski J, Czernicki Z, Jasielski P. Schwannoma of the common peroneal nerve. A differential diagnosis versus rare popliteal cyst. [Article in Polish] *Neurol Neurochir Pol* 2012; 46(4):396–402.

van Ark M, Zwerver J, van den Akker-Scheek I. Injection treatments for patellar tendinopathy. *Br J Sports Med* 2011; 45(13):1068–76.

Arumilli B, Adeyemo F, Samarji R. Bilateral simultaneous complete quadriceps rupture following chronic symptomatic tendinopathy: a case report. *J Med Case Rep* 2009; 8(3):9031.

Aydingoz U, Oguz B, Aydingoz O, Comert RB, Akgun I. Infrapatellar bursitis in children with juvenile idiopathic arthritis: a case series. *Clin Rheumatol* 2011; 30(2):263–7.

Bae DK, Kwon OS. Snapping knee caused by the gracilis and semitendinosus tendon. A case report. *Bull Hosp Joint Dis* 1997; 56(3):177–9.

Baker RL, Souza RB, Fredericson M. Iliotibial band syndrome: soft tissue and biomechanical factors in evaluation and treatment. *PMR* 2011; 3(6):550–61.

Bandinelli F, Fedi R, Generini S, et al. Longitudinal ultrasound and clinical follow-up of Baker's cysts injection with steroids in knee osteoarthritis. *Clin Rheumatol* 2012; 31(4):727–31.

Barber FA, Boothby MH, Troop RL. Z-plasty lengthening for iliotibial band friction syndrome. *J Knee Surg* 2007; 20(4):281–4.

Beltran J, Matityahu A, Hwang K, et al. The distal semimembranosus complex: normal MR anatomy, variants, biomechanics and pathology. *Skeletal Radiol* 2003; 32(8):435–45.

Borrero CG, Maxwell N, Kavanagh E. MRI findings of prepatellar Morel-Lavallée effusions. *Skeletal Radiol* 2008; 37(5):451–5.

Bylund WE, de Weber K. Semimembranosus tendinopathy: one cause of chronic posteromedial knee pain. *Sports Health* 2010; 2(5):380–4.

Choi HR. Patellar osteomyelitis presenting as prepatellar bursitis. *Knee* 2007; 14(4):333–5.

Ciaschini M, Sundaram M. Radiologic case study. Prepatellar Morel-Lavallée lesion. *Orthopedics* 2008; 31(7):626, 719–21.

Cook JL, Purdam C. Is compressive load a factor in the development of tendinopathy? *Br J Sports Med* 2012; 46(3):163–8.

Dawn B, Williams JK, Walker SE. Prepatellar bursitis: a unique presentation of tophaceous gout in a normouricemic patient. *J Rheumatol* 1997; 24(5):976–8.

Dean BJ, Reed DW, Matthews JJ, et al. The management of solitary tumours of Hoffa's fat pad. *Knee* 2011; 18(2):67–70.

Distel E, Cadoudal T, Durant S, Poignard A, Chevalier X, Benelli C. The infrapatellar fat pad in knee osteoarthritis: an important source of interleukin-6 and its soluble receptor. *Arthritis Rheum* 2009; 60(11): 3374–7.

Drac P, Köcher M, Utikal P, Cerna M, Kozak J, Bachleda P. Cystic adventitial disease of the popliteal artery: report on three cases and review of the literature. *Biomed Pap Med Fac Univ Palacky Olomouc Czech Repub* 2011; 155(4):309–21.

Dragoo JL, Johnson C, McConnell J. Evaluation and treatment of disorders of the infrapatellar fat pad. *Sports Med* 2012; 42(1):51–67.

Fairclough J, Hayashi K, Toumi H, et al. The functional anatomy of the iliotibial band during flexion and extension of the knee: implications for understanding iliotibial band syndrome. *J Anat* 2006; 208(3):309–16.

Fujimoto H, Shimofusa R, Shimoyama K, Nagashima R, Eguchi M. Sarcoidosis presenting as prepatellar bursitis. *Skeletal Radiol* 2006; 35(1): 58–60.

Ghate SD, Deokar BN, Samant AV, Kale SP. Tumor like swellings arising from Hoffa's fat pad: a report of three patients. *Indian J Orthop* 2012; 46(3):364–8.

Giombini A, Dragoni S, Di Cesare A, Di Cesare M, Del Buono A, Maffulli N. Asymptomatic Achilles, patellar, and quadriceps tendinopathy: A longitudinal clinical and ultrasonographic study in elite fencers. *Scand J Med Sci Sports* 2011. DOI: 10.1111/j.1600-0838.2011.01400.x.

Guha AR, Gorgees KA, Walker DI. Popliteus tendon rupture: a case report and review of the literature. *Br J Sports Med* 2003; 37:358–60.

Helfenstein M Jr, Kuromoto J. Anserine syndrome. *Rev Bras Reumatol* 2010; 50(3):313–27.

Huang YC, Yeh WL. Endoscopic treatment of prepatellar bursitis. *Int Orthop* 2011; 35(3):355–8.

Hudes K. Two cases of medial knee pain involving the medial coronary ligament in adolescents treated with conservative rehabilitation therapy. *J Can Chiropr Assoc* 2011; 55(2):120–7.

Iguchi Y, Ihara N, Hijioka A, et al. Calcifying tendonitis of the gastrocnemius. A report of three cases. *J Bone Joint Surg Br* 2002; 84(3):431–2.

Ingabire MI, Deprez FC, Bodart A, Puttemans T. Soft tissue chondroma of Hoffa's fat pad. *JBR-BTR* 2012; 95(1):15–7.

Izumi M, Ikeuchi M, Tani T. Septic arthritis of the knee associated with calf abscess. *J Orthop Surg (Hong Kong)* 2012; 20(2):272–5.

Karataglis D, Papadopoulos P, Fotiadou A, Christodoulou AG. Snapping knee syndrome in an athlete caused by the semitendinosus and gracilis tendons. A case report. *Knee* 2008; 15(2):151–4.

Karkos CD, Sampath SA, Bury R, Mohandas P, Forrest L. Arteriovenous fistula of the lateral superior and inferior geniculate arteries. A unique cause of a recurrent prepatellar bursa. *Int Angiol* 2002; 21(3):280–3.

Köroğlu M, Callıoğlu M, Eriş HN, et al. Ultrasound guided percutaneous treatment and follow-up of Baker's cyst in knee osteoarthritis. *Eur J Radiol* 2012; 81(11):3466–71. DOI: 10.1016/j.ejrad.2012.05.015.

Larsson ME, Käll I, Nilsson-Helander K. Treatment of patellar tendinopathy—a systematic review of randomized controlled trials. *Knee Surg Sports Traumatol Arthrosc* 2012; 20(8):1632–46.

Lavine R. Iliotibial band friction syndrome. *Curr Rev Musculoskelet Med* 2010; 3(1–4):18–22.

Longo UG, Garau G, Denaro V, Maffulli N. Surgical management of tendinopathy of biceps femoris tendon in athletes. *Disabil Rehabil* 2008; 30(20–2):1602–7.

Lougher L, Southgate CR, Holt MD. Coronary ligament rupture as a cause of medial knee pain. *Arthroscopy* 2003; 19(10):E19–20.

De Maio F, Bisicchia S, Potenza V, Caterini R, Farsetti P. Giant intra-articular extrasynovial osteochondroma of the knee: a report of two cases. *Open Orthop J* 2011; 5:368–71.

Malinowski K, Synder M, Sibiński M. Selected cases of arthroscopic treatment of popliteal cyst with associated intra-articular knee disorders primary report. *Orthop Traumatol Rehabil* 2011; 13(6):573–82.

Mann KJ, Edwards S, Drinkwater EJ, Bird SP. A lower limb assessment tool for athletes at risk of developing patellar tendinopathy. *Med Sci Sports Exerc* 2012.

Marcheggiani Muccioli GM, Zaffagnini S, Tsapralis K, et al. Open versus arthroscopic surgical treatment of chronic proximal patellar tendinopathy. A systematic review. *Knee Surg Sports Traumatol Arthrosc* 2012.

Michels F, Jambou S, Allard M, Bousquet V, Colombet P, de Lavigne C. An arthroscopic technique to treat the iliotibial band syndrome. *Knee Surg Sports Traumatol Arthrosc* 2009; 17(3):233–6.

Neubauer H, Morbach H, Schwarz T, Wirth C, Girschick H, Beer M. Popliteal cysts in paediatric patients: clinical characteristics and imaging features on ultrasound and MRI. *Arthritis* 2011; 2011:751593.

Ogilvie-Harris DJ, Gilbart M. Endoscopic bursal resection: the olecranon bursa and prepatellar bursa. *Arthroscopy* 2000; 16(3):249–53.

Pascarella A, Alam M, Pascarella F, Latte C, Di Salvatore MG, Maffulli N. Arthroscopic management of chronic patellar tendinopathy. *Am J Sports Med* 2011; 39(9):1975–83.

Shenoy PM, Kim DH, Wang KH, et al. Calcific tendinitis of popliteus tendon: arthroscopic excision and biopsy. *Orthopedics* 2009; 32(2):127.

Singh VK, Shah G, Singh PK, Saran D. Extraskeletal ossifying chondroma in Hoffa's fat pad: an unusual cause of anterior knee pain. *Singapore Med J* 2009; 50(5):e189–92.

Sivasubramanian H, Ee G, Srinivasaiah MG, De SD, Sing A. 'Not always a Baker's cyst'—an unusual presentation of a central voluminous posteromedial meniscal cyst. *Open Orthop J* 2012; 6:424–8.

Smith J, Sayeed YA, Finnoff JT, Levy BA, Martinoli C. The bifurcating distal biceps femoris tendon: potential pitfall in musculoskeletal sonography. *J Ultrasound Med* 2011; 30(8):1162–6.

Spinner RJ, Desy NM, Agarwal G, Pawlina W, Kalra M, Amrami KK. Evidence to support that adventitial cysts, analogous to intraneural ganglion cysts, are also joint-connected. *Clin Anat* 2012. DOI: 10.1002/ca.22152.

Stahnke M, Mangham DC, Davies AM. Calcific haemorrhagic bursitis anterior to the knee mimicking a soft tissue sarcoma: report of two cases. *Skeletal Radiol* 2004; 33(6):363–6.

Subhawong TK, Eng J, Carrino JA, Chhabra A. Superolateral Hoffa's fat pad edema: association with patellofemoral maltracking and impingement. *Am J Roentgenol* 2010; 195(6):1367–73.

Tennent TD, Goradia VK. Arthroscopic management of calcific tendinitis of the popliteus tendon. *Arthroscopy* 2003; 19(4):E35.

Tibrewal SB. Acute calcific tendinitis of the popliteus tendon—an unusual site and clinical syndrome. *Ann R Coll Surg Engl* 2002; 84(5): 338–41.

Tosti R, Kelly JD IV. Pigmented villonodular synovitis presenting as a baker cyst. *Am J Orthop (Belle Mead NJ)* 2011; 40(10):528–31.

Turhan E, Doral MN, Atay AO, Demirel M. A giant extrasynovial osteochondroma in the infrapatellar fat pad: end stage Hoffa's disease. *Arch Orthop Trauma Surg* 2008; 128(5):515–9.

Visnes H, Bahr R. The evolution of eccentric training as treatment for patellar tendinopathy (jumper's knee): a critical review of exercise programmes. *Br J Sports Med* 2007; 41(4):217–23.

van Wilgen CP, Konopka KH, Keizer D, Zwerver J, Dekker R. Do patients with chronic patellar tendinopathy have an altered somatosensory profile? A quantitative sensory testing (QST) study. *Scand J Med Sci Sports* 2011. DOI: 10.1111/j.1600-0838.2011.01375.x.

van der Worp H, van Ark M, Roerink S, Pepping GJ, van den Akker-Scheek I, Zwerver J. Risk factors for patellar tendinopathy: a systematic review of the literature. *Br J Sports Med* 2011; 45(5):446–52.

Chapter 39

Superior tibiofibular joint

Mark Batt and Gurjit Bhogal

Anatomy of the superior tibiofibular joint

The superior tibiofibular joint is a diarthrodial plane joint between the medial facet of the head of the fibula and the tibial facet on the posterolateral tibial condyle. The joint has a synovial lining and is closely related to the common peroneal nerve which runs posteriorly. It is recognized that there is a connection between the tibiofemoral joint and superior tibiofibular joint in 10–60% of individuals (Bozkurt et al. 2004). However, recently, a study using computed tomography (CT) and magnetic resonance (MR) arthrograms has suggested that this connection is a more consistent anatomical feature (Puffer et al. 2013). Consequently, the superior tibiofibular joint is also known as the 'fourth compartment of the knee' (van Seymortier et al. 2008).

The joint has a fibrous capsule reinforced by anterior and posterior superior tibiofibular ligaments and tendinous insertions. The stronger anterior superior tibiofibular ligaments are comprised of three bands, meaning that the anterior capsule is thicker than the posterior capsule, whereas the posterior superior tibiofibular ligament is a relatively weak single band. Additional stability is provided superiorly by the lateral collateral ligament, inferomedially by the interosseous membrane, anterolaterally by the biceps femoris tendon, and posteriorly by the popliteus tendon. The arcuate ligament, the fabellofibular ligament, and the popliteofibular ligament also contribute to the structural stability of this region. The superior tibiofibular joint is, therefore, an inherently stable articulation, especially when the knee is extended.

There is considerable variation in superior tibiofibular joint size, shape, and orientation. Ogden classified the joint as either horizontal or oblique after studying 84 cadaveric and fresh post-mortem knee specimens (Ogden 1974a,b). He defined 20° of inclination as being the division between the horizontal and oblique types. The oblique orientation is characterized by relative immobility and a smaller joint surface, which diminishes in size as the angle of inclination increases (Ogden 1974a). Therefore, the oblique type of superior tibiofibular joint is more vulnerable to rotational forces and injury.

Biomechanics of the superior tibiofibular joint

The superior tibiofibular joint moves during the gait cycle. Ogden (1974a) described three key functions of the superior tibiofibular joint:

(1) dissipation of torsional stresses at the ankle

(2) dissipation of lateral bending moments of the tibia

(3) tensile, rather than compressive, weightbearing.

The fibula externally rotates and the joint glides laterally as the ankle dorsiflexes. Additionally, there is distal migration secondary to contraction of muscles attached to the fibula. The joint does not sit in the true sagittal plane, so the gliding motions are anterolateral and posteromedial, the latter occurring naturally as the knee extends in response to the pull of biceps femoris and the lateral collateral ligament.

Injuries to the superior tibiofibular joint

Injuries to the superior tibiofibular joint are relatively uncommon and are typically acute rather than chronic in nature. Such injuries should be considered in the differential diagnosis of all cases presenting with lateral knee pain. However, it is recognized that superior tibiofibular joint pathology is misdiagnosed, potentially reflecting a lack of knowledge of this joint and associated injury (Ellis 2003).

If the principal joint stabilizers, or joint itself, are injured from direct or indirect, acute or chronic trauma, laxity of the joint may ensue. Laxity may progress to instability of the joint causing subluxation or dislocation (Smith et al. 2010).

Ogden described four types of injury affecting the superior tibiofibular joint: subluxation only (type I), anterolateral (type II), posteriosuperior (type III), and superior (type IV). The anterolateral, or type II, injury is recognized as being the most common type (Ogden 1974b). The anterolateral (type II) and posteriosuperior (type III) types are the most likely to also have a peroneal nerve injury associated with them (Ellis 2003).

Acute injuries

The joint may be injured by direct or, more commonly, indirect trauma. Acute injuries tend to be clear-cut, although delayed presentation and complication can make assessment problematic.

Mechanism

Indirect injuries may occur in combination with fracture of the tibia, or fibula, or fracture–dislocation of the ankle (producing superior laxity), but, more commonly, in the sporting setting, they occur when an athlete falls on a flexed, adducted leg with ankle inversion. This latter sliding mechanism is seen with the sliding tackle in soccer or base-slides in baseball or softball, or following awkward falls in water-skiing or parachuting. In this position, the knee is flexed, relaxing the biceps femoris tendon and the lateral collateral ligament, and the ankle is inverted and plantarflexed, producing tension on the muscle origins of the anterolateral muscle compartments. When combined with an external rotation torque on the tibia, anterolateral instability ensues. Anterolateral subluxation or dislocation (type II) is much the more common type of instability, occurring in 90% of patients. Direct injury to the joint is less common than indirect injury and results from a direct blow to the flexed knee when in a sitting position, as in horse riding or jet-skiing. This produces posteromedial dislocation and carries higher morbidity due to associated peroneal nerve injury and persistent instability.

A self-limiting, typically bilateral, atraumatic subluxation is also described in adolescents with generalized ligamentous laxity. This tends to resolve with skeletal maturation. A further injury specific to this age group is an epiphyseal fracture of the proximal fibula.

Evaluation

An awareness of these injuries and their mechanism will facilitate their recognition. The description by the patient of symptoms referable to the knee may lead to confusion as pain, giving way, and locking may occur at both the knee and the tibiofibular joint. However, the lack of knee joint effusion is a clue to superior tibiofibular joint injury. Additionally, patients may complain of ankle problems in association with lateral knee pain. Physical examination is crucial, as patients' symptoms may be vague, without recollection of a specific injury episode. Acutely, there may be a tender swelling over the proximal fibula with associated hypermobility and pain. Forced dorsiflexion of the ankle may cause pain, and care should be taken to exclude common peroneal nerve damage. Open-chain knee flexion may be reduced and painful with a 'pinch' at end of range. Closed-chain knee flexion, as a single leg mini-dip, may be impaired because of pain and instability. Comparison should be made with the normal limb, as these signs may be soft. Specific plain radiograph views for the superior tibiofibular joint have been described, but instability is commonly demonstrated on bilateral anteroposterior and lateral views, without resort to internal rotation, oblique, or fluoroscopic views.

Treatment

Acute dislocations require closed reduction by manipulation, which produces pain relief and sometimes audible relocation. This is achieved by flexing the knee to 90° with the ankle dorsiflexed and everted. After reduction, the joint is generally stable, but casting in near full extension (non-weightbearing) for 3 weeks may aid healing and prevent recurrence. After the cast is removed, structured rehabilitation should be undertaken, avoiding early hamstring work in the case of posteromedial laxity. A counterforce brace may be used during rehabilitation to aid subsequent return to sport, which should be possible at 6–12 weeks.

Chronic injuries

Chronic injuries may arise as complications of acute injuries or *de novo* as overuse injuries. As there may be no clear history of trauma, the diagnosis of chronic superior tibiofibular joint injury may be challenging. The differential diagnosis is extensive, including lateral meniscus tear and cysts, popliteus tendonitis, iliotibial band syndrome, lateral collateral ligament sprain, posterolateral knee instability, arthritis, fabella syndrome, and ganglions. Chronic superior tibiofibular joint injuries described by Wong and Weiner include recurrent subluxation or dislocation, idiopathic subluxation, and proximal tibiofibular synostosis (Wong and Weiner 1978).

Mechanism

Idiopathic subluxation may occur as an overuse injury due to training errors, in association with adverse lower limb biomechanics resulting in excessive fibular rotation. Posteromedial subluxation results from stretching of the anterior capsule and ligaments of the superior tibiofibular joint in conjunction with sustained posterior pull of biceps femoris and soleus muscles.

Evaluation

Assessment of chronic laxity of the superior tibiofibular joint requires the knee to be flexed to 90° with relaxation of the hamstrings. Comparing with the contralateral side, the examiner then attempts to translate the fibular head anterolaterally.

Treatment

Taping or use of a counterforce brace may help the unstable joint. Physiotherapy to strengthen the biceps femoris and activity modification may also provide satisfactory results (Halbrecht and Jackson 1991). When this fails and chronic debilitating instability persists, a variety of surgical procedures to either excise or stabilize the fibular head have been advocated. No large series comparing different surgical procedures exists, making informed comparisons impossible (Shapiro et al. 1993; Weinert and Raczka 1986). Resection of the fibular head is avoided in athletes because of the requirement to reattach the lateral collateral ligament and biceps femoris tendon. Similarly, fusion of the joint is avoided to prevent subsequent ankle symptoms.

Other pathology of the superior tibiofibular joint

Other disorders at the superior tibiofibular joint may occur.

Osteoarthritis

Chronic instability can stress the joint such that degenerative change leads to osteoarthritis. Commonly, this occurs in conjunction with osteoarthritis of the knee, but can occur in isolation. Typical features of osteoarthritis may be evident on X-ray, like loss of joint space, osteophytes, and subchrondral sclerosis/cysts.

Ganglions

Ganglions are cystic lesions that can arise from muscle, tendon sheaths, and joints too (Miskovsky et al. 2004). Up to 20% of ganglia occur in the lower limb and approximately a third occurs around the knee (Rozbruch et al. 1998). They may enlarge and extend into the neighbouring soft tissues. Ganglia that arise from the superior tibiofibular joint can compress the peroneal nerve; therefore patients may complain of numbness and tingling affecting the lateral aspect of the lower limb (Miskovsky et al. 2004). If they are large, the mass may be visible. It is recognized that symptoms of anterior chronic exertional compartment syndrome may, rarely, be caused by ganglia from the superior tibiofibular joint (Ward and Eckardt 1994).

Neoplasms

Osteochondromas, osteoblastomas, and osteosarcomas are known to present around the knee. If patients present with 'red flag' signs and symptoms, including a rapidly enlarging painless mass, night pain, and constitutional symptoms, urgent investigation is recommended.

References

Bozkurt, M., Yilmaz, E., Akseki, D., Havitcioglu, H., and Gunal, I. (2004) The evaluation of the proximal tibiofibular joint for patients with lateral knee pain. *Knee*, 11, 307–12.

Ellis, C. (2003) A case of isolated proximal tibiofibular joint dislocation while snowboarding. *Emergency Medicine Journal*, 20, 563–4.

Halbrecht, J. L. and Jackson, D. W. (1991) Recurrent dislocation of the proximal tibiofibular joint. *Orthopaedic Review*, 20, 957–60.

Miskovsky, S., Kaeding, C., and Weis, L. (2004) Proximal tibiofibular joint ganglion cysts—excision, recurrence, and joint arthrodesis. *American Journal of Sports Medicine*, 32, 1022–8.

Ogden, J. A. (1974a) Anatomy and function of proximal tibiofibular joint. *Clinical Orthopaedics and Related Research*, 101, 186–91.

Ogden, J. A. (1974b) Subluxation of proximal tibiofibular joint. *Clinical Orthopaedics and Related Research*, 101, 192–7.

Puffer, R. C., Spinner, R. J., Murthy, N. S., and Amrami, K. K. (2013) CT and MR arthrograms demonstrate a consistent communication between the tibiofemoral and superior tibiofibular joints. *Clinical Anatomy*, 26, 253–7.

Rozbruch, S. R., Chang, V., Bohne, W. H. O., and Deland, J. T. (1998) Ganglion cysts of the lower extremity: an analysis of 54 cases and review of the literature. *Orthopedics*, 21, 141–8.

van Seymortier, P., Ryckaert, A., Verdonk, P., Almqvist, K. F., and Verdonk, R. (2008) Traumatic proximal tibiofibular dislocation. *American Journal of Sports Medicine*, 36, 793–8.

Shapiro, G. S., Fanton, G. S., and Dillingham, M. F. (1993) Reconstruction for recurrent dislocation of the proximal tibiofibular joint. A new technique. *Orthopaedic Review*, 22, 1229–32.

Smith, J., Finnoff, J. T., Levy, B. A., and Lai, J. K. (2010) Sonographically Guided Proximal Tibiofibular Joint Injection Technique and Accuracy. *Journal of Ultrasound in Medicine*, 29, 783–9.

Ward, W. G. and Eckardt, J. J. (1994) Ganglion cyst of the proximal tibiofibular joint causing anterior compartment syndrome—a case-report and anatomical study. *Journal of Bone and Joint Surgery—American Volume*, 76A, 1561–4.

Weinert, C. R. and Raczka, R. (1986) Recurrent dislocation of the superior tibiofibular joint—surgical stabilization by ligament reconstruction. *Journal of Bone and Joint Surgery—American Volume*, 68A, 126–8.

Wong, K. and Weiner, D. S. (1978) Proximal tibiofibular synostosis. *Clinical Orthopaedics and Related Research*, 135, 45–7.

Chapter 40

Exertional lower leg pain

Gurjit Bhogal and Mark Batt

'Shin splints' and exertional lower leg pain

Many athletes (especially runners) and their coaches, and some clinicians, still use the term 'shin splints' to describe presentations of exertional lower leg pain, usually affecting the medial border of the tibia. 'Shin splints' is a non-specific, unhelpful term which should not be used. We recognize now that there are many causes of shin pain (Table 40.1) which may present to the musculoskeletal physician, some of which specifically present or worsen while exercising. Shin pain, and exertional lower leg pain specifically, is a diagnostic challenge and thorough history taking and examination skills are vital for successful diagnosis.

This chapter will concentrate on three pathologies that we believe must be understood to allow effective evaluation and management of patients presenting with exertional lower leg pain. These three pathologies are:

Stress fractures

Medial tibial stress syndrome (MTSS)

Chronic exertional compartment syndrome (CECS)

Abnormal biomechanics, increase in activity levels, and lower limb strength and flexibility imbalances are implicated with these three pathologies. These factors should be considered in the evaluation of any patient with exertional lower leg pain.

Bony stress injury, MTSS, and CECS may co-exist, to greater or lesser degrees, in patients presenting with exertional lower leg pain. The musculoskeletal physician must be aware of this and identify all pathologies present. If they do not, pain may be persistent due to incomplete management.

Stress fractures of the lower leg

Tibial stress fractures

Stress fractures are common overuse injuries that may account for 5–10% of all sports injuries. Running or marching are the most reported causes of stress fracture in the literature and 31–51% of such diagnosed fractures occur at the tibia (Ha et al. 1991). The majority affect the postero-medial aspect of the tibia; however, those that affect the anterior cortex of the tibia are of major concern because they are prone to delay or non-union (Brukner 2000).

Stress fractures may occur due to bony fatigue, where abnormal stress is placed on to normal bone, or bony insufficiency, where normal stress on abnormal bone results in fracture (McCormick et al. 2012).

Stress fractures due to bone fatigue occur due to repetitive loading, typically occurring in the athlete or military recruit who suddenly increases training load and/or volume. The normal response of bone to repetitive loading is to undergo physiological remodelling; however, this may become pathological if inadequate rest occurs between loading. Here, bony resorption (osteoclastic activity) outstrips the formation of new bone (osteoblastic activity). This imbalance causes bone marrow oedema and microfractures. On magnetic resonance imaging (MRI) bone marrow oedema may be noted reflecting a 'bone stress reaction'. This stress reaction is symptomatic and often presents with localized bone pain. If repetitive loading continues with inadequate rest, a bone stress as reaction will progress to a stress fracture, where there is true cortical disruption (Beck 1998). The process described is part of a spectrum and it is incorrect to consider a stress fracture as an all or nothing event. It is better to consider the spectrum of bone stress as being from physiological remodelling through to frank cortical disruption.

Stress fractures due to bone insufficiency occur in individuals in whom their bone is of abnormal quality, usually meaning they have low bone mineral density. Bone mineral density is affected directly by in adequate nutrition and, in females, by hormonal changes, which may present as menstrual irregularity.

Risk factors

Females are at higher risk of stress fractures than men. Females have an even higher risk if they have irregular or no periods (amenorrhoea). Amenorrhoea may be due to excessive exercise. These women have relatively low circulating oestrogen due to disruption of release of hypothalamic hormones that normally stimulate oestrogen production. Oestrogen influences osteoclasts, so lack of it in amenorrhoeic women disrupts physiological remodelling of bone after loading (Lloyd et al. 1986).

There is no good-quality data to indicate conclusively that age is related to stress fracture risk; however, there are suggestions that increasing age may increase risk. Racial variations are poorly studied, although Caucasians appear to have the highest risk of stress fractures from the limited literature available (Brunet et al. 1990). Stress fractures occur at a higher incidence in inexperienced exercisers compared to those used to high levels of activity (Goldberg and Pecora 1994).

Table 40.1 Selected causes of 'shin pain'

Common	Less common	Rare
Periosteal contusion	Popliteal entrapment syndrome	Primary bone malignancy, e.g. osteosarcoma
Fracture of tibia/fibula	Nerve entrapments—superficial peroneal nerve	
Stress fracture*	Lumbar radiculopathy	
Medial tibial stress syndrome*	Referred from ankle joint	
Chronic exertional compartment syndrome*	Referred from superior tibiofibular joint	
	Osgood-Schlatter's apophysitis	
	Intermittent claudication	

*Important causes of exertional lower leg pain

Smoking is strongly associated with stress fractures (Reynolds et al. 1994). Vitamin D and calcium are known to be important in bone homeostasis. Relatively few studies have prospectively examined the affect of calcium and vitamin D supplementation on the incidence of stress fractures. Overall, available data suggests supplementation of 2000 mg of calcium and 800 IU of vitamin D daily may confer some protective benefit against stress fracture development (Lappe et al. 2008).

Identification and modification of biomechanical abnormalities have traditionally been an important part of stress fracture evaluation. Leg-length discrepancies, excessive dynamic hip adduction when running, hind-foot eversion, and 'knock knees' have all been identified as specific biomechanical abnormalities that are linked to tibial stress fractures.

A change of running surface, use of old running shoes, and hill running are all risk factors for the development of stress fractures (Brunet et al. 1990). Shock-absorbing insoles used within running shoes reduce the risk of tibial stress fracture (Jones et al. 2002). Excessive running is a further risk factor; however, there is little in the literature to guide us on how much is too much and optimal recovery time after training.

Presentation

Tibial stress fractures present with the progressive onset of tibial pain, usually associated with a history of increased physical activity. In about 15% of cases, these injuries may occur bilaterally (Matheson et al. 1987). A typical history of 'crescendo pain' is described and this is associated with examination findings of localized tibial tenderness made worse by percussion or hopping. Occasionally, erythema and swelling may be noted. Most patients present with postero-medial tibial pain, although a small subgroup presents with anterior mid-tibial pain. Anterior mid-tibial stress fractures are liable to progress to non-union, with pain localized to the anterior crest of the tibia. The patient history may reflect training errors in addition to unforgiving running surfaces, inappropriate shoes, dietary issues, and, in women, poor bone health from menstrual irregularity (Table 40.2).

Table 40.2 Key points that should be elicited in the history of those with confirmed or suspected bony stress injury

	Key points from the history
1.	Dietary history—eating habits, any suggestion of an eating disorder
2.	Training patterns—intensity, frequency, terrain, or equipment (e.g. running shoes)
3.	Menstrual history—oligo- or amenorrhoea

Investigations

The usefulness of various radiographic techniques in the diagnosis and confirmation of tibial stress fractures is dependent upon the time course of the injury. Radiographs are widely available and relatively cheap, and are therefore the most frequently used initial investigation in the assessment of exertional lower leg pain. However, radiographs are insensitive in detecting early bony stress response (1–4 weeks). Positive findings of periosteal response may be detected radiographically after as little as 4–6 weeks of pain and suggest higher-grade bony stress injury. Subsequent plain radiograph findings may include cortical hypertrophy, medullary canal narrowing, and periosteal elevation. Typically, anteroposterior and lateral projections will suffice, although, on occasions, oblique projections may provide additional periosteal information.

MRI is a sensitive modality in the detection of bony stress injury. MRI does not expose the patient to potentially damaging radiation and provides detail of the surrounding soft tissues, aiding diagnosis of exertional lower leg pain. These advantages make MRI a popular and standard modality for clinicians. Fredericson et al. developed a classification system which grades bony stress injury severity between grades 1 to 4 on the basis of MRI findings (Table 40.3) (Fredericson et al. 1995). Grade 4 injuries represent a complete stress fracture, while grades 1 to 3 represent stages of worsening bony stress injury. The higher the grade of bony stress injury, the longer the recovery period is likely to be (Table 40.3).

Computed tomography (CT) is sensitive at detecting cortical abnormalities, more so than MRI, and is therefore useful in confirming the diagnosis of a complete stress fracture. CT is poor at differentiating earlier bony stress injury, thereby limiting its use in early diagnosis of exertional lower leg pain.

Traditionally, triple-phase bone scan (TPBS) was regularly used. TPBS is a very sensitive modality detecting subtle changes in bone

Table 40.3 MRI grading of bony stress injury of the tibia with estimated rest and recovery time

MRI radiological grade	MRI findings	Typical recovery time
1	Mild periosteal oedema	3 weeks' rest
2	Periosteal oedema and marrow oedema on STIR sequences	3–6 weeks' rest
3	Periosteal oedema and marrow oedema on STIR and T1 sequences	12–16 weeks' rest
4	Visible fracture line	>16 weeks' rest

Source: Arendt and Griffiths 1997; Fredericson et al. 1995

metabolism and therefore early bony stress injury. However, TPBS has fallen out of favour because of poor specificity and radiation exposure (often in younger patients). TPBS may still have a role when MRI is not available, or when there is an imperative to know that there is no active bony remodelling.

Management

Treatment should focus on two inter-related areas: first, management of the bony stress injury/fracture; and second, investigation and correction of precipitants.

Fracture management should include a period of relative rest where the objective is to ensure the patient is pain-free. In some, this may mean a period of non-weightbearing rest with crutches. However, for many, the use of a pneumatic leg brace controls pain effectively allowing for pain-free activity. Healing is typically accelerated with the use of a pneumatic leg brace (Swenson et al. 1997). It is often used for 1 to 2 weeks until the patient is pain-free. When pain-free, the patient may begin weightbearing without the brace and undertake a graduated return to lower limb loading. These same braces may too help the healing of difficult anterior cortex non-union stress fractures, which previously were treated surgically (Batt et al. 2001).

During the period of fracture healing, cardiovascular fitness may be maintained with cross-training; the use of non-impact activities such as cycling is encouraged. Anti-inflammatory medications should be avoided due to their adverse effects on bone healing. Intrinsic and extrinsic precipitants of these overuse injuries, like nutritional, biomechanical, and menstrual factors should be sought and corrected. Some advocate the use of bone stimulation (electrical or ultrasonic) to accelerate healing; however, limited literature exists supporting its use. Rarely, surgery is required for recalcitrant cases.

Fibula stress fractures

Fibula stress fractures are commonly reported, accounting for 12–20% of stress fractures in runners and 8% in the military. They are also reported to occur in figure skating, aerobics, and ballet. Once dubbed the 'runner's fracture', fibula stress fractures most commonly occur in the distal third of the fibula, although they have been described in the proximal third too. These fractures present typically with a history of crescendo pain and localized tenderness. Often, biomechanical abnormalities such as excessive pronation/supination of the foot are present. With modified rest and a graduated return to full activity once pain-free, the prognosis for these fractures is good.

Medial tibial stress syndrome

Medial tibial stress syndrome (MTSS) typically presents with chronic symptoms of posteromedial tibial pain. It has an incidence of up to 35% in athletes (Moen et al. 2009). Various authors have described this posteromedial diffuse presentation and have used a number of different terms including medial tibial syndrome, tibial stress syndrome, and 'shin splints'. Traction on the posteromedial periosteum of the tibia by the muscles of the calf may cause pain. Older studies have suggested the tibialis posterior and flexor hallucis longus as being the muscles most likely to be causing the tractional periosteal pain; however, more recent studies have implicated the flexor digitorum longus and soleus (Beck and Osternig 1994). Debate exists whether traction on the periosteum truly produces inflammation and pain, and this aetiology inadequately explains symptoms in the lower third of the tibial diaphysis. Histological studies have been inconclusive.

Risk factors

Sub-optimal biomechanics during the mid-stance phase of running appears to excessively load the plantarflexors and invertors of the foot and ankle eccentrically, which attempt to control foot pronation. The soleus in particular, which forms the majority of the medial component of the Achilles tendon, forcefully contracts eccentrically.

Important instrinsic risk factors increasing the risk of MTSS include female gender, excessive pronation of the foot, increased inversion, eversion, and plantarflexion of the ankle, excessive internal and external rotation of the hips, higher body mass index (BMI), lower bone mineral density, and inexperienced exercisers (Burne et al. 2004; Hubbard et al. 2009; Viitasalo and Kvist 1983). Those that have increased medial longitudinal arch deformation dynamically while walking or statically while standing are also at higher risk of MTSS (Bandholm et al. 2008). Other risk factors implicated include muscle fatigue, excessive training workload, training on hard surfaces, and training in poor, inadequate footwear. However, no well-designed studies specifically support these risk factors.

Broadly, the risk factors described contribute directly, or indirectly, to sub-optimal biomechanics causing eccentric overload of the plantarflexors and invertors of the foot and ankle. Repetitive eccentric overload leads to chronic traction on the muscular insertions onto the posteromedial tibial periosteum, which causes MTSS.

Presentation

Patients typically present with chronic, or acute on chronic, symptoms of posteromedial tibial pain (usually middle-distal third) that is diffuse, linear, and often bilateral and occurs during exercise. Usually, the patient can initially complete their exercise session but pain is often worse the next morning. As the condition worsens, the pain may be present throughout exercise and be present during rest.

On examination, there is diffuse tenderness on palpation of the distal two-thirds of the posteromedial border of the tibia, with or without mild oedema.

Focal pain may suggest a bone stress injury rather than MTSS. MTSS may concurrently present with tibial bony stress injuries and chronic exertional compartment syndrome creating a mixed presentation (Figure 40.1) (Brukner 2000). Careful history taking and examination is important in allowing the clinician to identify whether multiple pathologies exist.

Investigations

Initially, if the symptoms and signs are typical of MTSS and no other coexisting pathologies are suspected, formal investigation prior to treatment may not be required. Investigations are requested if there is clinical doubt. Plain radiographs of the shin are usually first performed and are typically normal; rarely, periosteal reaction is noted on the posteromedial tibia. MRI is an extremely useful modality in the investigation of MTSS. The features seen correspond closely to a grade 1 or 2 bony stress injury, with oedema seen on fluid-sensitive sequences (Arendt and Griffiths 1997; Fredericson

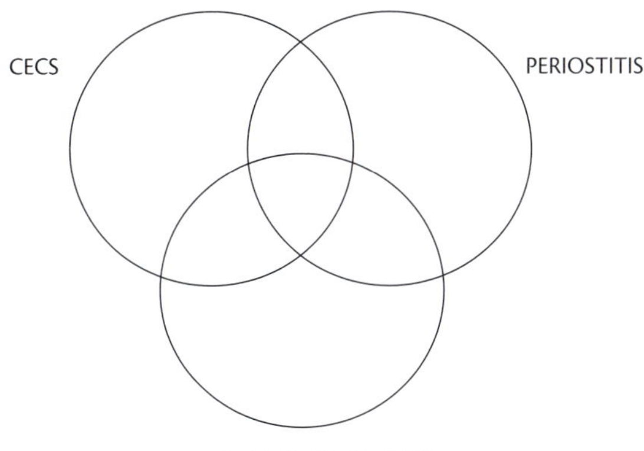

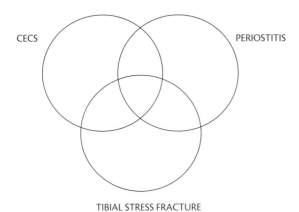

Figure 40.1 The interaction and overlap of the conditions that commonly cause exertional lower leg pain—namely, tibial stress fracture, chronic exertional compartment syndrome (CECS), and medial tibial stress syndrome (MTSS) (or 'periostitis').
(Reproduced with permission from Brukner, P. (2000) Exercise-related lower leg pain: an overview. *Medicine and Science in Sports and Exercise*, 32, S1–S3.)

et al. 1995). More severe MTSS presentations may also show periosteal, cortical, and bone marrow oedema, suggesting an overlap with bone stress reactions. Traditionally, TPBS was regularly used; however, MRI is recognized as having similar sensitivity and specificity and, as such, TPBS is now rarely performed.

It is worth noting that asymptomatic athletes may have MRI and TPBS findings in keeping with MTSS. Anderson et al. found 43% of the runners they studied had MRI features of MTSS despite being asymptomatic (Anderson et al. 1997). Indeed, 36% of the same runners studied, who had a clinical diagnosis of MTSS and had symptoms for over 46 months, had a normal MRI (Anderson et al. 1997). This further emphasizes that the history and examination are the most crucial aspects of the assessment of those with suspected MTSS.

High-resolution CT has also been evaluated in the diagnosis of MTSS and has been found to have high specificity but is rarely required with the widespread availability of MRI (Gaeta et al. 2006).

Management

Management of MTSS must include pain control, identification and optimization of risk factors, and training modification, although the evidence base is thin.

Rest, ice, compression, elevation, and oral analgesia often allow adequate pain control. For severe cases, a short period of immobilization in a pneumatic leg brace can help; however, studies have not found a significant benefit in their use. If weightbearing exacerbates pain, then low-impact cross-training, e.g. cycling, can help maintain cardiovascular fitness.

The risk factors should be identified and corrected if possible. Taping and orthotics have been used to control foot position by reducing excessive pronation. Few studies have shown a significant benefit. Loudon and Dolphino found that regular lower limb stretching and 'off the shelf' orthotics reduced MTSS symptoms by half in 3 weeks (Loudon and Dolphino 2010). The authors suggested that orthotics should be used as part of the management of MTSS.

Physical techniques to treat the pathology itself include fascial stripping with the use of ischaemic pressure, proprioceptive neuromuscular facilitation (PNF) stretching to optimize muscle lengths, and strengthening to improve the eccentric strength of the plantarflexors and invertors of the foot and ankle. Low-energy laser, ultrasound, iontophoresis, prolotherapy, and platelet-rich plasma injections have been tried but have no proven benefit. However, extracorporal shockwave (ECSW) therapy has some promising early results when combined with stretching and strengthening (Rompe et al. 2010).

Overall, it is unclear why patients improve, but it is thought that denervation may be responsible.

In recalcitrant cases, surgery which releases the structures along the posteromedial border of the tibia has proven successful (Jarvinnen et al. 1989), but is very rarely required. Effective denervation may be the reason why surgery has some positive results.

Chronic exertional compartment syndrome

The lower limb consists of four compartments, classically described as anterior, lateral, deep, and superficial posterior (Figure 40.2). The presence of separate posterior compartments is debated, and indeed some believe that tibialis posterior has its own fascial investment. Chronic exertional compartment syndrome (CECS) is defined as an 'overuse condition presenting as pain in the lower limb, associated with the muscles contained within the myofascial compartments of the shank' (Roberts and Franklyn-Miller 2012). CECS has been estimated as being the cause of exertional lower leg pain in up to 33% of cases (Styf 1988).

Traditionally, increased intra-compartmental pressure, within a closed compartmental space, causes reduced tissue perfusion and pain secondary to ischaemia (Black and Taylor 1993). However, increasingly, the precise pathophysiological mechanisms of CECS are uncertain. Some suggest that the symptoms of CECS are purely due to muscle overload (Franklyn-Miller et al. 2012). Others theorize that repetitive muscle overload within a compartment causes inflammation. This inflammation creates fibrotic hypertrophy of the fascia encasing a compartment, meaning the compartment itself becomes less compliant. Fascial defects have been implicated too and are noted in up to 40% of those diagnosed with CECS (Fronek

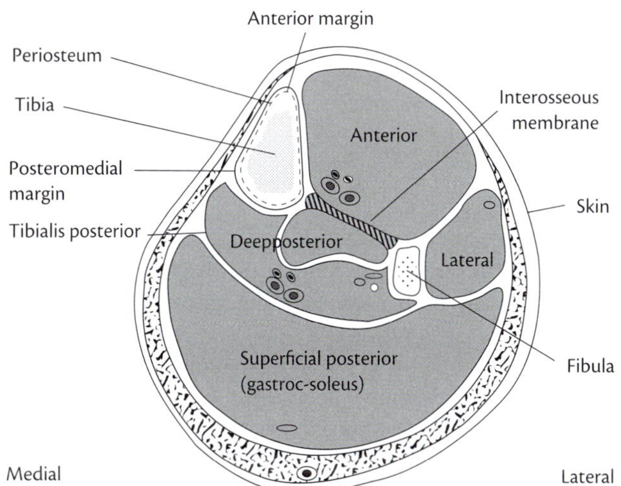

Figure 40.2 The cross-sectional anatomy of the lower leg.
(Reproduced with permission from Brukner, P. (2000) Exercise-related lower leg pain: an overview. *Medicine and Science in Sports and Exercise*, 32, S1–S3.)

et al. 1987). Some describe pain may be secondary to periosteal pain nociceptor involvement. Edmundsson et al. have published evidence to suggest the pathophysiology of CECS may be due to lower capillary density compared to muscle fibre size, as compared to asymptomatic controls, thereby causing reduced muscle microcirculation blood flow (Edmundsson et al. 2010).

There are reports in the literature of anterior, lateral, and deep posterior compartment syndrome. Chronic anterior compartment syndrome is most commonly reported and may be seen in running athletes as well as rowers. Lateral compartment syndrome is uncommon, and the existence of deep posterior compartment syndrome is subject to considerable debate.

Table 40.4 Comparison of three diagnostic criteria for intracompartmental pressure values for the diagnosis of chronic exertional compartment syndrome

Values	Reid	Pedowitz	Styf
At rest	>30 mmHg	>15 mmHg	Unreliable
1 min after exertion	>60 mmHg	—	>30–35 mmHg
2 min after exertion	>20 mmHg	>30 mmHg	—
5 min after exertion	—	>20 mmHg	>Rest values

Source: Pedowitz et al. 1990; Reid 1992; Styf 1995

Presentation

Those presenting with CECS are usually running athletes or military personnel under 30 years old. Males and females are affected equally and often symptoms are experienced bilaterally in the lower legs. The pain from anterior/lateral compartment syndrome is usually felt in the anterolateral aspect of the lower leg. The pain from the superficial deep compartment is often felt through the upper mid-posterior lower leg, while pain is isolated typically in the medial shin for deep posterior compartment syndrome (Blackman 2000).

The pattern of pain of CECS is different from that of a stress fracture. Crucially, there is no pain at rest, and significant relief on cessation of activity. The pain experienced by the patient with a stress fracture typically continues significantly after activity, whereas patients with CECS have initially an ache, burning, or tightness within the lower limb that develops into severe crescendo pain which typically resolves rapidly on stopping activity. A mild ache often persists post exercise. The recurrence of exertional pain in CECS when re-exercising is predictable. Occasionally, weakness or paraesthesia may be an additional presenting feature on exertion.

Classically, examination at rest is normal. Examination after activity that triggers symptoms may reveal muscle tenderness, areas of muscular tightness, or small muscle herniations. Neurological examination may identify motor weakness or areas of decreased sensation if a nerve passing through a compartment is affected.

Commonly, CECS may coexist with MTSS and/or bony stress injury (Brukner 2000), so clinical signs of MTSS or bony stress injury may be elicited too. The clinical signs of MTSS and bony stress injury are reviewed earlier in this chapter.

Investigations

Various investigations have been described in the literature to diagnose CECS. These include intracompartmental pressure measurements, ultrasound (Lynch et al. 2009), and spectroscopy (van den Brand et al. 2004). Typically, intracompartmental pressure measurements are undertaken to confirm the diagnosis of CECS and have traditionally been considered the gold standard in CECS investigation.

Measurement of intracompartmental pressure may be achieved via a variety of techniques including injection, infusion, non-infusion, and pressure transducer (Styf 1989). Along with this variability of standardized technique, there is wide variability in the protocol used to exercise the patient to reproduce their pain. Some recognized protocols include supine with resisted plantarflexion, calf raises, treadmill walking, and treadmill running. Table 40.4 shows a comparison of three different diagnostic criteria that have been described for CECS. It is difficult to meta-analyse normal and abnormal pressure recordings in the literature, as different equipment and techniques may give rise to different sets of baseline and exercise data. Furthermore, different lower leg compartments produce different results. Generally, only anterior compartment measurements are reliable, while the validity of deep posterior compartment measurements is uncertain (Styf 1988).

The wide variation in technique, protocol, and diagnostic criteria to measure intracompartmental pressure mean the process is not robustly reliable as universal standards do not exist. Hislop and Batt have comprehensively summarized the limitations of intracompartmental pressure measurements elsewhere (Hislop and Batt 2011). Further work must be done to truly mean intracompartmental measurements are the 'gold standard' investigation in the diagnosis of CECS.

Management

In the past, if abnormal pressures were measured within one or more compartments, the patient would be routinely referred for fasciotomy, with or without fasciectomy. Typically, this provides good results, with symptomatic relief and lowering of intracompartmental pressures. Before surgery, patients should be warned that there will be scarring of the legs and, in addition, some bulging of the released muscle compartment. However, with the lack of robust reliability of the technique, protocol, and diagnostic criteria to measure intracompartmental pressure, authors have suggested an initial conservative approach to management should be adopted prior to surgery (Roberts and Franklyn-Miller 2012).

Conservative management includes soft tissue massage, transverse frictions/dry needling of trigger points, modifying exercise workload, addressing strength and flexibility imbalances, and optimizing the patient's biomechanics. The biomechanical assessment should be done both statically and dynamically, while observing the patient running.

Biomechanical overload syndrome

Franklyn-Miller et al. have recently described a new clinical term for the presentation of exertional lower limb pain, namely 'biomechanical overload syndrome' (2012). This group have described CECS as due to muscle overload within one of the four compartments of the lower leg producing symptoms. They analysed running technique, rather than immediately proceeding to surgery, and attempt to coach a preferred running method, to reduce compartmental muscular overload. The authors favoured a mid-foot strike, over heel strike, in those with anterior compartment syndrome (Franklyn-Miller et al. 2012). Diebal has also found pain and function improve with this running method in those with anterior CECS (Diebal et al. 2012). A full description of this syndrome is found elsewhere (Franklyn-Miller et al. 2012); however, they also suggest MTSS may improve significantly with running analysis and re-education.

Bony stress injury, MTSS, and CECS may coexist in cases of exertional compartment syndrome (Figure 40.1) and sub-optimal biomechanics, especially when running, is a common aetiological factor in all three conditions, as previously described in this chapter. It follows, therefore, that running analysis and re-education may be an important aspect of the management in the majority of cases of exertional lower leg pain. However, further research must be conducted to confirm conclusively the effect of running re-education.

Other pathologies of exertional lower leg pain

Popliteal artery entrapment

This unusual syndrome occurs when there are changes in the usual arrangement of the anatomy of the popliteal artery and the medial head of gastrocnemius, and surrounding soft tissues, as the artery exits the popliteal fossa. Variations in the anatomy have been described (Figure 40.3) (Levien and Veller 1999). Patients are usually young men involved in physical activity who complain of progressive posterior lower leg exertional pain. Depending on the anatomy, walking may produce more profound symptoms than running, reflecting a more sustained gastrocnemius contraction trapping the popliteal artery. The majority of authors have described the progressive posterior lower leg pain on exertion as ischaemic in nature, producing a similar presentation as intermittent claudication and reflecting arterial entrapment. However, others feel that the pain perceived is neural in nature and reflects nerve, not artery, compression causing impingement against the lateral soleal fascia that forms a narrowed exit from the popliteal fossa (Turnipseed and Pozniak 1992). Consequently, the exact pathophysiology is still debated and some prefer the term 'popliteal entrapment' rather than 'popliteal artery entrapment'.

Initially, screening may be undertaken by duplex ultrasound, which is reliable and non-invasive, and ankle brachial index, which may be performed in 'stress positions' (forced plantar/dorsiflexion positions) to provoke popliteal entrapment. MR angiography is an important investigation, which can be performed in the 'stress positions' described, thereby providing information not only on arterial patency and flow, but also on the surrounding soft tissues.

The treatment of this condition involves release of the involved soft tissues and repair of the arterial lumen where appropriate. The prognosis depends on the anatomy and degree of arterial damage.

Fascial hernias

Most fascial defects are asymptomatic. They are most commonly seen involving the tibialis anterior, but may involve other compartments. Their occurrence is often associated with venous perforations of the fascia or at the site of the exit of the superficial peroneal nerve. Such fascial defects may give rise to symptoms, and indeed have been reported to be present in 20–60% of patients with chronic anterior compartment syndrome and 5% of patients with anterior lower leg pain from other causes (Styf 1989). Herniations may only become evident with physical activity and may result from muscle hypertrophy following intense training. They typically present as a painful tender mass that appears after activity, which is reducible. If bothersome, they are best treated by longitudinal fasciotomy of the compartment (Berlund and Stocks 1993). Closure of the fascial defects causing the local muscle herniation is not recommended as this may lead to decreased compartment size and subsequent compartment syndrome (Miniaci and Rorabeck 1986).

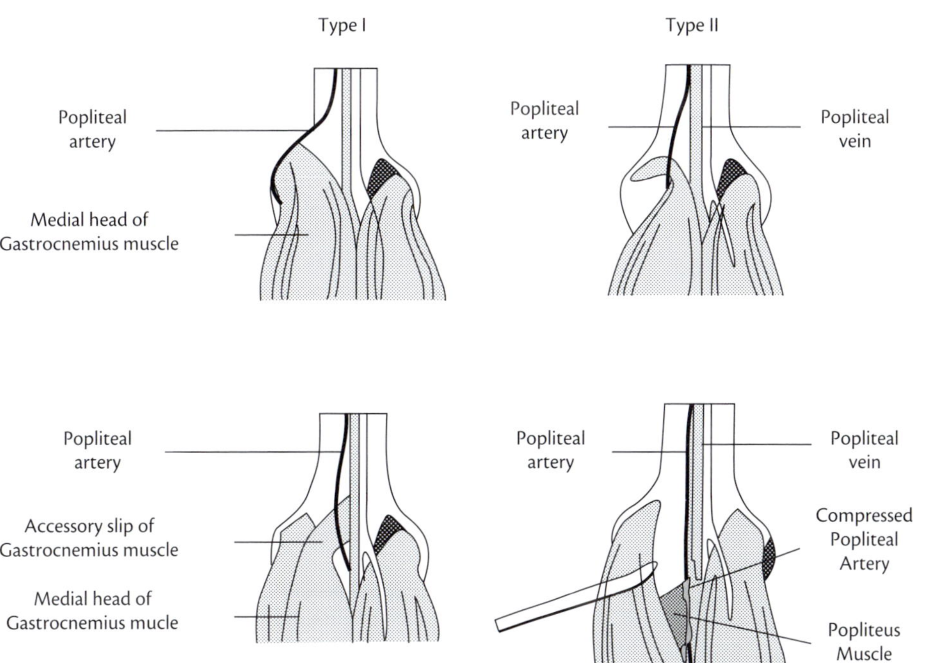

Figure 40.3 Classification of popliteal artery entrapment syndrome.
(Reproduced with permission from Levien, L. J. and Veller, M. G. (1999) Popliteal artery entrapment syndrome: more common than previously recognized. *Journal of Vascular Surgery*, 30, 587–598.)

Nerve entrapments

Peripheral nerve entrapments may give rise to lower leg pain and should be considered as part of the differential diagnosis of exertional lower leg pain. In a large series of patients with complaints of lower extremity pain with suspected lumbar radiculopathy, peripheral nerve entrapments were found as a sole cause of leg pain in over 1% of this group; 50% also had concomitant back pain. The peroneal nerve was the most commonly involved, followed by femoral and tibial nerves (Saal et al. 1988). Compression of the superficial peroneal nerve may be associated with a fascial defect and muscle herniation, or an anomalous course of a nerve. It may also arise after ankle sprain, or as a complication following fasciotomy of the anterior compartment (Styf 1989). Superficial peroneal nerve entrapment is characterized by sensory disturbance over the dorsum of the foot during exercise and some positional dysaesthesia at rest. The latter symptom is of particular diagnostic importance, as compartment syndrome never begins before exercise commences. There may be localized discomfort over the anterior intermuscular septum with an associated positive Tinel's sign. Pain may occur when the ankle joint is passively dorsiflexed and supinated. Evaluation of nerve conduction velocities may improve diagnostic specificity and is recommended prior to decompression. Surgical release of the lateral compartment may provide relief of symptoms in up to 50% of cases.

References

Anderson, M. W., Ugalde, V., Batt, M., and Gacayan, J. (1997) Shin splints: MR appearance in a preliminary study. *Radiology*, 204, 177–80.

Arendt, E. A. and Griffiths, H. J. (1997) The use of MR imaging in the assessment and clinical management of stress reactions of bone in high-performance athletes. *Clinics in Sports Medicine*, 16, 291–306.

Bandholm, T., Boysen, L., Haugaard, S., Zebis, M. K., and Bencke, J. (2008) Foot medial longitudinal-arch deformation during quiet standing and gait in subjects with medial tibial stress syndrome. *Journal of Foot & Ankle Surgery*, 47, 89–95.

Batt, M.E., Kemp, S., and Kerslake, R. (2001) Delayed Union stress fractures of the anterior tibia (Conservative management). *Br J Sports Med*, 35, 74–7.

Beck, B. R. (1998) Tibial stress injuries—an aetiological review for the purposes of guiding management. *Sports Medicine*, 26, 265–79.

Beck, B. R. and Osternig, L. R. (1994) Medial tibial stress syndrome—the location of muscles in the leg in relation to symptoms. *Journal of Bone and Joint Surgery–American Volume*, 76A, 1057–61.

Berlund, H. and Stocks, G. (1993) Muscle hernia in a recreational athlete. *Orthopedic Reviews*, 11, 1246–8.

Black, K. P. and Taylor, D. E. (1993) Current concepts in the treatment of common compartment syndromes in athletes. *Sports Medicine*, 15, 408–18.

Blackman, P. G. (2000) A review of chronic exertional compartment syndrome in the lower leg. *Medicine and Science in Sports and Exercise*, 32, S4–S10.

van den Brand, J. G. H., Verleisdonk, E. J. M. M., and van der Werken, C. (2004) Near infrared spectroscopy in the diagnosis of chronic exertional compartment syndrome. *The American Journal of Sports Medicine*, 32, 452–6.

Brukner, P. (2000) Exercise-related lower leg pain: an overview. *Medicine and Science in Sports and Exercise*, 32, S1–S3.

Brunet, M. E., Cook, S. D., Brinker, M. R., and Dickinson, J. A. (1990) A survey of running injuries in 1505 competitive and recreational runners. *Journal of Sports Medicine and Physical Fitness*, 30, 307–15.

Burne, S. G., Khan, K. M., Boudville, P. B., et al. (2004) Risk factors associated with exertional medial tibial pain: a 12 month prospective clinical study. *British Journal of Sports Medicine*, 38, 441–5.

Diebal, A. R., Gregory, R., Alitz, C., and Gerber, J. P. (2012) Forefoot running improves pain and disability associated with chronic exertional compartment syndrome. *American Journal of Sports Medicine*, 40, 1060–7.

Edmundsson, D., Toolanen, G., Thornell, L. E., and Stal, P. (2010) Evidence for low muscle capillary supply as a pathogenic factor in chronic compartment syndrome. *Scandinavian Journal of Medicine & Science in Sports*, 20, 805–13.

Franklyn-Miller, A., Roberts, A., Hulse, D., and Foster, J. (2012) Biomechanical overload syndrome: defining a new diagnosis. *British Journal of Sports Medicine*. 48, 415–416.

Fredericson, M., Bergman, A. G., Hoffman, K. L., and Dillingham, M. S. (1995) Tibial stress reaction in runners—correlation of clinical symptoms and scintigraphy with a new magnetic-resonance-imaging grading system. *American Journal of Sports Medicine*, 23, 472–81.

Fronek, J., Mubarak, S. J., Hargens, A. R., et al. (1987) Management of chronic exertional anterior compartment syndrome of the lower-extremity. *Clinical Orthopaedics and Related Research*, 220, 217–27.

Gaeta, M., Minutoli, F., Vinci, S., et al. (2006) High-resolution CT grading of tibial stress reactions in distance runners. *American Journal of Roentgenology*, 187, 789–93.

Goldberg, B. and Pecora, C. (1994) Stress-fractures—a risk of increased training in freshmen. *Physician and Sports Medicine*, 22, 68–78.

Ha, K. I., Hahn, S. H., Chung, M. Y., Yang, B. K., and Yi, S. R. (1991) A clinical study of stress fractures in sports activities. *Orthopedics*, 14, 1089–95.

Hislop, M. and Batt, M. E. (2011) Chronic exertional compartment syndrome testing: a minimalist approach. *British Journal of Sports Medicine*, 45, 954–5.

Hubbard, T. J., Carpenter, E. M., and Cordova, M. L. (2009) Contributing factors to medial tibial stress syndrome: a prospective investigation. *Medicine and Science in Sports and Exercise*, 41, 490–6.

Jarvinnen, M., Aho, H., and Niittymaki, S. (1989) Results of the surgical-treatment of the medial tibial syndrome in athletes. *International Journal of Sports Medicine*, 10, 55–7.

Jones, B. H., Thacker, S. B., Gilchrist, J., Kimsey, C. D., and Sosin, D. M. (2002) Prevention of lower extremity stress fractures in athletes and soldiers: a systematic review. *Epidemiologic Reviews*, 24, 228–47.

Lappe, J., Cullen, D., Haynatzki, G., Recker, R., Ahlf, R., and Thompson, K. (2008) Calcium and vitamin D supplementation decreases incidence of stress fractures in female navy recruits. *Journal of Bone and Mineral Research*, 23, 741–9.

Levien, L. J. and Veller, M. G. (1999) Popliteal artery entrapment syndrome: more common than previously recognized. *Journal of Vascular Surgery*, 30, 587–98.

Lloyd, T., Triantafyllou, S. J., Baker, E. R., et al. (1986) Women athletes with menstrual irregularity have increased musculoskeletal injuries. *Medicine and Science in Sports and Exercise*, 18, 374–9.

Loudon, J. K. and Dolphino, M. R. (2010) Use of foot orthoses and calf stretching for individuals with medial tibial stress syndrome. *Foot & Ankle Specialist*, 3, 15–20.

Lynch, J. E., Lynch, J. K., Cole, S. L., Carter, J. A., and Hargens, A. R. (2009) Noninvasive monitoring of elevated intramuscular pressure in a model compartment syndrome via quantitative fascial motion. *Journal of Orthopaedic Research*, 27, 489–94.

Matheson, G. O., Clement, D. B., Mckenzie, D. C., Taunton, J. E., Lloydsmith, D. R., and Macintyre, J. G. (1987) Stress fractures in athletes—a study of 320 cases. *American Journal of Sports Medicine*, 15, 46–58.

Mccormick, F., Nwachukwu, B. U., and Provencher, M. T. (2012) Stress fractures in runners. *Clinics in Sports Medicine*, 31, 291–306.

Miniaci, A. and Rorabeck, C. H. (1986). Compartment syndrome as a complication of repair of a hernia of the tibialis anterior—a case-report. *Journal of Bone and Joint Surgery–American Volume*, 68A, 1444–5.

Moen, M. H., Tol, J. L., Weir, A., Steunebrink, M., and De Winter, T. C. (2009) Medial tibial stress syndrome: a critical review. *Sports Medicine*, 39, 523–46.

Pedowitz, R. A., Hargens, A. R., Mubarak, S. J., and Gershuni, D. H. (1990) Modified criteria for the objective diagnosis of chronic compartment syndrome of the leg. *American Journal of Sports Medicine*, 18, 35–40.

Reid, D. (ed.) (1992) *Sports injury assessment and rehabilitation*. New York: Churchill Livingstone.

Reynolds, K. L., Heckel, H. A., Witt, C. E., et al. (1994) Cigarette smoking, physical fitness, and injuries in infantry soldiers. *American Journal of Preventive Medicine*, 10, 145–50.

Roberts, A. and Franklyn-Miller, A. (2012) The validity of the diagnostic criteria used in chronic exertional compartment syndrome: a systematic review. *Scandinavian Journal of Medicine & Science in Sports*, 22, 585–95.

Rompe, J. D., Cacchio, A., Furia, J. P., and Maffulli, N. (2010) Low-energy extracorporeal shock wave therapy as a treatment for medial tibial stress syndrome. *American Journal of Sports Medicine*, 38, 125–32.

Saal, J. A., Dillingham, M. F., Gamburd, R. S., and Fanton, G. S. (1988) The pseudoradicular syndrome: lower extremity peripheral nerve entrapment masquerading as lumbar dadiculopathy. *Spine*, 13, 926–30.

Styf, J. (1988) Diagnosis of exercise-induced pain in the anterior aspect of the lower leg. *American Journal of Sports Medicine*, 16, 165–9.

Styf, J. (1989) Chronic exercise-induced pain in the anterior aspect of the lower leg—an overview of diagnosis. *Sports Medicine*, 7, 331–9.

Styf, J. R. (1995) Intramuscular pressure measurements during exercise. *Operative Techniques in Sports Medicine*, 3, 243–9.

Swenson, E. J., Dehaven, K. E., Sebastianelli, W. J., Hanks, G., Kalenak, A., and Lynch, J. M. (1997) The effect of a pneumatic leg brace on return to play in athletes with tibial stress fractures. *American Journal of Sports Medicine*, 25, 322–8.

Turnipseed, W. D. and Pozniak, M. (1992) Popliteal entrapment as a result of neurovascular compression by the soleus and plantaris muscles. *Journal of Vascular Surgery*, 15, 285–94.

Viitasalo, J. T. and Kvist, M. (1983) Some biomechanical aspects of the foot and ankle in athletes with and without shin splints. *American Journal of Sports Medicine*, 11, 125–30.

Chapter 41

Biomechanics of the foot and ankle

Bryan English and Nat Padhiar

Introduction to the biomechanics of the foot and ankle

Understanding the biomechanics of the foot and ankle is of great importance when considering musculoskeletal complaints of the lower limb in particular. The search for structural pathology may be a fruitless exercise if the underlying aetiology is a functional problem. Because of the complexity of the structure, the biomechanics are different from individual to individual. In effect, the biomechanics of the foot are as unique as a fingerprint.

The foot and ankle consists of 26 bones, 57 joints, 32 muscles, and a network of ligaments. This complex has to work harmoniously to create bipedal ambulation. Any alteration in the biomechanics will result in an alteration of forces throughout the lower kinetic chain (the lower limb) that predominantly functions as a closed kinetic chain (i.e. the foot is in contact with the floor), and not as an open chain like the upper limb (i.e. the hand being free and not 'fixed' on a surface). This alteration of forces will therefore affect and possibly disrupt the biomechanics of the rest of the body. If the body is unable to adapt to an alteration or disturbance in biomechanics, then a normal or an abnormal compensation will take place somewhere in the chain. An abnormal compensation will lead to injury.

The foot/ankle complex provides:

- support and adaptation to terrain/surface
- balance
- shock absorbency, with differing landfall patterns depending on the activity
- force production/propulsion in a multitude of directions.

The forces that have to be absorbed in this area consist of:

- the body weight and the effects due to gravity
- the ground reaction force, i.e. the force that is generated by the ground against the body (Newton's third law: 'To each action there is an equal and opposite reaction')
- compressive forces applied across the complex due to muscle contraction producing a co-contraction of forces assisting in stability.

These forces are amplified up to five times during running. In a pes cavus foot type, which is a rigid structure and therefore a poor shock absorber, the ankle (which is the size of a postage stamp) has to absorb the force. This illustrates one of the functions of articular cartilage.

Before discussing the biomechanics, some terminology must be introduced:

- *rear foot*: loose term usually meaning the hind and midfoot, or purely as the calcaneus when viewed from behind
- *hindfoot*: the talus and the calcaneus
- *midfoot*: the navicular, cuboid, and cuneiforms
- *forefoot:* the metatarsal 'rays' and the phalanges.

Positions of the foot

Figures 41.1 and 41.2 show various rear and forefoot positions. Note that the terminology is used as though the foot is a vertical continuum of the lower leg (and not at right angles to the coronal/frontal plane; Figure 41.3). Therefore, abduction of the foot occurs in the transverse plane and not in the coronal plane, as is the case with abduction of the lower leg.

- Varus and valgus positions of the foot occur in the coronal plane.
- Inversion and eversion are the terms of movement that create a rear foot varus and valgus respectively, and therefore they occur in the coronal plane.
- Plantarflexion and dorsiflexion of the foot occur in the sagittal plane.
- Abduction and adduction of the foot occur in the transverse plane.

Pronation and supination

- A *supinated foot* is a rigid lever. This form is useful for stability and 'push off' and consists of plantarflexion combined with inversion and adduction of the foot. The appearance is of a high arched foot.

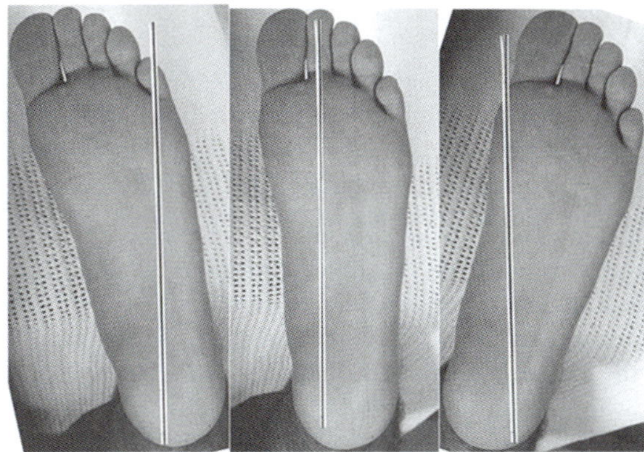

Figure 41.1 Positions of the left foot in the transverse plane: (left) adducted; (middle) midline; (right) abducted. The normal axis of the foot passes through the second ray. The diagrams should be visualized as though looking at the right lower limb from behind.

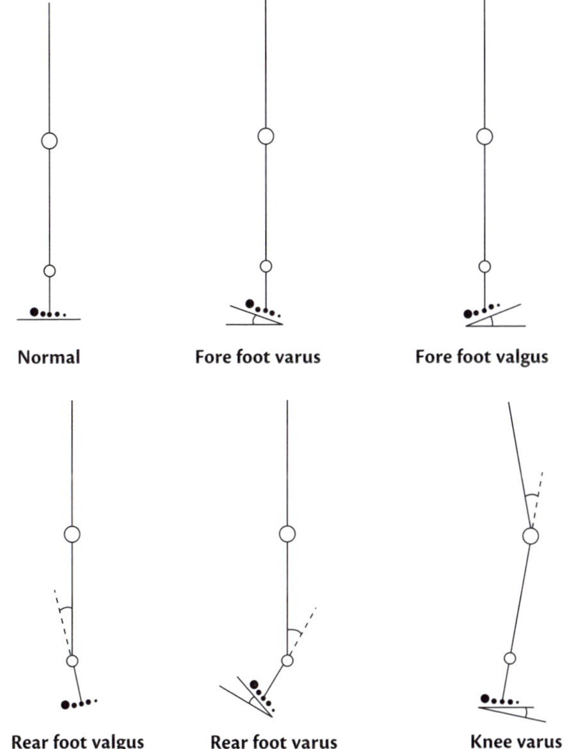

Figure 41.2 Varus and valgus positions of the foot.

- Pronation consists of dorsiflexion, eversion, and abduction of the foot. The *pronated foot* is a loose 'bag of bones', acting as an effective shock absorber. The appearance is of a flat foot.

Joint axes within the foot and ankle

This section provides a guide to the complexities involved within the moving foot. The reader should also appreciate how orthotic or surgical interference of the structure and mechanics of the foot will lead to an alteration of this refined system. A normal or abnormal adaptation may then take place. (Note that figures quoted for the angle of the axis of a joint are generalized, because of the variability of human structure.)

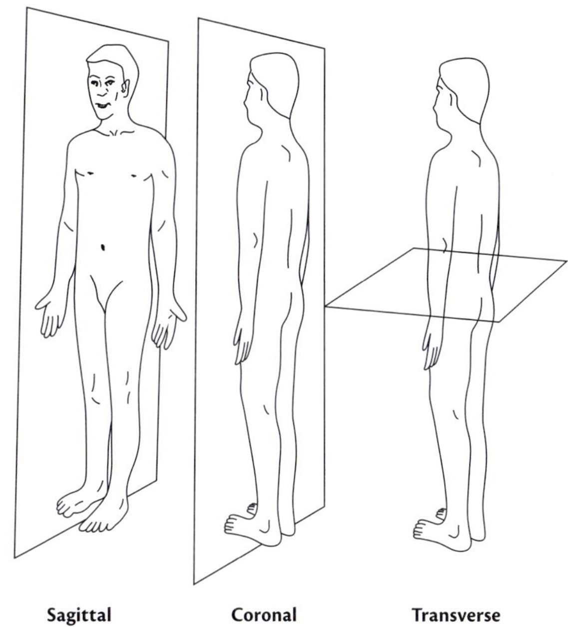

Figure 41.3 Anatomical positions.

- The complexity of lower limb biomechanics is partly predetermined by the axis of each joint as well as the levers that act across the joint.
- The closer a joint is to a body plane, the less movement will take place in that plane.
- The axis of the ankle joint descends at a 20° angle in the frontal plane, from the medial malleolus, through the talus, to the tip of the lateral malleolus. Therefore, dorsiflexion (20°) of the ankle joint is accompanied by abduction of the foot. Plantarflexion (45°) is accompanied by adduction of the foot.

Subtalar joint

The subtalar joint has a triplanar axis (as it does not run in any of the cardinal axes of the body). This runs from the posterolateral–plantar aspect to the anteromedial–dorsal aspect. It is angled at 16° medially from the sagittal plane, 42° upwards from the transverse plane, and, therefore, 48° and 74° from the frontal plane (Figure 41.4).

The only movement that is measurable, from a clinical point of view, is the degree of inversion and eversion (functionally, this is a rear foot varus and valgus respectively) that occurs (in the coronal plane).

Talo–calcaneo–navicular complex

This has a similar axis to the subtalar joint. The inclination and anterior angle is 40°, with a medial deviation of 30° from the sagittal plane. This axis allows pronation and supination to occur.

Transverse tarsal complex

This is an S-shaped structure created by the talonavicular joint and the calcaneocuboid joint. There are two axes about which the foot

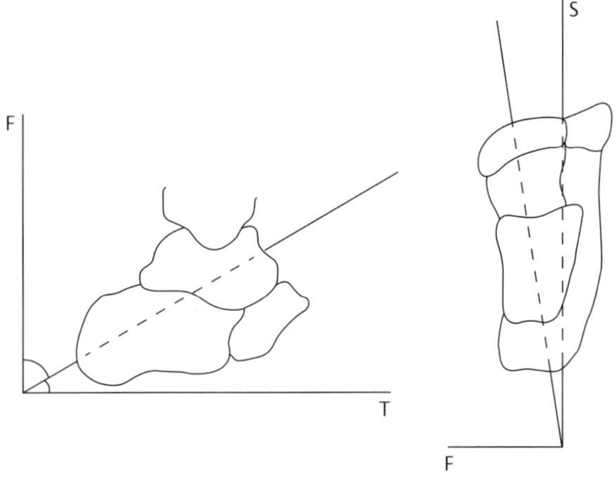

Figure 41.4 The triplanar axis of the subtalar joint.

pronates and supinates: the longitudinal axis, which inclines upwards and medially in the anteroposterior direction, and the oblique axis, which is at a similar angle to that of the talo–calcaneo–navicular joint.

When weightbearing, the cuboid does not move, but the calcaneus and talus move on the navicular and cuboid. Movement at the transverse tarsal complex, which can contribute up to one third of the pronation and supination of the talo–calcaneo–navicular complex, is dependent on subtalar position.

Tarsometatarsal joints and metatarsals (rays)

- The first three rays involve the first three metatarsals and the medial, intermediate, and lateral cuneiforms respectively. The fourth and fifth metatarsals form joints with the cuboid.
- The axis of the first ray is oblique and allows dorsiflexion with inversion and adduction, and plantarflexion with eversion and abduction. The fifth ray has an oblique axis nearly perpendicular to that of the first; hence, the movements are opposite in that dorsiflexion will be accompanied by eversion and abduction, plantarflexion with inversion and adduction.
- The second and fourth metatarsals have axes that are less oblique in that they are more perpendicular to the longitudinal axis of the foot. The axis of the third ray is perpendicular, so the movement is predominantly into plantar and dorsiflexion.
- The second tarsometatarsal joint is wedged in between the three cuneiforms and the first and third metatarsal. This is useful for stability, but may result in increased stress going through the second metatarsal (especially if it is longer than the first metatarsal, as in a Morton's foot) and the resulting susceptibility to a stress fracture (March fracture).

Metatarsophalangeal joints

These allow abduction and adduction. However, plantar and dorsiflexion are the main movements, creating the hinge type of movement during ambulation. The windlass mechanism involving these joints and the plantar fascia are discussed in the section on heel pain.

Arches of the foot

- The medial longitudinal arch is higher 'off the ground' and more flexible than the lateral arch. This flexibility allows pronation. The arch is supported by the bony configuration as well as the soft tissues, thereby creating a degree of elastic recoil as the foot returns to supination.
- The transverse arch is perpendicular to the longitudinal arch, and is most obvious in the mid- and forefoot. The bony configuration of the cuneiforms and the cuboid creates a concavity of the rays on the plantar aspect of the foot. This allows a fan-like spread of the forefoot during weightbearing, which contributes towards shock absorbency.

Muscles of the foot

- There are 13 extrinsic muscles and 19 intrinsic muscles of the foot. The details of their relative actions on the foot are discussed in greater detail elsewhere in this chapter.
- The extrinsic muscles of the posterior compartment act as plantarflexors (mainly via the gastrocnemius, soleus) and toe flexors (flexor digitorum longus and flexor hallucis longus), and provide stability to the ankle and the longitudinal arch (tibialis posterior).
- The lateral compartment muscles act as evertors of the foot and ankle; the peroneus longus also acts as a plantarflexor at the midtarsal joint.
- The anterior compartment muscles act as dorsiflexors of the foot (tibialis anterior) and extensors of the toes (extensor hallucis longus and extensor digitorum longus). The tibialis anterior contributes to inversion of the foot, extensor hallucis longus to eversion.
- The intrinsic muscles provide specific movements; for example, the flexor hallucis brevis flexes the proximal phalanx of the great toe, and its tendons house the sesamoid bones. The extensor digitorum brevis extends the medial four toes at the proximal phalanx.

Biomechanical analysis of the foot and ankle

The neuromuscular structures control foot and ankle movement about a predetermined axis. This can be assessed kinematically and kinetically, and has been extensively investigated and analysed in humans. The following paragraphs provide a brief generalization of the biomechanics that may be observed.

People vary a great deal in relation to how their foot comes into contact with the ground. For example, most runners will strike the ground with the heel, followed by distribution of force throughout the foot prior to toe off. This is called a *heel–toe technique* and will be used as the example in the following paragraphs. Other patterns include a *forefoot technique* (where the heel does not actually strike the floor, but descends sufficiently to allow eccentric stretch of the ankle dorsiflexors) and a *toe–heel–toe technique* (with the initial strike taking place at the midfoot or forefoot).

A functional model

The heel strikes the ground on the lateral border of the heel. The supinated foot, with an inverted rear foot, starts to pronate. The degree of pronation will be dictated by the subtalar joint. If no movement occurs here, then the only way the foot can pronate is by internal rotation of the lower leg. The subtalar joint is a *torque convertor* (see section on the subtalar joint). Movement here will unlock the foot for pronation and lock the foot for supination.

- As foot pronation occurs, there is internal rotation of the lower leg. This rotation increases if there is limited subtalar joint movement. This internal rotation results in a functional knee valgus and an increase in the Q angle of the knee (see Chapter 37).
  - Most causes of bilateral anterior knee pain are due to a high Q angle that is increased by excessive pronation.
- Excessive subtalar movement will put increased stress on the medial aspect of the ankle and/or lower leg.
  - Insertional tendonitis of the tibialis posterior and/or medial shin pain may be due to excessive pronation, with the action of the tibialis posterior being overcome by the body weight and the ground reaction force.
- Excessive pronation will also put increased stress on the medial aspect of the Achilles tendon.
  - Palpate the sore tendon of a distance runner. If the tendon is just tender medially, then excessive pronation is probably the cause of the excess strain.
- As the excessively pronated foot with limited subtalar movement and functional knee valgus now attempts to supinate, the lower leg will start to externally rotate, while the femur wants to stay internally rotating to create knee extension.
  - Could there be a mistiming of thigh on lower leg movements here? Is the knee being forced to perform a pivot shift manoeuvre? Is this a possible reason why 80% of anterior cruciate ligaments tear as a result of non-contact injuries?
- With the foot excessively pronated with a functional knee valgus, the abductor muscles of the buttock are attempting to abduct the adducted thigh.
  - Is pronation, aided by excessive weight, the reason why the sedentary population suffer from lateral buttock pain?
- Due to the aforementioned effects of pronation, functional shortening of the lower leg can occur causing a strain to the pelvis, lumbar spine, and beyond.
  - If people get pain in the lower back and lower limb that is aggravated by exercise, have a look at the lower limb biomechanics, i.e. examine them while they are experiencing their pain and not just standing or lying on a couch when they have told you that these positions do not cause pain.

All these components will be magnified with increased activity such as running. So often, we are dealing with functional problems caused by a functional and/or structural problem within the foot.

Kinematics

Kinematics can be defined as the branch of mechanics concerned with the motion of objects without reference to the forces which cause the motion.

Gait can be broken down to a stance phase and a swing phase (Figure 41.5). The stance phase lasts for approximately 65% of the gait cycle in walking. This percentage decreases with running. The phase consists of heel strike, flat foot, mid stance, heel off, and toe off. Each section of the phase is dependent on many factors such as foot anatomy, type of footwear, and type of surface.

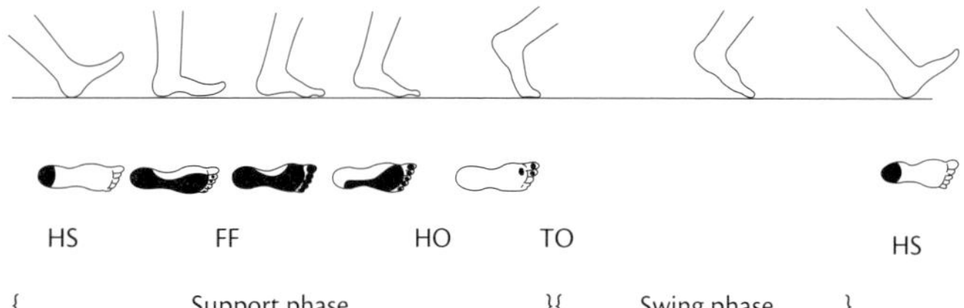

Figure 41.5 Gait cycle.

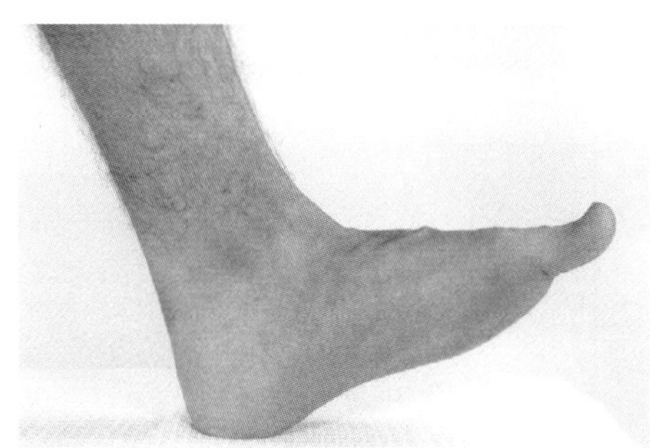

Figure 41.6 Heel strike.

Heel strike

Most muscular activity as the foot adapts to the surface occurs in the first 15% of the cycle that follows heel strike (Figure 41.6).

The graphs in Figure 41.7 are a simple representation of the activity within the peroneus longus, gastrocnemius, and tibialis anterior muscles during the cycle. The heel strikes the ground in a more or less vertical plane. The vectors of the ground force reaction are mentioned later in this chapter in the discussion of force plate studies.

The heel strikes on the lateral border of the rear foot as the leg is swinging towards the line of progression (external rotation of the thigh to counteract the transverse plane rotation of the pelvis, and also the foot is supinated at this point). Wearing out of the lateral border of a shoe is therefore a normal phenomenon. Soon after heel strike, the rear foot starts to move from an inverted towards an everted position, thus producing fairly rapid pronation (a useful way to absorb shock).

Flat foot

As pronation is starting to occur when approaching flat foot (Figure 41.8a), the lower leg is starting to internally rotate (due to the torque convertor effect of the subtalar joint). The timing of the joint movements during this phase is important as the foot adapts to the surface. Internal rotation of both the femur and tibia on a partly flexed knee incorporates more force down on to the talus, encouraging more pronation and an 'unlocking' of the foot.

After *mid stance* (where the lower leg is perpendicular to the ground), ankle dorsiflexion produces a degree of locking of its mortise. The lower leg starts to externally rotate on the ankle, resulting in a return towards supination (Figure 41.8b).

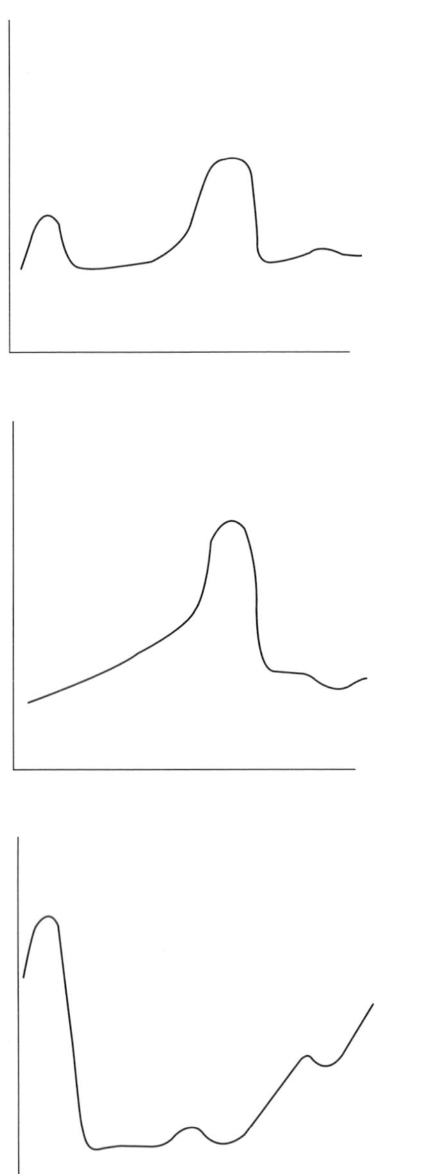

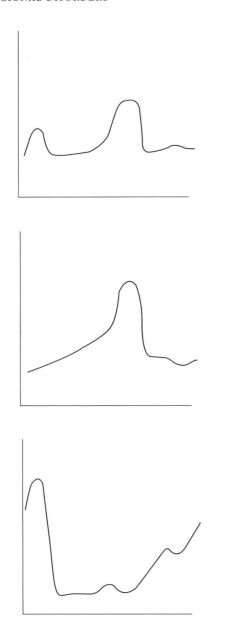

Figure 41.7 (Top) The activity of the peroneus longus, which is active at heel strike and toe off, acting as a stabilizer to the ankle joint; (middle) the gastrocnemius acting eccentrically during weightbearing before maximal activity at toe off; (bottom) initial high eccentric activity of the tibialis anterior to prevent foot slap and activity during the swing phase to keep the foot off the ground.

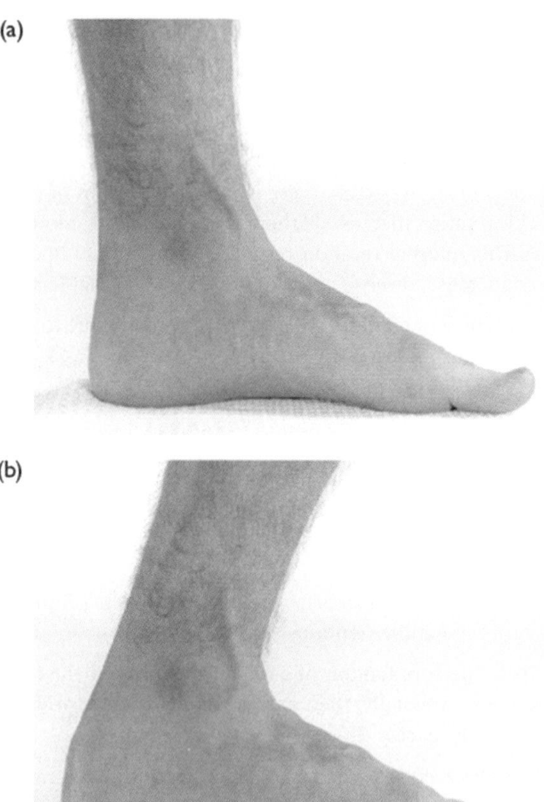

Figure 41.8 (a) Flat foot; (b) ankle dorsiflexion in flat foot.

Heel off

Plantarflexion is initiated along with dorsiflexion of the metatarsophalangeal joints which stretches the plantar fascia encouraging increased supination (Figure 41.9). This more rigid foot is ideal for the propulsive action that is about to take place. Ideally, the heel is in the neutral position at this stage to prevent excessive forces occurring on either the medial aspect (if the foot remains in pronation) or the lateral aspect (rapid movement over to supination with an inverted rear foot). *Toe off* is the end of the stance phase (Figure 41.10), and usually occurs at the great toe.

Swing phase

The main concern during this phase is to prevent the foot from catching the floor, so the ankle returns from a highly plantarflexed position at toe off, to a dorsiflexed position in the middle of the swing phase.

Normally, the ankle is in a more stable dorsiflexed position before heel strike. However, when landing from a jump, 80% of individuals have the foot plantarflexed. This position allows the foot and ankle to absorb the increased force of landing from a height (Valiant and Cavanagh 1985).

Figure 41.11 shows stick diagrams representing the biomechanics of a left lower limb viewed from the front (running towards the reader):

(a) a 4° forefoot varus, 4° rear foot valgus, and 8° tibial varus at heel strike;

(b) for the foot to reach the floor, 8° of rear foot valgus will be required, resulting in increased internal tibial rotation;

(c) the foot may start to supinate with tibial external rotation, while the femur is still internally rotating to create knee extension;

(d) the foot may remain pronated, so knee extension is possible only with increased internal rotation of the femur (i.e. self-inflicted pivot shift manoeuvre).

Is this a possible reason for the 'mistiming' of joints, considering that many ligamentous injuries to the knee are non-contact injuries? Using the aforementioned model, would an orthotic controlling rear and forefoot movement have a beneficial effect on abnormal knee rotation?

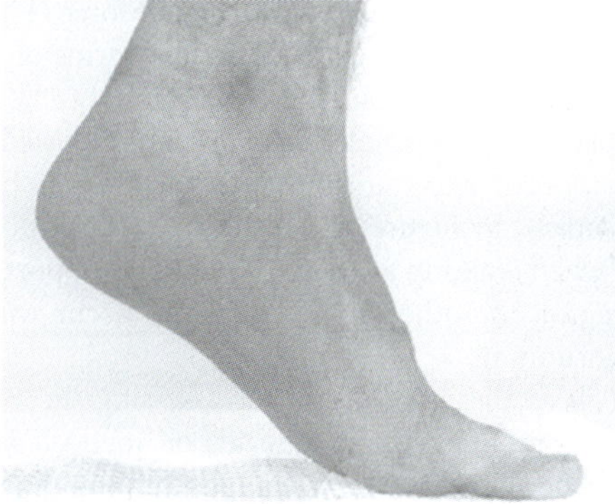

Figure 41.9 Heel off.

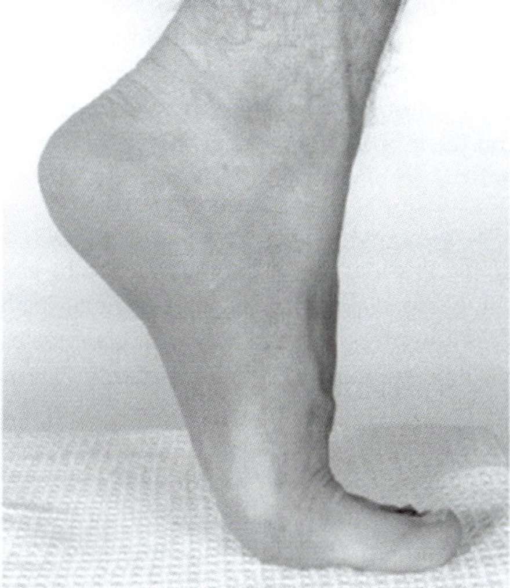

Figure 41.10 Toe off.

Methods for measuring kinematics

- *Observation*: Inexpensive, but very subjective.
- *Multiple exposure*: Inexpensive basic camera required with reflective markers on the patient. Gait cannot be observed.
- *Cinematography/television*: Relatively inexpensive cine camera with video playback analysis. The most commonly employed system for the clinician. Body markers may be placed on bony anatomical landmarks (to minimize the movement of the soft tissues), or the body can be marked with ink. This analysis, in its basic form, is subjective to an extent and useful for high-speed sporting activities, but tedious frame by frame visualization of playback is required if statistical analysis is to take place (in which case body markers need to be used). However, computer software systems are now available that will digitize from a video with markers.
- *Television/computer*: Expensive. Cameras emit infrared light on to reflective body markers, and the reflection is received by the same camera. Six cameras appear to be the minimum required for sophisticated analysis of all the body planes and ensuring that the body markers are always visible.
- *Active marker systems*: These markers emit their own characteristic signal so the cameras can easily tag each marker separately. A power source has to be carried by the patient.

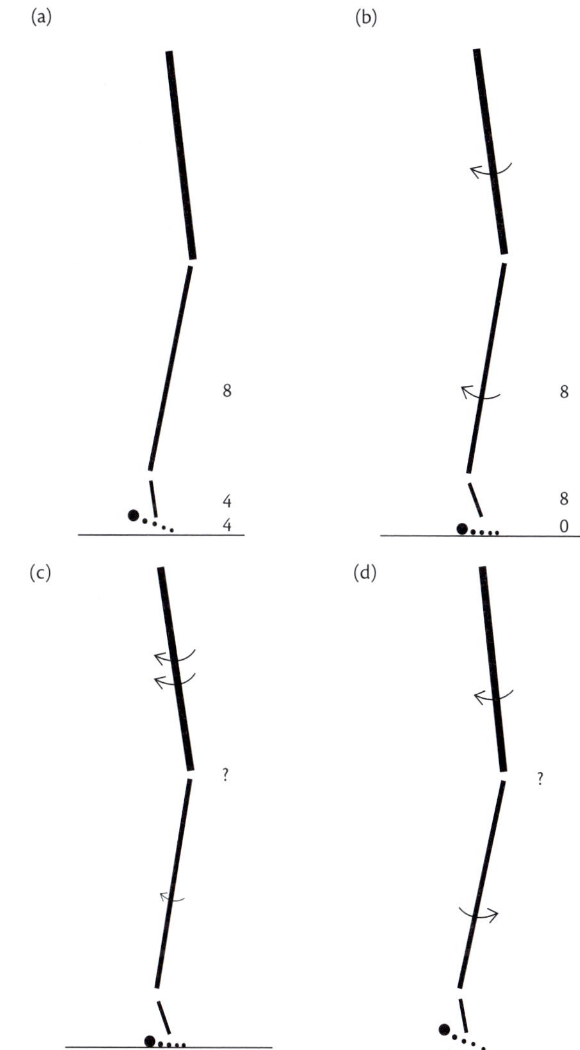

Figure 41.11 The biomechanics of a left lower limb (see text for details).

Kinetics

Kinetics can be defined as the branch of mechanics concerned with the motion of bodies under the action of forces.

Lower limb kinetics can be complex. It is still very much in the realms of research, and could form the subject of an entire textbook. The following few paragraphs are aimed at the clinician, as an introduction to the possibilities of scientific assessment and how these are best applied in the clinical setting.

When requesting dynamic computer-assisted analysis, it is best for the clinician to request that specific clinical questions be answered if at all possible. Scientific analysis will produce vast reams of data that may overcomplicate the situation if they are not communicated well for the benefit of the patient (Hamill and Knutzen 1995).

Types of force

Internal forces: muscle action; friction between soft tissues; elastic/stored energy

External forces: gravity; ground reaction force; external friction

Ground reaction force

This force can be measured with a rectangular force plate/platform which is embedded into the floor, so the patient is unaware that they are walking upon the 'chosen' surface. The plate has pressure transducers at each corner. Data collected will be the magnitude, direction, line of action, and point of application of the ground reaction force.

Newton's third law (quoted earlier) states that to each action there is an equal and opposite reaction. The force of the body hitting the floor is met by an equal and opposite ground reaction force. Since

$$\text{force} = \text{mass} \times \text{acceleration}$$

the ground force measured is, therefore, a measure of the acceleration of the centre of mass of the body (the mass being easily determined by body weight).

Vertical, horizontal, and translational forces can be measured (Figure 41.12). The vertical force (*FY*) is usually the greatest force and includes the effects due to gravity. The horizontal force (*FX*) includes forces in the direction of movement plus frictional forces. The translational force (*FZ*) is the sideways movement that occurs on contact with the ground, and obviously this also consists of a frictional force (enabling the body to change directions quickly without the foot slipping).

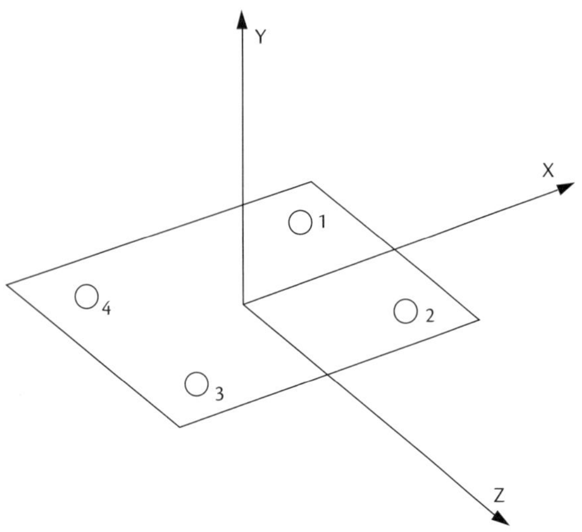

Figure 41.12 Measuring forces in three dimensions.

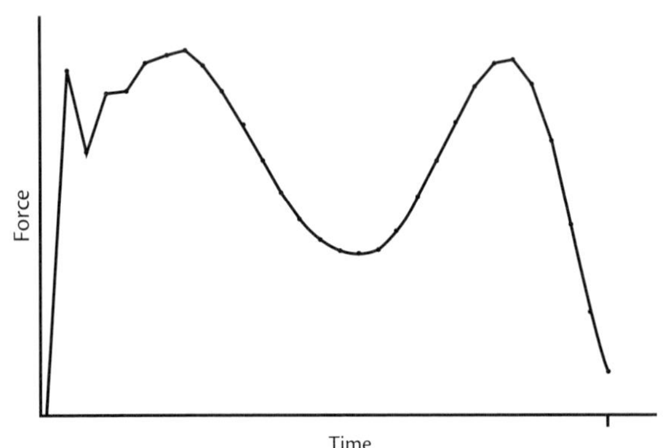

Figure 41.13 Ground reaction force.

The resulting graphs of the ground reaction force (Figure 41.13) are characteristic for human gait and certain forms of foot strike. With a heel strike, for example, there is an initial spike as the foot 'strikes' the plate (this is termed a passive peak) followed by a curve as the whole foot contacts the ground (this active peak being under muscular control). In Figure 41.13, the active peak occurs twice. This occurs when walking as there is a double support phase (i.e. weightbearing on the other leg). It does not occur with a stance phase during running.

Graphs such as these are useful for assessing the effectiveness of an amputee gait, for example (affected or unaffected limb). The prosthesis can be altered to recreate a relatively normal ground reaction force. These diagrams are not useful in determining what part of the foot is undergoing pressure, after the initial contact.

Excessive force on heel strike may also be a reason for athletic-induced injuries; for example, basketball players who land with a flat foot after a jump have been observed to produce a ground reaction force up to 30% greater than those who land toe to heel. Admittedly, one cannot rule out the effects of inertia (the effect that gravity has on the limb), but there may be a problem of technique. Runners can have problems with this, especially after an injury.

Vector forces

Knowing the direction of the forces that have to be absorbed is of particular value, especially when considering gait analysis of athletes as well as amputees and patients with cerebral palsy. Vector diagrams can be extrapolated to form 'butterfly diagrams' (directions of force throughout the stance phase) (Figure 41.14). These are useful to determine when the body's centre of gravity comes across the midline.

A vector is a force with a direction. In vector diagrams such as Figure 41.15, the length of the line is proportionate to the degree of force, relative to the other lines of the diagram (hence the line R is longer than *v* and *h*). For example, according to the equation of

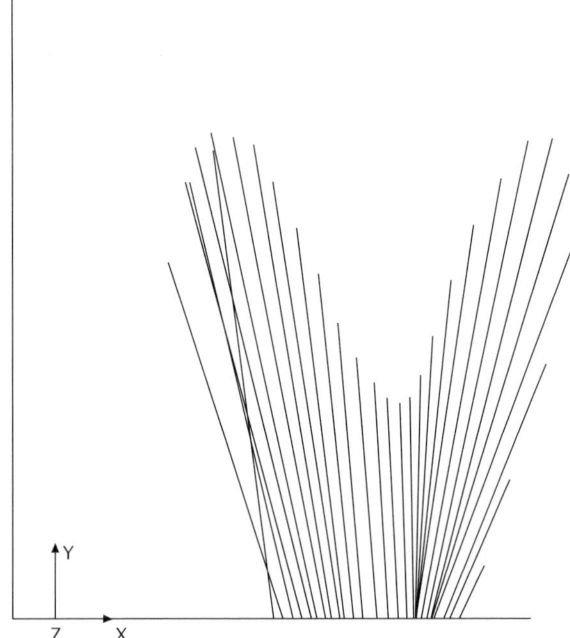

Figure 41.14 Butterfly diagram.

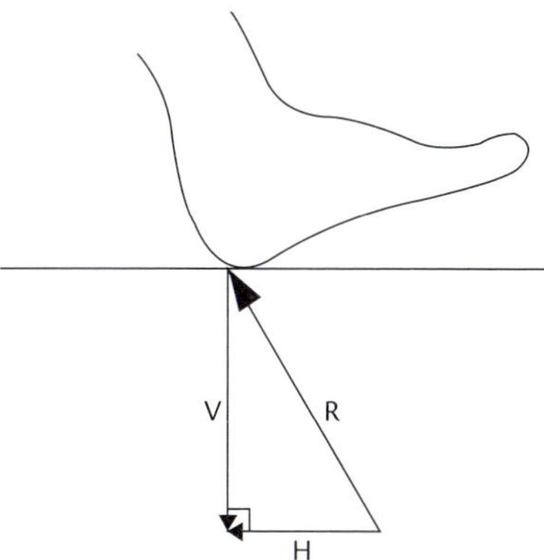

Figure 41.15 Vector of forces diagram.

a right-angled triangle, the resultant force vector R in Figure 41.15 can be derived using the following simple equation:

$$F_R = \left(\sum F_h^2 + \sum F_v^2\right)$$

where F_R is the resultant and ground reaction force and F_h and F_v are the horizontal and vertical forces that are detected by the force plate. Further algebraic manipulation will also reveal the angle of F_R.

The examples given here are for movements in the sagittal plane. Medial and lateral movement in the coronal plane can also be assessed. Details have been published elsewhere (Palastagna et al. 1994; Sammarco 1995; Subotnik 1989; Valiant and Cavanagh 1985).

Free-body diagrams

After the vector forces have been obtained, the effect of these forces on one body segment can be determined (Figure 41.16). In the Figure 41.16, R is the ground reaction force/vector, A is the muscle force required to resist plantarflexion (eccentric tibialis anterior work), and C is the weightbearing load. It can be seen from the diagram that R acts behind the centre of the ankle joint. This will result in a moment of force in the clockwise direction to produce plantarflexion.

If the compressive force C acts through the centre of the joint, then force A has to equal R in order to prevent a rapid plantarflexion manoeuvre.

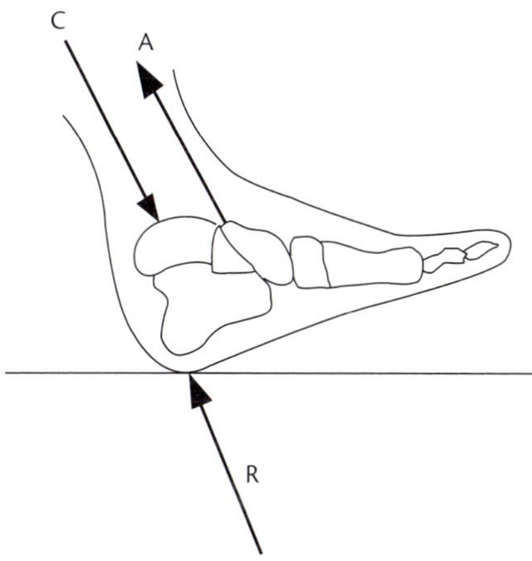

Figure 41.16 Free-body diagram. Moment = force × distance (measured in Newton metres).

Pressure measurement at the foot

So far we have only discussed the forces that are distributed to the ankle and leg.

Pressure-sensitive materials

Measurement of the pressure distribution at the foot can be performed with pressure-sensitive materials that, for example, will release a certain amount of ink onto the mat placed above them (the greater the pressure, the more ink is released).

Dynamic pressure measurement

A more sophisticated, dynamic method of measuring pressure distribution is to use a pedobarograph. This device consists of a layer of plastic placed above a sheet of glass. The plastic distorts under pressure, distorting the light passing through. The results are digitized and presented as a colour print-out. This is useful to determine time under pressure at a particular site; for example, when assessing the cause of undue pressure due to a 'dropped' metatarsal head.

Other devices for dynamic testing consist of materials made up of a few hundred isolated cells (each acting as its own pressure transducer), which react when weight is placed upon them. Shear forces make actual pressure transducer insoles difficult to employ. They also require the patient to be electrically linked to the recording device. Any device that the patient is aware of may alter the gait.

Treatment for abnormalities of lower limb biomechanics

History

There may be several pointers in the history that should lead the clinician to suspect the possibility of a biomechanical problem.

Bilateral pain

It would be unusual for a structural disorder to occur on both sides unless it is congenital or developmental in the growing years. Bilateral anterior knee pain, for example, is a biomechanical disorder until proved otherwise, in my opinion. Other examples would be bilateral tibialis posterior tendonitis and bilateral lateral buttock pain. Spinal pathologies may present with bilateral pain, but other aspects of the history will differentiate them.

Pain with exercise

With biomechanical problems, exercise is often the aggravating factor, but non-weightbearing exercise will be painless. Problems simply with going up and down stairs are suggestive of such problems. The clinician should therefore examine the patient when they are ambulant. Too often, the patient is examined standing and lying down only (i.e. when they do not have pain). Examination while the pain is being produced can produce a totally different set of observations.

Exercise-related pain may also be associated with other diagnoses, such as compartment syndrome or a stress fracture, that have been dealt with in Chapter 40.

No trauma

Often, the history is of an insidious onset when the musculoskeletal system has been subjected to increased demand. The body may adapt to biomechanical abnormalities until the stage is reached when an increased load will result in breakdown. This may be due to increased demand, increased weight, or a change in surface (such as a mountain runner starting to train on concrete).

Previous multiple assessments and investigations

The following clinical case represents such a scenario. A 22-year-old woman presented to the orthopaedic department with bilateral anterior knee pain of 4 years' duration. The pain was exacerbated by exercise. She had been given various forms of self-management exercises and several courses of manual and electrical physiotherapy. Following the lack of response to this treatment, she underwent the following investigations:

- skyline X-rays followed by serial skyline radiographs (20°, 40°, 60°)
- computed tomography (CT) scan of the patellofemoral joint followed by serial CT (0–20°)

As these investigations were normal, a decision was made to perform bilateral arthroscopies that demonstrated a normal knee and patellofemoral joint. Subsequently, surgical lateral release was undertaken bilaterally. This had no effect on the patient's pain. Before examination, the patient was asked if anyone had ever looked at her feet, or watched her walking or running. She answered that this had not been the case. Standing examination demonstrated a mild degree of overpronation that was notably exaggerated on walking, producing functional maltracking of the patella. The patient was provided with foot orthotics for walking and for exercise and became symptom-free within 2 months.

Not all cases will be as straightforward. However, a simple history and examination can avoid unnecessary investigations, unnecessary radiation, and unnecessary surgery.

Examination

Standing

Asymmetry is very common in the musculoskeletal system (Figure 41.17). Moderate asymmetry is obvious to the naked eye which can detect scoliosis, spinal movement asymmetry, pelvic level, internal femoral torsion, tibial varus, pronated or supinated feet, and a relaxed calcaneal stance position (when viewed from behind, as demonstrated in the middle photograph of Figure 41.18). A useful tip is to talk to the patient, allowing them to relax into a position that is normal for them. Pronation will occur as the patient relaxes and becomes used to being observed.

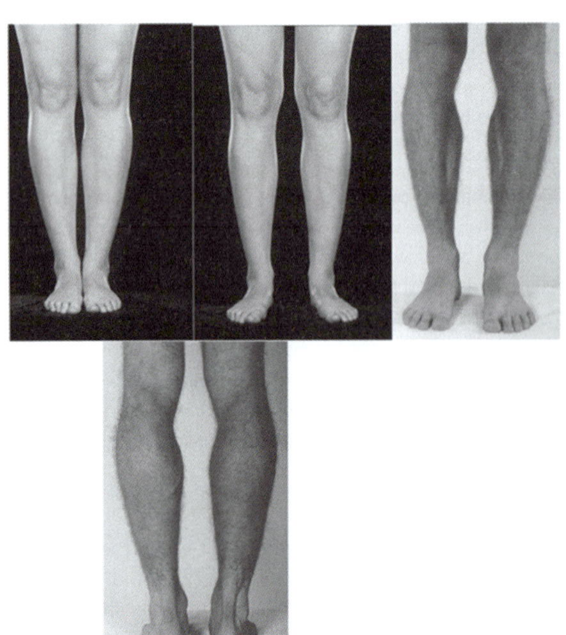

Figure 41.17 Asymmetry in the musculoskeletal system.

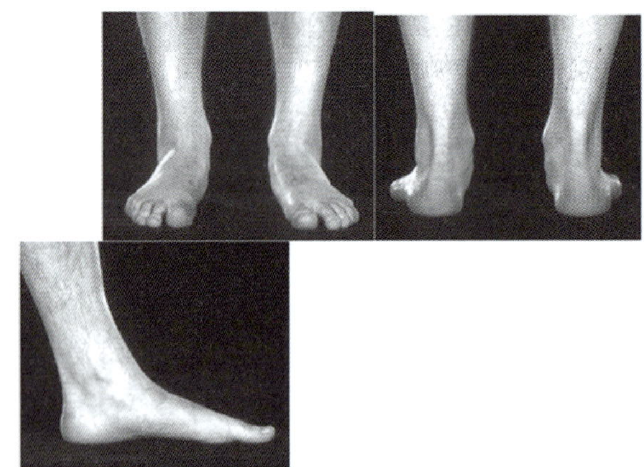

Figure 41.18 Pronated feet. Observe a medial talar bulge and flat arch.

When the patient is standing, the movements of the foot and especially the ankle can be observed by:

- *Standing on tiptoes:* This demonstrates plantarflexion of the ankle and hyperextension of the great toe (Figure 41.19). In this relatively supinated position, the arches of the foot and the soft tissues of the fascial layers may be observed for their integrity.
- *Flexing the knee and moving the knee joint as far over the front of the foot as possible:* This is useful to detect the degree of dorsiflexion of the ankle and the degree of pronation that may occur (Figure 41.20). To prevent the patient from avoiding pain-

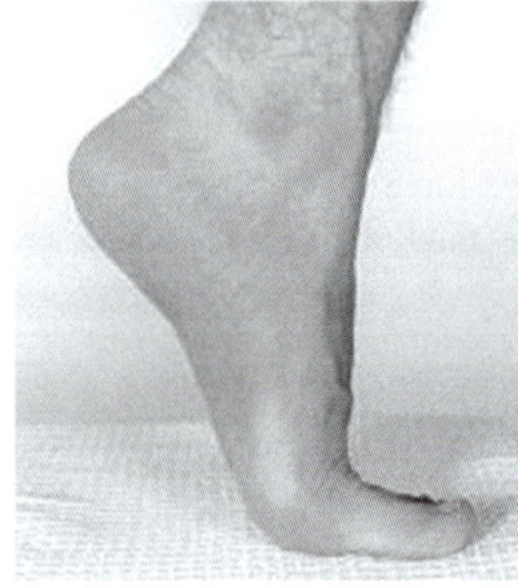

Figure 41.19 Standing on tiptoe.

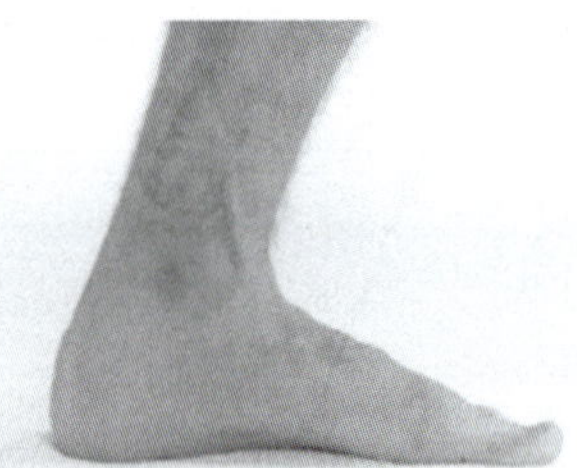

Figure 41.20 Ankle dorsiflexion.

ful anterior impingement of the ankle, the instruction should be to produce this movement in the sagittal plane initially and then to allow pronation with subtalar joint movement.

Sitting

A functional scoliosis will become straight if the pelvis becomes level as in sitting.

Supine

Pelvic level, hips, knees, and limb length deformity can be examined with the patient supine. The ankle and foot can be examined passively:

- *Malleolar position* should be approximately 13–18° but will be decreased, for example, by internal tibial torsion. This is an angle of inclination going from the lateral malleolus to the medial malleolus.
- *Ankle dorsiflexion* with the knee flexed (otherwise a tight gastrocnemius/soleus complex may limit the movement). This movement may be easier in the prone position.
- *Plantarflexion* of the ankle ensuring that the movement comes from the talocrural area and not the midfoot/forefoot.
- *Midfoot movement* is difficult to detect, but testing one side compared to the other is useful. Shearing (translatory) movements of the navicular, cuboid, and cuneiforms on their neighbouring bones may produce pain in a symptomatic patient.
- *Forefoot movement* consists of shearing movements of the metatarsals on one another. The first tarsometatarsal joint is the only one that has substantial movement (10–25°). There is relatively no movement of the second tarsometatarsal joint as it is fixed in position by the neighbouring bones. The movements of the metatarsophalangeal joints are of importance, especially that involving dorsiflexion of the first metatarsophalangeal joint.

Prone

Sacroiliac joints and pelvic level can be examined. This position is particularly useful for examining the relationship between the lower leg, rear foot, and forefoot (Figure 41.21). Lines bisecting the lower leg and rear foot may be drawn on the skin to assist with the visual inspection. Tibia varus of up to 8° is normal, and the range of subtalar joint movement can be detected using a protractor. The range of subtalar joint movement is divided into two-thirds inversion and one-third eversion. The rear foot to forefoot relationship is observed with the subtalar joint in the neutral position and the talus fixed into the mortise of the ankle joint. A typical forefoot varus is demonstrated in Figure 41.22.

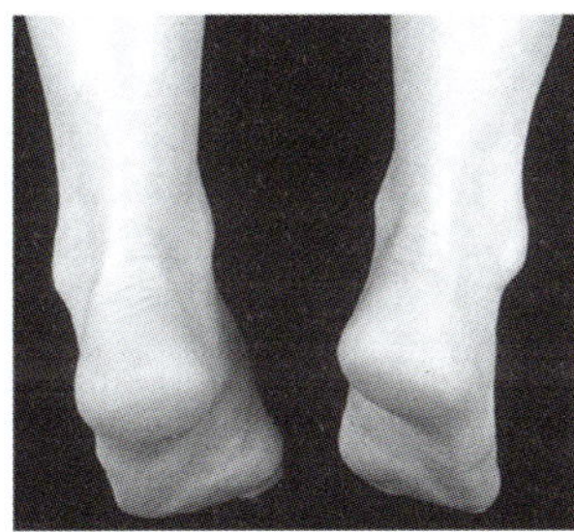

Figure 41.21 Lower leg, rear foot, and forefoot relationship.

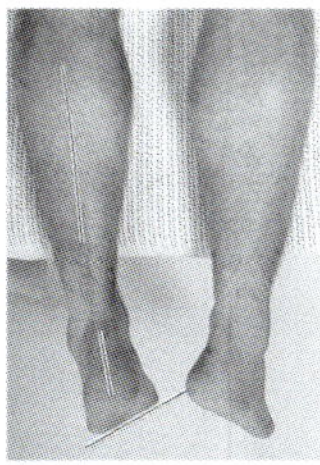

Figure 41.22 Lower leg, rear foot, and forefoot relationship.

Walking

Functional abnormalities may be highlighted by ambulation, which can take place in a consulting room, with or without a treadmill. The numerous possible observations include increased pronation, abduction of the feet on ambulation, early heel rise (due to a tight gastrocnemius), functional knee valgus/squinting of the patella, and excessive strain/bowing of the Achilles tendon due to rear foot valgus (Figure 41.23).

Running

Abnormalities on running may have to be detected by video analysis, as the more subtle problems cannot be detected by the naked eye at the speeds that may be involved. All of the aforementioned factors may be further pronounced because of the higher impact forces (up to five times body weight).

Assessment

The various forms of functional assessment have been discussed elsewhere in this section.

Radiographs of the foot and ankle with the patient weightbearing may be useful. The talar declination angle and the calcaneal inclination angle (Figure 41.24) will confirm the degree of supination/pronation that is present. Radiography may also detect congenital abnormalities such as tarsal coalition.

Treatment

Self-management

With any biomechanical disorder, the neuromuscular system is a determinant of movement of the structure. An individual may look

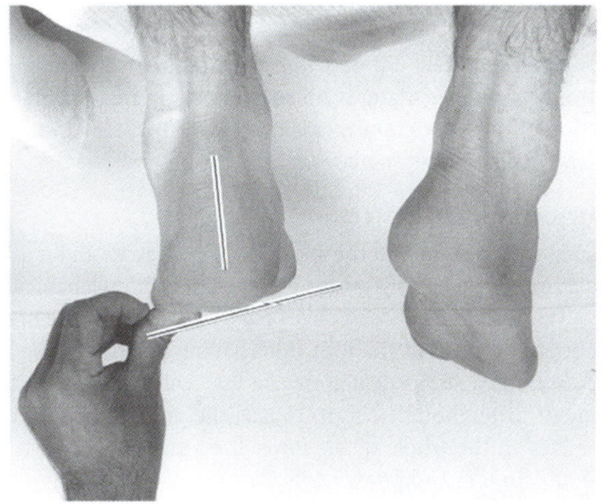

Figure 41.23 Typical forefoot varus.

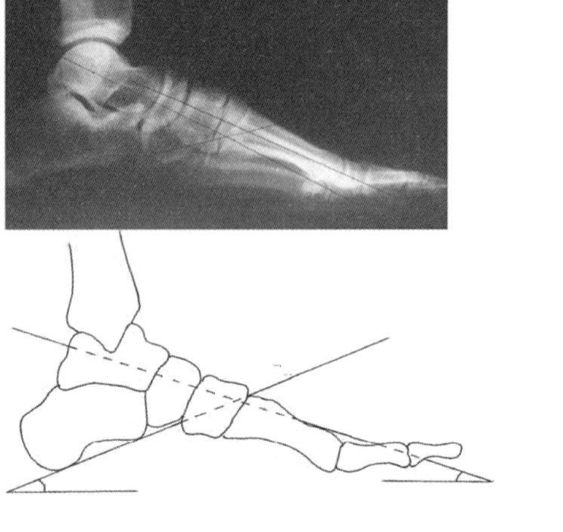

Figure 41.24 Calcaneal inclination angle and talar declination angle.

after their own system by complying with flexibility work and general body conditioning. A muscle will never produce 100% power without 100% flexibility. Neuromuscular stretches should be part of a daily routine for anyone who presents with biomechanical problems.

Physician advice: type of exercise, footwear, terrain, sport

Some individuals are not designed to run marathons. The morphology of an individual, plus various anthropometric measurements, may suggest that certain activities may lead to problems whether there is a biomechanical problem or not. The symptoms from a lower limb disorder may be aggravated by running on concrete, and the athlete would be advised to cross-train (i.e. spend some time doing other sports or competing on a different, more forgiving surface).

Footwear is also a crucial factor. A patient walking in a pair of worn-out shoes (specifically if they are worn out on the lateral aspect of the heel where heel strike occurs) will be liable to problems. Modern footwear can consist of sophisticated shock-absorbing material as well as providing 'support' for those with biomechanical problems.

Physiotherapy, muscle work, etc.

Self-management may not be sufficient. Manual work on areas of specifically tight musculature will be of benefit in releasing tension. Detection of muscle tightness and dysfunction will lead to a more prescriptive phase of post-injury rehabilitation.

Podiatry, orthotics

This area of treatment and the specialty of podiatry can be the key to most of the clinical dilemmas presenting as biomechanical disorders. The basis behind corrective orthotics is to bring the floor up to the foot and prevent the foot from having to drop to the floor. The orthotic is a sophisticated device that will control and guide movement throughout the foot. Hence, the effects of the orthotic will be 'felt' in the whole of the lower limb and beyond (McPhoil et al. 2000; Rodger and Leveau 1982).

Orthoses consist of shock-absorbing materials that also provide stability for support. Carbon fibre is used for those orthotics requiring a firmer degree of control.

There is a great deal of anecdotal evidence of benefit from the use of orthoses, but there is still a great deal of work to be done to prove their value scientifically (Nawoczenski et al. 1995; Stacoff et al. 2000). Precision making of the device is ruled out by the inter-observer error in measuring range of movement of the subtalar joint, for example. For this reason, 'off the shelf' orthotics for the most common abnormality (a forefoot varus) will often suffice, providing the gross adjustment and allowing the body to make the finer adjustments. For more unusual abnormalities, casting of devices by a practitioner experienced with the technique is recommended.

When orthoses have been prescribed, the patient should gradually be introduced to wearing them (e.g. 15 minutes on the first day, increasing by a further 15 minutes on subsequent days). The patient should be wearing walking orthotics for several weeks before running orthotics are prescribed. Wearing orthotics too much, too soon, may cause discomfort, blistering, and biomechanical problems elsewhere in the body if there has been insufficient time to adjust.

Surgical treatment

Structural adjustment of a biomechanical abnormality is required when all else has failed. Once surgery has been performed, the rehabilitation phase has to be carefully monitored as the body adjusts and hopefully adapts to the new forces to which it will be subject. The technical details of surgical correction for ankle and foot abnormalities are extensive and are dealt with in many other reference books (Baxter 1995; McGlamry et al. 1992; Subotnik 1989).

Surgery may sort out one problem only to cause another. The patient should be advised carefully before any form of surgery.

References

Baxter, D. E. *The foot and ankle in sport*. Mosby, St Louis, 1995.

Hamill, J., Knutzen, K. M. *Biomechanical basis of human movement*. Williams and Wilkins, Baltimore, MD, 1995.

McGlamry, E. D., Banks, A. S., Downey M. S. *Comprehensive textbook on foot surgery* (2nd edn). Williams and Wilkins, Baltimore, MD, 1992.

McPhoil, T. G., Cornwall, M. W. The effect of foot orthoses on transverse tibial rotation during walking. *Journal of the American Podiatry Association*, 2000, 90, 2–11.

Nawoczenski, D. A., Cook, T. M., Slatzman C. L. The effect of foot orthotics on three-dimensional kinematics of the leg and rear foot during running. *Journal of Orthopaedic and Sports Physical Therapy*, 1995, 21, 317–27.

Palastagna, N., Field, D., Soames, R. *Anatomy and human movement* (2nd edn). Butterworth-Heinemann, Oxford, 1994.

Rodger, M. M., Leveau, B. F. Effectiveness of foot orthotic devices used to modify pronation in runners. *Journal of Orthopaedic and Sports Physical Therapy*, 1982, 4, 86–90.

Sammarco, G. J. *Rehabilitation of the foot and ankle*. Mosby, St Louis, 1995.

Stacoff, A., Reinschmidt, C., Nigg B. M. Effects of foot orthoses on skeletal motion during running. *Clinical Biomechanics*, 2000, 15, 54–64.

Subotnik, S. (ed.) *Sports medicine of the lower extremity*. Churchill Livingstone, Edinburgh, 1989.

Valiant, G. A., Cavanagh, P. R. A study of landing from a jump: implications for design of a basketball shoe. In: Winter D. A. et al. (eds) *Biomechanics IX-B*. Human Kinetics, Champaign, IL, 1985.

Chapter 42

The ankle joint

Richard Higgins

Anatomy of the ankle joint

The ankle joint, or talocrural joint, is a hinged synovial joint consisting of a complex combination of articular surfaces. The stability of the joint is reliant on its position. In dorsiflexion, the talus is squeezed by the malleoli, as because of its shape, it spreads the mortice, tightening the interosseous and anterior and posterior tibiofibular ligaments, securely locking the joint. This contrasts with the relative instability experienced in plantarflexion. Contributing to the adjustment to uneven surfaces and assisting in shock absorption are additional important functions of the ankle joint.

During sporting activity, the lateral ankle complex is more frequently injured than any other major structure (Liu and Jason 1994). Forces generated when landing from a jump are absorbed through the kinetic chain via the foot and ankle complex, as it progresses from plantarflexion through to dorsiflexion and pronation. Landing flatfooted would therefore transmit most of these forces proximally to other structures. Situations in which this occurs are common in many sports, and with up to 80% of players landing in a significantly plantarflexed position (Valiant and Cavanagh 1985), any additional factors such as the player attempting a sudden turn or landing being affected by contact with another player, can increase lateral movement and further increase the chances of sustaining an inversion injury.

The talus, wider anteriorly than posteriorly, slots into the ankle mortice, formed by the distal tibial and fibular surfaces, articulating superiorly via its trochlear surface. Its medial and lateral surfaces bear facets that articulate with their respective malleoli.

Joint movements available are those of dorsiflexion, primarily produced by the tibialis anterior, during which the malleoli are forced slightly apart, and plantarflexion, with the gastrocnemius and soleus acting as the prime movers. In addition, rotation in the transverse plain, abduction, and adduction also occur in plantarflexion, with most inversion and eversion occurring at the subtalar joint.

The capsule derives its strength from local ligamentous structures. Medially, the deltoid ligament consists of three superficial and two deep components, fanning out in a triangular fashion from the medial malleolus, inserting into the navicular, calcaneum, and talus respectively, with each reflection being named accordingly. In addition to conferring significant stability to the medial side of the joint, the deltoid ligament provides support to the medial longitudinal arch while securing the calcaneum and navicular to the talus.

The lateral or tripartite ligament (Figure 42.1) is a less substantial structure. It comprises the relatively weak anterior talofibular ligament, a capsular thickening passing anteromedially to the talus, the stronger posterior talofibular ligament passing almost horizontally, and the cord-like calcaneofibular ligament, which passes posteroinferiorly, being crossed superficially by the tendons of the peroneous longus and brevis and blending with the medial wall of their tendon sheath.

The anterior and posterior portions of the capsule remain relatively thin and the synovial capsule is somewhat superficial in these areas, so if there is any swelling it is often evident here.

Inversion injuries of the ankle joint

Aetiology

Inversion injuries, or acute lateral ligament sprains, are the commonest form of sporting injury (Barker et al. 1997), accounting for, on average, 40% of all injuries and up to 85% of ankle sprains (Garrick 1977), which in themselves are responsible for over 15% of all time lost from sport (Liu and Jason 1994). The injury occurs when the athlete lands with the foot plantarflexed and slightly inverted, a position that unlocks the joint. Of factors thought to confer increased risk of sustaining an inversion injury, muscle imbalance, relating eversion to inversion strength, appears to be particularly significant.

Disruption of the anterior talofibular ligament is most frequently encountered and will involve capsular damage. A more severe injury includes damage to the calcaneofibular ligament, which is rarely injured on its own, and involving the peroneal tendon sheath because of its confluence. This is easily demonstrated on arthrography. Additional injury to the posterior talofibular ligament is the least common finding, occurring relatively infrequently.

Classification of lateral ligamentous injuries is variable. Injuries are described as primary, secondary, or tertiary or grade 1, 2, or 3, in order of increasing severity. Grading also reflects the combination of ligaments involved, progressing from a single-ligament injury to complete disruption.

Diagnosis

This is based on the clinical history, with the patient's description of mechanism of injury directing the clinician towards the possibility of associated damage, such as syndesmotic rupture. Clinical examination then helps to confirm suspicions. Rushed history taking,

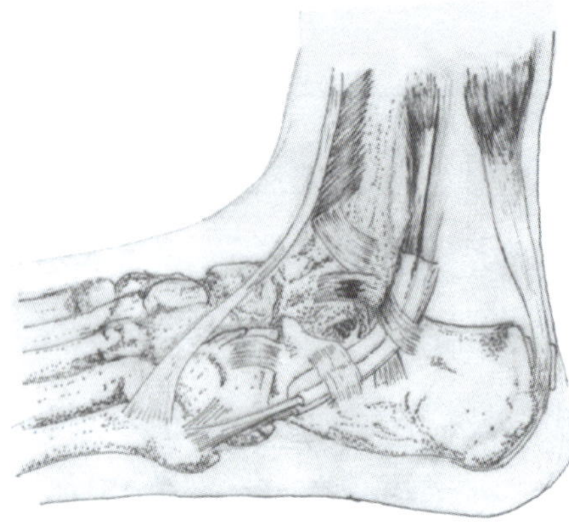

Figure 42.1 Anatomy of the lateral ligament.

and subsequent failure to accurately elucidate the mechanism of injury, often leads to the assumption that this is just another 'simple ankle sprain'. Associated injuries may be missed, at best leading to confusion and embarrassment when symptoms are slow to resolve, at worse leading to possible legal implications.

Most sports physicians enjoy having some involvement as a team physician to complete their professional development, and realize its necessity. However, it is in this environment that mistakes most often occur. Lunchtime visits, dealing with multiple complaints, tempt one to cut corners. Adequate time and private consultation facilities, away from interfering enthusiasts, are essential.

Examination findings

Associated swelling around the lateral malleolus is usually present even in grade 1 injuries, often extending proximally. Palpation will reveal tenderness over the respective ligaments and pain over the anterior joint line possibly suggests a talar dome injury. Inversion will often be painful when tested both actively and passively.

When an anterior drawer is undertaken (Figure 42.2), it should always be compared with the other side, as normal variations in ligamentous laxity may produce false positives. A movement of 5–10 mm is considered abnormal, with most of the research findings falling within this range, although, as with many tests, there is an element of subjectivity. Equipment cannot replace experience. A positive test undertaken in slight plantarflexion indicates a complete tear of the anterior talofibular ligament. Further investigations such as talar tilt are sometimes used in helping to confirm the diagnosis.

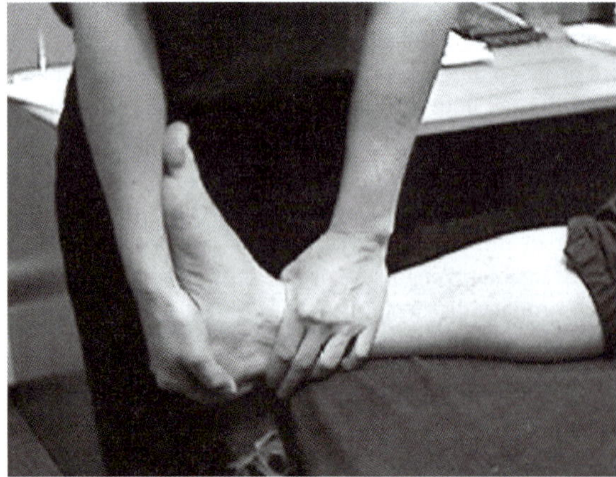

Figure 42.2 Anterior drawer sign.

The distal tibiofibular syndesmosis should be palpated. Specific tenderness in association with either a positive squeeze test (which compresses the fibula to the tibia above the midpoint of the calf, causing pain distally) or external rotation of the foot in dorsiflexion (the external rotation stress test), similarly causing local discomfort, are indicative of disruption. Always palpate the base of the fifth metatarsal to exclude an associated fracture.

Investigations

Plain radiographs should be undertaken if there is suspicion of a fracture. An inability to weightbear continuing on arrival in the emergency department, alongside bony tenderness on either malleolus, form the basis of the Ottawa rules, a scoring system which gives a good indication as to whether there may be an underlying fracture and has been shown to decrease requests for unnecessary investigations. At least two views should be requested, fields extending to include the base of the fifth metatarsal, with stress radiographs being undertaken if significant instability is suspected.

Talar dome injuries are best imaged using magnetic resonance imaging (MRI). Widening of the ankle mortice indicates a rupture of the syndesmosis; complete disruption indicating surgical intervention.

Treatment

Acute phase

Initial treatment of an acute inversion injury or simple ankle sprain follows the usual regime of *r*est, *i*ce, *c*ompression, *e*levation (RICE). This regime is often not undertaken aggressively enough. Ice is beneficial immediately after injury, decreasing swelling and helping with pain relief (Hocutt et al 1982). However, blood flow does not decrease significantly for about 10 minutes after the application of ice, by which time considerable bleeding may already have occurred, so the compressive element becomes equally important as an aid to restricting haemorrhage (Lehmann et al 1990). If sports-related, the athlete should be removed from the field of play without placing weight on the joint, the limb being elevated as soon as possible and compression applied. Cryocuffs (Figure 42.3) are often used in this situation and although some of the research is conflicting, experience shows that they are a useful adjunct in the initial 24–48-hour period. Non-steroidal anti-inflammatories are also of benefit at this time.

During the acute phase, compression is achieved by taping, with the addition of a U-shaped stirrup (Figure 42.4) to produce a more local application of pressure around the lateral malleolus; this has been shown to be more beneficial than non-specific compression (Wilkerson and Horn-Kingery 1993).

Air splints (Figure 42.5) are often used as rehabilitation progresses and have been shown to be protective against re-injury in many studies. The suggestion is that they should be worn for at least 6 months after moderate to severe injuries, although in many sports this is not practical (Bahr et al. 1997a).

Contrast baths are sometimes suggested as treatment after the acute phase, but research does not support this, in some cases indicating an increase in swelling after use (Cote et al. 1988), confirming the thinking that ice and compression are the most appropriate modalities during this phase.

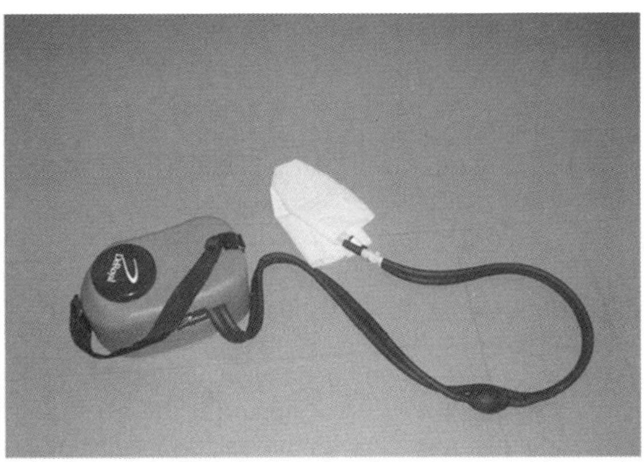

Figure 42.3 Cryocuff.

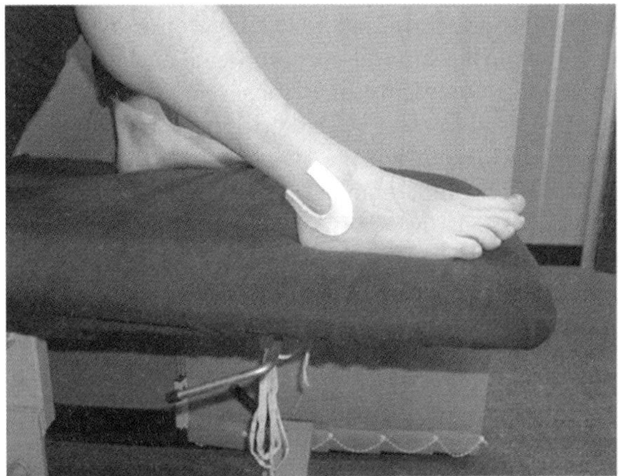

Figure 42.4 U-shaped stirrup.

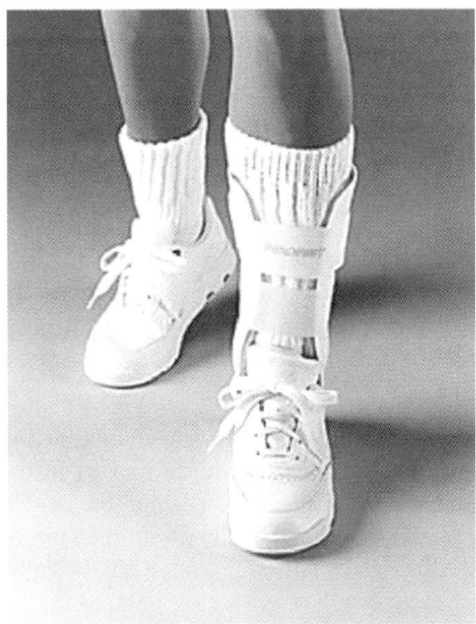

Figure 42.5 Aircast brace.

Heat produces analgesia and decreases muscle spasm, but should not be used while swelling is still present. Electrical treatments such as ultrasound are often used in the post-acute stage. Ultrasound has thermal effects which are probably responsible for most of the therapeutic benefit experienced (Coakley 1978). Its non-thermal effects are still not clearly understood and, although some research has been published to the contrary, it most probably provides little or no benefit.

The athlete should also be taken through passive and active assisted exercises, to improve range of motion. All these steps must be followed aggressively, each being of vital importance in the acute phase of the rehabilitation programme.

Unfortunately, it is still not uncommon to see an athlete hobbling into the clinic on crutches a week after an inversion injury; the local emergency department is often the culprit, with recovery already having been compromised. Management regimes comprising prolonged non-weightbearing or cast immobilization are still advised, but are unacceptable. Observation and review of these cases, backed by research (Kannus and Renstrom 1991), show that this approach leads only to ongoing pain and dysfunction.

Recovery phase

The recovery phase then begins, during which multidirectional activities are introduced. Weightbearing exercise is undertaken using an airbrace or taping as support, early mobilization being essential as it decreases recovery time. Proprioceptive exercises are added, which may begin as alphabet writing (balancing on the affected side while spelling out letters with the other foot) or heel walking, progressing to various wobble boards (Figure 42.6) with differing degrees of difficulty.

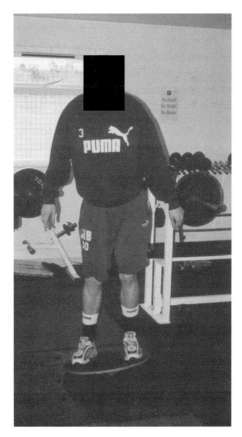

Figure 42.6 Wobble board.

Muscle strengthening is imperative at this stage, starting with isometric-type exercises, then gradually progressing to both closed and open kinetic chain exercises, strengthening of the peroneals proving very important in future ankle stability.

Functional phase

Finally, the athlete progresses through to the functional phase, which aims at restoring a full range of motion in all positions. Proprioceptive exercises are essential, with various techniques being used to increase load and difficulty by adding external forces. The activities undertaken aim to improve agility, with the intensity of exercise being increased. Eccentric loads are applied at this stage. The result is an increase in contractile strength of the peroneals and improved neuromuscular function, similar effects also having been demonstrated contralaterally, with speed of contraction increasing significantly after such a regime (Benjamin et al. 2000).

Once activities using equipment such as a wobble board or a pilates board or fitter (a curved board with foot plates on runners) have been completed, progression follows through to trampete exercises, then increasing eccentric loading and difficulty through various functional activities. Sandpit exercises (Figure 42.7) have been used successfully by an inventive physiotherapist involved with professional soccer.

After an initial injury, the risk of recurrence doubles (Milgrom et al. 1991), so only when all stages have been satisfactorily completed may the athlete return to competition. At this time, a full range of motion should be accompanied by adequate joint stability, proprioception, and muscle strength. Failure to achieve this can lead to recurrent injury with the possible sequelae being ankle instability due to ligamentous laxity and a 'chronic ankle sprain', a scenario that should never occur.

Many sportsmen tape their ankles prophylactically after an inversion injury. The usefulness of this practice is much debated. Although some research has shown taping to improve stability, it has also demonstrated that the supportive effect becomes negligible after approximately 20 minutes (Greene and Hillman 1990). The presumption therefore is that it works by improving proprioception, in much the same way that patella taping appears to produce a cure in anterior knee pain. The frantic demand for strapping in the treatment room before a professional soccer game lends weight to this theory. Although support is anecdotal in the main, it would not be wise to refute the practice; experience shows that the professional sportsman's intuition sometimes proves to be more informed than a plethora of conflicting and inconclusive research.

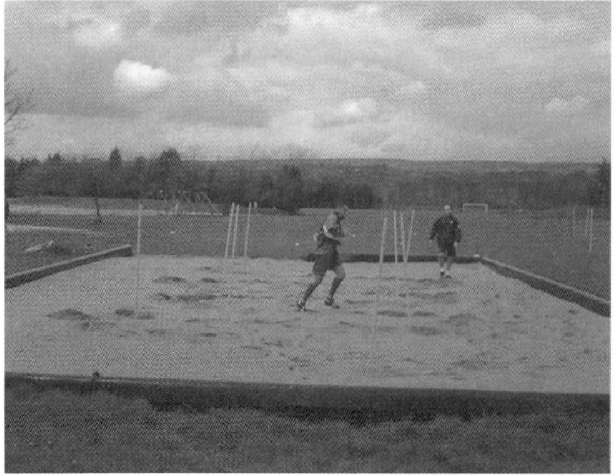

Figure 42.7 Training in sand. (Courtesy Dave Ferre, Blackburn Rovers F.C.)

Should it be advised that a career-long preventive programme should be the aim? Anecdotal evidence suggests that players seen in the gym after training seem to suffer fewer recurrences after their return to play than their less conscientious colleagues, who, though keen to return to competition, tend also to return to the physiotherapist's table at an earlier date. Supporting this observation, 'focused conditioning', involving specific exercises aimed at prevention alongside education, has been shown to produce a decrease in injury rate (Bahr et al. 1997b; Ekstrand et al. 1983).

Surgery

Osteochondral fractures of the talar dome can be a consequence of a severe inversion injury and are classified according to their severity and displacement, with lateral lesions proving more unstable and requiring surgical intervention at an earlier stage than medial lesions. Symptoms suggesting referral for arthroscopic examination are recurrent swelling, stiffness, instability, clicking or locking, and ongoing pain. Chondroplasty is undertaken for chondral lesions, with a number of procedures being available to correct ligamentous instability, an unnecessary sequela of inadequate rehabilitation.

Anterolateral impingement syndrome, described in the section 'Impingement syndromes', is sometimes associated and may require arthroscopic debridement.

Other associated injuries

Syndesmotic injury

This is most commonly caused during a collision in which the ankle is forcefully externally rotated or dorsiflexed, either individually or in combination. These injuries are thought to comprise up to 10% of 'ankle sprains'. Inversion injury can also cause disruption of the syndesmosis, with the anterior inferior tibiofibular ligament sometimes being torn (Cox 1985).

The syndesmosis consists of the anterior inferior tibiofibular ligament, posterior inferior tibiofibular ligament, transverse ligament, and interosseous ligament and membrane. Disruption follows a characteristic pattern, in a similar manner to lateral ligament tears, with damage occurring initially to the anterior inferior tibiofibular ligament followed by the interosseous ligament. Diagnosis is confirmed on clinical examination.

A Maisonneuve fracture, which is a fracture of the proximal fibula, is sometimes present in association with complete syndesmotic rupture.

Peroneal subluxation

This is a possible complication following an inversion injury. If recurrent, it may require surgery, both to prevent further episodes of subluxation and to repair any tear within the tendon or sheath that may have accompanied the injury, with the same occasionally happening to the tibialis posterior tendon after a significant eversion stress.

Sinus tarsi syndrome may also occur as a consequence of an inversion injury, sometimes complicating the picture (see Chapter 43).

Impingement syndromes at the ankle

Anterior and posterior

Aetiology

Anterior and posterior impingement syndromes, particularly common in soccer and ballet and often called 'footballer's ankle', may occur in any sport that entails forceful plantarflexion and dorsiflexion of the foot at the ankle joint. Initial impingement of the soft tissues progresses, with the development of osteophytes anteriorly and posteriorly at the articular margins, as a result of the bony impact in these regions. A sequela of this can be the production of associated loose bodies. Additional complications in relation to posterior impingement may be the presence of an os trigonum (Figure 42.8), an unfused ossification centre, posterior to the talus, present in 7–10% of the population. This may be the cause of the symptoms or an addition to them. Recent studies have shown an os trigonum to be present more frequently in soccer players, suggesting that the nature of the sport may be causal.

Examination

Clinical presentation is that of localized joint line tenderness, with passive plantarflexion reproducing the pain in posterior impingement, and dorsiflexion, the pain in anterior impingement.

Investigation

Plain radiographs demonstrate the abnormality quite clearly, with further investigation often being unnecessary, as damage to the articular cartilage is not a part of the pathology, the osteophytes being unrelated to an osteoarthritic process. An isotope bone scan is sometimes useful in helping to decide the contribution of an os trigonum to the athlete's posterior ankle pain.

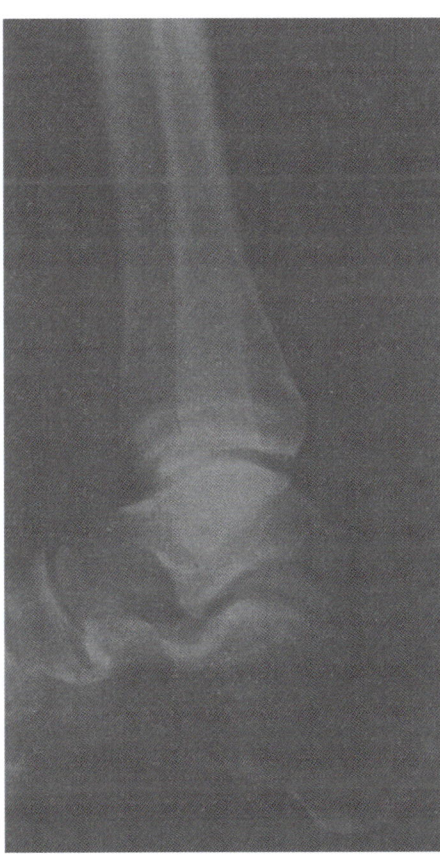

Figure 42.8 Radiograph of os trigonum.

Treatment

Initial management is conservative, with restriction of aggravating factors, non-steroidal anti-inflammatory medication, and localized physiotherapeutic modalities. If symptoms fail to resolve, a well-directed injection of a long-acting corticosteroid is often beneficial. In the more chronic cases, usually demonstrating radiographic changes, treatment tends to be surgical once symptoms become persistent and the osteophytes restrict movement. Arthroscopic removal of any loose bodies, with removal of the osteophytes, is undertaken. Persistent posterior impingement in the presence of an os trigonum may require its removal. Surprisingly, although gross radiographic changes are often noted incidentally in players in their early twenties, the majority remain asymptomatic, with surgery being less prevalent than one would expect. Although it is common practice to order plain radiographs of the ankles in pre-signing medicals for professional soccer clubs, this practice therefore appears to be unfounded.

Anterolateral

Anterolateral impingement syndrome occurs after injury to the lateral ligamentous structures (Jacobson and Lui 1992). Inadequate rehabilitation after an inversion injury may potentiate recurrent injury to the region, with the subsequent development of chronic inflammatory changes within the tissues, leading to the production of scar tissue, which is repeatedly trapped in the lateral gutter. The result is persistent lateral ankle pain. Again, the initial approach is physiotherapeutic, with the correction of any biomechanical abnormalities being important. Localized steroidal injection into the area, also injecting into the sinus tarsi in case of associated pathology, may achieve a cure. However, persistence of symptoms suggests that surgical intervention may be necessary. Arthroscopic debridement has a high success rate; most patients become symptom-free (Jacobson and Lui 1992).

Midfoot pain

Stress fractures occur as overuse injuries, with different sports producing this effect in different regions. One of the most important midfoot stress fractures is that of the navicular (Figure 42.9), because of its tendency to progress to fracture with non-union and with avascular necrosis being an unfortunate sequela. The navicular is easily located, with its prominent tuberosity medially, surrounded by the talus, cuboid, and three cuneiforms, and articulating with all.

Aetiology

Navicular stress fractures are found in a variety of sports, commonly those entailing forceful dorsiflexion of the foot as the athlete pushes off. They predominate in track and field athletes, and are not particularly common in soccer. In my experience, however, they are becoming increasingly common in rugby league as the pace and intensity of the game increase.

History and examination

Diagnosis is mainly a clinical one, with a history of pain on exercise, crescendoing if the athlete attempts to persist with their training

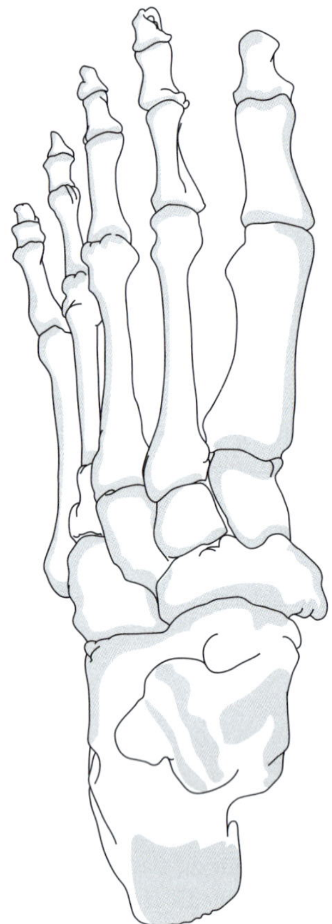

Figure 42.9 Anatomy of the navicular.

regime, and culminating in pain both at rest and at night. Any degree of discomfort on palpation in this region warrants caution and further investigation. Classically, tenderness is felt over the proximal portion of the navicular, in the midline, the region in which the stress fracture most commonly occurs and often described as the 'N' spot.

Investigation

An isotope bone scan will confirm the suspicion, though it often remains 'hot' long after healing has occurred. MRI is becoming the investigation of choice, revealing early stress reactions that may suggest caution, though plain radiographs and computed tomography (CT) should be used to image the bony disruption accurately in definite cases.

Treatment

An aggressive approach must be undertaken to prevent the debilitating sequelae associated with non-union. A non-weightbearing cast is applied for 6–8 weeks. Occasionally, even prolonged immobilization is unsuccessful and surgical intervention with bone grafting becomes necessary.

Cuboid syndrome

Ongoing discomfort in the lateral midfoot may indicate subluxation of the cuboid, the normal articulations of which are the navicular and lateral cuneiform medially, the calcaneum posteriorly, and the fourth and fifth metatarsals anteriorly. Often following an inversion injury and frequently presenting in ballet dancers, the cuboid is subluxed in a plantarwards direction, the medial portion occasionally being rotated dorsally. Using direct pressure over the bone and directing it upward in the reverse direction to the subluxation, manipulation often produces a successful reduction, the foot being simultaneously plantarflexed during the manoeuvre, with an associated clunk and an immediate relief of symptoms being the result. Taping techniques may help to prevent recurrence.

A differential diagnosis of cuboid stress fracture is rare but has been reported and so should be borne in mind, with cases sometimes mimicking peroneal tendinitis. Both CT and isotope bone scans have proved useful in helping achieve a diagnosis (Beaman et al. 1993: Mahler and Fricker 1993).

Occasional disorders at the ankle

- ***Talar stress fractures*** occur infrequently, presenting with ankle pain that is more severe when hopping.
- *Midtarsal sprains* quite commonly prove to be the cause of midfoot pain, either in association with an acute injury or due to more chronic biomechanical deficiencies.
- *Tarsal coalition* must be considered as a possible cause of midfoot or ankle pain, and although the cuneiforms are not often included in this, rarely, they may be implicated. I have experienced one case producing symptoms and findings on isotope bone scan that were markedly similar to those of a metatarsal stress fracture.

References

Bahr, R., et al. A two fold reduction in the incidence of acute ankle sprains in volleyball after the introduction of an injury prevention programme: a prospective cohort study. *Scandinavian Journal of Medicine and Science in Sports*, 1997a, 7, 172–7.

Bahr, R., et al. Incidence of acute volleyball injuries. *Scandinavian Journal of Medicine and Science in Sports*, 1997b, 7, 166–71

Barker, H. B., et al. Ankle injury risk factors in sports. *Sports Medicine*, 1997, 23, 69–74.

Beaman, D. N., Roeser, W. M., Holmes, J. R., Saltzman, C. L. Cuboid stress fractures: a report of two cases. *Foot and Ankle*, 1993, 14(9), 525–8.

Benjamin, S., et al. The benefit of a single-leg strength training programme for the muscles around the untrained ankle. *American Journal of Sports Medicine*, 2000, 28(4), 568–73.

Coakley, W. T. Biophysical effects of ultrasound at therapeutic intensities. *Physiotherapy*, 1978, 64, 166.

Cote, D. J., et al. Comparison of three treatment procedures for minimizing ankle sprain swelling. *Physical Therapy*, 1988, 68, 1072.

Cox, J. S. Surgical and nonsurgical treatment of acute ankle sprains. *Clinical Orthopaedics*, 1985, 188, 88–96.

Ekstrand, J., et al. Prevention of soccer injuries. *American Journal of Sports Medicine*, 1983, 11, 116–20.

Garrick, J. G. The frequency of injury, mechanism of injury and epidemiology of ankle sprains. *American Journal of Sports Medicine*, 1977, 5, 241–2.

Greene, T. A., Hillman, S. K. Comparison of support provided by a semirigid orthosis and adhesive ankle taping before, during and after exercise. *American Journal of Sports Medicine*, 1990, 18(5), 498–506.

Hocutt, J. E., et al. Cryotherapy in ankle sprains. *American Journal of Sports Medicine*, 1982, 10, 316.

Jacobson, K. E., Lui, S. H. Anterolateral impingement of the ankle. *Journal of the Medical Association of Georgia*, 1992, 81(6), 297–9.

Kannus, P., Renstrom, P. Treatment for acute tears of the lateral ligaments of the ankle. Operation, cast, or early controlled mobilisation. *Journal of Bone and Joint Surgery*, 1991, 73A, 305–12.

Lehmann, J. F., et al. Cryotherapy. In: *Therapeutic heat and cold* (4th edn). Williams and Wilkins, Baltimore, 1990.

Liu, S. H., Jason, W. J. Lateral ankle sprains and instability problems. *Clinics in Sports Medicine*, 1994, 13(4), 793–809.

Mahler, P., Fricker, P. Case report: cuboid stress fracture. *Excel*, 1993, 8(3), 147–8.

Milgrom, C., et al. Risk factors for lateral ankle sprain: a prospective study among military recruits. *Foot and Ankle*, 1991, 12, 26–30.

Valiant, G. A., Cavanagh, P. R. A study of landing from a jump. In: *Biomechanics IX-B*. Human Kinetics, Champaign, IL, 1985.

Wilkerson, G. B., Horn- Kingery, H. M. Treatment of the inversion ankle sprain: comparison of different modes of compression and cryotherapy. *Journal of Orthopaedic and Sports Physical Therapy*, 1993, 17(5), 240–6.

Chapter 43

The subtalar joint

Bryan English

Anatomy of the subtalar joint

The inferior aspect of the talus and the superior aspect of the calcaneum form this joint. Normally, the surface consists of three facets and an accessory joint along the mid sulcus of the calcaneum:

- *posterior facet:* biconvex calcaneum opposing biconcave talus
- *anteromedial facet:* biconcave calcaneum opposing biconvex talus
- *anterolateral facet:* concave calcaneum opposing convex talus.

Arthroscopy has demonstrated that although most people have three facets to this joint, a small proportion have only two (the anterior facets being combined). The three-facet joint in supination forms an osseous block. An interesting hypothesis is that the two-facet joint has a greater surface area and will allow more movement as the axis of the joint will move towards the transverse plane and away from the coronal plane (see the section 'Joint axes within the foot and ankle' in Chapter 41). It follows that people who pronate excessively may have a higher incidence of only one anterior facet. Anterior to the posterior facet is the sinus tarsi (which acts like an accessory joint). Two thickenings of the capsule of the joint at this site form the anterior and posterior interosseous ligaments, which provide the majority of support for the subtalar joint (Sarrafian 1983). They protect the joint during inversion and restrain possible joint separation. Other ligament supports to the joint are listed in Table 43.1.

Movements at the subtalar joint

No muscle inserts onto the talus, so any ankle movement has to be mediated via the subtalar joint. Closed kinetic chain movement occurs with heel strike. The movement at the subtalar joint will determine the action of the foot and the lower leg. It therefore acts as a torque convertor. If there is very little subtalar movement, the foot and lower leg will move early to compensate. If there is excessive subtalar movement, the movement of the lower leg and foot will be dragged along with the subtalar joint and lower limb joint movements may be mistimed.

As mentioned in Chapter 41, the subtalar joint has a triplanar axis, but the only axis of movement that can be detected on examination is that in the coronal plane, involving eversion and inversion. The range varies from 6° to 25°, with two-thirds of the movement being into inversion and one-third into eversion.

Injuries of the subtalar joint

Inversion injury

Considering the importance of its role, the subtalar joint is remarkably 'uncomplaining'. It is most commonly injured as a result of an inversion injury to the ankle. If the lateral collateral ligament of the ankle is ruptured, the subtalar joint may undergo ligament damage. Subsequent hypermobility of this joint will lead to ongoing symptoms and instability of the ankle during the rehabilitation process (Heilman et al. 1990). Strapping, temporary or permanent, may be required to 'ease' the joint. As with all joints, good proprioceptive function is important to assist in recovery.

Ligament damage may be difficult to detect clinically without the assistance of further imaging such as magnetic resonance imaging (MRI).

Stress fracture

The subtalar joint is a good shock absorber, but regular excessive loading may lead to stress fracture, presenting with diffuse heel pain that is worse at night (Eisle and Sammarco 1993). MRI is diagnostic, although computed tomography (CT) and isotope bone scans are still commonly used. If there is no obvious cause for the fracture, such as excessive loading, then further investigations of bone density and hormonal status should be considered.

Conservative treatment would be to avoid activity that causes pain, and the wearing of shock-absorbing insoles. Immobilization in a plaster of Paris slipper or non-weightbearing foot brace for up to 12 weeks is the treatment of choice, but may be viewed by some as too aggressive. Others would allow weightbearing if this was asymptomatic.

Sinus tarsi syndrome

This often follows trauma and occasionally presents as an overuse injury (Shear et al. 1993). The pathology of the condition is open to debate. Inflammation of the synovium, the interosseous ligaments, and the chondral surface of the joint have all been suggested, along with a further postulation of entrapment of a branch of the peroneal nerve (Heilman et al. 1990). My opinion is that chondral

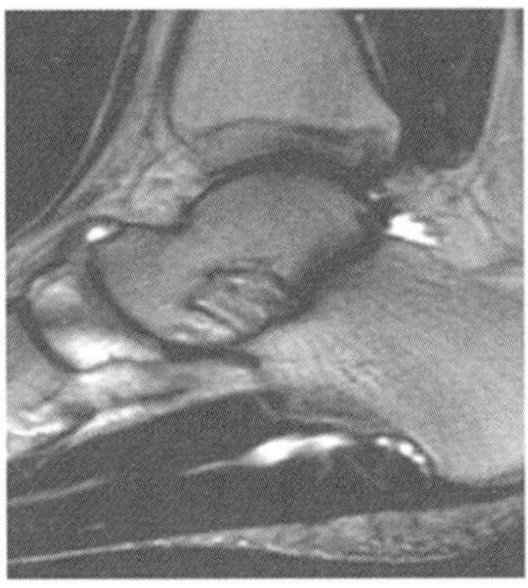
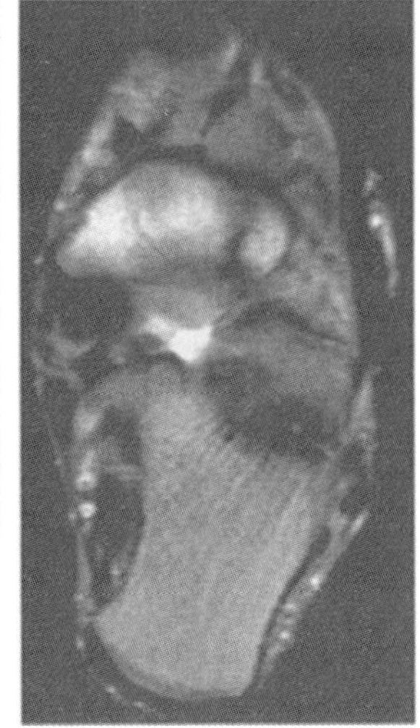
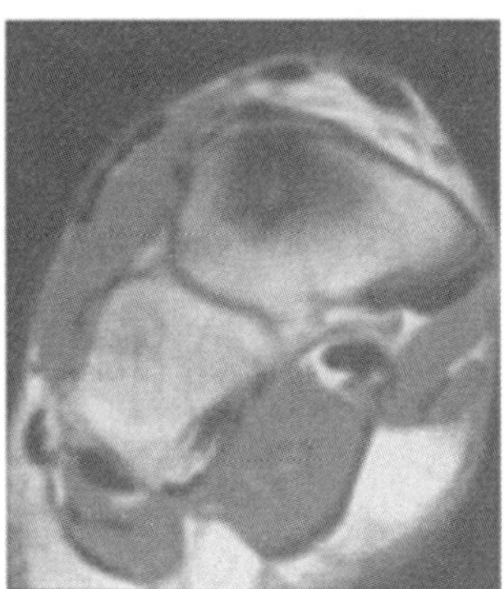

Figure 43.1 Chondral bruising of the subtalar joint.

Table 43.1 Ligament supports of the subtalar joint

Ligament	Protects joint from
Lateral talocalcaneal	Inversion and dorsiflexion
Anterior talocalcaneal	Inversion
Medial talocalcaneal	Eversion
Posterior talocalcaneal	Inversion and dorsiflexion
Calcaneofibular ligament (lateral collateral of the ankle)	Inversion and dorsiflexion
Deltoid/tibiocalcaneal ligament (medial collateral of the ankle)	Eversion and abduction

inflammation/bony bruising is the most common cause detected on MRI (Figure 43.1), further aggravated by hypermobility of the joint due to ligamentous damage.

The symptoms are diverse, but often consist of pain on weight-bearing with lateral and/or medial heel pain. There may be tenderness over the sinus tarsi, indicating inflammation of this accessory joint. The location is most easily palpated just above the sustentaculum talus (a projection of the calcaneum) and some way below the medial malleolus. Detection of the swelling and bony oedema within the area is best detected by MRI. Forced eversion of the ankle can cause pain, and hypermobility of the joint can be detected by passive movements, comparing subtalar movements of both limbs (Shear et al. 1993).

The treatment is conservative before considering immobilization. The use of an orthotic device may be of use if the rear foot demonstrates a chronic valgus deformity, for example (Wooten et al. 1990). Other anti-inflammatory modalities and medication should be considered, along with appropriate footwear.

A cortisone injection under radiographic screening can be diagnostic as well as therapeutic. One technique for injecting the joint is via the posterolateral approach. The point of entry is approximately 2.5 cm above the tip of the lateral malleolus and 1 cm medial to the posterior border of the fibula. The needle is introduced at a 55° angle until the resistance of the chondral surface is felt. Other approaches to the joint can be directly from the medial and lateral aspect of the subtalar joint, detecting the route via surface anatomy and checking the progress of the needle with imaging. These approaches are difficult because the bony contours vary from patient to patient (Cyriax and Cyriax 1993).

References

Cyriax, J. H., Cyriax, P. J. *Cyriax's illustrated manual of orthopaedic medicine* (2nd edn). Butterworth-Heinemann, Oxford, 1993.

Eisle, S. A., Sammarco, G. J. Fatigue fractures of the foot and ankle in the athlete. *Journal of Bone and Joint Surgery*, 1993, 75A, 290–8.

Heilman, A. E., Braly, W. G., Bishop, J. O., Noble, P. C., Tullos, H. S. An anatomic study of subtalar instability. *Foot and Ankle*, 1990, 10(4), 224–8.

Sarrafian, S. S. *Anatomy of the foot and ankle* (2nd edn). Lippincott, Philadelphia, 1983.

Shear, M. S., Baitch, S. P., Shear, D. B. Sinus tarsi syndrome. The importance of biomechanically based evaluation and treatment. *Archives of Physical Medicine and Rehabilitation*, 1993, 74, 777–81.

Wooten, B., Uhl, T., Chandler, J. Use of an orthotic device in treatment of posterior heel pain. *Journal of Orthopaedic and Sports Physical Therapy*, 1990, 11, 410–3.

Chapter 44

Plantar fasciitis and heel pain

Bryan English

Plantar fasciitis

The fascial layers within the foot have several functions:

- shock absorbency by limiting displacement of the fat pads under the calcaneum and metatarsal heads
- site for muscle attachments
- protection of the plantar vessels, nerves and muscles from excessive compressive forces
- facilitation of tendon movement and 'holding down' of muscles and tendons in the sole of the foot
- creation of optimal transmission of biomechanical forces.

The fascial layers consist of interdigitating fibrous tissue. The main fascial layer is the plantar aponeurosis, which consists of medial, lateral, and central portions. Only the central section is truly aponeurotic. The origin of this tissue, at the medial process of the medial calcaneal tuberosity, is the site of the most common type of plantar fasciitis (Figure 44.1). The fascia may also be inflamed elsewhere along its length, when it is painful on stretching with dorsiflexion of the toes. The insertion of the fascia is partly via the superficial stratum that inserts into the dermis (under and distal to the metatarsophalangeal joints) and partly via the deep stratum that inserts into the plantar ligaments of the metatarsophalangeal joints, the flexor tendon sheaths, and the periosteal layer of the proximal phalanges.

Aetiology

Table 44.1 lists causes of plantar fasciitis. The condition can be very resistant to treatment. It may occur in the flat (pronated) foot as well as the high-arched (supinated) foot. However, a common fault is a failure to address the biomechanical abnormalities or variants that may be present. As stated in Chapter 41, excessive strain can be put on the fascia by alteration of rear foot and/or forefoot mechanics. Excessive or repetitive stretch on the fascia will lead to microtrauma and inflammation.

The windlass mechanism (Figure 44.2) is widely mentioned in literature on the foot and ankle. The mechanical dynamics of this system are worth mentioning in this chapter in relation to heel pain. As a consequence of the sites of origin and insertion of the plantar fascia, there is supination of the foot during toe off in the gait cycle. At toe off, there is dorsiflexion of the metatarsophalangeal joints, thereby tensioning the plantar fascia, which in turn decreases the distance of the fascial length between the calcaneum and the metatarsophalangeal joints. The result is a supinated foot, which is a rigid lever and therefore the most appropriate structure to transmit forces during the propulsive phase of gait. Excessive dorsiflexion of the metatarsophalangeal joints may occur in an effort to maintain the duration of the weightbearing phase and to transmit the maximum forces possible. For example, decreased ankle dorsiflexion due to a tight gastrocnemius–soleus complex will result in an increased dorsiflexion of the metatarsophalangeal joints during gait. This excessive movement in turn results in extra stretch on the plantar fascia due to the windlass mechanism. The resulting microtrauma leads to inflammation at the calcaneal insertion of the fascia.

The valgus heel or excessive functional pronation of the foot can result in excess strain of the plantar fascia because of the increased distance between the origin and insertion. However, when the foot remains in pronation, excessive work is performed by the muscles to transmit the necessary forces. The pronated foot is a non-rigid lever. The mechanical inefficiency that is therefore present may also lead to microtrauma within the foot or lower leg.

Increased tension with great toe hyperextension encourages a supinated foot.

Diagnosis

This is confirmed by history and examination. The patient will describe pain and an inability to walk normally for several minutes on rising in the morning and after several minutes' sitting during waking hours. The pain will ease to an extent after walking for several minutes.

Examination demonstrates an area of specific tenderness at the insertion of the aponeurosis at the heel. It is common for stretching of the fascia to be painless, whereas palpation of the plantar fascia itself may detect other areas of tenderness due to microtrauma, and also tightness that can be visible (especially with passive dorsiflexion of the toes) and palpable comparing one side to the other (compared to a boggy sensation if there has been a medial band rupture). Interestingly, passive dorsiflexion of the toes does not cause pain at the insertion of the calcaneum; however, there is pain if there is a plantar fasciitis in the midfoot.

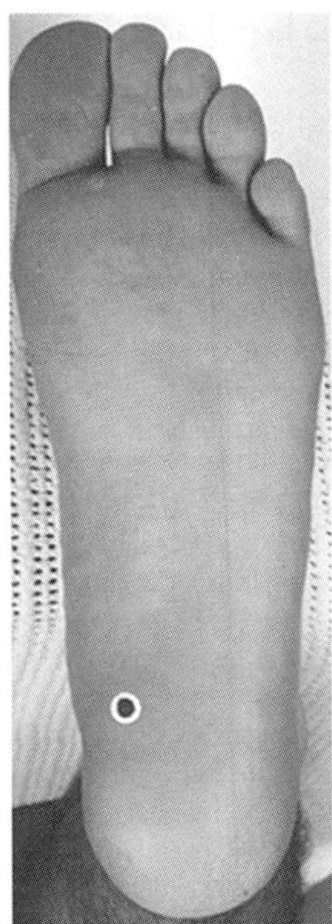

Figure 44.1 The classic site for plantar fasciitis is the anteromedial border of the calcaneum.

Investigations

These are of limited value for this condition. The presence of a calcaneal spur on a lateral radiograph is normally irrelevant, although a tumour or stress fracture of the calcaneum would be excluded as part of the differential diagnosis. The resistant fasciitis, however, may be due to the presence of a rheumatological disorder. An enthesopathy may be present in conditions such as the seropositive and seronegative arthritides. A plain radiograph will show furring at the site of inflammation and this pathology may be confirmed with appropriate serological investigations and an isotope bone scan, although this latter investigation may be positive with a purely trauma-induced periostitis.

Table 44.1 Causes of plantar fasciitis

Structural	Supinated foot with poor flexibility of fascia
	Excess weight
Structure leading to a functional disorder	Pronated foot due to rear/forefoot abnormality
	Tight plantar fascia
	Decreased dorsiflexion at the ankle
Functional disorder	Overuse injury due to excessive training/poor footwear/hard surface
	Hypertonic gastrocnemius–soleus complex
	Hypertonic deep flexors of the lower leg
Systemic	Enthesopathy due to rheumatological disorder

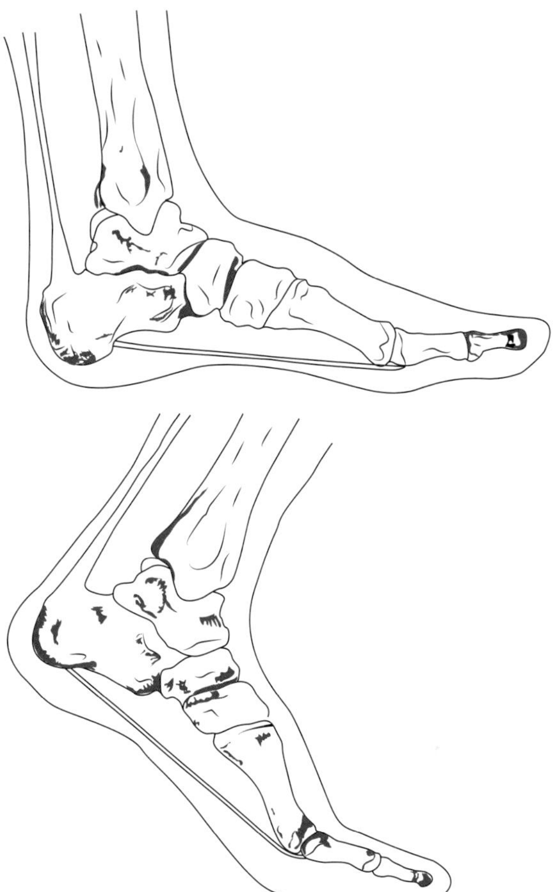

Figure 44.2 Windlass mechanism.

Treatment

This is related to the aetiology (Batt and Tanji 1995). It is important to establish realistic goal-setting; the individual may find it hard to accept that this 'injury' may take 6 months to heal. The basic principle here is to decrease the forces that go through the plantar fascia. Correction of biomechanical abnormalities has been discussed in Chapter 41. If the condition occurs as a result of overuse, then once again, temporary or permanent orthoses may be used to take the strain off the fascia. As this condition often proves resistant to treatment, a multidisciplinary approach is indicated, as is the case with most enthesopathies (e.g. compare with lateral epicondylitis).

Self-management

This may be the key. It consists of self-massage to the length of the fascia (with fingers or rolling the foot over a golf ball), self-articulation to the joints of the ankle and foot (to result in a more compliant and shock-absorbing structure), stretching of the calf muscles and deep flexors, decreasing excess body weight, and wearing shoes with good shock absorbency (such as marathon running shoes or devices with viscoelastic insoles). Avoiding aggravating factors (such as running on roads) must also be considered. Anti-inflammatory drugs may be prescribed for a 4-week period at a maximum dose.

If there is a degree of success with self-management, then the patient should be introduced to a rehabilitation programme that will gradually increase the stress on the fascia, so that it may remodel

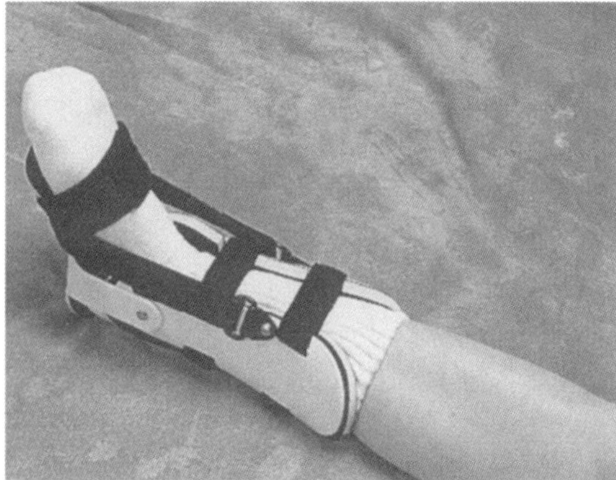

Figure 44.3 Night splint.

and begin to cope with increased force. Progress may seem painfully slow, especially for the impatient athlete. Long-distance walking should be employed well before running. Adequate explanation to the patient will often result in increased compliance. Use of a night splint (Figure 44.3) or strapping techniques will maintain fascial stretch when at rest.

Orthotics

These may then present a second line of treatment, used in conjunction with self-management. It must be pointed out that although examination of the foot may demonstrate no biomechanical abnormalities, visualization of the foot when walking or running may highlight notable overpronation that may be the cause of the plantar fasciitis.

Other methods of treatment

If there is no success with these treatments, then the use of a *cortisone injection* may have greater success than if it were used as a first line of treatment. The injection should be directed to the site of tenderness preferably from the medial aspect of the calcaneum, with an administration of 1.5 ml of local anaesthetic plus 10 mg of triamcinolone, for example. Injections directly into the inferior aspect of the foot can be very painful and cause degeneration of the shock-absorbing fat pads within the area.

Immobilization of the foot in a slipper cast is a method of alleviating forces through the fascia if the pathology appears to be purely chronic inflammation. A more popular method of 'scientific' immobilization is with the use of a night splint (Figure 44.3) that creates a stretch on the fascia when at rest.

Surgery to the plantar fascia must be avoided if at all possible. The alteration of the foot biomechanics in the absence of an effective aponeurosis will result in increased compressive forces in the midfoot, plus a decreased arch height and an increased susceptibility to metatarsalgia. Incision of the plantar fascia using a medial approach can be used, taking care to avoid damage to the medial calcaneal branch of the posterior tibial nerve (damage to the nerve may result in a painful neuroma) and the first branch of the lateral plantar nerve.

Other causes of heel pain

A number of conditions may give rise to heel pain (Doxey 1987; Leach et al. 1983).

Entrapment of the first branch of the lateral plantar nerve

This nerve innervates the medial aspect of the calcaneum, the long plantar ligament, and the muscles of flexor brevis and abductor digiti quinti (Henricson and Westlin 1984). The nerve may become trapped between the muscles of the quadratus plantaris, superiorly, and the muscles of the abductor hallucis and flexor brevis, inferiorly (Figure 44.4). These muscles may become particularly hypertonic in athletes such as sprinters. A calcaneal spur may also add a compression element in this narrow space, and the local inflammatory changes of a plantar fasciitis may also be a causative factor.

This pathology is differentiated from a plantar fasciitis on clinical grounds. The site of tenderness is medial and superior to the origin of the plantar fascia. Pressure at this site may also produce referred pain to the heel. Paraesthesia is rare, and not a reliable diagnostic feature. Correspondingly, nerve conduction studies are not sufficiently sophisticated to isolate this branch.

Treatment of this lesion is very similar to that of plantar fasciitis. Physical therapy to the relevant musculature can also be of great benefit. If self-management, manual treatment, orthotics, and injections have not succeeded, then surgical release of the nerve is indicated. This consists of release of the fascial layers of the muscles compressing the nerve, along with removal of a heel spur if present.

Tarsal tunnel syndrome

The posterior tibial nerve may be trapped as it passes beneath the flexor retinaculum due to the anatomical restrictions within the tarsal tunnel (Figure 44.5). The compression of the nerve is commonly due to increased pressure within the tunnel, this in turn being due to swelling or inflammation as a result of acute or chronic trauma. The symptoms are of a diffuse heel pain/burning plus paraesthesia or numbness of the lateral and plantar aspect of the foot

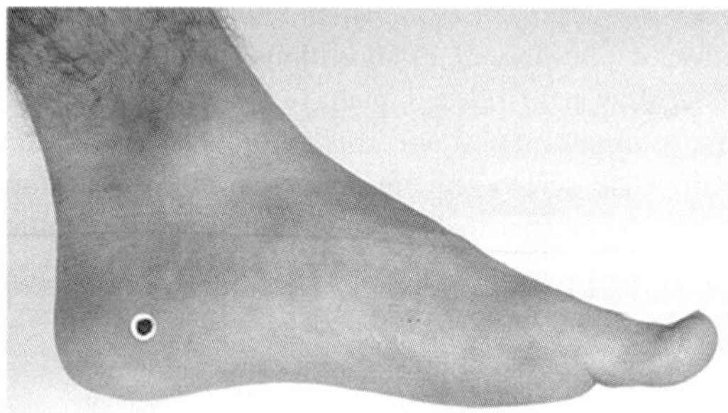

Figure 44.4 Site of tenderness and of entrapment.

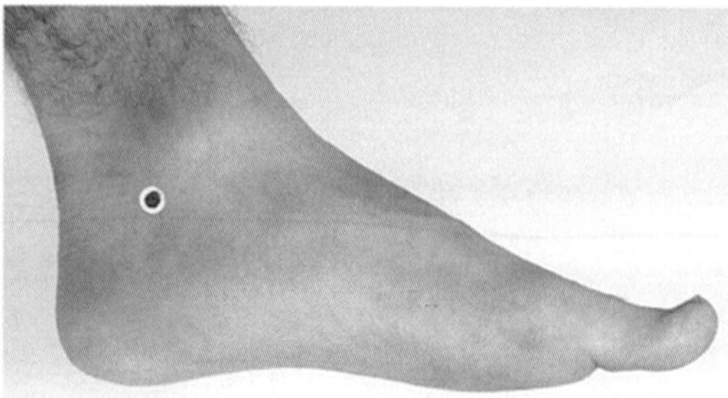

Figure 44.5 Tarsal tunnel syndrome.

and toes. The symptoms may be reproduced by percussion over the nerve (Tinel's sign). Tenderness over the heel is rare.

Other than pure compression, causes of tarsal tunnel syndrome comprise varicose vein, bony fracture/osseous encroachment, ganglion (or other space-occupying lesion), and systemic pathologies such as myxoedema.

The diagnosis tends to be made from the history and examination findings. Nerve conduction tests are unreliable and, if anything, are used to confirm a diagnosis, not to make one (as for carpal tunnel syndrome). An injection of local anaesthetic into the tarsal tunnel may alleviate the distal symptoms and further substantiate the diagnosis.

Treatment is initially by relieving the pressure on the nerve. In a patient who overpronates, the use of a corrective orthotic can solve the problem. Cortisone may be only a temporary measure. Surgical release of the retinaculum is the treatment of choice if other measures have failed. Once again, the benefit of a good history and precise examination, including a functional analysis, will assist the practitioner in differentiating one of the less common pathologies associated with heel pain.

Fat pad atrophy

The fat pad is a 'cushion' consisting of a series of spirals of vertically orientated elastic adipose tissue, connecting the calcaneum to the skin. The pad is an effective shock absorber that deteriorates with increasing age. The pain and tenderness are situated directly under the body of the calcaneum (Figure 44.6) but, in some patients, the pain and tenderness can be diffuse. Patients with atrophy or degeneration of the fat pad can be diagnosed by palpation. Rather than a density of 'rubbery' soft tissue under the heel, there is a sensation of a thin dermal layer overlying the bone. Indeed, the calcaneal tuberosities are easily palpable through this tissue.

Treatment for this condition is limited. Shock-absorbing heel cups are of benefit, with footwear that is made with highly attenuating material (that is, with viscoelastic properties).

Immobilization in a plaster of Paris slipper relieves the area of weightbearing for a period of 4–6 weeks. The concern over injecting cortisone into this area is the direct association with fat degeneration. Such a treatment can give marked relief, but there is a lack of controlled studies and long-term follow-up with this treatment. Injectable
anti-inflammatory homeopathic remedies, such as Traumeel, have been advocated by those who fear the adverse side-effects of cortisone.

Retrocalcaneal bursitis

This occurs due to repetitive motion of the Achilles tendon over the back of the calcaneum. Patients may have a prominence of the superior angle of the calcaneum (Figure 44.7).

Adequate stretching of the calf muscles is advised. A temporary heel raise may prevent excessive dorsiflexion. Injection therapy may be of benefit; otherwise, the superior angle of the calcaneum may be surgically removed.

Achilles (postcalcaneal) bursitis

Direct pressure of footwear over the back of the tendon, with the prominent bone beneath, may result in this condition (Figure 44.8). Avoiding pressure to the area is an obvious treatment, so removal of a heel tab on running shoes can provide a 'useful cure'. Injection therapy may alleviate the acute symptoms if more invasive treatment is sought. The lesion may become chronic and lead to the development of granulation/fibrous tissue and bone bossing, resulting in a lesion called a 'pump bump'. This disorder is common in sports such as ice hockey and with people who wear footwear that is too tight.

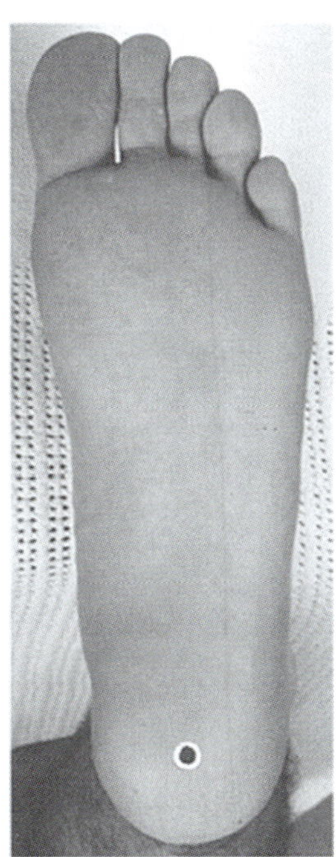

Figure 44.6 Central site for heel tenderness with fat pad atrophy.

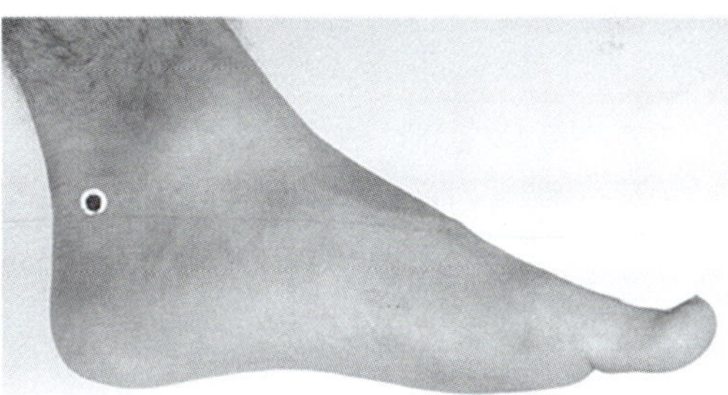

Figure 44.7 Retrocalcaneal bursitis.

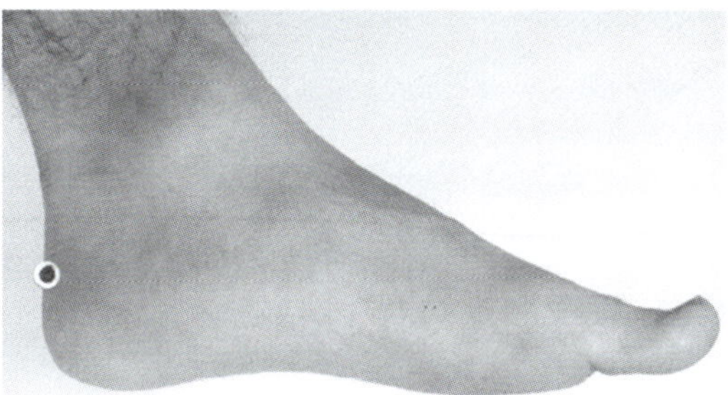

Figure 44.8 Achilles bursitis.

Surgical excision of the excess soft tissue, along with excision of the bony prominences, is sometimes the only way to restore comfort.

References

Batt, M. E., Tanji, J. L. Management options for plantar fasciitis. *The Physician and Sports Medicine*, 1995, 23, 77–86.

Doxey, G. E. Calcaneal pain: a review of various disorders. *Journal of Orthopaedic and Sports Physical Therapy*, 1987, 9, 25–32.

Henricson, A. S., Westlin, N. E. Chronic calcaneal pain in athletes. Entrapment of the calcaneal nerve? *American Journal of Sports Medicine*, 1984, 12, 152–4.

Leach, R. E., Delorio, E., Harney, R. A. Pathologic hindfoot conditions in the athlete. *Clinical Orthopaedics*, 1983, 177, 116.

Chapter 45

Tendinopathies and enthesopathies

Thomas Crisp

Structure and function of tendons

Ligaments and tendons are very similar collagenized structures with minor subtle differences. Studies on ligament structure give clear indications relevant to tendons and vice versa and will be considered as the same in this chapter. Adult tendons and ligaments are composed of largely type 1 collagen in tight bands, with very little type III collagen. The fluid between the fibrils contains proteoglycans and a small number of elastic fibres. There is a slightly wavy 'crimp' with a consequent ability to stretch built in. The number and type of collagen fibrils correlates closely with the tensile strength. The tendon is able to stretch up to about 4% without any loss of structure and tearing occurs after this point, up to complete rupture at about 10% stretch. The structure allows the Achilles, for example, to withstand 4000 Newtons in toe running and the patellar tendon accepts 8000 Newtons landing from a jump.

The effect of immobilization is to reduce the tensile strength; 12 weeks of immobilization of a rabbit's medial collateral ligament showed a 30% reduction in collagen mass (Amiel et al. 1983). In contrast, experiments on animals generally show an increase in ligament strength as a response to endurance exercise with, in some, an increase in collagen mass. Magnusson suggests that some of the effects of ageing on collagen mass, fibre size, and type are reversed by endurance exercise in humans (Magnusson et al. 2008). These changes are slow and, especially after either immobilization or surgery, experiments suggest it may be up to 6–12 months before strength is regained.

Blood supply is somewhat limited and is restricted to small vessels in the fascicular membrane around the fascicles arising from the musculo-tendinous junction and the bone insertion. There is no additional blood supply in the normal tendon along its length.

Pathology of a tendinopathy

Viidik (1973) has shown that tendons undergo increasing deformation with repeated loads, which are well below the area of the load–strain curve that indicates fibre disruption. It is therefore possible that some runners do not have Achilles tendons strong enough to withstand repetitive loading without disruption of some fibres, leading to accumulating damage and tendinopathy. Studies by Chun (1989) have also shown that there are differences in the ability of fibres to resist force—with the medial fibres of human patellar tendon failing at loads that the lateral fibres can withstand.

Constant turnover of collagen is carried out by tenocytes in the tendon and changes occur to this process in tendinopathy. There is increased production of type III collagen and changes to the proteoglycan molecules in the ground substance. Such changes may cause more water to be held in the tendon, thereby contributing to swelling of the tendon. Metalloproteinases, which show increased levels in painful tendinopathy, play an as yet undetermined role in this degradation process. There is also an increase in neuropeptides in degenerate tendons and this is thought to possibly play a part as well.

It is evident from these changes that the process is one of degeneration and not inflammation—hence a tendinosis (or tendinopathy), not tendinitis. There is no evidence of up-regulation of inflammatory cytokines in chronic tendinopathy, although they may play a part in short-term inflammation after a bout of exercise.

It has been suggested that there is a strict sequence of changes in the tendon as tendinopathy develops (Malliaras et al. 2010). The first finding in early tendinopathy is a change in the ground substance with increased water and changes in collagen—this is evident clinically with swelling and tenderness of the tendon. Diagnostic ultrasound at this stage (the investigation of choice) will show thickening of the tendon with maintenance of the normal striated pattern of the tendon. This stage is associated with changes in the proteoglycan molecules as already mentioned. It is not yet clear whether the dimensions of the tendon vary during the course of 24 hours in response to rest, exercise, stretching, etc.

As the degradation of collagen proceeds, areas of hypoechoicity appear on ultrasound and the pattern on magnetic resonance imaging (MRI) scanning shows some reduced signal on T1-weighted images and less homogeneity. At this stage, neovessels appear on Doppler scanning, arising deep to Achilles and patellar tendons and growing into the tendon. These vessels seem to be related to significant production locally of vascular endothelial growth factor (VEGF), stimulated by a combination of mechanical stress, hypoxia, and inflammatory cytokines and causing increased production of metalloproteinases (Pufe et al. 2005).

Associated with the neovessels are nerves, and it is possible that they do more than contribute to the sensation of pain. Equally, removing the nerves and arteries may be an important part of treating the condition. It is possible that a neural message alters the behaviour of the tenocytes, possibly by modulating the metalloproteinases and VEGF, but the alterations in tenocyte behaviour have been shown to continue *in vitro*, producing type III collagen if taken from a tendinopathic tendon. It has been suggested that there is a neural element to many chronic injuries and treating back dysfunction is an essential part of treating tendinopathy (Webborn 2008).

Aetiology of a tendinopathy

A number of factors have been identified as contributing to the risk of developing tendinopathy (Table 45.1). Adverse biomechanics and shock-absorbing properties of the lower limbs have been discussed as causes of lower limb tendinopathy and it is likely they contribute, but the evidence is not conclusive (Bartosik et al. 2010). More important probably is the amount of stress, often the miles run, and there is good evidence that the risk of repetitive stress injury increases with increasing running miles. Perhaps as important is the rate of increase—it is often found that repetitive stress injury is most likely to occur within 2 weeks after starting an activity or after a significant increase in load. McHugh found little convincing evidence that stretching affects risk of injury (McHugh and Cosgrave 2010), and there is even less evidence, at present, comparing forefoot striking with rearfoot strike. A lot is written about footwear and the need for shoes that conform to 'desirable' biomechanics, but this has yet to be proven (Richards et al. 2009). However, it is apparent that pronation is associated with a degree of torsion of the Achilles tendon and this may contribute to the stress and so to the damage to collagen fibres.

Recent studies have shown a possible relationship with fat distribution (Gaida et al. 2010) with central fat in men but peripheral fat in women being associated with tendinopathic changes in Achilles tendons, and there has been recent interest in possible relationship between bilateral Achilles tendinopathy and back dysfunction. Yet while we strive for evidence on which to base our medical practice, we are often left making assumptions—for example, that foot biomechanics affects the risk of developing Achilles tendinopathy.

Table 45.1 Aetiological factors for tendinopathy

Intrinsic factors	Extrinsic factors
Foot biomechanics	Footwear
Leg length discrepancy	Training load (speed and distance)
Flexibility	Training venue (hill running, etc.)
(a) Age	
BMI/fat distribution	
Back pain	
Running style (forefoot striking, etc.)	
Achilles structure and size	
Genetics/gender	
Age	

History of a tendinopathy

Tendinopathy, like most repetitive stress injuries, presents gradually in a patient who has been accustomed to exercise that includes running. Often, the first symptom is pain at the start of exercise, which eases with warm-up, to recur at the end of exercise, but as it progresses, it lasts longer during the exercise and for longer afterwards. Early morning stiffness is a relatively early symptom and, without this symptom, the diagnosis becomes less certain. Swelling is a relatively late symptom and may not be noticed at all; it can also vary depending on recent exercise. Clearly, high-impact exercise is more likely to produce symptoms than low- or non-impact. Symptoms may vary in different footwear; trainers that support the foot may cause less pain walking than court or work shoes that offer little support. A sudden onset of pain in a previously asymptomatic tendon implies a partial tear and demands investigation. Experience shows lengthy recovery if not diagnosed and treated aggressively, early; ultrasound scanning should be considered if there is any doubt.

In undiagnosed or inadequately treated partial tears, it is often found that secondary tendinopathy develops at a later stage. It is also not uncommon to find some tendinopathic changes in the asymptomatic limb that may occasionally become symptomatic when the other side is treated.

The patient should be asked about risk factors for inflammatory disease, which may be associated with tendinopathy—family history, presence of psoriasis, ulcerative colitis, urethritis, etc. There is also an association with recent antibiotic intake, especially of Ciprofloxacin.

Examination for a tendinopathy

Examination will reveal possible risk factors for tendinopathy such as anomalous foot biomechanics, leg length difference, etc. It may reveal stiffness in the ankle, triceps surae, or quadriceps. In some, there is a history suggestive of prior calf tears and this may be associated with tenderness or thickening of the calf musculature. The back should be examined and referred pain or a neural component excluded where possible.

Locally, there may be swelling of the tendon, and tenderness. Localized tenderness is almost always reduced by stretching the tendon, a feature that has been validated as being associated with tendinopathy at The London Hospital, Whitechapel. If there is no tenderness or if it is not reduced by stretching, the diagnosis must be called into question. There may be tenderness deep to the distal portion of the free tendon—at Haglunds bursa. In insertional tendinopathy, the swelling is at the portion of the tendon overlying the calcaneum; a superficial bursa may be evident. The tenderness associated with fascia crural tears is very localized and is evident usually on one side (commonly medial) of the tendon. There is no sign on examination that indicates involvement of the plantaris, although symptoms are often more medial.

Differential diagnosis of a tendinopathy

Many conditions may mimic tendinopathy and this varies with site. The following is not a comprehensive list but indicates areas of possible confusion:

- Partial or complete ruptures
- Inflammatory enthesopathy
- Bursitis
- Impingement syndromes (e.g. ankle or Hoffa's fat pad)
- Accessory soleus muscle
- Fascia crural tears (Achilles)
- Referred pain, neural entrapment
- Muscle tears (including plantaris)
- Stress fractures

Imaging for a tendinopathy

The modality of choice for tendinopathy in all sites is ultrasound. This gives greater detail of the striated pattern in the normal and variations in the pathological. With the advent of power Doppler, it provides the ability to monitor neovascularity. However, the assessment of vascularity is extremely subjective and variable. Mild tension in a tendon can cause the vessels previously evident to disappear. With patellar tendinopathy, extreme knee extension can have the same effect, maybe by compression. The presence of vessels is also blood pressure dependent and they can disappear with a mild vaso-vagal attack, for example. Ultrasound is particularly accurate at identifying small partial tears that need to be treated differently, as well as abnormalities in the fascia cruri that are seen to either side of the Achilles tendon. It can pick up ectopic calcification in the distal Achilles or proximal patellar tendon. The plantaris muscle can be seen on ultrasound scanning in the medial portion of the intermuscular fascia between the gastrocnemius and soleus and distally, closely associated with the medial border of the Achilles tendon. Ultrasound may show thickening and, occasionally, tears of the plantaris.

MRI can pick up some of the differential diagnoses as well as showing some of the tendinopathic abnormalities. It can reveal an accessory soleus—an abnormally low musculo-tendinous junction (and therefore short, free tendon) that can cause compression and a phenomenon similar to compartment syndrome. It will demonstrate bursae—both superficial and deep (Haglunds)—but no better than ultrasound. It may not show well the calcification that often occurs in insertional tendinopathy. However, it can demonstrate changes within the adjacent bones that can, rarely, cause tendinopathy-like symptoms.

X-ray will demonstrate calcification within the tendon and can show the sharp postero-superior angle of the calcaneum in Haglunds' syndrome where the bone impinges on the lower portion of the Achilles. However, it is rarely as useful as ultrasound.

Management of a tendinopathy

Eccentric loading has become the gold standard for non-invasive treatment of tendinopathy, whether in the Achilles or patellar tendon or common extensor origin at the elbow. Before Alfredson's team devised the heavy eccentric regime, there had been work by Stanish et al. (1985), among others, suggesting that eccentric loading may be more effective than concentric. Now, these exercises, performed with mild discomfort, are the gold standard. It is important to perform the exercises wearing shoes and with a straight knee for part of the exercise programme and slightly flexed for another. However, various alterations or additions have been tried to give greater efficacy. Dimitrios, for example, showed that stretching as well as eccentric loading was better than eccentrics alone for patellar tendinopathy (Dimitrios et al. 2012).

Eccentric exercises work slowly—Alfredson (2008) showed significant improvements over 12 weeks and, in some patients, disappearance of abnormalities on ultrasound, although in our experience the symptoms abate before the appearance of the tendon itself improves. Strengthening the quadriceps for the patellar tendon and calf, for Achilles tendinopathy, has been shown to have benefits. Anecdotally, improving core stability and thus shock absorption may be of benefit.

Treatment of identified predisposing factors is essential, as is reduction of training load during the treatment period. For those patients who have been unable to pursue their high-impact sport, we have advised them to return gradually and to take approximately half the time they have been out of sport to get back to pre-injury levels. So, for a runner unable to run for 6 months, we would advise 3 months to return to full training once treated and asymptomatic.

It is important to reduce the heel lowering to no further than neutral in insertional Achilles tendinopathy and to perform eccentric squats for the patellar tendon on a 20° decline (toes down) to reduce the load on the Achilles. Equally important though is to perform a complete rehabilitation programme to address any loss of function that has either contributed to or has resulted from the tendinopathy.

Other treatment modalities have been shown to have some benefit. Glyceryl trinitrate (GTN) patches reduce pain but there is little evidence that they affect healing. Acupuncture and dry needling have been used as an adjunct to rehabilitation. A small proportion of patients have an inflammatory process (and this may be evident on ultrasound), and this aspect must be addressed.

Injection therapy for a tendinopathy

In the past, it has been customary to inject corticosteroid around tendons in resistant cases. Concerns have been raised that this may lead to increased risk of rupture, but unless the injection is within the tendon, there is no hard evidence that this is so. However, there are now more effective treatments. Ohberg and Alfredson (2002) have demonstrated that removal of the neovessels can be beneficial. They injected a sclerosant (polidocanol) around the neovessels with some success, although this has not been reproduced elsewhere and the long-term results may be less successful.

A technique developed by Humphrey and colleagues (2010) involves injection of a high volume (40 ml) of normal saline and 10 ml of local anaesthetic deep to the Achilles tendon (slightly smaller volumes for the patellar tendon). This has produced the best published results (over 80% return to sport without symptoms). It has been possible to return to top-level sport, including Premier League football in the UK, 14 days after this procedure (Table 45.2). A recent multi-centre comparison (yet to be published) between this injection with a small dose of hydrocortisone and the same without shows no significant difference in results, and it is therefore reasonable to omit the steroid.

Results seem to be similar regardless of the stage of degeneration (as previously described) and irrespective of neovascularity, and it is still merely speculation what the local effect of these injections is. It has been proposed, however, that there is some denervation, since the early morning stiffness is very often lost the day after injection.

Table 45.2 Post-injection protocol for high-volume injection

Day 0	Injection
Days 1–3	No exercise
Days 4–6	Eccentric exercises only
Days 7–9	Non-impact exercise and strengthening
Day 10	Gradual start to impact exercise

Autologous blood and PRP (platelet-rich plasma) have received a large amount of publicity in recent years but the published results are variable and there is probably no difference between the two, as demonstrated in a study of tennis elbow (Creaney et al. 2011). Further, these injections are given into the substance of the tendon and could cause similar damage to that associated with other injections into the tendon, as well as being only possible if there is significant degeneration of the tendon. Further research is needed before these injections can be regarded as normal practice. There is also huge variation in the preparation methodology of PRP and, therefore, in the content of growth factors that are said to be the effective ingredient, and further standardization is needed before conclusions can be drawn about efficacy. A recent IOC (International Olympic Committee) consensus statement published in *Sports Medicine* in 2011 concluded that there was insufficient evidence to justify the expense of PRP injection into tendons, at present.

Other types of injections are carried out—including other forms of sclerosant—either around the vessels or into the tendon. Injections such as epidural steroid injections (to address possible neural components) have also been used. There is little data to support most of these treatments.

Surgical treatment for tendinopathy

Surgery for tendinopathy has become much less common due to the advances in non-surgical treatments over the last 10 years. Various studies have shown slow return of strength to tendons following surgery, even after minimally invasive procedures, taking over 26 weeks in many cases. There is also a significant infection risk after surgery to Achilles tendons, which cannot be totally avoided.

One simple treatment for Achilles tendinopathy is to separate the tendon from Kagar's fat by running a scalpel down the deep surface of the tendon. In more severe cases, it may be necessary to divide the tendon and remove degenerate tissue. Some surgeons are trying progressively less invasive treatments such as drawing a thread down the deep surface of the tendon. At present, however, no clear benefit has been demonstrated for these techniques over the various treatments outlined in this chapter.

Surgery addressing the shape of the patella tip or the superior calcaneum (in Haglunds' syndrome) has been used with success. Overall however, it is clear that surgery should be a late option.

References

Alfredson H, Cook J, (2007) A treatment algorithm for managing Achilles tendinopathy: new treatment options. B J Sports Med 41(4):211–216.

Amiel D, Akeson WH, Harwood FL, Frank CB. (1983) Stress deprivation effect on the metabolic turnover of MCL collagen. *Clin Orthop Related Res* 172:265–70.

Bartosik KE, Sitler M, Hillstrom HJ, Palamarchuk H, Huxel K, Kim E. (2010) Anatomical and biomechanical assessments of medial tibial stress syndrome. *Am Podiatr Med Assoc* 100(2):121–32.

Chun KJ. (1989) Spatial variation in material properties in human patellar tendon. *Trans Orthop Res Soc* 14:214.

Creaney L, Wallace A, Curtis M, Connell D. (2011) Growth factor-based therapies provide additional benefit beyond physical therapy in resistant elbow tendinopathy: a prospective, single-blind, randomised trial of autologous blood injections versus platelet-rich plasma injections. *J Sports Med* 45(12):966–71. DOI: 10.1136/bjsm.2010.082503.

Humphrey J, Chan O, Crisp T, et al. (2010) Short-term effects of high-volume image-guided injections in resistant non-insertional Achilles tendinopathy. *J Sci Med Sport* 13(3):295–8.

Dimitrios S, Pantelis M, Kalliopi S. (2012) Comparing the effects of eccentric training with eccentric training and static stretching exercises in the treatment of patellar tendinopathy. A controlled clinical trial. *Clin Rehabil* 26(5):423–30. DOI: 10.1177/0269215511411114.

Gaida JE, Alfredson H, Kiss ZS, Bass SL, Cook JL. (2010) Asymptomatic Achilles tendon pathology is associated with a central fat distribution in men and a peripheral fat distribution in women: a cross sectional study of 298 individuals. *BMC Musculoskelet Disord* 11:41. DOI: 10.1186/1471-2474-11-41.

Magnusson SP, Narici MV, Maganaris CN, Kjaer M. (2008) Human tendon behaviour and adaptation, in vivo. *J Physiol* 586(1):71–81.

Malliaras P, Purdam C, Maffulli N, Cook J. (2010) Temporal sequence of greyscale ultrasound changes and their relationship with neovascularity and pain in the patellar tendon. *Br J Sports Med* 44(13):944–7. DOI:0.1136/bjsm.2008.054916.

McHugh MP, Cosgrave CH. (2010) To stretch or not to stretch: the role of stretching in injury prevention and performance. *Scand J Med Sci Sports* 20(2):169–81.

Ohberg L, Alfredson H. (2002) Ultrasound guided sclerosis of neovessels in painful chronic Achilles tendinosis: pilot study of a new treatment. *Br J Sports Med* 36(3):173–5; discussion 176–7.

Pufe T, Petersen WJ, Mentlein R, Tillmann BN. (2005) The role of vasculature and angiogenesis for the pathogenesis of degenerative tendons disease. *Scand J Med Sci Sports* 15(4):211–22.

Richards CE, Magin PJ, Callister R. (2009) Is your prescription of distance running shoes evidence-based? *Br J Sports Med* 43(3):159–62.

Stanish WD, Curwin S, Rubinovich M. (1985) Tendinitis: the analysis and treatment for running. *Clin Sports Med* 4(4):593–609.

Viidik A. (1973) Functional properties of connective tissues. *Intern Rev Connect Tiss Res* 6:127–215.

Webborn AD. (2008) Novel approaches to tendinopathy. *Disabil Rehabil* 30:1572–7.

Chapter 46

Metatarsalgia

Bryan English

The true definition of metatarsalgia is 'pain in the forefoot in the region of the heads of the metatarsals'. The term is subject to abuse, and patients may present with a diagnosis of metatarsalgia with any forefoot pain.

Metatarsophalangeal joint capsulitis

This condition is often due to trauma, but inflammation and a capsulitis at this site can be the result of an underlying inflammatory arthropathy. A non-traumatic onset of problems at this site should alert the diagnostician to consider rheumatological investigations including radiographs and possibly an isotope bone scan.

Traumatic capsulitis of the joints is due to excessive forces being applied to this area. Sportspeople may develop this condition if their footwear lacks adequate shock absorbency. A sudden increase in mileage, a change of footwear, an alteration of terrain, and a recent increase in body weight are all factors that must be taken into account with sports-related overuse trauma. In the sedentary population, excessive body weight and unsuitable footwear (Figure 46.1) are the main causative factors.

As this type of capsulitis is due to excessive loading, any device that will decrease the shock that has to be absorbed will be of great assistance.

The assessment of metatarsal position is important, along with assessment of metatarsal length. A typical presentation of length (numbering the metatarsals from great toe to little toe) is 2 > 1 = 3 > 4 > 5 (Bjosen-Moller 1979).

Interdigital neuroma

Neuritic pain in the region of the metatarsal heads will suggest the presence of a neuroma between two of the metatarsal heads (usually between 2 and 3 or 3 and 4). The neuroma occurs at the anastomoses of the medial and lateral plantar nerves. Other symptoms are paraesthesiae spreading along the two toes that are supplied by the interdigital nerve. The symptoms are aggravated by walking with shoes on.

To confirm this diagnosis, a squeeze test may be performed by clasping the forefoot in one hand and applying pressure to compress the enlarged nerve between the metatarsal heads. Palpation may reveal tenderness over the nerve. This may recreate the pain and/or produce a click (Mulder's sign). The neuroma is a space-occupying lesion and may therefore separate the toes. This is called a 'Winston Churchill' sign, for obvious reasons.

One must also take care to elicit any signs of peripheral neuropathy or vascular insufficiency with neuritic pain. Instability of the metatarsal head may also present in a similar way. Finally, the diagnosis of neuroma may be confirmed by injecting local anaesthetic into the metatarsal space. Ultrasound and magnetic resonance imaging (MRI) investigation will demonstrate the pathology.

Treatment of an interdigital neuroma should initially be conservative. The patient must address the issue of footwear. Shoes that are ill-fitting, especially if they are too tight, may be the cause of the problem. A reduction in those activities that bring on the pain will help, along with a temporary orthotic placed just proximal to the affected interspace. If the pain is due to inflammation, then local infiltration of cortisone can be beneficial. Infiltration would be indicated on up to three occasions at 4-weekly intervals, with the access to the interdigital space being from the dorsal aspect of the foot.

If conservative therapy fails, surgical excision of the neuroma should be considered. The dorsal approach is preferable to the plantar approach. Although the former is technically a more difficult procedure, the latter may produce a painful scar on the weightbearing surface.

Metatarsophalangeal joint instability

This is not an easy diagnosis to make, especially in the early stages. The most common site for the lesion is the second metatarsophalangeal joint. The reason for this is that, in many people, the second metatarsal is longer than the first. This fact, plus excessive loading (for example, in long-distance runners with pronated feet) may lead to joint instability due to collateral ligamentous insufficiency and laxity/disruption of the volar plate (Coughlin 1993). The presentation is of a vague forefoot pain often exacerbated by weightbearing.

There will be tenderness over the joint involved, but no referred neuritic pain (differentiating this disorder from a neuroma) and no tenderness over other metatarsophalangeal joints (as would normally be the case with an inflammatory arthropathy). On examination, the drawer sign will stress the joint in the dorsiplantar direction. Not only will there be excessive movement, but also pain may be intense at the end of range when stretching the joint capsule and/or collateral ligaments. At a later stage, there will be deviation

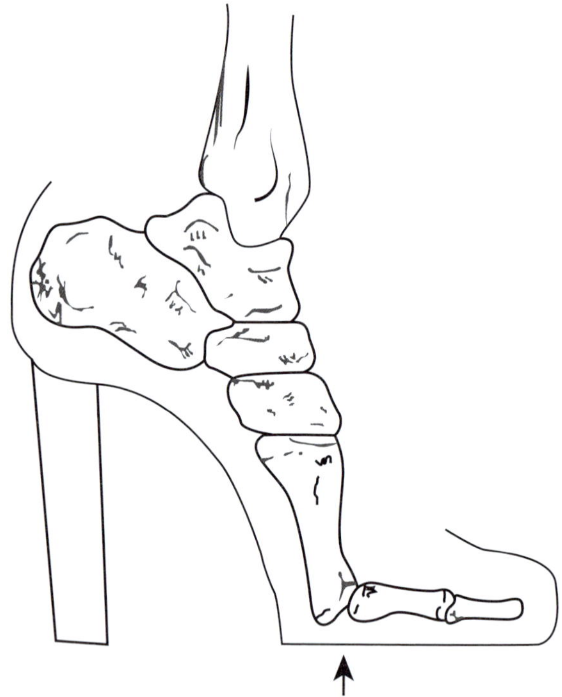

Figure 46.1 Footwear can have a profound effect on the pressure placed on the metatarsophalangeal joints.

of the second toe due to medial malalignment. The exact site of the pain can be determined by infiltrating local anaesthetic. Radiological investigation would consist of an arthrogram.

Treatment for this disorder is conservative if the condition is diagnosed in the early stages. A decrease in activity (if exercise has been an aggravating factor) will be part of the self-management for such a condition. Taping the toe to a neighbouring toe, or using a sling taping device which wraps around the base of the toe (Figure 46.2) may be helpful.

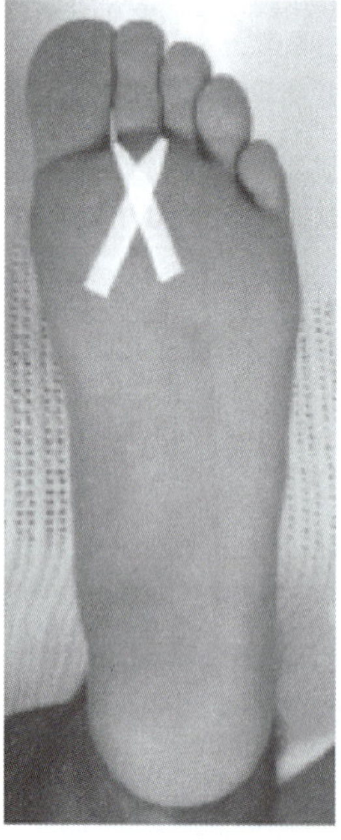

Figure 46.2 Sling taping device.

A metatarsal pad placed proximal to the metatarsophalangeal joint, or a more formal orthotic, will limit the degree of dorsal and plantarflexion, thereby providing a degree of stability. These devices may be used for several months. However, if the symptoms do not resolve, and if the patient undertakes a high level of activity, then surgery may have to be considered (Shereff and Baumhauer 1998). This would take the form of capsular reefing (with a flexor tendon transfer if hyperextension/dorsiplantar instability persists) which tightens the part of the capsule of the joint that has been overstretched. This procedure may not be advisable for a serious athlete, as a return to previous function and the demands of weightbearing sport may not be possible. Surgery would normally be withheld until the end of the athlete's career.

Disorders of the great toe

Hallux rigidus

Degenerative change of the first metatarsophalangeal joint occurs insidiously in some individuals. Various predisposing factors have been suggested, such as osteochondritis of the metatarsal head, a flattened metatarsal head, an overpronated foot, and metatarsus primus elevatus.

The more dramatic presentation follows trauma. An acute synovitis occurs with tenderness, specifically over the dorsal and lateral aspect of the joint. Later, there is bony overgrowth that causes painful impingement, again specifically at the dorsal and lateral aspect of the joint where an exostosis will be visible and palpable. The exostosis may cause discomfort because it forms a pressure point against footwear. Hyperextension of the interphalangeal joint is present.

Decreased dorsiflexion of the first metatarsophalangeal joint can be due to bony proliferation at the superior aspect of the joint, as well as to arthritic degeneration.

The decreased range of movement is very restricting to ambulation and effective use of the foot as an energy return system. This condition is disastrous for athletes, because of the functional restrictions it imposes on jumping, turning, accelerating, etc. Other problems may occur as the individual attempts to compensate for the restriction by walking on the outside of the foot, or by externally rotating the lower limb, i.e. walking with the foot in an abducted position, thereby avoiding a dorsiflexion strain on the first metatarsophalangeal joint.

Diagnosis may be confirmed by radiography. However, in the early stages of the condition, one must rely more on clinical evaluation as the chondral changes will not be evident. Bony spurs or exostoses will appear later, along with a decreased joint space of a degenerate joint. Care is necessary in making the diagnosis, in order to take into account other pathologies that occur in this area, such as gout, sesamoiditis, or a fracture within the joint.

Treatment may be conservative. Orthoses may be used to aid dorsiflexion, but firm insoles will decrease the function of the foot as a loading structure. Mobilization by a manual therapist will help in the mild forms before a cortisone injection into the joint is considered. The footwear must be addressed: shoes that are too small compress the first metatarsalphalangeal joint, further aggravating the symptoms.

Surgical intervention is often successful if the restriction to movement is bony. There are joint-preserving or joint-destroying surgical techniques. The latter, typically consisting of an arthrodesis, have been extensively studied (Shereff and Baumhauer 1998). However, the joint-preserving procedures such as cheilectomy (Hattrup and Johnson 1988) and/or osteotomy should not be overlooked (Thomas and Smith 1999). A cheilectomy removes the bony growth that is causing the impingement, and this is the operation of choice as a percentage of joint range of movement will be restored. The individual may return to full function, although the degenerative change will continue. Joint replacement, such as a Keller's excisional arthroplasty, is considered in more elderly patients (Kilmartin 2000).

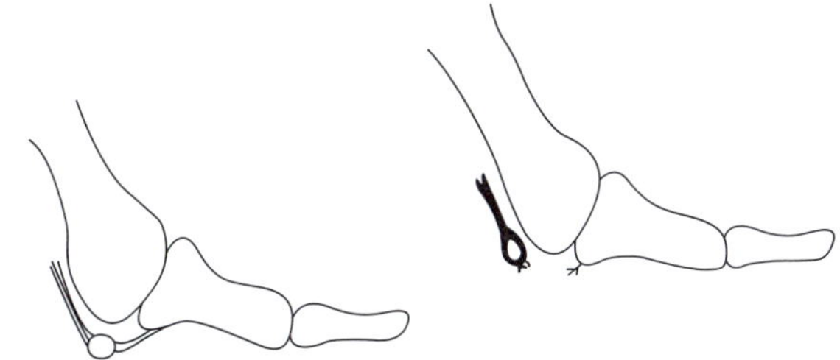

Figure 46.3 Lateral radiograph of the great toe can demonstrate avulsion of the sesamoid ligament complex.

Turf toe

This term was introduced by Bowers and Martin in their 1976 study into shoe-related injuries in American football (Bowers and Martin 1976). They found that up to 45% of players had sustained an injury to the great toe at some stage of their career. The term 'turf toe' is open to excessive use, as with other non-specific terms such as 'shin splints' and 'frozen shoulder'. I prefer to use this term to apply to inflammation of the capsule of the first metatarsophalangeal joint, with damage to the capsuloligamentous structures more commonly on the plantar aspect (Haverstock 1998). I would also prefer to rename it 'astroturf toe' as the greatest incidence appears to occur in sports that are played on this surface (Ekstrand and Nigg 1989). An important consideration is that arthritis of this joint (and restricted range of movement) is not necessarily a painful condition. However, a painful capsulitis can be an extremely disabling condition and will cause greater morbidity than many other injuries around the foot and ankle complex.

The cause of turf toe is trauma. Hyperextension, forced abduction, forced adduction (and occasionally hyperflexion; Frey et al. 1996) can result in excess strain to the strong supportive capsuloligamentous complex that supports this joint (Coker et al. 1978). The sesamoid ligaments are part of this complex and will be addressed later in this section. Compression injury (stubbing of the toe) and a direct blow (kicking the side of the joint against a post, for example) are other mechanisms of injury.

The effects of trauma may also be exacerbated by certain types of footwear that apply excessive pressure to the joint (footwear that is too small) or lack adequate support (flimsy, lightweight shoes such as running spikes). Football boots may aggravate the condition because of the location of the screw-in stud.

The training surface is also important. Astroturf is an unforgiving surface that allows little or no foot movement once the foot is planted on the ground. The compressive forces and effects of body loading therefore have to be absorbed throughout the musculoskeletal system. As the first metatarsophalangeal joint is the first and last point of contact in speed sports, and most pivotal manoeuvres emanate from this area when the joint is in hyperextension, it is not surprising that turf toe can be a career-threatening injury. Anything that can dissipate these forces, such as playing sport on a grass surface with adequate shock absorbers within the shoe, will be of use in preventing injury.

Diagnosis begins with a concise history. The biomechanics of the injury should be ascertained, if possible. The more chronic presentations are characterized by pain and stiffness of the joint after rest. Pain after exercise may be profound, and the athlete will point to the site of the pain. There may be a degree of swelling around the joint. The end of range of movement in all directions may be painful, especially if there has been a capsuloligamentous injury. Valgus and varus testing will detect collateral instabiltity. Crepitus on movement will raise the question of a possible bony injury. Palpation will reveal if the area affected is localized (such as a collateral ligament injury) or whether another pathology of close proximity is suspected (such as a sesamoiditis). The differential diagnosis of pain in this area includes sesamoiditis/fracture and osteochondritis/fracture.

If a bony pathology is suspected, then radiographs of the area (anteroposterior, lateral, oblique, and sesamoid views) should be requested. Fracture, degenerative change, or bony avulsion (due to ligamentous injury) may be present. The sesamoid views will be addressed in the next section. The lateral view, in neutral position and hyperextension of the joint, may indicate if there has been ligamentous avulsion of the sesamoid ligamentous complex (Figure 46.3).

Initial treatment is aimed at decreasing the inflammation and stress placed on the joint, such as the NICER regime (*n*on-steroidals, *i*ce, *c*ompression, *e*levation, and *r*elative rest). A rigid, full-length orthotic will be of great benefit to prevent the joint being forced into hyperextension on general ambulation. Immobilization should be considered if significant ligamentous damage has occurred (3–6 weeks) or if a chondral pathology or sesamoid fracture has been detected (6 weeks). Gradual return to exercise is then advised with a graded, carefully planned rehabilitation package. At all stages, if the area is not being totally immobilized, the joint should be gently mobilized by the therapist and the athlete. This involves passive movements towards the end of range, employed with and without a gentle traction force applied across the joint (some practitioners will call this a distraction technique). Biomechanical evaluation may suggest the use of temporary or permanent orthotics. Finally, the prescription of 'sensible' footwear is essential, along with advice on how to avoid further stress and injury.

Sesamoiditis

This condition can be confused with turf toe. Indeed, the symptoms may be similar, although examination findings should easily differentiate one condition from another. The end of range of movement of the first metatarsophalangeal joint does not cause pain with a sesamoiditis, except possibly at the end of range of hyperextension. With sesamoiditis, the tenderness is specifically on the plantar aspect of the joint, and indeed the sesamoid itself may be palpable. Inflammation of this area results from excessive loading. Therefore, as with turf toe, orthotics, local therapy, and corrective footwear may be helpful. A local cortisone injection may resolve particularly resistant cases.

Sesamoid radiographic views are useful, especially if fracture is suspected (Figure 46.4). Bipartite sesamoids are not unusual, and

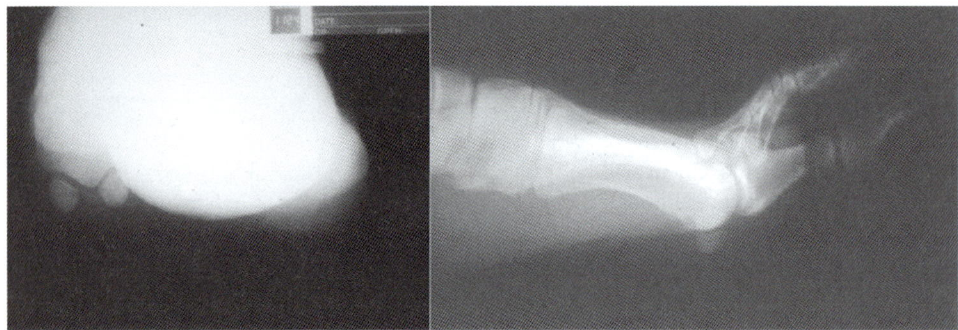

Figure 46.4 Sesamoiditis.

may occur on both sides of the great toe (Frankel and Harrington 1990). The smooth appearance of the bones will suggest that the structure is bipartite and not fractured. If the clinical suspicion is of a fracture or stress fracture, an isotope bone scan is diagnostic (van Hal et al. 1982). The treatment of a fracture is a minimum of 6 weeks' immobilization or surgical removal of the bone.

Hallux valgus

The normal range of valgus for this joint is up to 12°. In hallus valgus, the great toe is displaced laterally and rotated medially in a valgus position. The first metatarsal is displaced medially in a varus position. In this position, the abductor hallucis longus is displaced inferiorly, resulting in its action becoming that of a flexor rather than of an abductor. The flexor and extensor hallucis longus and the flexor hallucis brevis muscles are displaced laterally, increasing abduction.

Collectively, the alteration in forces causes increased valgus strain on the great toe (Shaw 1974). Encroachment on the second toe may then occur as the hallux causes dorsal subluxation of the second metatarsophalangeal joint. The base of the second proximal phalanx is then displaced superiorly and lies over the metatarsal head, and the pull of the lumbricals and dorsal interossei then causes hyperextension of the metatarsophalangeal joint and flexion of the proximal and distal interphalangeal joint (i.e. a 'claw toe'). Incidentally, if flexion does not occur at the distal interphalangeal joint, the deformity is termed a 'hammer toe'.

Associated with a valgus deformity is the development of inflammation of the medial collateral ligament of the metatarsophalangeal joint, the joint capsule, and the medial soft tissues. The swelling is called a bunion. The partly exposed medial metatarsal head and a resulting exostosis are also aggravating factors leading to a bunion.

Hallux valgus is all too often an acquired condition that will lead to increased stress on the joint and the progression of degenerative change (Figure 46.5). Inappropriate, tight-fitting footwear can cause this deformity. Court shoes were designed with fashion in mind, with no consideration for the anatomy of the foot. If a patient stands barefoot next to their shoes, and the feet are wider than the shoe, then obviously there will be compressive forces applied throughout the forefoot. Therefore, useful advice to the patient is that there should be space (approximately the width of the thumb) at the end of the shoe to allow movement, backed up by appropriate width.

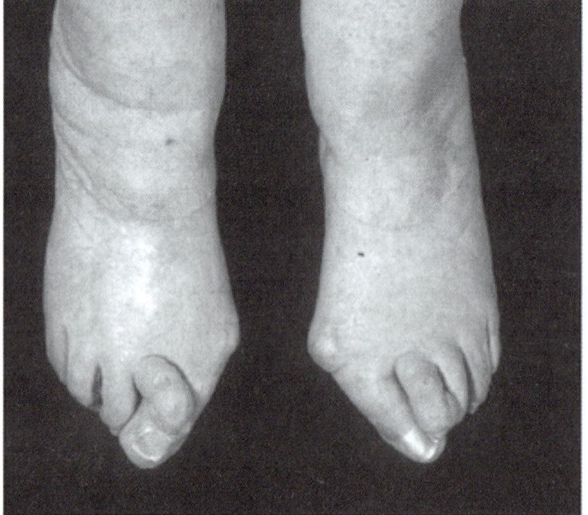

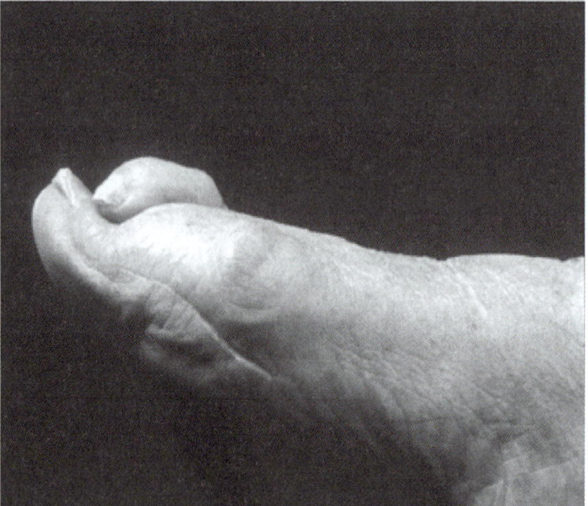

Figure 46.5 Hallux valgus.

Treatment

Preventing this condition is the ideal; hence, the benefit of good footwear advice from a young age. An excessively pronating foot may result in hallux valgus, and the use of foot orthotics may prevent this. Orthoses may also be used to prevent the worsening of an established case of this condition. However, should the deformity accelerate, then surgical intervention should be considered to prevent disorders spreading to other toes within the foot. Various osteotomy procedures are available, such as the techniques of Reverdin and Austin (Austin and Leventen 1981; Beck 1974). A concise text on forefoot surgery is the book by Dalton McGlamry, Banks, and Downey (2001); Hetherington (1994) is also recommended.

References

Austin, D. W., Leventen, E. O. A new osteotomy for hallux valgus. *Clinical Orthopaedics*, 1981, 157, 25–30.

Beck, E. L. Modified Reverdin technique for hallux abducto-valgus (with increased proximal articular set angle of the first metatarsophalangeal joint). *Journal of the American Podiatry Association*, 1974, 64, 657–66.

Bjosen-Moller, F. Calcaneocuboid joint and stability of the longditudinal arch of the foot at high and low gear push off. *Journal of Anatomy*, 1979, 129(1), 165–76.

Bowers, K. D., Martin, R. B. Turf toe: a shoe related football injury. *Medicine Science Sports and Exercise*, 1976, 6, 81–3.

Coker, T. P., Arnold, J. A., Weber, D. L. Traumatic lesions of the metatarsophalangeal joints in athletes. *American Journal of Sports Medicine*, 1978, 6, 326–34.

Coughlin, M. J. Metatarsophalangeal joint instability in the athlete. *Foot and Ankle*, 1993, 14, 309.

Dalton McGlamry, E., Banks, L., Downey, M. *Comprehensive textbook of foot surgery: volume 1* (3rd edn). Williams & Wilkins, Baltimore, 2001.

Ekstrand, J., Nigg, B. M. Surface related injuries in soccer. *Sports Medicine*, 1989, 8, 56–62.

Frankel, J. P., Harrington, J. Symptomatic bipartite sesamoids. *Journal of Foot Surgery*, 1990, 29, 318–23.

Frey, C., Anderson, G. D., Feder, K. S. Plantarflexion injury to the first metatarsophalangeal joint (sand toe). *Foot and Ankle International*, 1996, 17, 576–81.

van Hal, M. E., Keene, J. S., Lange, T. A., Clancy, W. G. Stress fractures of the great toe sesamoids. *American Journal of Sports Medicine*, 1982, 10, 122–8.

Hattrup, S. J., Johnson, K. A. Subjective results of hallux rigidus following treatment with cheilectomy. *Clinical Orthopaedics*, 1988, 226, 182–5.

Haverstock, B. D. Turf toe—injury of the first metatarsophalangeal joint. *British Journal of Podiatry*, 1998, 2(1), 46–9.

Hetherington, V. J. (ed.) *Hallux valgus and forefoot surgery*. Churchill Livingstone, Edinburgh, 1994.

Kilmartin, T. Metatarsal osteotomy for hallux rigidus. An outcome study of three different osteotomy techniques compared with Keller's excisional arthroplasty. *British Journal of Podiatry*, 2000, 3(4), 95–101.

Shaw, A. H. The biomechanics of hallux valgus in pronated feet. *Journal of the American Podiatry Association*, 1974, 64, 193–201.

Shereff, M. J., Baumhauer, J. F. Hallux rigidus and osteoarthrosis of the first metatarsophalangeal joint. *Journal of Bone and Joint Surgery*, 1998, 80**A**, 898–908.

Thomas, P. J., Smith, R. W. Proximal phalanx osteotomy for the surgical treatment of hallux rigidus. *Foot and Ankle International*, 1999, 20, 3–12.

Chapter 47

Podiatry (podiatric medicine and surgery)

Nat Padhiar and Bryan English

Introduction to podiatry (podiatric medicine)

Podiatry (or podiatric medicine as it is currently known) is a specialty devoted to the study of disorders of the foot, ankle, and lower extremity including diagnosis, investigations, and medical and surgical treatment. The term *podiatry* came into use in the early twentieth century in the USA and is now widely used worldwide, including in countries such as the United Kingdom and Australia.

This chapter primarily focuses on common conditions encountered in podiatric practice and introduces injection intervention of the foot and ankle, describing techniques used, with and without imaging modality. The musculoskeletal conditions that afflict the foot and ankle are tabulated (Table 47.1) and some of the common conditions described only briefly, as these are covered in other chapters of this textbook.

Anatomy of the foot and ankle

Leonardo da Vinci (1490), who combined art and science, described the foot as a *masterpiece of engineering*. Surprisingly, our present-day understanding of the biomechanics and function of the foot still remains the same (Mason 1962)—a mixture of art and science, with little change in the level of knowledge but greater progress in technology to assess the biomechanics and function of the lower extremity.

The human foot is a complex anatomical structure (Figure 47.1) consisting of 28 bones, including sesamoids; 33 joints; hundreds of ligaments, tendons, and muscles; and a network of nerves and blood vessels. The human foot is uniquely designed to withstand forces exerted during walking and standing. Shock absorption is an important component of loading response, when the swinging foot rapidly decelerates from initial contact to foot-flat. While the foot plays an important role, the entire limb contributes to shock absorption. Extrinsic muscles (Figure 47.2) of the foot also play an important role in providing shock absorption. For example, dorsiflexion muscle action, essentially of the tibialis anterior, provides muscular shock absorption during ankle motion.

Biomechanics, gait, and functional lower limb characteristics

Generally, the lower limb works as an integrated functional unit, each limb consisting of segments with specific capabilities and limitations. The lever system of the long bones in the lower limb transmit the body weight and must operate through the foot which has the capacity to sustain the stresses put upon it and to absorb and transmit considerable forces involved in locomotion.

'Normal' relationships between body segments are a prerequisite for 'normal' function. Any significant deviation in position, structure, or function may lead to abnormal compensation. This usually leads to mistiming of joint motion in the gait cycle, misalignment of joints, altered angle of muscle function, and reduced capacity to withstand forces acting on that part.

The foot becomes a rigid lever at the point of initial contact with the ground, a flexible lever at a point of forefoot loading, and again a rigid lever at a point of propulsion (toe-off phase). The series of lower limb joint motions transforms the lower limb and specifically the foot and ankle complex into a loose packed structure that accepts weightbearing and provides shock absorption. Meanwhile, the medial longitudinal arch remains effective at absorbing energy and adapting to uneven surfaces and variable ground reaction forces. After the midstance phase, a series of alignment changes occur between the hip, knee, and tibia that reverse from internal rotation to external rotation. As loading continues from midstance to late stance and upon heel rise, the metatarsophalangeal joints undergo increasing dorsiflexion, which creates tension upon the plantar fascia to effectively shorten its length. As the plantar fascia shortens, it produces the windlass effect, which lifts the medial longitudinal arch and transforms the talonavicular and calcaneocuboid joints (mid-tarsal joint) into a close packed alignment where the navicular, cuneiforms, and cuboid align similar to the trusses of a bridge. At the end of the stance phase, forefoot dorsiflexion reaches a peak, maximizing the windlass effect.

The foot and ankle demonstrate a Type 2 lever system where the resistance is located between the fulcrum and the force. For

Table 47.1 List of common conditions that affect the foot and ankle

Forefoot	Midfoot	Hindfoot and ankle
Morton's neuroma	Osteoarthritis	Tendinopathy, e.g. tibialis posterior tendon, FHL
Bursitis	Stress fractures, e.g. navicular	Mid-portion Achilles tendinopathy
Synovial cysts (ganglion)	Metatarsal stress fracture and fracture, e.g. 2nd metatarsal, 5th metatarsal base	Insertional Achilles tendinopathy
Osteoarthritis of MTPJ	Cuboid compression syndrome	Haglund's deformity
Synovitis of MTPJ	Crisp-Padhiar syndrome	Retro-calcaneal bursitis
Gout	Chronic exertional compartment syndrome	Anterior and posterior ankle impingement syndromes
Freiberg's infraction/ disease		Lateral ankle ligament injury, e.g. ATFL
Plantar plate tear		Sinus tarsi syndrome
Stress fracture		Plantar fasciitis/plantar fascia partial tears
Digital deformities, e.g. hallux valgus, hammer toes		Tarsal tunnel syndrome
Sesamoiditis/sesamoid stress fracture/ avascular necrosis		Osteochondral defect and lesion
		Fractures
		Syndesmotic joint pathology

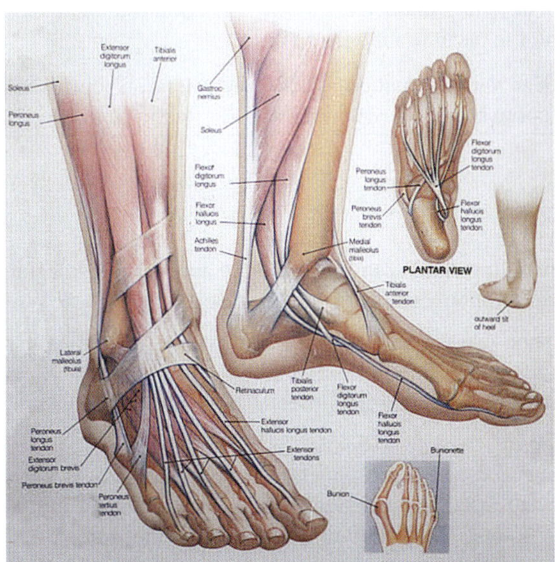

Figure 47.1 Complex anatomy of the foot and ankle. (http://www.footankleinc.com/foot-and-ankle-anatomy.html)

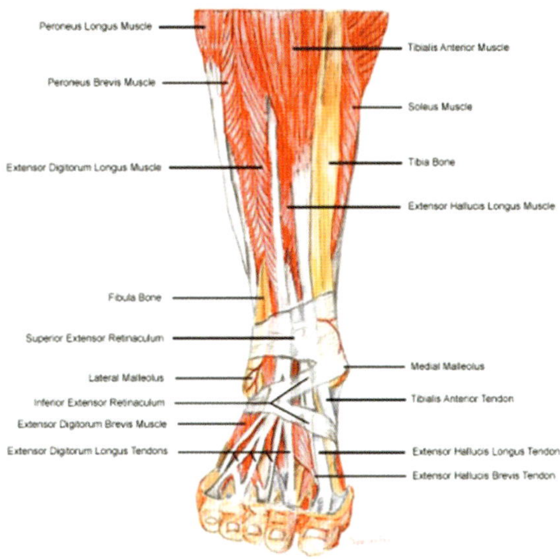

Figure 47.2 Extrinsic muscles of the foot. (http://www.healthcommunities.com/running-injuries/overview.shtml)

example, when a person stands on their toes, the calf muscles act as force generators and pull the heel (end of the lever) to elevate the foot and the weight of the entire body, with the ball of the foot acting as the fulcrum.

All of these biomechanical, gait, and functional components work together in unison to provide the body with support, balance, and mobility. A structural flaw or malfunction in any one part can result in the development of problems elsewhere in the body. Conversely, abnormalities in other parts of the body ultimately can lead to problems in the feet.

Common foot and ankle problems

The process of assessing foot and ankle problems starts with making a diagnosis, for which it is useful to think of oneself as a detective. This process primarily depends on the following.

History

'A clinician who cannot take a good history and a patient who cannot give one are in danger of giving and receiving bad treatment' (Paul Dudley White). The principal component of making a diagnosis of foot and ankle problems is a good history.

Anatomical knowledge and examination

The foot and ankle have many small structures; a good tip would be to ask the patient to put one finger where it hurts. This will identify the anatomy under the finger and also narrow the area of examination. Examination will also include special tests, e.g. Tinel test.

Biomechanical examination

This is an important examination. In some conditions that affect the foot and ankle, biomechanical and functional factors may either predispose or contribute to the pathology. In certain circumstances, orthoses are prescribed as part of the treatment, especially in chronic recurrent conditions or when the pathology is due to mechanical overload, e.g. Achilles tendinopathy and medial tibial stress syndrome. In such circumstances, it is worth conducting a static and observational gait analysis. Biomechanical examination should be simple, concise, and meaningful. In the main, the assessment is carried out to identify factors that may cause abnormal or excessive pronation and supination (Boxes 47.1 and 47.2). An attempt may then be made to associate any abnormal biomechanics with the pathology (Boxes 47.3 and 47.4). Pronation and supination play an important role in the gait cycle (Box 47.5) and it is therefore very important to understand and assess these two motions very carefully.

Investigations

Investigations have to be appropriate and will be based on structures or systems that may be involved. For example, there is no point in requesting an X-ray for a history that suggests plantar fasciitis; ultrasound scan may be more appropriate. Imaging modalities commonly used in podiatry include:

(a) *X-ray*—always request two views as one view alone may not give enough information (Figures 47.3 and 47.4). X-rays are very good as a first-line investigation where bone pathology is suspected.

(b) *Magnetic resonance imaging (MRI) scan*—this is becoming widely used and provides a good assessment of all relevant pathology, thus defining the severity. However, MRI scans should be interpreted in conjunction with the clinical picture. MRA (magnetic resonance angiography) is very useful to assess vascular pathology, e.g. popliteal artery entrapment syndrome.

Box 47.1 Common causes of abnormal pronation (eversion, abduction, and dorsiflexion)

- Hereditary and congenital
- Obesity
- Growth spurts
- Systemic, e.g. rheumatoid arthritis
- Cerebral palsy
- Scoliosis
- Limb length discrepancy
- Genu varum/valgum
- Tibial varum/valgum
- Ankle equinus
- Subtalar joint evertus
- Supinatus
- Dorsiflexed first ray
- Tibialis posterior dysfunction
- Poor proximal pelvic control, e.g. weak gluteal muscles
- Tarsal coalition
- Crisp-Padhiar syndrome

Box 47.2 Common causes of abnormal supination (inversion, adduction, and plantarflexion)

- Congenital pes cavus
- Limb length discrepancy
- Genu varum
- Tibial varum
- Subtalar joint invertus
- Plantarflexed first ray
- Foot orthoses

Box 47.3 Common problems associated with abnormal pronation

- Overuse injuries
- Low back pain
- Sciatica
- Greater trochanteric bursitis
- Medial knee pain
- Retro-patellar pain
- Patellafemoral dysfunction
- Medial tibial stress syndrome
- Achilles tendinopathy
- Plantar fasciitis
- Stress fracture
- Hallux valgus
- Digital deformity

Box 47.4 Common problems associated with abnormal supination

- Decreased shock absorption
- Osteoarthritis
- Stress fractures
- Lateral knee pain
- Lateral ankle sprain
- Digital deformity
- Ilio-tibial band frictional syndrome (ITBFS) and orthoses

Box 47.5 Effect of pronation and supination of the subtalar joint

Subtalar joint *pronation*—'unlocks' the midtarsal joint, allowing the foot to become a mobile adapter.

Subtalar joint *supination*—'locks' the midtarsal joint, allowing the foot to become a *rigid lever*.

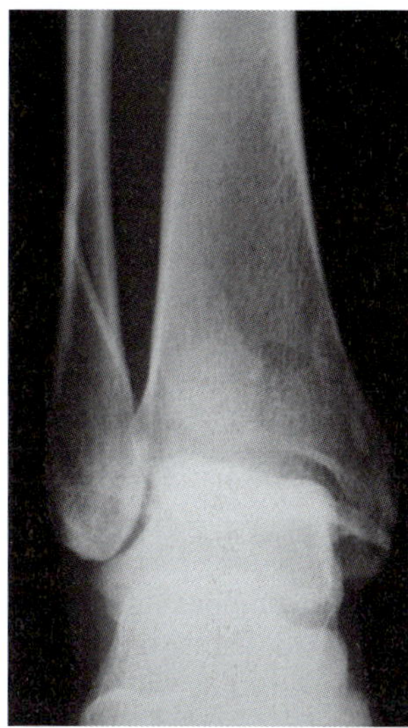

Figure 47.3 AP view of an ankle following trauma. There is a spiral fracture of the distal fibula and diminished joint space.

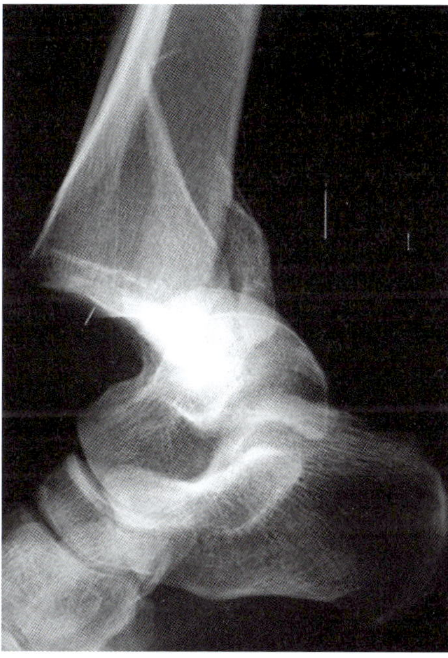

Figure 47.4 Lateral view of the same ankle as seen in Figure 47.3, showing partial but substantial dislocation of the ankle.

(c) *Computed tomography (CT) scan*—current high-tech CT scans can provide greater detail not just of the bone but also of soft tissue and especially tendons.3-D dynamic reconstructions are extremely useful in assessing impingement syndrome or fracture non-union.

(d) *Ultrasound scan (USS)*—this is considered by some to be the ultimate tool for clinicians and is often referred to as a 'clinician's stethoscope'. It is dynamic and useful to show patients their problem. USS is widely used for image-guided injections, aspirations, and taking biopsies.

(e) Other—EOS imaging system, Dexascan, and isotope bone scan.

Blood tests are primarily requested when infection or systemic and local inflammatory aetiology is suspected, e.g. rheumatoid arthritis, gout.

Additional investigations that are sometimes utilized include electromyography (EMG), nerve conduction test, histology, dynamic intra-compartment pressure test, Doppler study, and Duplex scan.

Where there is uncertainty in making a diagnosis, *local anaesthetic* as a diagnostic test is very useful. It is probably best performed under image guidance to ensure that the anaesthetic is infiltrated accurately at the site of the presumed problem.

Treatment

Even though injection intervention is highlighted in this chapter, it is vital and very important to consider all the other treatment options identified in Box 47.6. The list is by no means exhaustive. A multidisciplinary team (MDT) approach is advocated for many of the conditions that affect the foot and ankle.

Injection intervention for foot and ankle conditions

Traditionally, injections have been performed using clinical, anatomical landmark, and palpation skills, but in the last two decades, image-guided injections have become more popular. Nevertheless, the evidence for and benefits of performing image-guided injections remain unclear and open to debate. Bloom et al. (2012) conclude in their review paper that although ultrasound guidance may improve the accuracy of injection to the putative site of pathology, it is not clear that this improves its efficacy to justify the significant added cost. Schiffer et al. (2013) also conclude in their retrospective review of injection therapy in Morton's neuroma that no advantage has been demonstrated in this survey of ultrasound-guided injection versus palpation-guided injection. Further studies are needed to prove the effectiveness of ultrasound-guided corticosteroid injection. Nam et al. (2014) in their study showed no statistical difference in clinical outcomes but image-guided injection had a higher accuracy of needle placement compared to palpation-guided.

Box 47.6 Treatment modalities (not an exhaustive list)

- P.R.I.C.E.
- Injury-specific rehabilitation programme
- Braces and splints
- Plaster of Paris and Scotch casts
- Physiotherapy
- Functional foot orthoses
- Image-guided injections
- Percutaneous procedures, e.g. osteochondral defect (OCD) decompression, Achilles tendon repair
- Arthroscopy
- Open surgery
- Post-injury rehabilitation programme

It is clear from evidence that exists and the author's own extensive experience in this field that because of a higher accuracy of needle placement, image-guided injections should be the preferred choice.

Imaging modality

The choice of imaging modality (Figure 47.5) is very much dependent on the anatomical structures that are being injected and also on the experience of the clinician. Generally speaking, CT scanning and fluoroscopy are utilized for joints and bony structures, and USS for soft tissue structures. In the author's opinion, fluoroscopy is a better imaging modality for long tendons as it provides a global view of tendon and muscle with areas of adhesions, sheath distensions, etc. It is important to have a radiographer present or in the vicinity for technical help with scanners.

Injectable therapeutic drugs

Steroid and local anaesthetic (LA) remain the main substances that are utilized for foot and ankle conditions. There are no strict guidelines on choice or dosage of steroid and LA. The choice of steroid still remains anecdotal and empirical (Table 47.2). The main reasons for using steroid are:

(1) To suppress inflammation in joints and connective tissue
(2) To suppress inflammatory flares in degenerative joint disease
(3) To break up the cycle of inflammatory response in low-grade re-injury of soft tissue.

Patients often ask if there is a risk of tendon rupture after steroid injection. Although a complete tendon rupture with loading after steroid injection has been reported, no reliable proof exists of the deleterious effects of peritendinous injections; conclusions in the medical literature are based mainly on uncontrolled case reports that fail under scientific scrutiny, whereas scientifically rigorous studies have not been performed (Paavola et al. 2002).

Some of the common adverse effects of corticosteroids are documented in Box 47.7 and contraindications in Box 47.8.

The amide anaesthetic agents are usually the preferred choice, with the two most popular being 1% and 2% Lignocaine and 0.25% and 0.5% Bupivacaine. Other LA agents include Ropivacaine, Prilocaine, and Mepivacaine. The LA has the following therapeutic benefits:

(1) Pain reduction by immediate inflammatory pain inhibition
(2) Widens the field of steroid effect by increasing the volume of the injection

Table 47.2 Choice of steroids (adapted from British National Formulary)

Generic drug	Anti-inflammatory potency	Approx. effective time-scale
Hydrocortisone acetate	+	36 hours
Methylprednisolone	++++	Weeks & months
Triamcinolone acetonide	+++++	Weeks & months
Triamcinolone hexacetonide	+++++	Weeks & months

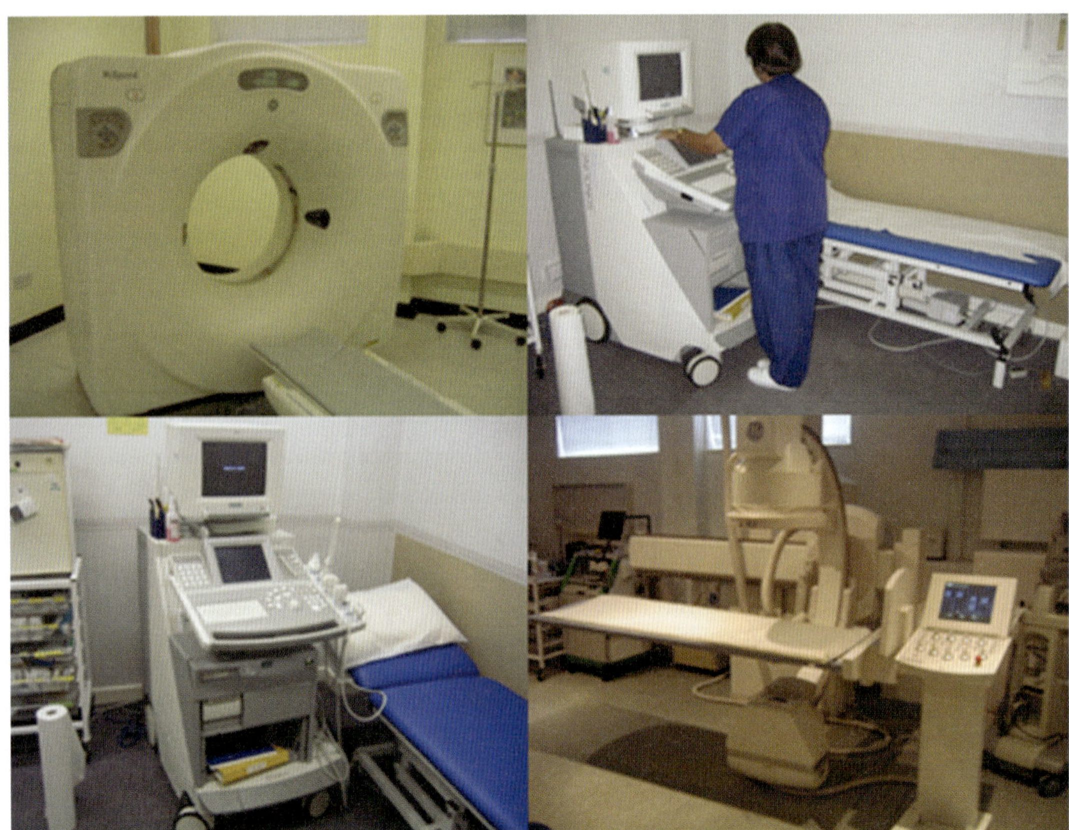

Figure 47.5 Clockwise from top left: CT scanner, radiographer, USS unit, and fluoroscopy unit.

Box 47.7 Adverse effects of corticosteroid injection

1 Facial flushing
2 Alteration in glycaemic control (relevant to diabetics)
3 Joint sepsis
4 Soft tissue infections
5 Subcutaneous atrophy/skin depigmentation
6 Post-injection pain
7 Tendon rupture
8 Steroid arthropathy

Box 47.8 Contraindications to steroid injection

1 Infection
2 Allergy to injectable drugs
3 Coagulation disorders
4 Recent trauma
5 Psychological overlay
6 Diabetes

(3) Dilutes the steroid which in turn may reduce the risk of tissue toxicity and atrophy
(4) Alleviates steroid-induced tissue irritation which may occur in the 24 hours post injection.

LA can also be used as a diagnostic agent, with immediate resolution of pain aiding the making of a diagnosis and differential diagnosis.

The other therapeutic agents which are widely used in podiatry include hyaluronic acid/hyaluronan (joints, tendons, and myofascial scars), injectable saline (Achilles tendon), Traumeel (for various musculoskeletal conditions), and prolotherapy (15–25% glucose for syndesmotic joints, ligaments, and subperiosteal space).

Informed consent

Good clinical practice demands provision of appropriate information to and consent from the patient. Box 47.9 outlines some of the important factors that should be considered as part of the consenting process. Informed consent should include information about the diagnosis or differential diagnosis, information about the injection procedure, and, more importantly, verbal and written information about potential complications.

Conditions of the forefoot

Forefoot metatarsalgia is an umbrella term, which should be discouraged. There are five common conditions that are often the cause of forefoot pain:

(1) Morton's neuroma
(2) stress fracture of a metatarsal
(3) Freiberg's infraction

Box 47.9 Informed consent

1 Nature of their condition
2 Details of proposed treatment and alternatives
3 Nature of drugs to be given
4 Possible side-effects and incidence
5 Likely benefits
6 Plans for follow-up and after care

(4) synovitis of the metatarsophalangeal joints (MTPJ)
(5) plantar plate tear.

There are other conditions that affect the first MTPJ including hallux valgus, hallux limitus and rigidus, sesamoiditis, sesamoid fracture, and avascular necrosis (AVN) of a sesamoid.

Morton's neuroma

This is the most common condition encountered as a cause of forefoot pain and a common foot problem seen in a podiatry clinic. The condition is also known as Morton's metatarsalgia, Morton's neuralgia, plantar neuroma, and intermetatarsal neuroma. It is a nodular enlargement of an intermetatarsal plantar nerve, most commonly, the nerve between the proximal heads of the third and fourth metatarsal bones. Although Morton's neuroma was originally described in 1876 by Thomas Morton, it is argued that this condition was first described by a foot clinician named Durlacher (1845). Although labelled as a 'neuroma', the nodule is actually a perineural fibroma (fibrous tissue formation around nerve tissue). It is believed that this fibrous formation is the result of thickening and nerve enlargement due to repeated insult during physical activities (Hassouna and Singh 2005; Mulder 1951).

The diagnosis of this condition is largely dependent on clinical presentation and examination:

(1) pain on weightbearing
(2) sharp shooting pain affecting either the second and third or third and fourth toes
(3) feeling of having a stone in the shoe
(4) burning sensation
(5) paraesthesia
(6) numbness.

USS is the imaging modality of choice when Morton's neuroma is suspected. It is however very much user-dependent and, therefore, close co-operation between clinicians and radiologists is recommended. USS will identify the location of the neuroma in the intermetatarsal space and the size, which can vary from 2.5 mm to 12 mm. The prevalence of sonographic presence of Morton's neuroma in an asymptomatic general population remains unknown. Symeonidis et al. (2012), in their study of 48 asymptomatic subjects, showed that 54% of their subjects had bilateral interdigital neuroma measuring 5 mm or more and 35.4% had enlarged nerves. They also recommended that clinical examination still remains the gold standard for diagnosis of Morton's neuroma. USS is also used as modality of choice for performing the injection for all soft tissue abnormities that affect the lower extremity (Hassouna and Singh

2005; Sharp et al. 2004). Gadolinium-enhanced MRI scan (Sharp et al. 2004; Zanetti and Weishaupt 2005) is an alternative.

There is no real evidence to suggest that one treatment works better than the other. The choice of treatment is very much what works in individual hands, and individual clinicians will have their preference.

(a) Padding, orthotic, and footwear adjustment to relieve pressure and compression on the interdigital nerve.

(b) Physiotherapy, manipulations, acupuncture, and stretch exercises to relieve the pressure on the forefoot by improving flexibility.

(c) Non-steroidal anti-inflammatory drugs (NSAIDs), e.g. ibuprofen.

(d) Cryotherapy and radio-frequency ablation.

(e) Surgery (Figure 47.6). When all conservative management has failed and the condition remains symptomatic with substantial disability, surgery should be considered. The mainstay surgical choices involve either decompressing the interdigital space and releasing the nerve or excising the nerve (dorsal or plantar approach). The outcome varies between patients and is very much dependent on patient's expectation. Womack et al. (2008) concluded that the long-term result following excision of neuroma is not as successful as previously reported. They also found the only significant ($p = 0.027$) difference in outcome was the location of the neuroma: second web space had worse outcomes than third web space neuromas on both the Visual Analogue Scale (VAS) and neuroma score. The stump neuroma is the worst complication following surgery and it is estimated that 30% of patients will develop post-operative stump neuroma. Amis et al. (1992) suggest the potential cause of stump neuroma to be the presence of plantarly directed nerve tetherings which are found mostly in the second/third intermetatarsal space.

(f) Injections of local anaesthetic, steroid, and alcohol can be administered either under image guidance (USS) or via palpation method. The choice of steroid and local anaesthetic varies between clinicians and no recommendations are made in this chapter. Alcohol injections have become more popular in the last 10 years but, even though the short-term results were promising, long-term prognosis has remained poor (Gurdezi et al. 2013).

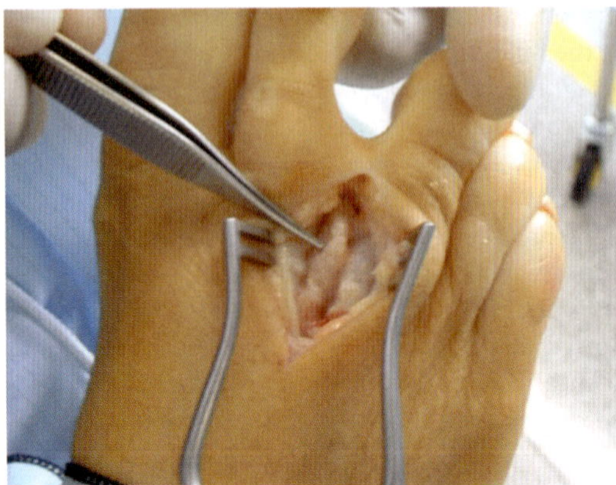

Figure 47.6 Excision of neuroma from dorsal approach.

Image-guided injection

This is a very simple procedure. An ultrasound scanner is used to locate and identify the lesion (Figure 47.7) and the needle is inserted from the dorsal aspect under real-time USS guidance (Figure 47.8). Usually, three injections of 50 mg hydrocortisone acetate and 4 ml 0.5% marcaine are planned, allowing 2-week intervals between injections. VAS scale is useful in assessing pain, which is judged against what induces that pain, e.g. high heel shoes. A second injection is performed if either there is no change or there is less than 50% decrease in symptoms. In some cases where steroid injection fails to produce the desired outcome, alcohol is used, but this is a very painful injection.

Where there is no imaging facility, Morton's neuroma can be injected utilizing the anatomical landmarks. The interdigital nerve usually lies plantar to the intermetatarsal ligament (IML), so by marking the metatarsal heads (Figure 47.9), entry into the IM space is facilitated. A blue needle (90° to the skin) is introduced from the dorsal aspect and progressed until resistance offered by the IML is felt. Once through this structure, the needle point will be on top of the neuroma. Sometimes, the patient may complain of paraesthesia in the toes, which is a sign that the needle is correctly placed.

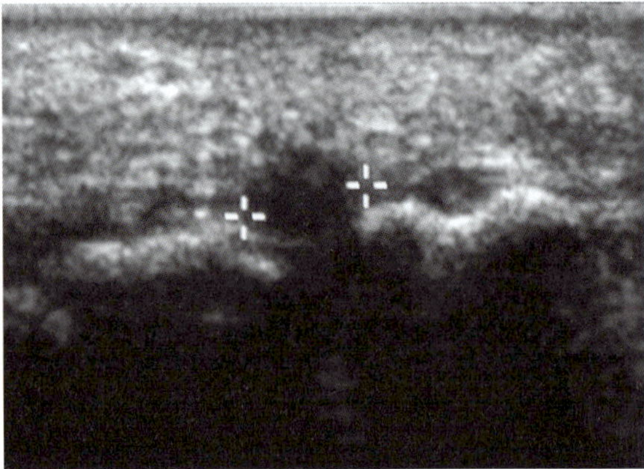

Figure 47.7 Inverted USS image in a transverse plane.

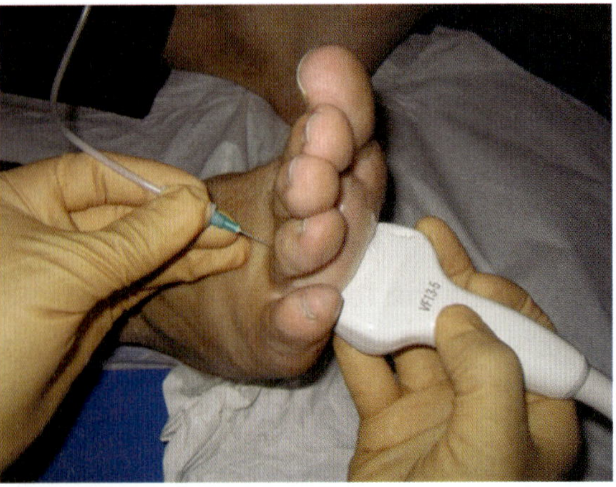

Figure 47.8 Ultrasound-guided Morton's neuroma injection from dorsal approach.

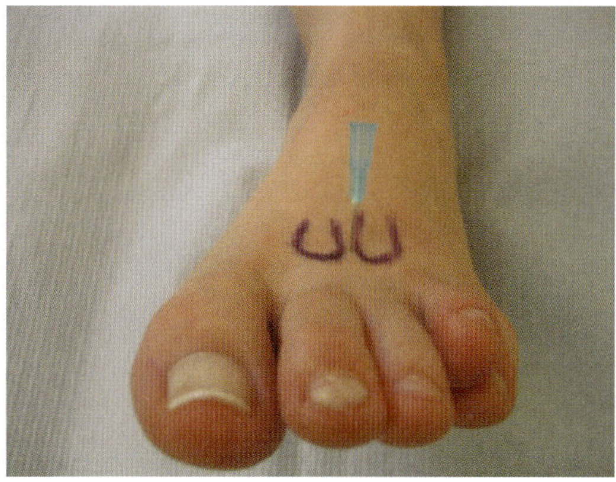

Figure 47.9 Mark the metatarsal heads and insert a blue needle from the dorsal aspect keeping it 90° to the skin, between the metatarsal heads.

Metatarsophalangeal joint (MTPJ) pathology

The common conditions encountered are identified in Table 47.1 and covered in some detail in Chapter 46. In this section, the focus is on the injection technique used for MTPJs.

Fluoroscopy guided injections are recommended for all MTPJs, even though it is possible to inject the first MTPJ by using the palpation method. Use of a fluoroscopy or image intensifier is specifically useful when there is suspicion of either capsular or plantar plate tear. The main indication for injection is pain. Hyaluronic acid is now widely used in degenerate joints, with the benefit of improving range of motion (ROM) by its lubricating property; it is also thought to be chondroprotective by inhibiting hydrogen peroxide and superoxide (Yu et al. 2014).

The most common cause of pain in the first MTPJ is osteoarthritis (Figure 47.10). Pain around the first MTPJ may also occur due to sesamoiditis, sesamoid fracture (Figure 47.11), and AVN of a sesamoid. An antero-posterior (AP) X-ray view of the sesamoids may be misleading when bipartite sesamoids are present; skyline views of both feet should be requested. With a long history of sesamoid-related pain, MRI scan is useful in excluding AVN (Figures 47.12a and b).

A vicious cycle often develops where a degenerative joint causes pain, which further limits active and passive movement with resultant stiffness and protective antalgia. As a result, small structures around the joint (Figure 47.13) develop adhesions and also shorten, thus limiting ROM further. By reducing pain, an injection may inhibit further chondral degeneration and reduce restriction. In such a scenario, high-volume injection is recommended and should include 25 mg hydrocortisone acetate, hyaluronic acid, and 5 ml 0.5% marcaine.

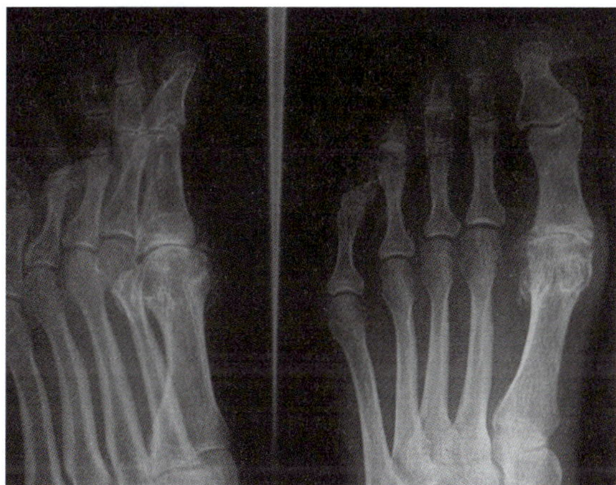

Figure 47.10 AP and oblique X-ray views. Osteoarthritis of the first MTPJ.

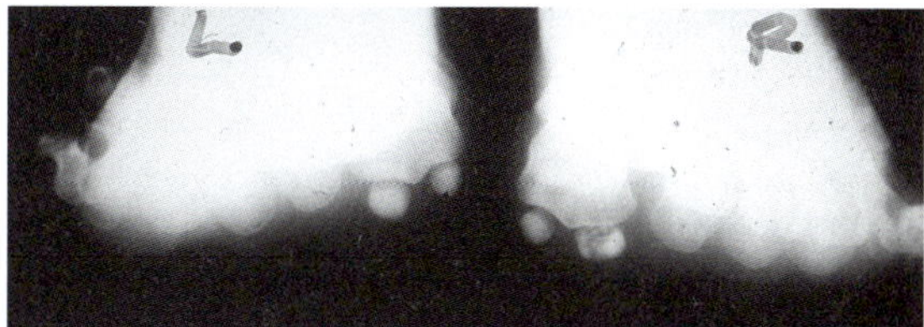

Figure 47.11 Skyline view of both feet with fracture of the right lateral sesamoid.

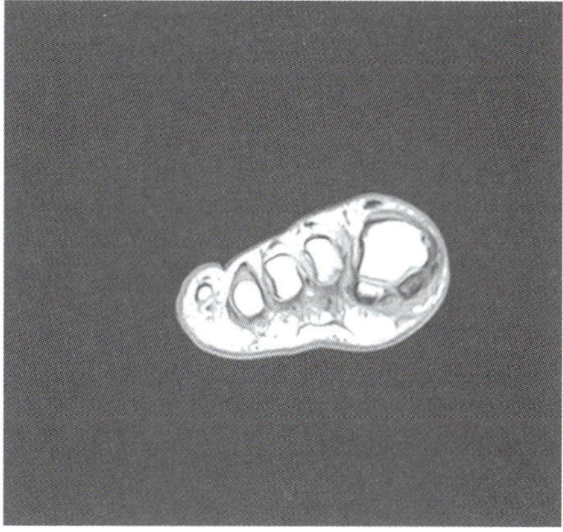

Figure 47.12a T2-weighted sequence of MRI scan showing AVN of the medial sesamoid.

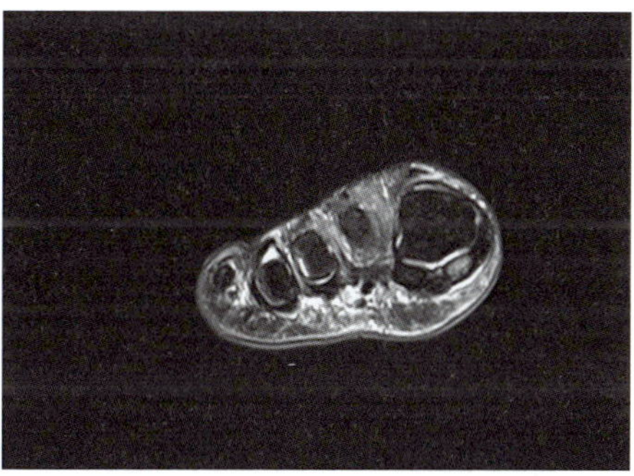

Figure 47.12b STIR sequence of MRI scan showing AVN of the medial sesamoid.

The patient is positioned in a supine position with the knee flexed to 90° and foot flat on the fluoroscopy table (Figure 47.14). Images are acquired and a blue or an orange needle placed over the metatarsal head, near the joint line, but not necessarily in the joint as it may cause more joint damage. The needle is then inserted and provided it is within the joint capsule, the therapeutic agent will infiltrate the whole of the MTPJ–sesamoid complex. Contrast is infiltrated to confirm flow in the joint (Figure 47.15) which is then

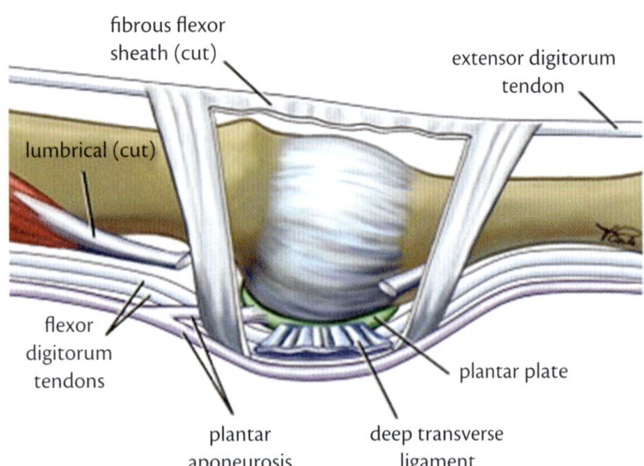

Figure 47.13 Anatomy around the first MTPJ. (http://www.aapsm.org.au/articles/plantar-plate-injury)

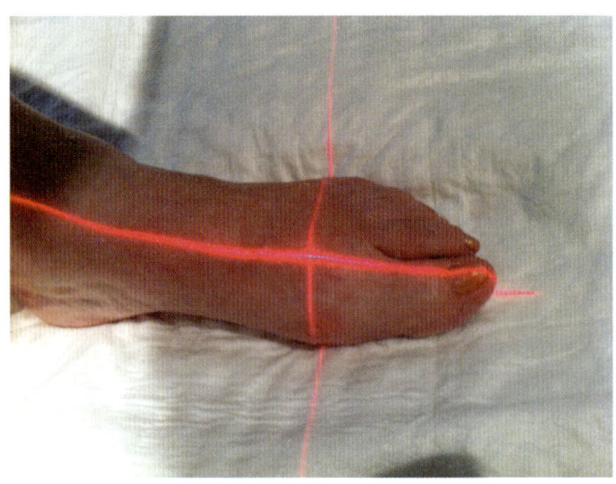

Figure 47.14 Position of the foot on the fluoroscopy table, with laser marker.

followed by infiltration of therapeutic drugs. A high- volume injection of the first MTPJ–sesamoid complex is carried out in the same way for sesamoid abnormalities. Post injection, the patient is to remain non-impact for up to 72 hours, after which they can slowly and gradually resume their physical activity, monitoring pain and disability.

The main indication for a lesser MTPJ injection is pain due to synovitis, Freiberg's infraction, or plantar plate tears. The injection procedure is exactly the same as for the first MTPJ, except smaller volumes are used. Steroid injections are very effective in treatment of synovitis but repeated injection may cause subluxation (Gray and Gottlieb 1983; Reis et al. 1989) of the digits due to weakening and atrophy of the capsule.

Freiberg's disease/infraction

Freiberg's disease is a form of osteochondrosis affecting the lesser metatarsal heads, most commonly, the second and third. When first described by Freiberg in 1914, the aetiology was thought to be trauma, but now it is generally agreed that it is multi-factorial. There are a number of classification systems described in the literature which are mainly based on radiological

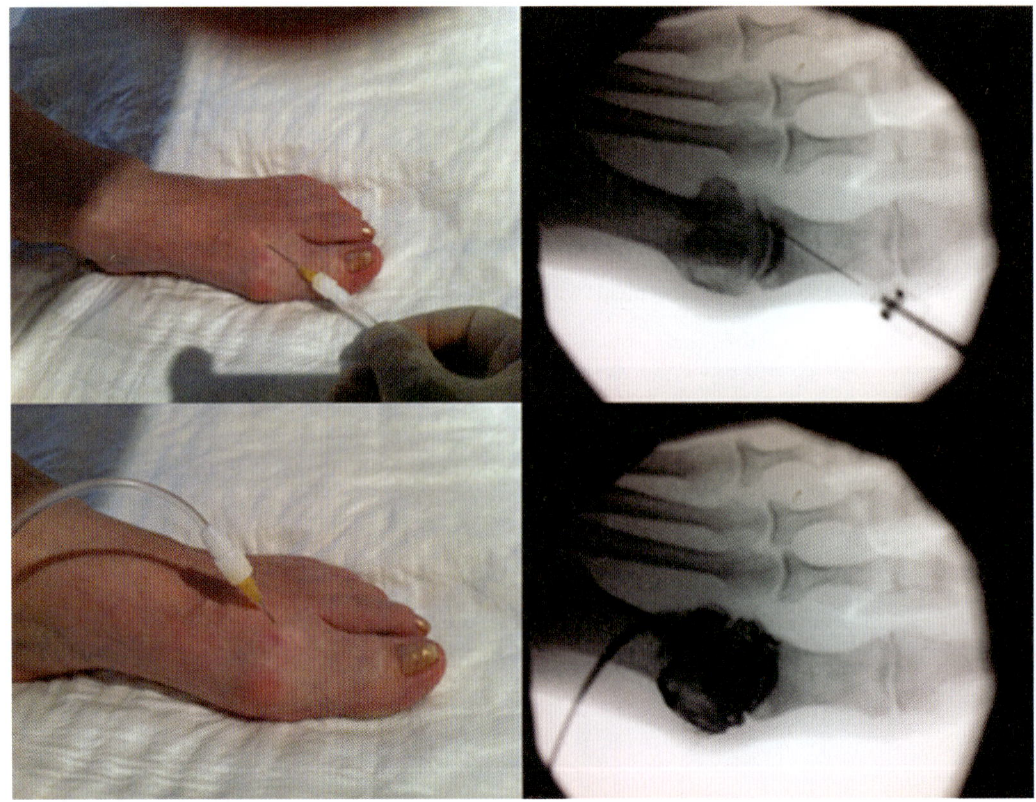

Figure 47.15 Fluoroscopy-guided first MTPJ injection—Omnipaque 300 contrast confirming correct needle placement.

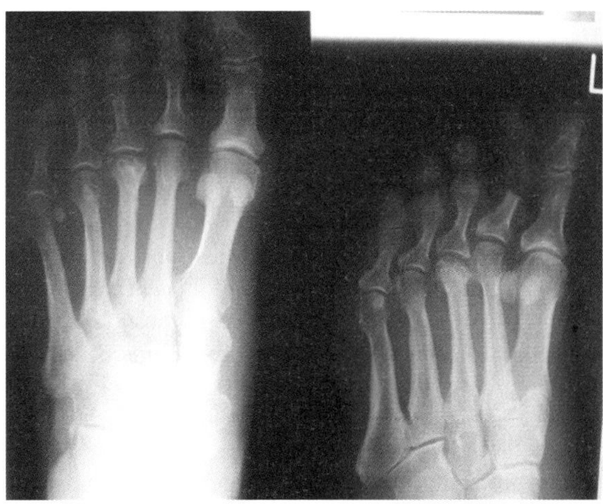

Figure 47.16 X-ray presentation of Frieberg's disease: flattening and cystic lesions of the affected metatarsal head, widening of the MTPJ, sclerosis and flattening of the bone, and increased cortical thickening.

findings (Gauthier and Elbaz 1979; Katcherian 1994; Smillie 1957; Thompson 1987).

The patient will usually complain of pain with corresponding swelling over the affected MTPJ. The pain is worse with weightbearing activity. Pain is induced on direct pressure over the metatarsal head and often it is pin-point specific. There is also loss of ROM due to swelling and, as a result, there may be a plantar callosity over the affected metatarsal.

X-ray (Figure 47.16) is the most common imaging modality used for diagnosis and can be used to classify the stage of the disease. MRI scan has the advantage of detecting early changes of the condition and some authors have used it to classify the condition (Torriani et al. 2008).

First line of management is conservative, with the aim of reducing pain and the progression of the disease. This may include a period of immobilization, physiotherapy, orthoses, footwear modification with a rocker sole, and gradual return to physical activity. Palamarchuck et al. (2000) found the use of orthoses to be most effective and beneficial in treatment of the elite athlete who suffered from this condition. NSAIDs and steroid injections can be used to help reduce swelling. If conservative treatment fails, then surgical correction may be required. Various surgical procedures are described, including joint preserving closing wedge osteotomy (Gauthier-Elbaz 1979), hemi-phalangeal arthroplasty, simple debridement and small joint implant.

Plantar plate tear

The plantar plate is a deep fibrocartilaginous structure, which originates from the metatarsal head and attaches to the proximal phalanx through the joint capsule (Figure 47.13). Its function is to stabilize the MTPJ and to dissipate compressive forces during the forefoot loading phase of the gait cycle (Kirby 2009).

Plantar plate injury is probably more common than it is diagnosed, and it is probably the most common cause of pain under the second MTPJ.

The main cause of this injury is repetitive loading of the metatarsal with excessive dorsiflexion at the affected MTPJ, e.g. long-distance running, tennis. Biomechanical factors include deformities of the first ray, e.g. hallux valgus and metatarsus primus varus, with resultant overloading of the lesser MTPJ, long second metatarsal, abnormal metatarsal ratio, pes cavus, and excessively pronated feet. There are extrinsic factors that can cause the condition, e.g. high heel shoes.

The patient will complain of pain on both the dorsal and plantar aspect of the MTPJ, which is exacerbated and made worse on weightbearing but mostly relieved with some residual ache with rest. There may be some swelling on the plantar aspect and sometimes patients present with a bruise on the dorsal aspect.

Clinically, the condition can be evaluated by performing a vertical stress test (Thompson and Hamilton 1987) which is also referred to as a digital Lachmann's test. This test assesses the instability of the digit with dorsal excursion greater than 2 mm. MRI and USS have a part to play but the gold standard investigation of choice is an arthrogram (Figures 47.17 and 47.18).

In less severe cases, treatment is mostly conservative, with the aim of reducing pain and stabilizing the deformity. This may include RICE (rest, ice, compression, elevation), NSAIDs, addressing the biomechanics with orthoses to reduce the dorsiflexion moment at the MTPJ, footwear modifications, and taping to stabilize the digit in more plantarflexion.

Fluoroscopy-guided injection of either steroid or 25% glucose, following arthrogram confirmation, can provide pain relief and early return to recreational or sporting activities. It is a useful adjunct to other conservative measures but repeated injections are to be discouraged as there is risk of digit subluxation (Freiberg 1914; Reis et al. 1989).

If the deformity is severe, chronic, and unmanageable, surgery is indicated. Surgical procedures include primary repair, adjunct surgery to hammer toe or subluxation of digits, and metatarsal osteotomies to relocate the digits.

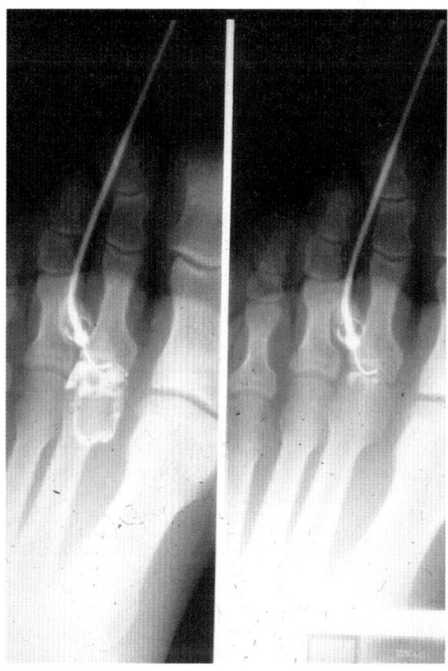

Figure 47.17 Normal arthrogram with contrast remaining within the joint.

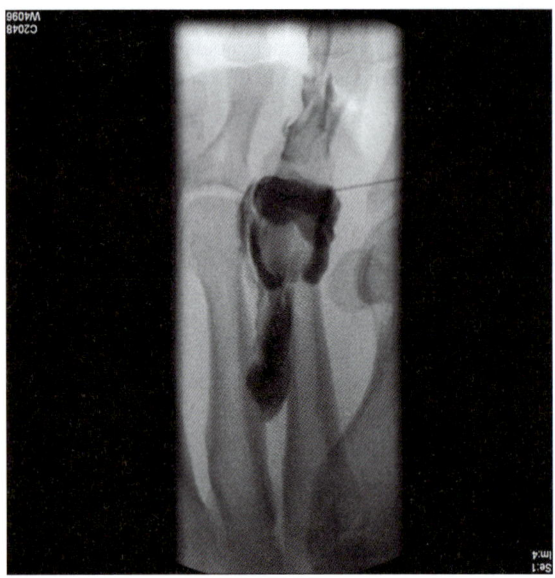

Figure 47.18 Positive arthrogram for plantar plate tear with contrasts leaking into the soft tissue.

Conditions of the midfoot

Anatomy

The midfoot plays an important role in providing stability and support during the gait cycle. The anatomy consists of three cuneiforms, which form the only true architectural arch in the foot, navicular, and cuboid. The navicular and cuboid articulate with the talus and calcaneum respectively (midtarsal joint); the three cuneiforms and cuboid articulate with the forefoot via the bases of the five metatarsals (Lisfranc joint). The midfoot has syndesmotic fibrous joints, which are linked together like brickwork. Along with the unique position between the hindfoot and forefoot, the midfoot plays a pivotal role during walking and standing. It has many ligaments, which stabilize the construct along with intrinsic and extrinsic muscle (Figure 47.19).

Common problems that occur in the midfoot are tabulated in Table 47.1. The most common problem encountered is osteoarthritis of the midfoot joints and, in particular, the Lisfranc joint.

Tarsometatarsal joint (TMTJ) osteoarthritis (OA)

TMTJ OA is a debilitating condition, which causes midfoot instability, severe dysfunction, pain, and antalgic gait. The most common cause is primary TMTJ OA (Patel et al. 2010) which mostly occurs in the sixth decade and affects the second and third TMTJs

COMPLEX ANATOMY OF THE MIDFOOT

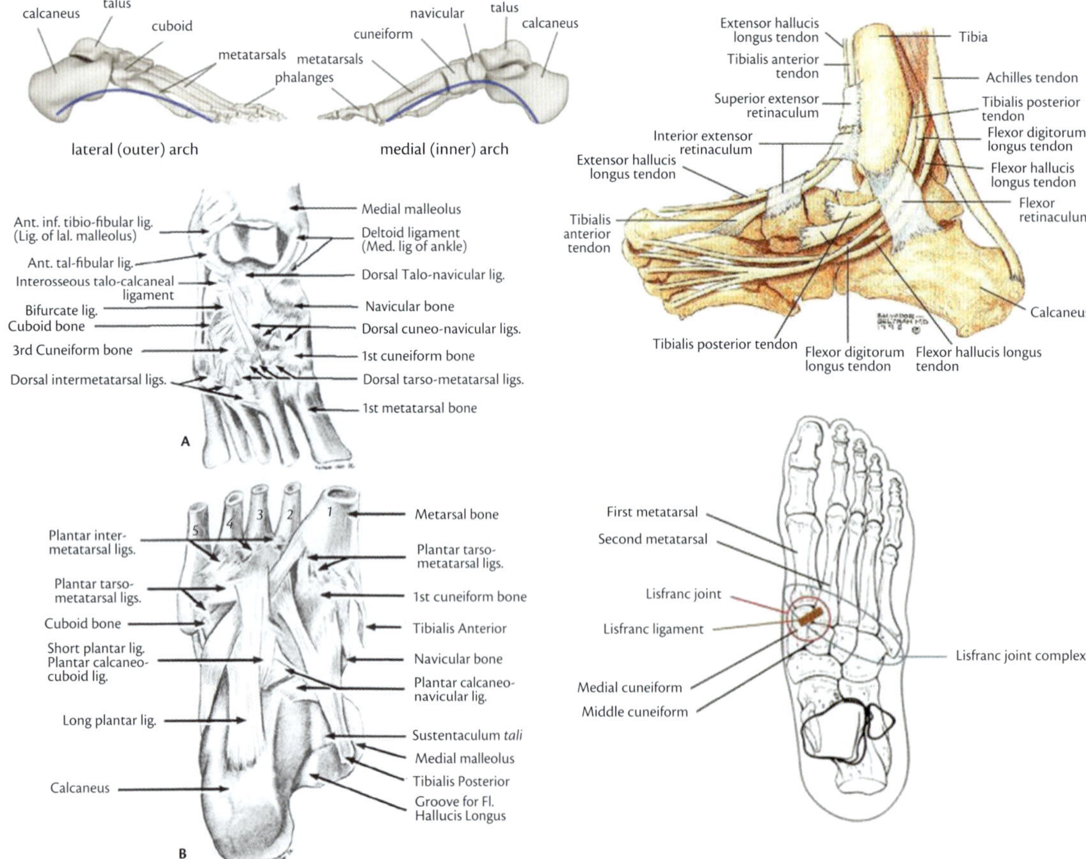

Figure 47.19 Midfoot anatomy.

(a) Reprinted with permission of Bandha yoga, http://www.BandhaYoga.com;

(b) http://www.orthoteers.com; (c) *Rockwood and Green's Fractures in Adults*, Bucholz, Robert W., Lippincott Williams and Wilkins; 6th revised edition (1 Dec. 2005); (d) reprinted from *Osteopath Family Physician* Hardy, Melanie, and Park, David J, Case report: An Atypical Presentation of a Lisfranc Fracture, p. 85–87. Copyright (2012) with permission from Elsevier.

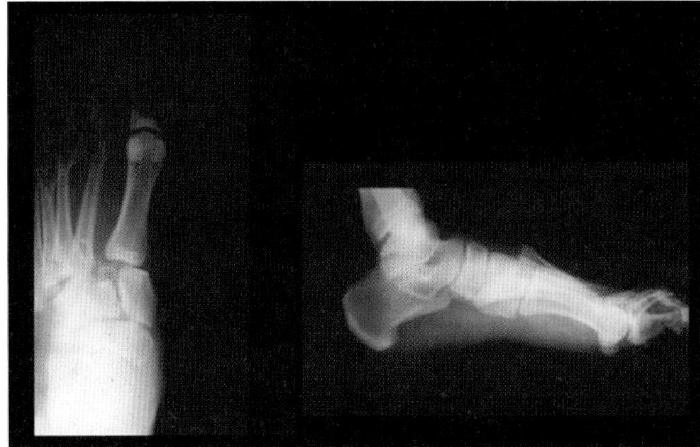

Figure 47.20 Lisfranc injury: common cause of secondary midfoot OA.

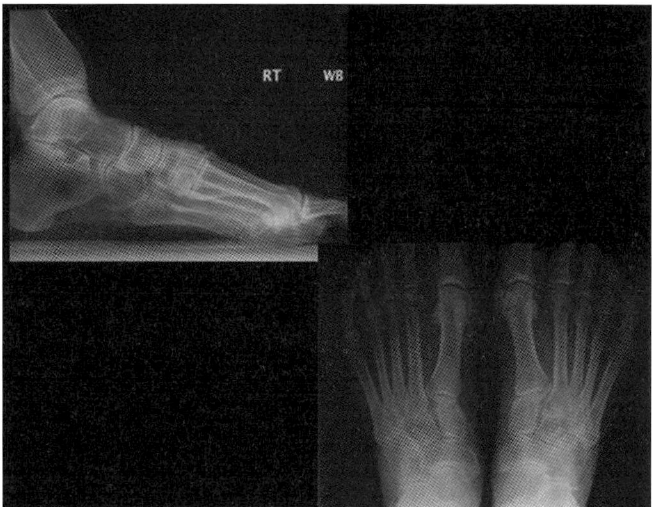

Figure 47.21 Primary OA of the midfoot.

predominantly. Patients with secondary degeneration (Myerson et al. 1986; Rao 2008) following trauma (Figure 47.20) become symptomatic usually in the fourth decade with the first, second, and fourth TMTJs mostly affected.

The plantar and dorsal ligaments provide the stability of these joints with the Lisfranc ligament being the strongest. The TMTJ has a reduced ROM in the sagittal plane (Ouzounian and Shereff 1989) (Table 47.3), a property which provides its stability. It is of interest that the motion of the medial (1–3) midfoot is much less than the lateral (4–5). There is greater ROM required during the heel-strike phase of the lateral column and more stability required during the medial rotation of the foot which would be starting to progress into pronation. The predisposing factors for primary OA are hindfoot valgus, loss of longitudinal arch, forefoot valgus, and acquired midfoot flatfoot.

Symptoms are pain and disability with activity, acquired flatfoot, with difficulty with shoes.

Weightbearing AP and lateral view X-rays of the foot are the primary investigation (Figure 47.21). CT scan is sometimes useful, especially 3-D reconstruction to provide positional assessment of the foot joints.

Treatment is aimed at reducing the pain and maintaining stability of the midfoot. This is never fully achieved and patients need to be counselled regarding their expectations and future limitations. Conservative measures include NSAIDs, orthoses, braces, footwear modification with possible rocker system, physiotherapy, acupuncture, manipulations and mobilization, and injections.

Fluoroscopy-guided injections allow accurate placement. Injections without imaging are discouraged. Figure 47.22 is self-explanatory and the process of injection is the same regardless of condition injected.

Table 47.3 Sagittal plane motion of tarsometatarsal (TMT) joints

TMT joint	Motion
1ST	1.6°
2ND	0.6°
3RD	3.5°
4TH	9.6°
5TH	10.2°

Cuboid syndrome

This is a difficult condition to diagnose and hence it is often overlooked when pain occurs over the inferior antero-lateral aspect of the ankle radiating over the lateral column of the foot.

'Cuboid syndrome' includes cuboid subluxation, locked cuboid, dropped cuboid, cuboid fault syndrome, cuboid compression, lateral plantar neuritis, and peroneal cuboid syndrome (Newell and Woodle 1981; Subotnick 1989). It is, however, difficult to envisage and even more difficult to prove that cuboid ever dislocates or subluxes as it is anatomically (shape and position) in a stable and safe location. It does, however, undergo compressive forces, thus possibly causing cuboid complex disruption and hence pain.

The condition usually occurs following acute or chronic ankle inversion injury and also as a result of overuse. It is more common in feet that excessively pronate and in hypermobile syndromes, but it is also reported to occur in pes cavus feet. The main mechanism appears to be an increase in mechanical advantage of the peroneus longus as it courses under the cuboid (Newell and Woodle 1981). Overcorrected foot orthoses and poor footwear are also thought to be predisposing factors.

The main symptom is pain, which is often intense with activity, especially over uneven terrain, but can also present as a dull ache in the area of the fifth metatarsal/cuboid/calcaneum. In severe cases, the pain is intense enough to make the patient limp and can radiate along the peroneus longus tendon. There are no physical signs but pain can be provoked by palpation, often specific to metatarsal–cuboid and cuboid–calcaneum articulations.

The diagnosis is based on history and physical examination. Imaging modalities are usually unhelpful, even though MRI scans with smaller slices may pick up high signal within the soft tissue or bone bruising around cuboid articulations. Two clinical tests (midtarsal adduction and supination tests) have been described (Durall 2011) which may further aid the diagnosis of this often misdiagnosed condition.

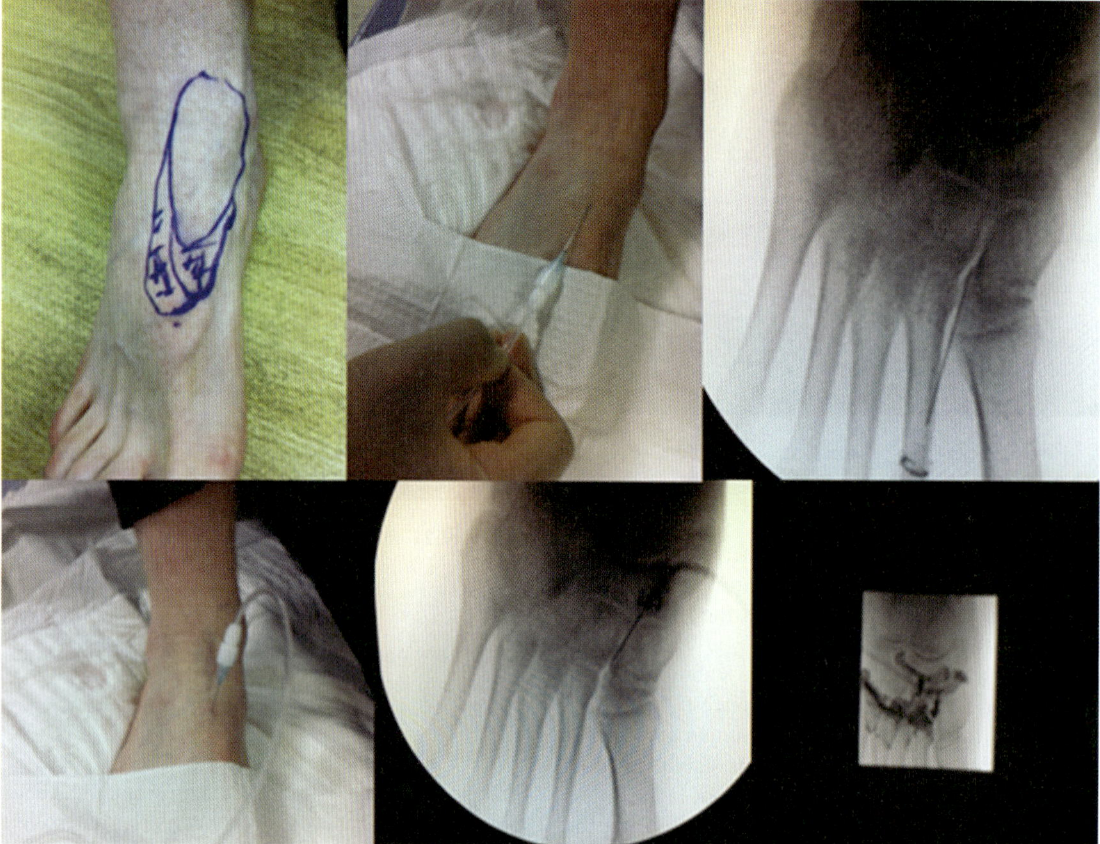

Figure 47.22 Fluoroscopy-guided midfoot injection.

Conservative treatment includes addressing the predisposing factors using taping, orthoses, footwear modifications, intrinsic and extrinsic muscle strength work, improving proprioception and balance, manipulation, and fluoroscopy-guided injections (Figure 47.23). Surgery is very rarely performed and may involve fusing the joints.

Crisp-Padhiar syndrome

The common causes of medial midfoot pain following acute trauma are navicular stress fracture, Lisfranc injury, tibialis posterior tendinopathy with dysfunction, and os naviculare syndrome. These are disabling conditions, which are often described and treated in isolation.

Crisp-Padhiar syndrome (series of 42 cases) (Crisp et al. 2011) highlights the complexity of the problem when a patient presents with post-traumatic medial midfoot pain. Following an acute pronatory or supinatory sprain, patients present with pain. There is often swelling and bruising around the navicular with pin-point tenderness over the os naviculare, which is made worse by resisted supination of the foot. On history and physical examination, there is a combination of the following:

(1) trauma

(2) presence of os naviculare

(3) tibialis posterior tendinopathy

(4) tibialis posterior dysfunction

(5) acquired flatfoot

(6) os naviculare synchondrosis

(7) anomalous tibialis posterior tendon attachment on the os naviculare with only around 20% attached to the main body of the navicular.

A plain X-ray is often sufficient to confirm the presence of an os naviculare (Figure 47.24) but an MRI scan (Figure 47.25) will provide added information regarding anomalous tibialis posterior tendon attachment and sometimes a high signal of synchondrosis.

The initial treatment, in more severe cases, is immobilization in a knee-high walker for 2 weeks, followed by stabilization of the medial structures in a posterior tibial tendon dysfunction (PTTD) brace for 4 weeks, followed by intensive physiotherapy. Depending on reduction of symptoms and degree of flat footedness, fluoroscopy-guided tendon distension injection and the introduction of customized carbon-fibre foot orthoses may be considered.

Surgery is only performed in patients who were either misdiagnosed, and therefore have a more chronic condition, or did not respond to conservative management. Surgical procedures are:

(1) Removal of os naviculare, shortening and advancing the tendon to the main body of the navicular (Figure 47.26)

(2) Fusing the os naviculare to the navicular.

Patients remain in a below-the-knee Scotch cast for between 4–6 weeks, after which they follow a strict post-operative and return to sport specific rehabilitation programme.

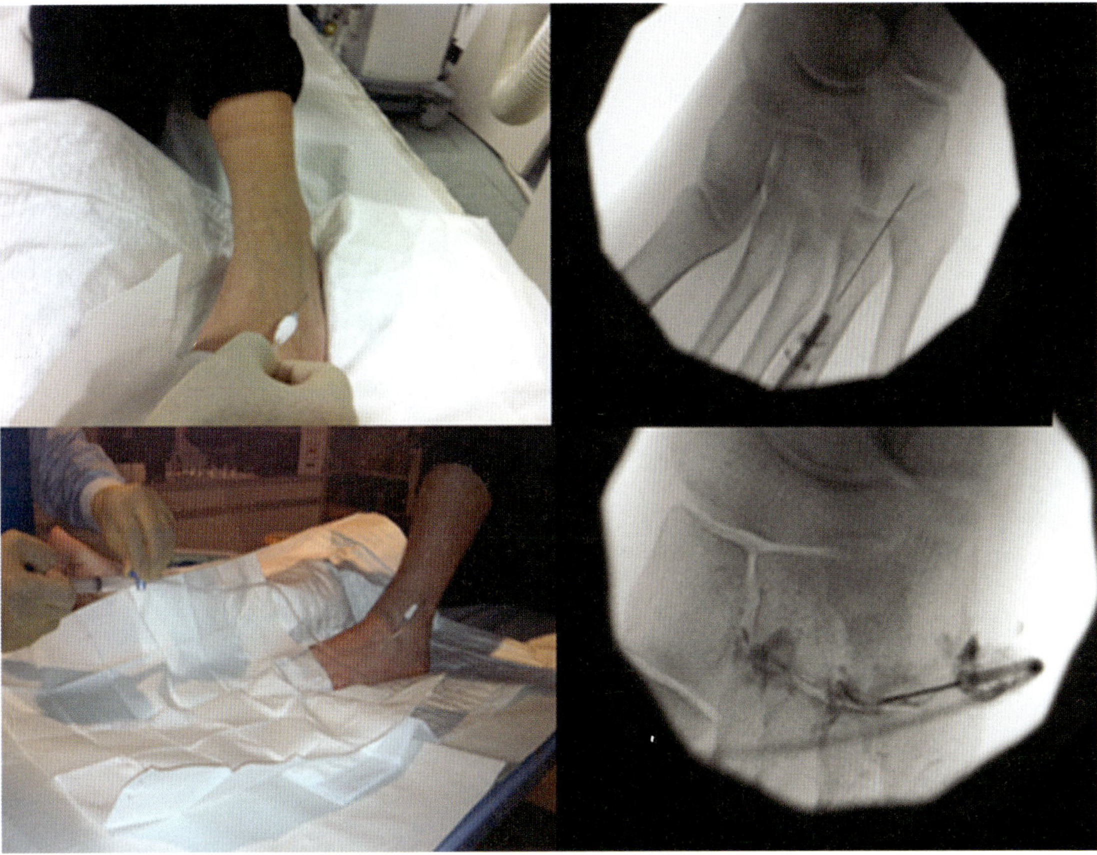

Figure 47.23 Fluoroscopy-guided injection for cuboid syndrome.

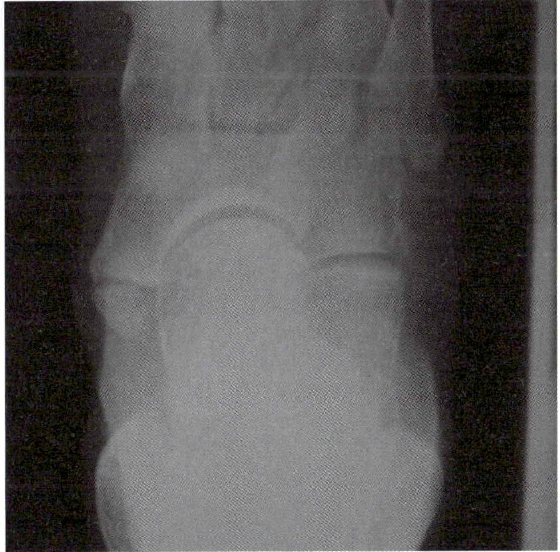

Figure 47.24 X-ray showing presence of os naviculare in Crisp-Padhiar syndrome.

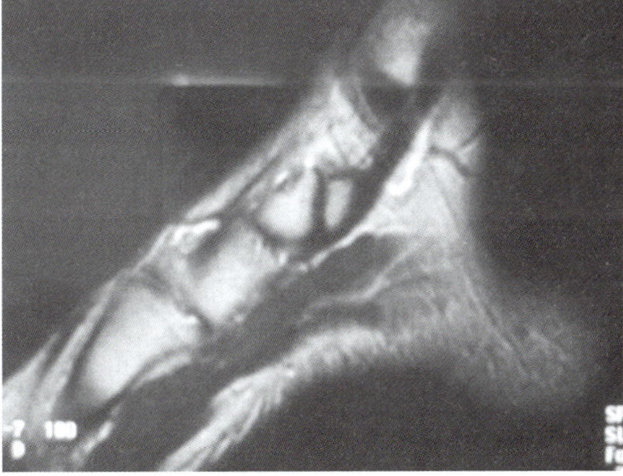

Figure 47.25 MRI scan showing anomalous tibialis posterior tendon attachment of os naviculare.

Chronic exertional compartment syndrome

Chronic exertional compartment syndrome (CECS) (Padhiar et al. 2009) usually refers to myoneural ischaemia from a reversible increase in tissue pressure within a myofascial compartment. Although CECS of the leg is well documented, its first description being by Mavor in 1956, CECS of the foot remains under-diagnosed and under-recognized, and there is very little in the literature to guide clinicians to make this diagnosis.

Wood Jones (1944) proposed that there are four compartments in the foot, but Manoli and Weber (1990) suggest that there are nine separate compartments. They propose five separate forefoot compartments (four interossei and one adductor hallucis), a medial compartment (abductor hallucis and flexor hallucis brevis), a lateral compartment (adductor digiti minimi and flexor digiti minimi

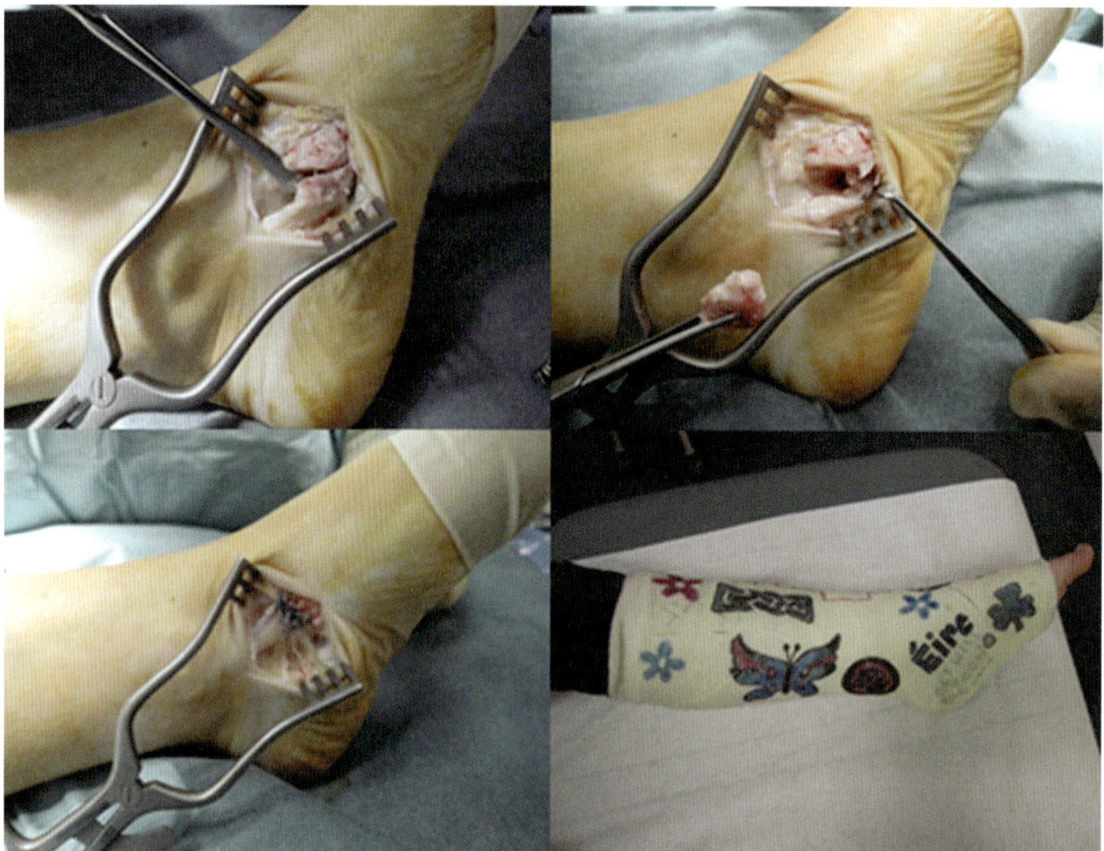

Figure 47.26 Surgery for Crisp-Padhiar syndrome.

brevis), a superficial central compartment (flexor digitorum brevis), and a deep central or calcaneal compartment (flexor digitorum accessorius). There is one more extensor compartment, which has not been mentioned in the literature.

The incidence is unclear as very little is reported in the literature. It is a condition that affects young, active, competitive individuals, but can occur in any age.

The clinical signs and symptoms of CECS of the foot remain vague, diverse, and lack the consistency of its counterpart in the leg. Patients complain of 'cramp-like' pain in the foot (which may be bilateral or unilateral) during exercise, relieved by variable periods of rest, usually within minutes of stopping, after which they can continue again. In some cases, there is a dull ache, which can last for hours. Pain may be non-specific in its anatomical location but usually in the heel and medial longitudinal arch (medial compartment). In some cases, examination may provoke pain at the medial attachment of the plantar fascia and more distal. Swelling, tension, cramps, tightness, paraesthesia, numbness, cyanosis, and soft tissue induration may be present (Lokiec et al. 1991; Miozzari et al. 2008; Mollica 1998; Muller and Masquelet 1995).

The preferred method of investigation is by a real-time dynamic intra-compartment pressure (DICP) test, with tracings of pressure variables in the patient's exercise that provokes the symptoms (Padhiar and King 1996) (Figure 47.27). Tracing interpretation is vital for the reasons given in Box 47.10.

Diagnosis of CECS of the foot remains one of exclusion. In most cases, conditions such as plantar fasciitis, tarsal tunnel syndrome, flexor hallucis longus tendinopathy, fat pad contusion, have been investigated and excluded before considering CECS.

The most effective treatment is a fasciotomy (Figure 47.28a and b).

Conditions of the hindfoot

The hindfoot is a complex part of the foot, both in function as well as anatomy (Figure 47.29). The subtalar and ankle joints provide the starting point of the gait cycle with the first two levers occurring at heel strike. This part of the foot provides the 'gear mechanism'. If it fails, nothing moves efficiently. The midfoot forms the stable part to take the impact of the force that is generated with medial rotation of the foot before forefoot loading. The forefoot provides the 'spring board' after foot pronation (shock absorption) for the toe-off phase.

The talus is probably the most important bone in the body. It has no muscle or tendon attachments and therefore sits freely between the foot and the leg. It allows for the foot and leg to move appropriately over uneven or elevated terrain, whereby progression is maintained in a straight line with the talus having the property to accommodate ever-changing positions of the foot and the leg, without any detrimental effect on the limb. Damage to this bone has the potential to end careers in sport. A list of conditions that are common are tabulated in Table 47.1.

This section focuses on image-guided injection for sinus tarsi syndrome, tendinopathy of the extrinsic tendons of the foot (Figure 47.29), and plantar fasciitis.

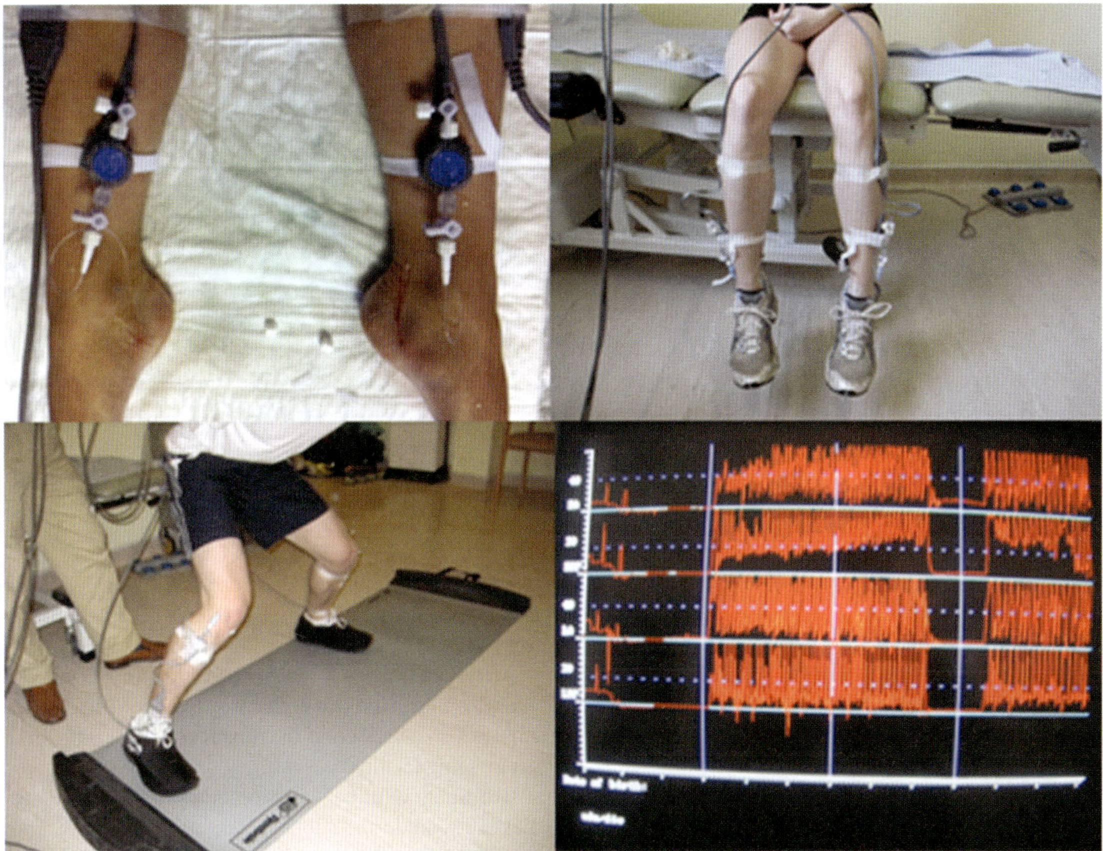

Figure 47.27 Clockwise from top left: DICP of medial foot compartment; resting position; tracing vital for various aspects of pressure interpretation; exercise-specific (Padhiar and King 1996) on-line collection of ICP.

Box 47.10 Importance of intra-compartment pressure tracing

- It allows an opportunity to check whether the catheter is in the right compartment and that the catheter is patent by squeezing the compartment that is being investigated.
- One can measure maximum, mean, relaxation, and resting pressures.
- It can detect blockage at the tip of the catheter or a kink in the catheter, as the wave form changes.
- It can detect whether the catheter has slipped and is sitting under the skin, as the wave form changes.
- It can detect whether the catheter is part or fully in the blood vessel, as the wave form changes.
- In some patients, the increase in ICP is exercise-specific (Padhiar and King 1996). DICP with tracing and long leads allows for comparison between different exercises at the time of testing, e.g. forearm CECS (rowing, cycling, tennis, typing, guitar playing, weightlifting), and lower limb and foot CECS (treadmill, cycling, walking, skating, ballet).

Sinus tarsi syndrome (STS)

STS (Pisani et al. 2005) is a secondary clinical condition, which usually occurs following trauma (acute inversion injury of the ankle). It can also occur in patients with chronic instability of the ankle with periodic ankle sprains. It is characterized by pain over the anterolateral hindfoot.

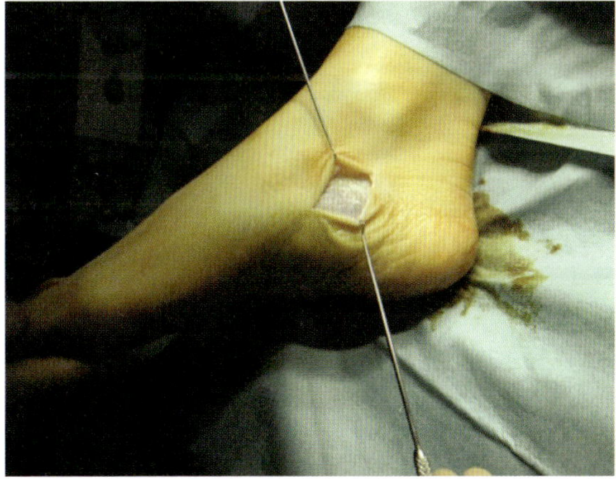

Figure 47.28a Superficial fasciotomy.

The sinus tarsi is a conical cavity between the anterior and posterior talocalcaneal joint, with the widest point of the cone lying in the anterolateral aspect of the inferior ankle (Figure 47.30). It is stabilized by extrinsic (calcaneofibular, anterior talofibular, lateral talocalcaneal) and intrinsic (cervical and interossei) ligaments. Tears, partial tears, and laxity of intrinsic ligaments lead to instability of the ankle joint as a result of increased ROM of the subtalar joint.

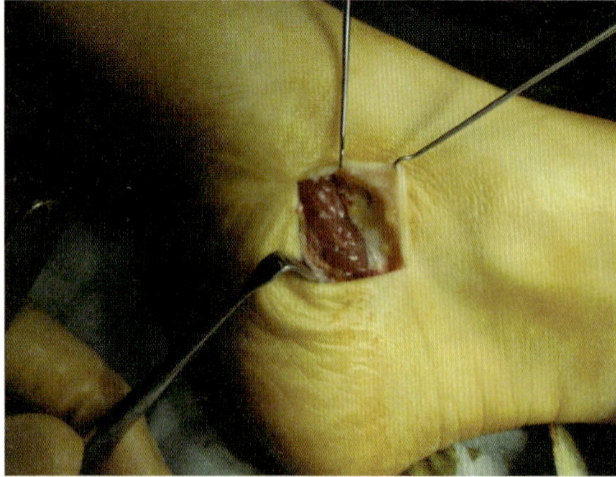

Figure 47.28b Superficial fasciotomy.

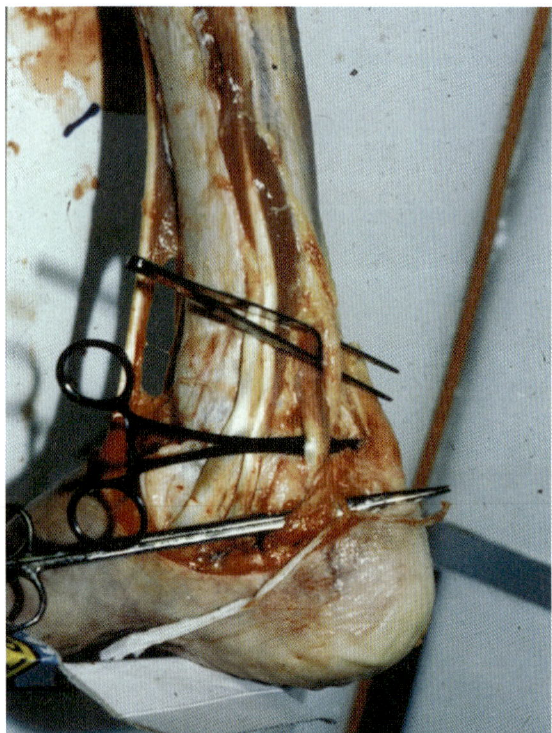

Figure 47.29 Complex anatomy around the ankle and subtalar joint.

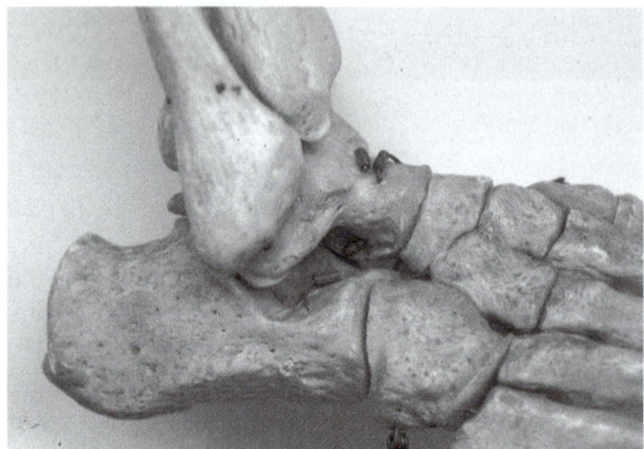

Figure 47.30 Anatomical position of conical-shaped sinus tarsi between the talus and calcaneum.

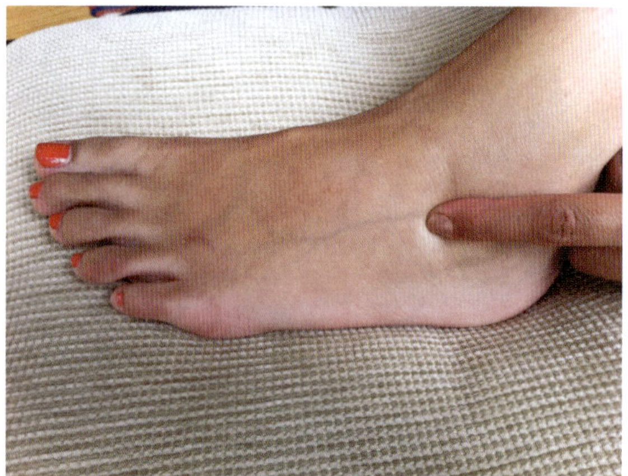

Figure 47.31 Sinus tarsi is a clinical diagnosis.

Pain and instability are experienced with possible hindfoot valgus. It is a clinical diagnosis assisted by the patient putting one finger over the sinus tarsi opening (Figure 47.31).

MRI scan is the most useful investigation and may show high signal within the sinus tarsi. Local anaesthetic infiltrated into the sinus tarsi is also a very good diagnostic test, especially in the absence of an imaging facility.

Treatment is initially physiotherapy to improve muscular strength, flexibility, ankle and subtalar joint proprioception, and balance, and to address any other more proximal functional deficit, e.g. core issues. Bracing, taping, and foot orthoses all have a part to play in stabilizing the subtalar joint. NSAIDs, cryotherapy, and steroid injections can help to reduce inflammation. Surgery is indicated if all conservative measures fail; arthroscopy has become more popular recently.

Injections are often used to break the pain cycle so that sport-specific rehabilitation can proceed before a return to sport and they are an important aspect of management. They are mainly performed under imaging to accurately place the needle at the apex of the sinus tarsi. CT scan is the modality of choice, even though fluoroscopy with contrast can be utilized. The best image is identified and used to insert the needle into the sinus tarsi, aimed at the apex on the medial aspect of the foot (Figure 47.32); 9 ml 0.5% marcaine and 40 mg triamcinolone acetate is then infiltrated. A bandage or ankle brace is applied and the patient advised to refrain from high-impact activity for 72 hours, after which they can start a rehabilitation programme. It is possible to inject the most arthritic and inaccessible joints using this CT-guided technique (Figure 47.33).

Clinically guided STS injection is performed as described in Figure 47.34.

Tendon distension tenogram for tibialis posterior, flexor hallucis longus, and peroneal tendon tendinopathy

Tendinopathies of the extrinsic tendons are common (Gluck et al. 2010; Heckman et al. 2009; Lee et al. 2013; Lynch and Pupp 1990; Simpson and Howard 2009) and covered in other chapters of this textbook. This section describes tendon distension tenogram as an investigative and therapeutic procedure (Na et al. 2005).

USS has been used extensively to inject tendons as it is widely available, easy to use, and dynamic. It has some minor disadvantages which include:

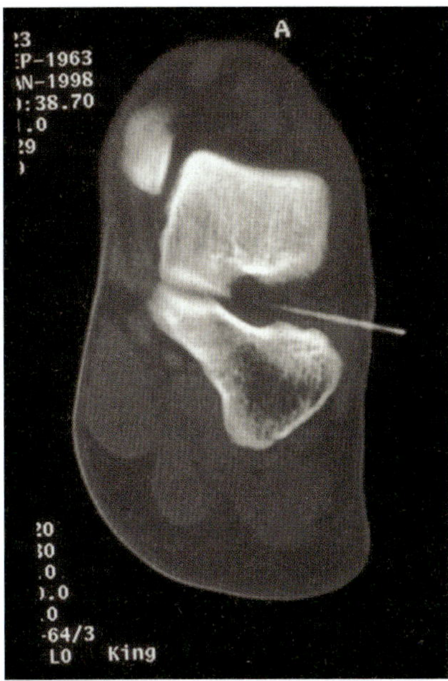

Figure 47.32 Needle inserted and aimed at the apex of the sinus tarsi.

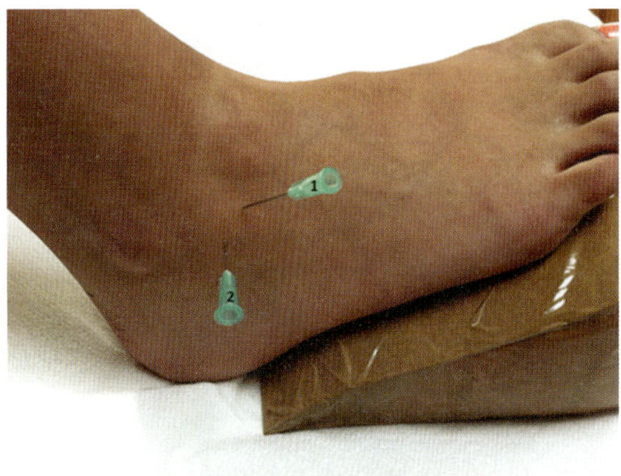

Figure 47.34 Clinically guided sinus tarsi injection. Patient positioned supine, knee flexed to 90°, foot resting 45° in supinated and adducted position, and knee slightly internally rotated. Incorrect: needle 1 inserted in the anatomical direction of the sinus tarsi which may not penetrate to apex. Correct: needle 2 is inserted 90° to the skin at the inferior aspect of the sinus tarsi.

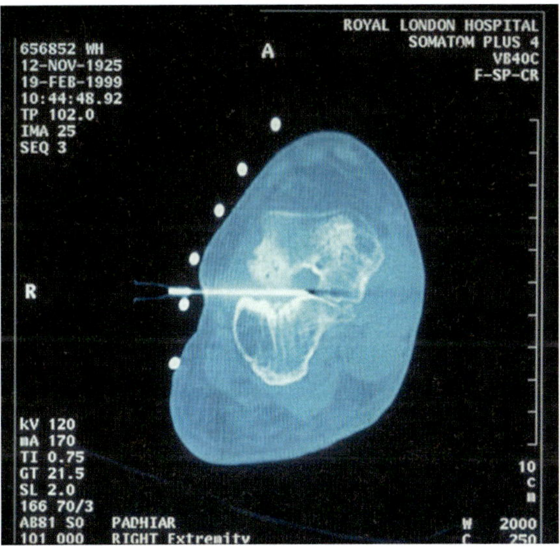

Figure 47.33 Using CT guidance most arthritic joints can be accessed easily.

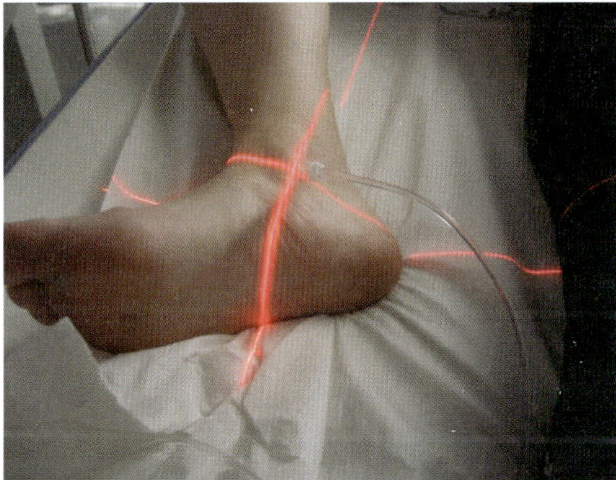

Figure 47.35 Needle introduced into the tendon under image guidance.

1) It is difficult to maintain a sterile or aseptic field due to the gel. Sterile covers and other accessories are available but add to the cost and often reduce the resolution of the image.
2) The needle visibility is only possible in the longitudinal plane; it appears as a dot in the transverse plane (as with Morton's neuroma injection).
3) The field of vision is limited to the size of the probe; therefore it is difficult to assess the whole tendon–muscle patho-anatomy.

Fluoroscopy-guided tendon distension tenogram is the procedure of choice for all long tendons, as it meets all the requirements. It provides additional information on the patho-anatomy of the tendon, which is very useful in defining the pathology and also helps in the planning of future treatment.

Figures 47.35 and 47.36 are of a young long-distance runner who presented with a history highly suggestive of tarsal syndrome which was confirmed by a diagnostic injection of 1 ml of 2% lignocaine under USS guidance, confining it to the tibialis posterior nerve. The pain was totally abolished and she was able to run without any symptoms. She underwent steroid injection along with modification to her sports footwear and had foot orthoses. She remained totally pain-free for 6 months after which she had a recurrence of the same symptoms. An MRI scan did not show any cystic lesion within the tarsal tunnel but showed fluid within the tibialis posterior tendon (Figure 47.37). This was thought not to be relevant at this stage and a second injection for tarsal tunnel syndrome was administered. She experienced a recurrence of her symptoms within 4 weeks, and tendon distension tenogram was performed.

The procedure is performed in a sterile or aseptic field. A blue needle is introduced into the tendon (Figure 47.35) and contrast infiltrated (Figure 47.36), demonstrating a distended synovial sheath, especially within the tarsal tunnel, with multiple adhesions.

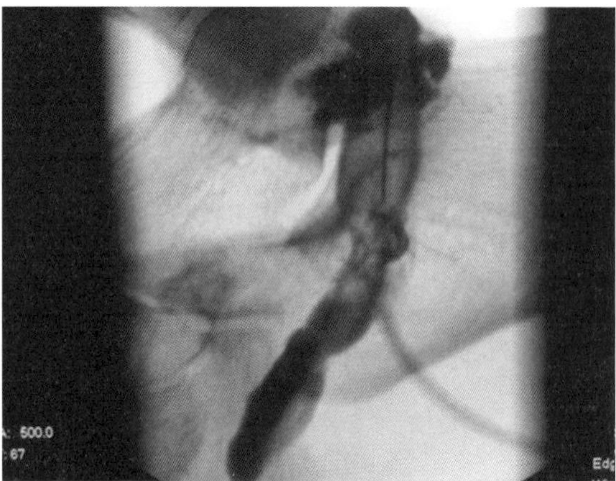

Figure 47.36 Contrast infiltrated to show severely distended tibialis posterior tendon sheath with accumulation of fluid causing secondary tarsal tunnel syndrome.

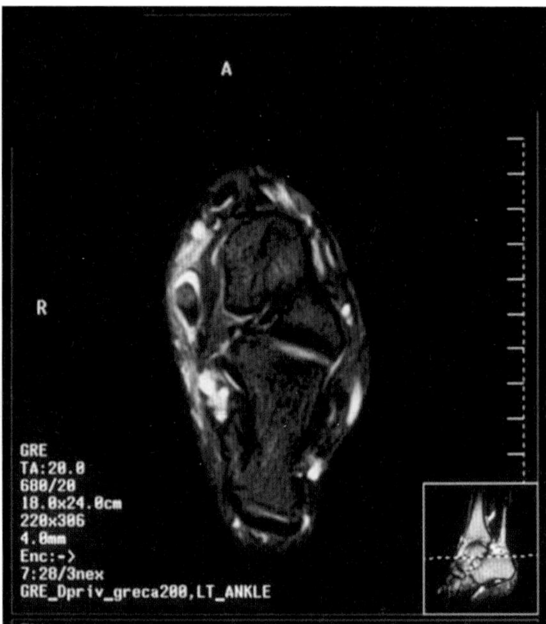

Figure 47.37 MRI scan showing fluid within the tibialis posterior tendon.

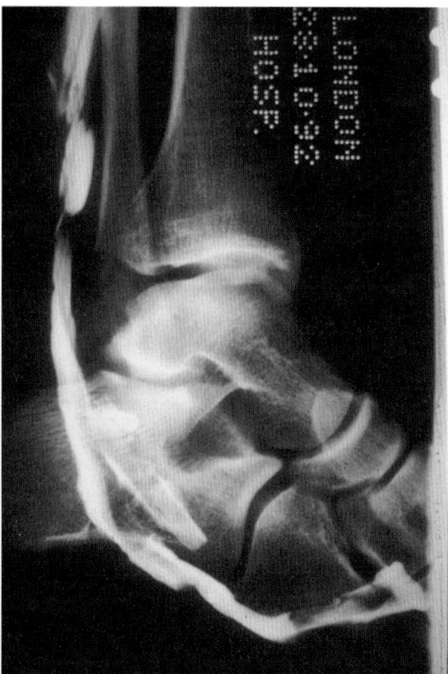

Figure 47.38 Tendon distension tenogram—peroneal tendinopathy. Note the shared tendon sheath and divergence of the brevis and longus inferior to the lateral malleolus.

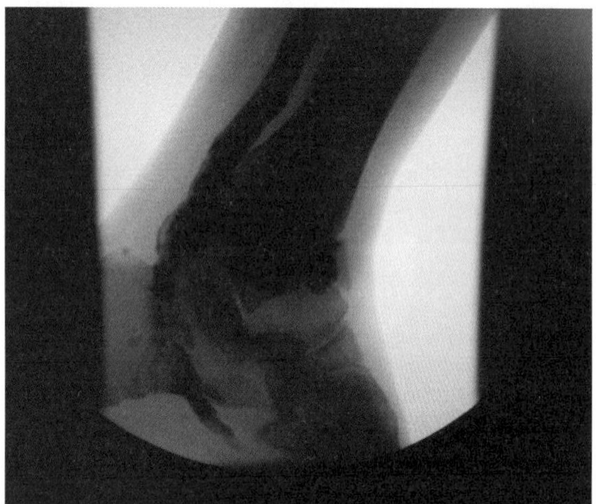

Figure 47.39 Tendon distension tenogram—flexor callucis longus tendinopathy.

Normal tendons and tendon sheaths are linear structures, which maintain the same width thoughout their course. The findings were discussed with the patient and treatment of choice was surgery. She made a full recovery and return to sport.

The same procedure is performed for peroneal tendinopathy (Figure 47.38) and flexor hallucis longus tendon (Figure 47.39).

A brace or ankle bandage is applied post injection and the patient advised to remain relatively non-impact for up to 72 hours, after which they can resume their physical activity under physiotherapy supervision.

Plantar fasciitis

Plantar fasciitis (enthesiopathy) (Schwartz and Su 2014) is a common cause of heel pain and it is characterized by pain first thing in the morning and after a period of rest at the medial plantar aspect of the heel, which improves with activity. There are different treatment options that are available (Cutts et al. 2012; Orchard 2012) and injection therapy remains the most popular.

Image-guided injection is performed under USS guidance (Figure 47.40) and it is a very simple procedure with good visualization and easy needle access; 6 ml 0.5% marcaine and either 50 mg hydrocortisone acetate or 40 mg depomedrone is infiltrated.

Palpation-guided injection is an equally easy procedure but is reliant on anatomical knowledge (Figure 47.41). Important considerations are the nerves, medial calcaneal tuberosity (MCT), and the

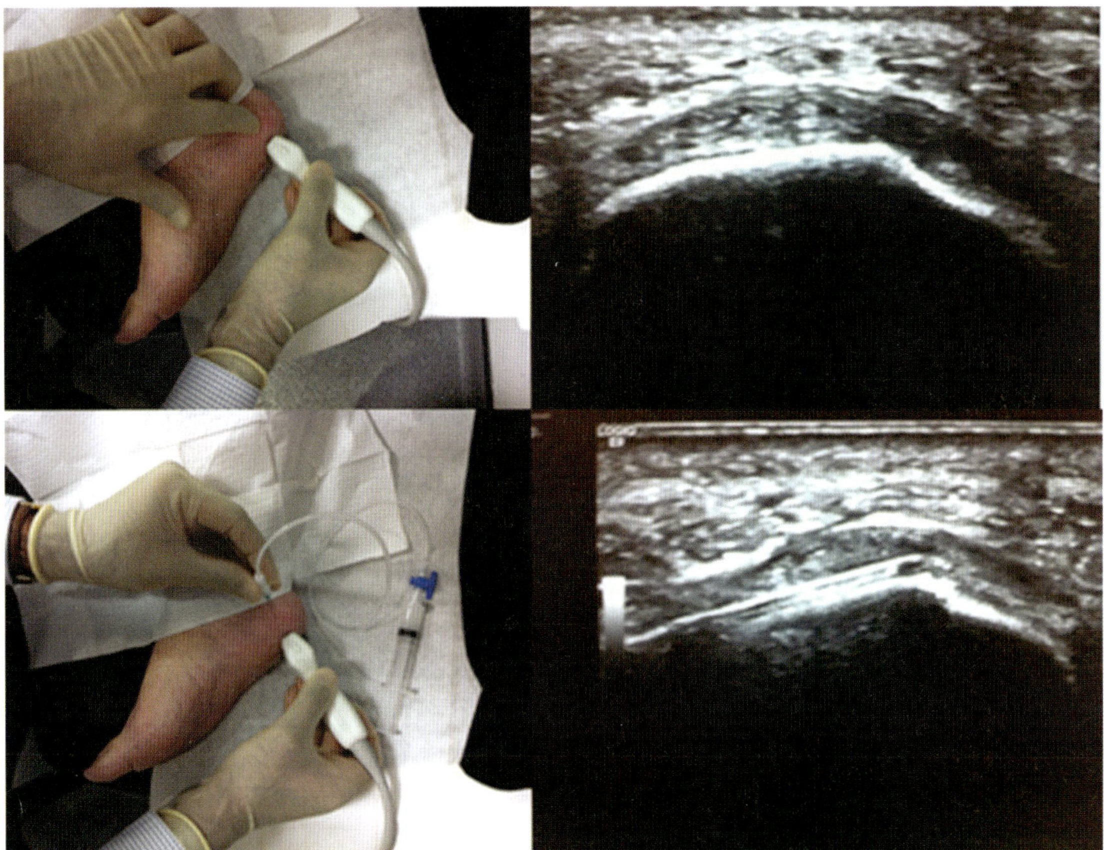

Figure 47.40 Ultrasound-guided plantar fascia injection.

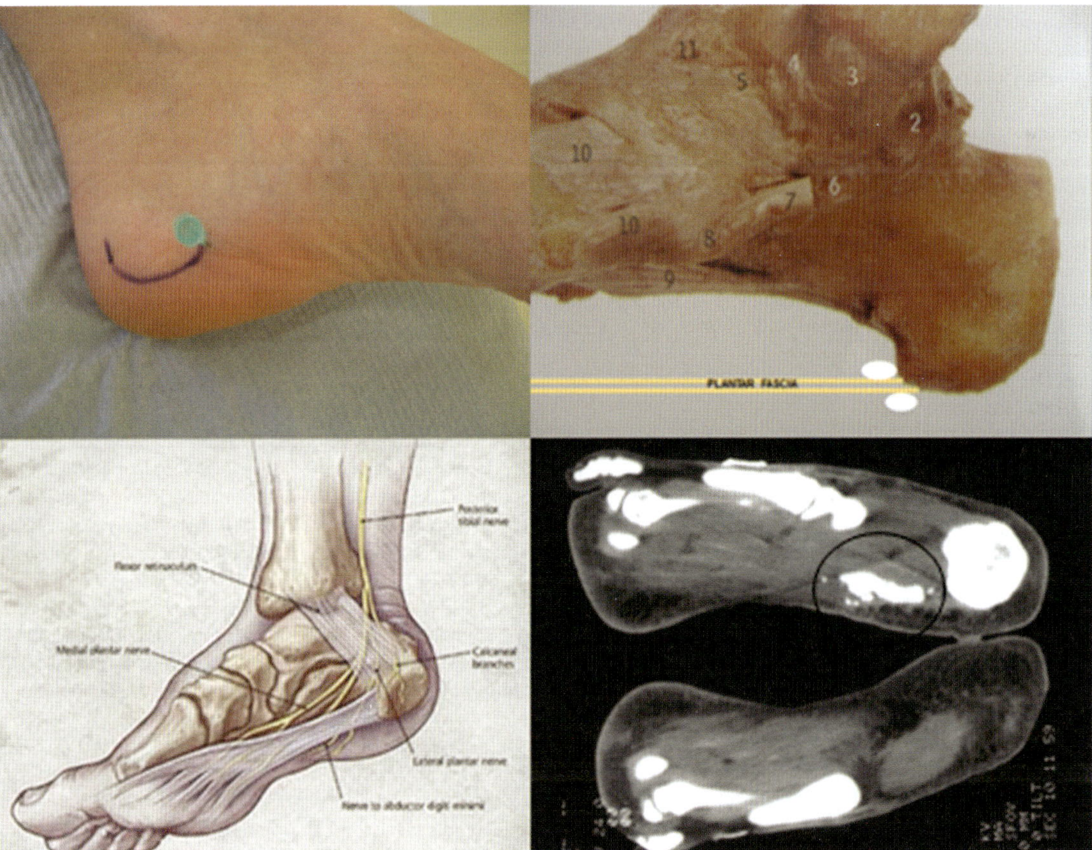

Figure 47.41 Clinically guided plantar fascia injection. Clockwise from top left: needle inserted from the medial aspect; plantar fascia used as an anatomical marker and infiltrated as shown; CT scan showing myositis ossificans following aggressive injection; anatomy around plantar fascia. (http://www.heelspurs.co.uk/diagnosing_heel_pain_anatomy.htm)

attachment of the medial band of the plantar fascia. The needle is inserted by feeling the most distal end of the MCT and directed superior and inferior to the plantar fascia simultaneously (Figure 47.40), taking care to infiltrate slowly to reduce trauma to soft tissue. It is possible to cause a bleed and, in some cases, myositis ossificans (Figure 47.41). 3 ml 0.5% marcaine and 25 mg hydrocortisone acetate is infiltrated at each site. Injection hydrostatic pressure can be reduced by using a 30-cm connecting tube and smaller syringes.

Acknowledgement

I would like to acknowledge the contributions of Dr O. Chan, Dr R. Jalan, and Dr M. Ahmad, who over the last two decades have worked closely with clinicians and are instrumental in setting protocols and standards for all image-guided injections discussed in this chapter. We continue to work closely to develop better, safer, and efficient techniques by auditing and being innovative. High-volume image-guided injection for mid-portion Achilles tendinopathy is the product of this close working relationship and is now the gold standard treatment of choice for this condition.

References

Amis JA1, Siverhus SW, Liwnicz BH. An anatomic basis for recurrence after Morton's neuroma excision. *Foot Ankle* 1992; 13(3):153–6.

Bloom JE1, Rischin A, Johnston RV, Buchbinder R. Image-guided versus blind glucocorticoid injection for shoulder pain. *Cochrane Database Syst Rev* 2012; 8:CD009147.

Crisp TA, King JB, Chan O, Padhiar N. Crisp-Padhiar syndrome. *Br J Sports Med* 2011; 45:e1.

Cutts S, Obi N, Pasapula C, et al. Plantar fasciitis. *Ann R Coll Surg Engl* 2012; 94(8):539–42.

Durall C. Examination and treatment of cuboid syndrome: a literature review. *The University of Wisconsin* 2011; 514–9.

Durlacher L. *Treatise on corns, bunions, disease of nails, and the general management of the feet*. London, UK: Simpkin and Marshall, 1845, p. 52.

Freiberg AH. Infraction of the second metatarsal bone. *Surg Gynecol Obstet* 1914; 19:191.

Gauthier G, Elbaz R. Freiberg's infraction: a subchondral bone fatigue fracture a new surgical treatment. *Clin Orthop* 1979; 142:93.

Gluck GS, Heckman DS, Parekh SG. Tendon disorders of the foot and ankle, part 3: the posterior tibial tendon. *Am J Sports Med* 2010; 38(10):2133–44.

Gray RG, Gottlieb NL. Intra-articualar steroids: an updated assessment. *Clin Orthop* 1983;177–235.

Gurdezi S, White T, Ramesh P. Alcohol injection for Morton's neuroma: a five-year follow-up. *Foot Ankle Int* 2013; 34(8):1064–7.

Hassouna H, Singh D. Morton's metatarsalgia: pathogenesis, aetiology and current management. *Acta Ortop Belg* 2005; 71:646–55.

Heckman DS, Gluck GS, Parekh SG. Tendon disorders of the foot and ankle, part 1: peroneal tendon disorders. *Am J Sports Med* 2009; 37(3):614–25.

Katcherian DA. Treatment of Freiberg's disease. *Orthop Clin North Am* 1994; 25:69.

Kirby KA. *Foot and lower extremity biomechanics III. Precision Intricast Newsletters, 2002–8*. Payson, AZ: Precision Intricast Inc., 2009, pp. 107–8.

Lee SJ, Jacobson JA, Kim SM, et al. Ultrasound and MRI of the peroneal tendons and associated pathology. *Skeletal Radiol* 2013; 42(9):1191–200. DOI: 10.1007/s00256-013-1631-6.

Lokiec F, Sievner I, Pritsch M. Chronic compartment syndrome of both feet. *J Bone Joint Surg* 1991; 73–B:178–9.

Lynch T, Pupp GR. Stenosing tenosynovitis of the flexor hallucis longus at the ankle joint. *J Foot Surg* 1990; 29(4):345–8.

Manoli A, Weber TG. Fasciotomy of the foot: an anatomical study with special reference to release of the calcaneal compartment. *Foot Ankle* 1990; 10:267–75.

Mason SF. *A history of the sciences*. New York, NY: Collier Books, 1962, p. 550.

Mavor GE. The anterior tibial syndrome. *J Bone Joint Surg*1956; 38–B: 513–7.

Miozzari HM, Gerad R, Stern R, et al. Exertional medial compartment syndrome of the foot in a high level athlete. A case report. *Am J Sports Med* 2008; 36:983–6.

Mollica MB. Chronic exertional compartment syndrome of the foot. *J Am Podiatr Med Assoc* 1998; 88:21–4.

Morton TG. A peculiar and painful affection of the fourth metatarsal articulation. *Am J Med Sci* 1876; 71:37–45.

Mulder JD. The causative mechanism in Morton's metatarsalgia. *J Bone Joint Surg Br* 1951; 33B:94–5.

Muller GP, Masquelet AC. Chronic compartment syndrome of the foot. A case report. *Rev Chir Orthop Reparatrice Appar Mot* 1995; 81:549–52.

Myerson MS, Fisher RT, Burgess AR, Kenzora JE. Fracture dislocations of the tarsometatarsal joints: end results correlated with pathology and treatment. *Foot & Ankle* 1986; 6:225–42.

Na JB, Bergman AG, Oloff LM, Beaulieu CF. The flexor hallucis longus: tenographic technique and correlation of imaging findings with surgery in 39 ankles. *Radiology* 2005; 236(3):974–82.

Nam SH, Kim J, Lee JH, Ahn J, Kim YJ, Park Y. Palpation versus ultrasound-guided corticosteroid injections and short-term effect in the distal radioulnar joint disorder: a randomized, prospective single-blinded study. *Clin Rheumatol* 2014 Dec;33(12):1807–14.

Newell SG, Woodle A. Cuboid syndrome. *Phys Sports Med* 1981; 9:71–6.

Orchard J. Plantar Fasciitis. *BMJ* 2012; 345:e6603.

Ouzounian TJ, Shereff MJ. In vitro determination of midfoot motion. *Foot & Ankle* 1989; 10:140–6.

Paavola M, Kannus P, Jarvinen TA, Jarvinen TL, Jozsa L, Jarvinen M. Treatment of tendon disorders. Is there a role for corticosteroid injection? *Foot Ankle Clin* 2002; 7(3):501–13.

Padhiar N, Allen M, King JB. Chronic exertional compartment syndrome of the foot. *Sports Med Arthrosc* 2009; 17(3):198–202.

Padhiar N, King JB. Exercise induced leg pain—chronic compartment syndrome. Is the increase in intra-compartment pressure exercise specific? *Br J Sports Med* 1996; 30(4):360–2.

Palamarchuk HJ, Oehrlein CR. Freiberg's infraction in a collegiate heptathlete. *J Am Podiatr Med Assoc* 2000; 90(2):77–80.

Patel A, Rao S, Nawoczenski D, Flemister AS, DiGiovanni B, Baumhauer JF. Midfoot arthritis. *J Am Acad Orthop Surg* 2010; 18:417–25.

Pisani G, Pisani PC, Parino E. Sinus tarsi syndrome and subtalar joint instability. *Clin Podiatr Med Surg* 2005; 22(1):63–77, vii.

Rao SBJ. Nonoperative options and decision making for fusion. *Tech Foot Ankle Surgery* 2008; 7:188–95.

Reis ND, Karkabi S, Zinman C. Metatarsophalangeal joint dislocation after local steroid injection. *J Bone Joint Surg Br* 1989; 71(5):864.

Schiffer G, Chan O, Jalan R, Padhiar N. Retrospective review of injection therapy in Morton's neuroma. *Br J Sports Med* 2013; 47(10):e3.

Schwartz EN, Su J. Plantar fasciitis: a concise review. *Perm J* 2014; 18(1): e105–7.

Sharp RJ, Wade CM, Hennessy MS, Saxby TS. The role of MRI and ultrasound imaging in Morton's neuroma and the effect of the size of lesions on symptoms. *J Bone Surg* 2003; 85–B(7):999–1005.

Simpson MR, Howard TM. Tendinopathies of the foot and ankle. *Am Fam Physician* 2009; 80(10):1107–14.

Smillie IS. Freiberg's infraction. *J Bone Joint Surg Br* 1957; 39:580.

Subotnick SI. Peroneal cuboid syndrome. *J Am Pod Med Assoc* 1989; 79(8): 413–4.

Symeonidis PD, Iselin LD, Simmons N, Fowler S, Dracopoulos G, Stavrou P. Prevalence of interdigital nerve enlargements in an asymptomatic population. *Foot Ankle Int* 2012; 33(7):543–7.

Thompson FM, Hamilton WG. Problems of the second metatarso-phalangeal joint. *Orthopedics* 1987; 10:83.

Thompson FM, Hamilton WG. Problems of the second metatarsophalangeal joint. *Orthopaedics* 1987; 10(1):83–9.

Torriani M, Thomas BJ, Bredella, Ouellette H. MRI of metatarsal head subchondral fractures in patients with forefoot pain. *Am J Roent* 2008; 190:570–5.

Womack JW1, Richardson DR, Murphy GA, Richardson EG, Ishikawa SN. Long-term evaluation of interdigital neuroma treated by surgical excision. *Foot Ankle Int* 2008; 29(6):574–7.

Wood Jones F. *Structure and function as seen in the foot*. Baltimore: Williams & Wilkins, 1944, pp. 60–3.

Yu CJ, Ko CJ, Hsieh CH, et al. Proteomic analysis of osteoarthritic chondrocyte reveals the hyaluronic acid-regulated proteins involved in chondroprotective effect under oxidative stress. *J Proteomics* 2014; 99:40–53.

Zanetti M,Weishaupt D. MR imaging of the forefoot: Morton's neuroma and differential diagnosis. *Semin Muscluloskelet Radiol* 2005; 9:175–86.

Part 4

Management strategies

Chapter 48

Musculoskeletal triage—a physiotherapist's perspective

Angela E. Clough

The changing face of physiotherapy within the National Health Service

UK patients have often experienced inadequate or inequitable access to musculoskeletal physiotherapy services since the inception of the National Health Service (NHS), for a variety of reasons (Foster et al. 2011).

I am approaching 30 years in physiotherapy practice and have participated in many initiatives to enhance access to improved musculoskeletal services during that time. Approximately 18 years ago in Leeds, as a precursor to the now well-established extended scope practitioner (ESP) roles for physiotherapists, a colleague, Steve Young (now a respected consultant physiotherapist) and I were tasked by our physiotherapy service manager with 'blue letter screening' or triaging as it is now known. The blue letters were the referral letters from general practitioners (GPs) to orthopaedic consultants for a musculoskeletal opinion on their patients. Physiotherapists working in NHS musculoskeletal out-patients at that time faced increasing pressure regarding waiting time for patients' access to physiotherapy, as orthopaedic consultant referrals requesting physiotherapy had risen sharply. Orthopaedic consultants, in the main, were the 'gatekeepers' to free physiotherapy treatment. There was limited direct GP access to physiotherapy through service contracts with the NHS. If patients did not pay for private physiotherapy, the majority could only access physiotherapy by attending their GP who could make a referral for an orthopaedic consultant opinion. If the musculoskeletal condition did not require surgical intervention, the orthopaedic consultant would refer the patient for physiotherapy. Physiotherapists, tasked with reading, reviewing the content, and filtering the 'blue letters', arranged for the patients to attend an assessment with an experienced senior physiotherapist. Steve and I had the clinical freedom to assess, treat, and also 'fast track' an appointment for an orthopaedic consultant review for the patient if we reasoned it clinically to be an appropriate course of action. It was a very successful project and it is a long-held regret that we did not publish our success with the trial project at the time. Our legacy is that it led to the establishment of several ESP roles for physiotherapists in Leeds—a positive move to develop physiotherapy practice.

Physiotherapy had undergone considerable development at that time. It had moved from a nationalized, standardized, diploma course based in schools of physiotherapy to a university-based, all-degree profession. As physiotherapy training places were still embedded in NHS hospital clinical placements, it was an unwritten rule, or certainly an expectation, that all graduating physiotherapists would seek employment in the NHS.

Professional autonomy had long since been established and the referrals now had a clear diagnosis with a request for assessment and treatment, rather than a prescriptive request for 'heat and exercise please' that I recall from my own student days. Senior/experienced physiotherapists attended specialist clinics to work jointly with orthopaedic consultants. I had previously worked in the South of England in an NHS soft tissue injury clinic, with an inspirational accident and emergency (A&E) consultant. I was motivated to spend 16 years in university educational roles before returning again to clinical practice. In Leeds where I had worked alongside a well-admired shoulder surgeon. It was a privilege to work with two consultants who cared so passionately about patients' well-being and best outcome.

Trust in each other's respective clinical skills and a very clear network of professional support for physiotherapists were both evident and valued qualities in the NHS at that time. Strong teamwork was embedded in the NHS and seen as a valued strength; no junior would work without the support of a senior experienced colleague. In the main, it would be a senior clinical specialist physiotherapist who would attend clinics and be the named link and liaison person for the rest of the physiotherapy out-patient team. A simple phone call to the consultant's secretary would result in a review at the next available appointment as there was mutual respect, providing increased job satisfaction. Now (in 2015), this style of service is sometimes provided but there is more diversity in practice (Stanhope et al. 2011) and a significant rise in administrative paper exchanges. These administrative duties often interfere with clinical service provision.

The foundation of musculoskeletal triage

In 2006, the Department of Health published a report 'The Musculoskeletal Services Framework—a joint responsibility: doing it differently'. This recognized the demographic realities of the musculoskeletal pressures of disability, with an increase in the number and proportion of older people in the population—a trend that was set to rise. A creative, open-minded approach was required in order to deal appropriately with this demographic challenge and enable patient access to effective and timely advice in order to maximize their health potential to remain independent, while having a limited budget to provide adequately for the increasing demand on services.

The increasing cost of providing musculoskeletal healthcare is a key reason to explore a different clinical practice. In 1998, the total direct costs of back pain were £1.6 billion, of which physiotherapy accounted for £251 million (Maniadakis and Gray 2000). Estimates are that these costs have risen by at least 30% (Savigny et al. 2009).

Impacting factors on musculoskeletal triage

- The possibility of a non-surgical, conservative intervention that may benefit the referred patient with a musculoskeletal problem.
- Contract/commissioning targets.
- 'Acute' versus 'routine' criteria for referrals to physiotherapy.
- An 'acute' patient may be one who needs an appointment within, for example, 2 weeks. Examples may be:
  - a soft tissue injury screened in the A&E department
  - an elective protocol patient who may require:
  - arthroscopic subacromial decompression (ASAD)
  - manipulation under anaesthetic (MUA)
  - rotator cuff repair
  - anterior cruciate ligament (ACL) reconstruction
- 'routine' patient may be one whose condition would not be expected to significantly deteriorate if they were not seen within 2 weeks. The average target waiting time for 'routine' patients is 6 weeks, but commissioning of service contracts may vary and stipulate different time frames.
- Prevention of:
  - chronicity
  - fear avoidance
  - reduced function, loss of independence
- Staffing—appropriate skill and expertise; appropriate staffing level to meet service needs.

PhysioDirect—one model of telephone-based musculoskeletal triage

In the UK, the triage process within PhysioDirect offers a way of providing timely access to physiotherapy for patients that may benefit. There are several variations of PhysioDirect. They all involve patients being invited to telephone a physiotherapist for initial assessment and advice. Many patients are posted generalized information on self-management and exercise (Foster et al. 2011).

PhysioDirect and similar initiatives contribute towards the NHS modernization agenda, which looks at more convenient approaches to providing timely access to appropriate care. Concerns raised about these telephone-based services are:

- Potential inequity of service.
- Potential de-skilling of physiotherapists; fear that important diagnoses might be missed and that physiotherapy might turn into an office-based profession (Gamlin and Duffield 2001; Lyall 2007).
- Conflict in studies. Turner (2009) found that 71% of patients assessed over the phone required further assessment or 'hands-on' treatment. This would undermine the cost effectiveness of this approach.

Evidence to support the development of services like PhysioDirect includes:

- Audits undertaken, using telephone consultation, identified that approximately 60% of callers are managed by telephone assessment alone. Non-attendance rates reduce from more than 15% to less than 1%. GPs have fewer musculoskeletal consultations, and patients have quicker access to secondary care consultants (Gamlin and Duffield 2001).
- A study showed that physiotherapists came to the same clinical decision when using telephone triage as they did with a face to face intervention (Turner 2009).
- Patient satisfaction on the whole is good (Clayson and Woolvine 2004; Taylor et al. 2002).
- GP satisfaction also appeared to be good (Clayson and Woolvine 2004).

SWOT analysis of musculoskeletal triage: strengths, weaknesses, opportunities, threats

Strengths

- Contract/commissioning (if based on quality issues, with appropriate senior, experienced physiotherapists and sufficient staffing levels to meet service needs).
  - Recognition for highly skilled, professional ESP role models in musculoskeletal practice.
  - Patients receive timely advice, from the most appropriate health professional, with scope to refer on in a timely manner.
- Improved patient well-being; decreased anxiety if timely and appropriate consultation and advice are provided.

Weaknesses

- Contract/commissioning (if based on inexperienced/newly qualified graduates or minimum staffing levels, with minimum peer support)
  - Potential erosion of professional autonomy as may have to follow an algorithm rather than professional judgement and reasoning.

- Often bureaucratic, contract-led services rather than based on clinically reasoned assessment of need.

- Electronic records may be more 'efficient' but valuable eye contact and verbal cues might be overlooked as the professional focuses on tapping a screen rather than on observation, active listening, and rapport with the patient in front of them.

Opportunities

- Contract/commissioning (if based on quality issues and evidence service development needs, e.g. mindfulness/cognitive functional therapy based programmes to deal with psychosocial impacting factors on musculoskeletal patients).
- 'Informatics'—scope for creative ways forward with musculoskeletal practice and consultations, as highlighted by Karen Middleton, Chief Executive Officer of the Chartered Society of Physiotherapy.

Threats

- Contracts/commissioning of services:
  - Uncertainty, job insecurity, lack of job satisfaction. Is service contract being renewed? A respected colleague expressed fear and concern over the future of their job as a well-known business mogul might be their new boss and service contract holder. Health is seen as a business and as such there may be a conflict of interest for health professionals between keeping a job and meeting targets and making the best decision for a patient, using best clinical judgement based on clinical reasoning.
  - Threat to professional autonomy if contract based on 'time-bound' restricted assessment and number of attendances rather than professional judgement and patient needs.
  - Lack of clarity on minimum staffing and appropriate experience of staffing.

Implications for musculoskeletal triage in practice: a discussion of the literature

In their 2011 systematic review, Stanhope and Grimmer-Somers identified 1071 studies. Most were of low quality on the hierarchy of evidence scale. This followed their disappointing finding of a paucity of additional clarity from their earlier systematic review. They still found large differences in autonomy and clinical decision making. However, the literature suggested that ESP physiotherapists were comparable with medical doctors in terms of decision making. There was no high-quality evidence, however, in support of increased efficiency of out-patient management pathways using ESPs.

Suckley (2012) identified 104 clinical competencies of ESPs working in musculoskeletal settings in a Delphi study. Of those, 85 were agreed by consensus. This work should inform the skills, knowledge, attitudes, and behaviours of ESP roles.

Dunbar (2009), a GP and associate Dean, reported on the work in his clinic, which was run jointly with a physiotherapist ESP. The approach had been the 2006 winner of the Royal College of General Practice (RCGP) Paul Freeling award for innovative practice. Dunbar identified five key areas of musculoskeletal problems:

1 back and neck pain

2 osteoarthrosis

3 tendinopathy

4 joint pain and injury

5 chronic pain.

He captured the essence of how successful the process of their working practice was:

> . . . perform a thorough assessment and then provide the patient with the information and explanation about their condition. We try to involve the patients in the management of their problems and hopefully enable self-management. Much of this work might be categorised as in the cognitive and behavioural domain. (Dunbar 2009, p. 88)

In a study of two physiotherapists and three surgeon participants, there was agreement on 91.8% of musculoskeletal assessments of patients with reported hip and knee problems. There was 85.5% agreement on whether and if a patient was a candidate and willing to have a total joint replacement. They concluded that further research was required to establish added value and most appropriate use of ESPs (McKay et al. 2009).

Bath and Janzen (2012), in their Canadian questionnaire-based study, found that spinal triage service which was delivered by physiotherapists was a shift in traditional practice boundaries. There was high satisfaction with the service provided. The negatives that the study highlighted were a perceived lack of detail and time to follow up, and issues related to access to services either due to cost or lack of local availability. There were other impacting themes that the study highlighted that would be worthy of further research: persisting or chronic symptoms, comorbidities. It was noted that these 'other' issues impact upon pain, function, and quality of life.

Key points in relation to musculoskeletal triage

- Need for further definitive evidence from high-quality randomized controlled trials prior to more widespread roll out of PhysioDirect across the NHS.
  - Some services using PhysioDirect only employ experienced band 6 or 7 staff to do telephone triage (Foster et al. 2011).
- More research is required into measurement of the quality of the intervention:
  - Large differences in autonomy and decision making from a recent systematic review of the literature of ESP roles in out-patients (Gilmore et al. 2011; Stanhope and Grimmer-Sommers 2011).
  - The value added and most appropriate ESP (McKay et al. 2009).
  - A shift in focus from stakeholder need to an awareness of additional measures to investigate well-being, e.g. Short Form 36 (SF36), Hospital Anxiety and Depression Scale (HADS).
  - Recognition of psychosocial factors when educating on self-management, reassuring, and reducing anxiety by the therapist.
  - Cognitive functional therapy approach.
  - Mindfulness.

- Consideration of professional autonomy:
  - Good support network with the Chartered Society of Physiotherapy.
  - Special interest group for ESPs.
- Whatever the approach taken to triage, the initial assessment should include appropriate patient-specific as well as condition-specific advice.

References

Bath, B., Janzen, B. (2012) Patient and referring health care provider satisfaction with a physiotherapy spinal triage assessment service. *J Mulitidis Health Care*, 5, 1–15.

Clayson, M., Woolvine, M. (2004) Back pain direct clinic: a collaboration between general practitioners and physiotherapists. *Work Based Learn Prim Care* 2, 38–43.

Dunbar, A. (2009) Craven Musculoskeletal Clinic. *Int Musc Med* 31(2), 88–9.

Foster, N.E., Williams, B., Grove, S., Gamlin, J., Salisbury, C. (2011) The evidence for and against 'PhysioDirect' telephone assessment and advice services. *Physiotherapy* 87(1), 78–82.

Gamlin, J., Duffield, K. (2001) *PhysioDirect*. Cambridgeshire, UK: Huntingdonshire NHS Primary Care Trust.

Gilmore, L.G., Morris, J.H., Murphy, K., Grimmer-Somers, K., Kumar, S. (2011) Skills escalation in allied health: a time for reflection and refocus. *J Healthcare Lead* 3, 53–8.

Lyall, J. (2007) Physiotherapy direct worries. *Physiother Frontline* 13(6), 7, March.

Maniadakis, N., Gray, A. (2000) The economic burden of back pain in the UK. *Pain* 84, 95–103.

McKay, C., Davies, A.M., Mahomed, M., Badley, E.M. (2009) Expanding roles in orthopaedic care: a comparison of orthopaedic surgeon recommendations for triage. *J Eval Clin Prac* 15(1), 178–83.

Savigny, P., Kuntze, S., Watson, P., Underwood, M., Ritchie, G., Cotterell, M. (2009) *Low back pain: early management of persistent non-specific low back pain*. London: National Collaborating Centre for Primary Care and Royal College of Practitioners.

Stanhope, J., Grimmer-Somers, K. (2011) Extended scope physiotherapy roles for orthopaedic out-patients: an updated systematic review of the literature. *J Multidisc Healthcare* 5, 37–45.

Suckley, J.E. (2012) *Core clinical competencies for extended scope patients working in musculoskeletal interface clinics based in primary care: a Delphi consensus study*. Unpublished PhD thesis; University of Salford.

Taylor, S., Ellis, I., Gallagher, M. (2002) Patient satisfaction with a new physiotherapy telephone service for back pain patients. *Physiotherapy* 88, 645–57.

Turner, D. (2009) An exploratory study of physiotherapy telephone assessment. *Int J Ther Rehabil* 16, 97–105.

Chapter 49

Patient education and self care

Jennifer Klaber Moffett and Angela E. Clough

Appropriate patient education is an essential part of managing musculoskeletal conditions effectively. If someone has insight into their problem and how to deal with it, the disorder is likely to improve more quickly. Effective patient education is likely to depend as much on the method of delivery as the content (di Blasi and Kleinen 2000; Butler 2012; Critchley et al. 2007; Fersum et al. 2011; Hurley et al. 2007, 2012; Klaber Moffett 1989; Nordin 1995; Williams 2009).

The first part of this chapter deals with the problem of successfully delivering the message. In the remainder of the chapter, the content of the message is then addressed, using research-based evidence and personal clinical experience. Many of the examples are directly related to back pain, which often forms at least 50% of a musculoskeletal workload. Since 2007, there have also been significant cost-effective self-care problems with patients with chronic knee and hip pain. Much of the wealth of research knowledge relating to the back and resulting principles could often safely be transferred to the peripheral joints and applied to other conditions (Roland et al. 1996; Williams et al. 2009).

Unfortunately, patient education, care, and self care are not always optimal because individuals may:

- have *inappropriate beliefs and misconceptions* about their condition
- not have *understood* exactly what the clinician wanted them to do
- believe the advice was not *relevant* for them, and anyway would not help
- not feel able to carry out the advice because it seemed *impractical*, i.e. there are physical barriers
- find it would be too much effort.

If people are not doing as much as they might to help themselves, then the efforts of clinicians, regardless of expertise and skill, will be largely wasted.

Patient's perspective on education and self care for musculoskeletal problems

Inappropriate beliefs and misconceptions

One of the first aims of patient education is to dispel misconceptions that may act as a barrier to recovery. Frequently, this may relate to the attribution or cause of the condition about which the individual is consulting. Misconceptions need to be replaced with an explanation that is credible and will provide the patient with the confidence to carry out an active rehabilitation programme and encourage them to return to normal activities as soon as possible.

The cause of pain and pain mechanisms

Misconceptions about the cause of pain need to be addressed. Some insight into how pain is perceived and sustained can be helpful, especially in chronic pain. The individual needs to understand that pain is not processed through a simple mechanical pathway, but is a complex process that can be modified at many different levels of the nervous system. The pain experienced is modulated in the higher centres of the brain by such factors as distraction and suggestion. A large series of fascinating experiments have confirmed the powerful effect of such psychological variables on the reporting of physical symptoms (Pennebaker 1982, 1984). Patient education could include a simple description of the pain gate theory (Melzack and Wall 1982), which provides an explanation of how the mind influences the pain experience.

Most people have a working hypothesis, and if they do not, they will be searching for an explanation for their condition. If the clinician's explanation is in conflict with the individual's expectations, it will be seen as irrelevant and any advice will probably be rejected. A very useful question to ask is, 'What is it that concerns you about the pain?'. This is not a loaded question, and could be asked of anyone. It is a useful way of eliciting beliefs that might otherwise remain hidden.

Fear of movement and re-injury

If the individual believes that their back pain is due to an injury received at work, they may well believe that continuing with this work would be damaging. Similarly, if someone has apparently damaged their back while rowing, they may be afraid of returning to this activity. Back pain is now considered more often than not to be accumulative strain, influenced by psychosocial factors, rather than a simple one-off biomechanical problem (Burton 1997; Waddell 1998).

The appropriate use of positive terminology has been the focus of research. Williams (2009) highlighted the issue of words that harm and words that heal. Butler (2012), at the International

Federation of Orthopaedic and Manipulative Physical Therapists in Quebec, Canada, 2012, explained the role of a manual therapist as a linguist. He suggested that advances in our understanding of the concept of neuroplasticity have exposed dated metaphors that require challenging, for example, 'it's just your age'. Instead, enriching metaphors, such as 'motion is lotion' may help with the integration of active exercise. Introduction of positive philosophical metaphors, such as 'you are not your thoughts', helps to establish the concept of mindfulnesss and living in the moment.

It has therefore been suggested that it is better not to use the term 'back injury', as this is inaccurate and encourages the avoidance of movement (Hadler 1987, 1997). The individual may be afraid of movement that appears to reproduce the pain, associating it with further damage and preventing healing. Compare this to the sportsperson's attitude when recovering from an injury: she/he will expect movements to be sore until the full range of movement is gained and will not be surprised to find that unaccustomed exercise is usually slightly painful. With a coach, she/he will work through a carefully prepared training package. Such sportspeople—who of course also have the advantage of being highly motivated—generally recover even from quite major trauma much faster than other people. It is necessary for individuals to understand and believe that any advice to exercise will actually assist the healing process.

Research is emerging which shows that people who can overcome a fear of movement and physical activity have better outcomes (Burton et al. 1999; Indahl et al. 1998; Vlaeyen and Linton 2000). Overcoming fear with clear, educationally based rehabilitation programmes is an approach that has also been transferred to peripheral joints, producing better outcomes in the knee and hip (Critchley et al. 2007; Hurley et al. 2007, 2012; Jessop 2014).

Fear of wear and tear

People who have been told they have arthritis or 'wear and tear' may believe that they should reduce their levels of physical activity in order to save the joints. Most people appreciate that exercise can strengthen muscles, but they do not realize that exercise and movement also play a very important role in the healing of other structures such as ligaments and even bone. Wear and tear is an inadequate description of osteoarthritis; it is far too passive (Williams 2009). Rather than the movement, like a worn-out ball-bearing, the process is more dynamic with the potential for some cartilage repair and remodelling of the underlying bone.

People with arthritis need to be told that the right sort of exercise increases the lubrication in the joint space rather than wearing down the joint surfaces. For each condition, an explanation to suit that individual needs to be offered in the context of the person's own belief patterns.

Fear of a progressive condition

Another fear and misconception that may hinder recovery, especially if the person does not relate the pain to a physical incident or injury, is the unspoken possibility of the presence of some dreaded progressive disease. An individual may fear ending up in a wheelchair, or suspect that their pain must be due to cancer. Since these fears may not be voiced, it is incumbent on the clinician to elicit any such beliefs so that they can be dispelled.

Epidemiological studies show that the prognosis, in terms of pain and disability, is not inevitably gloomy, as roughly one-third get worse, one-third stay the same, but one-third improve (Peters et al. 2005). The words we use to describe illness are very important—'wear and tear' and 'degenerative change' speak to me of inevitable decline, with the patient powerless to change their situation; but we know this is not the case. Health psychologists tell us that our coping response to illness is governed by our beliefs about the nature of the illness: how well we understand the symptoms, its chronicity, its controllability, its cause, and the seriousness of its consequences (Cameron and Leventhal 2003; Horne 1999).

After a brief but appropriate history taking and examination, the clinician is then in a good position to offer a credible and non-threatening explanation of the condition to reassure the person. In some cases, no further treatment will then be required. However, for most people, the rehabilitation process can then begin. For someone who is suitably motivated, much of this can be carried out at home with appropriate guidance. Educational interventions should emphasize that control is possible and within individuals' capabilities. The level of physical activity in older adults in the UK is low (NHS 2006) and reduced further by pain-related fear of movement in those with osteoarthritis (Hendry et al. 2006; Heuts et al. 2004). This will be considered further in the section 'Home exercise programmes'.

Understanding the message

The commonest reason for not 'complying with advice' may be to do with how the message is received and interpreted. The clinician may believe that they have clearly asked the person to carry out a few simple exercises and given specific advice about activities or positions to avoid. However, if the receiver is on a different waveband from the one the message was sent out on, the advice will not be received. Generally, patients want to please and certainly do not want to look foolish, so they will usually appear to cooperate. It is maybe only when they get home that they realize how blurred the message was. An anxious person who feels insecure in the presence of the 'expert' may be unable to take in any details at all. The more relaxed and at ease an individual feels with the clinician, the more likely they are to be receptive to the message.

Language or jargon may be a problem. Words that are familiar to a clinician may be meaningless to a lay person, or be interpreted in quite a different way from how they were meant (Williams 2009). A different problem arises when the clinician provides a message that conflicts with the patient's beliefs. In this case, the individual may find it difficult to make sense of information because of their prior mindset and beliefs.

Advice perceived not to be relevant

If the advice given does not fit with the individual's understanding of their problem, commitment to it will be lacking. The individual will perceive that the advice is irrelevant and will not believe that the effort involved will be worthwhile. The advice must be credible in the patient's eyes. This may be achieved after assessment of the condition, which includes asking appropriate questions and a physical examination, followed by a brief non-threatening explanation of the problem.

Impractical advice: physical and perceived barriers

Practical reasons for not following the advice given could include:

Forgetting to do it

This could be because the person leads a busy life with many work and/or domestic commitments. The suggested programme may have a low priority on their schedule and thus may be overlooked. For others, including older people, memory may be a problem, and methods of reminding themselves to do things may be necessary. The home programme needs to be written down and appropriate times negotiated and set by the patient. The time for doing the exercises then becomes part of a daily routine, with specific cues to aid memory; for example, 'I do this postural correction while the kettle boils' or 'I stand up and do my stretches every time someone leaves my office'. The chances of continuing with a programme of exercises long term increases if they are always done at the same time of the day and linked with another activity. The habit or behaviour is reinforced if it is followed by an activity that the person enjoys or finds rewarding, such as having a cup of tea.

Exercise or advice is difficult to follow for a physical reason, e.g. obesity, ill health

It is important that the clinician does not ask someone to carry out an activity without checking that it is within their perceived capability.

Time not available

The clinician should be realistic in prescribing how much exercise to expect someone to carry out. If an individual is asked to carry out an exercise programme every hour while they are at work, not only may this be unrealistic but also it could be disadvantageous because the person has to focus on their disorder rather than on their work. Another major disadvantage in making excessive demands is that the therapist may lose credibility in the patient's eyes.

Too expensive

Using a special facility such as a gym may be expensive. If an individual does not rate the activity as being very important or desirable, they will not think it is worth the money.

Lack of transport

For someone without a car, the additional effort of walking and using public transport may be perceived as an impossible barrier.

Lack of suitable space

It may difficult for someone to find space and privacy to carry out a routine conveniently. A mother with young children and little support at home may not have the necessary space and time to carry out the programme. People at work may have similar difficulties.

Lack of social support

In addition to any or all of the previously discussed reasons for not complying with an exercise programme, social support is an important factor. If family, friends, and work colleagues understand the importance of carrying out the routine, they are more likely to be encouraging. In contrast, if they do not perceive the exercise programme to be important, they may very easily act as a major antagonist.

In order to encourage family and friends to be supportive, it can be very helpful to involve them in the rehabilitation process. Commonly, the individual's family and work colleagues may be overprotective and may provide more sympathy than is helpful. They may encourage the individual in an invalid role by regularly offering to do tasks for them. This does not aid the rehabilitation process, and can also be quite demoralizing for the individual. If they understand the issues better, family, friends, and colleagues may be able to support and help the person in a much more appropriate way. They should at least have access to written information, which the individual should be encouraged to show them. A useful example of this is *The Back Book* (see later section 'Encouraging early return to activity'). This provides evidence-based information and positive messages to encourage recovery.

Effort and motivation

The aim of patient education is to provide people with information and increase their knowledge and understanding of their condition. It can influence their attitude to their disorder. However, although knowledge and attitudes are important, they do not necessarily predict behaviour. An individual may have been told that they should do exercises and know that this could be helpful, but for a number of different reasons, there may be barriers, both mental and physical, that prevent them from doing the prescribed exercises. This is a key issue that health professionals need to address more closely. It is essential that the individual believes that it is worth putting the effort into doing the exercises. The chances of carrying out a new programme and maintaining it can be predicted using the 'health beliefs' model (Becker 1985; Janz and Becker 1984). The key variables included in this model are:

- the perceived costs and effort required, balanced by
- the perceived benefit likely to be achieved, and
- the seriousness of the condition as perceived by the individual, and
- perceived barriers.

Techniques such as motivational interviewing can be used to improve the chances of a person taking on a new programme (Rollnick et al. 1992; Smith et al. 1997) and will be discussed in the following section.

Clinician's perspective and approach to patient education and self care for musculoskeletal problems

Effective communication

Effective patient education depends on effective communication. Most of us like to believe that we are good communicators, even though we may have had little or no training in this skill. Research into communication, words used, and motivational interviewing, as part of a more effective communication strategy, has been highlighted in recent years (Butler 2012; O'Sullivan 2012; Williams 2009). A skilfully conducted interview is an essential starting point for optimal management of a musculoskeletal condition. If this is not done well, subsequent advice and management may well be inappropriate.

Time may be a real barrier for clinicians, but if patient education is considered to be an essential part of treatment intervention rather than a nice extra (Lorig 1995), it might be given greater priority. In the longer term, it has been shown that effective communication can cut down on the use of healthcare resources, improving both patient satisfaction and treatment outcomes. In a study by Daltroy et al. (1992), it was found that if a rheumatologist made a clear statement about the purpose of a non-steroidal anti-inflammatory drug (NSAID), 79% of patients were compliant, compared with 33% where no clear statement was made. Also, it has been shown that after a consultation, the *doctor's perception* of what they told the patient may vary significantly from the *patient's perception* of what they have been told. The way in which information is provided is at least as important as the content of the information. Some clinicians may believe they should give each patient as much information as possible, whereas others commonly underestimate the amount of information that patients want. In either case, the best approach is to find out what the individual's current understanding is and what other information they require. Open-ended questions such as 'what do you know about your condition?' may be a useful starting point.

A number of benefits may result from improved communication (Ley 1988) including:

- increased patient understanding and recall
- increased patient satisfaction
- less ill-informed consent
- increased patient compliance
- quicker and less stressful recovery from illness and surgery.

A change in emphasis to a patient-centred approach (Mead and Bower 2000) and awareness of words that harm and words that heal (Butler 2012; Williams 2009), in a cultural shift to more of a motivational interviewing approach (O'Sullivan 2012), enhances patient–clinician rapport.

Patient–practitioner interaction

The health professional can influence the outcome of treatment by shaping beliefs, and providing support alongside physical care. These concepts have been highlighted in a couple of systematic reviews (di Blasi and Kleinen 2000; Mead and Bower 2000), the former linked into Leventhal's self-regulatory model (Leventhal 1985; Leventhal and Cameron 1987). A combination of cognitive care, emotional care, and physical care has been reported to improve recovery in surgical cases and cardiac patients and probably applies also to people with musculoskeletal disorders. It seems likely that how the practitioner provides the information is as important as what material is provided. Di Blasi and Kleinen (2000) postulate that accompanying supportive care is an important aspect that is under-researched and could have an impact on successful outcome of treatment.

The aim of the systematic review by Mead and Bower (2000) was to explore relationships between the concept of patient centredness and its measurement. The search covered a 30-year time span. The term 'patient centredness' covers many different concepts which may compromise its scientific utility. A five-dimension framework was proposed:

- Dimension one—the degree to which a clinician uses a *biopsychosocial perspective*
- Dimension two—relates to the clinician's understanding of the *patient as a person*
- Dimension three—*sharing power and responsibility*
- Dimension four—*therapeutic alliance*
- Dimension five—the *doctor as a person*; awareness of personal qualities and aspects of the relationship particular to the individual clinician–patient dyad.

Mead and Bower (2000) highlighted the complexity of influences, identifying key factors that affect the five dimensions of patient centredness:

- *Time*
- '*Shapers*'—cultural norms and societal expectations, socioeconomic background, formal and informal learning (e.g. the media, personal experience, training), and experience.
- *Clinician factors*—attitudes, values, knowledge, personality, gender, age, ethnicity, knowledge of patient.
- *Professional context influences*—professional norms, performance, incentives and targets, accreditation, government policy and initiatives.
- *Patient influences*—attitudes, expectations, knowledge, personality, gender, age, ethnicity, nature of problems, and knowledge of clinician.
- *Consultation-level influences*—communication barriers, physical barriers, interruptions, presence of third parties, time limitations, workload pressures.

Overall, they found the term 'patient centredness' to be multifactorial and therefore ambiguous in terms of specifics. However, they did provide some support for the view that specific evidence of how we can appropriately measure the benefits of patient centredness is lacking at present, and this should be considered, caution exercised, and context borne in mind when setting standards (Mead and Bower 2000, 2002). Patients' views of general practitioners (GPs) may be of some value in setting standards, but while access to services is an important issue in itself, evidence concerning the cost benefit of rapid access is important in the wider debate (Gulliford et al. 2002).

The most important goal in arthritis patient education, according to Daltroy (1993), is to develop a cooperative relationship between the physician and patient so that the patient will adhere to a mutually agreed regimen and the regimen is guided by accurate feedback from the patient. In this way, the symptoms can be monitored and managed most effectively. The patient needs to be asked what they see as their goal of treatment. The clinician needs to explain what is possible, including implications and limitations. The patient's preferences need to be taken into account, so alternative possibilities need to be discussed. In this way, an adult–adult relationship is encouraged rather than a child–adult relationship implying undue dependency on the clinician (Klaber Moffett and Richardson 1997).

Providing the information

There is notable disparity about doctors' information-giving to patients (Street 1992) which distinguishes patient centredness from doctors' information-giving behaviour; while Roter et al. (1987) consider information-giving as a patient-centred skill. However, in contrast, Mead and Bower (2002) consider the exchange of psychosocial information, by either party, is treated as patient centredness, whereas biomedical information exchange is not.

When providing patient education and advice, it is very tempting to think that the 'best' education is providing the individual with all the information that is available. However, this is a mistake—albeit one that some of us have taken many years of practice to appreciate. We have tended to spend time imparting a great deal of information and may have, at times, been surprised and disappointed at the result. The information is generally designed to provide a background and explanation to the person's disorder, in order to encourage them to carry out an exercise programme or modify their lifestyle or posture in some way. However, the key is not to give too much information. The person is likely to remember the first or the last piece of information they are given; most of the rest will be forgotten, or may never even have been processed.

It is essential to find out what the person would like to know. They should be given only strictly relevant information, and it should not be thrust upon them. It is likely to be much more useful to provide people with a small piece of information at each visit rather than a large amount of information at one visit.

Supplementary information to complement clinician advice, that can be referred to, was shown to be a useful adjunct in the UK BEAM trial for low back pain and led to the development of the 'Back Book'. The principles have been ultilized and transferred for peripheral joints of the hip and knee (Klaber Moffett et al. 1999; Roland et al. 1996; Williams et al. 2009).

> Knowledge, if it does not determine action, is dead to us. (Plotinus, Roman philosopher, 205–270 CE)

People learn better if they take an active role in seeking information. For this reason, techniques such as motivational interviewing may be useful, where a change in behaviour would be desirable but may be difficult to achieve.

Labels, explanations, and the meaning of words

Both in an individual situation and in a group situation (such as a 'Back School'), explanations about the anatomy, biomechanics, and pathology can be provided in a simplified form. Great care and consideration needs to go into this process. Words may often be interpreted in a way that was not intended (Cameron and Leventhal 2003; Horne 1999; Williams 2009). People are very keen to have a label to attach to their condition, so that they can tell their neighbour what is wrong with them. They will then behave in a way that seems to fit the label, and the recovery rate may therefore hinge on the patient's understanding of their problem.

Radiographs

These are very frequently taken unnecessarily, but people who believe that a radiograph would show exactly what is wrong with them will be very keen to have one. It is therefore important for the practitioner to explain the limited usefulness of radiography. The clinical guidelines produced by the Royal College of General Practitioners on the management of low back pain recommend that radiographs should not be routinely taken unless there is a specific indication (Waddell et al. 1996), and this is consistent with the recommendations of the Royal College of Radiologists (Chisholm 1991). In fact, it has been estimated that 19 lives per year are sacrificed to the effects of unnecessary radiation. Many people are unaware that lumbar spine radiographs involve 120 times more radiation than chest radiographs. Less dramatically, radiography may have negative effects because the individual may understand that the radiograph shows they have a 'degenerative spine' and infer from this that their spine is nearly 'worn out'. The message can be a powerful and very negative one if the corollary is understood as 'I had better save my back and not do too much physical activity or exercise in case I damage it further'.

Compliance or concordance?

The term 'compliance' is an unfortunate one, implying that the health professional is in a superior position, as the expert, and the patient is the recipient. It implies an unfortunate adult–child relationship rather than the adult–adult one which is desirable if the person is to not to become dependent on the health professional. The word 'patient' itself implies helplessness and long suffering and is therefore a very unfortunate term, for which a more positive one should be substituted wherever possible.

The interaction of the relationship between the health professional and the individual is very important in successful treatment outcomes (Mead and Bower 2000; Bower et al. 2003; Butler 2012; Klaber Moffett and Richardson 1997; Mead and Bower 2002; O'Sullivan 2012). The term 'adherence' or 'concordance' is more consistent with a relationship based on an equal partnership. It is then acknowledged that the health professional is an expert in one respect but the patient is the expert relating to their own particular condition and is the only person who knows what it feels like. Someone with a failed knee replacement that needs to be revised and is currently causing excessive swelling, loss of range of movement, and pain, may not welcome the well-meaning physiotherapist saying, 'I know just how it feels'. In one particular case, the response to this was direct and educational: 'You do *not* know how it feels'. A more appropriate way of expressing empathy might have been to say, 'It must be really very unpleasant/difficult for you'.

Having decided what to tell the patient, the problem in the clinician's mind remains 'how am I going to get them to do it?'. It is known, from the literature on compliance with taking drugs, that often less than 50% of the tablets prescribed are taken. This could be partly because many people do not like taking drugs. On the other hand, it is often much easier to swallow a pill than to follow an exercise programme. In a study of exercise compliance, it was found that providing written information as well as oral information increased compliance from 33% to 77%. Many other studies have shown the importance of providing written material (Ley 1988).

A number of other factors are likely to influence whether a person carries out an exercise programme and maintains it over a longer period of time: the latter is much less likely. 'Concordance' implies that a programme has been discussed and negotiated with the full involvement of the individual, so its likelihood of successful uptake and maintenance is much greater. As far as longer-term maintenance is concerned, ownership of the programme is important. It is also more likely to be tailored to the needs of the individual as it has been agreed through discussion and is therefore more likely to be acceptable and realistic for that person.

Motivational interviewing

The basis of this counselling technique, which has been developed for use by busy doctors during short (5–15-minute) consultations, is that the interview is not dominated by the clinician but rather appears to be led by the patient. Motivational interviewing was originally developed in the field of addiction, for helping people deal

Box 49.1 An example of motivational interviewing

You ask 'On a scale of 0–10, how ready would you say you are to change?'

If the person says 3, then you ask 'Why 3 and not 0?'

He may say 'Because I know that going for a swim three times a week, like I used to, would help my shoulder problem.'

You say 'So why 3 and not 10?'

He then replies 'Well, it's 3 and not 10 because I couldn't have the car when I would like to go swimming immediately after work.'

Then you would explore what other options there might be.

with ambivalence about behaviour change (Rollnick et al. 1992). It is based on the premise that many people are not ready to change when they consult a healthcare professional. It can be applied to educational messages such as those concerning physical activity and exercise. The technique is to ask the individual about their readiness to change (or carry out a particular change in lifestyle) (see Box 49.1).

If the individual is not ready to change at present, it may be most sensible for the clinician and patient to openly accept this. Through this non-judgemental discussion, the door is left open for the person to return when they feel ready to change. *Confidence of success*, which is another key concept to successful adherence in making lifestyle changes, is also explored in a similar way, asking them how confident they are that they could succeed in bringing that change about, or taking up a new activity and sticking with it.

Information-giving is a central part of the motivational interviewing technique, but is patient-centred and maximizes the freedom of choice for the individual. It avoids a judgemental or authoritarian approach. It can also be more satisfying for the practitioner who does not need to feel he has failed if the person is not able to take on the suggested advice at present. It is often argued that the technique is too time-consuming but, in fact, time can be saved as soon as the practitioner accepts that not all patients will be receptive to advice all the time.

Home exercise programmes for musculoskeletal disorders

Home programmes form an essential part of most patient education and often include exercises (Critchley et al. 2007; Hurley et al. 2007, 2012; Jessop et al. 2014; Klaber Moffett 1989; Williams et al. 2009) These need to be carefully taught: each exercise should be demonstrated, and then tried out with guidance from the practitioner. The purpose of each exercise should be clearly explained, and the programme should be written down and illustrated.

A home programme should be developed by the practitioner together with the patient and will be based on certain guiding principles such as:

(1) setting specific and realistic goals

(2) working in a disciplined way, gradually increasing the amount of exercise or activity and its grade of difficulty

(3) using positive support systems to provide encouragement and feedback.

Setting realistic goals

The first task is to find out what it is that the individual would like to achieve. Specific and realistic goals need to be set. These should also be fulfilling, and if possible enjoyable, for the person who needs to carry them out. Once the goals (not more than three) have been arrived at, they need to be written down. It is important also to write down *when* the activity will be carried out, i.e. how many times a week or times a day, and for *how long, how far*, etc.

The task—say, doing the shopping—may need to be broken down into components, looking at what is required in order to carry out that activity. This may include, for example, walking to the bus stop, waiting at the bus stop, getting on to the bus, walking to the shops and round the shops, carrying shopping, and so on. Similarly, other activities, such as playing a round of golf, can be broken down into smaller components that the person can be guided to achieve gradually, over a period of several weeks or months.

With any exercise or activity, it is essential to start at a very low baseline that is certain to be manageable, in order to avoid failure, which can be detrimental. Clear quotas of gradually increasing activity levels are then set. The person should keep careful records, noting exactly what they have achieved, each day and each week. It is helpful if the activity can be easily measured in distance and/or time, so that even small improvements can be recognized. Immediate feedback is a very important factor in encouraging and motivating an individual to continue with an activity.

Graded activity

Any new exercise or activity needs to be introduced in a graded fashion (see Box 49.2). Advice needs to be quite carefully thought through, and details need to be carefully explained in order to avoid confusion.. The same principles of graded activity can be applied to gardening, tennis, walking, running, and even housework. All these activities need to be built up in a stepwise fashion, while successively spreading the load and effort to different parts of the body and different areas of soft tissue (muscle and its associated tissue as well as ligaments) and bone and cartilage. Walking on hard, regular surfaces such as pavements repetitively loads the same part of the joint, and can be uncomfortable. Experience shows that joints may more happily tolerate walking longer distances in the countryside than on pavements.

Box 49.2 Introducing exercise gradually

A woman tells her physiotherapist that she was advised to go swimming, but found it made her neck and back pain worse. On closer questioning, it turns out that she had attempted to do 15 lengths of the pool, although she had not done any swimming for several years. When asked what stroke she swam, she explained that she could only do breast stroke and did not like to get her hair wet, so swam with her head and trunk held in extreme extension. Advice to alternate different strokes, or to devise a simple programme that includes different positions, is important. This woman can be advised to intersperse her breast stroke with walking in chest-deep water and floating on her back. She may be encouraged to join classes, which are now widely available for adults of all levels of ability, to improve her swimming technique.

Use of positive support systems to provide rewards

Long-term adherence with exercise is dependent on perceived benefits and rewards. Positive feedback and a sense of self-efficacy are predictors of outcome (Bandura 1982; Butler 2012; Dolce 1987; Dolce et al. 1986; Jensen et al. 1991; Kores et al. 1990; O'Leary 1985; Williams 2009).

Social support from family or friends can help a great deal. Without the possibility of encouragement and rewards for the effort, success with a home programme is less likely. Even worse than lack of support is a situation that actually discourages the individual from carrying out their home programme. For example, if the person perceives that the family is laughing at their efforts, the chances of adherence are very slim. This is a reason why it may be helpful to involve the partner in the self-management programme; to get their support in encouraging the patient. This is especially important for long-term adherence.

Patient education for an acute musculoskeletal problem

Rest

Rest may be necessary because of pain or a very extensive injury or surgical wound, but very rarely for more than 24 hours. For upper and lower limb extremities, the advice to apply ice, compression, and elevation is still sensible. For the back, in very severe cases, as much as 3 days' bed rest may be needed, but generally it is better to allow as much movement as the individual can tolerate. For the neck, a collar may be worn to provide the person with a feeling of protection, but not for more than a day or two, and only if the pain is very acute. European evidence-based guidelines advise against prescribing rest (van Tulder et al. 2006).

Ice

In the presence of heated or inflamed tissue, ice may be more useful than heat. Bleakley et al. (2004), in a systematic review of randomized controlled trials (RCTs), showed marginal evidence that ice plus exercise is more effective than exercise alone. The individual may wish to purchase an ice pack from a local sportshop or pharmacy, which can be kept in the freezer between uses. Instructions for its safe use need to be given: applying an ice pack directly to the skin can easily cause a burn, but this can be avoided by placing the ice pack in a wet towel. As many experienced clinicians, sportspeople, and others will know, the application of ice can have quite a dramatic effect; for example, in reducing an Achilles tendon swelling. It is more likely to be effective if the painful and inflamed tissue is fairly superficial.

In some instances, ice may be a good substitute for anti-inflammatories, particularly for people who tend to suffer from the common side-effects of these drugs. It is worth discussing this point with the individual, in order to check that they have not developed gastrointestinal symptoms. They may not be aware why they had developed pains in this region, possibly together with loss of appetite. It is does not appear to be common knowledge that NSAIDs, if taken over a long period of time, can cause bleeding and gastrointestinal ulcers in more vulnerable people (Rodriguez and Jick 1994). It should never be taken for granted that the GP has found the time to discuss these side-effects.

Heat

Applying heat, in the form of a hot shower, has some advantages over soaking in a bath, since the heat can be directed onto the painful area while the person can move, rather than being restrained in a fixed and possibly awkward position in the bath tub. Another method is to apply heat via a small towel soaked in hand-hot water, wrung out, and placed over the painful area. It should be placed directly in contact with the skin with a dry towel over it, to prevent the loss of heat being too rapid. Some people prefer to use a hot-water bottle, although this is not so malleable. Superficial heating is often more effective than no heating. Heat may often be used as a substitute for painkillers and should be used before stretching exercises.

Stretching exercises

Stretching exercises are an important part of the rapid recovery process and need to be taught very carefully. Most people carry out their stretches too quickly, as most of us are far too impatient! Each stretch should be held for at least 15 seconds and repeated three times. A cold muscle should not be stretched; warm tissue has more elastic properties and is less likely to be injured. There are several different methods of stretching each muscle group in the body, but whichever method is chosen, it is important to do it correctly. The individual needs to be shown exactly how to do it, pointing out common errors such as turning the foot out when carrying out a calf muscle stretch instead of pointing the toes straight ahead (Herbert and Gabriel 2002). They should also be provided with diagrams and detailed instructions of when and how often to carry out the exercises. A well-illustrated book on the subject can be very useful (Anderson 1981).

Patient education and self care: posture and ergonomic advice

Posture

A great deal of emphasis is often put on this aspect of patient education, without considering how effective it is likely to be. Ergonomic advice on its own may not be sufficient, as psychosocial aspects may be more important (Burton et al. 1997; Liddle et al. 2007).

It is difficult to change an individual's habitual posture, and attempts to do so may even be counterproductive. Successful techniques use training methods which involve repeating movements and positions over and over again, over a long period of time, with guidance and encouragement. Fast results are not expected but high levels of motivation, patience, and persistence are necessary. One such technique is the Alexander technique, which can be used to improve the posture and use of the spine and rest of the body. Oriental teachings, such as yoga and tai chi, can also train better posture. A clinician attempting to correct a poor posture in the course of a conventional consultation is less likely to succeed in making changes to the habitual stance of the individual.

It is often forgotten that posture is likely to be influenced by other factors:

- *Emotional status*: If a person is unhappy or insecure, they may tend to fold their arms and stoop, whereas a happy confident person is more likely to be upright and maintain a more relaxed posture. The clinician treating a person with a musculoskeletal disorder should take this into account. It is important to be sensitive to body language. It may be counterproductive to tell a person who is depressed that their posture is bad and that they should stand up straighter; at the least, it may just be a waste of time.

- *Genetics*: Observation shows us that members of some families tend to have a very hollow lumbar spine, with a marked forward incline of the pelvis. Others have a much more flat lumbar spine. This is at least, in part, due to tight hamstrings. Teaching the person to do effective hamstring stretching exercises may be the key to helping them.
- ***Habits***: Posture is habitual, and training plays an important role if maintained over a long enough period of time. Ballet dancers, army personnel, and Alexander technique teachers are examples of people who can be recognized by their 'good' posture, which is learned over many years.

Strengthening and training specific muscle groups

Theoretically, it should be possible to improve posture by strengthening particular muscles that help to maintain the body in a state of equilibrium. Some specific techniques put a great deal of emphasis on training individual muscles, such as the transversus, abdominus, and multifidus muscles, which are deep segmental muscles of the trunk and are considered to act as trunk stabilizers (Hides et al. 1995, 1996; Jull and Richardson 1994). Pilates, which is currently very popular, aims to teach control of pelvic, abdominal, and trunk muscles by 'zipping and tucking' the pelvic area in order to maintain a neutral position of the pelvis. Data suggests that pilates, used as a specific core stability exercise incorporating functional movements, can improve non-specific chronic low back pain (LBP) in an active population compared to no intervention. In addition, pilates can improve general health, pain level, sports functioning, flexibility, and proprioception in individuals with LBP (Gladwell et al. 2006).

The workplace

It is important that the practitioner should explore the patient's work circumstances, both physical and psychosocial. For those in paid employment, recent guidance produced by the Faculty of Occupational Medicine could be useful (Carter and Birrell 2000; Waddell and Burton 2000). Liaison with the workplace (the occupational health department or the supervisor) can make a huge difference in helping the person to get back to work.

Office environment

It may be possible, through simple advice, to improve, for example, the working position of an individual who spends their whole day at a desk. A few very basic rules are worth considering. Ideally, it is helpful to observe the individual in their working situation, in order to be able to make specific recommendations. One visit to the workplace may be worth half a dozen sessions in a clinic. If a visit is not possible, a detailed discussion is necessary to find out whether there could be some simple adaptation of the working environment. Unless the changes are very small, it will be necessary to involve the supervisor or human resources department. UK health and safety at work legislation makes it the duty of the employer to respond to reasonable requests for new equipment to make the employee more comfortable. It is now accepted by most employers that this is actually to their advantage, as it may avoid the person having to take time off sick. They should appreciate that buying a new chair for a sedentary worker could represent a cost saving if the alternative is for that employee to be off work for 6 months.

Seating at work

Making sure that the chair is at a suitable height relative to the desk and the computer is a basic necessity that is sometimes overlooked. Someone who is shorter or taller than average is more likely to have problems achieving a good position. A taller person may require the desk to be raised.

Mandal (1985), in an interesting little book on seating, analyses different postures in children and adults seated in a variety of different chairs. He argues that the traditional furniture found in schools and offices does not meet the requirements of most people. Rather, he has found most people would benefit from higher chairs that tilt forward. He emphasizes that lumbar supports, when provided, are rarely used and are not a realistic requirement. Furthermore, he recommends the use of a tilting chair that moves with the person. My personal experience has been that the use of such an office chair (which tilts forward and backwards through about 15°) immediately reduced longstanding backache and referred pain in the hip area. It has continued to be comfortable over a period of 5 years—a fact emphasized by the discomfort I feel when sitting in long meetings in ordinary chairs. There has been considerable interest in 'alternative seating' such as kneeling chairs, which originated from Scandinavia. Some people find these useful, but few people are comfortable on them for long periods. The design was thought to reduce stress on the spine because the angle between the thighs and the trunk is greater than 90°, making it easier to maintain a lordosis. More recent research (Althoff et al. 1992) does not support this theory.

Physiotherapists and doctors have used findings based on the work of Nachemson (1960) to advise patients that standing puts less strain on the spine than sitting. They also have advised people to sit up straight. However, recent research challenges these principles (Althoff et al. 1992; Wilke et al. 1999). Althoff and colleagues used a stadiometer to measure stature for assessing spinal loading. These researchers validated a technique previously developed by Eklund and Corlett (1984). The research by Althoff is very interesting as it appears to contradict some of the widely accepted findings published by Nachemson (1960) four decades ago. Nachemson inserted a needle in the L3/4 disc space and measured intradiscal pressure in different postures. Classically, he reported that the intradiscal pressure was 30% greater in unsupported sitting than in standing. Althoff's more recent work refutes this and, furthermore, two other recent studies support these findings (Rohlmann et al. 1995; Wilke et al. 1999). Wilke and colleagues used a more refined method of measuring intradiscal pressure by surgical implantation (see Figure 49.1). The latest research continues to support the idea that pressure on the spine is reduced by keeping the load closer to the body and bending the knees rather than the back.

It is commonly recommended, by physiotherapists and other practitioners, that a good posture of the spine requires a lordosis to be maintained all the time (McKenzie 1981). This is not easy to do when sitting. However, a relaxed sitting posture has been shown to put less pressure on the disc than sitting upright (Baird et al. 2000; Wilke et al. 1999). This is probably related to muscle tension. The most important advice is probably to avoid maintaining any fixed posture for longer than necessary. The body, and especially the spine, likes movement, and this needs to be encouraged.

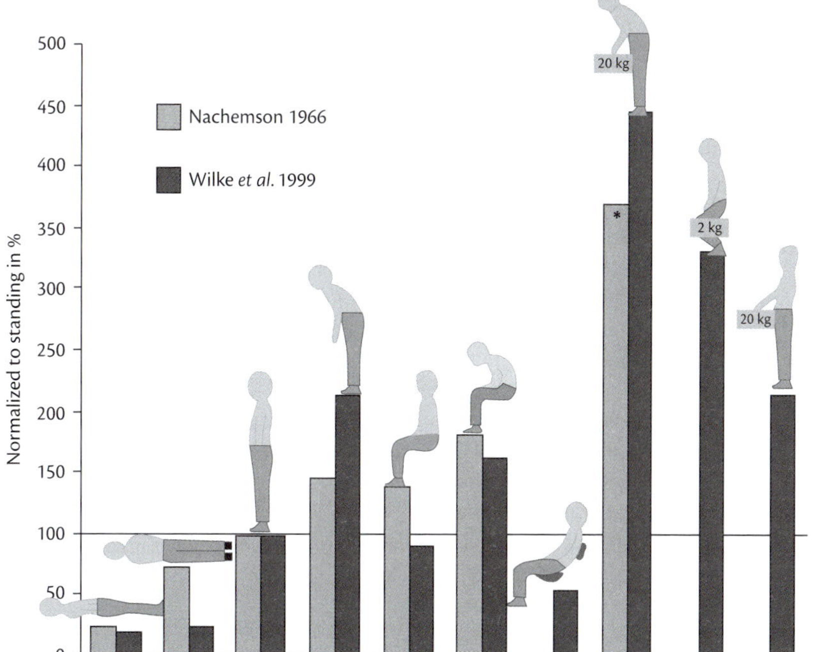

Figure 49.1 Effect of body position on intradiscal pressure.
Nachemson (1966) and Wilke (1999).

For many people, physical activity is becoming less and less a part of their lives. Particularly in later life, people who are total 'couch potatoes' may have to pay the price of being much less able-bodied, overweight, and generally more at risk of most life-threatening conditions. As a greater proportion of desk-based jobs are seated and there is more passive leisure time, spent in a prolonged seated position, there should be a greater emphasis on seating (Baird et al. 2000).

Manual handling

There is evidence that heavy and frequent lifting of loads in excess of 50 kg can lead to a reduction in overall disc height in the entire lumbar spine (Brinckmann et al. 1998). Workers lifting in cramped conditions or on uneven ground are also at risk. Further, research on miners has shown that whole-body vibration can result in damage to the discs.

The UK Health and Safety Executive guidance on regulations for manual handling does not set specific requirements such as weight limits (HSE 1992). It simply advocates that hazardous manual handling should be avoided where possible. It recommends the threshold limits of weights and related manoeuvres which, if exceeded, require individual assessments. These depend not only on the weight of the object but also the height and distance from the body. Physiotherapists and doctors have traditionally recommended that people always lift with a straight back and bent knees and, theoretically, this can reduce pressure on the discs. However, workers often find this technique is not feasible. Indeed, for many women and older people of both genders, the 'squat' technique is impossible, as it requires considerable strength in the quadriceps muscle to raise the weight of the body as well as of the external load. It requires good flexibility of the ankles, knees, and hips. Finally, it requires skill, together with good balance and coordination. A recent review of the literature has examined the data on spinal compression, bending moments, net moments, and shear forces during 'stoop' lifting and 'squat' lifting (van Dieen et al. 1999). These authors confirm that the biomechanical literature does not support recommending the use of the squat lift which did not reduce the net moments and compression forces—the main problem being that the load is usually some distance from the body. The actual energy expenditure and the perceived exertion is greater for the squat lift (Welbergen et al. 1991). In any case, this technique is unlikely to be complied with.

Group education programmes for musculoskeletal problems

Back schools

A back school is a popular method of providing group education for people with back pain. It was first described by a physiotherapist in Sweden (Zachrisson-Forsell 1980) and is popular with physiotherapists throughout the Western world. Some back schools, particularly in the US and Scandinavia, are multidisciplinary in their approach; the programme is delivered by a physiotherapist, an occupational therapist, a psychologist, a nurse, and a doctor. In the UK, back schools are usually run by physiotherapists. They were originally set up and evaluated in a Volvo factory, and found to be effective (Berquist-Ullman and Larsson 1977). Since then, a number of other trials have been conducted, with varied findings, and these have been evaluated in several systematic reviews of the literature on back schools (Cohen et al. 1994; Keijsers et al. 1991; Koes et al. 1994; Linton and Kamwendo 1987).

The evidence for their effectiveness is unclear. This is not too surprising, as back schools vary considerably; their success will depend on both the contents and the method of delivery (Klaber Moffett 1989; Nordin 1995; Nordin et al. 1992). Back schools which are based in the occupational setting are more likely to be effective. This could be because the advice is likely to be seen to be more relevant to the individual's needs in the workplace, and also because the employers are seen to be interested and involved in the workers' problems. Having a supervisor or employer who care appears to be an important variable in the equation.

A back school is more likely to be successful if it includes an exercise programme encouraging normal activity and fitness (Frost et al. 1995, 1998). Just telling people to become more active and exercise more may not be sufficient. Trying to change people's attitudes and behaviour is difficult, especially in the longer term. Knowledge on its own does not necessarily bring about a change in attitudes or behaviour (Mazzuca 1982). Young people often know about the serious health risks associated with smoking, but this does not stop them doing it. Similarly, people with back pain may know that sitting in front of a computer all day and then slumping onto a sofa to watch television may not help their back problem, but they often continue to do so. Conversely, a new behaviour can influence attitudes. Experience shows that if people carry out exercises at a class and find—to their surprise—that the exercises, although they may hurt a bit at the time, do not make the back pain worse, their attitude and beliefs may be radically altered. They may re-evaluate their problem and realize that they can function normally again, and no longer think of themselves as a person with a serious problem. Long-term adherence, in particular, needs to be addressed when setting up a programme.

Back to fitness programmes

Over the past 15 years, exercise programmes for people with back pain have been developed which are an important substitute or adjunct to back schools. They aim to help participants overcome the fear of damaging their spine by using cognitive-behavioural principles to restore confidence in using the back normally. Research on these programmes, which are now referred to as 'back to fitness programmes', is promising. Maintenance of beneficial effects of the exercise classes has been demonstrated 1 year and even 2 years later (Frost et al. 1995, 1998; Klaber Moffett et al. 1999). The programme is led by physiotherapists and the manual for setting it up has been published (Klaber Moffett and Frost 2000).

Other forms of group education

Considerable clinical experience has now been documented showing the value of self-management programmes for back pain, chronic arthritis, and other chronic diseases, particularly knee and hip, in recent years. The development of these programmes and their evaluation is described in a 12-year case study (Lorig and Gonzalez 1992). The key to the success of the programmes seems to be that they are patient-centred. Indeed, all patient education needs to be patient-centred so that individuals can receive the advice and information that they require rather than the information the health professional perceives they require.

This appears to be a very promising area for further research and development, particularly as demands for healthcare continue to increase. It could also be a way of reducing the gap between the public's expectations of health and healthcare and what is actually possible in reality (Coulter 2000; Klaber Moffett and Frost 2000).

The work of Klaber Moffett and Frost has been transferred to peripheral joints and principles have been applied to the knee and hip (Critchley et al. 2007; Hurley et al. 2007, 2012; Jessop et al. 2014; Williams et al. 2009).

The multidisciplinary and cross-continent team looking at managing chronic knee pain has also included cost effectiveness in their publications, an area of increasing focus in recent years (Critchley et al. 2007; Hurley et al. 2007, 2012; Jessop et al. 2014).

Pain and discomfort at night or on rising: positioning at night

Personal experience, over many years, has shown that providing relevant advice about placing pillows to provide suitable support during the night can make a big difference to a person's comfort and dramatically reduce pain. The individual may be suffering disturbed and uncomfortable nights, with a lot of stiffness or pain on awakening. This can often be reduced if the following tips are carefully conveyed and the principle of keeping the joints in neutral positions is understood.

Neck pain

Many acute neck problems result from sleeping in an awkward position such as:

(1) sleeping with the head in extreme flexion (too many pillows)

(2) sleeping on the side with too few pillows to support the head

(3) worst of all, sleeping face down with a pillow which puts the head in an extreme position of extension and rotation.

Different possibilities will suit different people, and the following may be suggested:

- If using a feather pillow, tie it in the middle to make a 'butterfly' pillow. Use the 'wings' of the pillow to support the head and prevent it rolling into an awkward position.
- Explain the principle that pillows can be used to maintain a comfortable position and avoid putting structures into a stretched or stressed position. If this happens, the person will either be woken up by discomfort or find that the pain may be bad in the morning.

Sleeping prone—face down

Some people say they cannot get to sleep unless they sleep face down. This seems to be one of the commonest causes of neck pain, as the head is forced into rotation. Using pillows under the head makes it worse, as the head is then also forced into extension. These are positions that most people's cervical spines cannot tolerate, especially in middle age.

Careful placing of two pillows can reduce the ill-effects of sleeping prone. One is placed lengthways under the person's torso. The other is under the head, but mostly under the ear, allowing the nose to point down into the mattress. This provides two important advantages: the neck is only slightly rotated, and the person can breathe easily.

Foam pillows

These are better for anyone who suspects they may be allergic to feathers. It is important that they are put in the correct place, and are of the right proportion to suit the individual. Once the principle of support is understood, the person should be able to find out what suits them best.

Pillows are available in various shapes, but the principle is always the same—the purpose of the pillow is to support the neck and head in a neutral position while maintaining a cervical lordosis. They can be purchased as a large foam roll which is placed under the neck. A thin pillow may be used to support the head.

Shoulder disorders, e.g. adhesive capulitis, 'frozen shoulder', or rotator cuff syndrome

These conditions can be very painful, especially at night-time, causing distress and all the problems associated with a sleep deficit. Advice about placing pillows can be very useful. The aim is mainly to avoid the arm falling backwards into extension in the night and to maintain it in a neutral position. The individual can be advised to use a substantial pillow under the arm, with the arm flexed at the elbow to 90° and slightly flexed at the shoulder. It can be helpful to put the arm inside the pillowcase so that a restless sleeper will still maintain the support of the pillow even when moving around in the night. Advice on exercise, distraction techniques, relative rest, and management (Atkins et al. 2010; Neviaser and Hannaji 2011) should be given.

Lower limb disorders

Painful hips or knees can similarly be supported on a pillow to maintain the joints in a neutral position. A pillow between the legs can usefully support the upper leg when the individual mostly sleeps on their side. The thickness of the pillow is important, and the individual should be encouraged to experiment with different-sized pillows.

A painful foot may not be able to tolerate any weight of bedclothes. A cradle can be improvised at home using a cardboard box with two sides cut out and placed over the feet under the bedclothes. Personal experience of working on orthopaedic wards has shown that nurses are often unhappy for a patient to use pillows under the leg, possibly because of a fear of putting extra pressure on the leg and especially the calf. This does not seem relevant for anyone who is moving around during the day.

Relaxation

The inclusion of relaxation techniques can improve well-being and body awareness. The Laura Mitchell method of physiological relaxation is a personal favourite. The reader is directed to *Relaxation; a physiotherapist's perspective* (Clough 2012).

Back pain

If sleep is disturbed by back pain, positioning needs to be considered. The mattress might need changing to provide suitable support to the spine. A heavier person needs a firmer mattress; couples may each require mattresses of different densities. If one mattress is shared in a double bed, an adaptation can be made by removing some of the slats under the mattress of the lighter partner. This will have a similar effect to lying on a softer mattress. It is not essential to spend large sums of money on new mattresses or beds. An orthopaedic bed is certain to be very expensive, but is not certain to bring relief of pain and a good night's sleep. Better shops will encourage beds and mattresses to be tried out in the shop. They will also allow them to be loaned out for a couple of nights for a trial.

Some people with back pain find that a roll or thin pillow under the waist is useful, especially for side-lying positions. A larger pillow will be needed for women if the hips are much wider than the waist, in order to maintain the spine in a neutral position. A large pillow may also be needed under the upper leg, to avoid it dragging on the lumbar spine and causing discomfort.

Early return to activity after a musculoskeletal disorder

Management guidelines emphasize the central role of exercise (National Collaboration Centre for Chronic Conditions 2008; Roddy et al. 2005; Royal College of Physicians 2008). However, the level of physical activity in older adults in the UK is low, as identified by the NHS (2006). An early return to activity is reduced further by pain-related fear of movement in those with osteoarthritis (Hendry et al. 2006; Heuts et al. 2004) There is a culturally conditioned response to pain that encourages rest. How can primary care clinicians be helped to encourage more patients to increase their physical activity, within a 10-minute consultation? One approach is to refer patients to exercise prescription schemes; however, 17 sedentary people need to be referred for one to become moderately active (Williams et al. 2007). Also, referral by primary care clinicians to these schemes is extremely variable.

In aiming to help patients take responsibility and cope with acute back pain, the Royal College of General Practitioners in the UK, in conjunction with the Department of Health, have produced a booklet called *The back book* (Roland et al. 1996). It is written by a multidisciplinary group of back pain researchers and contains very simple messages. Based on the research evidence for the management of back pain and linked with UK clinical guidelines (Royal College of General Practitioners 1996), it is designed to be given to patients by GPs and therapists. It has been carefully designed to be easily read and accessible to most of the population. It encourages positive attitudes, and emphasizes the benefits of an early return to activity. Preliminary surveys of users of this booklet show that they understand the messages and that it can result in a positive shift in attitudes towards back pain (Burton et al. 1996). Also, it has been shown in a RCT that it can alter patients' knowledge and beliefs about back pain (Burton et al. 1999). It is likely to be most effective if it is used as a back-up to oral advice on back care encouraging a return to physical activity. The booklet also provides advice on how to cope with an acute attack of back pain.

The advice to return to normal activities is probably relevant for conditions other than back pain, including, for example, ankle sprains, knee problems, and shoulder problems. However, of course, the clinician will need to provide individual advice depending on the particular condition and the patient's situation. It is important for the clinician to bear in mind that the reported pain is only one factor in the equation predicting outcome. Many other factors are influential, including psychosocial factors such as attitudes and beliefs, and the patient's circumstances and their environment (Burton et al. 1994; Kovacs et al. 2007; Waddell 1987).

Aiming to prevent recurrences of musculoskeletal conditions—learning to cope

It may be difficult to prevent recurrences. However, disciplined approaches to exercise, physical activity, and sport can help to cut down on recurrences. Learning to cope with recurrences is of fundamental importance. Much of this is about building self-confidence.

Longer-term maintenance is very often forgotten, but is important if one aim is to avoid repeated referrals and visits.

Conclusions about patient education and self care for musculoskeletal problems

Patient education is a key part of the management of musculoskeletal conditions. Its success will depend on how it is delivered, and this requires some thought.

Simple advice that is appropriate to the needs of the individual can make the difference between long, drawn-out periods of treatment with slow recovery, and a quick return to optimal function. One of the main advantages of effective patient education is that a sense of self-efficacy and coping will be achieved. Passive dependency can then be translated into a sense of control and acceptance of responsibility for dealing with the problem.

Acknowledgement

Thanks are due to Kim Burton, Director of the Spinal Research Unit, Huddersfield, for his helpful comments and for providing additional evidence on biomechanical issues.

References

Althoff, I., Brinckmann, P., Frobin, W., Sandover, J., Burton, K. (1992) An improved method of stature measurement for quantitative determination of spinal loading. Application to sitting postures. *Spine*, 17, 682–93.

Anderson, J. (1981). Low back pain—cause and prevention of long-term handicap (a critical review). *International Rehabiliation Medicine*, 3, 89–93.

Atkins, E., Kerr, J., Goodlad, E. (2010) *Orthopaedic medicine—a practical approach*. Elsevier, Edinburgh: Butterworth-Heineman.

Baird, A., Malyan, V., Heaton, N. (2000) Seating in the real world. In P.T. McCabe., M.A. Hanson and S.A. Robertson *Contemporary Ergonomics*, 396–400. Taylor and Francis: London.

Bandura, A. (1982) Self-efficacy mechanism in human agency. *American Psychologist*, 37(2), 122–47.

Becker, M. (1985) Patient adherence to prescribed therapies. *Medical Care*, 23, 539–55.

Berquist-Ullman, M., Larsson, U. (1977) Acute low back pain in industry. *Acta Orthopaedica Scandinavica (Suppl)*, 170, 1–117.

Bleakley, C., McDonough, S., MacAuley, D. (2004) The use of ice in the treatment of acute soft tissue injury. A systematic review of randomised controlled trials. *American Journal of Sports Med*, 32, 251–62.

Bower, P., Roland, M., Mead, N. (2003) Setting standards based on patients views on access and continuity: secondary analysis of data from the general practice assessment survey. *British Medical Journal*, 1(326), 258.

Brinckmann, P., Frobin, W., Biggemann, M., Tillotson, M., Burton, K. (1998) Quantification of overload injuries to thoracolumbar vertebrae and discs in persons exposed to heavy physical exertions or vibration at the workplace: part II. Occurrence and magnitude of overload injury in exposed cohorts. *Clinical Biomechanics*, 13(Suppl 2), 1–36.

Burton, K. (1997) Spine update. Back injury and work loss. Biomechanical and psychosocial influences. *Spine*, 22(21), 2575–80.

Burton, K., Symonds, T., Zinzen, E., et al. (1997) Is ergonomic intervention alone sufficient to limit musculoskeletal problems in nurses? *Occupational Medicine*, 47, 25–32.

Burton, A., Tillotson, K., Main, C., Hollis, S. (1994) Psychosocial predictors of outcome in acute and sub-chronic low-back trouble. *Spine*, 20, 722–8.

Burton, A., Waddell, G., Burtt, R., Blair, M. (1996) Patient education material in the management of low back pain in primary care. *Bulletin of Hospitals for Joint Diseases*, 55(3), 138–41.

Burton, A. K., Waddell, G., Tillotson, K. M., Summerton, N. (1999) Information and advice to patients with back pain can have a positive effect. A randomized controlled trial of a novel educational booklet in primary care. *Spine*, 24(23), 2484–91.

Butler, D. (2012) Manual therapy in a neuroplastic world. *Journal of Science and Technology*, 42,10, A17–A21.

Cameron, L. D., Leventhal, H. (2003) *The self-regulation of health and illness behaviour*. New York: Routledge.

Carter, J., Birrell, L. (2000) *Occupational health guidelines for the management of low back pain at work—principal recommendations*. London: Faculty of Occupational Medicine.

Chisholm, R. (1991) Guidelines for radiological investigations. *British Medical Journal*, 303, 797–800.

Clough, A. (2012) Relaxation: a physiotherapist`s perspective. In: P. Clough and D. Strycharczyk, *Developing Mental Toughness. Improving performance, wellbeing and positive behaviours in others*. London: Kogan Page.

Cohen, J., Goel, V., Frank, J., Bombardier, C., Peloso Guillemin, F. (1994) Group education interventions for people with low back pain. An overview of the literature. *Spine*, 19, 1214–22.

Coulter, A. (2000) [Editorial] Promoting realistic expectations. *Health Expectations*, 3, 159–60.

Critchley, D. J. Ratcliffe, J., Noonan, S., Jones, R. H., Hurley, M. V. (2007) Effectiveness and cost-effectiveness of three types of physiotherapy used to reduce chronic low back pain disability. A pragmatic randomized trial with economic evaluation. *Spine*, 32(**14**), 1474–81.

Daltroy, L. (1993) Doctor–patient communication in rheumatological disorders. *Bailliere's Clinical Rheumatology*, 7(2), 221–39.

Daltroy, L., Katz, J., Liang, M. (1992) Doctor–patient communication and adherence to arthritis treatments. *Arthritis Care and Research*, 5, S19.

Di Blasi, Z., Kleinen, J. (2000). *Patient–practitioner interactions: a systematic review*. York: University of York.

van Dieen, J., Hoozemans, M., Toussaint, H. (1999) Stoop or squat: a review of biomechanical studies on lifting technique. *Clinical Biomechanics*, 14, 685–96.

Dolce, J. (1987) Self-efficacy and disability beliefs in behavioral treatment of pain. *Behavioural Research and Therapy*, 25, 289–99.

Dolce, J., Crocker, M., Moletierre, C., Doleys, D. (1986) Exercise quotas, anticipatory concern and self-efficacy expectations in chronic pain: a preliminary report. *Pain*, 24, 365–72.

Eklund, J., Corlett, E. (1984) Shrinkage as a measure of load on the spine. *Spine*, 9, 184–94.

Fersum, K. V., O'Sullivan, P. B., Kvale, A., Smith, A., Skouen, J. (2011) *Classification based cognitive functional therapy for the management of non-specific low back pain (NSLBP)—a randomised control trial*. Melbourne International Forum XI: Primary Care Research on Low Back Pain; March 8–15, Melbourne, Australia.

Frost, H., Klaber Moffett, J., Moser, J., Fairbank, J. (1995) Randomised controlled trial for evaluation of fitness programme for patients with chronic low back pain. *British Medical Journal*, 310, 151–4.

Frost, H., Lamb, S., Klaber Moffett, J., Fairbank, J., Moser, J. (1998) A fitness programme for patients with chronic low back pain: 2 year follow-up of a randomised controlled trial. *Pain*, 75, 273–9.

Gladwell, V., Head, S., Hagger, M., Benek, R. (2006) Does a program of pilates improve chronic LBP. *Journal of Sport Rehabilitation*, 15, 338–50.

Gulliford, M., Figueroa-Munoz, J., Morgan, M., Hughes, D., Gibson, B., Beech, R. (2002) What does access to healthcare mean? *Journal of Health Services Research & Policy*, 7, 186–188.

Hadler, N. (1987) Regional musculoskeletal diseases of the low back. Cumulative trauma versus single incident. *Clinics in Orthopaedics and Related Research*, 221, 33–41.

Hadler, N. (1997) Workers with disabling back pain. *New England Journal of Medicine*, 337(5), 341–3.

Hendry, M. A., Williams, N. H., Wilkinson, C., Markland, D., Maddison, P. (2006) Motivation to exercise in arthritis of the knee: a qualitative study in primary care patients. *Family Practice*, 23, 558–567.

Herbert, R.D., Gabriel, M. (2002) Effects of stretching before and after exercise on muscle soreness and risk of injury: systematic review. *British Medical Journal*, 31, 325.

Heuts, P. H. T. G., Vlaeyen, J. W. S., Roelofs, J. (2004) Pain-related fear and daily functioning in patients with osteoarthritis. *Pain*, 110, 228–35.

Hides, J., Richardson, C. A., et al. (1995) *Multifidus inhibition in acute low back pain: recovery is not spontaneous*. MPAA Ninth Biennial Conference Proceedings, Gold Coast, Queensland, Australia.

Hides, J., Richardson, C. A., et al. (1996). Multifidus muscle recovery is not automatic after resolution of acute, first episode low back pain. *Spine*, 21, 2763–9.

Horne, R. (1999) Patients' beliefs about treatment: the hidden determinant of treatment outcome? *Journal of Psychosomatic Research*, 47, 491–5.

Health and Safety Executive (HSE) (1992) *Manual handling operations regulations. Guidance on regulations*. Sheffield: Health and Safety Executive.

Hurley, M. V., Walsh, N. E., Mitchell, H., Nicholas, J., Patel, A. (2012) Long term outcomes and costs of an integrated rehabilitation program for chronic knee pain: a pragmatic, cluster randomized, controlled trial. *Arthritis Care & Research*, 64, 2, 238–47.

Hurley, M. V., Walsh, N. E., Mitchell, H. L., et al. (2007) Clinical effectiveness of a rehabilitation program integrating exercise, self management and active coping strategies for chronic pain: a cluster randomized trial. *Arthritis & Rheumatism (Arthritis Care & Research)*, 57(7), 1211–9.

Indahl, A., Halderson, E. H., Holm, S., et al. (1998) Five-year follow-up study of a controlled trial using light mobilisation and an informative approach to low back pain. *Spine*, 23, 2625–30.

Janz, N., Becker, M. (1984) The health belief model: a decade later. *Health Education Quarterly*, 11, 1–47.

Jensen, M., Turner, J., Romano, J. (1991) Self-efficacy and outcome expectancies: relationship to chronic pain coping strategies and adjustment. *Pain*, 44, 263–9.

Jessop, D.C., Sparks, P., Buckland, N., Harris, P.R., Churchill, S. (2014) Combining self- affirmation and implementation intentions: evidence of detrimental effects on behavioural outcomes. *Annals of Behavioural Medicine*, April, 47(2): 137–47.

Jull, G., Richardson, C. (1994) Rehabilitation of active stabilization of the lumbar spine. In: Twomey, L., Taylor, J. (eds) *Physical therapy of the low back*. Edinburgh: Churchill- Livingston. pp. 251–73.

Keijsers, J., Bouter, L., Meertens, R. (1991) Validity and comparability of studies on the effects of back schools. *Physiotherapy Theory and Practice*, 7, 177–84.

Klaber Moffett, J. (1989) Backschools. In: Roland, M., Morris, J. (eds) *Back pain. New approaches to rehabilitation and education*. Manchester: University of Manchester Press.

Klaber Moffett, J., Frost, H. (2000) Back to fitness programme. The manual for physiotherapists to set up the classes. *Physiotherapy*, 86, 295–305.

Klaber Moffett, J., Richardson, P. (1997) The influence of the physiotherapist–patient relationship on pain and disability. *Physiotherapy Theory and Practice*, 13, 89–96.

Klaber Moffett, J., Torgerson, D., Bell-Syer, S., et al. (1999) A randomised trial of exercise for primary care back pain patients: clinical outcomes, costs and preferences. *British Medical Journal*, 319, 279–83.

Koes, B., van Tulder, M., et al. (1994) The efficacy of back schools: a review of randomised clinical trials. *Journal of Clinical Epidemiology*, 47, 851–62.

Kores, R., Murphy, W., Rosenthal, T., et al. (1990) Predicting outcome of chronic pain treatment via a modified self-efficacy scale. *Behavior Research and Therapy*, 28(2), 165–9.

Kovacs F. M., Abraira V., Santos S. (2007) A comparison of two short education programs for improving low back pain related disability in the elderly: a cluster randomised controlled clinical trial. *Spine*, 32, 1053–9.

Liddle, S. D., Gracey, J. H., Baxter, D. (2007) Advice for the management of LBP; a systematic review of randomised controlled trials. *Manual Therapy*, 12, 310–27.

Leventhal, H. (1985) The role of theory in the study of adherence to treatment and doctor–patient interactions. *Medical Care*, 23, 556–63.

Leventhal, H., Cameron, L. (1987) Behavioral theories and the problem of compliance. *Patient Education and Counseling*, 10, 117–38.

Ley, P. (1988) *Communicating with patients. Improving communication, satisfaction and compliance*. London: Croom Helm.

Linton, S., Kamwendo, K. (1987) Low back schools. A critical review. *Physical Therapy*, 67(9), 1375–83.

Lorig, K. (1995) Patient education: treatment or nice extra. *British Journal of Rheumatology*, 34, 703–6.

Lorig, K., Gonzalez, V. (1992) The integration of theory with practice: a 12-year case study. *Health Education Quarterly*, 19(3), 355–68.

Mandal, A. (1985) *The seated man*. Klampenborg: Dafnia Publications.

Mazzuca, S. (1982) Does patient education in chronic disease have therapeutic value? *Journal of Chronic Disability*, 35, 521–9.

McKenzie, R. (1981) *The lumbar spine*. New Zealand: Spinal Publications.

Mead, N., Bower, P. (2000) Patient centredness: a conceptual framework and review of empirical literature. *Social Science and Medicine*, 51(7), 1087–110.

Mead, N., Bower, P. (2002) Patient centred consultations and outcomes in primary care: a review of the literature. *Patient Education and Counselling*: 48, 51–61

Melzack, R., Wall, P. (1982) *The challenge of pain*. Harmondsworth: Penguin.

Nachemson, A. (1960) Lumbar intradiscal pressure. *Acta Orthopaedica Scandinavica Suppl*, 43, 1–93.

Royal College of Physicians (2008) *National clinical guideline for the care and management of osteoarthritis in adults*. London: Royal College of Physicians.

National Health Service (NHS) (2006) *Health survey for England 2006 latest trends*. Available at: www.hscic.gov.uk/pubs/hse06trends

National Collaboration Centre for Chronic Conditions (2008) Available at: www.nice.org.uk/guidance/cg79/documents

Neviaser, T. J., Hannaji, J. A. (2011) Adhesive capsulitis. *Journal of the American Academy of Orthopedic Surgeons*, 19(9), 536–42.

Nordin, M. (1995) Back pain: lessons from patient education. *Patient Education and Counseling*, 27, 67–70.

Nordin, M., Cedraschi, C., et al. (1992). Back schools in prevention of chronicity. *Clinical Rheumatology*, 6, 685–703.

O'Leary, A. (1985) Self-efficacy and health. *Behavior Research and Therapy*, 23(4), 437–51.

O`Sullivan P. (2012) A classification-based cognitive functional approach for the management of low back pain. *Journal of Science and Technology*, 42(10), A17–A21.

Pennebaker, J. (1982) *The psychology of physical symptoms*. New York: Springer-Verlag.

Pennebaker, J. (1984) Accuracy of symptom perception. In: Baum, A., Tayler, S., Singer, J. (eds). *Handbook of psychology and health*. New Jersey: Lawrence Erlbaum Associates.

Peters, T. J., Sanders, C., Dieppe, P., Donovan, J (2005) Factors associated with change in pain and disability over time: a community-based prospective observational study of hip and knee osteoarthritis. *British Journal of General Practice*, 55, 205–11.

Roddy, E., Zhang, W., Doherty, M., et al. (2005) Evidence based recommendations for the role of exercise in the management of osteoarthritis of the hip or knee—the MOVE consensus. *Rheumatology*, 44, 67–73.

Rodriguez, L., Jick, H. (1994) Risk of upper gastrointestinal bleeding and perforation associated with individual non-steroidal anti-inflammatory drugs. *Lancet*, 343, 769–72.

Rohlmann, A., Bergmann, G., Graichen, F., Weber, U. (1995) In vivo measurement of implant loads in a patient with a fractured vertebral body. *European Spine Journal*, 4, 347–53.

Roland, M., Waddell, G., Klaber Moffett, J., Burton, K., Main, C., Cantrell, E. (1996) *The back book*. London: The Stationery Office.

Rollnick, S., Heather, N., Bell, A. (1992) Negotiating behaviour change in medical settings: the development of brief motivational interviewing. *Journal of Mental Health*, 1, 25–37.

Roter, D., Hall, J., Katz, N. (1987) Relations between physicians' behaviour and analogue patients' satisfaction recall and impressions. *Medical Care*, 25, 437–51.

Royal College of General Practitioners (1996) *Clinical guidelines for the management of low back pain*. London: Royal College of General Practitioners.

Smith, D., Heckemeyer, C., Kratt, P., Mason, D. (1997) Motivational interviewing to improve adherence to a behavioural weight-control program for older obese women with NIDDM. *Diabetes Care*, 20(1), 52–4.

Street, R. (1992) Analyzing communication in medical consultations: do behavioural measures correspond to patients perceptions? *Medical Care*, 30, 976–88.

van Tulder, M., Becker, A., Bekkering, T., Breen, A., et al. (2006) European guidelines for the management of acute non-specific low back pain in primary care. *European Spine Journal*, 15(Suppl.2), S169–91.

Vlaeyen, J., Linton, S. (2000) Fear-avoidance and its consequences in chronic musculosketal pain: a state of the art. *Pain*, 85, 317–32.

Waddell, G. (1987) A new clinical model for the treatment of low back pain. *Spine*, 12(7), 632–44.

Waddell, G. (1998) *The back pain revolution*. Edinburgh: Churchill Livingstone.

Waddell, G., Burton, K. (2000) *Occupational health guidelines for the management of low back pain at work—leaflet for practitioners*. London: Faculty of Occupational Medicine.

Waddell, G., Feder, G., McIntosh, A., Lewis, M., Hutchinson, A. (1996) *Low back pain evidence review*. London: Royal College of General Practitioners.

Welbergen, E., Kemper, H., Knibbe, J., Toussaint, H., Clijssen, L. (1991) Efficiency and effectiveness of stoop and squat lifting at different techniques. *Ergonomics*, 34, 613–24.

Wilke, H., Neef, P., Caimi, M., Hoogland, T., Claes, L. (1999) New in vivo measurement of pressures in the intervertebral disc in daily life. *Spine*, 24, 755–62.

Williams, N. H. (2009) Words that harm. Words that heal. *International Musculoskeletal Medicine*, 31(3), 99–100.

Williams, N. H., Amoakwa, E., Burton, K. (2009) *The hip and knee book: helping you cope with osteoarthritis*. London: TSO.

Williams, N. H., Hendry, M. A., France, B., Lewis, R., Wilkinson, C. A (2007) Systematic review of the effectiveness of exercise referral schemes to promote physical activity in adults. *British Journal of General Practice*, 57, 979–86.

Zachrisson-Forsell, M. (1980) The Swedish back school. *Physiotherapy*, 66, 112–4.

Chapter 50

Manual treatment of somatic dysfunction

Michael L. Kuchera

The role of manual techniques in the management of somatic dysfunction

The medical history of manipulation dates back to the ancients and is a part of every culture's healing tradition even today. Manipulation, under anaesthesia, of the shoulder (as in adhesive capsulitis) and of the low back (as in specific disk disorders) is part of the current armamentarium of the modern orthopaedic surgeon. Likewise, manual reduction of various anatomically displaced somatic structures—fractures, dislocations, and subluxations—are common conservative treatment modalities. The use of manual treatment techniques to improve muscle function and balance, reduce fibrous adhesions or contractures, and relieve pain and joint dysfunction figures strongly in today's physical medicine and rehabilitation strategies. As an internal medicine specialist, Janet Travell pioneered the use of manual and needling techniques to address myofascial pain and dysfunction—even to modify somatovisceral reflex phenomena. In their first 4 years of training, all American-trained osteopathic physicians are taught the diagnostic and manual treatment skills (osteopathic manipulative treatment) to identify, differentiate, and address primary or secondary somatic dysfunction in patients with somatic, somatovisceral, or viscerosomatic complaints.

Worldwide, physician practitioners of musculoskeletal medicine are exploring optimum roles for the use of manual techniques in the conservative management of somatic dysfunction and pain. In the right hands and used for the proper reasons, these techniques can increase patient satisfaction and lead to symptomatic relief. They can remove the underlying somatic component maintaining a significant patient problem with pain or dysfunction. And they can be a significant option in part of a total physician-directed treatment programme to enhance health and well-being.

Manual technique alone does not constitute manual medicine. Manual techniques applied to the musculoskeletal system may be delivered by any number of lay people (e.g. coaches or sports trainers), by a variety of therapists in a systematic manner, or even by well-meaning family members. Furthermore, a number of allied health therapists spend a significant portion of their training using their hands applying manual techniques. Manual techniques are applied by therapists as 'massage therapy', or 'physical therapy', or as a specific school of therapy (e.g. Rolfing). Conversely, manual techniques applied by physicians constitute 'manual medicine'. Physicians treat, therapists provide therapy.

Physicians incorporate the choice of treatment—manual or otherwise—into a complex algorithm of diagnostic and treatment choices, incorporating differential diagnoses followed by assessment of indications and contraindications (see Chapter 60). Physicians employing manual medicine incorporate manual techniques into a larger field of medicine such as 'physical medicine and rehabilitation', 'neuromusculoskeletal medicine', or 'orthopaedic medicine', or, in the case of American osteopathic physicians, incorporate manual diagnostic and treatment techniques as an integral approach throughout primary patient care. Various descriptions of the scope of physician training and use for manual techniques were developed and published in 2014 by the International Federation of Manual/Musculoskeletal Medicine as *Guidelines for Basic Training and Safety in Manual Medicine* and are recommended (FIMM 2014).

Unfortunately, the proliferation of various practitioners with varying educational backgrounds employing an expanding portfolio of hands-on techniques with variable therapeutic (and less than therapeutic) results has been the source of growing confusion. The public has difficulty in differentiating between 'manual medicine' and use of a manual technique by a non-physician. A further complication, beyond physician delivery of a given manual 'manoeuvre or technique', is the issue of whether the physicians themselves have the training or ability to apply manual techniques within the larger field of medicine, or even the background to recognize somatic dysfunction requiring such treatment. Other than members of the International Federation of Manual/Musculoskeletal Medicine (FIMM) and American-trained osteopathic physicians and surgeons, few fully licensed physicians have adequate training in the palpation of somatic dysfunction; even fewer have skills in effectively delivering manipulative techniques. (FIMM physicians generally receive their manual medicine training after receiving their professional degree; US-trained osteopathic physicians have integrated training throughout both their professional degree programme and afterwards.)

In the wrong hands, manipulative techniques can be benignly ineffective; at worst, they could be dangerous, even lethal (Kuchera 2002). In the absence of a well thought-out treatment plan, manipulative techniques alone are only manoeuvres with little likelihood of prolonged benefit. The confusion raises serious implications ranging from standardization of nomenclature to issues dealing with training, licensing, certification, research, reimbursement, and allocation of resources.

Nomenclature issues

Confusion in nomenclature is the easiest area to address. Manipulation is a generic word that in medicine historically denoted the use of 'therapeutic application of manual force' (ECOP 2011). Different connotations are now associated with this and other 'hands-on' terms. 'Manipulative *treatment*', in contradistinction to 'manual *therapy*', was one attempt to make a semantic distinction between physician-applied 'treatment' rather than a therapist applying a technique. In some circles, 'manipulation' is specifically reserved as a term for a high-velocity, low-amplitude (HVLA) thrust-type technique, but in other circles it remains a generic term for all forms of hands-on therapeutic technique. The chiropractic profession (from the Greek root *chiros*, meaning hand) refers to its manipulative techniques as 'chiropractic adjustments'; not to be confused with the manual medicine techniques performed by German physicians, known as 'chiropraktikers', who incorporate 'chiropraxis'.

Osteopathic physicians in the USA employing 'osteopathic manipulative treatment' (OMT) sought to convey, through specific nomenclature, that guiding osteopathic principles and therapeutic goals were a component part of the manual techniques they delivered. The difference between a physical therapist applying a counterstrain technique and an osteopathic physician performing OMT using that same counterstrain technique lay in the physician-level differential diagnosis, weighing of treatment options, and integration of the technique and its outcome with the ongoing plan applied during a patient visit. It is this difference that practitioners of musculoskeletal medicine seek to convey in their management. Throughout this chapter, I will refer to MMMT (musculoskeletal medicine manipulative treatment) in recognition of the physician-level differential diagnosis and therapeutic choice that precedes each MMMT prescription for and delivery of manual techniques.

The musculoskeletal medicine manipulative treatment (MMMT) prescription

The MMMT prescription is best directed by a physician working towards definitive goals. In order to do this properly, a working diagnosis derived from historical, physical, and palpatory findings is essential (see Chapter 27). As with any prescription, the physician must select the best therapeutic agent for the situation, must calculate the appropriate dose and frequency for the agent, and must both educate the patient and be prepared to deal with any potential side-effects or untoward results.

The MMMT prescription consists of:

- **Setting goals:** What area would benefit from MMMT? What general indications are being addressed and what contraindications need to be avoided? What physiological or biomechanical end result is desired?
- **Choosing methods:** What form of MMMT is indicated? Is the tissue texture change associated with an underlying physiological status that is acute, chronic, or mixed? What techniques are most likely to accomplish the goal(s) with the fewest side-effects?
- **Determining dose:** How long should each MMMT session last? What is the homeostatic reserve of the patient available to respond to the choice of method?
- **Prognosticating frequency:** How frequently should the MMMT be repeated? When, can, and should the patient return? When should the patient be re-evaluated?
- **Recognizing potential side-effects or complications:** Are there potential risk factors posed by underlying host factors (age, health status, concomitant pathology, etc.)? Might the technique or its outcome lead or mislead the patient to ignore other important factors in their presenting or ongoing condition?

Common MMMT-related questions and clinical experiences are outlined in Table 50.1.

The most commonly used methods are defined as being either direct or indirect. In *direct method techniques*, the set-up engages the restrictive barrier of the somatic dysfunction and then the physician applies an activating force that moves through the barrier to re-establish motion. In *indirect method techniques*, the set-up requires the physician to move away from the barrier to a specific site ('balance point') where various physiological or inherent mechanisms cause the somatic dysfunction barrier to dissipate.

The *exaggeration method* is essentially an exaggerated indirect method wherein the set-up moves in the direction of freedom, past the balance point, to the normal physiological barrier opposite the motion loss barrier. At this point, an activating force is applied. The exaggeration method may be seldom used in some systems of manual medicine while in others, activating forces (typically thrust) may be applied only in the direction of pain-free motion.

Physiological response method techniques depend upon careful patient positioning and movement to obtain a therapeutic result. The lumbosacral junction, for example, may be positioned to encourage physiological motion of the sacrum towards a single desired response. Motion induced actively or passively would then cause the sacrum to move in the specific direction needed to restore its normal motion characteristics.

Sometimes a single technique incorporates more than one of the aforementioned methods. For example, the technique may start by loading the tissues with the restrictive barrier being engaged in the manner of a direct method technique but then the regional soft tissues are moved to maintain the indirect balance point. Thus, the description of this form of myofascial release (MFR) technique, also called 'myofascial unwinding' because of its appearance, best fits a *combined method technique* classification. Combined method techniques include integrated neuromusculoskeletal release and MFR techniques (Ward 2002) as well as the Still technique (named after its originator) (van Buskirk 2002).

Activating forces include:

- HVLA or thrust (Kappler and Jones 2002)
- low-velocity, moderate-amplitude springing or articulation (Patriquin and Jones 2002)

Table 50.1 Clinical experiences modifying musculoskeletal medicine manipulative treatment

Question or option	Clinical experience (generalities and guidelines only)
Selection of direct or indirect method	Indirect or direct techniques are of no value to a physician who lacks the skill to use that technique (Kappler and Kuchera 2002)
	Indirect techniques may be especially helpful in somatic dysfunction manifesting acute, oedematous tissue texture changes
	Direct techniques may be especially helpful in somatic dysfunction with chronic changes such as fibrosis
How much force should be used in an HVLA thrust?	'... enough to affect a physiological response (increased joint mobility, produce a vasomotor flush, produce palpable circulatory changes in periarticular tissues, and/or provide pain relief) but not enough to overwhelm the patient.' (Kimberly 1980)
Parameters modifying dose or frequency in the MMMT? (Kappler and Kuchera 2002)	The sicker the patient, the less the dose
	Paediatric patients can be treated more frequently
	Geriatric patients require a longer interval between treatments to respond
	Acute cases should have a shorter interval between treatments initially
General guidelines for treatment order based upon	In the chest cage, generally treat somatic dysfunction in this order: thoracic vertebrae, ribs, sternum
	In the pelvis, generally treat 'non-physiological' somatic dysfunctions (shears) before other dysfunctions
	For **very** acute somatic dysfunction, it may be necessary to treat secondary or peripheral areas first to allow access to the acute site
	In lymphatic goals, open fascial drainage pathways before enhancing the effects of diaphragmatic or augmented lymphatic pumps; local effleurage or other local tissue drainage is best done after other lymphatic techniques designed to achieve tissue drainage
What side-effects alert the clinician to modify the MMMT?	If the patient reports a flare-up of discomfort for more than 24 hours, modify the dosage, choice of activating method, and/or duration of treatment as needed
	In set-up and activating phases, it is best to avoid certain positions that aggravate otherwise intermittent radiculopathic signs (cervical or lumbar spine) in patients with spinal DJD or herniated nucleus pulposus
	Care must be paramount if HVLA is selected in a patient suspected to harbour significant osteoporosis; often, forward-bending pressures should be avoided as well
Guidelines: how long to treat?	Caring, compassionate novices often err on the side of over-dosage
	Chronic conditions usually require chronic treatment; one rule of thumb suggests that it may take as many treatment sessions as years of dysfunction
Risk to benefit issues	An appropriate assessment and diagnostic examination before, during, and after an MMMT permits accurate risk to benefit decision making regarding indications, relative contraindications, and absolute contraindications
	Manipulative treatment is among the safest treatments that a physician can administer (serious adverse response report 1:400,000 to 1:1,000,000—Kuchera et al. 2002)

DJD = degenerative joint disease; HVLA = high-velocity, low-amplitude (thrust) manipulation

- various patient-assisted, physician-directed muscle energy applications (including post-isometric relaxation, reciprocal inhibition, concentric ('move the bone') and rhythmic resistive duction) (Ehrenfeuchter 2011)
- respiratory co-operation or force (inhalation causing spinal curves to straighten and extremities to externally rotate; exhalation causing spinal curves to accentuate and extremities to internally rotate)
- inherent forces or the body's tendency towards balance and homeostasis (certain positioning seems to enhance inherent activities associated with normal breathing, vascular pulsations, proprioceptive resetting, central response to reduction of afferent load, enhancement of lymphatic return, and other homeostatic mechanisms to dissipate barriers to functional motion)
- patient cooperative reflex activities (including eye movements and activation of other specific muscles in specific directions and/or at a specific time).

As with the set-up positions used in various combined methods, a combination of activating forces may be more effective than repeated use of a single activating force. For example, in a direct method upper cervical technique using combined activating forces, the somatic dysfunction restrictive barrier should be optimally engaged. The initial activating force may be a request for one to three 3-second isometric muscle energy activations in a direction away from the barrier, with the physician carefully re-engaging the 'new' direct barrier site after each muscle energy activation. Combining forces simultaneously, by having the patient look in the same direction in which they are pushing, engages oculocervicogyric reflex connections to the small suboccipital muscles. Immediately after the last relaxation of muscle energy, the physician may apply an HVLA through any remaining barrier. Approaching the same evolving barrier with a single technique employing this combination of activating forces may be more effective (and certainly more time-efficient) than attempting three separate direct-method techniques with three separate activating forces.

Selection of methods and activating forces to accomplish specific physiological goals often depends on whether the tissue texture changes reflect acute, chronic, or mixed pathophysiological findings. Such tissue texture changes influence the underlying viscoelastic properties of tissues and seem to affect the postulated mechanisms of action in manual medicine approaches, including tissue decongestion, viscoelastic creep, muscle guarding, central neurological gate phenomena, and mechanotransduction.

In addition to the choice of method and activating force, the dose and frequency used in an MMMT prescription are also often determined by host factors, including their underlying constellation of pathophysiological changes. Key considerations include the age and health status of the patient, individual homeostatic reserve, accompanying systemic or regional rheumatologic or vascular pathophysiology, and prior response to particular MMMT methods or activating forces. The most common response to a less than optimal choice of method, activating force, or dose is a flare-up of muscle soreness or whatever symptoms brought the patient to the office. Although this is the most common side-effect of an MMMT, it is usually a minor annoyance to the patient and, in capable hands, not a frequent occurrence. A flare-up is rarely desirable, and any flare-up lasting more than 24 hours probably warrants reconsideration of the MMMT prescription. Usually modifications of the activating force, method, and/or dose during the next visit eliminate the problem.

Finally, one other major variable plays into the ability to deliver an appropriate MMMT prescription—the physician. The ability of a physician to safely, effectively, and efficiently accomplish the treatment procedures includes many factors. Among these factors are:

- personal stature, strength, and sense of balance
- palpatory ability to sense subtle tissue texture, symmetry, and motion changes in tissues before, during, and after treatment
- training level and mastery of a variety of techniques, methods, and activating forces
- knowledge of functional anatomy, physiology, and pathophysiology
- level of experience in problem-solving situations involving patients with primary and compensatory somatic dysfunction.

Other issues

The discussion of other issues identified in the introduction to this chapter—training, licensing, certification, research, reimbursement, and allocation of resources—is beyond the scope of this chapter. Throughout this chapter, the use of MMMT and discussion of manipulative techniques are presented in the context of their use by fully trained, fully licensed physicians and/or surgeons. MMMT integration with musculoskeletal medicine management approaches will represent, whenever possible, peer consensus of specialists, research evidence, and/or cost-effective perspectives.

Musculoskeletal medicine manipulative treatment (MMMT) techniques

The bulk of this section of the chapter consists of individual MMMT techniques which must be applied within the context of a larger physician-level field of knowledge such as musculoskeletal medicine, neuromusculoskeletal medicine, orthopaedic medicine, osteopathic medicine, physical medicine, rehabilitation medicine, orthopaedic surgery, and family practice. The assorted technique examples selected here are not meant to be all-inclusive; rather, each is illustrative of manual medicine applications employing various combinations of technique methods and activating forces in different regions with the patient in different positions. Unless otherwise noted, all illustrations used in this Chapter have been selected from either the Kimberly manual (Kimberly and Funk 2000) or teaching slides associated with the Nicholas manual (Nicholas and Nicholas 2012).

Head region

Basilar decompression technique (direct method)

Diagnosis: Occipitoatlantal backward bending somatic dysfunction with compression of the occipital condyles. Tension is palpated at the base of the skull. There is freedom of backward bending of the occiput upon the atlas with restriction to forward bending.
Patient position: Supine.
Operator position: Seated at head of table/bed.
Contact: Middle fingers placed at base of skull (occiput) pointed anteromedial in line with the occipital condyles (Figure 50.1).
Position to initiate technique: Patient is asked to draw chin towards chest as the operator's fingers are drawn posterolateral to hold the point of tissue tension.
Activation: Operator brings wrists together, pulling occipital condyles posterolateral in the direction of the facet motion allowed. As the tissues soften, slack is gradually taken up, drawing the head further into forward bending on the neck.

Temporomandibular joint (TMJ) muscle energy technique

Diagnosis: Left TMJ restricted; jaw deviates to the left when opened.
Patient position: Supine.
Operator position: At head of table/bed.
Contact: Operator's right hand supports right side of patient's head; left hand contacts left mandible (Figure 50.2).
Position to initiate technique: Patient instructed to open mouth until mandible first begins to deviate to the left. Operator's left hand applies pressure to the right until the 'feather edge' of the dysfunctional barrier is reached.

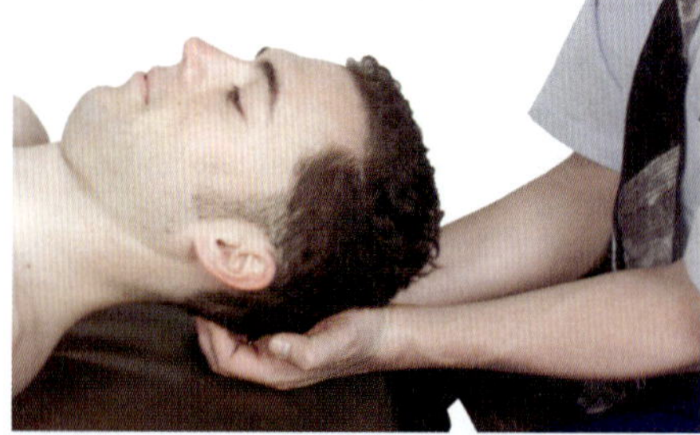

Figure 50.1 Basilar decompression technique (direct method). (Kimberly and Funk 2000)

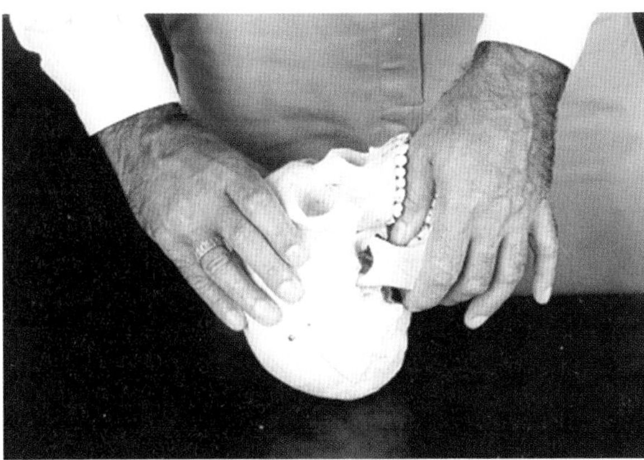

Figure 50.2 TMJ muscle energy technique. (Nicholas and Nicholas 2012)

Activation: Patient is instructed to gently push the chin for approximately 3 seconds to the left against isometric pressure from the operator's hand and then relax. During relaxation phase, a new barrier is engaged by removing slack by increasing pressure to the right. Repeat three times.
Follow-up: Re-evaluate S.T.A.R. characteristics (see Chapter 10). Instruct avoidance of repetitive asymmetrical chewing activities (e.g. gum).

Occipitomastoid (OM) sutural V-spread technique

Diagnosis: Tenderness and bogginess over OM suture on the right.
Patient position: Supine.
Operator position: At head of table/bed.
Contact: Operator's right index and middle finger pads on opposite sides of OM suture at site of maximum tenderness and tissue texture change; left index and middle finger pads resting gently over left frontal eminence (Figure 50.3).
Activation: Right finger pads create tension across suture site by operator attempting to spread index and middle fingers apart into a 'V'; left fingers place 10–40 g pressure in synchrony with extension phase of the cranial mechanism. Distracting tension maintained on right with rhythmic on–off pressure on left until right side releases.
Follow-up: Recheck S.T.A.R. characteristics.

Sphenobasilar synchondrosis (SBS) indirect technique (e.g. right SBS torsion)

Diagnosis: SBS prefers right torsion and is restricted in left torsion.
Patient position: Supine.
Operator position: Seated at head of table/bed.
Contact: Vault hold with index finger pads bilaterally over greater wings of sphenoid; middle and ring fingers straddling the ear with respective volar metacarpophalangeal joints over the squamous portion of the temporal bones; pads of the fifth digit over the squamous occiput (Figure 50.4).
Position to initiate technique: Right index and left fifth digits drawn superiorly; left index and right fifth digits drawn inferiorly to point of balanced membranous tension.
Activation: Patient instructed to hold respiration in inhalation or exhalation (whichever provides greatest tension release) as long as possible with continuous minor adjustment of hands to maintain balance point as release is accomplished.
Follow-up: Recheck asymmetry and motion characteristics.

Sphenopalatine ganglion (lateral pterygoid) pressure technique

Diagnosis: Tension and tenderness over left lateral pterygoid muscle; excessive maxillary sinus secretion.
Patient position: Seated.
Operator position: Standing, facing patient.
Contact: Operator's gloved or sheathed right fifth digit is passed along the outside of the patient's gum line, beyond the last molar, and tipped superior, posterior, and medial to contact the left lateral pterygoid muscle (Figure 50.5).
Activation: Patient tips head to the left against the operator's fingertip for 2–3 seconds. This procedure is repeated three times.
Follow-up: Observe for unilateral lacrimation indicative of parasympathetic stimulation and then repeat on opposite side.

Frontal lift

Diagnosis: Restricted motion of the frontal bone; dural imbalance; ethmoidal–frontal restriction.
Patient position: Supine.
Operator position: Seated, at head of patient.
Contact: Operator's index fingers are placed at glabella with thumbs placed in the midline immediately anterior to the coronal suture; middle fingers hook around the orbital process of the frontal bone (at the edge of the brow) (Figure 50.6).

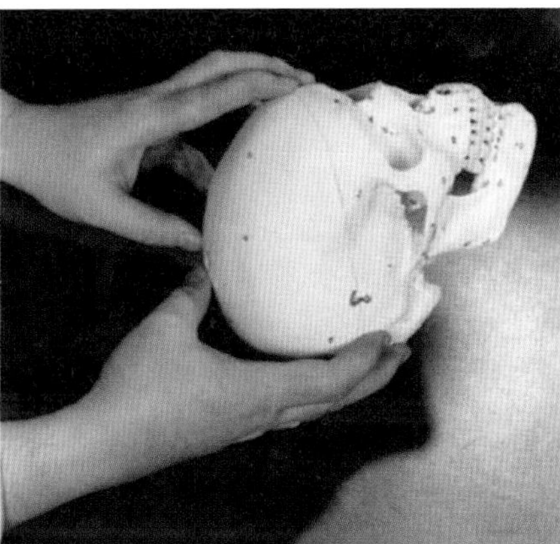

Figure 50.3 OM sutural V-spread technique. (Nicholas and Nicholas 2012)

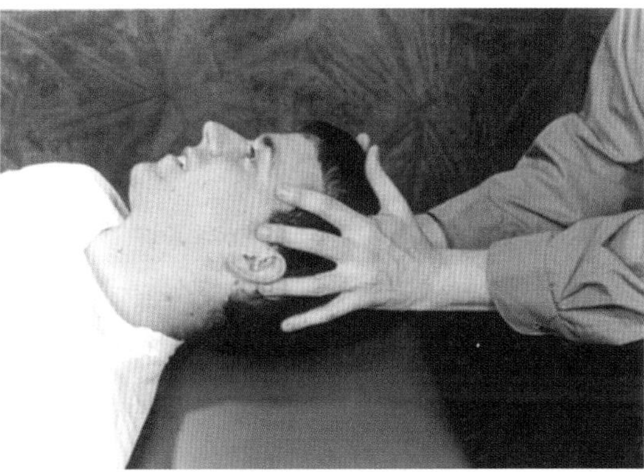

Figure 50.4 SBS indirect technique (e.g. right SBS torsion). (Nicholas and Nicholas 2012)

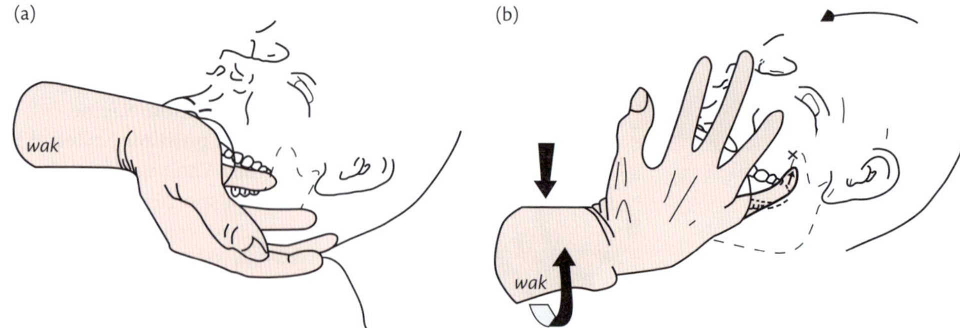

Figure 50.5 Sphenopalatine ganglion (lateral pterygoid) pressure technique.

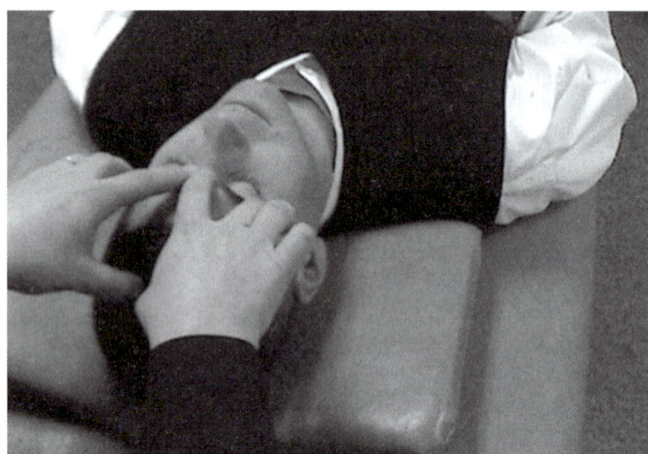

Figure 50.6 Frontal lift. (Nicholas and Nicholas 2012)

Position to initiate technique: Operator lightly compresses middle fingers medially to disengage the frontals from the parietals.
Activation: Lift the frontal bone anteriorly (towards the ceiling) and seek balanced membranous tension.
Follow-up: Recheck overall motion characteristics with frontal and vault holds.

'CV 4'

Diagnosis: Low-amplitude or asymmetrical cranial rhythmic impulse (CRI). Technique used also for homeostatic enhancement.
Patient position: Supine.
Operator position: Seated at head of table/bed.
Contact: Operator's hands are gently overlapped to place thenar eminences over the squamous occiput bilaterally, immediately medial to each mastoid process (Figure 50.7).

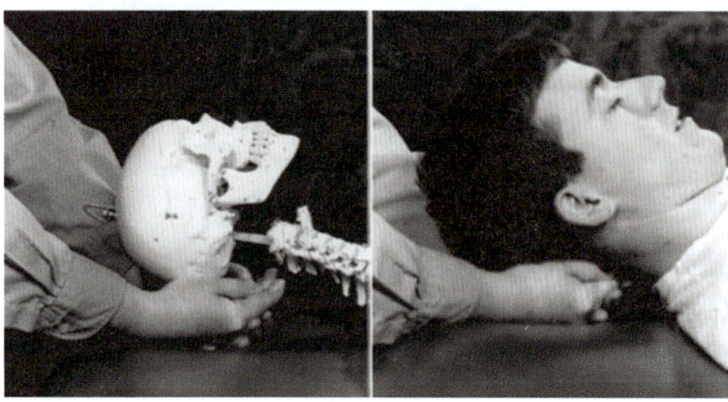

Figure 50.7 'CV 4'. (Nicholas and Nicholas 2012)

Position to initiate technique: Gentle pressure from each thenar eminence triangulating the anatomical location of the fourth ventricle.
Activation: Compression dampening CRI with progressive exaggeration of the extension phase continues until a 'still point' is reached; increased warmth is often felt and the patient will often express a sigh at this point. Pressure is then released.
Follow-up: Reassess the CRI; specifically rule out iatrogenic introduction of cranial extension somatic dysfunction.

Craniocervical junction and cervical region

Superior cervical segment

Occipitoatlantal (OA) muscle energy with post-isometric relaxation oculocervical reflex muscle energy activation

Diagnosis: OA sidebending left, rotation right.
Patient position: Supine.
Operator position: Seated at head of table.
Contact: One hand forms a 'V' with the thumb and index finger of one hand and supports the posterior arch and lateral masses. Use other hand to control the head (Figure 50.8).
Position to initiate technique: Adjust flexion/extension to localize at the dysfunctional segment; induce right sidebending and left rotation of the occiput to engage the restrictive barrier and provide counterforce.
Activation: Activate the oculocervicogyric reflex by instructing the patient to look to the right while the operator offers isometric counterforce for 3–5 seconds. The patient ceases the directed gaze force and the operator simultaneously ceases the counterforce.
Follow-up: Operator waits for tissue relaxation and then moves the head to the new restrictive barrier (all three planes), repeating activation and follow-up until normal motion is returned (typically 3–5 times).

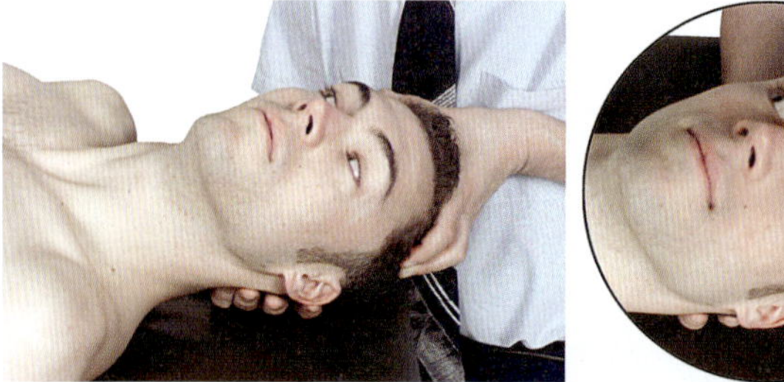

Figure 50.8 OA muscle energy with oculocervical reflex muscle energy activation ($S_L R_R$). (Kimberly and Funk 2000)

OA indirect method with respiratory co-operation

Diagnosis: OA flexion, sidebending left, rotation right.
Patient position: Supine.
Operator position: Seated at head of table.
Contact: Hand resting on the table forms a 'V' with the thumb and index finger supporting the posterior arch and lateral masses. Use other hand to control the head (Figure 50.9).
Position to initiate technique: Using the head, flex, sidebend the OA joint to the left and rotate it to the right to the point of balanced ligamentous tension.
Activation: Test respiratory phases and instruct patient to hold breath as long as possible in the phase that provides the best ligamentous balance. Make minor adjustments in all three planes as needed to maintain ligamentous balance.
Follow-up: Repeat activating step as needed until the best motion is obtained.

OA HVLA

Diagnosis: OA sidebending left, rotation right.
Patient position: Supine.
Operator position: Standing at head of table.
Contact: Right hand contacts patient's right posterior occiput posterior to, but not on, the mastoid process. Physician's left hand cradles the head (Figure 50.10).

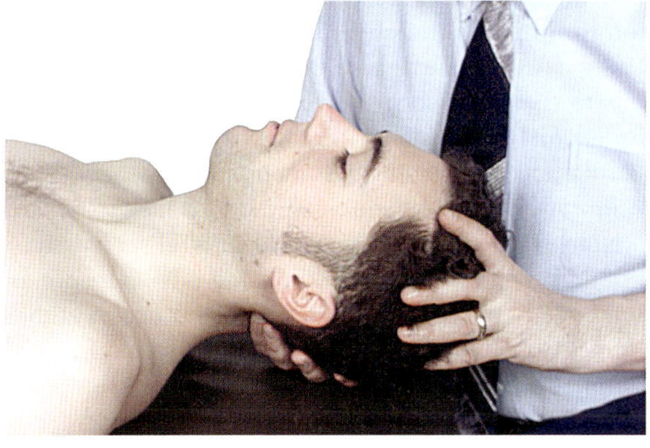

Figure 50.9 OA indirect method with respiratory cooperation (e.g. $S_L R_R$). (Kimberly and Funk 2000)

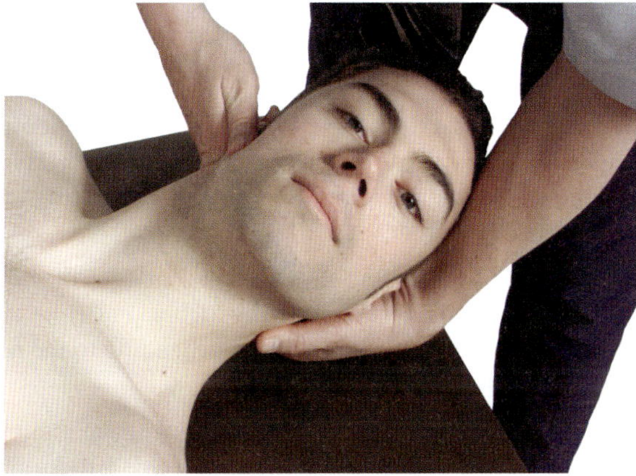

Figure 50.10 AA muscle energy (e.g. AA rotated left). (Kimberly and Funk 2000)

Position to initiate technique: Regardless of flexion or extension preference, flex slightly. Sidebend the occiput to the right on the atlas and minimally rotate it (1–3°) to the left to localize at the restrictive barrier.
Activation: A HVLA left sidebending thrust is applied, directed medially, anteriorly, and superiorly (towards opposite eye).
Follow-up: Recheck motion characteristics.

Atlantoaxial (AA) post-isometric relaxation muscle energy

Diagnosis: AA left rotation.
Patient position: Supine.
Operator position: Standing at head of table.
Contact: Place palms on each side of the patient's head and contact both lateral masses of the atlas with the lateral margin of the index or middle fingers (Figure 50.11).
Position to initiate technique: Extend head minimally over contact fingers and rotate the atlas to the 'feather edge' of the restrictive barrier.
Activation: Patient is instructed to turn the head to the left while the physician offers isometric counterforce for 3–5 seconds, sensing that the patient's contractile force is localized at the AA joint.
Follow-up: After the patient ceases the directive force and the operator simultaneously ceases the counterforce and moves the head and atlas to the new restrictive barrier, repeating until the best motion is obtained (typically 3–5 times).

AA indirect method with respiratory co-operation

Diagnosis: AA left rotation.
Patient position: Supine.
Operator position: Seated at head of table.
Contact: Cradle the patient's head in both palms and contact both lateral masses of the atlas with the fingertips (Figure 50.12).
Position to initiate technique: Rotate the atlas to the left to the point of balanced ligamentous tension (slight regional adjustments of sidebending and flexion or extension may be needed).
Activation: Test respiratory phases and instruct to hold breath as long as possible in the phase that provides the best ligamentous balance (make minor regional adjustments in all three planes as needed to maintain ligamentous balance).
Follow-up: Recheck and repeat as needed to achieve optimal motion.

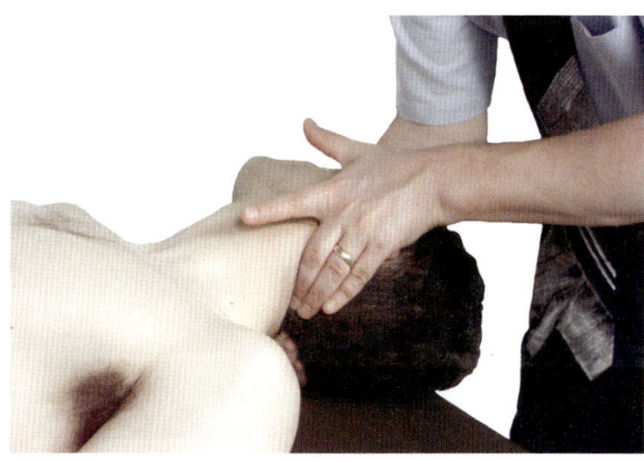

Figure 50.11 OA HVLA (e.g. $S_L R_R$). (Kimberly and Funk 2000)

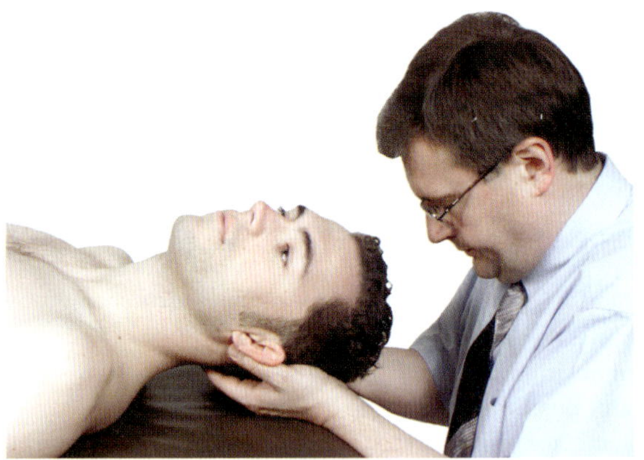

Figure 50.12 AA indirect method with respiratory co-operation. (Kimberly and Funk 2000)

Lower cervical segment

Typical cervical HVLA (rotation activation)

Diagnosis: C2–3 extension, rotation left, sidebending left.
Patient position: Supine.
Operator position: Standing at head of table.
Contact: Support head with wrists/forearms while contacting both articular pillars of the dysfunctional vertebra with the index fingers (Figure 50.13).
Position to initiate technique: Flex head/neck until motion is localized at the dysfunctional segment. Operator maintains flexion at the dysfunctional segment and extends the vertebral segments above. (This isolates the dysfunctional segment to enable rotation while the fingers act as fulcrums.) Sidebend the neck slightly to the left to lock the vertebrae above the dysfunction; then rotate the neck to the right to the feather edge of the restrictive barrier.
Activation: HVLA rotational thrust is applied through both hands with the force directed along the plane of the facets. (Note: rotation in the typical cervical spine is automatically accompanied by sidebending to the same side; therefore, correction of the sidebending component automatically occurs at the localized segment when the rotational thrust is applied.)
Follow-up: Recheck motion characteristics; if no improvement, then consider a sidebending activation alternative.

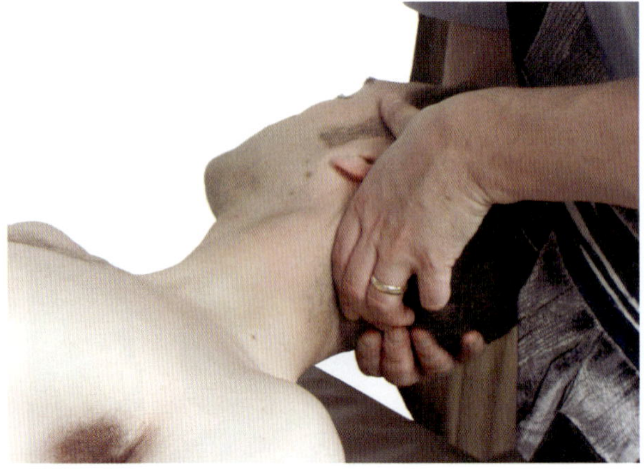

Figure 50.13 Typical cervical HVLA rotation activation (e.g. C2 ER_LS_L). (Kimberly and Funk 2000)

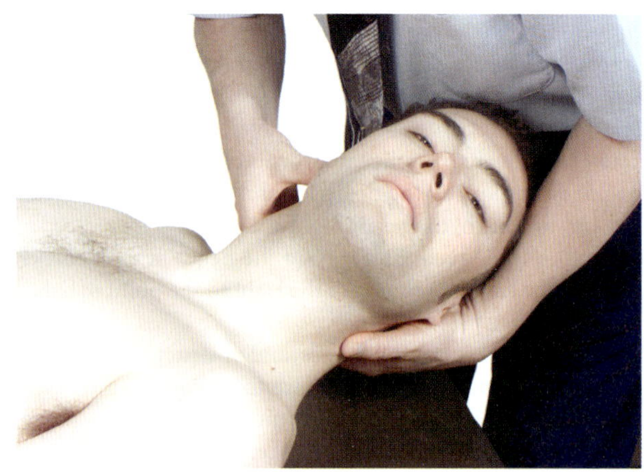

Figure 50.14 Typical cervical HVLA sidebending activation (e.g. C4 NR_LS_L). (Kimberly and Funk 2000)

Typical cervical HVLA (sidebending activation)

Diagnosis: C4–5 neutral rotation left, sidebending left.
Patient position: Supine.
Operator position: Standing at head of table.
Contact: Support the head with wrist/forearm while contacting the articular pillars of the dysfunctional vertebra with the lateral margin of the index fingers (Figure 50.14).
Position to initiate technique: Lift the head to flex the neck and sidebend the neck to the right to the restrictive barrier. Then rotate the neck to the left to lock the vertebrae above the dysfunction. (Adjust flexion or extension within the neutral range as needed to localize all three planes at the dysfunctional segment.)
Activation: A HVLA sidebending thrust is applied to the articular pillar. (Note: sidebending in the typical cervical spine is automatically accompanied by rotation to the same side; therefore, correction of the rotational component automatically occurs at the localized segment when the sidebending thrust is applied.)
Follow-up: Recheck motion characteristics; if no improvement consider rotational activation alternative.

Typical cervical muscle energy

Diagnosis: C3 neutral rotation left, sidebending left.
Patient position: Supine.
Operator position: Seated at head of table.
Contact: Sidebending is introduced at the dysfunctional segment using one of the following:

- Reach under the cervical spine to contact the right side of the articular column with the finger pads. Pull the cervical spine towards the left, inducing right sidebending to the feather edge of the restrictive barrier; **or**
- Place the pad of the thumb on the lateral margin of the right articular pillar of the dysfunctional vertebra. Push the articular column to the left, inducing right sidebending to the feather edge of the restrictive barrier.

Position to initiate technique: In addition to sidebending right, rotate right and flex or extend the neck as needed to localize to the dysfunctional segment; other hand grasps the head for counterforce (Figure 50.15).

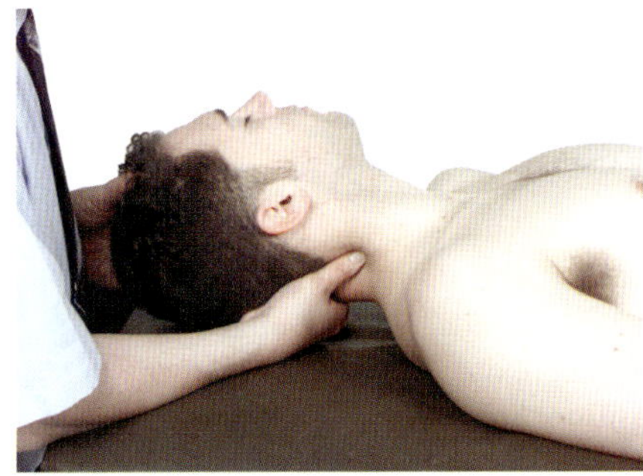

or

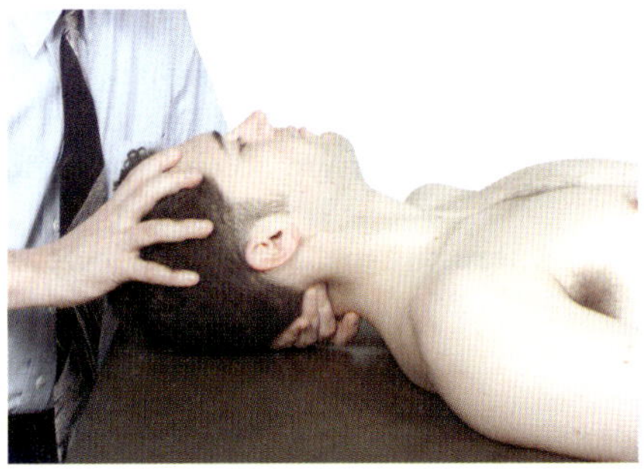

Figure 50.15 Typical cervical muscle energy (e.g. C3 NR_LS_L). (Kimberly and Funk 2000)

Activation: Instruct to gently rotate left or sidebend left down to that vertebral unit for 3–5 seconds. Then cease the directive force and simultaneously cease counterforce.
Follow-up: Sidebend, rotate, and adjust the sagittal plane to the new barrier, repeating activating force until best motion is obtained (typically 3–5 times).

Typical cervical counterstrain

Diagnosis: Tender right AC5 (located on the anterolateral aspect of the transverse process of C5).
Patient position: Supine.
Operator position: Seated at head of table.
Contact: Right finger over tender AC5 site; left hand cupping and controlling the posterior aspect of the skull (Figure 50.16).

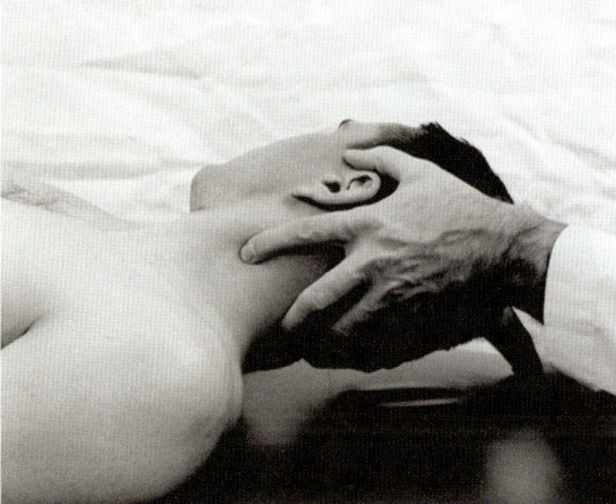

Figure 50.16 Typical cervical counterstrain (e.g. AC5). (Nicholas and Nicholas 2012)

Position to initiate technique: Flex the patient's neck to the level of the tender point. Sidebend and rotate the patient's neck away (left, in the example shown in Figure 50.16) until the patient expresses at least 70% reduction of tenderness to pressure palpation.
Activation: Hold position for 90 seconds and slowly return the head and neck to the neutral position.
Follow-up: Confirm at least 70% reduction to pressure palpation in the neutral position.

Typical cervical indirect method with respiratory co-operation

Diagnosis: C3 neutral, rotation left, sidebending left.
Patient position: Supine.
Operator position: Seated at head of table.
Contact: Support the head with palms, wrists, or forearms; contact the articular pillars bilaterally with the index fingers (Figure 50.17).
Position to initiate technique: Sidebend neck left, rotate it left, and flex/extend as needed to balance ligamentous tension (BLT) in all three planes at the dysfunctional segment.
Activation: Test respiratory phases and instruct to hold breath as long as possible in the phase that provides the best ligamentous balance. (Make continuous minor adjustments in all three planes as tissue balance dictates to maintain ligamentous balance.) Await tissue release.
Follow-up: Recheck motion for success.

Cervicothoracic junction and upper thoracic cage

Cervicothoracic junction, superior thoracic inlet

Superior thoracic inlet HVLA (two-step technique)

Diagnosis: Thoracic inlet sidebent and rotated right.
Patient position: Supine.
Operator position: Standing at head of table (Figure 50.18).
Step 1 contact (sidebending component): Cradle patient's head with the right palm and place the web between the left thumb and index finger on the soft tissues at the cervical–thoracic junction (as a fulcrum).
Step 1 position to initiate technique: Sidebend the neck and thoracic inlet over the fulcrum to the fascia's restrictive barrier while rotating the head and neck in the opposite direction to lock the cervical spine. Add flexion or extension to localize to the restrictive barrier.

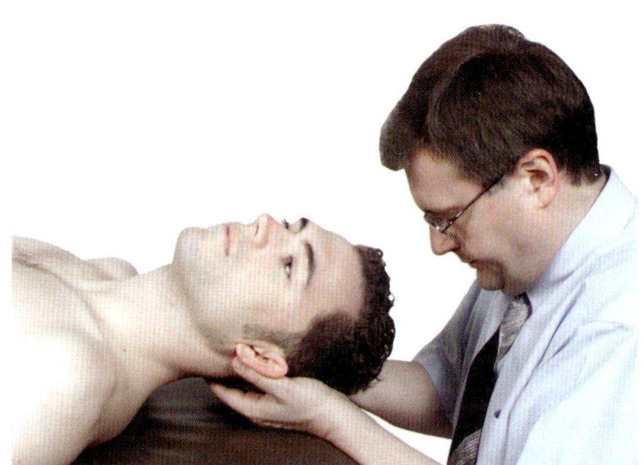

Figure 50.17 Typical cervical indirect method with respiratory co-operation (e.g. C3 NR_LS_L). (Kimberly and Funk 2000)

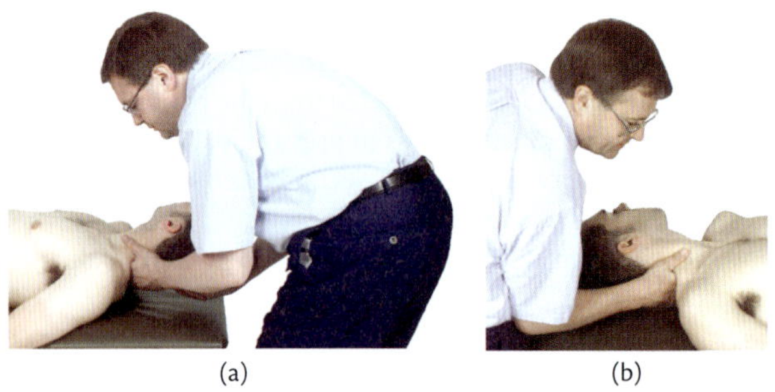

Figure 50.18 Superior thoracic inlet HVLA (two-step technique S_RR_R): (a) sidebending component; (b) rotation component. (Kimberly and Funk 2000)

Step 1 activation: HVLA thrust is applied through the left hand inferiorly and slightly medial.
Step 2 contact (rotation component): Transfer support of the patient's head to the left hand placing the web between the right thumb and index finger over the soft tissues at the cervical–thoracic junction.
Step 2 positioning: Rotate the neck and thoracic inlet to the left to engage the fascial restrictive barrier; sidebend the head and neck to the right to lock the cervical spine, adding flexion or extension to localize to the restrictive barrier.
Step 2 activation: HVLA thrust is applied through the right hand carrying the thoracic inlet in a rotational direction anteriorly and medial (the left hand on the head maintains tissue tension only as the region is rotated).

Superior thoracic inlet indirect technique with respiratory co-operation

Diagnosis: Thoracic inlet sidebent and rotated right.
Patient position: Supine.
Operator position: Seated at head of table.
Contact: Place hands over the thoracic inlet with fingers spread over the anterior thorax and thumbs over the posterior thorax (Figure 50.19).
Position to initiate technique: Carry the thoracic inlet region into right rotation and right sidebending (with left translation); add flexion or extension until tension in all three planes are at ligamentous balance.
Activation: Test respiratory phases and instruct the patient to hold breath as long as possible in the phase that provides the best BLT until maximal tissue response has been obtained. Continuously adjust to follow tissue release.

Thoracic spine T1–4

Upper thoracic HVLA

Diagnosis: T2 flexed, sidebent left, rotated right.
Patient position: Supine with elbows together.
Operator position: Standing on the patient's left side.
Contact: Contact the right transverse process of the dysfunctional segment with the left thenar prominence near the proximal phalanx of the thumb (Figure 50.20).
Position to initiate technique: Sidebend right down to the restrictive barrier and lift the head with the left hand (or ask patient to lift their own head) until pressure accumulates at the operator's left hand.
Activation: HVLA thrust is applied through the patient's elbows into the operator's thenar eminence to induce vertebral rotation to the left.

Upper thoracic muscle energy

Diagnosis: T3 neutral, sidebent left, rotated right.
Patient position: Supine.
Operator position: Seated at head of table.
Contact: Place the pad of a finger of the right hand on the left side of the spinous process of the dysfunctional segment to monitor and to induce left rotation and extension (Figure 50.21).
Position to initiate technique: Left hand is placed on patient's head and upper neck so that the neck can be moved into left rotation and right sidebending down to the dysfunctional segment.
Activation: Patient is instructed to gently sidebend their head to the left against an isometric counterforce for 3–5 seconds.
Follow-up: After the patient and operator cease mutual isometric counterforces, the segment is sidebent right and rotated left to engage the new restrictive barrier. Slight flexion or extension adjustment may also be required. Repeat 2–4 times.

Upper thoracic indirect with respiratory co-operation

Diagnosis: T3 neutral, sidebent left, rotated right.
Patient position: Supine (Note: this technique is especially useful in acute traumatic situations and can also be performed in the

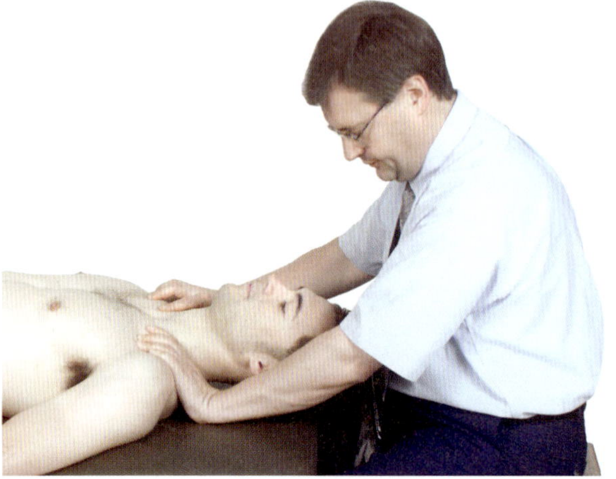

Figure 50.19 Superior thoracic inlet indirect technique with respiratory co-operation (e.g. inlet S_RR_R). (Kimberly and Funk 2000)

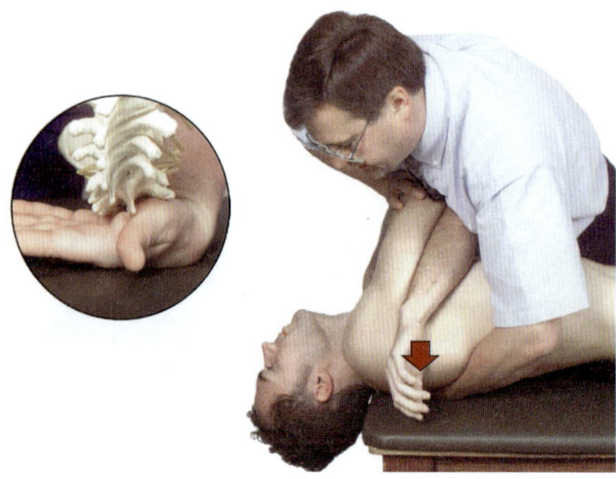

Figure 50.20 Upper thoracic HVLA (e.g. T2 $N_FS_LR_R$). (Kimberly and Funk 2000)

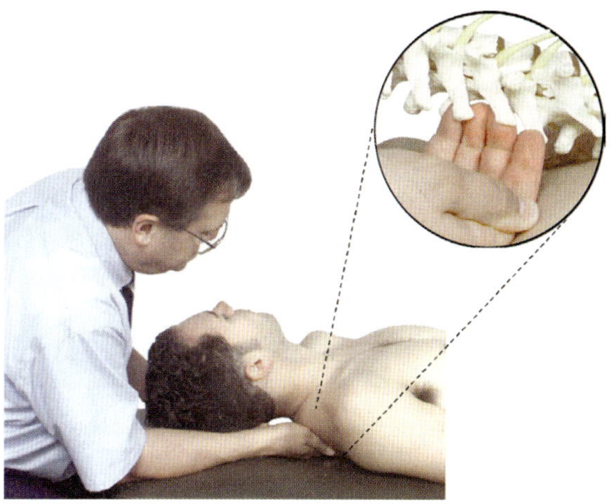

Figure 50.21 Upper thoracic muscle energy (e.g. T3 N $S_L R_R$). (Kimberly and Funk 2000)

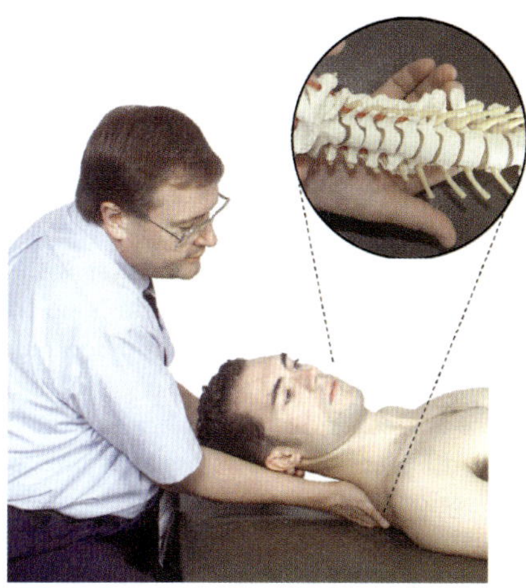

Figure 50.22 Upper thoracic indirect with respiratory co-operation (e.g. T3 N $S_L R_R$). (Kimberly and Funk 2000)

seated position. The technique can also be used with the patient supine and the patient's head supported beyond the end of the table if additional extension is required.)

Operator position: Seated at head of table.

Contact: Support the head with left hand and reach under the neck to place the pad of the right index or middle finger on the left transverse process of the dysfunctional segment (Figure 50.22).

Position to initiate technique: Position in neutral using minor flexion or extension motions as needed to localize forces to T3. Introduce rotation and right translation (left sidebending) to the point of BLT.

Activation: Test respiratory phases and instruct to hold breath as long as possible in the phase that provides the best ligamentous balance. Make minor adjustments in all three planes, as needed, to maintain ligamentous balance.

Upper thoracic counterstrain

Diagnosis: Right posterior third thoracic (PT3)—tenderness over T3 spinous process or right transverse process of T3.

Patient position: Prone.

Operator position: Standing on same side as tender point with knee on table to support the patient's right shoulder.

Contact: Right finger monitoring most tender point (Figure 50.23).

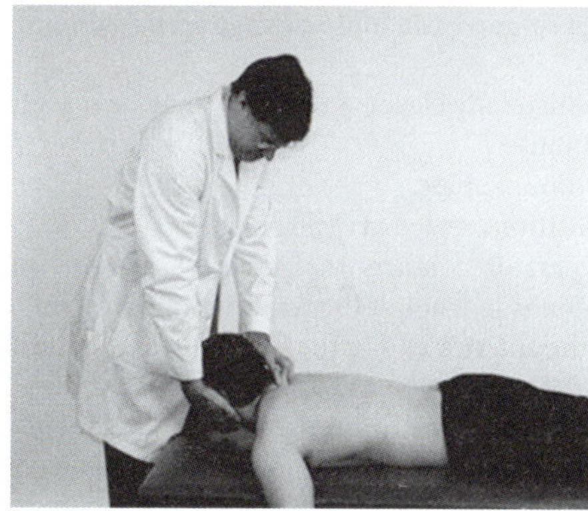

Figure 50.23 Upper thoracic counterstrain (e.g. PT3). (Nicholas and Nicholas 2012)

Position to initiate technique: Extend, rotate away, and sidebend slightly away from the tender point until patient expresses at least a 70% reduction of tenderness in pressure palpation.

Activation: Hold the position for 90 seconds and then slowly return the patient to the neutral position.

Follow-up: Reconfirm at least a 70% reduction in tenderness to pressure palpation.

Rib cage R1–2

Rib 1: HVLA

Diagnosis: Right first rib elevated posteriorly.

Patient position: Seated (may be modified for supine patients).

Operator position: Standing behind patient.

Contact: Physician contacts the superior part of the posterior surface of the right first rib with the metacarpophalangeal joint of his/her index finger. The physician's elbow is elevated and directed inferiorly towards the dysfunctional rib. The elbow of the other hand rests on the patient's shoulder with the hand controlling head motion (Figure 50.24).

Position to initiate technique: Move neck into sidebending towards and rotation away from the dysfunctional rib. Tension is increased with both hands until the rib is carried to the restrictive barrier.

Activation: A HVLA thrust is applied to the rib inferiorly, anteriorly, and medially to the rib (in a direction towards the opposite nipple).

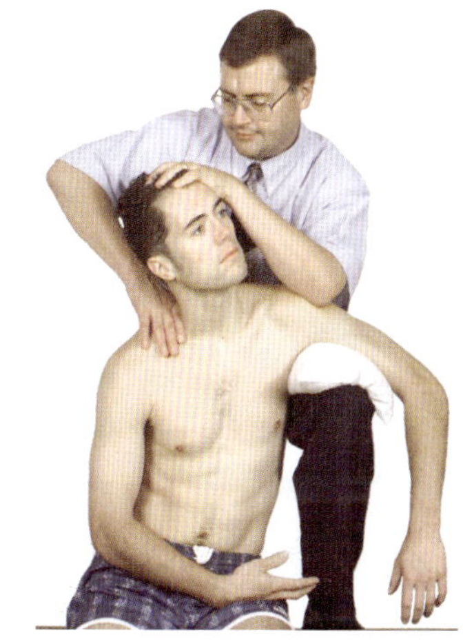

Figure 50.24 HVLA (elevated right first rib). (Kimberly and Funk 2000)

Rib 1: Patient co-operation muscle energy with respiratory co-operation

Diagnosis: Bilaterally elevated first ribs (may be modified for unilateral elevation).
Patient position: Supine.
Operator position: Seated at head of table.
Contact: Operator contacts the posterior margins of both first ribs with thumbs in front of the trapezius and the pad of the index finger over the anterior end of the first rib near the sternoclavicular joints (Figure 50.25).
Position to initiate technique: To modify for unilateral elevated first rib, sidebend patient's neck towards the involved rib (to remove scalene pull) and rotate head away from involved rib (to free costovertebral articulation).
Activation: Patient is instructed to shrug shoulder(s) towards ears while inhaling as operator maintains firm caudad pressure. The patient exhales and relaxes shoulders as the operator follows the first ribs caudally. Repeat for a total of 3–5 times.

Thoracic cage

Thoracic spine T4–12

Mid–lower thoracic: HVLA

Diagnosis: T7 neutral, sidebending left, rotation right.
Patient position: Supine.
Operator position: Stand on the side opposite the rotation (for this diagnosis, on patient's left side).
Contact: Patient crosses arms across the chest with the opposite arm on top. (For this diagnosis, the right arm is on top.) Operator's right hand lifts and rolls the patient forward, placing the left thenar eminence (as a fulcrum) posterior to the right transverse process and articular facets of the dysfunctional segment. Fingers are extended over the left paraspinal region. Patient is rolled back onto the table, resting on the fulcrum (Figure 50.26).
Position to initiate technique: Patient's elbows are placed in the operator's epigastric region (or on the sternum or in the left axilla). The spine is extended at the level of the dysfunction while maintaining flexion above. Sidebend right to engage the restrictive barrier. Transfer tension through the patient's elbows into the fulcrum hand while maintaining localization of extension, right sidebending, and left rotation at the dysfunctional segment.

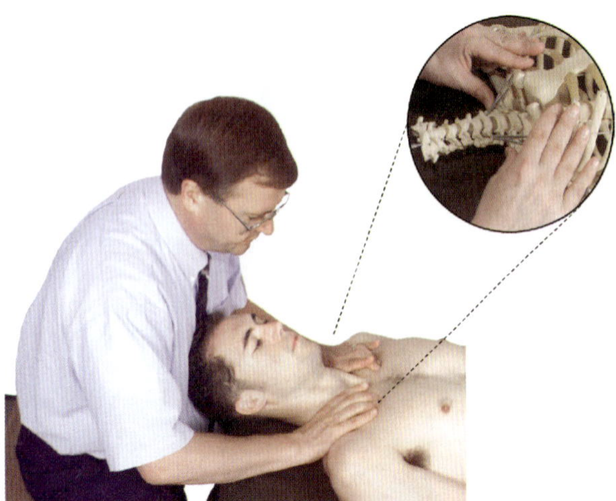

Figure 50.25 Rib 1: patient co-operation muscle energy with respiratory co-operation. (Kimberly and Funk 2000)

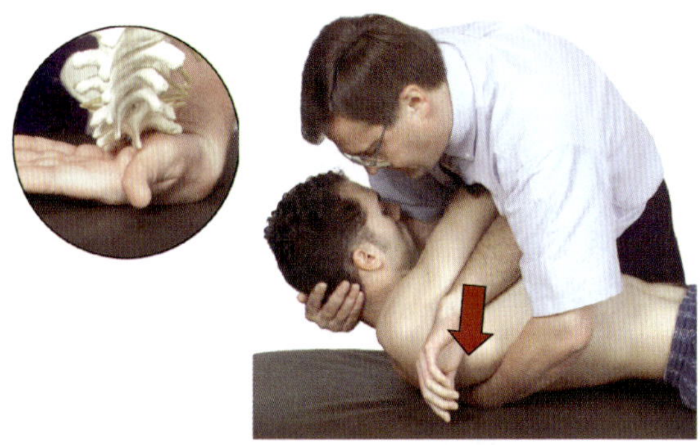

Figure 50.26 Mid–lower thoracic: HVLA (e.g. T7 N $S_L R_R$). (Kimberly and Funk 2000)

Activation: A HVLA thrust is applied through the patient's elbows into the fulcrum. This will result in left rotation, right sidebending, and extension of the dysfunctional unit.

Mid–lower thoracic: HVLA

Diagnosis: T7 extended (non-neutral), rotation and sidebending left.
Patient position: Supine.
Operator position: Stand on the side opposite the rotation (patient's right side, in this example).
Contact: Patient crosses arms across the chest with the opposite arm on top. (For this diagnosis, the left arm is on top.) Operator uses the left hand to grasp patient's left shoulder and rolls the patient into flexion to place the right thenar eminence posterior to the left transverse process and articular facets of the dysfunctional segment. Extended fingers are laid across the spine to the patient's right paraspinal region (Figure 50.27).
Position to initiate technique: Patient's elbows are placed in the operator's epigastric region (or on the sternum or in the left axilla). The patient is rolled back onto the table until flexion is localized at the dysfunctional unit. Flexion is maintained while the head and neck are used to introduce right sidebending down to the dysfunctional segment. The operator's body weight is applied through the epigastrium, sternum, or axilla to induce right rotation into the restrictive barrier.
Activation: A HVLA thrust is applied posterosuperiorly through the patient's elbows into the fulcrum at approximately a 45–60° angle to the table.

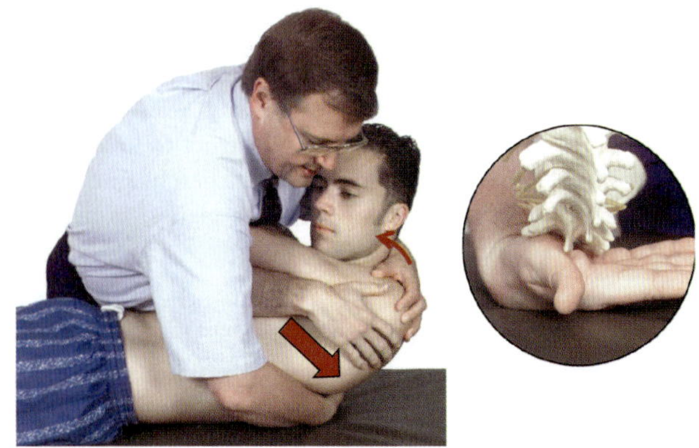

Figure 50.27 Mid–lower thoracic: HVLA (e.g. T7 E $R_L S_L$). (Kimberly and Funk 2000)

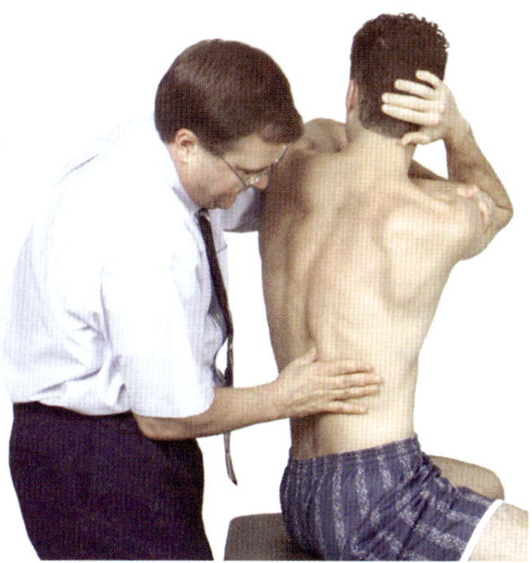

Figure 50.28 Mid–lower thoracic: muscle energy (e.g. T11 N S_LR_R). (Kimberly and Funk 2000)

Mid–lower thoracic: muscle energy

Diagnosis: T11 neutral, sidebending left, rotation right.
Patient position: Seated on table.
Operator position: Standing behind patient.
Contact: Patient places right hand behind head or neck and grasps the elbow with the other hand. Operator reaches under patient's left arm, across the chest, grasping the right shoulder or mid-humeral region. The operator's right thumb is placed over the right transverse process of the dysfunctional segment (Figure 50.28).
Position to initiate technique: The thoracic spine is flexed or extended within the neutral range, as needed, to localize the sagittal plane to the vertebral unit to be addressed. The patient is then sidebent right and rotated left until the restrictive barrier is engaged in all three planes.
Activation: Patient is instructed to turn to the right and/or sidebend to the left while the operator offers isometric resistance. The operator has the patient maintain the force long enough to sense that the patient's contractile force is localized at the dysfunctional segment (typically 3–5 seconds).
Follow-up: After simultaneously discontinuing isometric counterforces, the operator waits for the tissues to relax completely (1–2 seconds) and then moves the dysfunctional segment to the new restrictive barrier. Activation and follow-up are repeated until best motion is obtained (typically 3–5 times).

Mid–lower thoracic: indirect with respiratory co-operation

Diagnosis: T6 neutral, sidebending left, rotation right.
Patient position: Seated.
Operator position: Seated or standing behind patient.
Contact: Right thumb contacts the right transverse process of the lower vertebra of the dysfunctional unit; left thumb contacts the left transverse process of the upper vertebra of the dysfunctional unit (Figure 50.29).
Position to initiate technique: Patient leans backwards at the hips to establish firm contact, then sits up straighter or slouches forwards slightly to localize the sagittal plane at the dysfunctional vertebral unit. The patient is instructed to lean left or right in small increments until all three planes are at the point of BLT.
Activation: Test respiratory phases and instruct patient to hold breath (as long as possible) in the phase providing the best

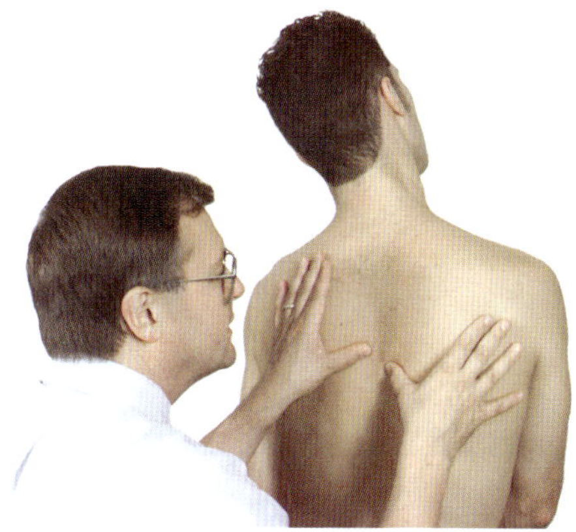

Figure 50.29 Mid–lower thoracic: indirect with respiratory co-operation (e.g. T6 N S_LR_R). (Kimberly and Funk 2000)

ligamentous balance. The physician makes continuous minor adjustments in the patient's position to maintain tissue balance.

Rib cage R3–12

Rib cage: HVLA

Diagnosis: Rib 4 exhalation somatic dysfunction on the right.
Patient position: Supine.
Operator position: Standing on opposite side.
Contact: Cross patient's arms in front of the chest, with the patient's forearm opposite the physician placed on top of the other forearm (Figure 50.30).
Position to initiate technique: Grasp patient's arms, roll patient to place thenar eminence, as a fulcrum, on the superior margin of the posterior angle of the rib involved, if single. In rib groups, the thenar eminence is placed on the highest rib of the group. Roll patient back onto the fulcrum hand which should apply caudal traction on the rib. Compress through the patient's upper arm to the fulcrum.
Activation: A HVLA thrust is applied from above while a caudal force on the angle of the rib is created by a quick wrist abduction or caudal motion.

Rib cage: muscle energy

Diagnosis: Rib 5 exhalation somatic dysfunction on the right.
Patient position: Supine.
Operator position: On same side as involved rib.
Contact: Hook fingers of caudad hand over the superior margin of the angle of the dysfunctional rib, or the upper rib of a group of exhalation ribs, and apply caudad tension (Figure 50.31).

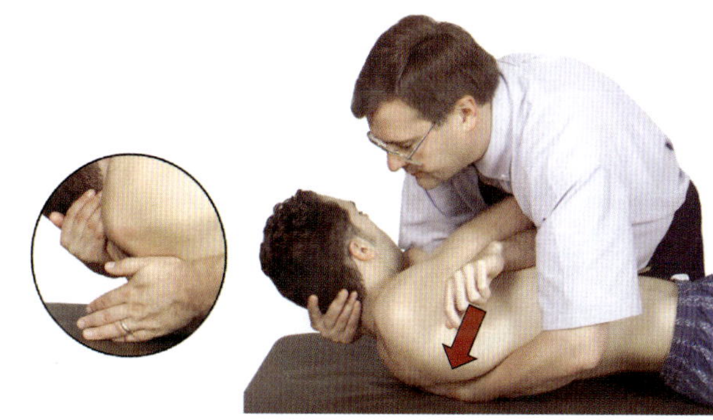

Figure 50.30 Rib cage: HVLA (e.g. right exhalation rib 4). (Kimberly and Funk 2000)

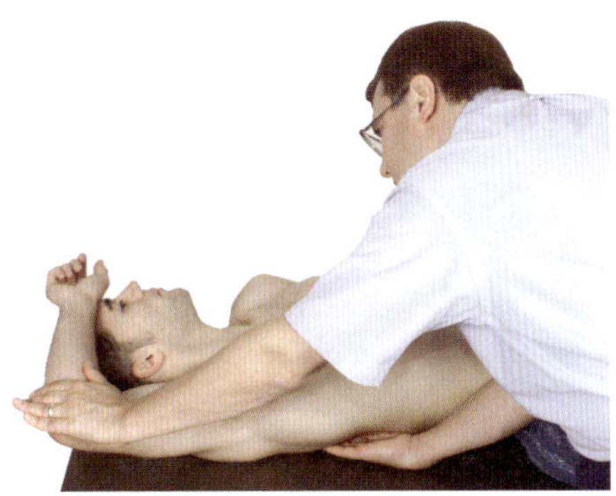

Figure 50.31 Rib cage: muscle energy (e.g. right exhalation rib 5). (Kimberly and Funk 2000).

Position to initiate technique: Patient's head is turned away from the dysfunctional rib; forearm is abducted and externally rotated to place the dorsal hand over the forehead on the side of the dysfunction; operator's cephalad hand holds patient's elbow and forearm.
Activation: Patient is instructed to press elbow into operator's hand at a vector that transfers the most muscle tension to the dysfunctional rib, while the physician offers isometric counterforce. (The direction of muscle energy activation is anteromedial to activate the pectoralis minor for treatment of ribs 3–5, anteroinferior to activate serratus anterior for treatment of ribs 6–9, and inferior towards hip to activate the latissimus dorsi to treat ribs 9–11.) Hold for 3–5 seconds, wait for tissues to relax completely, and then take up the slack with the caudad hand at the rib angle to the new restrictive barrier. Repeat a total of 3–5 times.

Rib cage: muscle energy

Diagnosis: Rib 6 inhalation somatic dysfunction on the right.
Patient position: Supine.
Operator position: Near head of table on same side as involved rib.
Contact: Hook fingers of cephalad hand over the inferior margin of the angle of the dysfunctional rib, or the lower rib of a group, and apply cephalad tension (Figure 50.32).

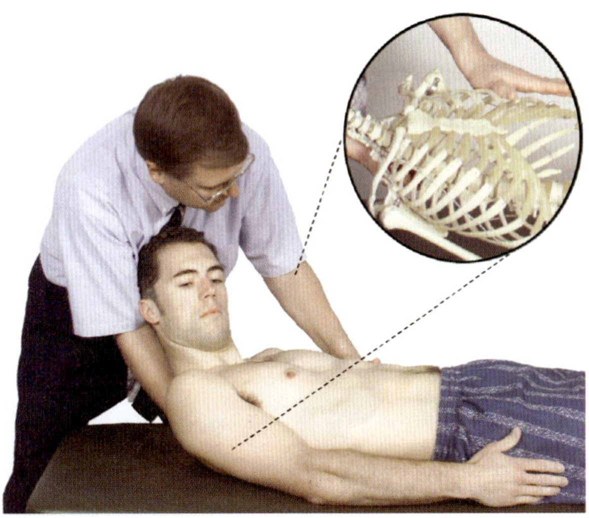

Figure 50.32 Rib cage: muscle energy (e.g. left inhalation rib 6). (Kimberly and Funk 2000)

Position to initiate technique: Patient's head is turned away from the dysfunctional rib with forearm placed along lateral or anterolateral thigh on the side of the dysfunction; operator's caudad hand contacts the anterolateral rib involved.
Activation: The patient exhales and reaches with the left hand towards the foot of the table at a vector that puts the most muscle tension on the dysfunctional rib. The physician offers isometric counterforce. Hold for 3–5 seconds.
Follow-up: As patient relaxes, wait for tissues to relax completely, and then take up the slack with both rib contacts to the new restrictive barrier. Repeat 3–5 times.

Rib cage: indirect with respiratory co-operation

Diagnosis: Rib 4 dysfunction (inhalation or exhalation).
Patient position: Supine or seated.
Operator position: Seated beside patient on side of involved rib.
Contact: Pass posterior hand behind the patient and contact the inferior aspect of the angle of the involved rib with the lateral margin of the index finger. Place lateral margin of index finger of the anterior hand on the superior aspect of the dysfunctional rib at the midclavicular line. The thumbs are on the shaft at the midaxillary line (Figure 50.33).
Position to initiate technique: Use both hands to simultaneously move the rib angle medial and anterior to the point of BLT. (Adjust towards inhalation in that dysfunction and towards exhalation in an exhalation dysfunction.)
Activation: Patient is instructed to inhale for an inhalation dysfunction (or exhale for exhalation dysfunction) with operator continuously adjusting tension as needed to maintain ligamentous balance until tissues release and dysfunction resolves.
Follow-up: Repeat as needed.

Sternum

Sternum: indirect 'stacking' technique

Diagnosis: Somatic dysfunction in sagittal, coronal, and horizontal planes of the manubrium and of the sternal body; manubriosternal dysfunction; (useful after motor vehicle accident with seat harness, after sternotomy, and after cardiopulmonary chest compressions).
Patient position: Supine.
Operator position: Standing beside patient.
Contact: Place the heel of one hand on the manubrium and the palm of the other hand on the sternal body with the fingers along its long axis (pointing towards the sternal angle) (Figure 50.34).

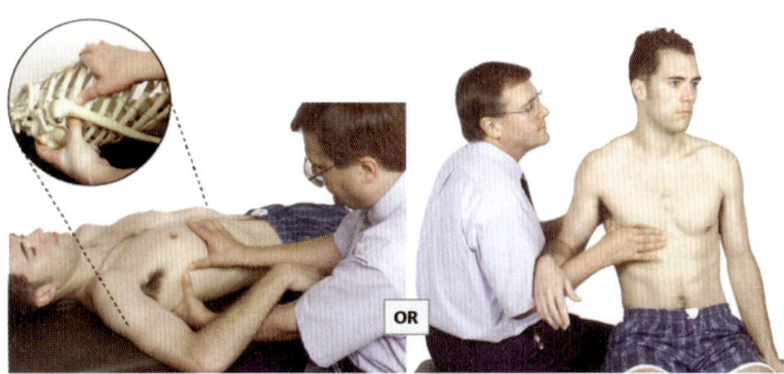

Figure 50.33 Rib cage: indirect with respiratory co-operation. (Kimberly and Funk 2000)

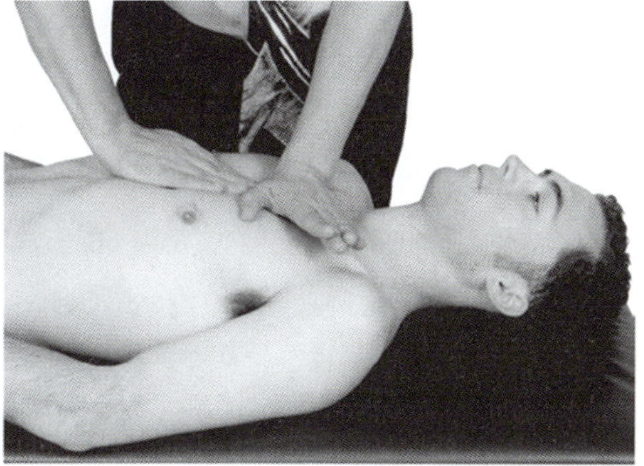

Figure 50.34 Sternum: indirect 'stacking' technique. (Kimberly and Funk 2000)

Position to initiate technique: Simultaneously carry both the sternal body and manubrium to the point of BLT.
Activation: Test respiratory phases instructing patient to hold the breath as long as possible in the phase that provides the best ligamentous balance. Make continuous minor adjustments between hands as the tissues release, to maintain ligamentous balance.

Sternum: 'plastic hand' indirect technique

Diagnosis: Restricted sternal motion within chest cage; (this is also a treatment for the superior mediastinum). **Patient position:** Supine.
Operator position: Seated at head of table.
Contact: Palm of one hand is placed over the sternum (heel of hand over the manubrium and the fingers on the sternal body along its long axis). The other hand is placed on the back extending from T1 to T4. Patient's head is supported by operator's forearm (Figure 50.35).
Position to initiate technique: Sternal hand carries sternum and overlying soft tissues to the point of BLT in three planes. The posterior hand provides counterforce and assists in positioning to ligamentous balance.
Activation: Test respiratory phases instructing patient to hold the breath as long as possible in the phase that provides the best ligamentous balance. Make continuous minor adjustments between hands as the tissues release, to maintain ligamentous balance.

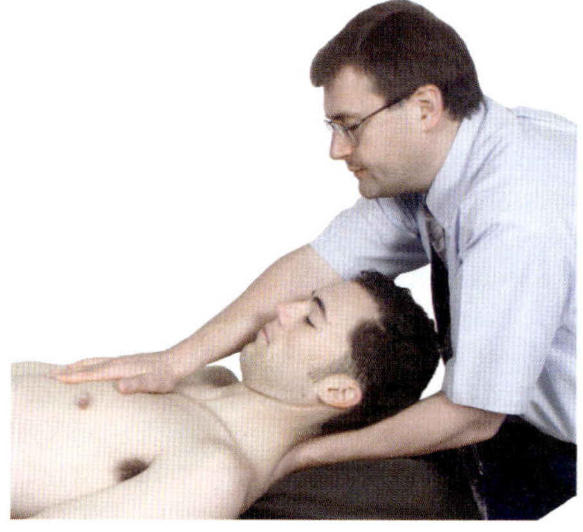

Figure 50.35 Sternum: 'plastic hand' indirect technique. (Kimberly and Funk 2000)

Thoracolumbar junction, inferior thoracic outlet, and lumbar spine

Thoracolumbar junction/inferior thoracic outlet

Thoracolumbar regional (indirect loading) myofascial release (including diaphragm redoming)

Diagnosis: Fascial dysfunction (left rotation and sidebending) of the inferior thoracic outlet region with or without diaphragm dysfunction.
Patient position: Supine.
Operator position: Standing on either side of the patient (Figure 50.36).
Contact no. 1 (lateral): Grasp the lateral sides of the patient's rib cage with palms, fingers spread apart.
Alternate contact no. 2 (anteroposterior): Place one hand posteriorly to cup L1–3 vertebral column, with fingers contacting paraspinal muscles on one side and the heel of the hand contacting the opposite muscles; fingers of the anterior hand broadly contact the subxiphoid region.
Position to initiate technique:

- **No. 1—lateral hand hold:** Carry the lower chest cage fasciae to the point of BLT by rotating and sidebending further to the left. Translate tissues right to create left sidebending while simultaneously rotating the lower chest cage and fasciae to the left.
- **No. 2—anteroposterior hand hold:** Rotate one hand clockwise and the opposite hand counterclockwise (whichever is indicated by testing fascial drag); also add any superior–inferior and left–right translation of the soft tissues needed to establish a sense of balance between anterior and posterior hands.

Activation: Closely monitor tissue balance with normal respiration and follow the tissues in their ease of motion as the patient exhales continuously, adjusting minor motions as the tissues release.
Follow-up: Hold through several respiratory cycles until tissues under both hands release completely (both hand holds) and there is a sense of equal motion during inhalation from both sides of the diaphragm (lateral hold).

Quadratus lumborum soft tissue/twelfth rib technique

Diagnosis: Left twelfth rib somatic dysfunction in downward pincer position **or** tight left quadratus lumborum muscle without rib dysfunction.
Patient position: Prone with the left arm extended and resting alongside their head; lower extremities moved to the patient's right to induce lumbar sidebending and traction to place the left quadratus lumborum muscle on tension.

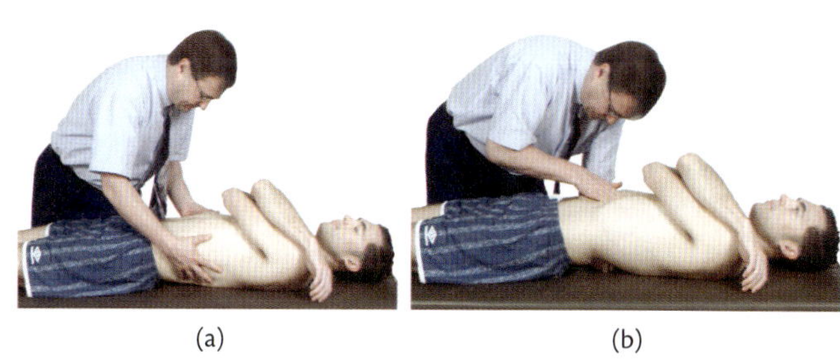

Figure 50.36 Thoracolumbar regional (indirect loading) myofascial release (including diaphragm redoming): (a) lateral hold; (b) anteroposterior hold. (Kimberly and Funk 2000)

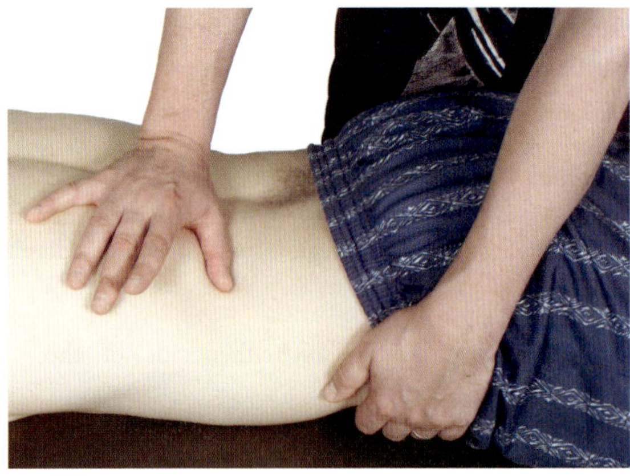

Figure 50.37 Quadratus lumborum soft tissue technique (e.g. hypertonic quadratus lumborum muscle or twelfth rib dysfunction in downward pincer position) (Kimberly and Funk 2000). Contact entire twelfth rib.

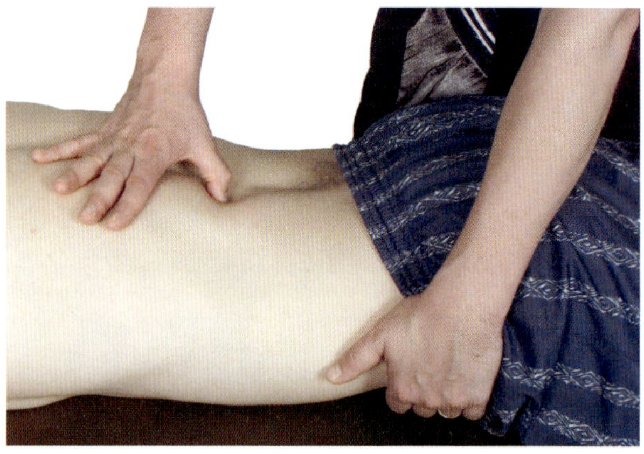

Figure 50.38 Thoracolumbar region/twelfth rib: muscle energy technique (left twelfth rib in upward pincer position) (Kimberly and Funk 2000). Contact costotransverse junction with thumb tip.

Operator position: On side opposite the involved rib (right side).
Contact: Contact the inferior margin of the shaft of the left twelfth rib with the full length of the right thumb to stabilize the entire rib. Grasp the anterior superior iliac spine (ASIS) with the left hand (Figure 50.37).
Position to initiate technique: Lift the pelvis with the left hand while the right thumb maintains an anterior and superior pressure against the twelfth rib at the restrictive barrier.
Activation: Instruct the patient to pull their ASIS towards the table, against isometric resistance.
Follow-up: After activation, the patient relaxes and new barriers are engaged to repeat the procedure until the quadratus releases the rib (typically 3–5 times).

Thoracolumbar region/twelfth rib: muscle energy technique

Diagnosis: Left twelfth rib in upward pincer position.
Patient position: Prone with lower extremities positioned to induce right lumbar sidebending and traction to place the left quadratus lumborum muscle on tension.
Operator position: Standing on side opposite involved rib (patient's right side in this example).
Contact: Place right thumb pad near the costotransverse joint of rib 12 to serve as a fulcrum; left hand grasps the left ASIS (Figure 50.38).
Position to initiate technique: Lift pelvis until tension is palpated at fulcrum.
Activation: As patient exhales, operator further lifts the hip posteriorly (to new tissue tension). The quadratus lumborum will pull the rib shaft in a caudad direction rotating around the fulcrum into an exhalation position.
Follow-up: Repeat until the best motion is obtained (typically 3–5 times).

Lumbar spine L1–5

Lumbar: HVLA

Diagnosis: L2 neutral, sidebending left, rotation right (L2 N_E S_LR_R).
Patient position: Left lateral recumbent.
Operator position: Standing in front of the patient.
Contact: Fingers of right hand monitor motion, contacting the interspinous ligament of the dysfunctional segment (Figure 50.39).
Position to initiate technique: Draw the patient's knees and hips into flexion until motion is palpated at the dysfunctional segment (Figure 50.39a). Grasp patient's ankles and lift them towards the ceiling to sidebend the lumbosacral region until localized at the dysfunctional segment (Figure 50.39b). This introduces right sidebending below the dysfunction. Ask the patient to straighten the left lower extremity (Figure 50.39c). Pull the patient's left shoulder superiorly (Figure 50.39d) to maintain right sidebending. Without increasing or decreasing the sagittal plane position, pull the shoulder anteriorly (Figure 50.39e) to rotate the thoracic and upper lumbar spine down to the dysfunctional site. As shown in Figure 50.39f, the physician's right forearm is placed in front of the patient's right shoulder with the patient's right forearm resting over the physician's. Tension is focused on the dysfunctional segment by rolling the lower half of the patient slightly forwards while maintaining posterior pressure against the patient's right shoulder and simultaneous anterosuperior pressure against the patient's pelvis behind the greater trochanter. Optimally, this will be accomplished by the physician's upper torso turning as a unit in a counterclockwise direction around the fingers localized at the site of dysfunction.
Activation: A sidebending HVLA thrust is applied anterosuperiorly to the pelvis while providing counterforce through the patient's shoulder. Because the patient is rolled slightly forwards to vertically align the plane of the facet joints, this allows the activating force to be directed towards the floor.

Lumbar: HVLA

Diagnosis: L2 non-neutral, flexion, rotation left, sidebending left (L2 NN_F R_LS_L).
Patient position: seated straddling table, maintaining shoulders over hips as much as possible for balance throughout procedure.
Operator position: standing behind and to patient's right.
Contact: The physician's left hypothenar eminence is placed on the left transverse process of the dysfunctional segment, bracing the left elbow on the left hip for support (Figure 50.40).
Position to initiate technique: The physician's right axilla or anterior shoulder is placed over the cap of the patient's right shoulder while reaching across the chest to grasp the patient's left shoulder. Pull the patient's left shoulder forwards to induce the varying increments of right rotation needed for individualized localization. Introduce right sidebending to the barrier by depressing the patient's right shoulder and by simultaneously translating the lumbar

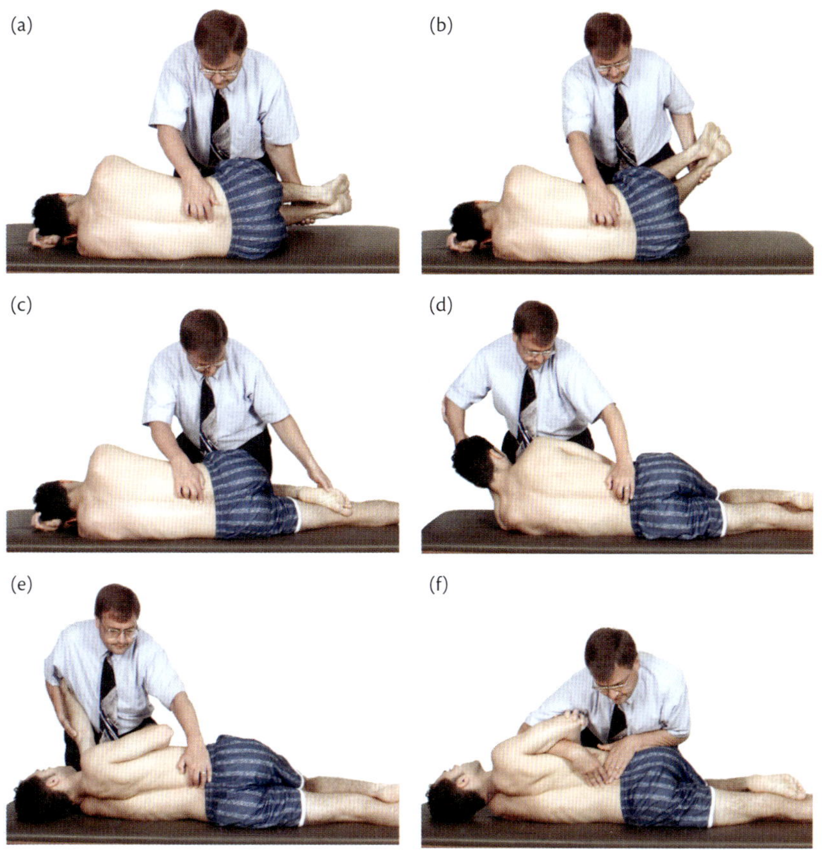

Figure 50.39 Lumbar: HVLA. See text for details. (Kimberly and Funk 2000)

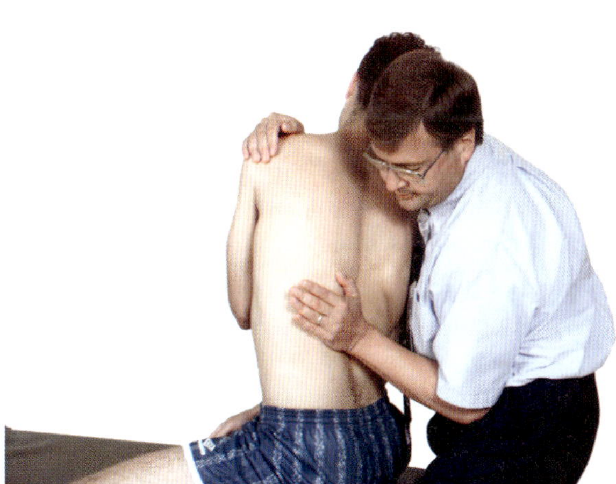

Figure 50.40 Lumbar: HVLA (e.g. L2 F $R_L S_L$). (Kimberly and Funk 2000)

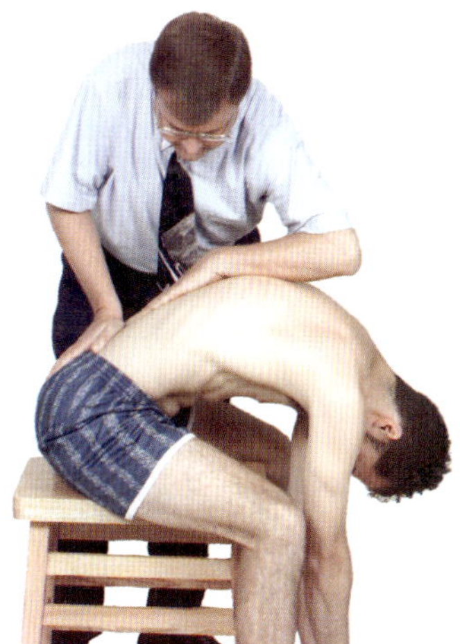

Figure 50.41 Lumbar: muscle energy (e.g. L3 E). (Kimberly and Funk 2000)

region using the hypothenar eminence of the left braced arm. Add sagittal plane localization to fully engage the restrictive barrier.
Activation: HVLA thrust is directed anteriorly and superiorly by introducing a full body motion through the left braced hypothenar eminence.

Lumbar: muscle energy

Diagnosis: L3 extension (L3 E).
Patient position: Seated on stool with knees apart.
Operator position: Standing beside the patient.
Contact: Physician's caudad hand contacts the lumbar spine (or sacrum) one segment below the dysfunctional segment. Physician uses the other hand to apply superior traction in the midline and to tap the patient's back over the spine of the dysfunctional segment to inform the patient where to concentrate their attempts at motion (Figure 50.41).
Position to initiate technique: Patient bends forwards allowing hands to fall towards the floor.

Activation: Patient is instructed to 'arch your back like a cat' to push the identified site posteriorly while the physician provides isometric counterforce (typically 3–5 seconds).
Follow-up: Upon simultaneous relaxation, wait for tissues to relax completely and then increase flexion to the new restrictive barrier. Repeat until the best motion is obtained (typically 3–5 times).

Lumbar: muscle energy

Diagnosis: L2 neutral, sidebending left, rotation right (L2 $N_E S_L R_R$).
Patient position: Seated on stool or straddling table, maintaining shoulders over hips as much as possible for balance throughout procedure.
Operator position: Standing behind and to patient's left side.
Contact: Place right thumb pad on transverse process of the dysfunctional segment to monitor motion and provide a fulcrum; reach across the patient's chest with left hand to grasp the patient's right shoulder or arm (Figure 50.42).
Position to initiate technique: Use patient's left shoulder to induce varying increments of left rotation, right sidebending, and flexion or extension to fully engage the restrictive barrier.
Activation: Patient is instructed to gently bend to the left **or** turn to the right, localized against an isometric counterforce through the physician's thumb (typically 3–5 seconds).
Follow-up: Upon simultaneous relaxation, wait for tissues to relax completely, reposition all planes to the new restrictive barrier, and repeat until the best motion is obtained (typically 3–5 times).

Lumbar: muscle energy

Diagnosis: L2 non-neutral with flexion, rotation left, sidebending left (L2 $NN_F R_L S_L$).
Patient position: Seated straddling table, maintaining shoulders over hips as much as possible for balance throughout procedure.
Operator position: Standing or seated behind.
Contact: Left thumb pad contacts the right side of the spinous process of the dysfunctional segment to induce right rotation (Figure 50.43).
Position to initiate technique: Physician's right hand grasps the patient's right shoulder and guides the patient's lumbar spine into right sidebending, right rotation, and extension, as needed, until all three planes are localized at the restrictive barrier.

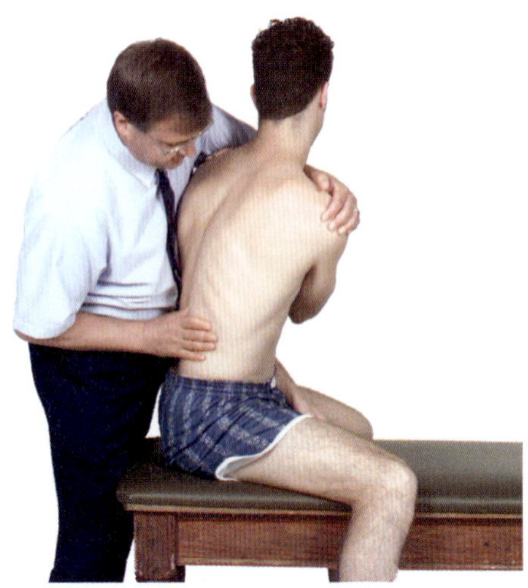

Figure 50.42 Lumbar: muscle energy (e.g. L2 N $S_L R_R$). (Kimberly and Funk 2000)

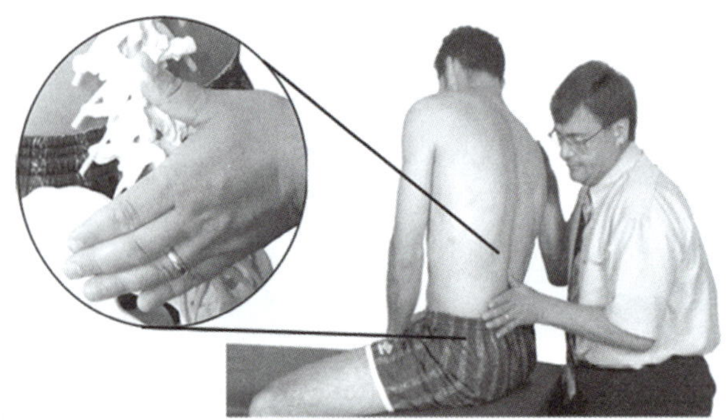

Figure 50.43 Lumbar: muscle energy (e.g. L2 $NN_F R_L S_L$). (Kimberly and Funk 2000)

Activation: Patient is instructed to gently bend to the left **or** turn to the left, localized against an isometric counterforce through the physician's thumb (typically 3–5 seconds).
Follow-up: Upon simultaneous relaxation, wait for tissues to relax completely, reposition all planes to the new restrictive barrier, and repeat until the best motion is obtained (typically 3–5 times).

Lumbar: indirect with respiratory co-operation

Diagnosis: L1 neutral, sidebending left, rotation right (L1 $N_E S_L R_R$).
Patient position: Supine
Operator position: Seated to patient's right.
Contact: Reach under patient and place the pad of a finger on the left transverse process of the dysfunctional segment (Figure 50.44).
Position to initiate technique: Patient is instructed to arch or flatten back to BLT in the sagittal plane. Physician applies anterior pressure against the left transverse process (creating right rotation) and pulls the area gently towards him/her (creating left sidebending) to the point of BLT.
Activation: The respiratory phases are tested and the breath is held as long as possible in the phase providing optimal ligamentous balance. The physician continuously makes minor adjustments in all three planes, as needed, to maintain BLT as release is palpated.
Follow-up: Positioning and activation may be required through more than one respiratory session to reintroduce motion.

Lumbar: indirect with respiratory co-operation

Diagnosis: L2 non-neutral, rotation left, sidebending left (L2 $NN_F R_L S_L$).

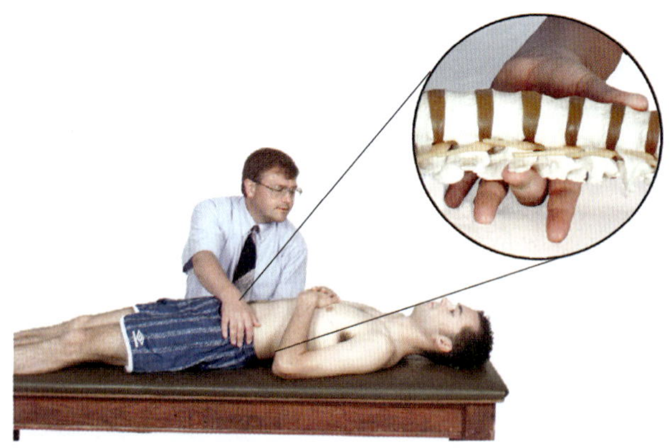

Figure 50.44 Lumbar: indirect with respiratory co-operation (e.g. L1 $N_E S_L R_R$). (Kimberly and Funk 2000)

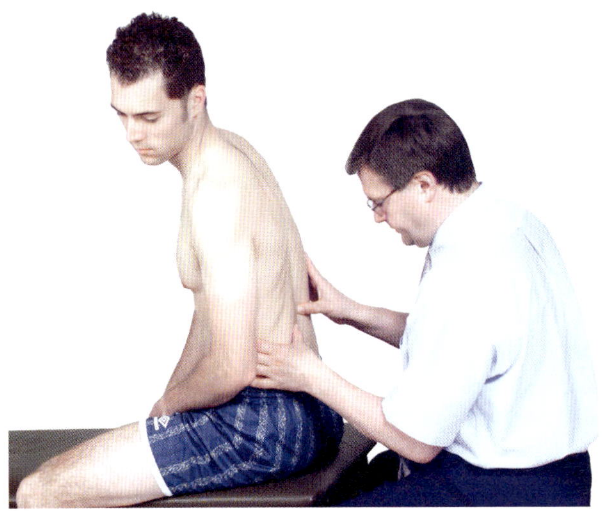

Figure 50.45 Lumbar: indirect with respiratory co-operation (e.g. L2 $NN_F R_L S_L$). (Kimberly and Funk 2000)

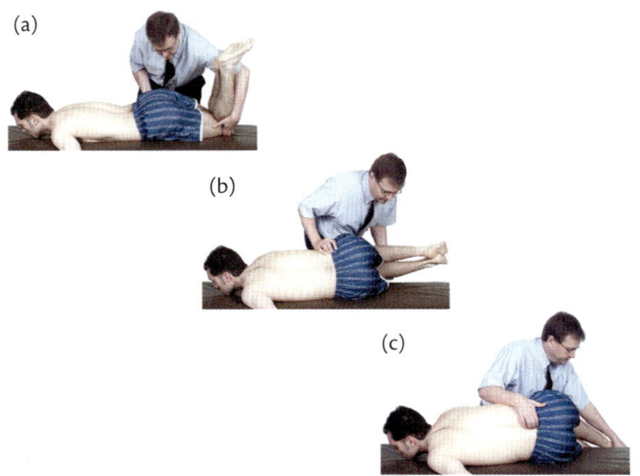

Figure 50.46 Lumbopelvic region: muscle energy or springing (low-velocity, moderate-amplitude) physiological method (e.g. left sacral torsion). (Kimberly and Funk 2000)

Patient position: Seated.
Operator position: Seated behind patient.
Contact: Physician's left thumb pad contacts the left transverse process of the lower segment of the dysfunctional unit; the right thumb pad contacts the right transverse process of the upper segment (Figure 50.45).
Position to initiate technique: Patient is instructed to lean backwards against both thumbs and then to slump slightly to localize the sagittal plane. Further patient instruction to slightly bend to the left and/or to turn to the left accompanies slight additional pressure through the right thumb (to create left rotation of the dysfunctional segment). Fine-tune these minor positional and pressure changes to achieve optimal BLT.
Activation: The respiratory phases are tested and the breath is held as long as possible in the phase providing optimal ligamentous balance. The physician continuously makes minor adjustments in all three planes, as needed, to maintain ligamentous balance as release is palpated.
Follow-up: Positioning and activation may be required through more than one respiratory cycle to reintroduce motion.

Lumbopelvic junction and pelvis

Lumbopelvic junction

Lumbopelvic region: muscle energy or springing (low-velocity, moderate- amplitude) physiological method

Diagnosis: Left on left lumbosacral 'torsion' (this is a combined diagnosis of L5 $NS_L R_R$ **and** the sacrum rotating left around a left oblique sacral axis).
Patient position: Prone.
Operator position: Standing at patient's right side.
Preparation for technique: Patient flexes knees and raises the right hip (Figure 50.46a) as the physician flexes the hips to at least 90° and guides the knees to the right side of the table (Figure 50.46b).
Contact: Physician supports the patient's knees on his/her right thigh to provide a fulcrum for the activating force and to protect the patient's thigh from the edge of the table.
Position to initiate technique: Physician monitors motion and flexes the hips until motion localizes at the lumbosacral junction. Physician grasps the spinous process of L5 with the fingers of the right hand to induce left rotation of vertebral bodies and lets the legs drop over the fulcrum, inducing left sidebending.
Activation: Low-velocity, moderate-amplitude springing is applied towards the floor to the patient's feet or legs. Physician uses right hand to pull the spinous process of L5 into rotation left. (Alternatively, activation may benefit from respiratory activation in which the patient inhales and upon exhalation, reaches for the floor with the right hand; **or** the patient is instructed, 'Lift your feet towards the ceiling' while the physician offers isometric counterforce for 3–5 seconds.)
Follow-up: Repositioning to the new barrier in all three planes is usually required with 2–4 repeated activations. Physician carefully assists the patient to the prone position again, with the legs extended on the table.

Lumbopelvic region: springing (low-velocity, moderate-amplitude) or muscle energy physiological method

Diagnosis: Right on left lumbosacral torsion (this is a combined diagnosis of L5 $NNR_L S_L$ **and** the sacrum rotating right around a left oblique sacral axis).
Patient position: Left lateral recumbent.
Operator position: Standing in front of the patient.
Position to initiate technique: Patient's left shoulder is drawn forwards to induce right rotation down to the lumbosacral junction and the physician's right forearm stabilizes the patient's upper body. Patient's knees and hips are flexed just enough to allow the legs and feet to drop downwards over the edge of the table. (Alternatively, the top lower extremity alone might be dropped over the edge of the table.) Flexion must be slight so that non-neutral sacral mechanics will not be induced.
Contact: Fingers of the right hand monitor the lumbosacral junction and sacral base (Figure 50.47).
Activation: Patient is instructed to breathe in. As they subsequently exhale, the physician pushes the patient's right shoulder further posteriorly and springs the feet towards the floor, increasing the left sidebending. Alternatively, the physician may instruct the patient to lift their ankles towards the ceiling against isometric resistance (held 3–5 seconds) localized to the physician's monitoring hand.

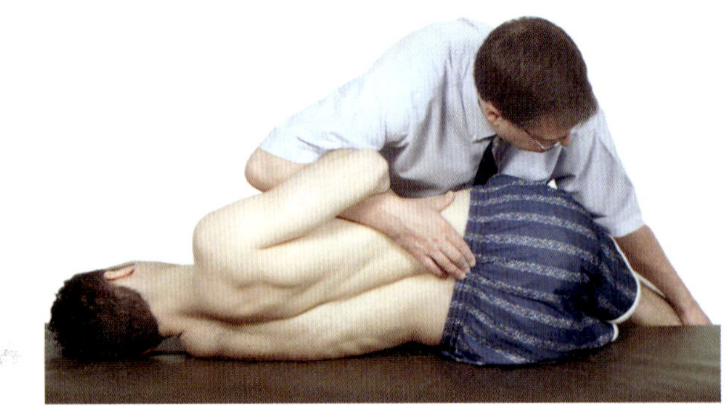

Figure 50.47 Lumbopelvic region: springing (low-velocity, moderate-amplitude) or muscle energy physiological method (e.g. right rotation on left oblique axis or right backwards torsion). (Kimberly and Funk 2000)

Follow-up: repeat one or both activating forces until the best motion is obtained (typically 3–5 times). Assist back to lateral recumbent position.

Sacrum

Sacrum: HVLA

Note: This technique is contraindicated in a patient with primary or metastatic bone cancer, severe arthritis of the hip or knee, or an artificial knee or hip.
Diagnosis: Left unilateral sacral flexion **or** left superior (upslipped) innominate shear.
Patient position: Supine.
Operator position: Standing at foot of the table.
Contact: Physician places a pressure pad (such as a small rolled towel) under the left inferolateral angle (ILA) so the patient's body weight moves the left ILA anteriorly and stabilizes the sacrum. Physician grasps the left leg just above the ankle with both hands (Figure 50.48).
Position to initiate technique: Physician abducts (tight packs) the leg slightly and internally rotates (loose packs) the hip to gap the sacroiliac joint. With the patient relaxing, traction along the long axis of the lower extremity is applied to localize forces up to the pelvis. The patient is instructed to take a very deep and full breath but with pelvic and lower extremity muscles relaxed. (Sometimes, mildly shaking the patient's leg along with the continued traction helps the physician to sense relaxation of the patient's muscles and localization to the restrictive barrier.) **Activation:** An HVLA longitudinal tug is applied through the lower extremity to gap the sacroiliac joint and glide the innominate inferior in relation to the sacrum.

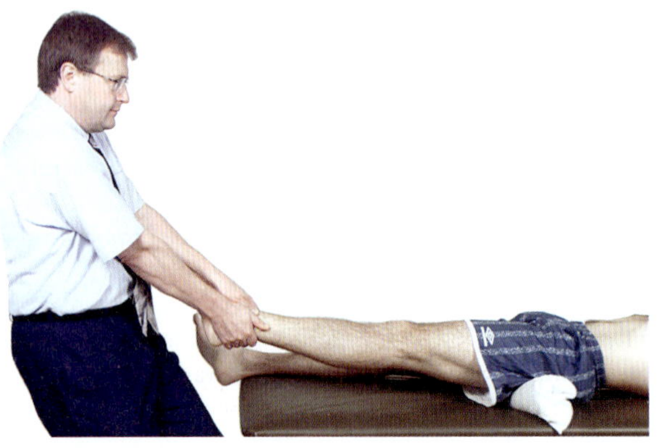

Figure 50.48 Sacrum: HVLA (e.g. left sacral shear or left superior innominate shear). (Kimberly and Funk 2000)

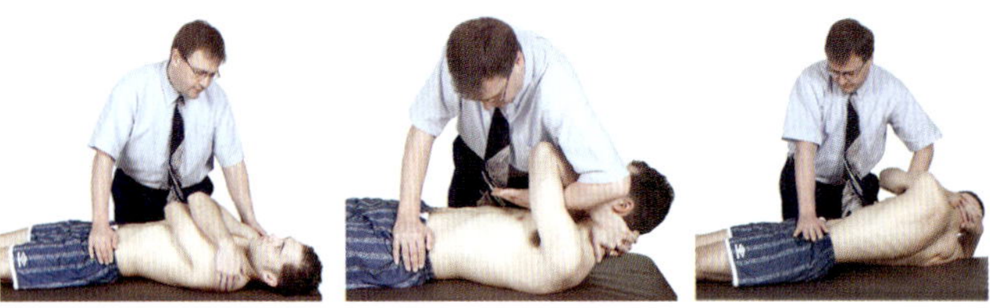

Figure 50.49 Sacrum: HVLA (e.g. left sacral margin posterior). (Kimberly and Funk 2000)

Sacrum: HVLA

Diagnosis: Left sacral margin posterior.
Patient position: Supine with hands clasped behind neck.
Operator position: Standing on the side opposite the dysfunction (the right side, in this example).
Initial positioning: Pull the patient's hips towards the operator and push their legs and shoulders away to create left sidebending (concavity on the side of the posterior sacral margin).
Contact: Physician bends over the patient, reaches across to insert the cephalad (left, in this example) hand and forearm, from lateral to medial, into the space between the patient's arm and forearm, resting the dorsum of the left hand on the patient's chest. Physician's other hand cups the patient's ASIS on the side of the posterior margin (Figure 50.49).
Position to initiate technique: Physician rotates the patient's torso towards him/her to induce right rotation of the spine and sacrum sufficiently to just initiate a lift of the innominate off the table. The innominate is carried posteriorly by the physician's right hand to reach and maintain a restrictive barrier.
Activation: At the moment the innominate starts to lift, an HVLA thrust is applied posteriorly through the ASIS. (Note that the initial sidebent positioning assures that the thoracolumbar spine will be essentially vertical to the sacrum and pelvis at the time that the thrust is applied.)

Sacrum: HVLA

Diagnosis: Bilateral sacral extension (sacral base posterior).
Patient position: Prone, supporting upper trunk on elbows (the patient's chin may be cradled in the palms of their hands to increase lumbar extension).
Operator position: Standing at the side of the table near the patient's knees.
Contact: Physician places the heel of the cephalad (left, in this example) hand on the sacral base; the other hand provides a counterforce with placement on the patient's ankle or leg (Figure 50.50).
Position to initiate technique: The sacral base is carried anteriorly to the restrictive barrier as the physician leans simultaneously onto the sacrum and lower extremity to apply a traction counterforce between both contact hands. The patient is instructed to take a very deep breath while the physician resists the posterior motion of the sacral base and then exhale while the physician follows the sacral base anteriorly.

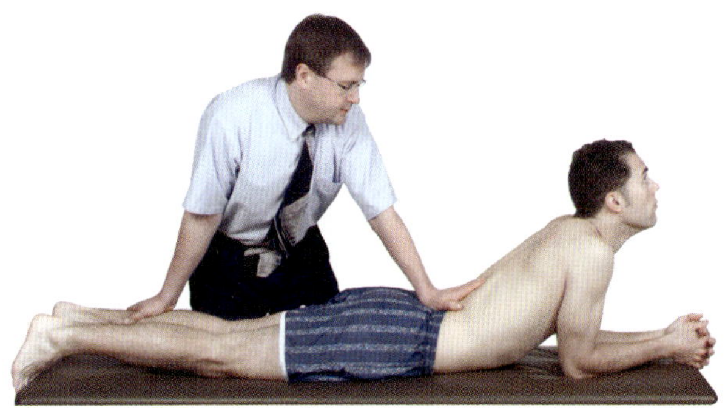

Figure 50.50 Sacrum: HVLA (e.g. sacral base posterior). (Kimberly and Funk 2000)

Activation: At full exhalation, while maintaining traction between both contact hands, the physician applies a HVLA anterior thrust to the sacral base.

Sacrum: muscle energy

Diagnosis: Bilateral sacral extension (sacral base posterior).
Patient position: Seated with knees apart; the lumbosacral junction is flexed and the patient's arms are allowed to hang freely.
Operator position: Standing beside patient.
Contact: Physician places his/her caudad (left, in this example) hand on the patient's sacrum with the heel of that hand below the middle transverse axis of the sacrum. (It helps if this hand can grasp the edge of the stool with fingertips to allow better stabilization of the sacrum.) Physician places cephalad (right, in this example) forearm along the vertebral column.
Position to initiate technique: Traction is applied through the cephalad arm, and caudad hand stabilizes the sacrum.
Activation: Patient is instructed to push the lowest portion of their back backwards (localized at the lumbosacral junction) while the physician offers isometric counterforce (typically for 3–5 seconds).
Follow-up: Physician waits for the tissues to relax completely (1–2 seconds) and then flexes the lumbosacral joint to the new restrictive barrier. The technique is repeated until the best motion is obtained (typically 3–5 times).

Sacrum: indirect with respiratory co-operation

Diagnosis: Sacrum left on a left oblique axis.
Patient position: Supine.
Operator position: Seated at the patient's left side (Figure 50.51b).
Initial positioning: Physician has the patient flex the right leg. Physician grasps the right knee, further flexes it and pulls it towards him/her, rolling the patient's hips towards the side of the table. This allows the physician to easily place a left hand under the sacrum. The patient is rolled back to a supine position with both legs extended.
Contact: The physician's fingers are specifically placed at the sacral base (typically with the index and ring fingers over the right and left aspects of S1 respectively) and the palm cupping the sacral apex. The physician's cephalad (right, in this example) hand may be used with the same forearm to bridge and compress the ASISs towards one another, attempting to 'gap' both sacroiliac joints (Figure 50.51a), or may alternatively be placed under the sacrum to reinforce the left lifting fingers (Figure 50.51c).
Position to initiate technique: Physician lifts the index (and possibly the middle) finger of the left hand, applying anterior pressure to the right sacral base (at S1) to the point of BLT. This rotates the sacrum to the left on the left oblique axis. Adjustments of flexion and extension may also be needed to obtain the best ligamentous balance. **Activation:** The respiratory phases are tested and the patient is instructed to hold the phase that provides the best ligamentous balance for as long as possible. As tissues release, the physician continuously modifies finger/hand pressures to ensure that the minor motions of the joint are maintained at the shifting point of BLT.
Follow-up: The technique may be repeated until the best possible motion is obtained.

Sacrum: indirect with respiratory co-operation

Diagnosis: Sacrum right on a left oblique axis.
Patient position: Supine.
Operator position: Seated at the patient's right side (Figure 50.52b).
Initial positioning: Physician has the patient flex the left leg. Physician grasps the left knee, further flexes it and pulls it towards him/her, rolling the patient's hips towards the side of the table. This allows the physician to easily place a right hand under the sacrum. The patient is rolled back to a supine position with both legs extended. **Contact:** The physician's fingers are specifically placed at the sacral base (typically with the index and ring fingers over the left and right aspects of S1 respectively) and the palm cupping the sacral apex. The physician's cephalad (left, in this example) hand may be used with the same forearm to bridge and compress the

(a) (c) (b)

Figure 50.51 Sacrum: indirect with respiratory co-operation (e.g. left rotation on a left oblique axis). (Kimberly and Funk 2000)

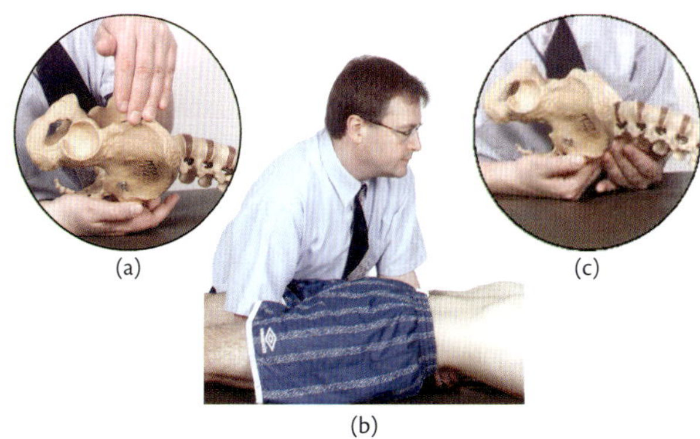

Figure 50.52 Sacrum: indirect with respiratory co-operation (e.g. sacral rotation right on a left oblique axis). (Kimberly and Funk 2000)

ASISs towards one another, attempting to 'gap' both sacroiliac joints (Figure 50.52a), or may alternatively be placed to reduce lumbosacral pressure (Figure 50.52c).
Position to initiate technique: Physician lifts the thenar eminence of the right hand, applying anterior pressure to the left ILA, encouraging right rotation on the left oblique axis to the point of BLT. Adjustments of flexion and extension may also be needed to obtain the best ligamentous balance.
Activation: The respiratory phases are tested and the patient is instructed to hold the phase that provides the best ligamentous balance for as long as possible. As tissues release, the physician continuously modifies finger/hand pressures to ensure that the minor motions of the joint are maintained at the shifting point of BLT.
Follow-up: The technique may be repeated until the best possible motion is obtained.

Sacrum: counterstrain

Diagnosis: Tender point over one sacral pole.
Patient position: Supine.
Operator position: Standing at the patient's side.
Contact: While contacting the tender pole with one finger, place the heel of the opposite hand (pisiform or thenar) in point contact with the sacrum over the pole diagonal to the involved pole; for example, for left lower pole tenderness, contact the right upper pole.
Position to initiate technique: Pressure is applied through the heel of the hand until pressure with the monitoring single digit elicits tenderness at the original point that is reduced by 70% or more.
Activation: Maintain for a period of 90 seconds that amount of pressure through the heel of the hand needed to reduce the point tenderness by 70%, with no pressure through the digit monitoring the tender point. After 90 seconds, gradually release the pressure.
Follow-up: Recheck to ensure that there is only 30% or less tenderness at the original site. It is possible to repeat the technique or select another approach to affect arthrodial somatic dysfunction. Alternatively, the possibility of a posterior sacroiliac ligament strain might be considered.

Sacrum: direct method—respiratory force and low-velocity, medium-amplitude (springing)

Diagnosis: Left unilateral sacral flexion (left inferior sacral shear).
Patient position: Prone.
Operator position: Standing on the side of the dysfunction (patient's left, in this example).
Contact: Physician places his/her thumb or fingers over the left sacroiliac joint to monitor motion. Physician positions self against the medial aspect of the patient's flexed leg to maintain internal rotation at the hip and left innominate. Physician places his/her right hypothenar eminence on the inferior aspect of the patient's left ILA and applies superior and anterior pressure (avoid pressure on the coccyx). The right hand may be reinforced with the left or, alternatively (as shown in Figure 50.53), the left fingers may pull laterally on the posterior superior iliac spine (PSIS) to enhance gapping of the sacroiliac joint (Figure 50.53).
Position to initiate technique: Physician flexes the patient's knee, then abducts and internally rotates the hip until gapping is palpated at the left sacroiliac joint. The knee is placed back onto the table at that point.
Activation: Patient is instructed to take a very deep breath. When they think they have taken a full breath, challenge them to add even further inhalation to completely encourage the sacral base to move

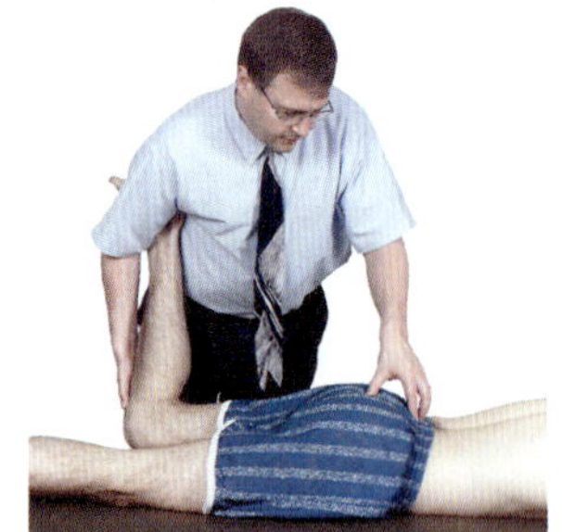
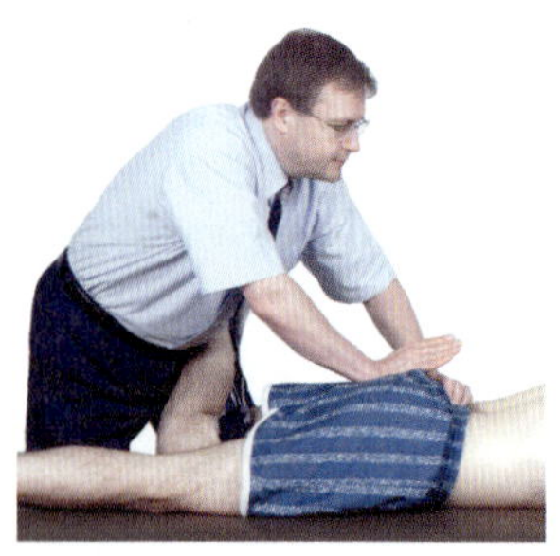

Figure 50.53 Sacrum: direct method— respiratory force and low-velocity, medium-amplitude (springing) (e.g. left unilateral sacral flexion). (Kimberly and Funk 2000)

posteriorly and engage the restrictive barrier. While relaxed but still holding the breath at full inhalation, the physician applies a superior and anterior low-velocity, medium-amplitude springing force through the left ILA.
Follow-up: The physician instructs the patient to exhale while maintaining a superior and anterior pressure on the left ILA. The activation procedure is repeated immediately another two times or until motion and better symmetry are re-established.

Sacrum: articulatory technique with respiratory co-operation

Note: This technique is especially useful in the severe sacral base anterior somatic dysfunction that may complicate late-term pregnancy or the postpartum period.
Diagnosis: Bilateral sacral flexion (anterior sacral base).
Patient position: supine with knees and hips flexed, feet flat on the table, and knees slightly apart.
Operator position: Standing at the side of the patient.
Preparatory positioning: Patient lifts the pelvis off the table to allow the physician to place a hand between the thighs and under the sacrum.
Contact: The physician's index, middle, and ring fingers of one hand contact on the sacral base above the middle transverse axis with the palm positioned at the sacral apex. The opposite forearm and fingertips bridge the ASIS, applying compression to bring the ASISs together and to attempt to 'gap' the sacroiliac joints bilaterally (Figure 50.54).
Position to initiate technique: After physician hand and arm placements, the patient's pelvis is lowered to the table and the knees are allowed to fall laterally and the soles of the feet are brought together (sometimes called the 'frog' position).
Activation: Patient is instructed to take a deep breath and hold it as the physician applies long axis traction down the arm holding the sacrum. This directly rotates the sacrum posteriorly. While the physician maintains traction, the patient (with knees hanging laterally) is instructed to exhale while rapidly sliding both feet simultaneously towards the foot of the table. The final position will result

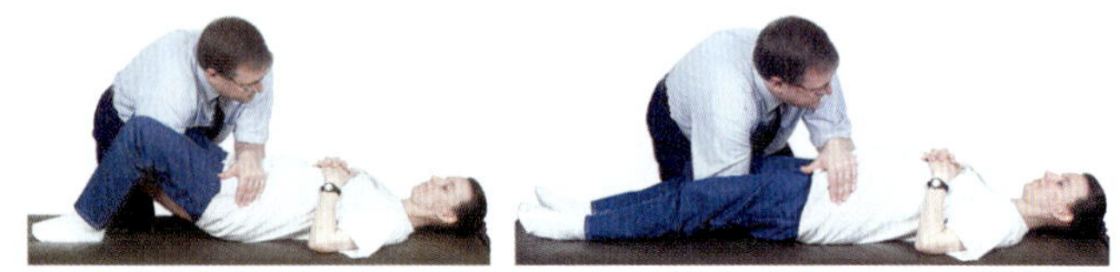

Figure 50.54 Sacrum: articulatory technique with respiratory co-operation (e.g. anterior sacral base). (Kimberly and Funk 2000)

in the physician still maintaining traction (to encourage a posterior position of the sacral base) and the patient will have an anatomical supine position with both lower extremities fully extended.

Follow-up: The patient can be instructed in a sacral gapping exercise in the supine position, hips and knees bent with feet on the floor spaced slightly more than shoulder width, but knees together. The patient's long, deep breaths help to rock the sacrum around transverse axes.

Pubic symphysis

Pubic symphysis: muscle energy

Diagnosis: Left inferior pubic shear.

Patient position: Supine.

Operator position: Standing on side of dysfunction (patient's left).

Contact: Patient's left knee is placed against the physician's chest. Physician cups the right hand over the patient's left ASIS and grasps the left ischial tuberosity with the other hand (Figure 50.55).

Position to initiate technique: The left lower extremity is flexed at the knee and hip and the thigh is abducted with just enough tension to gently 'gap' at the pubic symphysis. Rotate the innominate posteriorly (which carries the pubic ramus superiorly to the restrictive barrier) using the physician's hand contacts with the ASIS and ischial tuberosity and the chest contact with the patient's knee.

Activation: Patient is instructed to try to reposition their lower extremity back to the resting position by pushing inferiorly and medially through their knee against an isometric counterforce provided by the physician's chest (typically for 3–5 seconds). Concentric contraction of the hamstrings into the ischial tuberosity helps rotate the pelvis, while contraction of the ipsilateral adductor helps focus a gapping force at the pubic symphysis. (If the pelvis starts to roll, the ischial tuberosity hand can be shifted to stabilize at the opposite ASIS.)

Follow-up: Physician waits for tissues to relax completely (1–2 seconds) and then rotates the innominate posteriorly to the new restrictive barrier using both contact hands and chest. This carries the pubic ramus superiorly. Repeat until the best motion is obtained (typically 3–5 times).

Pubic symphysis: muscle energy

Diagnosis: Right superior pubic shear.

Patient position: Supine with the dysfunctional side near the edge of the table.

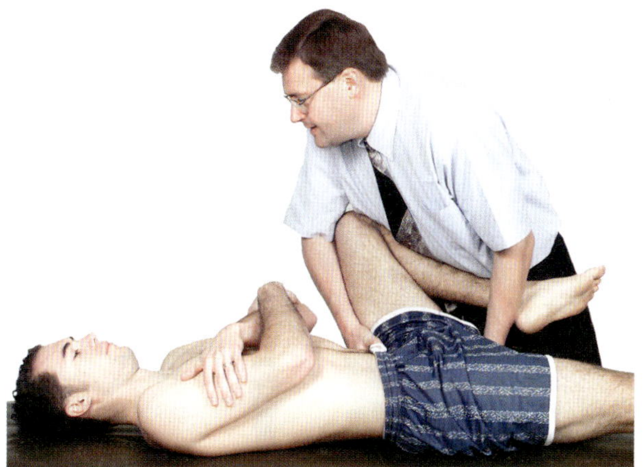

Figure 50.55 Pubic symphysis: muscle energy (e.g. left inferior pubic shear). (Kimberly and Funk 2000)

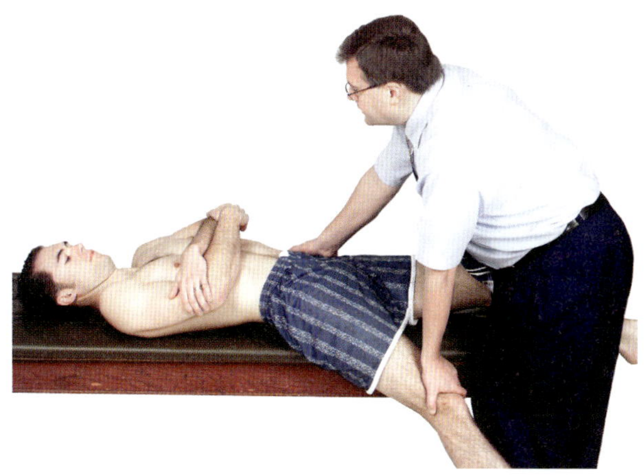

Figure 50.56 Pubic symphysis: muscle energy (e.g. right superior pubic shear). (Kimberly and Funk 2000)

Operator position: Standing on the side of the dysfunction (patient's right).

Contact: Physician instructs the patient to move to the edge of the table until the right ischial tuberosity is over the edge and then contacts the opposite (left) ASIS to stabilize the left hemipelvis. The patient may feel the need to 'hold on' to the table with one or both hands for stability. Physician's left hand is placed above the knee of the right (dysfunctional) extremity (Figure 50.56).

Position to initiate technique: Physician abducts the right lower extremity to localize 'gapping' at the pubic symphysis. The thigh is extended off the table to tissue tension. (This rotates the innominate anteriorly and carries the pubic symphysis inferiorly to the restrictive barrier.)

Activation: Patient is instructed to push with the knee towards the ceiling and medially against an isometric counterforce provided by the physician's left hand (typically for 3–5 seconds). The resulting concentric contraction of the rectus femoris muscle helps rotate the right hemipelvis, while contraction of the ipsilateral adductor helps focus a gapping force at the pubic symphysis.

Follow-up: Physician waits for tissues to relax completely (1–2 seconds) and then rotates the innominate anteriorly to the new restrictive barrier using the contact hand above the knee. This carries the right pubic ramus inferiorly. Repeat until the best motion is obtained (typically 3–5 times). The patient's extremity is passively returned to the table.

Pubic symphysis: indirect method, respiratory co-operation

Diagnosis: Inferior or superior pubic shear.

Patient position: Supine.

Operator position: Standing beside table.

Contact: Physician grasps each pubic bone with thumbs on the lower margins of each inferior ramus and index fingers on the superior margin of each superior ramus (Figure 50.57).

Position to initiate technique: Introduce appropriate superior and inferior glides by moving the pubic bones in opposite directions to the point of BLT.

Activation: The respiratory phases are tested and the patient's breath is held as long as possible in the phase that provides the best ligamentous balance. During this time the physician makes continuous minor adjustments of the pubic bones to maintain BLT.

Follow-up: Repeat if needed to obtain the best motion.

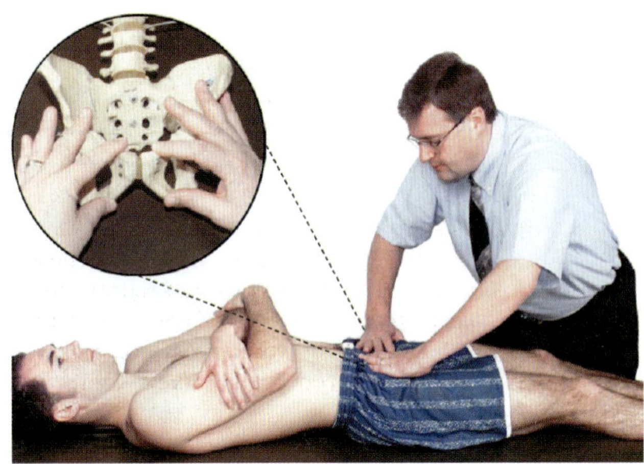

Figure 50.57 Pubic symphysis: indirect method, respiratory co-operation (e.g. inferior or superior pubic shear). (Kimberly and Funk 2000)

Pubic symphysis: muscle energy, direct method

Diagnosis: Compression of the pubic symphysis.

Patient position: Supine with the hips and knees flexed 25–30 cm apart and the feet flat on the table.

Operator position: Standing at the side of the table near the patient's hips.

Preparatory action: Physician grasps both knees, holds them together, and instructs the patient to gently try to abduct both knees against an isometric counterforce (held approximately 3 seconds and repeated an average of three times). This prepares the adductor muscles and the pubic symphysis for the pending activating portion of the corrective technique.

Contact: The heel of the physician's cephalad hand is placed on the medial side of the knee opposite him/her. The palm of the other hand is placed on the medial aspect of the other knee with the thumb abducted, grasping the other forearm (Figure 50.58).

Position to initiate technique: Physician spreads the knees 25–30 cm apart and adjusts the forearm grasp to brace the knees.

Activation: Patient is instructed to try to adduct both knees together against a simultaneous isometric counterforce. Physician has the patient maintain the force long enough to sense that the patient's contractile force is localized at the pubic symphysis (typically 3–5 seconds). An audible release may or may not occur during this procedure. **Follow-up:** Physician waits for the tissues to relax completely (1–2 seconds) and then moves the feet and the knees a few centimetres further apart. The technique may be repeated as needed to achieve return of motion and reduction of symphyseal tenderness.

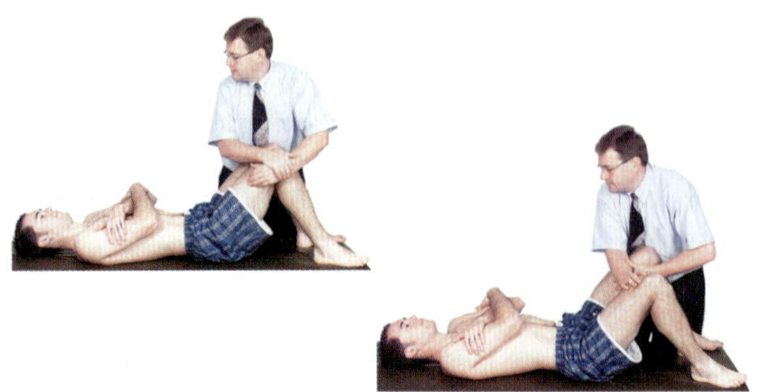

Figure 50.58 Pubic symphysis: muscle energy, direct method (e.g. pubic compression). (Kimberly and Funk 2000)

Innominate

Innominate: HVLA

Note: This technique is contraindicated in a patient with primary or metastatic bone cancer, severe arthritis of the hip or knee, or an artificial knee or hip.

Diagnosis: Left superior (upslipped) innominate shear or left unilateral sacral flexion.

Patient position: Lateral recumbent.

Operator and assistant positions: Physician stands at the foot of the table; an assistant stands in front or behind the patient (Figure 50.59).

Assistant contact: Places the hypothenar eminence of one hand on the inferior aspect of the inferolateral angle on the side of the dysfunction, applying a firm cephalad pressure. The assistant's other hand contacts the superior margin of the iliac crest, pulling it inferiorly and compressing it against the cephalad sacral pressure to the restrictive barrier.

Physician contact: Grasps the patient's leg above the ankle on the dysfunctional side.

Position to initiate technique: Physician abducts and internally rotates the patient's leg slightly (tight packing the hip joint and loose packing the sacroiliac joint) and applies steady traction along the long axis of the extremity to localize forces into the pelvis. The patient is instructed to take a very deep and full breath but with pelvic and lower extremity muscles relaxed. (Sometimes, mildly shaking the patient's leg along with the continued traction helps the physician to sense relaxation of the patient's muscles and localization to the restrictive barrier.)

Activation: An HVLA tug is applied longitudinally through the lower extremity to gap the sacroiliac joint and glide the innominate inferior in relation to the sacrum.

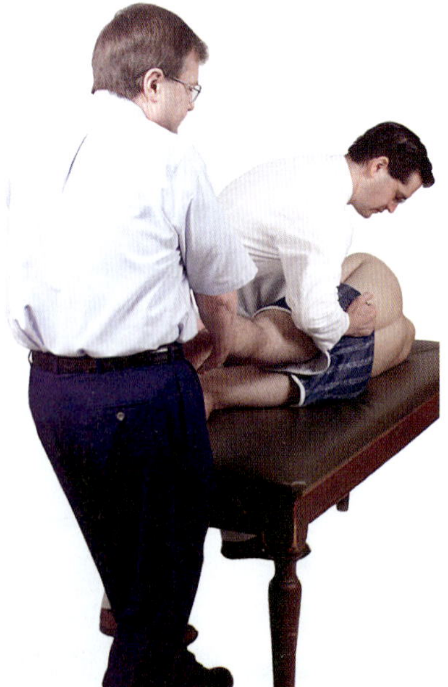

Figure 50.59 Innominate: HVLA (e.g. left upslipped innominate or left sacral shear). (Kimberly and Funk 2000)

Innominate: muscle energy

Diagnosis: Anteriorly rotated right innominate.
Patient position: Supine, lower extremity on the side of the dysfunction is flexed at the knee and hip to bring the knee over the patient's abdomen.
Operator position: Standing on the side of the dysfunction (the right side, in this example).
Contact: Physician holds the patient's flexed knee in that position with his/her shoulder against the leg while contacting the inferior surface of the ASIS with the cephalad thumb (the left, in this example). The fingers of the other hand grasp the posterior aspect of the right ischial tuberosity (Figure 50.60).
Position to initiate technique: Tension is increased at all contact points and the innominate is rotated posteriorly to the restrictive barrier.
Activation: To create concentric contraction of the hamstrings, the patient is instructed to push the knee against the physician's chest that, along with hand contacts, offers isometric counterforce for 3–5 seconds.
Follow-up: The physician waits for the tissues to relax completely (1–2 seconds) and then slightly flexes the hip while concentrating on rotating the innominate posteriorly to the new restrictive barrier with both hand contacts. Activation and follow-up steps should be repeated until the best motion is obtained (typically 3–5 times).

Innominate: muscle energy

Diagnosis: Posteriorly rotated left innominate.
Patient position: Supine. The patient is positioned at the edge of the table, close enough to permit the ischial tuberosity to be clear of the edge. (The patient may feel the need to grasp the table for stability.) The leg is allowed to hang freely.
Operator position: Standing on the side of the dysfunction (the left, in this example).
Contact: Physician reaches across the patient with one hand to cup the patient's opposite ASIS (for stability on the table) and places the other hand on the thigh of the dysfunctional extremity, just above the patient's knee. If necessary, the physician's foot is placed under the patient's foot to prevent it from touching the floor.
Position to initiate technique: Tension and a force directed towards the floor is applied to the thigh, rotating the innominate anteriorly to the restrictive barrier. The opposite hand restrains the pelvis from rolling up off the table.

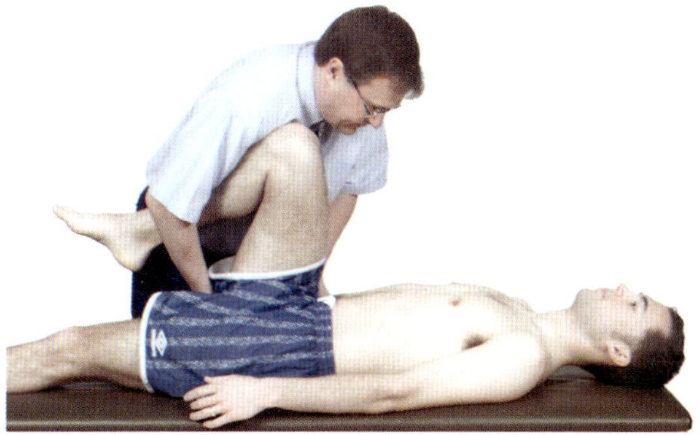

Figure 50.60 Innominate: muscle energy (e.g. anterior right innominate rotation). (Kimberly and Funk 2000)

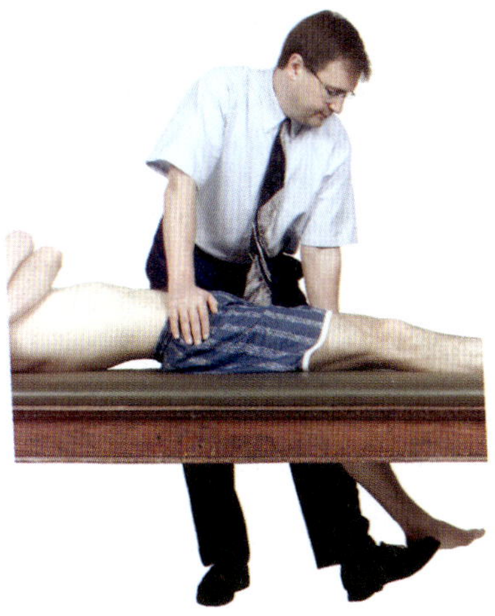

Figure 50.61 Innominate: muscle energy (e.g. posterior left innominate rotation). (Kimberly and Funk 2000)

Activation: Patient is instructed to pull the knee up towards the ceiling while the physician simultaneously offers isometric counterforce for 3–5 seconds through the thigh–hand contact (Figure 50.61).
Follow-up: The physician waits for the tissues to relax completely (1–2 seconds) and then slightly extends the hip while concentrating on rotating the innominate anteriorly to the new restrictive barrier. Activation and follow-up steps should be repeated until the best motion is obtained (typically 3–5 times).

Pelvic floor and coccyx

Ischiorectal fossa technique

Diagnosis: Tight pelvic floor with poor motion.
Patient position: Supine with knees and hips flexed and feet flat on the table or bed.
Operator position: Seated beside patient.
Contact: Physician's fingers are extended well into the ischiorectal fossa, travelling along the inner aspect of the ischial tuberosity to avoid midline structures (Figure 50.62).
Position to initiate technique: The physician uses extended fingers to compress the ischiorectal fat against the pelvic floor muscles. Compression is increased until the muscular barrier is encountered.
Activation: The patient is instructed to take in a big breath while the physician's fingers resist the inferior excursion of the pelvic floor that this initiates. During exhalation, the extended fingers press superiorly to 'take up the slack' until encountering the new barrier.

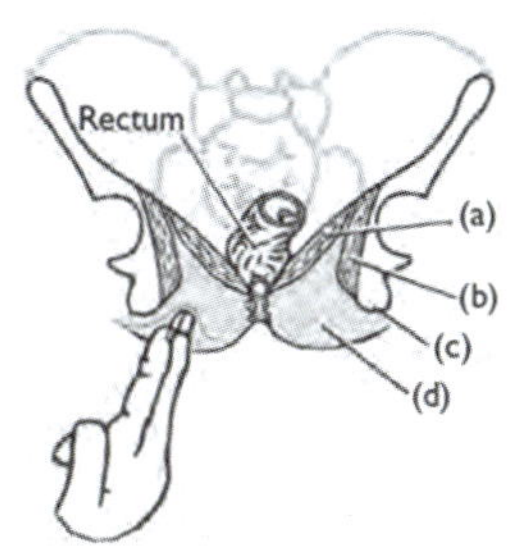

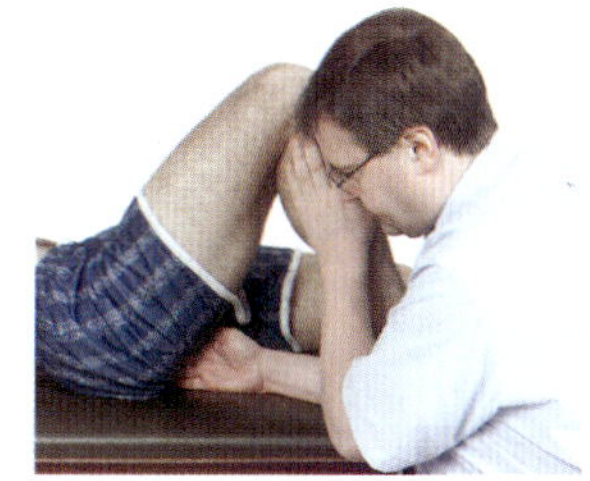

Figure 50.62 Ischiorectal fossa technique: (a = pelvic floor; b = obturator internus; c = ischial tuberosity; d = ischiorectal fat). (Kimberly and Funk 2000)

Follow-up: Repeat three or more times as needed to release the pelvic floor and then recheck the excursion allowed. (At the end of the last cycle of inhalation, the patient may be instructed to cough against a continuous finger pressure to stretch the pelvic floor more completely. This latter manoeuvre should not be attempted if there is a history or palpatory evidence of significant pelvic floor irritable hyperreactivity.)

Coccyx: indirect

Diagnosis: Coccygeal somatic dysfunction. (Diagnosis and treatment are done simultaneously in this technique. Please note that treatment of the coccyx is most effectively performed after treating all other pelvic dysfunction, including the pelvic floor, as just described for the ischiorectal fossa technique. If this technique is used, treatment of the coccyx should follow completion of inhibition over areas of the pelvic floor palpated to have tension or pelvic floor myofascial trigger points.)
Patient position: Lateral recumbent position with knees and hips comfortably flexed.
Operator position: Seated behind patient.
Contact: Using caudal gloved hand, a lubricated finger (usually the index) is passed into the rectum to contact the anterior surface of the coccyx. The thumb of the cephalad hand is placed externally over the skin covering the posterior coccyx. (For some patients and physicians, respective sizes allow the physician to contact these two sites with the same caudad hand.)
Position to initiate technique: The physician gently checks flexion–extension, right–left sidebending, and right–left rotation of the coccyx on the sacrum. Somatic dysfunction permits motion in one direction of each paired motion and a restricted barrier in the other. Maintaining the finger–thumb contacts, each permitted motion is simultaneously stacked to the point of ligamentous balance.
Activation: The respiratory phases are tested and the breath is held as long as possible in the phase that provides the best ligamentous balance. During this time, the physician makes continuous minor adjustments of the coccyx to maintain BLT.
Follow-up: Recheck motion and consider repeating until the best motion is obtained.

Abdominal region

Somatic

Mesenteric lift techniques: fascial release

Diagnosis: Poor lymphatic drainage within mesenteries containing the small and/or large intestines; sensation of bloating.
Patient position: Supine with knees bent and feet on table/bed; alternatively, side-lying positions, if possible, may allow the operator to better access the bowel and/or to use gravity to assist in the release.
Operator position: Standing on patient's right side.
Contact: Pads of operator's fingers (or edges of entire fifth digits) creating soft tissue slack in superficial abdominal tissues to allow deeper contact to viscera involved (small bowel; cecal area; ascending colon; or descending colon) (Figure 50.63).
Position to initiate technique: Draw viscera (contacted as previously described) in the direction towards its mesenteric attachment

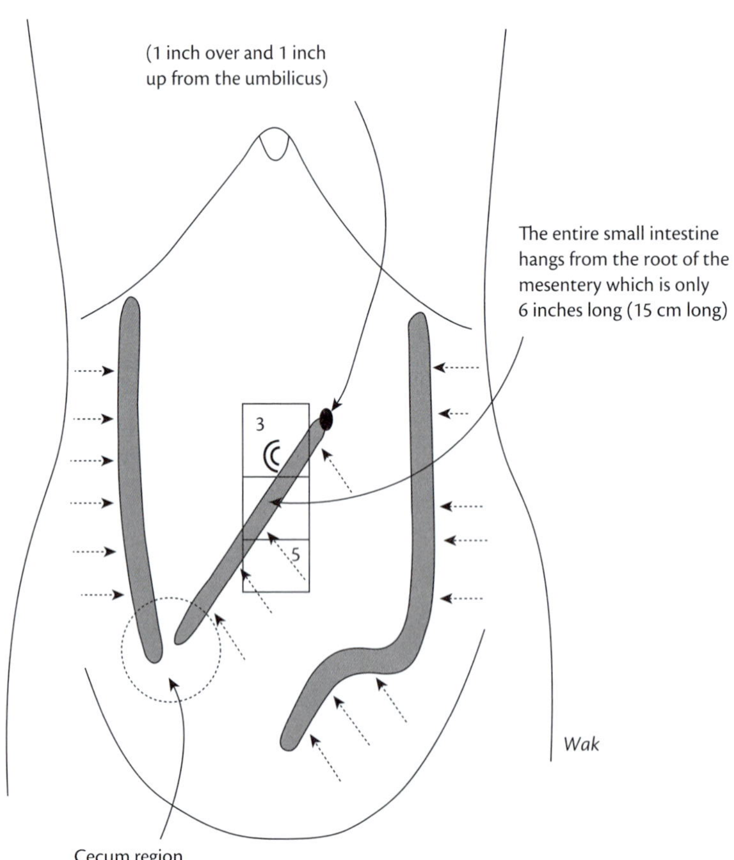
(1 inch over and 1 inch up from the umbilicus)
The entire small intestine hangs from the root of the mesentery which is only 6 inches long (15 cm long)
3
5
Cecum region
Wak

Figure 50.63 Mesenteric lift technique (fascial release): lift each intestinal region towards its respective mesenteric attachment.

to a point of balanced fascial tension; a small amount of torsion may need to be instituted for optimum softening.
Activation: Hold tissues at balance point and follow any viscoelastic creep.
Follow-up: Check other areas; often, follow through with each mesentery throughout the gastrointestinal tract for a clinical effect in patients with bloating, constipation, or with irritable bowel syndrome.

Visceral reflex

Collateral ganglion inhibition techniques

Note 1: This technique is contraindicated in the presence of an abdominal aneurysm, certain other visceral pathologies, or in the immediate post-operative healing stages; it is expected that a preliminary palpatory diagnosis of the abdomen shall have been made.
Diagnosis: Tension over one of three midline abdominal sites between the xiphoid process and umbilicus (see Figure 50.64: a = celiac ganglion site; b = superior mesenteric ganglion site; c = inferior mesenteric ganglion site). **Note 2:** In the viscerosomatic reflex model, these sites may correspond with viscerosomatic reflexes from (a) T5–9; (b) T10–11; (c) T1–L2, respectively. Assessing other palpatory clues including somatic clues (Chapman's reflexes and/or related spinal somatic dysfunction) and visceral clues (organ palpation and other traditional physical examination) might be warranted or advisable before treating.
Patient position: Supine with knees bent and feet flat on the table/bed.
Operator position: Standing at patient's side.
Contact: Maintaining all fingers the same length by gently bending several, compress gently in the midline over the involved ganglion/ganglia towards the abdominal aorta (Figure 50.64).
Position to initiate technique: Compress with enough pressure that the tissues gently resist, then ask the patient to take a half-breath to increase the tension to their tolerance.
Activation: Hold the inhibitory pressure as they hold their breath and when they exhale, follow the tissue tension in the direction of tissue release and then repeat the cycle a few more times or until the area over the site softens. **Follow-up:** If the problem was truly viscerosomatic in nature (due to a primary visceral pathology), the reflex findings will typically recur. While treatment of the secondary recurrent somatic findings in a viscerosomatic reflex may play an adjunctive role in MMMT, the underlying primary cause of this type of reflex should be sought and treated appropriately according to the accepted standard of medical care.

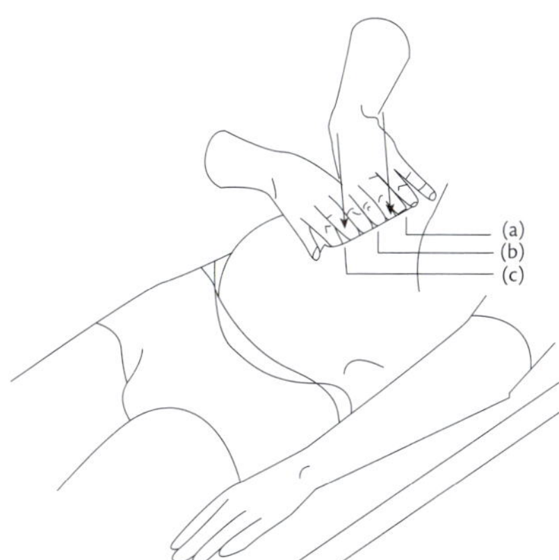

Figure 50.64 Collateral ganglion inhibition techniques. (From Kuchera M.L., Kuchera W.A. *Osteopathic considerations in systemic dysfunction*, 2nd edn, Greyden Press, Columbus, OH, 1994.)

Conclusion to manual treatment of somatic dysfunction

The examples of manual medicine techniques in this chapter are illustrative of general principles as they might be applied by manual medicine physicians to correct single somatic dysfunctions palpated and deemed clinically relevant. These and other manual medicine techniques can be integrated and used as valuable adjunctive tools in the complete management of patients with a wide variety of complaints. They have been shown to be capable of playing a role in reducing pain and improving function within the neuromusculoskeletal system as well as in supporting certain self-healing mechanisms.

An integrated musculoskeletal manipulative medicine treatment (MMMT) is most commonly prescribed within the context of its risk to benefit therapeutic ratio. It is deemed to be adjunctive or primary to the care of the patient (or sometimes contraindicated) by physicians who have undertaken at least several hundreds of additional hours learning palpatory diagnosis and manual treatment. Such physicians can appropriately make this determination based upon the entirety of the clinical context, the host factors involved, and the range of approaches available. The Fédération Internationale de Médecine Manuelle (FIMM) and its national physician groups acknowledge a range of specific training in skills which are considered necessary to safely and effectively administer manual techniques and integrated regimens to remove somatic dysfunction (FIMM 2014). The form that the treatment protocol may take, the goals selected, and the choice of techniques used to accomplish those goals are part of the science, philosophy, and art of the attending physician and the clinical specialty in which he or she is practicing.

Acknowledgements

The author gratefully thanks his father, William A. Kuchera, DO (professor emeritus), for the design and clarity of all of the line drawings in this chapter.

The author extends his thanks to the Kirksville College of Osteopathic Medicine (KCOM) for their permission to use the many illustrations of the author applying techniques. The original colour photographs and more detailed treatment directions, for these and many more techniques, can be found in the text from which they were originally taken: Kimberly, P., Funk, S.F. (eds) *Outline of osteopathic manipulative procedures: the Kimberly manual* (millennium edition, 2000), Walsworth Publishing Company, Marceline, MO. This text is available from the Department of Osteopathic Manipulative Medicine of KCOM at 800 W. Jefferson, Kirksville, MO 63501, USA.

Gratitude is also extended by the author to the Philadelphia College of Osteopathic Medicine (PCOM) for the permission of departmental chairperson, Professor Alexander Nicholas, D.O., F.A.A.O., to release some of the pictures taken for the earliest edition of the Nicholas manual, now in its second edition and published by Lippincott, Williams & Wilkins as the *Atlas of osteopathic techniques* (2012).

References

van Buskirk, R.L. Treatment of somatic dysfunction with an osteopathic manipulative method of Dr Andrew Taylor Still. Chapter 70 in: Ward, R.C. (ed.) *Foundations for osteopathic medicine* (2nd edn). (2002) Lippincott, Williams & Wilkins, Baltimore, MD, pp. 994–1114.

Education Council on Osteopathic Principles (ECOP). Glossary of osteopathic terminology. In: Chila, A.G. (ed.) *Foundations for osteopathic medicine* (3rd edn). (2011) Lippincott, Williams & Wilkins, Baltimore, MD, pp. 1087–110.

Ehrenfeuchter, W.C. Muscle energy. Chapter 46 in: Chila, A.G. (ed.) *Foundations for osteopathic medicine* (3rd edn). (2011) Lippincott, Williams & Wilkins, Baltimore, MD, pp. 682–97.

FIMM Health Policy Board. *Guidelines on basic training and safety in manual medicine*. (2014) Fédération Internationale de Médecine Manuelle (FIMM), Belgium.

Kappler, R.E., Jones, J.M. Thrust (high-velocity/low-amplitude) techniques. Chapter 56 in: Ward, R.C. (ed.) *Foundations for osteopathic medicine* (2nd edn). (2002) Lippincott, Williams & Wilkins, Baltimore, MD, pp. 852–80.

Kappler, R.E., Kuchera, W.A. Diagnosis and plan for manual treatment: a prescription. Chapter 40 in: Ward, R.C. (ed.) *Foundations for osteopathic medicine* (2nd edn). (2002) Lippincott, Williams & Wilkins, Baltimore, MD, pp. 574–9.

Kimberly, P. Forming a prescription for osteopathic manipulative treatment. *Journal of the American Osteopathic Association*, 1980, 79, 512.

Kimberly, P., Funk S.F. (eds). *Outline of osteopathic manipulative procedures: the Kimberly manual* (millennium edn). (2000) Walsworth Publishing Company, Marceline, MO.

Kuchera, M.L., DiGiovanna, E.L., Greenman, P.E. Efficacy and complications. Chapter 72 in: Ward, R.C. (ed.) *Foundations for osteopathic medicine* (2nd edn). (2002) Lippincott, Williams & Wilkins, Baltimore, MD, pp. 1143–52.

Nicholas, A.S., Nicholas, E.A. *The Nicholas atlas of osteopathic manipulative technique* (2nd edn). (2012) Lippincott, Williams & Wilkins, Philadelphia, PA.

Patriquin, D.A., Jones, J.M. Articulatory techniques. Chapter 55 in: Ward, R.C. (ed.) *Foundations for osteopathic medicine* (2nd edn). (2002) Lippincott, Williams & Wilkins, Baltimore, MD, pp. 834–51.

Ward, R.C. Integrated neuromusculoskeletal release and myofascial release. Chapter 60 in: Ward, R.C. (ed.) *Foundations for osteopathic medicine* (2nd edn). (2002) Lippincott, Williams & Wilkins, Baltimore, MD, pp. 931–68.

Chapter 51

Soft tissue injections

John Tanner

Rationale for soft tissue injections

There is no doubt that the careful placement of a small dose of local anaesthetic with corticosteroid in a painful and inflamed soft tissue can provide early and effective symptomatic relief. Other soft tissue injection treatments are discussed later in this section, including trigger point injection and intramuscular needling. Steroid injections are the most commonly used, however, and are the best researched.

Mason et al. (1980), Nevelos (1980), and Staff and Nilsson (1980) report on the use of corticosteroids in the treatment of a variety of soft tissue inflammatory conditions with a high success rate. Staff reported the success of treating iliotibial band friction syndrome in long-distance runners with betamethasone. He emphasized, however, that the use of steroid medication is to give temporary relief of symptoms. It does not afford lasting relief unless the mechanical problem that is causing the symptoms is alleviated. Goupille and Sibilia (1996) reviewed all controlled studies between 1955 and 1993 on the efficacy of local corticosteroid injections in the treatment of rotator cuff tendinitis (excluding capsulitis and calcific tendinitis). They concluded that local corticosteroid injections were more effective than placebo and oral non-steroidal anti-inflammatories (NSAIDs), especially for pain. However, they raised the question of whether local corticosteroid injections have a deleterious long-term effect on the rotator cuff, and it would seem logical to limit the number of local corticosteroid injections. Watson (1985) showed that poor surgical results were associated with a greater number of preoperative steroid injections, especially five or more. However, it is likely that the worse results are more closely correlated with the intensity or severity of the rotator cuff lesions, justifying more frequent symptomatic relief. Chard et al. (1988) showed that the natural history of non-operated rotator cuff tendinitis revealed no worse clinical outcome in those patients who had received a greater number of local steroid injections.

Muscle injections

Infiltrations of local anaesthetic alone are more commonly used for trigger point deactivation in myofascial dysfunction. The alternative to the use of local anaesthetic is to dry-needle the muscle trigger point with an acupuncture needle; many authorities would regard this as at least as effective, if not more so (see Chapter 58). There is no known indication for the use of depot steroid or hydrocortisone directly into muscle tissue other than its use for systemic effects.

Ligaments, tendon sheaths, and bursae

These are the structures most commonly treated by direct corticosteroid infiltration. It has long been known that the direct intratendinous injection of corticosteroid can cause weakening and necrosis of collagen, significantly increasing the chance of tendon disruption, particularly in athletes. Perhaps one of the most commonly injected sites in entire musculoskeletal practice is the musculotendinous origin, the enthesis of the common extensor origin, at the lateral epicondyle for the treatment of 'tennis elbow'. Other entheses commonly treated are the common flexor origin at the medial elbow epicondyle ('golfer's elbow'), the plantar fascia origin on the calcaneal tubercle, and the insertion of the external hip rotators to the posterior greater trochanter.

However, in most instances, the role of such infiltrations should be seen as ancillary to the overall therapeutic strategy. Better results will be achieved if account is taken of the functional and biomechanical factors involved in pathogenesis, which will indicate the underlying regimen for rehabilitation.

The rationale that lies behind the use of corticosteroids is based on the observation that many soft tissue lesions, which have traditionally been regarded as self-limiting, continue to cause symptoms long after normal healing should have occurred. As a result of the poor vascularity of dense collagenous tissue found in ligaments and entheses, the healing process is delayed or inadequate, leading to a chronic low-grade inflammatory response.

An anti-inflammatory agent such as corticosteroid blocks this response, reducing pain and allowing earlier motion. Earlier mobilization is believed to accelerate healing. This theory is both supported and contradicted by various authors who have looked at the effect of steroid on ligaments and tendons in the laboratory. Steroids are known to inhibit collagen synthesis (McCoy et al. 1980; Oikarinen et al. 1988) but we do not know whether the anti-inflammatory effect of corticosteroid can be separated from the collagen inhibition effect. Furthermore, we know that inflammation is the first phase of healing for collagenous tissues and if this is inhibited by steroids, we do not know whether the repair process is simply delayed or permanently altered. The anti-inflammatory action is mediated by inhibition of phospholipase A2 which catalyses the breakdown of membrane phospholipid to arachidonic acid. In contrast, NSAIDs inhibit inflammation at the next step by blocking the enzyme cyclo-oxygenase. Hence, corticosteroids inhibit both cyclo-oxygenase and lipo-oxygenase pathways and therefore inhibit the synthesis of leukotrienes in addition to prostaglandins and thromboxanes.

Corticosteroids: animal experiments

Wiggins et al. (1994) examined the healing characteristics of the New Zealand white rabbit medial collateral ligament after transection. One group was injected with saline, the second group with a dose of betamethasone, which from an earlier study had been shown to be sufficient to inhibit fibroblastic collagen synthesis, and the third group with a human-equivalent dose of betamethasone. The animals were killed at 10 days and 3 weeks postoperatively and were then subjected to biomechanical testing, collagen ratio analysis, and histological analysis. At 10 days, all injected groups showed biomechanical properties significantly inferior to those of non-injected controls. At 3 weeks, the human-equivalent steroid group continued to demonstrate significantly inferior properties. The histological appearance of the non-injected specimens at 10 days typically represented the late inflammatory healing phase, i.e. plump fibroblasts predominated, which under electron microscopy contained abundant rough endoplasmic reticulum indicating that they were synthesizing collagen actively. The higher-dose steroid group demonstrated minimal healing with fewer fibroblasts, more disorganization, and substantial oedema. In other words, the inflammatory phase appeared to be delayed or halted. At 3 weeks, all the non-injected rabbits demonstrated the typical appearance of remodelling with alignment of collagen fibres and reduced vascularity. The lower-dose steroid group remained hypercellular with immature cells consistent with the proliferative phase of healing. The higher-dose steroid group were even more delayed and less mature than the 10-day low-dose steroid specimens.

Wiggins et al. concluded from this study that the anti-inflammatory and collagen-inhibiting properties of steroids cannot be separated and that loss of the inflammatory phase of healing occurs with corticosteroid treatment. This probably represents only delay in healing and not true irreversible inhibition of healing, and what happens in the later phases of remodelling and maturation cannot be determined from this study. One might criticize this study on the basis that surgical transection of a ligament is not typical of the usual kinds of trauma treated in medical practice.

McWhorter et al. (1991) investigated the effect of hydrocortisone acetate injected around the Achilles tendon of the adult male rat after blunt trauma. He used 135 rats assigned to three groups. Groups 1 and 2 received a blunt trauma (a weight dropped on to the Achilles tendon). In Group 1, hydrocortisone in a dose of 12.5 mg was given either once or five times, at weekly intervals, adjacent to the tendon but not intrasubstance. Group 2 received trauma only. Group 3 received neither trauma or injections. The animals were killed at 3, 6, and 9 weeks, and histological and biomechanical analyses were performed. Hydrocortisone did not adversely affect the strength of the Achilles tendon of animals in this study except during week 6, when the control group demonstrated greater tendon strength than animals that had received trauma but no injections. Histologically, McWhorter et al. found that the use of steroids inhibited the presence of some cell types associated with healing. They concluded that if corticosteroid injections are used to treat acute tendinitis, their study recommends temporary immobilization and protection of the tendon from stress allowing for natural healing to occur. However, the results of this study seriously question the claims of Wrenn et al. (1954), Sweetnam (1969), and Halpern et al. (1977), that corticosteroids inhibit the healing process of tendons.

In a follow-up study of the long-term effects of a single injection of corticosteroid on ligament healing in rabbits, Wiggins et al. (1995) examined the remodelling and maturation phases and found that the tensile strength of the specimens that had been injected with steroids returned to a value that was equal to that of the controls; however, the resistance to repeated deformation and load remained inferior to that of the controls. This was accompanied by a lag in histological maturation. These studies were performed 84 days after collateral ligament transection and injection with steroid. They concluded that acute corticosteroid treatment of an injured ligament is detrimental to the healing process in both the early and the later phase of healing.

Whether these animal experiments have direct relationship to clinical practice remains uncertain. In reviewing the literature on the use of steroids for Achilles tendon pain, Read and Motto (1992) concluded that steroids can be used safely.

Guidelines for soft tissue injections

Any practitioner who is willing to perform local anaesthetic and/or corticosteroid infiltrations should be fully conversant with the physicochemical properties such as time of onset, duration of action, degree of sensory and motor blockade, potency, and lipid solubility. They should be aware of the pros and cons of the use of a vasoconstrictor such as epinephrine (adrenaline), and the potency and potential to cause toxic reactions affecting the central nervous system and cardiovascular system, and to cause allergy. Any practitioner performing injections needs to observe strict aseptic technique and be fully prepared to deal with the possible and occasionally life-threatening complications which can occur such as anaphylaxis, cerebral convulsions, and hypotension. Oxygen, basic resuscitation equipment, airways, intravenous fluids, and emergency drugs such as chlorpheniramine, epinephrine, hydrocortisone succinate, atropine, and diazepam should be available in the treatment room.

With our present state of knowledge, it is possible to recommend the following basic guidelines when considering the appropriateness of local corticosteroid injection:

1 Perform a full functional assessment of the region concerned including the governing spinal segments. Search for evidence of proximal and distal dysfunctions. Identify biomechanical factors that may predispose to the condition or delay recovery.

2 Consider a trial of physical therapy including mobilization and manipulation, local anaesthetic trigger point needling, and other approaches before resorting to a steroid injection. If active mobilization is not possible because of acute inflammation, judicious use of a small dose of corticosteroid to the affected site may allow earlier graduated progression of exercise.

3 Use the minimum dose necessary to achieve the therapeutic effect, i.e. no more than 10–20 mg of triamcinolone or 25–50 mg of hydrocortisone for ligament/bursa injection. It is important to

use water-soluble corticosteroid, rather than depot steroid which is lipophilic in superficial injections, to avoid subcutaneous lipoid atrophy. Increase volume where necessary with local anaesthetic dilution.

4 Avoid intratendinous injection.

5 Consider ultrasound-guided injection if available, where anatomy is difficult, and/or to improve accuracy in needle placement in joint, bursa, or tendon sheath.

6 Recommend avoidance of vigorous exercise of the temporarily weakened tissue for at least 2–3 weeks following injection. However, functional movement of the area encourages new collagen formation with orientation in the lines of stress, to make a more effective repair.

7 As a rule, no more than a series of three injections is advised without a review of the diagnosis and treatment (Woo et al. 1975). If relief provided is no more than temporary and the condition continues to relapse, other forms of therapy should be sought, but if there has been good remission for some months or years, then a further 1 or 2 injections could be considered.

Local corticosteroid therapy

Injectable corticosteroid preparations suitable for joint or soft tissue injection are listed in Table 51.1. It is generally recommended that the longest-acting preparations are not injected into tendon sheaths as they are less soluble and cause more soft tissue atrophy or chance of tendon rupture. The longest-acting, least-soluble preparations are typically used for intra-articular injections where a more powerful and long-lasting effect is sought.

Guidelines for the appropriate dose of corticosteroid to be injected are given in Table 51.2. Anaesthetic preparations can be safely combined or mixed with a corticosteroid preparation. However, if the corticosteroid preparation contains a paraben compound as a preservative, flocculation of the suspension is likely to occur. In practice, for the examples given in Table 51.2, it is recommended to use 1% lidocaine (lignocaine) either with hydrocortisone or triamcinolone, since flocculation or precipitation of the particle does not occur with this combination.

Entheses

Injection of musculotendinous attachments, such as the common extensor origin at the lateral epicondyle, is a useful adjunctive therapy in the management of these common musculoskeletal conditions. A maximum of 10–20 mg of depot steroid such as triamcinolone acetonide or 25 mg hydrocortisone, which may be mixed with 1–2 ml of 1% lidocaine (lignocaine), is delivered by meticulous infiltration in a 'peppering' fashion to the site of maximum tenderness. A small-gauge needle is used to deliver 0.1 ml at a time to the length, breadth, and depth of the involved tissue.

The patient should be advised that there may be a temporary exacerbation of pain lasting 12–24 hours; this occurs in a proportion of patients. If severe, this can be treated with application of ice and anti-inflammatories. Care must be taken to ensure that the dose is not delivered in the subcutaneous tissue to avoid the complications of fat atrophy. The patient should be advised to avoid heavy use of the structure for the following 2 weeks. When all or most of the pain has cleared, a programme of stretching and strengthening exercises should be instituted, as well as attention to occupation or sports that may involve activities which could cause a recurrence.

Ligaments

Ligament sprains, whether acute or chronic, can be treated effectively with local corticosteroid infiltration. If clinical examination reveals signs of an unstable joint, then it is wise to avoid the use of corticosteroids, since further weakening of the soft tissue restraints may occur. Such injections are therefore best reserved for first-degree strains of ligaments of peripheral joints, such as the knee or ankle, which are not settling with physiotherapy. A similar dose and method of administration is used as already described, with the needle directed towards the ligament attachment to the bone rather than mid substance. This is the area of the ligament that is most richly innervated with pain receptors. In the spine, interspinous ligaments, supraspinous ligaments, and iliolumbar and sacroiliac ligaments all respond well to this form of therapy; at peripheral joints, the commonest ligaments to be injected are those of the lateral ankle, the meniscotibial ligaments of the knee, the medial collateral ligaments, the ligaments of the wrist, and those of the

Table 51.1 Injectable corticosteroid preparations suitable for joint or soft tissue injection

Preparation	Strengths (mg/ml)	Prednisolone equivalent (mg)
Short acting, soluble		
Dexamethasone sodium phosphate	8	40
Hydrocortisone acetate	25	5
Long acting, less soluble		
Methylprednisolone acetate	20, 40, 80	25, 50, 100
Dexamethasone acetate	8	80
Longest acting, least soluble		
Triamcinolone acetonide	10, 40	12.5, 50
Triamcinolone hexacetonide	20	25
Betamethasone sodium phosphate	6	50

Table 51.2 Guidelines for the appropriate dose of corticosteroid to be injected

Site	Prednisolone equivalent dose (mg)
Bursa	10–20
Tendon sheath	10–20
Small joints of hands and feet	5–15
Medium-sized joints	15–25
Large joints	20–50

acromioclavicular joint. An alternative approach is the use of prolotherapy (see Chapters 54 and 55).

After injection with corticosteroid, a period of up to 2 weeks relative rest of the affected part should be advised before progressing with stronger rehabilitation programmes.

Peritendinous injections

Perhaps the most commonly treated condition in this category is De Quervain's tenosynovitis of the wrist, but all the flexor and extensor tendons of the wrist and fingers can be successfully treated by corticosteroid injections, when inflamed. The siting of the injection can be more contained in the portions surrounded by the synovial sheath, often affected where it is under a retinaculum, but small doses can be placed alongside the tendons in other areas. Around the ankle, the peroneal tendons, medial tibial tendons, and extensor tendons of the ankle slide within their sheath, showing swelling, heat, and tenderness when inflamed. Using a 23-gauge needle is often ideal; it may be bent to a 25° angle in order to allow insertion into the skin and then to follow a direction parallel with the tendon, so that a bolus dose of 1–2 ml of corticosteroid with local anaesthetic can be given. Patients should be warned of a possible flare-up for 24 hours after the injection, followed by a gradual resolution of symptoms. During the first 2 weeks, the affected region should be rested as far as possible in order to avoid undue physical stresses on the tendons.

Bursae

Many of the common sites of bursitis, both superficial and deep, can be identified through standard clinical examination and palpation techniques. In some cases, such as the prepatellar bursa or the olecranon bursa, aspiration of fluid should be attempted and if there is any suspicion of infection, corticosteroids should be withheld and the fluid sent for microscopy and culture. Less superficial bursae rarely become infected and respond very promptly to appropriate corticosteroid treatment, since these conditions clearly demonstrate the classic signs of acute inflammation. In large bursae such as the subgluteal bursa, up to 20 ml of low-concentration local anaesthetic, such as 0.5% lidocaine (lignocaine), should be administered with 10–20 mg of depot steroid in order to ensure spread of the fluid throughout the bursa. In conditions such as trochanteric bursitis, it is rarely possible to aspirate fluid since this is commonly recognized as a 'dry bursitis', except in the instance of rheumatoid or other inflammatory disease.

A stretching routine for the adjacent musculature appears to increase efficacy.

Complications following soft tissue injections

- *Infection* is rarely encountered with the use of sterile disposable syringes and needles and strict aseptic technique. The frequency of infection is probably the same as with joint injection.
- *Exacerbation of pain:* This is usually temporary, settling in 1–2 days; it occurs more frequently at entheses where ligaments or tendons insert.
- *Steroid flush* of the face may occur for 24–48 hours with higher doses, particularly in women of perimenopausal age.
- *Menstrual irregularities* may follow the use of higher-dose corticosteroid injections or where the series of injections is given over a relatively short period of time. It is important to be aware of this possibility, particularly when the patient is postmenopausal and complains of a bleed for the first time in some years, since it may precipitate gynaecological investigations.
- *Systemic effects of corticosteroids:* These are rarely seen with the low dosages used in this form of injection therapy.
- *Diabetics* should be warned that because of the small amount of steroid that can be absorbed, the blood glucose level will increase slightly for 2–3 days but it is not normally necessary to adjust the insulin regime.
- *Allergy:* This is a rare complication and may be due to the local anaesthetic (more commonly, the esters such as procaine), the corticoids, and any or all of the preservatives contained in the preparations
- *Haematoma:* Danger of haematoma formation is increased by anticoagulant therapy, which is a relative contraindication to the treatment.
- *Lipoid atrophy:* This occurs particularly with the use of the less soluble steroids rather than hydrocortisone, and is most likely in superficial injections where some of the solution may track back under the skin. In a series of 53 tennis elbow injections, Hay et al. (1999) reported that two cases showed evidence of skin atrophy at 6 months, and 1 case at 12 months. It is associated with hypopigmentation (more noticeable if the adjacent skin is sun-tanned), thinning of the subdermal tissue, and telangiectasiae.

References

Chard, M. D., et al. (1988) The long term outcome of rotator cuff tendinitis. A review study. *Br J Rheumatol*, 27, 385–9.

Goupille, P., Sibilia, J. (1996) Local corticosteroid injections in the treatment of rotator cuff tendinitis, except for frozen shoulder and calcific tendinitis. *Clin Exp Rheum*, 14, 561–6.

Halpern, A. A., et al. (1977) Tendon ruptures associated with corticosteroid therapy. *West J Med*, 127, 378–82.

Hay, E. M., Paterson, S. M., Lewis, P., et al. (1999) Pragmatic randomised trial of local corticosteroid injection and naproxen for treatment of lateral epicondylitis of elbow in primary care. *BMJ*, 319, 964–8.

Mason, J. O., et al. (1980) The management of supraspinatus tendinitis in general practice. *J Irish Med Assoc*, 73(1), 23–4.

McCoy, B. J., et al. (1980) In vitro inhibition of cell growth collagen synthesis and prolylhydroxylase activity by triamcinolone acetonide. *Proc Soc Exp Biol Med*, 163, 216–22.

McWhorter, J. W., et al. (1991) Influence of local steroid injections on traumatized tendon properties: a biomechanical and histological study. *Am J Sports Med*, 19, 435–9.

Nevelos, A. B. (1980) The treatment of tennis elbow with triamcinolone acetonide. *Curr Med Res Opin*, 6, 507–9.

Oikarinen, A. I., et al. (1988) Modulation of collagen metabolism by glucocorticoids. Receptor mediated effects of dexamethasone on collagen biosynthesis in chick embryo fibroblasts and chondrocytes. *Biochem Pharmacol*, 37, 1451–62.

Read M. T. F., Motto, S. G. (1992) Tendo achillis pain: steroids and outcome. *Br J Sports Med*, 26, 15–21.

Staff, P. H., Nilsson, S. (1980) Tendoperiostitis in the lateral femoral condyle in long distance runners. *Br J Sports Medicine*, 14, 38–40.

Sweetnam, R. (1969) Corticosteroid arthropathy and tendon rupture. *J Bone Joint Surg*, 51B, 397–8.

Watson, M. (1985) Major ruptures of the rotator cuff. *J Bone Joint Surg*, 67B, 618–24.

Wiggins, M. E., et al. (1994) Healing characteristics of a type 1 collagenous structure treated with corticosteroids. *Am J Sports Med*, 22, 279–88.

Wiggins, M. E., et al. (1995) Effects of local injection of corticosteroids on the healing of ligaments. *J Bone and Joint Surg*, 77A, 1682–90.

Woo, S. L-Y., Matthews, J., Akeson, W., Amiel, D., Convery, R. (1975) Connective tissue response to immobility: correlative study of the biomechanical and biochemical measurements of normal and immobilised rabbit knees. *Arthritis Rheum*, 18, 257–64.

Wrenn, R. N., et al. (1954) An experimental study of the effect of cortisone on the healing process and tensile strength of tendons. *J Bone Joint Surg*, 35A, 588–601.

Chapter 52

Epidural injections

Keith Bush

Introduction to epidural injections

The epidural space is the potential space surrounding the theca in the vertebral canal and runs from the foramen magnum to the sacral hiatus. It therefore forms a useful route whereby drugs that may influence the theca or surrounding tissues can be specifically delivered.

Traditionally, epidural injections have been associated with childbirth and surgical procedures, when local anaesthetic is injected to block the appropriate spinal nerve roots. However, the use of epidural injections in the management of spinal pain goes back to 1901 when Sicard described the introduction of cocaine through the caudal hiatus at the base of the spine (Sicard 1901). There follows an extensive and enthusiastic literature primarily documenting the use of local anaesthetic and normal saline (Bhatia and Parikh 1966; Cyriax 1984; Gupta et al. 1970; Malthotra et al. 2009) until the addition of corticosteroids in the 1950s (Bush and Hillier 1991, 1996; Bush et al. 1992; Carette et al. 1997; Cuckler 1986; Dilke et al. 1973; Klenerman et al. 1984; Koes et al. 1995; Manchikanti et al. 2012; Parr et al. 2011; Ridley et al. 1998; Snoek et al. 1977; Watts and Silagy 1995).

Some important clinical syndromes best managed by epidural injections are:

- sciatica
- cervical radiculopathy
- spinal claudication
- acute discogenic back pain
- acute discogenic neck or thoracic spinal pain.

Since writing this chapter for the first edition, almost a decade ago, a review of the world literature discovers 268 papers addressing epidural injections in the management of spinal pain syndromes. They confirm the increasing enthusiasm for performing these techniques. Most papers support their efficacy, although some controversy remains (Parr et al. 2011; Manchikanti et al. 2012; McGrath et al. 2011).

The safety and relatively low incidence of side-effects is also confirmed (McGrath et al. 2011). However, with such widespread usage, the small incidence of side-effects has been magnified, reminding us to remain vigilant. For instance in the USA, over 14,000 epidural injections were performed over a few months with contaminated deposteroids. This led to hundreds of catastrophic spinal infections and dozens of deaths.

The other serious complication of note is in relation to cervical transforaminal injections (dorsal root ganglion blocks), with dozens of neurological complications, including a few deaths, being reported (Malthotra et al. 2009). This, along with suggested precautions, will be addressed in the section on side-effects.

Pathology of spinal pain

In broad terms, much spinal pain can be attributed to either mechanical or inflammatory pathology. Mixter and Barr (1934) first drew attention to nerve root compression by a disc herniation as the cause for sciatica in 1934. Subsequently, Rydevick et al. (1984) expanded upon the pathoanatomy and pathophysiology of nerve root compression. However, access to non-invasive imaging such as computed tomography (CT) and magnetic resonance imaging (MRI) has demonstrated that many people with no symptoms may have apparent compressive pathology such as intervertebral disc herniations (Jensen 1994; Wiesel et al. 1984). There are, therefore, alternative pathologies to pure compression. Recent research has demonstrated that inflammation can play a major role (McCarron et al. 1987). Olmarker et al. (1993) have demonstrated that nuclear cell membranes from the nucleus pulposus are neurotoxic, both producing inflammatory and neurophysiological changes. Furthermore, these reactions are blocked by corticosteroids (Olmarker et al. 1994).

Thus, nuclear material which herniates into the vertebral canal through a crack in the annulus fibrosus may both compress and irritate the nerve roots and dura, resulting in back pain or sciatica and, of course, neck pain or brachialgia. Furthermore, repeat scanning has demonstrated that a high proportion of large disc herniations naturally regress with time (Bozzao et al. 1992; Bush et al. 1992, 1997; Delauche-Cavalier et al. 1992; Maigne and Deligne 1994; Maigne et al. 1992; Saal et al. 1990). Therefore, it is perfectly rational to place corticosteroids at the disc–nerve root interface to control inflammation, and thus pain, while nature deals with the mechanical issues. However, surgical decompression is still required in some patients.

Indications for epidural injections

Most controlled studies addressing the efficacy of epidural injections for disc lesions have related to the management of sciatica (Bush and Hillier 1991; Carette et al. 1997; Cuckler 1986; Dilke et al. 1973; Klenerman et al. 1984; Koes et al. 1995; Manchikanti et al. 2012; Parr et al. 2011; Ridley et al. 1998; Snoek et al. 1977). Results remain conflicting, but meta-analysis supports the use of epidural corticosteroids in the management of sciatica (Manchikanti et al. 2012; Parr et al. 2011; Watts and Silagy 1995). Their positive effect is in the intermediate term, over weeks and months (Bush and Hillier 1991; Carette et al. 1997).

There is therefore a place for repeating epidural injections over several months to control inflammation and thus pain. When this philosophy was applied to the management of 165 patients with sciatica, 86% made a satisfactory recovery, without the need for surgical decompression, with an average of three injections (Bush et al. 1992). When managing 68 patients with cervical radiculopathy, the non-surgical outcome was satisfactory in all patients, with an average of 2.5 injections (Bush and Hillier 1996).

Thus, in broad terms, all patients with radicular syndromes or dural irritation manifesting as spinal pain are suitable candidates for a trial of epidural injections. Indeed, these injections are useful diagnostically, as well as therapeutically, in that during the procedure, if the diagnosis is correct, the patient's symptoms may be replicated and then immediately blocked by the anaesthetic.

Patients with cauda equina syndrome (with bowel or bladder dysfunction) or cervical/thoracic myelopathy (with long tract symptoms or signs) may require urgent decompression, but in the common types of sciatica, surgical intervention does not influence the ultimate neurological outcome (Hakelius 1970; Weber 1983). So, neurological signs, in the form of reduced sensation, power, or reflexes, are not a contraindication to conservative management. However, we obtain a surgical opinion in cases with acute and complete foot drop, as urgent decompression may offer the best chance of recovery.

Epidural injection techniques

Asepsis

When performing epidural injections, it is important to have a fastidious aseptic technique. Although infection is very rare, epidural abscess has been reported, leading to severe and permanent neurological deficit. A solution of 0.5% chlorhexidine in 70% alcohol has been shown to be effective against the usual flora to be found on the back. Both the vial tops and the skin should be swabbed with this and allowed to dry before the drugs are aspirated and then injected. A non-touch technique is perfectly adequate; however, sterile gloves should be worn for more intricate, protracted procedures such as transforaminal epidurals/dorsal root ganglion blocks (DRGB). In addition to further protecting the patient from infection, the gloves protect the physician from the occasional flow-back of blood through the needle.

Caudal approach

For lumbar lesions, the caudal epidural injection technique has several advantages. Because the theca generally terminates several centimetres above the sacral hiatus, there is very little chance of intrathecal injection which is more of a hazard with the interlaminar approach. If 0.5% lidocaine without preservative is used, only the unmyelinated, nociceptive C fibres are blocked. There is therefore no loss of sensation or power and the blood pressure is not influenced (Cyriax 1984). The procedure can therefore safely be performed on an out-patient basis, with patients being able to get up and walk out shortly afterwards. Nevertheless, it is useful to monitor the patients with pulse oximetry, which will draw early attention to a vasovagal attack or other complication. Furthermore, facilities to resuscitate the patient should be available in case of anaphylaxis or spinal block.

Up to 20 ml 0.5% lidocaine, with the addition of a corticosteroid such as 40 mg triamcinolone, is commonly used for the caudal route: this volume should spread to L1–2, covering the usual levels of pathology (Burn et al. 1973). 10 ml will normally cover to L4–5, thus reaching 90% of discs responsible for sciatica.

Although epidural steroid injections have been performed as a standard procedure over the past five to six decades, no steroid preparation has actually been licensed for use in the epidural space. Methylprednisolone has been extensively used and triamcinolone, to a lesser extent. Some controversy has arisen as to whether epidural corticosteroids or the additional constituents of the preparations may be detrimental. However, an extensive report prepared on behalf of the Australian National Health and Medical Research Council (1994) has vindicated their use in the epidural space. There is, however, some evidence to suggest that intrathecal corticosteroids may occasionally produce arachnoiditis.

Interlaminar approach

The interlaminar approach is the route preferred by many anaesthetists. However, there is certainly a higher incidence of inadvertent thecal puncture because the distance between the ligamentum flavum and the dura is only millimetres. This should of course be recognized by the experienced injector, but a small dural tear may not be, so that a 'spinal' headache will result. If the injection solution contains anaesthetic, this technique should therefore be only practiced in a hospital setting, for fear of a spinal block.

Use of imaging

Accuracy of epidural needle placement can be tested by contrast media and imaging. Stitz and Sommer (1999) reported a 74% success rate overall, but higher correct positioning in cases with easily identified bony landmarks. Intravenous injection occurred in 3.7% of their cases. Poor needle placement may be one of the explanations for the lack of efficacy reported by some researchers. There is therefore an argument for performing epidural injections under fluoroscopic control (image intensifier C arm or CT) with the use of contrast media to confirm that the drug has reached the suspected pathology. Either the caudal (Figure 52.1) or interlaminar (Figure 52.2) route can be used. Furthermore, the transforamenal route/DRGB may also prove to be very useful, particularly in cases of lateral recess stenosis and far lateral disc herniation (Figure 52.3).

Choice of technique

Image-guided techniques are obviously more time-consuming and expensive. For this reason, it has been our practice first to perform a standard caudal epidural injection when managing appropriate lumbosacral pathology. However, if the response is unsatisfactory, a more specific approach can be performed under radiographic

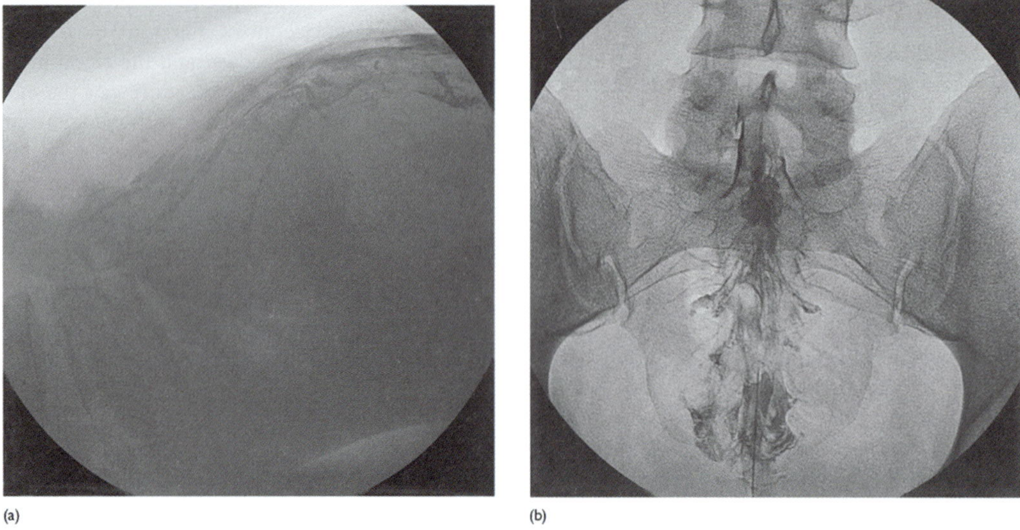

(a) (b)

Figure 52.1 Caudal epidurogram demonstrating the satisfactory spread of 5 ml of contrast medium to L5; (a) lateral view; (b) anteroposterior view.

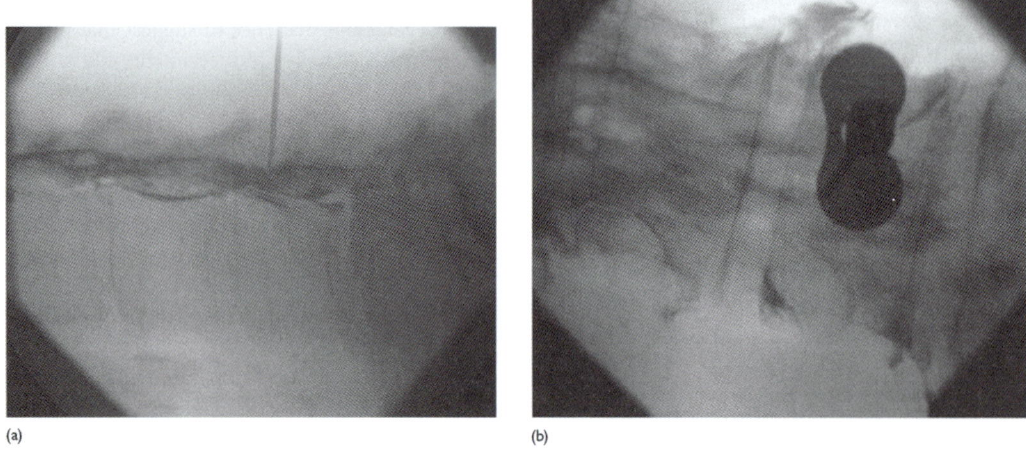

(a) (b)

Figure 52.2 Lumbar L3/4 interlaminar epidurogram in a patient with a degree of spinal stenosis: (a) lateral view; (b) anteroposterior view.

control once MRI or CT has been performed to localize the pathology. This allows for a higher concentration of drug to be introduced: 1 ml of lidocaine 1%, without preservative, with 40 mg triamcinolone being appropriate for a transforaminal epidural/DRGB after confirming position with 0.5–1 ml of contrast medium (Figure 52.3). We have debated whether MRI should precede all epidural/steroid injections or not (Bush 2012).

In managing a series of 165 patients with sciatica, we found it necessary to resort to more specific injection techniques under radiographic control in 24% of cases (Bush et al. 1992). However, of 68 cervical radiculopathies, less than 30% responded to the simple paravertebral block approach, with over 70% responding to more specific injection techniques, either interlaminar (Bush and Hillier 1996) or transforaminal (Figure 52.4).

The cervical radiculopathies seem to respond even better than the sciaticas, possibly because the cervical root canals are relatively larger than the lumbar root canals, the cervical nerve roots being surrounded by venous sinuses. Radiological contrast improves safety and efficacy of transforaminal epidurals/DRGBs in the cervical spine, where inadvertent intravenous/intra-arterial injection occurs more easily and frequently (Malthotra et al. 2009).

Besides steroid and local anaesthetics, other drugs such as morphine, clonidine, and hyaluronidase have been introduced into the epidural space. At present, the literature does not present a convincing case for their use.

Caudal epidural injection technique

Caudal epidural injections are best performed with the patient lying prone. This allows for easy identification of the sacral hiatus in the midline. A pillow placed under the pelvis, or breaking the couch to raise the pelvis, is also helpful in bringing the sacral hiatus to prominence. This position is also more comfortable for the

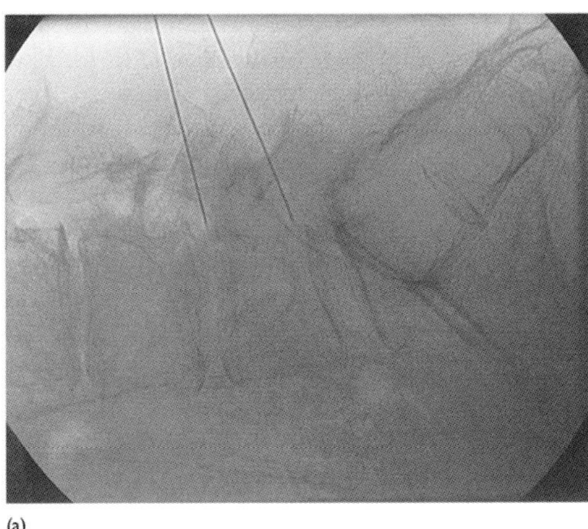

(a)

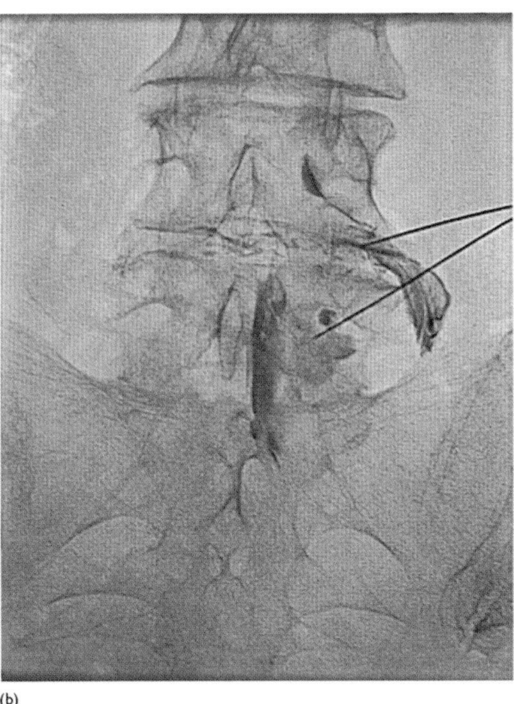

(b)

Figure 52.3 Lumbar selective epidurogram/DRGB two-needle approach to introduce drugs to the L4/5 intervertebral disc/L5 nerve root interface. Note that the needle posterior to the L4/5 intervertebral disc has entered the herniation and, initially, the introduction of contrast has resulted in a discogram until the needle was withdrawn. The lower needle is placed at the 6 o'clock position, just below the L5 pedicle: (a) lateral view; (b) anteroposterior view.

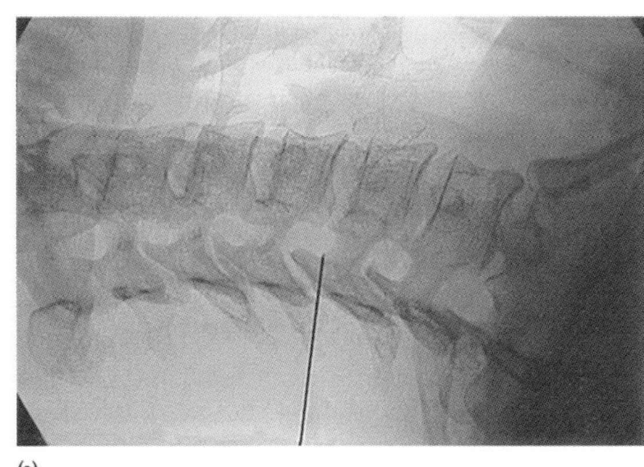

(a)

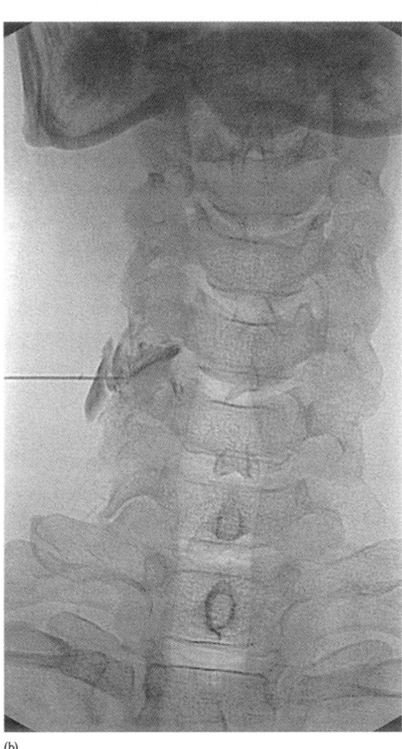

(b)

Figure 52.4 Cervical transforaminal epidurogram/DRGB at the C6 level: (a) oblique view—note that the needle is along the posterior surface of the root canal; (b) anteroposterior view—note that contrast has initially spread into the paravertebral tissues until the needle was introduced further up the root canal, ensuring placement of drugs at the intervertebral disc/nerve root interface.

occasional patient whose pain is aggravated by spinal extension, but some will still have to lie in the lateral decubitus position to achieve reasonable comfort. In this position, the soft tissues fall laterally, making identification of the sacral hiatus more difficult.

The sacral cornua can usually be palpated with the left thumb, bringing the thumb cephalad up the natal cleft. The skin is then marked with a thumbnail imprint which remains evident after the skin is swabbed with antiseptic. A small amount of local anaesthetic (e.g. 1 ml lidocaine 0.5%) is injected when introducing a 21-gauge 50-mm needle or a 22-gauge 90-mm spinal needle. The needle is introduced with the bevel facing down. This allows it to slide up the sacral canal without embedding into the periosteum. It is usually possible to feel the needle penetrating the membrane over the hiatus, and it is then introduced a further 1 cm or so.

Once the needle is in place, the syringe of local anaesthetic and steroid is connected. There is usually a moderate resistance to injection. However, resistance may be very high if the needle is subperiosteal, and this can usually be relieved by turning the needle through 180°. It is not uncommon for the needle to be intravenous, and it is therefore most important to aspirate and disconnect the syringe to check for blood flow-back. This problem can usually be resolved by introducing the needle further or slightly retracting it. It is very rare for it to be intrathecal, because the theca usually terminates several centimetres above the sacral hiatus, but if there is any doubt, the procedure should be abandoned and repeated with care a few days later (with minimal distance insertion, possibly using imaging).

The drugs are introduced slowly, but can often exacerbate the patient's back pain or sciatica. This is a good sign, indicating that they have reached the appropriate disc–dural interface. The patient should be told that the faster the injection, the sooner it will be over but the more it may hurt, and so a balance needs to be struck. Palpating over the sacrum with the left hand can detect an extrasacral injection. If there is any doubt, a 'woosh' test should be performed: once it has been ascertained that the needle is not intravenous, a 10-ml syringe filled with air is connected and this is introduced while auscultating with a stethoscope over the midlumbar spine. A clear `woosh' should be heard if the needle is correctly in the epidural space. Epidurography is the ultimate confirmation (Figure 52.1).

During the procedure, conversation with the patient and additional pulse oximetry leads to early detection of complications. The level of monitoring should reflect the potential for problems (for example, in the dosage and siting of local anaesthetic used) with this generally benign procedure. Maximum safety will be achieved by pulse oximetry, blood pressure and cardiac monitor, intravenous line, and the availability of resuscitation equipment and drugs. If there is any concern about the patient's reaction, the procedure should be terminated. The inadvertent intravenous injection of lidocaine leads to a feeling of panic with ringing in the ears, which passes rapidly if identified early. We avoid the use of bupivacaine because it has cardiotoxic properties.

It usually takes no more than 5 minutes to introduce 20 ml of steroid and local anaesthetic, except in patients with very severe sciatica. As already stated, a smaller volume such as 10 ml will give added safety and probably adequate effect. On completion, the patient should remain lying down for 10–30 minutes. If straight leg raises were limited, these can then be re-tested to detect improvement due to the anaesthetic effect (and some authors believe this is therapeutic). Although the patient may feel some numbness of the buttocks for half an hour with 0.5% lidocaine, it is very rare for there to be any weakness of the legs. If this does occur, the patient will have to rest until it resolves. The patient must not drive for a few hours.

Patients are instructed to proceed with care and lead a mobile but quiet lifestyle if the back condition allows. They are warned that when the anaesthetic wears off, there may be an initial exacerbation of symptoms for up to a few days. There is potential for improvement over a few weeks when using a depot steroid such as triamcinolone. If some improvement is achieved, but not enough, the procedure can be repeated on several further occasions ranging from a few weeks to a few months.

Interlaminar epidural injection technique

Lumbar and thoracic interlaminar epidural injections are best performed with the patient lying in the lateral decubitus position with the symptomatic side lowermost. Cervical epidural injections are best performed with the patient lying prone and the neck in flexion, which is aided by a break in the table. Radiographic control can confirm the spinal level and contrast medium can illustrate correct position in the epidural space (Figure 52.2).

Using a non-touch technique, 5 ml of 1% lidocaine is introduced into the soft tissues, confirming the level with lateral and anteroposterior screening. After the operator has scrubbed up and put on sterile gloves, a 16-gauge Tuohy needle (18-gauge with cervical epidurals) is then introduced using a loss of resistance technique with normal saline. Up to 5 ml of contrast medium is then introduced to absolutely confirm position before introducing 40–80 mg triamcinolone acetonide (40 mg/ml) and 5 ml 0.5% lidocaine (without preservative)—or normal saline if preferred. In the cervical spine, a mixture of 1 ml 1% lidocaine and 50 mg (5 ml) triamcinolone acetonide (10 mg/ml) is used.

There is no need to introduce a catheter in the lumbar and thoracic spines, but in the cervical spine it is best because the needle is not so well supported and the epidural position may be lost when changing syringes. It is advisable for the patient to rest and be monitored for 2 hours after the procedure, but otherwise, the same post-injection instructions apply as for caudal epidural injections.

Lumbar transforaminal epidural injections

Transforaminal epidural injections/DRGBs are best performed with the patient lying in the prone position and screening in the anteroposterior, oblique, and lateral planes. A butterfly needle serves as a marker to aim for the '6 o'clock' position just caudad of the appropriate pedicle, in the intervertebral foramen. The marker is positioned with appropriate screening in the saggital plane of the segment (cephalad/caudad) and then with 15°–45° of obliquity in the axial plane.

In selecting the level to be injected, we target above and below the intervertebral disc herniation (e.g. L4 and L5 for an L4/5 herniation).

Using an appropriate aseptic technique, a 22-gauge 90-mm spinal needle is introduced with screening in the oblique and lateral planes. Occasionally, a 125-mm needle is required. The needle can be steered away from the bevel to achieve correct position before introducing 0.5–1 ml contrast medium, which may exacerbate the patient's sciatica when screening in the anterior/posterior plane (Figure 52.3). Additionally, 1% lidocaine is introduced into the paraspinal tissues, but great care must be exercised not to injure the nerve root. It is therefore not appropriate to introduce local anaesthetic too close to the root canal until the needle is in place, and when close to the root canal, the needle is introduced very slowly. For the S1 nerve root, commonly affected by an L5/S1 disc prolapse, the approach is almost vertically into the first sacral foramen. Because the sacrum usually tilts forward, best visualization of the foramen may need up to 45° angle of the X-ray beam. A mixture of just 1 ml 1% lidocaine without preservative with 40 mg (1 ml) triamcinolone acetonide is injected around the appropriate nerve root and a similar injection is made at the next foramen up (e.g. L5), giving a double chance of reaching the disc–nerve root interface (Figure 52.3). Occasionally, patients experience some leg numbness and weakness from the local anaesthetic.

Cervical transforaminal epidural injection technique

Cervical transforaminal epidural injections/DRGBs are best performed with the patient lying supine with the head and neck on a completely radiolucent table to allow for oblique as well as anteroposterior and lateral screening. The cricoid is a guide to the C6 level and the C7 transverse process can usually be palpated in the interscalene space between scalenus anterior and scalenus medius.

Using an appropriate aseptic technique, a 22-gauge 90-mm needle is introduced laterally at the appropriate level into the interscalene space, avoiding the external jugular vein. It is directed slightly posteriorly and the level checked by screening in the lateral plane. The root canals are best viewed in the oblique plane, about 30° from the lateral plane (Figure 52.4).

The needle is introduced until it abuts the posterior canal wall. The bevel is then turned to face posteriorly and the needle is stepped over the edge and introduced very slowly along the posterior surface of the root canal so as to avoid piercing the nerve root. It is introduced about halfway down the canal as assessed in the anteroposterior plane. It is very common for the needle to be intravenous, and it needs to be adjusted in or out until contrast flows up the root canal (it may exacerbate the patient's arm symptoms) (Figure 52.4). Aspiration and observation is made for flow-back of venous or arterial blood and cerebrospinal fluid. Then, a test dose of 0.5 ml lidocaine 1% is introduced and the patient is observed for a few minutes before slowly introducing 1 ml lidocaine 1% plus 40 mg (1 ml) of triamcinolone acetonide (a non-particulate steroid such as dexamethasone 6.6 mg (2 ml) is an alternative). This may also exacerbate the patient's usual arm symptoms.

After the procedure, the patient may experience some arm numbness and weakness for half an hour or so.

Side-effects of epidural injections

In reviewing over 10,000 epidural procedures before 1982, Corrigan et a1. (1982) point out that reports of major complications are exceedingly rare. Abram and Connor also confirmed this in their 1996 review of the literature, as did McGrath et al. in 2011. This has certainly been my experience in performing some 30,000 procedures over the past three decades. However, technique should be fastidious. Anyone intending to perform these techniques should seek appropriate instruction and only attempt injections in the cervical spine under supervision. This is paramount because with increasing popularity, several dozen major neurological complications, including deaths, have been reported in recent years. ISIS (The International Spinal Intervention Society) advocates the use of non-particulate steroid in the cervical spine to avoid posterior fossa or cord infarcts due to inadvertent vertebral or radicular artery injection, respectively. Other measures to avoid complications mentioned in the literature include a test dose of local anaesthetic before the injection of steroids, live fluoroscopy, digital subtraction, no to light sedation, use of true lateral view to supplement frontal and oblique views in fluoroscopy, use of blunt needles, and CT guidance. As already stated in the section on techniques, we advocate the use of a test dose of local anaesthetic and we never use sedation.

There are a number of minor side-effects, such as initial exacerbation of symptoms (usually for a few hours to a few days), and menstrual irregularity. The incidence of side-effects was calculated by Tanner (1996) in a survey of almost 75,000 epidural procedures (see Table 52.1). Side-effects can be broadly classified into those resulting from the corticosteroid, those from the local anaesthetic, and those from the physical effects of the procedure. Some physicians choose to avoid the potential for side-effects of local anaesthetic by using normal saline for making up the solution to be injected epidurally. As already alluded to, ISIS advocates the use of non-particulate steroid in the cervical, thoracic, and upper lumbar spine.

Table 52.1 Complications of epidural injections

Anaphylaxis	0.01%
Hypersensitivity	0.01%
Prolonged hypotension	0.02%
Epidural abscess	0.005%
Headaches	0.07%
Severe aggravation of pain - for under 24 hours	1%
- for over 72 hours	0.29%

Diabetes

People with diabetes should be warned that their blood sugar may increase for a few days or weeks, according to the corticosteroid dose and preparation. Insulin may need to be increased over this period. Some authorities have also suggested the use of prophylactic antibiotics in diabetics.

Anticoagulants

Patients on warfarin should stop this for 4 days before the injection, to reduce the international normalized ratio (INR) to below 1.5, if their specialist agrees. This precaution reduces the chances of an epidural haematoma.

Concluding thoughts about epidural injections

Epidural steroid injection remains a most useful procedure when dealing with carefully selected spinal syndromes, but the benefit to the individual seems poorly conveyed by the controlled trials. A grateful ENT (ear, nose, throat) surgeon crystallized this sentiment: 'I am hard pushed to think of one procedure in my specialty which has such a dramatic and immediate benefit with so few possible side-effects. I envy you.'

References

Abram, S. E., O'Connor, T. Complications associated with epidural steroid injections. *Regional Anaesthesia*, 1966, 21(2), 149–62.

Bhatia, M. T, Parikh, L. C. J. Epidural saline therapy in lumbo-sciatic syndrome. *Journal of the Indian Medical Association*, 1966, 47(11), 537–42.

Bozzao, A., et al. Lumbar disc herniation: MR imaging assessment of natural history in patients treated without surgery. *Radiology*, 1992, 185, 135–41.

Burn, J. M., et al. The spread of solutions injected into the epidural space. *British Journal of Anaesthesiology*, 1973, 45, 338–45.

Bush, K. When should you order an MRI scan before performing an epidural injection for lower back pain? *International Musculoskeletal Medicine*, 2012, 34(4), 131–2.

Bush, K., Hillier, S. A controlled study of caudal epidural injections of triamcinolone plus procaine in the management of intractable sciatica. *Spine*, 1991, 16, 572–5.

Bush, K., Hillier, S. Outcome of cervical radiculopathy treated with periradicular/epidural corticosteroid injections: a prospective study with independent clinical review. *European Spine Journal*, 1996, 5, 319–25.

Bush, K., et al. The natural history of sciatica associated with disc pathology. A prospective study with clinical and independent radiologic follow-up. *Spine*, 1992, 17, 1205–12.

Bush, K., et al. The pathomorphologic changes that accompany the resolution of cervical radiculopathy. *Spine*, 1997, 22, 183–6.

Carette, S., et al. Epidural corticosteroid injections for sciatica due to herniated nucleus pulposus. *New England Journal of Medicine*, 1997, 336(23), 1634–40.

Corrigan, B., et al. Intraspinal corticosteroid injections. *Medical Journal of Australia*, 1982, Mar 6, 224–5.

Cuckler, J. M. The use of epidural steroids in the treatment of lumbar radicular pain. *Journal of Bone and Joint Surgery*, 1986, 67A, 6306–12.

Cyriax, J. *Textbook of orthopaedic medicine, Vol 1* (8th edn). Bailliere Tindall, London, 1984, pp. 319–26.

Delauche-Cavalier, M. C., et al. Lumbar disc herniation. Computed tomography scan changes after conservative treatment of nerve root compression. *Spine*, 1992, 17, 927–32.

Dilke, T. F. W., et al. Extradural corticosteroid injection management of lumbar nerve root compression. *British Medical Journal*, 1973, 2, 635–7.

Gupta, A. K., et al. Observations on the management of lumbosciatic syndromes (sciatica) by epidural saline. *Journal of the Indian Medical Association*, 1970, 54, 194–6.

Hakelius, A. Prognosis in sciatica. *Acta Orthopaedica Scandinavica (Suppl)*, 1970, 129, 1–76.

Jensen, M. C. Magnetic resonance imaging of the lumbar spine in people without back pain. *New England Journal of Medicine*, 1994, 331, 69–73.

Klenerman, C., et al. Lumbar epidural injection in the treatment of sciatica. *British Journal of Rheumatology*, 1984, 23, 35–8.

Koes, B. W., et al. Efficacy of epidural steroid injections for low back pain and sciatica: a systematic review of randomized clinical trials. *Pain*, 1995, 63, 279–88.

Maigne, J. V., Deligne, L. Computed tomographic follow-up study of 21 cases of non-operatively treated cervical intervertebral soft disc herniation. *Spine*, 1994, 19, 189–91.

Maigne, J. V., et al. Computed tomographic follow-up study of forty eight cases of non-operatively treated lumbar intervertebral disc herniation. *Spine*, 1992, 17, 1071–8.

Malthotra, G., et al. Complications of transforaminal cervical epidural steroid injections. *Spine*, 2009, 34(7), 731–9.

Manchikanti, L., et al. Effectiveness of therapeutic lumbar transforaminal epidural steroid injections in managing lumbar spinal pain. *Pain Physician*, 2012, 15(3), E199–245.

McCarron, R. F., et al. The inflammatory effect of the nucleus pulposus. *Spine*, 1987, 12, 758–64.

McGrath, J., et al. Incidence and characteristics of complications from epidural steroid injections. *Pain Medicine*, 2011, 12(5), 726–31.

Mixter, W. J., Barr, J. A. Rupture of the intervertebral disc with involvement of the spinal canal. *New England Journal of Medicine*, 1934, 211, 210–5.

National Health and Medical Research Council Australia. *Epidural use of steroids in the management of back pain*. National Health and Medical Research Council Australia, 1994, pp. 1–76.

Olmarker, K., et al. Autologous nucleus pulposus induced neurophysiologic and histologic changes in porcine cauda equina nerve roots. *Spine*, 1993, 18, 1425–9.

Olmarker, K., et al. Effects of methylprednisolone on nucleus pulposus¬ induced nerve root injury. *Spine*, 1994, 19, 1803–8.

Parr, A., et al. Caudal epidural injections in the management of chronic low back pain: a systematic appraisal of the literature. *Pain Physician*, 2011, 15(3), E159–98.

Ridley, M. G., et al. Out-patient lumbar epidural corticosteroid injection in the management of sciatica. *British Journal of Rheumatology*, 1998, 27, 295–301.

Rydevick, B., et al. Patho-anatomy and pathophysiology of nerve root compression. *Spine*, 1984, 9, 7–17.

Saal, J. A., et al. The natural history of lumbar disc extrusions treated non-operatively. *Spine*, 1990, 15, 683–6.

Sicard, A. Les injections medicamenteuses extra-durales par voie sacro¬ coccygienne. *Comptes Rendus Hebdomadaires des Seances et Mernoires de la Societe de Biologie*, 1901, 53, 396–8.

Snoek, W., et al. Double blind evaluation of extradural methylprednisolone for herniated lumbar discs. *Acta Orthopaedica Scandinavica*, 1977, 48, 535–41.

Stitz, M. Y., Sommer, H. M. Accuracy of blind versus fluoroscopically guided caudal epidural injection. *Spine*, 1999, 24, 1371–6.

Tanner, J. A. Epidural injections. A new survey of complications and analysis of the literature. *Journal of Orthopaedic Medicine*, 1996, 18, 78–82.

Watts, R. W., Silagy, C. A. A meta-analysis on the efficacy of epidural corticosteroids in the treatment of sciatica. *Anaesthesia and Intensive Care*, 1995, 23, 564–9.

Weber, H. Lumbar disc herniation: a controlled prospective study with ten years of observation. *Spine*, 1983, 2, 131–40.

Wiesel, S. W., et al. A study of computer assisted tomography. 1: The incidence of positive CAT scans in an asymptomatic group of patients. *Spine*, 1984, 9, 549–51.

Chapter 53

Guided (and anatomically landmarked) spinal injections

John Tanner and Michael Hutson

Spinal injections under fluoroscopic control

Introduction from John Tanner

Anyone considering performing spinal injections needs proper training to achieve a defined level of competence. This is usually available within a specialty or may be provided by a multidisciplinary organization (such as the British Institute of Musculoskeletal Medicine (BIMM) in the UK, or the International Spine Intervention Society in Europe and the USA).

Spinal injections usually involve the use of local anaesthetics within or close to the epidural space, and so entail potential risks. The operator therefore needs to have available a skilled nurse or assistant, intravenous fluids, oxygen, emergency drugs including adrenaline (epinephrine), hydrocortisone succinate, diazepam, and others, as well as resuscitation equipment, and needs to regularly update via advanced life support courses (run by the Resuscitation Council in the UK).

The descriptions of techniques outlined in this chapter, although detailed, are no substitute for proper training under supervision.

Cervical facet joint injection under fluoroscopic control

These joints can be approached posteriorly or laterally. (Injection of the atlanto-occipital and atlantoaxial joints requires special knowledge and skills which will not be covered in this section.)

Indications

'Mechanical' pain, i.e. pain on active movement felt in the cervicoscapular/upper thoracic area that is resistant to manual therapy and postural re-training, in the absence of disc signs such as radicular pain, with positive evidence of tenderness over specific levels in the articular column. These joints can be readily palpated between the posterior and lateral muscles of the neck and refer pain in typical reproducible patterns (Figure 53.1).

Materials

Two 5-ml syringes, a 22-gauge or 25-gauge 90-mm spinal needle, 1% lignocaine (lidocaine), depot steroid, contrast medium.

Technique: posterior approach

The patient lies prone with a pillow under the sternum to flex the neck.

Anteroposterior screening with intensifier directed craniad will identify the characteristic corrugated lateral edge of the articular columns. The joint margins lie at the convex points and the medial branches of the posterior primary ramus at the concave or waisted areas.

Raise a bleb over the midpoint of the designated facet joints viewed under this anteroposterior cranially oriented angle. Direct the needle to the posterior aspect of the joint. If these are not well visualized because of the mandible and metalware in the mouth, rotate the patient's head and jaw to the contralateral side. This also helps 'open' the lateral margin of the joints.

The needle tip should be insinuated carefully and slowly between the articular processes; a 25-gauge needle may be easier in very degenerated joints. The needle should not be passed too far into the joint, to avoid traversing it entirely and penetrating the root canal space or dura. A test dose of contrast (0.1–0.2 ml) should be used to obtain an arthrogram before injecting 1 ml or so of local anaesthetic and steroid (Figures 53.2, 53.3, and 53.4).

Technique: lateral approach

This is more comfortable for the patient, and makes it easier to visualize the joints. If it is possible to get a view straight through both joints, then placement is easy. If not, rotate the C-arm of the image intensifier a few degrees, and the uppermost level will move towards the same side of the rotation, separating the two sets of joint margins. C2–3 is often approached more easily in this way (Figure 53.5).

Lumbar facet joint injection under fluoroscopic control

Indications

'Mechanical' pain in the absence of signs of disc prolapse or radicular irritation, not responsive to manual therapy or therapeutic exercise. Pain usually refers only to the back or pelvic area, occasionally more distally into the limb. Features of the history include pain on

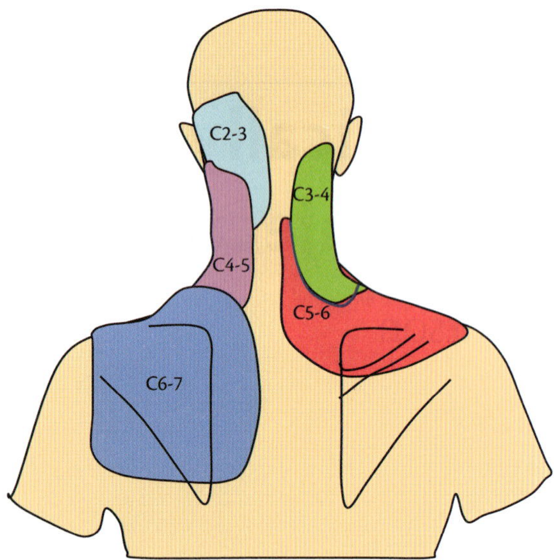

Figure 53.1 Pain referral patterns from cervical facet joints.

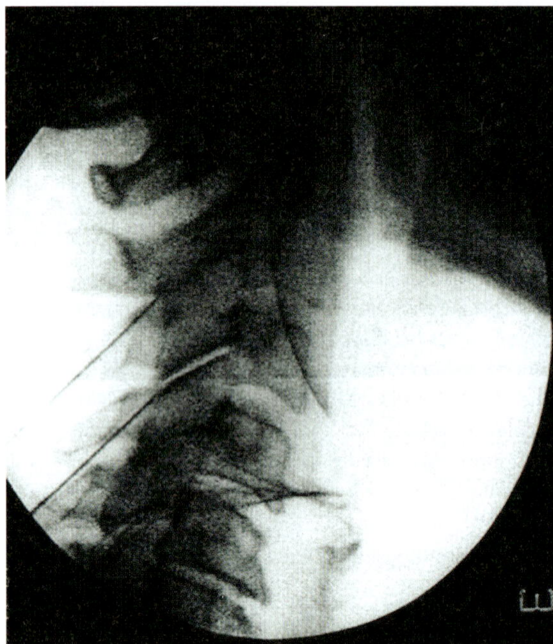

Figure 53.2 Posterior approach to C2–3 and C3–4.

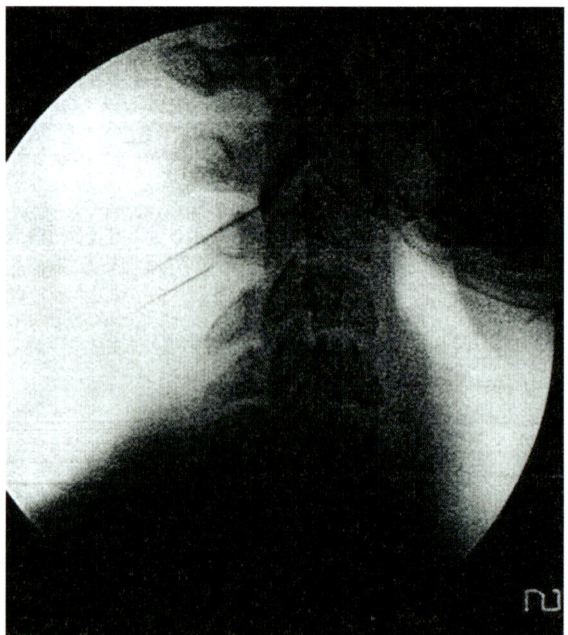

Figure 53.3 C2–3 arthrogram—right.

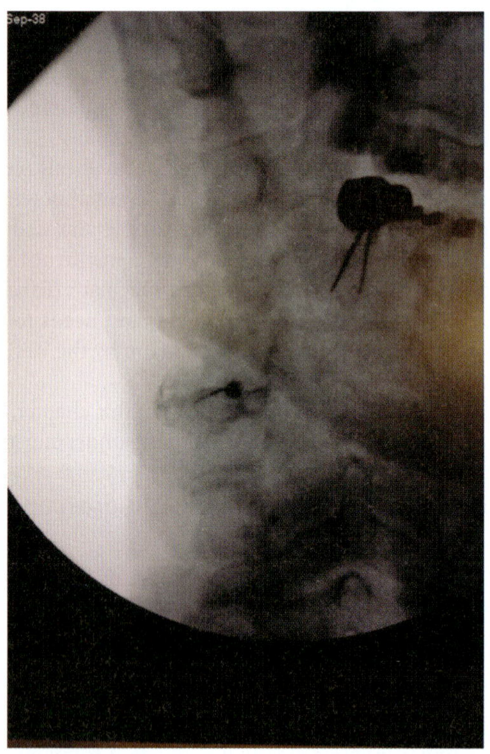

Figure 53.4 Arthrogram of degenerate mid cervical facet joint.

upright activity, relief with recumbency, and older age group. Contrary to widely held beliefs, pain on active extension and/or rotation is no predictor of response to facet joint blocks.

Tenderness may be found directly on deep palpation of the affected levels or by performing the Mennell facet rock test. Radiological changes of degeneration are not helpful in determining the affected levels, but single-photon emission computed tomography (SPECT) may be.

Meticulous intra-articular blocks using double-blinded, double-block design (one trial with short-acting, another with long-acting anaesthetic) suggests that facet joint pain is responsible for between 15% and 40% of a population with chronic 'non-specific' low back pain.

Materials

Two 5-ml syringes, 22-gauge 90-mm spinal needles, 1% lignocaine (lidocaine), depot steroid, water-soluble contrast medium.

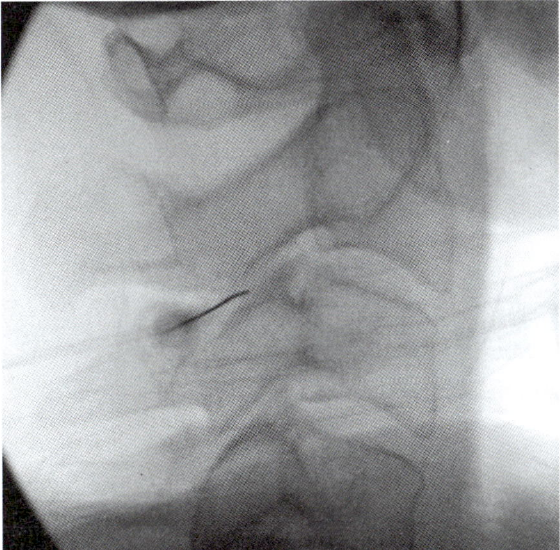

Figure 53.5 Needle placed in R C2-3 facet joint.

Technique

The patient lies prone. Take an anteroposterior view initially and raise a bleb overlying the inferior aspect of the designated facet joints. The sagittal plane of the joint is easy to identify in the upper lumbar levels but is usually oblique and not readily visualized at L4–5 and L5–S1. Follow the line of the lamina down to the tip of the inferior articular process and mark the entry point there.

Direct the spinal needle perpendicularly down to bone and directly into the inferior recess of the capsule. The characteristic feel of the tip snicking into this cleft is reassuring, but not always reliable. Inject a test dose of contrast (0.2 ml) and screen. If a facet arthrogram is obtained, inject 1–1.5 ml of steroid and local anaesthetic against the usual high resistance. At the lower lumbar levels, once the needle tip is on bone but no arthrogram has been obtained, rotate the C-arm of the image intensifier obliquely to the respective side while screening until the plane of the joint is visualized, and inject a test dose of contrast to obtain an arthrogram.

At L5–S1 you may need more than 45° rotation to see the parallel joint surfaces of the articular processes. Occasionally, even when in the joint, the contrast does not show. This indicates that the needle is intravascular. Reposition the needle towards the superior recess, taking care not to pass too far over the top and into the lateral root canal (Figures 53.6 and 53.7).

Cervical medial branch block under fluoroscopic control

As an alternative method to diagnose neck pain arising from the facet joint (zygapophyseal joint), this is preferable to intra-articular injection since it leads on to a proven method of semi-permanent pain relief—radio-frequency facet denervation. It is easier to perform than the latter, requires a good knowledge of neuroanatomy and fluoroscopic imaging, but has no therapeutic value. It does, however, have greater predictive validity. The facet joints are innervated by medial branches arising from the segmental spinal nerve above and below the target joint. Choosing the appropriate levels to 'block' is decided clinically from the referred pain pattern

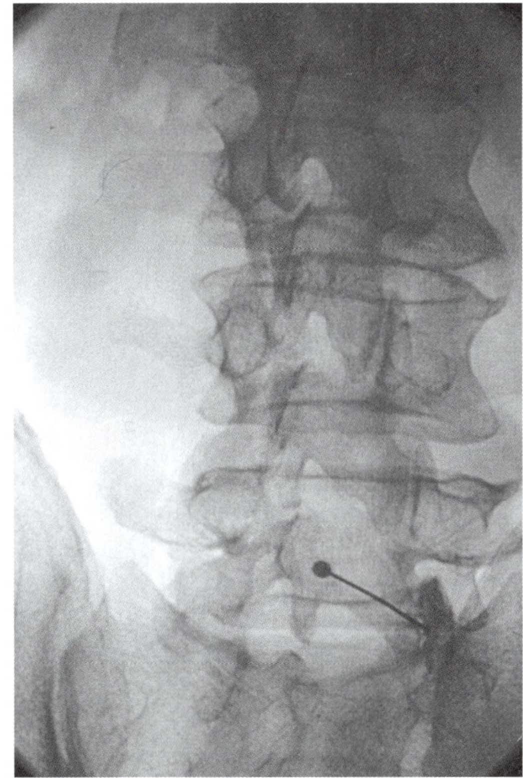

Figure 53.6 Right L5–S1 facet joint arthrogram.

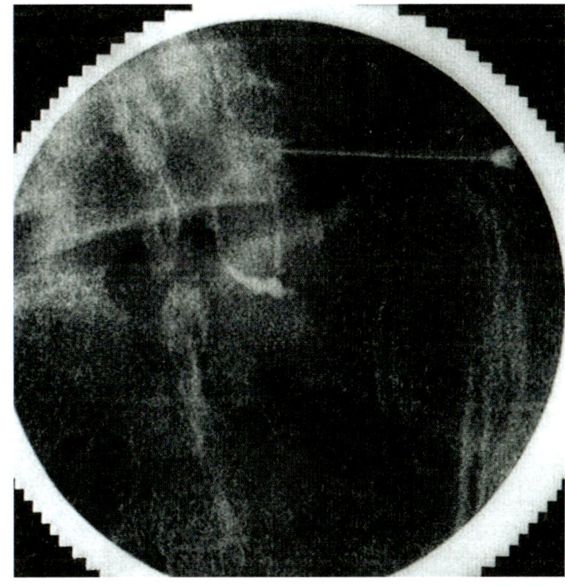

Figure 53.7 Facet arthrogram—L5–S1 superior approach.

(see Figure 53.1) and level of tenderness on palpation of the articular column.

Method

The patient lies on their side with the upper shoulder rotated back and the lower, forwards, to obtain optimal view of the cervical spine. The position will enable the operator to obtain a clearer view

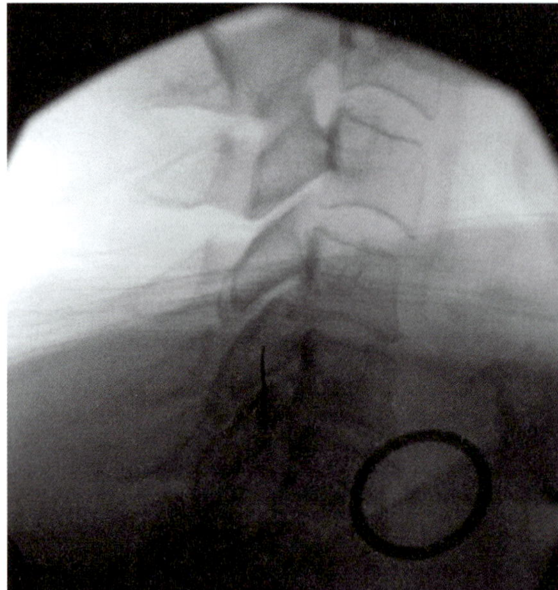

Figure 53.8 Needle placement at right C5 medial branch to block nerve.

of the cervical spine, although it will require a degree of rotation of the image intensifier to obtain a pure lateral view. This way, a direct perpendicular approach down the beam of the image intensifier through the lateral tissues of the neck, with a 25-guage paediatric spinal needle, can be achieved (Figure 53.8).

The nerve in the mid cervical levels lies in the centre of the articular pillar, midway between the joints. At C7, it is further up the superior articular process or out over the transverse process, and at C2–3, the innervation is more complex (Figure 53.9).

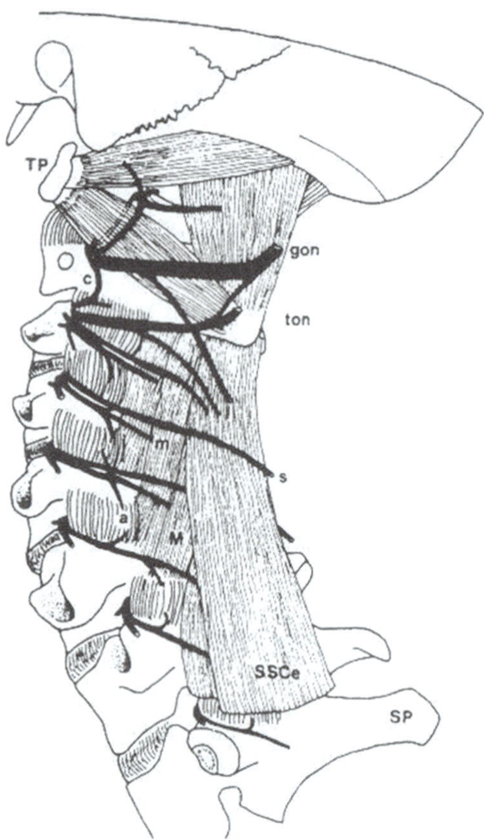

Figure 53.9 Gon – greater occipital nerve; ton – third occipital nerve; remaining medial branch innervation of joint and muscles.

The aim is to contact bone at these locations and inject a test dose of contrast medium, 0.2–0.5 ml maximum, to confirm local spread only and no intravascular spread or run-off into the foramen. Once achieved, 0.5 ml of either 2% lidocaine or 0.25% marcaine is injected. This is done at all the target levels selected, which should not be more than five in one sitting. The patient is then observed, with a pain diary or chart to ascertain the degree of pain relief in the subsequent hour(s) following the block, which should vary according to the chosen anaesthetic's duration of action. More than 80% relief is required on two separate occasions to make a satisfactory diagnosis of zygapophyseal joint pain.

Materials

Contrast agent, 2% lidocaine or 0.25% marcaine, 25-guage spinal needle of 50–100-mm length (according to size of patient).

Cervical radio-frequency facet denervation

This is undertaken when a patient has had a good temporary response to two medial branch block or intra-articular facet joint injections—that is, more than 80% pain relief.

The most effective way to achieve adequate long-term pain relief is to place the thermocouple within an insulated cannula, with a 10-mm exposed tip parallel to the course of the nerve along the 'waist' of the relevant articular pillar (Figure 53.10), and to perform three separate lesions, after minor adjustment of the cannula tip position along the course of the nerve, parasagittally and obliquely, to ensure adequate neurotomy (Figure 53.11) (Lord et al. 1996). Use of the traditional direct perpendicular approach is inadequate and larger diameter electrodes of 18–20G will bring better results.

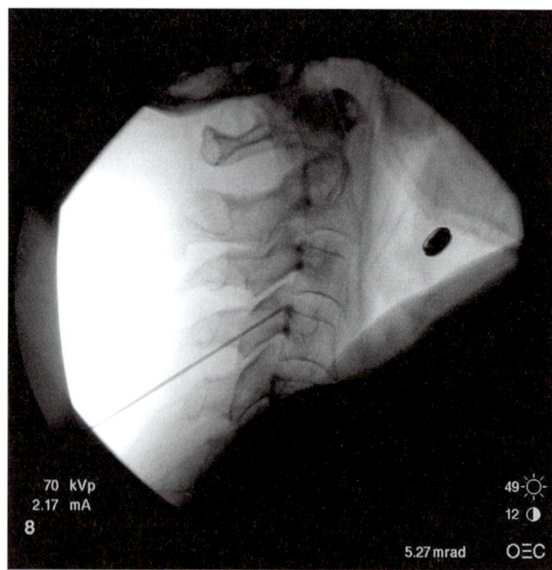

Figure 53.10 Parallel placement of electrode along C4 medial branch for RF denervation.

Once positioning has been checked in anteroposterior (AP) and lateral views, and sensory and motor stimulation checked to

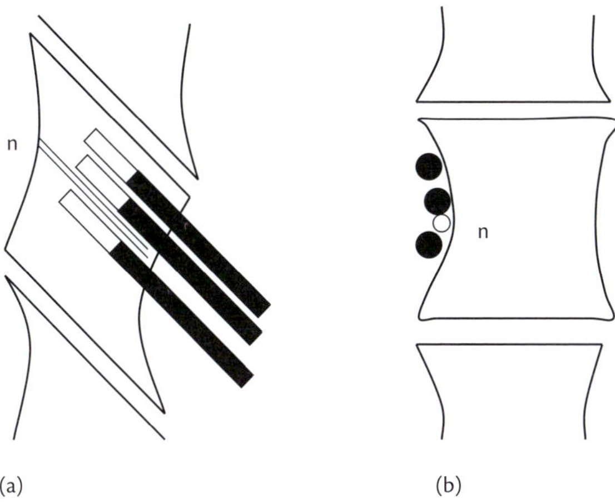

Figure 53.11 Electrode placement to obtain complete thermal denervation of medial branch shown in lateral and posterior views.

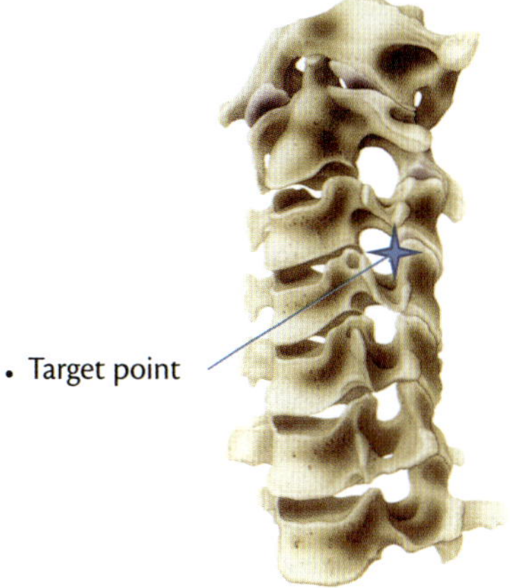

Figure 53.12 STAR marks optimum needle placement for cervical transforaminal injection (just anterior to articular pillar in lower half of foramen).

exclude segmental nerve proximity, 1 ml of local anaesthetic is administered through the cannula. After lesioning at 80–85°C for 60–90 seconds at three adjacent placements, many practitioners inject a small dose of steroid and anaesthetic to minimize post-procedural pain.

Results should be assessed in one month and over the longer term. Regeneration does occur in the longer term, so attention to optimal posture and conditioning is important to reduce the risk of recurrence.

Materials

A radio-frequency lesion generator, lidocaine or marcaine, 16–20 -gauge cannula with 10-mm exposed tip, suitable length electrodes (diameter is less important).

Cervical transforaminal (intraforaminal) nerve root block under fluoroscopic control

Indications

Cervical nerve root foraminal encroachment; compression or irritation due to disc protrusion.

Materials

Two 5-ml syringes, a 5-cm 25-gauge spinal needle, 1% lignocaine (lidocaine) or saline (preservative free), non-particulate steroid, connection tubing, and contrast medium.

Technique

The patient lies supine on a radiolucent trolley, with the head and neck supported on an extended section.

Identify target level under lateral screening. Rotate the C-arm to an oblique position until the foramina are well visualized. This may require rotating the intensifier caudally 10° or more to 'look up' the foramina.

Mark the entry point directly over the anterior margin of the superior articular process. Slowly direct the spinal needle 'down the beam' to the articular process. Once you have contacted bone, rotate the C-arm to the anteroposterior position and redirect the needle slightly anteriorly to slip off the posterior column into the foramen. The ideal position is in the posterior part of the foraminal floor (Figure 53.12).

Under real-time screening, inject 0.5–1 ml contrast through the connection tubing to display dorsal root ganglion and root. Ensure that the needle tip is not intravascular and has not strayed medially past the mid-zygoapophyseal 'line', as viewed under anteroposterior screening. This reduces the chance of intrathecal injection, although it does not eliminate it.

It is vitally important to ensure that the needle is not intradural or intravascular before injecting medication, particularly if local anaesthetic is being used. Contrast medium should always be used (Figure 53.13). Inject the medication only if you are secure in these matters.

Complications

- Avoid lignocaine (lidocaine) with adrenaline and particulate steroids in all spinal nerve blocks because of the risk of radicular spinal artery injection causing cord ischaemia.

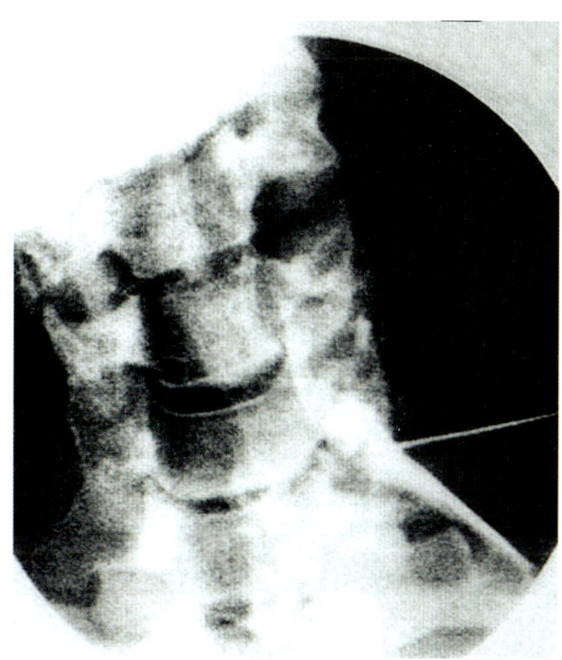

Figure 53.13 C7 neurogram.

- Intradural injection, leading to spinal hypotension and cardiac arrest.
- Intravascular injection, leading to toxicity or cord ischaemia.
- Haematoma of soft tissues, leading to airways obstruction.

Lumbar medial branch block under oblique imaging

These are performed solely for diagnostic purposes to determine the anatomical pain generator which ranges from 15–40% in the adult population, with chronic mechanical back pain sometimes referred to as 'non-specific back pain' until due diligence is applied.

Pragmatically, each facet joint is supplied by the medial branch of the segmental spinal nerve above and below the joint, although small ramifications may extend two segments below (i.e. the L3–4 joint is innervated by the medial branch of the dorsal primary ramus of L3 and L4).

The diagnostic block is performed with oblique imaging of the 'scotty dog' view, aiming the 22-guage spinal needle down the beam to hit bone at the 'eye' of the scotty dog (i.e. the junction of the superior articular process and transverse process). A small dose of 0.2–0.5ml contrast is injected to ensure local spread only (Figure 53.14). Once satisfied it is remaining local and not intravascular, inject 0.5 ml 2% lidocaine or 0.5% marcaine.

The patient should be observed immediately afterwards for abolition of pain on performing any provocative manoeuvres or standing or walking. Greater than 80% relief of pain for the duration of the anaesthetic is required, preferably on two separate occasions, to justify proceeding to radio-frequency lesioning of the nerve for semi-permanent relief. It is useful to provide a pain diary for the following 12–24 hours. Incomplete relief may mean that only one or two of the relevant levels have been successfully identified.

Materials

22-guage spinal needle, 2% lidocaine or 0.5% marcaine, contrast agent.

Lumbar transforaminal (intraforaminal) nerve root block under fluoroscopic control

Indications

Radicular irritation or compression by disc material. (Note: use of the term 'selective nerve root block' should be reserved for small-volume extraforaminal injection.)

In the foramen, the injected solution clearly spreads to more than one level, anaesthetizing the sinuvertebral nerve and, at L2, the afferents from most of the anterior spinal column in the lumbar region. A positive analgesic response does not necessarily inculpate that particular segment as the sole or main pain generator.

Materials

Two 5-ml syringes, a 22-gauge spinal needle, 1% lignocaine (lidocaine) or saline (preservative-free), water soluble steroid, 90-mm 22-gauge spinal needle, contrast medium.

Technique

The patient lies prone with lumbar spine flattened. Use anteroposterior fluoroscopy to identify target level, and tilt the beam either caudad or craniad, depending on the level, to obtain a parallel view through the superior end plate of the relevant vertebra (L5 for L5 root), and rotate the C-arm obliquely to the required side to about 30–45°.

The superior articular process (SAP, 'scotty dog's ear') points to the target of the emerging nerve root under the pedicle (Figure 53.15). Mark the skin, and direct the 22-gauge spinal needle down the tunnel of the beam. Once you have passed the SAP, that is, passed over the top of the zygoapophyseal joint, or when you have reached sufficient depth (in larger patients you may need a 120-mm or even a 150-mm needle), redirect the C-arm to anteroposterior viewing.

Guide the needle carefully to the supra neural 6 o'clock position, just under the face of the pedicle. Check position on a lateral view. Ideally, 1 ml of contrast injection should flow centrally and peripherally to outline the nerve root (Figure 53.16).

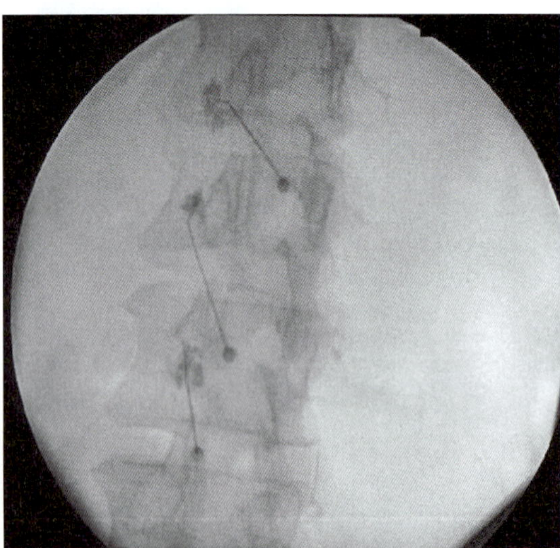

Figure 53.14 Lumbar medial branch blocks at 'eye of scottie dog' with contrast.

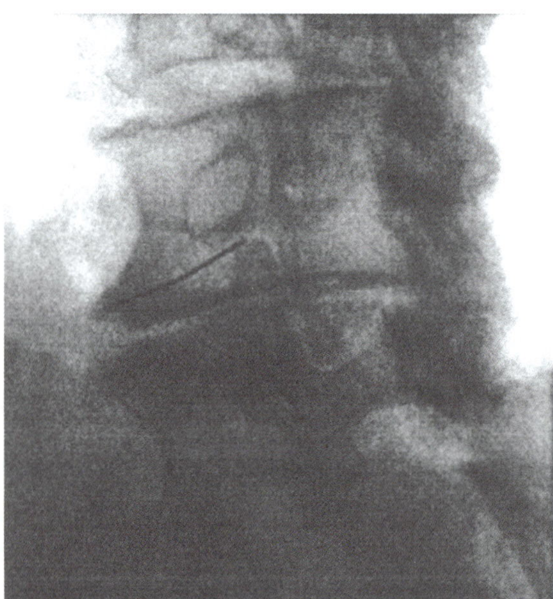

Figure 53.15 Needle tip between SAP and pedicle.

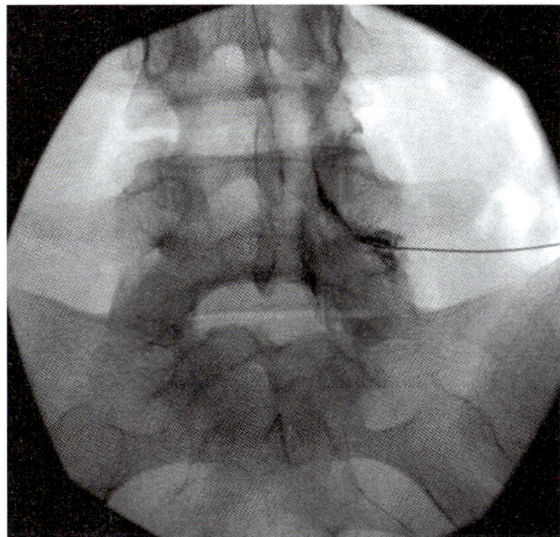

Figure 53.16 Right L5 transforaminal contrast injection outlining root.

Any pain or resistance to injection requires adjustment of the needle tip position. (In stenotic canals or where there is fibrosis, it may not be possible to eliminate these obstructions entirely. Sometimes an infra neural or retro neural needle tip placement is necessary)

Once you are satisfied with the 'neurogram' obtained, inject 2–3 ml of local anaesthetic mixed with corticosteroid. Injection of larger volumes or concentrations is not necessary, and increases the risk of complications.

Complications

- *Intravascular injection*: Recent reports of spinal cord ischaemia from inadvertent injection of the radicular artery with particulate steroids at all lumbar levels, including S1, indicate that extreme caution should be taken to ensure that there is no vascular flow, using adequate doses of contrast and digital subtraction angiography, if necessary, to avoid complications. Above level L3, it is advisable to use non-particulate steroid, since the risk of anterior spinal artery syndrome is higher.
- *Intraneural injection*: nerve damage (avoid by adjusting needle position if painful).
- *Intradural injection*: can be avoided by checking contrast flow and not passing needle medial to the 6 o'clock position under the pedicle.

Lumbar radio-frequency facet denervation

This is embarked on only if a patient has had good or excellent relief from comparative diagnostic blocks or intra-articular blocks, although it should be said that the two methods are not synonymous.

To achieve effective radio-frequency neurotomy of the lumbar medial branches, parallel electrode placement with higher gauges (up to 16-gauge) will bring better results. Parallel placement involves tilting the beam craniad for a variable angle of up to 45° and up to 25° oblique orientation, to place the 10-mm tip in the groove where the medial branch lies and avoid the mamillo accessory ligament which restrains the nerve under the joint (Figure 53.17).

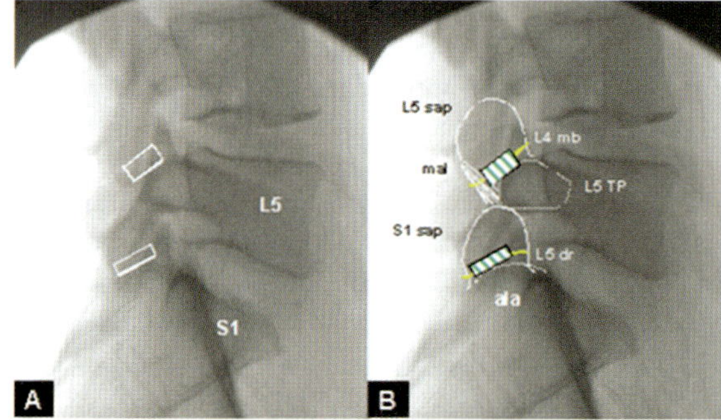

Figure 53.17 A marks target for L4 and L5 medial branch RF denervation; B shows mal – mammillary accessory ligament, sap – superior articular process.

Again, safe and correct anatomical placement is confirmed fluoroscopically and stimulation parameters checked if there is any doubt, before anaesthetizing the nerve with 1 ml of anaesthetic and performing the lesion. The lesion is performed in three locations, to cover variations in the nerve anatomy, at 80C for 60–90 seconds (Figure 53.18).

The patient is followed up at 1 month and longer term. A simple exercise programme to reduce the lumbar lordosis, incorporating posterior pelvic tilts, both lying and sustained in standing, will reduce the risk of recurrence due to regeneration of the nerves.

Materials

A radio-frequency lesion generator, lidocaine or marcaine, 16/18-gauge cannula with 10-mm exposed tip, suitable length electrodes (diameter is less important).

First sacral root block (with fluoroscopic control)

Indications

As for paralaminar (paravertebral) lumbar nerve root block when the first sacral root is irritated or compressed.

Materials

As for lumbar nerve root block.

Technique

The patient lies prone. Use anteroposterior screening, and screen caudally until the S1 translucent shadow is identified. It is significantly smaller than the S2 foramen which, in contrast, is easily identifiable. If the S1 foramen cannot be seen equidistant from the L5 pedicle and S2 foramen, rotate the C-arm 5–10° to the side being sought. This often identifies the foramen. Too oblique a view may

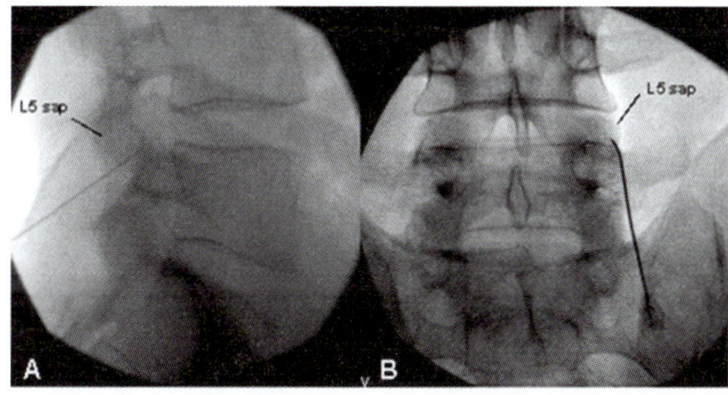

Figure 53.18 A – lateral, and B - posterior view of electrode placement for L4 branch.

result in the posterior superior iliac spine obscuring direct passage of the needle. Direct the spinal needle down the tunnel of the beam until you have contacted bone adjacent to the foramen. Note the depth. Withdraw slightly and bend the needle towards the foramen (using curved needle technique). Once the needle has entered by 1.5 cm, check a lateral view to ensure that the needle tip is neither too superficial or too deep, and then inject contrast to ensure placement is not intravascular and that the S1 root is outlined. Inject medication slowly. No more than 20–40 mg of steroid and 2 ml local anaesthetic or normal saline is required (Figures 53.19 and 53.20).

Complications

- Intravascular, intrathecal, or intraneural injection can occur (see complications in 'Lumbar transforaminal (intraforaminal) nerve root block under fluoroscopic control' section).

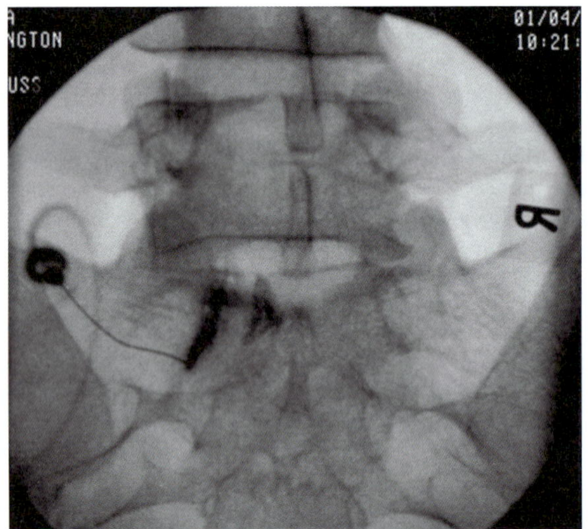

Figure 53.19 S1 transforaminal injection of contrast lateral view.

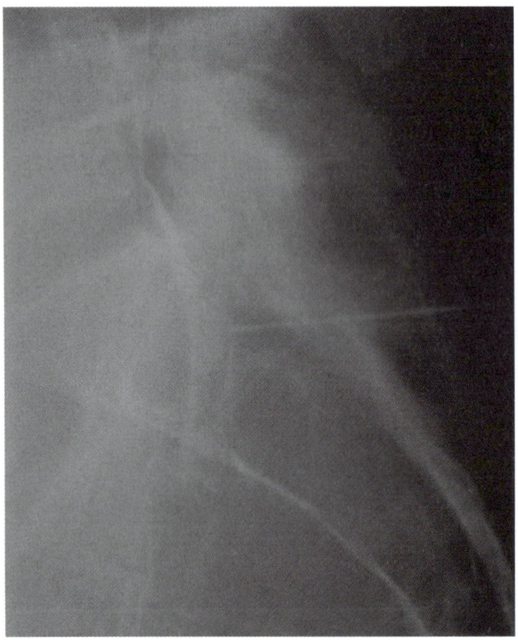

Figure 53.20 S1 transforaminal injection of contrast posterior view.

- There is a theoretical complication of large bowel perforation through passing the needle right through the sacrum into the pelvis. As far as I am aware, this has never actually happened.

Sacroiliac joint (with fluoroscopic control)

Indications

Pain deemed to be generated by the sacroiliac joint on history and examination

Materials

As for first sacral root block, but 50-mm 25-gauge needle plus contrast medium.

Technique

Patient lies prone. Use anteroposterior screening. Identify inferior pole of joint and mark the skin directly over the lower end of the posterior joint line (this should lie slightly medial). Direct the 25-gauge needle directly to the lower end of this medial line and into the joint. Having entered the lower limb of the L-shaped joint, there is high resistance to contrast injection: 0.2–0.5 ml should be enough to demonstrate an arthrogram (Figure 53.21).

Rotate the C-arm 30° to the same side to obtain an 'en face' view to visualize for contrast leakage indicating capsular rupture (Figure 53.22). This is relatively common. Injection of 2–2.4 ml medication is all an intact joint will allow.

Complications

Minor: haematoma.

General points

- Complications of these procedures, such as nerve damage, are extremely rare when performed correctly and competently. However, these descriptive accounts are included by way of introduction rather than an instruction manual. Proper training is required by a recognized professional body before starting to treat patients, particularly since the current evidence does not fully support the efficacy, due to earlier studies using flawed techniques. A more recent review, excluding these studies, shows varying levels of evidence to support it (Bogduk 2009).

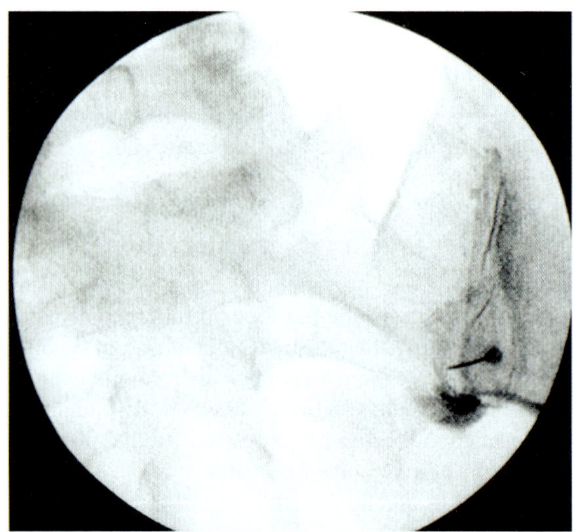

Figure 53.21 Sacroiliac joint arthrogram.

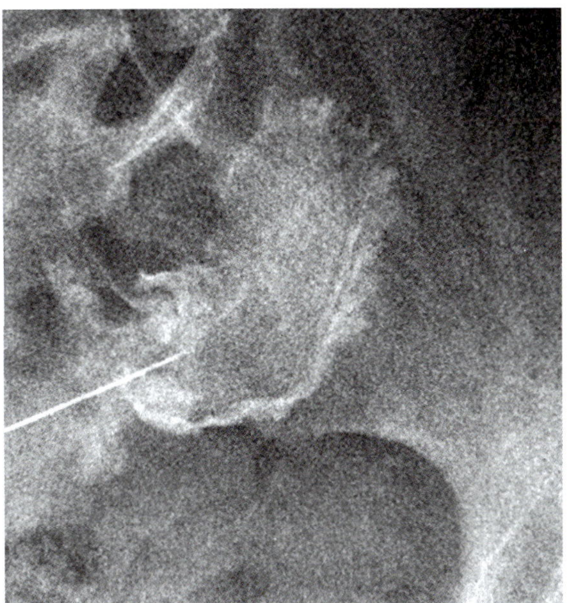

Figure 53.22 Right sacroiliac— 'en face' view (note: anterior capsular leakage).

- The author acknowledges the contribution that the International Spine Intervention Society has made to this field and strongly recommends attending their instructional courses in the USA or Europe (<http://www.spinalinjection.org> for details) and reference to the second edition of *Practice guidelines for spinal diagnostic and treatment procedures* (edited by Nikolai Bogduk) for a full account of the evidence base underpinning these methods.

Spinal injections using anatomical landmarks

Introduction from Michael Hutson

In the first edition of this textbook, my (longstanding) colleague, Dr John Tanner, wrote the chapter on spinal injections. For this second edition, Dr Tanner has undertaken an update of all musculoskeletal injection procedures, other than those spinal injections carried out without fluoroscopic control (that is, not guided, usually referred to as 'blind'). In view of his concern, over recent years, about the safety of spinal injections without such control, relying on bony landmarks only, Dr Tanner has suggested that I undertake this part of the chapter. For the reader's benefit, I confirm that I am happy to do so, as I continue to provide the following described injections in my clinical practice. I confirm that I do *not* consider these injections without fluoroscopic control to be a significant risk to the patient, assuming appropriate training and competence, the usual precautions of the availability of a skilled nurse or assistant, and resuscitation equipment. To the contrary, my experience from the use of these injections over 40 years is that they are safe and often very helpful.

I am grateful to Dr Tanner for allowing me to use some of his text from the first edition as the basis for this chapter, with my amendments. Training to achieve a defined level of competence should be undertaken under supervision.

Cervical perifacetal injection

These joints can be readily palpated between the muscles and the tender levels identified.

Indications

The described injections may be used for non-specific ('mechanical') neck pain (i.e. pain on active movement felt in the cervicoscapular/upper thoracic area that is resistant to manual therapy and postural re-training), in the absence of disc signs such as radiculopathy, with positive evidence of tenderness over specific levels in the articular column (common in limited chronic whiplash-associated disorders). Extension, rotation, and side-bending of the cervical spine may be painful and limited. When performing cervical perifacetal injections 'blind' (without fluoroscopic control), levels above C2/3 should not be attempted, for obvious reasons.

Materials

2-ml syringe, 0.8×40-mm 21-gauge hypodermic needle, 5–10 mg depot steroid, 1% lignocaine (lidocaine).

Technique

The patient leans over the side of a raised treatment table so as to flex the neck, with the head supported on the back of their hands or a firm pillow. If the patient is liable to faint, a prone position should be adopted over a couch with a breathing hole and the upper chest supported to achieve neck flexion. Even with the neck flexed in this way, the cervical laminae overlap to such an extent that providing the lateral articular column is approached from a perpendicular angle, there is no chance of passing between the articular processes and into the spinal canal.

A thorough working knowledge of anatomy is required, in particular, identification of bony landmarks such as the C2 and C7 spinous processes. With the cervical lordosis flattened, the *C2/3 facet joint* lies on a line drawn between the C2 and C3 spinous processes. Because of the increasing length and slope of the distal spinous processes, the interarticular line tends to lie closer to the line drawn at the level of the lower end of the upper spinous process (Figure 53.23).

The skin is prepared with full aseptic technique. The needle and attached syringe containing local anaesthetic and steroid is directed perpendicularly through skin and overlying muscle, at least one fingerbreadth (patient's finger size) from the midline, until it contacts bone. A total of 2 ml of steroid with local anaesthetic is injected into the 'peri-facetal' intracapsular area, after careful aspiration with the needle tip touching bone by 'walking up and down' the articular column, staying parallel to the midline; 0.2–0.3 ml is injected at each point. Care must be taken not to stray medially or laterally off the imaginary line parallel to the spinous processes, injecting only when in contact with bone.

Complications

- *Intravascular injection:* The posterior route is unlikely to risk vertebral artery trespass unless the needle strays above C2.
- *Dural puncture:* A possible complication if the needle strays towards the midline. It should be recognized early if slow and careful aspiration is performed regularly. No injection should be made unless the needle is in contact with bone.

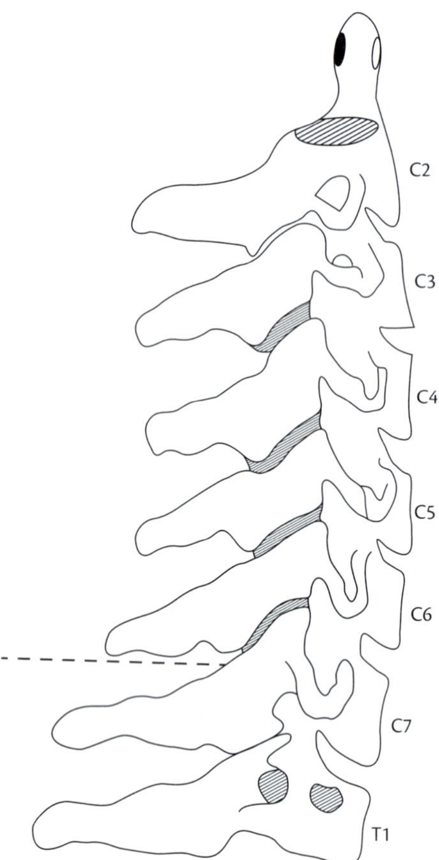

Figure 53.23 With the cervical lordosis flattened, the increasing length and slope of the distal spinous processes affect the interarticular lines of the facet joints.

- *Post-operative care:* Loss of balance and dizziness may occur if too many joints are injected in one session. This is due to local anaesthesia of joint proprioceptors. The patient should then be escorted home and not permitted to drive.

Lumbar perifacetal injection

Indications

As for the cervical spine, the described injections may be used for non-specific ('mechanical') pain in the absence of signs of disc prolapse or radicular irritation that is not responsive to manual therapy or therapeutic exercise. Pain usually refers only to the back or pelvic area; occasionally, more distally into the limb. Features of the history include pain on upright activity and on active extension (particularly) and/or rotation, relief with recumbency, and older age group. Pain on extension and tenderness on selective deep palpation over the underlying facet joints (usually, though not inevitably, L4/5 and L5/S1) are good predictors of response to perifacetal injections of steroid and local anaesthetic. Radiological changes of degeneration are not helpful in determining the affected levels.

Research using meticulous intra-articular blocks of double-blinded, double-block design (one trial with short-acting, another with long-acting anaesthetic) suggests that facet joint pain is responsible for no more than 15% of a population with chronic 'non-specific' low back pain. However, perifacetal blocks, as outlined here, being less specific, may ameliorate a wider range of problems related to the posterior spinal column.

Materials

5-ml syringe, 0.8×50-mm 21-gauge needle, 1% lignocaine (lidocaine), 10–20 mg triamcinolone (per joint).

Technique

The patient lies prone over a pillow or wedge to flatten out the lumbar region. The spinous processes are palpated and intersecting lines marked between them (Figure 53.24). The facet joints lie approximately 2–2.5 cm from the midline at their intersections, slightly less at the upper lumbar levels, and slightly more at the lumbosacral level, taking into account the size of the patient.

The needle and attached syringe containing local anaesthetic and steroid is directed perpendicularly through skin and overlying muscle, at least one fingerbreadth (patient's finger size) from the midline, until it contacts bone. Using the same technique as for cervical perifacetal injections, of 'walking' the needle up and down a line parallel to the midline, verification can be made of whether the needle tip is on the articular processes, which lie more superficial, or on the lamina, which lies deeper ('up the mountain, down the valley'). In this way, the periarticular tissues are infiltrated with a total of 2–3 ml of a 50:50 mixture of local anaesthetic and triamcinolone. By this means, the facet joints can be reached at two adjacent levels. It is inadvisable to angle the needle too far cranially, since it increases the risk of straying medially and through the ligamentum flavum.

If at first the needle does not contact bone, indicating that it is positioned too laterally, it should be withdrawn almost to the skin and re-directed at a perpendicular angle, rather than simply angling the needle more medially. If high resistance is met on attempting to inject, it indicates a high probability that an intra-articular facet injection has been achieved. Whether this is desirable or not with respect to a good outcome has not been established, but there is no reason for concern. The joint normally admits no more than 1–1.5 ml, unless there is capsular rupture.

Maintenance of the needle perpendicular to the plane of the lumbar spine, avoiding penetration medially or too far cranially, provides safety. As always, it is wise to aspirate slowly before injecting and to withhold the injection until the needle tip is on bone.

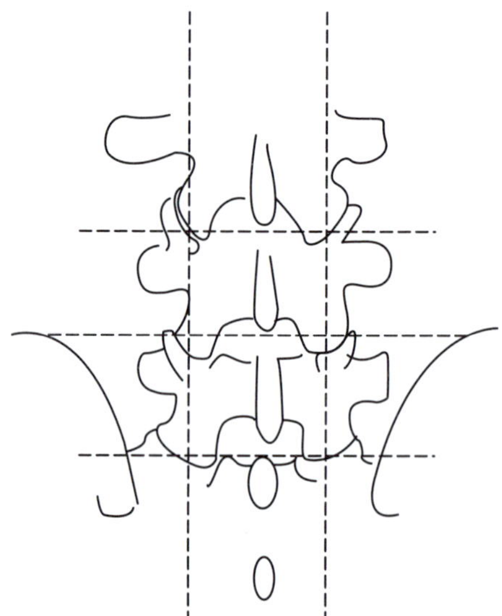

Figure 53.24 'Blind' lumbar facet joint approach, grid drawing.

Periforaminal lumbar nerve block

Indications

This injection may be used as an alternative to epidural steroid injection for leg pain due to radicular irritation or compression, lateral canal stenotic syndrome, or far lateral disc herniation. It is useful to have magnetic resonance imaging (MRI) confirmation of the nerve root involved, although imaging does not always provide conclusive information, and diffusion of injectate may be beneficial at the levels adjacent to that injected. The intention is to infiltrate around the foramen with steroid and local anaesthetic.

Materials

5-ml syringe, 0.8×50-mm 21-gauge needle, 1% lignocaine (lidocaine), 30 mg triamcinolone, 40-mm needle (if often too short).

Technique

The patient lies prone over a pillow. Mark out the intersecting horizontal lines between the spinous processes (as identified for facet injections). The spot approximately 4 cm lateral to the midline that lies midway between these lines on the relevant side should be marked. This should be slightly lateral to the edge of the lamina, just below the origin of the transverse process. The needle is directed downwards, medially, and caudally where it meets little or no resistance in this extraforaminal plane. If it contacts bone, the lamina of the vertebra of the relevant emerging spinal nerve, the needle should re-positioned slightly, advancing very slowly for the last 1 cm as the nerve is close by. Aspiration is attempted, as always. Injection occasionally evokes paraesthesiae, though other neurological symptoms are not expected.

Complications

Needle penetration of the dura surrounding the nerve root has occasionally been reported.

Sacroiliac 'joint' injection (without radiographic control)

Indications

Pain in the sacroiliac region or referred from that region which has not responded to manual/manipulative therapy or other treatment to the lumbar–pelvic region. Clinical diagnosis of sacroiliac dysfunction is not always a certain diagnosis. Refractory pain may respond to intra-articular steroid injections using the 'ex juvantibus' principle (see Chapter 60). Prolotherapy or denervation, rarely fusion surgery, may be logical steps in treatment for difficult cases. Radiographic, computed tomographic (CT), or MRI evidence of inflammatory changes may lead to a trial of local treatment when systemic treatment is not indicated, as for example in bilateral sacroiliitis.

Materials

5-ml syringe, 0.8×50-mm 21-gauge needle, 1% lignocaine (lidocaine), 30 mg triamcinolone.

Technique

The patient lies prone over a pillow to reduce lumbar lordosis. The L5 spinous process and the posterior superior iliac spine (PSIS) are marked. The needle is directed from the L5 spinous process laterally to the PSIS and about 45° caudally, at an angle of 30–45° to the skin, aiming to achieve the greatest depth through the posterior ligamentous tissue, into the cleft between the ilium and sacrum. It is rarely possible to enter the joint proper in this way, but in cases of sacroiliitis, a good therapeutic result is usually obtained. Injection of 3–4 ml of a mixture of local anaesthetic and steroid (30 mg triamcinolone) is quite adequate.

Complications

Minor: haematoma.

Other spinal injections

For techniques of injecting the thoracic spine, zygoapophyseal joints, and spinal nerve roots, the reader is referred to other texts such as that by Lennard (2000). The principles, however, are the same. Other diagnostic and therapeutic techniques rightfully constitute the domain of a musculoskeletal specialist's work—namely, the diagnosis and treatment of benign spinal pain, whether acute or chronic. These include sympathetic blocks, medial branch blocks of the posterior primary ramus, thermal denervation of facet joints, provocative discography, and diagnostic and therapeutic intradiscal procedures. For more detailed description of these topics, the reader is referred to texts written by specialist anaesthetists, interventional radiologists, and spinal surgeons.

References

Bogduk N, Dreyfuss P, Govind J. A narrative review of lumbar medial branch neurotomy for the treatment of back pain. *Pain Med* 2009, 10, 1035–45.

Lennard TA. *Pain procedures in clinical practice*. Hanley and Belfus, 2000.

Lord SM, Barnsley L, Wallis B, McDonald GM, Bogduk N. Percutaneous radio-frequency neurotomy for chronic cervical zygapophyseal joint pain. *N Eng J Med* 1996, 335, 1721–6.

Chapter 54

Prolotherapy in the USA

Thomas Dorman †

I am pleased to include this chapter by Tom Dorman in this edition. It was initially commissioned for the first edition of this textbook, and I believe that it complements the following chapter on prolotherapy in the UK by Simon Petrides in this edition.

Michael Hutson

Historical review of prolotherapy

The first description of the intentional provocation of scar formation is found in the writings of Hippocrates two and a half millennia ago. Hippocrates describes the insertion of searing needles into the anterior capsule of the shoulder in order to stabilize shoulders in javelin throwers, the warriors of Sparta. The irritant can be introduced in a more sophisticated manner by injection through a hollow needle to the appropriate site. The modern use of *sclerotherapy* hails from the herniologists of the era that antedated antiseptic surgery. In 1837, Valpeau of Paris described the use of scar formation for the repair of hernias. The genealogy of herniology, and later, the management of hydroceles and a variety of vein sclerosis techniques, was extensively reviewed by Yeomans (1939), and the tradition of vein sclerosis persists into contemporary medical times. Earl Gedney (1937), an osteopath from Philadelphia familiar with the sclerosing techniques of herniologists and venologists, was the first to introduce injection techniques for ligaments. Gedney injected a 'hypermobile sacroiliac joint (SIJ)' first, with salutary results. The term 'sclerotherapy' continued to be used until the mid-1950s, when the great organizer of prolotherapy, George Hackett, acquired the skills of injection techniques from the osteopathic profession, evaluated their benefit in an initial series of studies, and published a number of articles about his experiences. This culminated in a short textbook, the third edition of which was published in 1958—and the tradition of his textbook has been maintained into modern times.

Optimal healing

Scar tissue has a number of mechanical properties which differ from those of normal connective tissue and are considered disadvantageous. Scars can be recognized histologically as different from normal connective tissue. It was Hackett who realized that in situations where ligaments are 'relaxed' (his term for ligament insufficiency), hypertrophy of the ligament represented an advantage, contrasting with scar formation which would be a disadvantage.

The therapeutic window

Following this 'road map,' there evolved quite rapidly, in the 1940s and 1950s, a series of informal empiric trials, first in animals and later in patients with injured ligaments, of the use of a number of sclerosing agents which were now renamed *proliferant agents* by Hackett. It transpired that a great deal of benefit could be achieved clinically by the use of a number of agents which included extracts from several plants, the least unfamiliar being psyllium seed extract or Sylnasol (a product no longer available) and sodium morrhuate, an extract from fish oil (still available in the pharmacopeia). As judged by the frequency of usage, the chief proliferant agents are (1) glucose, (2) glycerin, and (3) phenol. They are usually used in combination (1.25% phenol, 12.5% glucose, 12.5% glycerin) made up with 0.5% lidocaine (lignocaine), for local analgesia, in water. This preparation is also called P25G or P2G.

Klein (1993) and Banks (1991) have classified the injectable proliferating solutions that initiate the wound-healing cascade as follows:

- *Irritants*, which cause a direct chemical tissue injury that attracts granulocytes. Phenol, quinine, and tannic acid come into this category.
- *Osmotic shock agents*, which cause bursting of cell membranes leading to local tissue damage. Hyperosmolar dextrose (12.5–15% maximum) and glycerin are examples of the most commonly used agents in this category.
- *Chemotactic agents*, which activate the inflammatory cascade. Sodium morrhuate is a prototype of this group. These compounds are the direct biosynthetic precursors of the mediators of inflammation, i.e. prostaglandins, leukotrienes, and thromboxanes.
- *Particulates*, such as pumice flour: these are small particles of the order of 1 μm, which lead to longer-lasting irritation and the attraction of macrophages to the site.

Several other materials were previously used, including zinc, Sylnasol, and sodium morrhuate. None of these offer any advantage and several have some distinct disadvantages, particularly the risk of allergic reactions.

Evidence of proliferant effect

George Hackett (1958) reported on the histological changes of the Achilles tendon of rats treated with proliferant therapy. These were uncontrolled studies. The next landmark in the study of prolotherapy was a blinded animal study combining histology, electron microscopy, and mechanical evaluation of rabbit ligaments. King Liu and his team (1983) used sodium morrhuate in the medial collateral ligaments of rabbit knees. The histological and mechanical beneficial effects of proliferant therapy in this experimental model were established categorically. The parallel effect on human tissues was established by taking biopsies of posterior SI ligaments which were performed before and after treatment in three patients with chronic low back pain (Oliver and Coughlin 1985). Treatment consisted of a series of six weekly injections into lumbar and SI ligaments, fascia, and facet capsular sites using a connective tissue proliferant (dextrose–glycerine–phenol) combined with mobilization and flexion/extension exercises. Biopsies carried out 3 months after completion of injections demonstrated fibroblastic hyperplasia on light microscopy and increases in average ligament diameter on electron microscopy from a pre-treatment value of 0.055 ± 0.26 µm to 0.087 ± 0.041 µm after treatment ($P < 0.001$). Range of motion significantly improved, after treatment, in rotation ($P < 0.001$), flexion ($P < 0.015$), and side flexion ($P < 0.001$), as did visual analogue pain ($P < 0.001$) and disability ($P < 0.001$) scores. Figure 54.1 illustrates the histology of human ligaments before and after prolotherapy.

The use of the dextrose–glycerine–phenol proliferant, as practiced by a number of doctors in California, was found to have a salutary effect, and a double-blind clinical study was conducted. This study confirmed the initial clinical impression of the experimenters of its benefit (Ongley et al. 1987). A criticism (which in my view was inapplicable) levelled at the study was that it combined four components of treatment: manipulation, local anaesthesia, select use of triamcinolone, and prolotherapy. I believe that the study evaluated a method, so a logical separation of the components is inappropriate. Nevertheless, the criticism was accepted by two of the co-authors, and a second double-blind study was conducted to evaluate prolotherapy as a single variable. These results were also statistically meaningful, but the disparity between the groups was much less than in the first study (Klein et al. 1993).

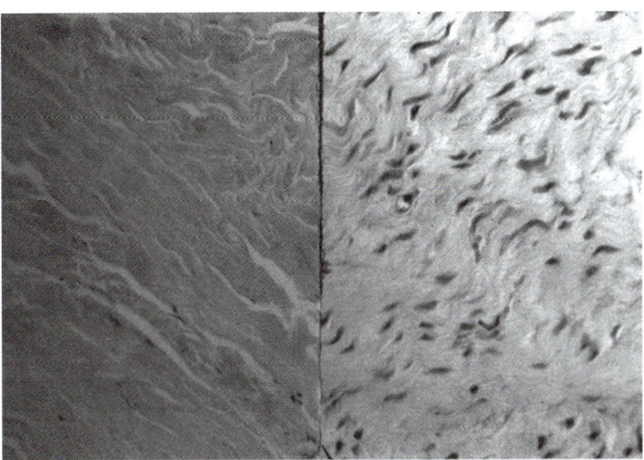

Figure 54.1 The histology of human ligaments (a) before and (b) after prolotherapy.

Low back syndromes: treatment by prolotherapy

Orthopaedic physicians recognize a large inventory of syndromes—clusters of symptoms and signs usually matching distinct pain diagrams which characterize specific mechanical dysfunctions. Some of these syndromes are dominated by symptoms which are secondary to the underlying mechanical cause. Many of these have been outlined by Cyriax (1983) or Dorman (1991) and are not considered in detail in this chapter.

Common to the sacroiliac dysfunction syndromes is one underlying phenomenon—that of ligament relaxation and *asymlocation* in the pelvis. This is the term used to convey the concept that in the *tensegrity model*, which we call the human pelvis, the sacrum is held or trapped between the ilia. It is prone to being held in a somewhat asymmetric position between them. This tends to place an asymmetric strain on the soft tissues, the fasciae, and ligaments. With a certain degree of relaxation of the ligaments, this asymmetry tends to advance to a point of exaggeration, akin to the phenomenon of fault propagation in mechanics. When this threshold is passed, recurrent entrapment of the sacrum asymmetrically amounts to a mechanical dysfunction, i.e. to *somatic dysfunction* in musculoskeletal terminology. This, in turn, is apt to provoke secondary phenomena which have been listed here as the 'mini' syndromes characteristic of the human pelvis. Some of these show themselves with ligament symptoms alone, some by muscle dysfunction or spasm, and some, through the phenomenon of transfer of torque through the axial skeleton, are manifested in the neck or the thoracolumbar junction.

Patients with these dysfunctions frequently report that manipulation in the hands of a manual therapist allows them temporary, intermittent relief from pain. Not infrequently, the situation worsens gradually over the years, so that patients seen after one or two decades of recurrent episodes of pain report that the pain has become continuous. Nonetheless, the hallmark of this syndrome is that the pain was intermittently, temporarily relieved early in the history. The improvement from manual therapy is due to a realignment of the pelvic bones. The recurrences are due to ligament relaxation which allows recurrent dysfunctions. The specific characteristic of the dysfunction at any one time might vary. It is proposed here, however, that the episodic improvement with manipulation is the hallmark of the ligament dysfunction in the axial skeleton, usually in the pelvic ring. A few examples of these syndromes are given here.

Recurrent sacroiliac strain

In this syndrome, patients report episodes where unexpectedly and suddenly following a slight movement—most characteristically rising from a stooped position with a slight degree of rotation in a casual manner and without a great weight—they feel severe, sudden-onset, asymmetric back pain, usually with radiating pain via one buttock down the leg. They are unable to stand straight. When examined acutely, these individuals are unable to form the normal lumbosacral lordosis, are able to flex forward, have marked asymmetry in sidebending and rotation at the lumbopelvic level, frequently suffer from marked limitation of straight leg raising on the painful side, may have secondary weakness due to pain, but do not suffer reflex suppression or sensory deficits. These individuals are frequently responsive to manipulative therapy. In its absence, the episodes typically recover in 2 weeks to 2 months, but are liable to recur. On detailed musculoskeletal examination, marked dysfunctions in the pelvis are always identifiable in the acute state.

It is the thesis of this chapter that the phenomenon is one whereby the sacrum becomes entrapped asymmetrically. Forces acting in the soft tissues, particularly in the upright human, are adducting. (This becomes obvious in viewing the sacrum as suspended between the ilia.) The pelvis, being a tensegrity ring, functions as a whole. When pain occurs, secondary muscle spasm disallows relaxation and restoration of symmetry of the sacrum between the ilia. Such an episode typically resolves in about 2 weeks. It is proposed here that the mechanism(s) of this resolution include one or more of the following factors:

(1) bone and ligament moulding occurring within 2 weeks

(2) natural slippage of the displaced parts *or*

(3) parts returning to normal through relaxation of the soft tissues *or*

(4) through manipulation *or*

(5) through a combination of all of these.

Sacrotuberous ligament

This ligament, or distal 'stay' of the pelvis, is often strained in SIJ dysfunction because it is further out in the radius of the pelvis (Figure 54.2). There is more than one pattern of pain, and individuals may vary as to how it affects them, although the repertoire of patterns is small. The diagnosis is made by the combination of local tenderness and the pain referral pattern.

Iliolumbar ligament sprain

This ligament, being the major stay of the relationship of the pelvis to the lower lumbar vertebrae, is frequently involved as a source of pain in pelvic dysfunctions. Marked local tenderness suggests the diagnosis. Of interest is that an asymmetry in physical findings is usual on examination when the subject is tested standing. It will be found that sidebending to one side provokes the pain, while rotation to the other side does so. (Note that I have not specified in which direction it is provoked. The ligament is a twisted three-dimensional structure, and the only consistent finding is that sidebending is painful in the direction opposite to that of rotation.)

Sciatica

This term implies pain in the low back with radiation down the lower limb posteriorly, via the buttock. It is well recognized that *radiculopathy*, usually due to pressure on the dural sleeve of one of the lumbar nerve roots, can be responsible for this pain. On the other hand, 'sciatica' is more often due to referred pain from the sacrotuberous ligament. In this case, the pain may 'skip' the popliteal space, but often the patterns of pain are indistinguishable on pain diagrams. Straight leg raising is also not a useful discriminant, although stretching the sciatic nerve in the popliteal fossa or through dorsiflexing the foot at a strategic position of straight leg raising is a better differentiator. (Both manoeuvres stretch the fascial sleeve of the leg and the branches of the sciatic nerve.) The absence or presence of neurological signs, the presence of tenderness at the attachment of the sacrotuberous ligament at the inferolateral angle of the sacrum, as well as clues from the medical history, are more useful.

Gluteus medius syndrome

As the gluteus medius has a specific role in locking the sacroiliac articulation on the stance side, it is subject to reflex inhibition when the ilium on the affected side is in a forwards position (DonTigny 1993). This can be manifested clinically by an alteration in its contraction, visible over the buttocks as an individual bends forwards, but is also identifiable on examination in the side-lying position (Dorman 1994). Tenderness is found on deep palpation just under the rim of the upper portion of the iliac crest as well.

Piriformis syndrome

As the piriformis muscle plays a major role in stabilizing the pelvis and is an important muscle traversing the SIJ, it is not surprising that it is strained at times when the pelvis is dysfunctional. The patient reports pain in the middle of the buttock, down the middle aspect of the thigh to the level of the popliteal fossa, affected by certain movements. Testing the muscle when maximally stretched provokes severe pain and yields the diagnosis.

Slipping clutch syndrome

This newly recognized syndrome is characteristic of about 15% of subjects suffering from back pain due to SI ligamentous dysfunction (Dorman 1994). Patients report episodes of one leg giving way. This

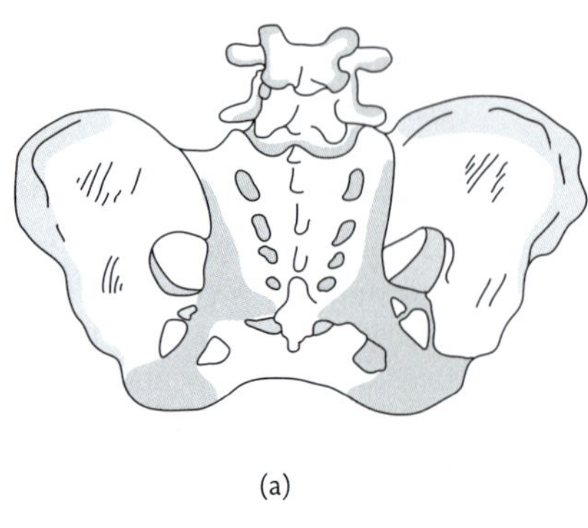

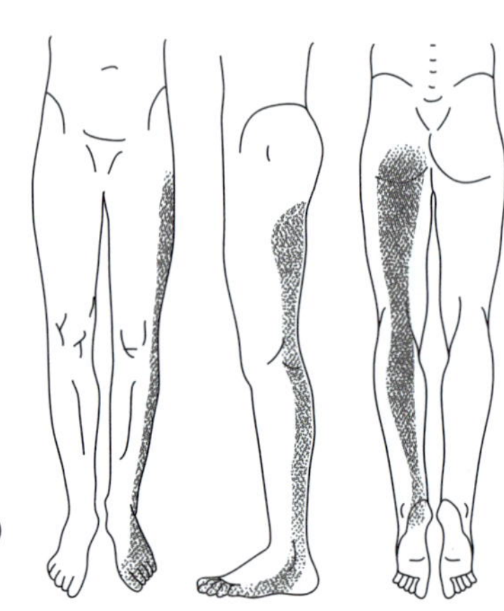

Figure 54.2 Sacrotuberous ligament strain in sacroliliac joint dysfunction.

is painless, although occasionally patients are injured after a fall. They may not fall down, as they often catch themselves. The phenomenon of the limb giving way occurs invariably as the affected side enters into stance and is thought to represent slight slippage due to failure of the *force closure* of the joint which should occur normally at this moment. As force closure is dependent, amongst other things, on the normal elastic function of the posterior SI ligaments, it is not surprising that relaxation of these structures can be responsible for mechanical dysfunction, as well as a source of pain.

The response to manipulation for low back dysfunction

Most of the syndromes surrounding the pelvis, as well as those created remotely—through the axial skeleton, the tensegrity, and fault propagation phenomena discussed earlier—are due to a single cause: relaxation of the ligaments controlling the tensegrity unit we call the pelvis. This is the source of all mechanical dysfunctions. The dysfunctions themselves lead to, or aggravate, strains of fasciae and ligaments. A vicious cycle develops. Muscle spasm is secondary. Its manifestations are well recognized in pain management circles.

Ongley's technique

From the discussion in this chapter so far, the reader will have drawn the logical conclusion that the optimal management should be restoration of symmetry followed by some measure to maintain the improved position. This, indeed, is exactly what is achieved with Ongley's technique. It goes without saying that the steps in this routine start with diagnosis. The diagnosis has to be based on a clinical assessment of the cause of the back pain, followed by a manipulation that should be so vigorous as to restore the pelvis to full symmetry and abolish any tendency for recurrence, which might be due to adhesions. Accordingly, it is an advantage if the patient can be maximally relaxed. A manipulation by the more popular and more gentle techniques of muscle energy, or even gentle thrust techniques, might be quite sufficient to restore a patient to temporary comfort but, in my opinion, might not restore the joint to optimal alignment nor completely release any adhesions which might have formed from prolonged malalignment. With this technique, therefore, the manipulation is vigorous.

In order to facilitate this manipulation (and it is intended to be performed once only), there is an advantage if dilute lidocaine (lignocaine) is injected into the soft tissues guarding the pelvis, particularly the posterior SI articulation, but also the ligaments around the lumbosacral junction, the iliolumbar ligaments, and the capsules of the zygoapophyseal joints at the two lowest levels of the spine. The details of the injection routine are detailed elsewhere (Dorman 1991). At times, individuals suffer from marked pain from a peripheral fascial strain, such as the fascia overlying the gluteus medius muscle as along the iliac crest. This can be relieved with a local anaesthetic injection, usually including small amounts of triamcinolone. It is important, however, not to place steroid injections into mechanically essential ligaments such as the posterior SI ligaments.

A manipulation, which is a modification of an osteopathic technique, is used next, restoring the pelvis to as much symmetry as possible, and in turn, this treatment is followed with proliferant therapy injections to the stabilizing ligaments of the pelvis, and in particular, the three layers of the posterior SI ligaments, with special attention to the deepest and central part. Droplet infiltration of proliferant injections is also placed along the iliolumbar ligaments, the zygoapophyseal joint capsules of the two lowest levels of the lumbar spine, and the transverse processes to make contact with the intertransverse ligaments at their periosteal attachments; and into the supraspinous and interspinous ligaments of the lowest levels; and the fascia over the erector spinae at the upper level of the sacrum is also treated. This can be achieved through a single needle insertion point in the midline opposite L5.

A treatment session

Light conscious sedation is used. After a general review of the status of the patient's health and establishing normal vital signs, the patient is sedated with an intravenous injection of 3 mg midazolam and 25 mg ketamine. The patient is placed in the prone position and continuously monitored with oximetry for pulse rate and oxygen saturation.

A total of 50 ml 0.5% lidocaine (lignocaine) is used by droplet infiltration. The operator utilizes a 10-ml Luer-Lock syringe with refills. The medication is distributed by droplet via one needle insertion point, at the spinous process of L5 in the midline, with the patient lying prone. The needle is advanced first by stepwise movements with droplet infiltration down the lateral aspect of the spinous process on the left side, making contact with the lamina, and with each needle contact, a droplet of the anaesthetic is dispensed (0.1–0.2 ml). Six such steps are made until the step-off at the zygoapophyseal joint. Here, a manoeuvre is performed to aim the needle into a somewhat more anterior direction as it is advanced. To achieve this, pressure is placed with the operator's left thumb over the skin at the estimated site of the tip of the needle. During this time, the syringe and needle are curved by a flexing manoeuvre of the syringe-holding hand while advancing the syringe and needle. This causes the needle to curve forwards, and contact can be made with the tip of the transverse process of L5 at an appropriate depth. Another droplet of anaesthetic is deposited here. The needle is then withdrawn to the subcutaneous situation. The operator's hands are reversed and the manoeuvre repeated on the patient's right side.

This being completed, the needle is again withdrawn to the subcutaneous level and the needle is now directed at an angle of about 45° caudad and laterally to the left and about 30° anteriorly. The palpating (left) thumb is held over the skin of the iliac crest as it curves from horizontal to vertical and anteriorly, aiming at the insertion of the iliolumbar ligament at the top of the iliac crest. Droplet infiltrations are deposited here. This having been completed, the needle tip is again withdrawn to a subcutaneous level and the procedure repeated (with reversed hands) to the right side. The needle is again withdrawn to the subcutaneous level and aimed at the posterior SI ligaments, first on the left side by a similar manoeuvre, again with a sentinel (left) thumb over the posterior superior iliac spine. The needle is aimed in the crevasse (cave) consisting of the dorsal attachment of the superficial layer of the posterior SI ligament. Droplet infiltration of local anaesthetic is deposited at this site, and by withdrawal and reinsertion, the needle is manoeuvred not only along the several points of insertion against the overhanging ilium but also against the deeper recessed sacral attachment of the posterior SI ligaments in three layers. About 20 droplet infiltrations are deposited on this side by these manoeuvres. Now, the needle is again withdrawn to the subcutaneous level, still being inserted at the midline at the spinous process of L5, the hands are reversed, and a similar manoeuvre is performed on the right. This routine takes about 40 ml lidocaine (lignocaine). The needle is now withdrawn and a suitable dressing applied at the needle insertion site.

In cases where an injection is required for a ligament causing pain, such as the sacrotuberous ligament, a separate injection is performed. In the case of the sacrotuberous ligament, this is best done in the side-lying position. The use of some triamcinolone at these sites is discretionary. After this is completed, the patient is returned into a supine position and mobilization undertaken. On this occasion, the patient is rolled onto one side, say the right, with the shoulder remaining supine, so torque can be applied to the torso. An assistant, standing on the patient's left, applies a cushion across the patient's chest and places her body in such a position as to maintain firm contact between the patient's left shoulder and the couch. The physician places his/her right hand so the tip of the middle finger is at the lumbosacral junction. The patient's lower (left) thigh remains stretched out on the couch close to its margin on the side close to the physician. The physician's right hand flexes the thigh until tension is noted at the lumbosacral junction by the palpating hand. With the thigh in this position, adduction is now applied to it until the slack of the thoracic and lumbar spine is completely taken up, the forces concentrating at the lumbosacral junction and below, predominantly at the SIJ. The left hand is now placed over the patient's left greater trochanter and the right hand over the knee, the leg remaining flexed at the knee. At a moment of body relaxation at the end of expiration, force is applied firmly along the line of shear of the left SIJ, the assistant maintaining firm control of the patient's shoulder and upper torso.

After this is done, the patient is placed in the supine position and, if no substantial change in the alignment of the low back is achieved, as judged by apparent leg length discrepancy, the manoeuvre is repeated on the other side. This usually achieves satisfactory mobilization of the SIJs.

Flexion manoeuvre

The assistant places him/herself at the patient's feet. The patient's outstretched hands are grasped by the assistant's one hand and the knees firmly held flat on the couch with the other. The physician brings the patient to the sitting position and, with the hands over the low lumbar spine, induces gentle repeated flexion movements. This usually increases the range of flexion of the patient's lumbar spine. The patient is restored to the supine.

The routine prolotherapy follow-up described next is typically used on the first day after the local anaesthesia and mobilization and weekly for a total of six sessions. It consists of 20 ml P2G distributed by droplet infiltration through one needle insertion point at the spinous process of L5 in the midline, with the patient lying prone. The needle is advanced first by stepwise movements, with droplet infiltration down the lateral aspect of the spinous process on the left side, making contact with the lamina, and with each needle contact, a droplet (0.1–0.2 ml) of proliferant is dispensed. Six such steps are made until the step-off at the zygoapophyseal joint. Here, a manoeuvre is performed to aim the needle into a somewhat more anterior direction as it is advanced. To achieve this, pressure is placed with the operator's left thumb over the skin at the estimated site of the tip of the needle. During this time, the syringe and needle are curved by a flexing manoeuvre of the syringe-holding hand while advancing the syringe and needle. This causes the needle to curve forwards and contact is made with the transverse process of L5 at an appropriate depth, by careful manipulation. Another droplet of proliferant is deposited here. The needle is then withdrawn to the subcutaneous situation. The operator's hands are reversed and the manoeuvre repeated on the patient's right side.

It is usual, at this time, to repeat the manoeuvre at the L4 level. It is not always necessary to make another cutaneous needle insertion. There is usually enough laxity in the skin to slide it cephalad, while holding the tip just deep enough to pass through the upper dermis. The interspinous ligaments of the two to three lowest lumbar levels need to be infiltrated at this time. The operator will have gained a sense of the depth of the lamina. On no account should an injection stray into the lumbar theca. It is best to place the tip of the needle onto the inferior surface of the spinous process above and the superior surface of the spinous process below, at each level. This can be facilitated by having the prone patient positioned passively for this portion of the injection, into trunk flexion. Many suitable treatment couches are available for this; some practitioners use an inflatable pillow. Next, the iliolumbar ligament is injected as already described for infiltration of the local anaesthesia. The needle is again withdrawn to the subcutaneous level and aimed at the posterior SI ligaments. The routine here also follows that already described. This is the most important part of the proliferant injection. Particular care must be given to reach the deep innominate SI ligaments. It is important not to exceed about 20 ml P2G in any one session to the back.

Finally, the patient is encouraged to perform a full range of movement 'exercises' to encourage healing in the natural lines of strain.

The special case of manipulation for neck pain

Though prolotherapy has been used for cervical and referred upper thoracic pain since the 1950s, this difficult area of treatment has received even less attention than the low back. Nonetheless, a few practitioners, who have followed an analytic process outlined here for the identification of the ligamentous structures responsible for pain after whiplash and allied cervical injuries, have had excellent results (Kayfetz et al. 1963). In whiplash injuries, where the integrated function of the motion segments is disturbed by damage (e.g. to the capsules of the zygapophyseal joints and/or the attachments of the annulus of the disc to the vertebral end plate), there is likely to be associated ligament injury.

The asymmetry in range of movement at the segment can frequently be improved by manipulation, with slight cervical extension under traction by the methods developed in the Cyriax school. However, when the correction is only temporary, consideration should be given to refurbishing the ligaments with prolotherapy. As in the case of the sacral dysfunction in the low back, Ongley has developed a routine for the neck.

Prolotherapy to the neck

The routine for light conscious sedation outlined in the previous section 'The response to manipulation for low back dysfunctions' is followed.

For the initial treatment of the neck, the patient lies prone, with the assistant sitting at the head of the treatment table which is elevated to the mid-waist level of the operator. It is best to use a treatment table with an appropriate opening for breathing. Local anaesthesia is applied with an air gun to the midline opposite the spinous process of C2 and another bleb opposite the spinous process of C5. A total of about 50 ml 0.5% lidocaine (lignocaine) can be used.

The superior segment is treated first. A 19-gauge 75-mm needle attached to a 10-ml Luer-Lock syringe is charged with 0.5% lidocaine (lignocaine). Needle contact is first made with the spinous process of C2 opposite the anaesthetic bleb. For accuracy of fine manual control, the neck is flexed, the assistant using his/her right hand on the back of the patient's head in the prone position. The assistant maintains pressure so that the neck remains flexed. His/her left hand is placed flat in the midline, palm down, opposite T1 and T2, so that the operator can grasp the assistant's index finger, for stability, with the medial fingers of the left hand, the fifth finger serving as a sensory prod close to the site of the needle insertion. The operator's right hand is braced on the patient's right shoulder or, as appropriate, the forearm is braced, and the right hand serves for needle placement. With this routine, the whole injection procedure is undertaken.

Initially, 20 ml 0.5% lidocaine (lignocaine) is infiltrated into the upper cervical segment. The needle is first carefully passed through the skin at the C2 level and then directed to multiple sites of ligament attachment to bone in the neck. It is first directed anteriorly until contact is made at a depth of about 3 mm with the spinous process of C2. When the site has been defined, a droplet of local anaesthetic is inserted here and a further droplet cephalad into the interspinous ligament at this depth. The needle is withdrawn marginally and directed laterally to the patient's left.

After passing over the lateral component of the bifurcate spinous process, the needle is now curved by a combined manoeuvre of the right (syringe-holding) hand and the palpating tip of the operator's left fifth finger, pressing over the skin lateral to the site of the insertion. This directs the needle anteriorly so it makes contact with the lateral aspect of the spinous process of C2. Here, another droplet of local anaesthetic is deposited and the needle is advanced stepwise, contact with bone being made at each step, until a change of angle is encountered—the lamina. Further droplets of local anaesthetic are deposited at these sites and the needle is advanced to the prominence of the zygoapophyseal joint of the C1–2 level. Here, further droplets of local anaesthetic are applied and the needle is then passed more laterally, so it just passes over the bulge of the joint. The small transverse process of C2 is palpated with the needle tip and a final droplet of local anaesthetic is applied here.

This being established, the needle is withdrawn to the subcutaneous level and an equivalent manoeuvre is performed on the right side. The needle is then again withdrawn subcutaneously and directed cephalad, the palpating tip of the operator's left fifth finger being applied firmly to the posterior prominence of the atlas. By gentle encroachment at a superficial level, the needle is brought in contact with the arch of the atlas. A droplet of local anaesthetic is applied here and the needle is carefully 'walked' across the arch of the atlas until the lateral side, or mass of the atlas, is reached. At this point, advancement is stopped (because of the vertebral artery) and the needle is applied more superficially, advanced beyond the expected site of the vertebral artery, and then directed anteriorly to the tip or posterior surface of the lateral mass, curving over the expected site of the vertebral artery. Another droplet of local anaesthetic infiltration is applied here and the needle is withdrawn to the midline subcutaneous position. The equivalent manoeuvre is performed on the right-hand side.

Throughout, the assistant is holding the neck in a firmly flexed position with his/her right hand, the left hand remaining on the dorsal aspect of the patient's upper thoracic spine as an anchor for the operator's directing left hand, the index finger being grasped between thumb and forefinger.

This manoeuvre having been completed, the needle (again withdrawn to the subcutaneous site) is directed caudad to the spinous process of C3. A similar manoeuvre of walking down the spinous process and lamina to the zygoapophyseal joint is performed, first to the patient's left and, finally, to the patient's right. This having been accomplished, the needle is withdrawn entirely from the C2 insertion site. A cotton swab and dressing are applied.

The patient's neck is maintained in flexion and the needle is introduced (with a second syringe containing 10 ml of local anaesthetic) opposite C5. An analogous manoeuvre is performed at the C5 level. The needle is then again withdrawn subcutaneously and now applied cephalad from this insertion site to the spinous process of C4, and the whole manoeuvre is repeated along this vertebra. This is facilitated by the skin gliding technique, allowing the operator to bring the dorsal cutaneous needle insertion site opposite the spinous process of the relevant vertebra to limit the number of cutaneous penetrations.

Finally, the needle is withdrawn, again subcutaneously, and now directed caudad towards the spinous process of C6 and then C7. In this position, it is not possible to slide the skin inferiorly and a diagonal approach is made to the (much larger) lamina and zygoapophyseal joints of the C6–7 and C7–T1 vertebrae. Contact is also made with the root of the first portion of the first rib from this particular manoeuvre. The remainder of the 10 ml of anaesthetic is again applied to this whole area by droplet infiltration distributed to the two sides. The use of some local anaesthesia with triamcinolone is discretionary, if the physician has made a diagnosis of a particularly inflamed area. The needle is now withdrawn. Suitable dressings are placed over the puncture site (there is no bleeding) and the patient is now placed in the supine position. The height of the couch is adjusted for mobilization.

Initial mobilization is performed by Cyriax's technique, with the assistant holding the lower limbs to avoid slippage and the patient positioned so that the shoulders are flush with the upper end of the couch. A straight pull is applied by Cyriax's technique. Firm continuous traction is applied to the cervical spine, the operator cradling the occipital portion of the head in the left hand and ensuring control with the right hand under the mandible. After traction is applied for about 10 seconds and the slack taken up, with slight maintenance of extension, the head is gently rotated to the unrestricted side and over-pressure is applied with very little movement. The manoeuvre is repeated to the other side and the patient then restored to the normal lying position (supine) on the couch. After this is completed, the height of the couch is readjusted and a lateral tilt chiropractic-style mobilization applied in each direction to mobilize the atlanto-occipital joints. The patient is restored to the supine position and head-rolling exercises initiated on the low pillow. After recovery from the light conscious sedation, the patient should be instructed in cervical exercises which facilitate complete movement of all the joints of the neck.

Prolotherapy is initiated the next day by a similar routine, also with light conscious sedation. The injection technique is the same as just described. It is not usual to exceed 20 ml P2G for any one session.

The skill of performing this rather delicate routine can only be learned by apprenticeship. It is recorded here for information only.

Mechanics and ligament proliferation of prolotherapy

Prolotherapy has been shown to provoke hyperplasia of ligament tissue, with an increased amount of collagen. The mechanical effects of prolotherapy in human ligaments were studied through the treatment of the joint capsule and injured ligaments of the knees of athletes who had suffered injuries. During the enrolment period, 30 patients with knee pain were seen, but in the cases of only five knees (in four patients) was it possible to obtain measurements after treatment, because the equipment was available only for 9 months and many of the athletes, after clinical improvement, failed to return for repeat measurements. All the selected subjects had substantial ligament instability. All measurements were taken by one researcher. The patients underwent multiple injections and were followed routinely; within 9 months, repeat measurements were obtained. Subjective symptoms were obtained at entry and exit from the study. Ligament stability was measured by a commercially available computerized instrument that measures ligament function objectively and reliably in three dimensions (Oliver and Coughlin 1985; Selsnick et al. 1986). It consists of a chair equipped with a six-component force platform and an electrogoniometer with six degrees of freedom. With computer-integrated force and motion measurements, a standardized series of clinical laxity tests can be performed and an objective report obtained. Earlier studies have compared clinical testing with objective tests (Daniel et al. 1985) and have established reproducibility (Highgenboten 1986).

The proliferant solution used in these cases was P25G. The proliferant injections were 'peppered' into the lax ligament(s), usually at 2-weekly intervals, each offending ligament being treated an average of four times. A total of 30–40 ml of the proliferant solution was injected into the appropriate portion of the joint ligaments. Details of the injection technique can be found in the original publication (Ongley et al. 1988).

Prolotherapy in other parts of the body

It will be evident to the reader, from the start of this chapter, that prolotherapy is a suitable injection treatment for treating any part of the fascioligamentous organ. Style of needle placement, the selection of the needle, the volume to be injected at any one site, and so on, vary, and details have been given elsewhere (Dorman 1991).

References

Banks, A. (1991) A rationale for prolotherapy. *Journal of Orthopaedic Medicine*, 13, 54–9.

Cyriax, J. (1983) *Textbook of orthopaedic medicine* (11th edn). W. B. Saunders, Baltimore, MD.

Daniel, D. M., Malcolm, L. L., Losse, G., Stone, M. L., Sachs, R., Burks, R. (1985) Instrument measurement of anterior laxity of the knee. *Journal of Bone and Joint Surgery*, 67A, 720–5.

DonTigny, R. L. (1993) Mechanics and treatment of the sacroiliac joint. *Journal of Manual and Manipulative Therapy*, 1, 1.3–12.

Dorman, T. (1991) *Diagnosis and injection techniques in orthopedic medicine.* Williams & Wilkins, Baltimore, MD.

Dorman, T. (1994) Failure of self bracing at the sacroiliac joint: the slipping clutch syndrome. *Journal of Orthopaedic Medicine*, 16, 49–51.

Gedney, E. H. (1937) Hypermobile joint. *Osteopathic Profession*, 4, 30–1.

Hackett, G. S. (1958) *Ligament and tendon relaxation treated by prolotherapy* (3rd edn). Charles Thomas, Springfield, IL.

Highgenboten, C. L. (1986) *The reliability of the Genucom knee analysis system.* 2nd European Congress of Knee Surgery and Arthroscopy, Basel, Switzerland.

Kayfetz, D. O., Blumental, L. S., Hackett, G. S., et al. (1963) Whiplash injury and other ligamentous headache—its management with prolotherapy. *Headache*, 3, 21–8.

King Liu, Y., Tipton, C., Matthews R. D., et al. (1983) An *in situ* study of the influence of a sclerosing solution in rabbit medial collateral ligaments and its junction strength. *Connective Tissue Research*, 11, 95–102.

Klein, R. G., Eek, B. J., DeLong, B., Mooney, V. (1993) A randomised double-blind trial of dextrose-glycerine-phenol injections for chronic low back pain. *Journal of Spinal Diseases*, 6, 22–3.

Oliver, J. H., Coughlin, L. P. (1985) *An analysis of knee evaluation using clinical techniques and the Genucom knee analysis system.* American Orthopedic Society for Sports Medicine Interim Meeting, Las Vegas, Nevada.

Ongley, M. J., Dorman, T. A., Eek B. C., et al. (1988) Ligament instability of knees: a new approach to treatment. *Manual Medicine*, 3, 151–4.

Ongley, M. J., Klein, R. G., Dorman, T. A., et al. (1987) A new approach to the treatment of chronic back pain. *Lancet*, 2, 143–6.

Selsnick, H., Oliver, J., Virgin, C. (1986) *Analysis of knee ligament testing—Genucom and clinical exams.* Presented at the American Orthopedic Society for Sports Medicine Annual Meeting, Sun Valley, Idaho.

Yeomans, F. C. (ed.) (1939) *Sclerosing therapy, the injection treatment of hernia, hydrocele, varicose veins and hemorrhoids.* Williams & Wilkins, Baltimore, MD.

Chapter 55

Prolotherapy in the UK

Simon Petrides

History of prolotherapy

Hippocrates first used the concept of connective tissue proliferation when treating soldiers by thrusting hot pokers into their shoulder joint capsules to prevent recurrent subluxations. Prolotherapy as an injection treatment has been used for musculoskeletal pain in several different forms for almost a century. George Hackett, an American surgeon, initially used the technique on hernias and then developed some of the musculoskeletal protocols used today (Hackett et al. 1993). Gustav Hemwall joined his practice and further disseminated his knowledge of the technique. Milne Ongley, a New Zealand physician, took Hackett's work further when he described the technique in association with systematic clinical evaluation developed by James Cyriax. Cyriax's principles of musculoskeletal examination and injection techniques are still being taught in the UK, with regular refinements to keep the educational knowledge base up to date with the constantly evolving literature.

Prolotherapy has become an accepted intervention in the UK for a variety of musculoskeletal complaints including back pain, despite its controversial 80-year history and failure, so far, to enter mainstream practice. This is not because of the lack of research or reasonable proof of its safety and efficacy but, more likely, due to its development outside the National Health Service (NHS), since the profession of musculoskeletal medicine is not widespread as a career pathway within the current NHS system.

Prolotherapy injections are used in the UK, USA, Australia, and New Zealand for a broad range of subacute and chronic recalcitrant musculoskeletal disorders. Although evidence for its effectiveness is reported to be inconclusive, anecdotal evidence of success has maintained the profile of this increasingly popular treatment. Evidence-based medicine demands that clinical trials demonstrate the effectiveness of medical interventions, but all back pain research is fraught with methodological difficulties.

A plethora of literature exists to analyse the effectiveness of prolotherapy in low back pain (Dechow et al. 1999; Klein et al. 1993; Mathews et al. 1987; Ongley et al. 1987; Yelland et al. 2004). Some of these trials support its effectiveness, while others are less convincing. However, there are significant shortcomings in the methodological scores for all of the trials such that overall evidence is still considered inconclusive by the Cochrane collaboration (Dagenais et al. 2010). More recently, progress has been made in the literature demonstrating the success of prolotherapy in peripheral tendinopathy and osteoarthritis (Maxwell et al. 2007; Rabago et al. 2009, 2010; Reeves and Hassanein 2000; Scarpone et al. 2008).

Terminology of prolotherapy

Originally, the injections using early solutions were called 'sclerosant therapy', on the assumption of scar formation, but this has been superseded by the term 'prolotherapy' which is now widely used since it implies a proliferation of normal connective tissue, which more closely represents the regeneration effect of the injections. Other terms used are 'fibro-proliferative therapy' or 'regenerative injection therapy' (Linetsky et al. 2002).

Other forms of prolotherapy include autologous blood injection, platelet-rich plasma injection, autologous conditioned plasma injection, dry needling, and stem cell therapy.

Proliferants used in prolotherapy

There are three major classes of proliferants commonly used in prolotherapy:

- *Irritants:* phenol. This acts by either damaging cells directly or by rendering the cells antigenic through alteration of surface proteins.
- *Chemotactics:* sodium morrhuate. This acts by attracting inflammatory cells.
- *Osmotics*: glucose/dextrose, glycerine, and zinc sulphate. These act by causing an 'osmotic shock' to cells, thus resulting in the release of pro-inflammatory substances (Banks 1991).

Two different solutions, with different modes of action, are commonly in use in the UK:

- *Hyperosmolar dextrose* (12.5–25%): causes osmotic damage to cell walls triggering release of inflammatory mediators.
- *Dextrose/glycerol/phenol mixture 'P2G'*: an osmotic and cellular irritant.

Another sclerosing agent in use in Europe is polidocanol, which causes sclerosing of pathological neovascularization which is associated with tendinopathy. Its usefulness has been particularly studied in the Achilles (Alfredson and Lorentzon 2007; Alfredson and Ohberg 2005), patellar, and wrist extensor tendons.

(a)

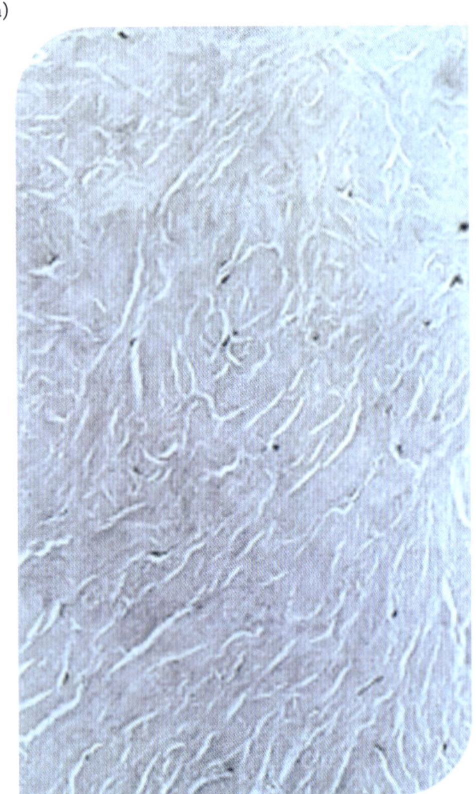

(b)

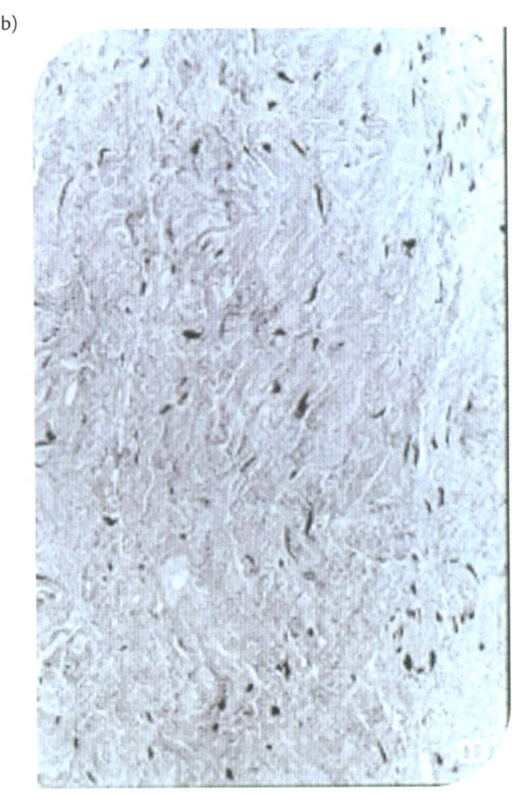

Figure 55.1 Normal collagen (a) and the appearance after prolotherapy (b) showing fibroblast hyperplasia.
(Liu Y, Tipton C, Matthes R, Bedford T, Maynard J, Walmer H. An in-situ study of the influence of a sclerosing solution in rabbit medial collateral ligaments and its junction strength. *Connective Tissue Research* 1983;11:95–102.)

Mode of action

Hypertonic dextrose and glycerol act by initiating an osmotic trauma by dehydrating cells. The more concentrated solution outside the cell attracts water from inside the cell across the semi-permeable cell membrane. The resulting membrane and cellular fragmentation attracts granulocytes and macrophages, initiating the 'healing cascade' through these cellular mediators. The macrophages phagocytose cellular debris and dying granulocytes; they secrete polypeptide growth factors which attract and activate fibroblasts. Some researchers have postulated that release of growth factors such as 'collagen derived growth factor (CDGF)' and 'transforming growth factor β (TGFBβ)' are responsible for the resulting 'fibro-proliferation', thickening, and strengthening of collagen fibres (Kim et al. 2004). Others have suggested that 'glycosylation of proteins' may be responsible in the same way that sclerodactyly, Dupuytren's contracture, and adhesive capsulitis are more common and more severe in diabetes.

Those cells not killed immediately by the osmotic trauma initiated by the hyperosmolar environment release prostaglandins, leukotrienes, and thromboxanes (derived from cell membrane arachidonic acid) which are humoral mediators of inflammation.

Anecdotally, most prolotherapy exponents have observed that aspirin or ibuprofen reduce the discomfort associated with prolotherapy but that the clinical effect is also diminished. This is because the drugs inhibit the enzyme, cyclo-oxygenase, which is important in the prostaglandin synthetic pathway (Oates et al. 1988).

The augmentation and fibro-proliferation of collagen fibres after injection of a sclerosing/proliferative solution (sodium morrhuate) has been demonstrated histologically (Liu et al. 1983) (Figure 55.1). An increase in mass and thickness in animal and human sacroiliac ligaments has been demonstrated in response to repeated injections of dextrose, glycerol, phenol, and lidocaine (Klein et al. 1989). Dextrose has been studied in rat models showing that injured medial collateral ligaments injected with 15% dextrose had a significant increase in cross-sectional area compared to non-injured and injured saline-injected controls (Jensen 2006). The resulting strengthening of collagen fibres is presumed to have a stabilising effect on the intervertebral segments, improving mechanical function and thus reducing pain.

Indications for prolotherapy

The indication for spinal prolotherapy is for subacute, chronic, or recurrent axial or referred pain. Clinically determined (as well as functional/radiological) instability can respond well to prolotherapy. The diagnoses in which prolotherapy is known to help are diverse but they all correlate with the theme of inadequate spinal or peripheral joint support mechanisms. Lumbar, sacroiliac, cervical, and thoracic instability are the main indications for use in the spine. However, while the treatment may help prevent progression to a more unstable state, it may also help avoid fusion surgery.

Lumbar instability

Although there is no 'gold standard' test to identify lumbar instability, the concept has been studied widely and several definitions have been proposed. Panjabi stated that instability is defined as:

> A significant decrease in the capacity of the stabilising system of the spine to maintain the intervertebral neutral zones within the

physiological limits so that there is no neurological dysfunction, no major deformity, and no incapacitating pain.

The neutral zone is the range of flexibility within which intervertebral motion is produced with minimal resistance. The 'elastic zone' exists from the end of the neutral zone up to the physiological limit and within which movement is available against significant resistance (Panjabi 1992, 2003).

Structural/radiological lumbar instability

Several radiographic criteria have been proposed as indicators of lumbar intervertebral instability and the topic remains controversial (Pitkänen 2002; Posner et al. 1982; Shaffer et al. 1990; Yone and Sakou 1999). Flexion/extension radiographs and more recently, videofluoroscopy, have been used in assessment (see Figures 55.2–55.5).

Sagittal rotation: Varying ranges of radiographic intervertebral sagittal rotation (tilt or flexion/extension) measurements have been proposed as indicators of instability: >10° (Dupuis et al. 1985), >15° (Nachemson 1985; White and Panjabi 1990), >20° (Hayes et al. 1989) have all been proposed as flexion/extension ranges suggesting instability.

Sagittal translation: The following measurements have also been suggested as indicators of instability: >3 mm (Dvorak et al. 1991; Knutsson 1944), >4 mm (Dupuis et al. 1985), and >5 mm (Hayes et al. 1989; Shaffer et al. 1990). Others have suggested that sagittal translation of >8–15% of the anteroposterior (AP) vertebral body diameter is indicative.

Instability measurements may be different at each level of the lumbar spine. Panjabi proposed that sagittal rotation range of more than 15° existing at L1–4, 20° at L4/5, and 25° at L5/S1 were more relevant (2003).

Evaluation of symptomatic sagittal translation (Figures 55.3 and 55.4) seems to be more revealing in the recumbent position, whereas a symptomatic sagittal rotation (Figure 55.5) is better revealed in standing flexion/extension views (Cabraja et al. 2012).

In the author's opinion, the variation between individuals is so large that 'normal' ranges are difficult to interpret and that it can be more useful to compare range of sagittal translation and sagittal rotation with the other levels in the same patient and also to assess sequencing of movement on video fluoroscopy. There is also a measurement error of a few degrees due to factors associated with the X-ray beam, imaging equipment, patient movement, etc. This error can be minimized using stereophotogrammetric X-ray analysis or quantitative fluoroscopy, although these are impractical for everyday use.

Functional lumbar instability

This is determined by three subsystems:

1) The '*passive stabilizing system*' includes the vertebrae, ligaments (supraspinous, iliolumbar, interspinous, posterior/anterior longitudenal, ligamentum flavum), discs, joint capsules, and facet joints. The passive stabilizers are effective at the limits of the neutral zone and into the elastic zone.
2) The '*active stabilizing system*' includes the tonic (transversus abdominis and multifidus) and phasic (external oblique, erector spinae, rectus abdominis) muscles. The active stabilizers are effective within the neutral zone.
3) The '*neuromuscular system*' co-ordinates the timing, balance, magnitude, and control of all movements through proprioceptive afferent input from mechanoreceptors, with output producing muscle activation depending on need. Poor control may explain why low back pain (LBP) can occur without significant load (Cholewicki and McGill 1996).

(a)
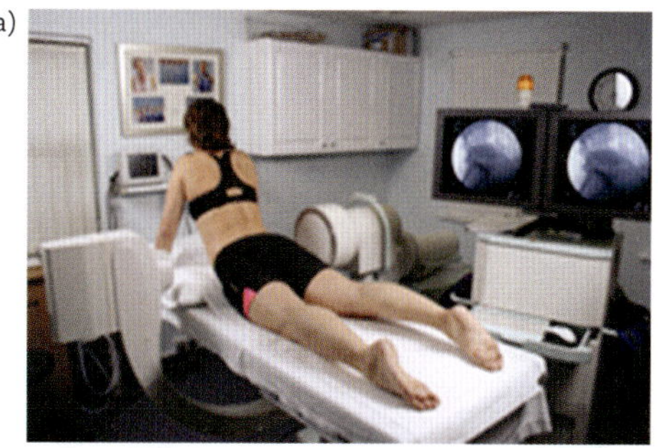
(b)
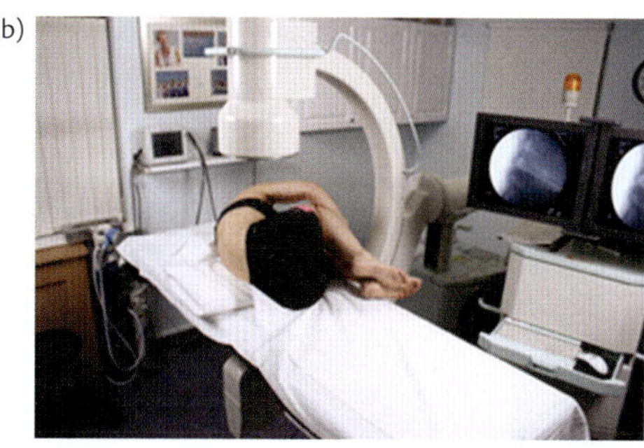
(c)
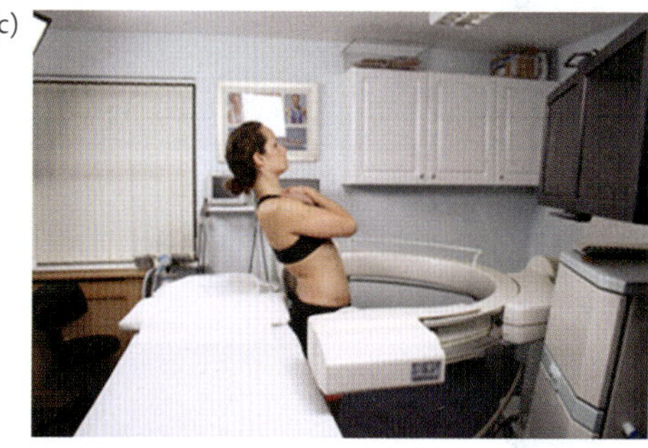
(d)
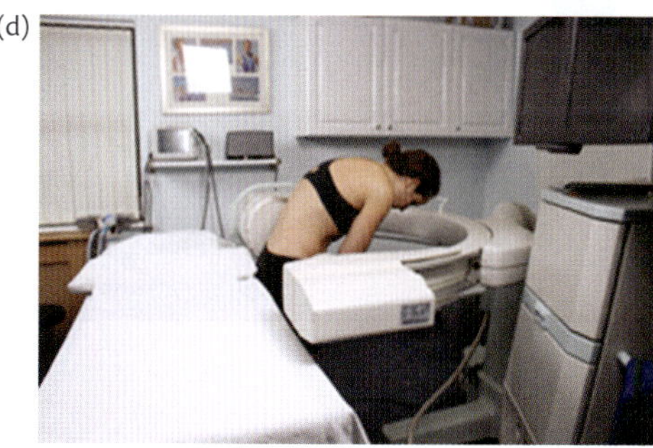

Figure 55.2 C-arm assessments of lumbar flexion and extension while (a,b) recumbent (passive) and (c,d) standing (active). The standing flexion and extension movements can also be viewed under videofluoroscoy to assess movement sequencing.

These three subsystems are functionally interdependent. Many patients have been expertly managed by experienced physical therapists such that the 'active' and 'neuromuscular' systems have been

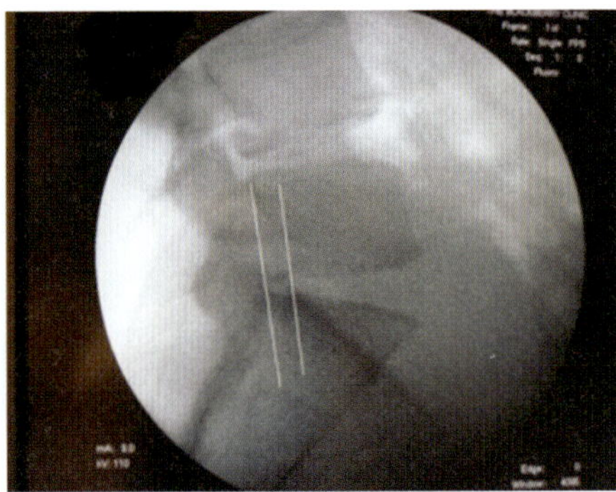

Figure 55.3 Extension radiograph showing excessive sagittal translation posteriorly at L5/S1.

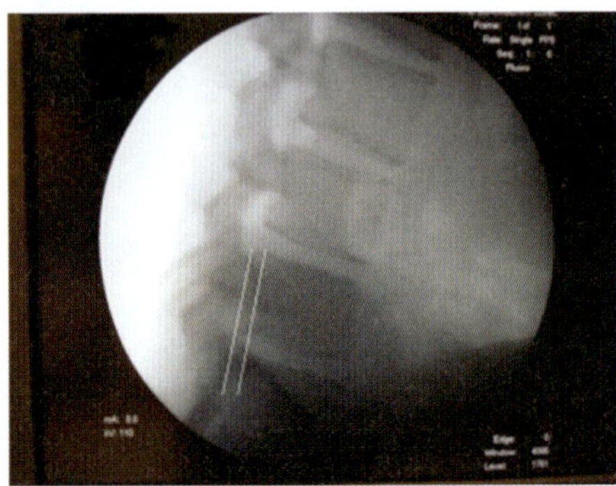

Figure 55.4 Flexion radiograph of the same patient as in Figure 55.3, showing reduction in posterior sagittal translation at L5/S1.

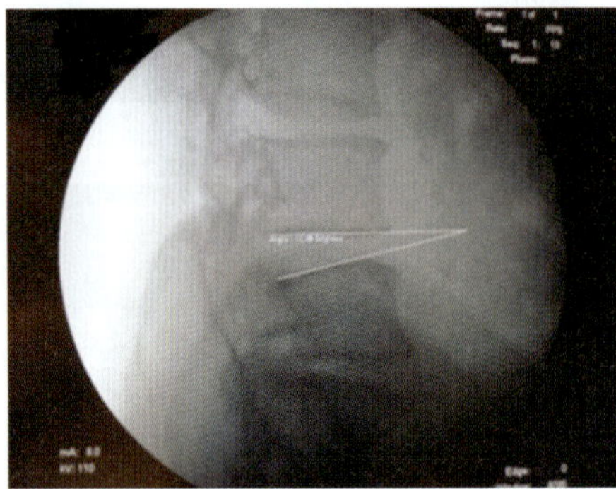

Figure 55.5 Flexion radiograph showing an excessive sagittal rotation angle of 12° at L4/5. The end-plate angle in flexion at all levels should be 0–5°.

optimized. Prolotherapy can play an important role in augmentation of the ligamentous component of the 'passive' subsystem such that not only do the ligaments exhibit increased size and strength (narrowing the neutral zone), but they also allow earlier firing of mechanoreceptors enabling the 'active' and 'neuromuscular' systems to control movement more finely within the neutral zone.

Diagnostic features of lumbar instability

History

Features on direct questioning which suggest lumbar instability include episodic LBP and episodes of the back 'going out', pain on prolonged postures, pain on transition from sitting to standing, diminishing effectiveness of manipulation, and episodic sacroiliac dysfunction or sacroiliac hypermobility.

Examination

Clinical tests of instability in regular use include:

- *Generalized ligamentous laxity scale (LLS):* The Beighton LLS for generalized ligamentous laxity shows high inter-examiner reliability.
- *Abberrant motion with trunk range of movement (ROM):* This demonstrates higher levels of reliability.
- *Instability catch sign* on flexion or deflexion.
- *Gower sign:* hand walking up the legs on deflexion.
- *Painful arc on flexion or deflexion.*
- *Reversal of the lumbopelvic rhythm.*
- *Prone instability test:* The patient is prone with the upper torso on the couch and the feet on the floor. The practitioner performs passive intervertebral motion testing. The patient then lifts his/her legs just off the floor and passive tests are repeated. The test is positive when the patient reports pain before the leg lift and no pain after. It is assumed that lumbopelvic stabilizers contract to stabilize the segment (Hicks et al. 2003).
- *Passive lumbar extension test:* The patient is prone and is asked to keep the knees extended while the practitioner lifts the legs 30 cm above the couch and exerts a small amount of traction. Reproduction of pain is a sign of a positive test. When measured against radiological evidence of instability, the sensitivity is 84.2% and the specificity, 90.4% (Kasai et al. 2006).
- *Motion palpation tests:* Passive physiological intervertebral motion (PPIVM) tests (Figure 55.6) and passive accessory intervertebral motion (PAIVM) tests (Figure 55.7) are used, to varying degrees, by many different manual therapists.

These tests have a reasonably high *specificity* but low *sensitivity* when validated against structural measurements of radiological instability. The passive lumbar extension test (Figure 55.8) has a high degree of sensitivity and specificity. The prone instability test (Figure 55.9), use of the generalized Beighton LLS, and aberrant motion with trunk ROM demonstrate high levels of reliability (Hicks et al. 2003).

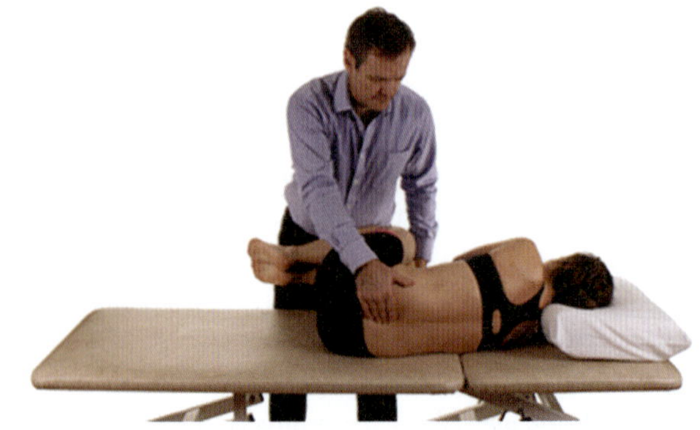

Figure 55.6 Passive physiological intervertebral motion (PPIVM) testing.

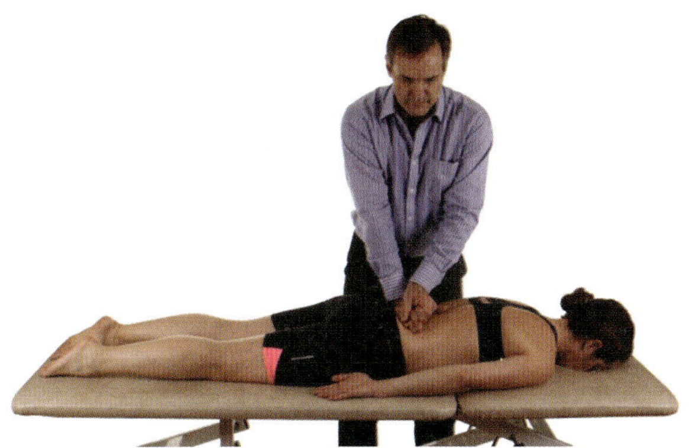

Figure 55.7 Passive accessory intervertebral motion (PAIVM) testing.

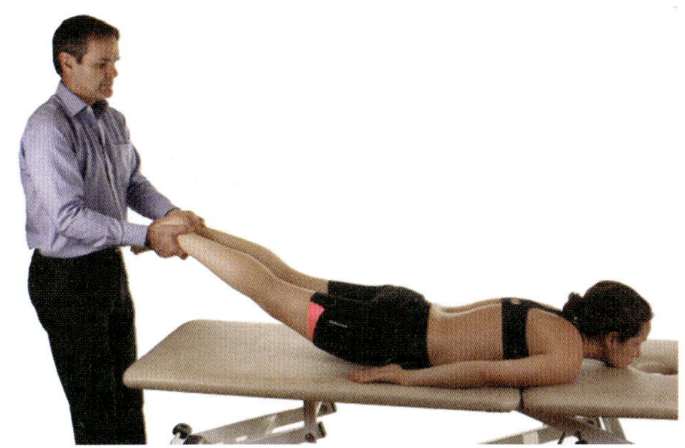

Figure 55.8 The passive lumbar extension test. For a positive test, pain is experienced during the manoeuvre.

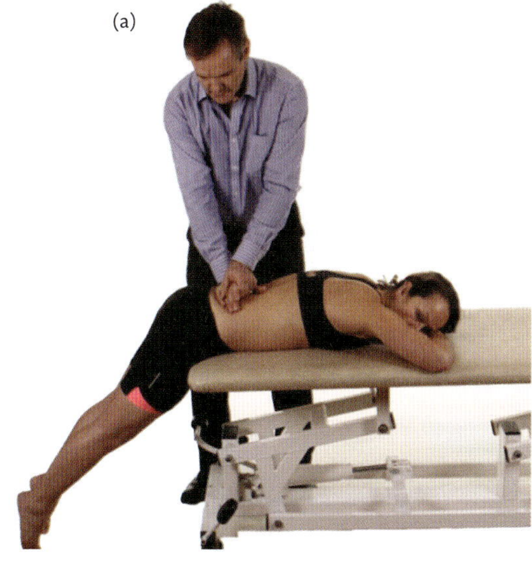

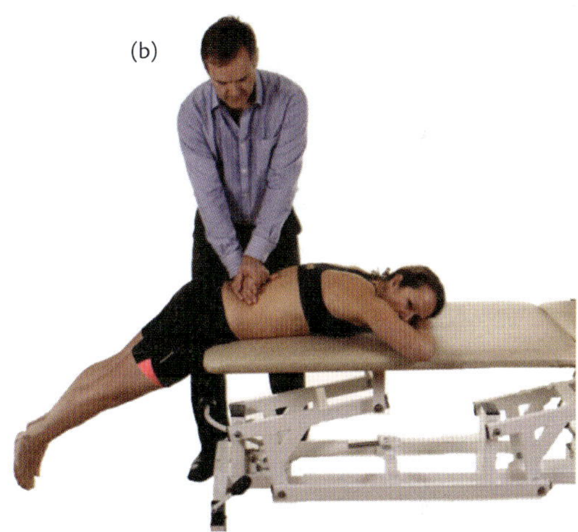

Figure 55.9(a) and (b) The prone instability test. Firstly, a PAIVM antero-posterior shear is used to reproduce *pain*; the test is considered positive if this pain is reduced significantly after lifting the toes off the floor and repeating the PAIVM test.

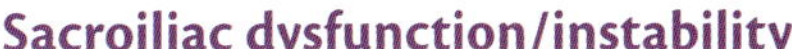

Sacroiliac dysfunction/instability

Sacroiliac (SI) instability tests have been described in Chapter 35 and include several which imply SI joint instability, particularly the 'active straight leg raise' test (Figure 55.10) which has been extensively studied, especially in pregnancy-related pelvic girdle pain (PGP).

Investigations

The following investigations can contribute to the holistic evaluation of the patient with suspected instability when considering whether prolotherapy may be a relevant approach:

- *MRI (magnetic resonance imaging) and CT (computed tomography) scan*: Existence of degenerative disc and facet joint disease is not diagnostic of instability but can help in the work-up of a patient in whom instability is a possible diagnosis.
- *Flexion/extension radiographs:* Have been previously described. Measurements of *sagittal rotation* and *sagittal translation* can help to implicate levels that may be symptomatic.
- *Videofluoroscopic kinematic analysis*: Can be useful for discriminating between subjects with and without LBP based on movement parameters on videofluoroscopy. According to one author, abnormalities in 'how' the motion occurred in mid-range (rather than total range) seems to be associated with LBP. The variables used in this study described a disruption in the rate of attainment of angular or linear displacement during mid-range postures (Teyhen et al. 2007). Assessments can be made of extent of movement along with quality and sequencing of movement.
- An intersegmental motion lag is observed in the lumbar spine during flexion in normal subjects. Lumbar flexion initiates at the L3/4 segment. The L4/5 segmental motion is delayed from the L3/4 motion and precedes the L5/S1 motion. In extension, L3–L5 segmental motion is small, and the L5/S1 segment contributes most of this movement (Kanayama et al. 1996). In the author's view, this fluoroscopic assessment can help differentiate segments with abnormal movement and can contribute to the overall diagnostic pathway in determining the extent or level of instability which may respond to prolotherapy.
- *Provocation/anaesthetic discometry and discography*: The presence of painful discs can be demonstrated by these methods, although there was previously some concern as to the diagnostic validity. According to a meta-analysis in 2008, discography

(a)

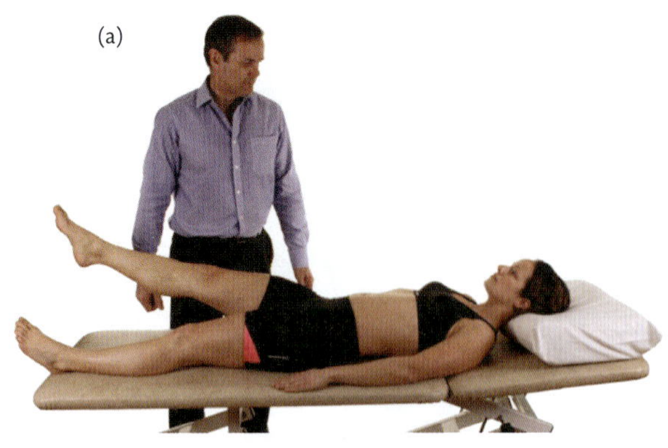

(b)

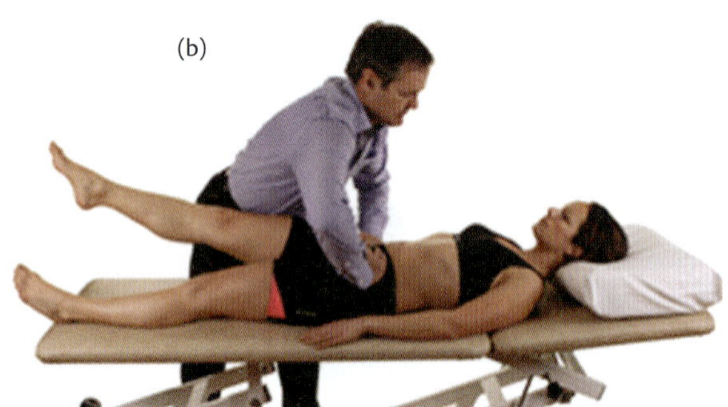

Figure 55.10 The active straight leg raise test and reinforcement of pelvis on retesting.

has a low false positive rate for the diagnosis of discogenic pain (Wolfer et al. 2008). Now, discography has applications in a number of clinical settings and has been well studied. Provocation discometry relies on the ability of increased intradiscal pressure to produce pain and thereby identify a painful disc. This allows treatment to be based at a specific level.

- *Medial branch block injections*: The validity, specificity, and sensitivity of these facet joint nerve blocks are considered strong in the diagnosis of facet joint pain (Manchikanti et al. 2003). They have been shown to be able to identify painful facet joints. The presence of painful facet joints may implicate existing and pre-existing segmental instability as a precursor.

Protocol for prolotherapy in the UK

Small volumes of a solution containing hyperosmolar dextrose or a solution called P2G (25% dextrose, 25% glycerol, and 2% phenol) are injected around ligamento-periosteal junctions, teno-osseous junctions, or into joints. A common proliferant injectate used in the UK is a 50/50 mixture of P2G and 1% lidocaine. A weaker solution that can be used is 50% dextrose diluted with 1% lidocaine to form a 12.5–25% dextrose solution.

Prolotherapy is usually performed on three occasions initially, with 1–3 weeks between each treatment. A further course of three treatments is used if the first course is subjectively or objectively helpful on a visual analogue scale (VAS) for pain and/or the Oswestry Disability Index (ODI) but if the improvement is incomplete.

Prolotherapy technique in the UK

Verbal or written consent is obtained. Then with the patient in the prone position (Figure 55.11), injection is made, under fluoroscopic X-ray guidance, into 13 sites around the L4/5 and L5/S1 intervertebral segments (Figure 55.12). In the UK, most practitioners use 5 ml P2G mixed with 5 ml 1% lidocaine or a solution of dextrose with lidocaine. The sites injected are as shown in Figure 55.13.

Frequently, the S1 spinous process is not visible or may exhibit a spina bifida occulta, so it is not routinely injected.

After-care

There is frequently a flare of pain for 1–2 days after the injection and patients are warned about this. They are asked not to take non-steroidal anti-inflammatory drugs (NSAIDs) for the duration of the course of treatment. Patients are usually advised to walk for 20–30 minutes per day for 2 weeks after the last injection. This is assumed to encourage functional orientation of newly augmented collagen fibres. Research shows that best results for back pain are when the course of injections is accompanied by active rehabilitation and advice on self-management.

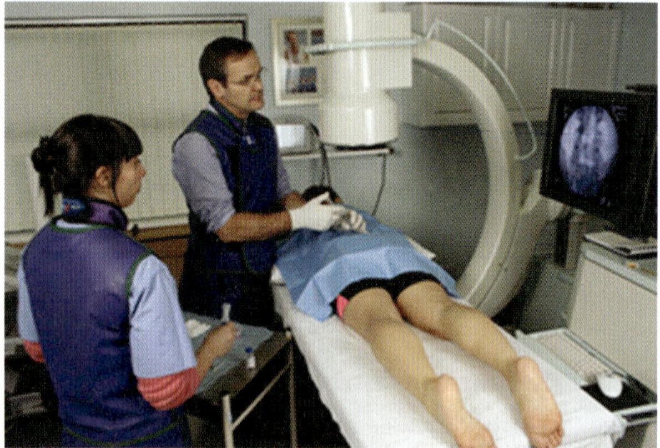

Figure 55.11 Prolotherapy in a fluoroscopy theatre. (Blackberry Clinic with permission)

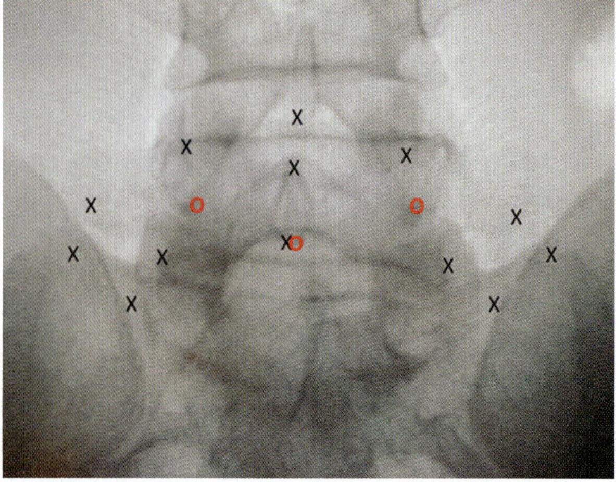

Figure 55.12 The red circles represent skin puncture sites and the black crosses represent the target points.

(a)

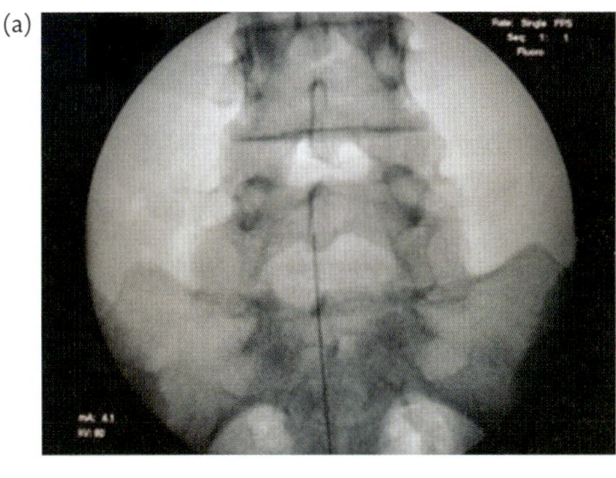

(b)

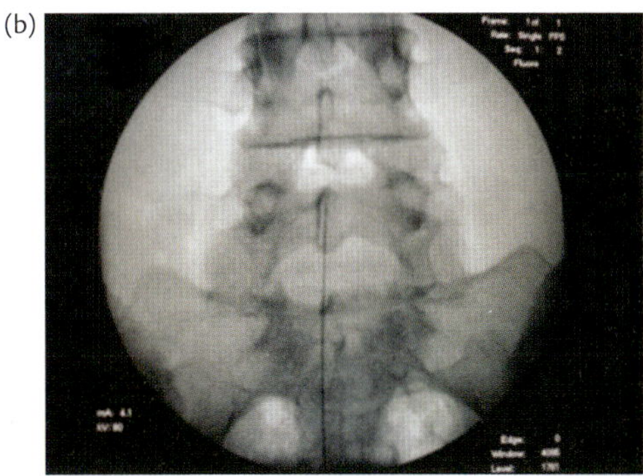

(c)

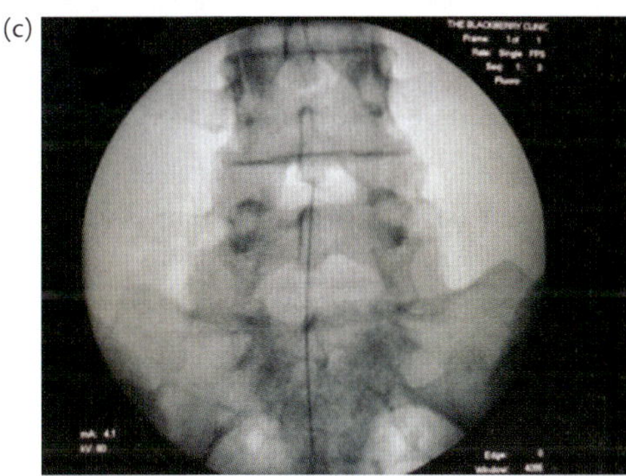

(d)

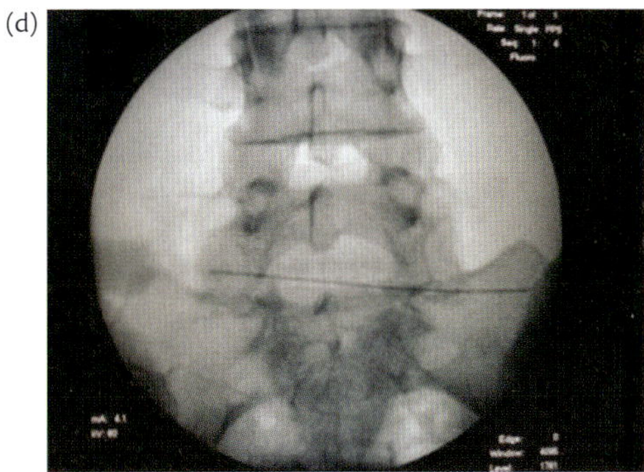

Figure 55.13 Target points: (a) caudal aspect of L5 spinous process (supraspinous ligament insertion); (b) cephalad aspect of L5 spinous process (supraspinous ligament insertion); (c) caudal aspect of the L4 spinous process (supraspinous ligament insertion); (d) inside the posterior iliac crest bilaterally (iliolumbar ligament insertion); (e) sacral insertion of the posterior sacroiliac ligaments bilaterally; (f) L4/5 and L5/S1 facet joint capsules bilaterally; (g) inferior margin of the tip of the L5 transverse processes (iliolumbar ligament origin) bilaterally.

(e)

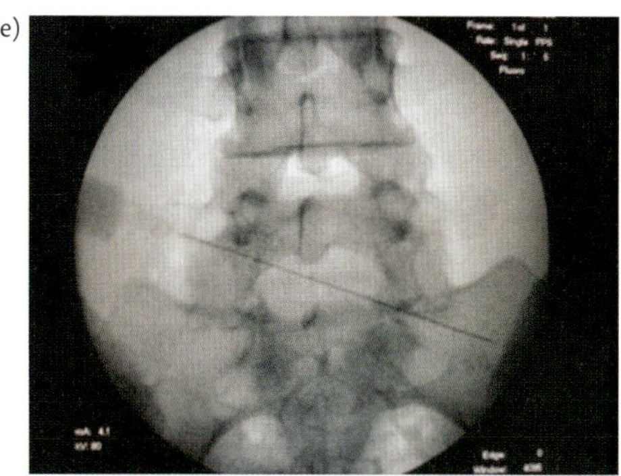

(f)

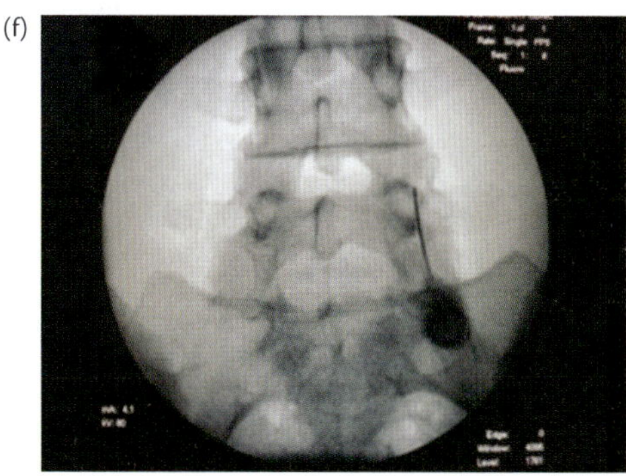

(g)

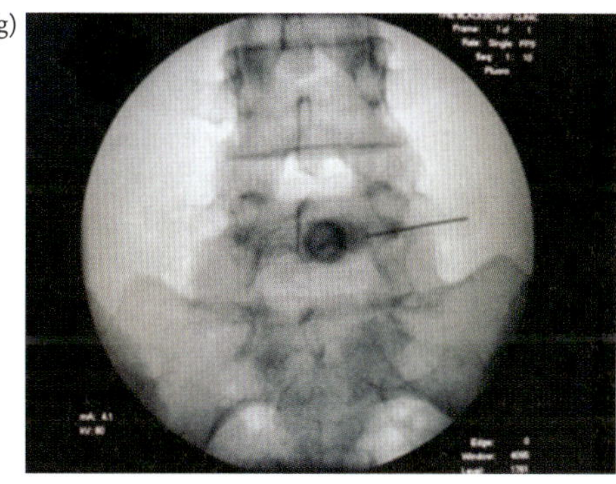

Figure 55.13 *(continued)*

In those patients for whom the technique is successful, there is usually a period of greatly reduced pain and infrequent or rare attacks of back pain for several years. Pain relief should be accompanied by steadily increasing levels of activities. Some patients, especially those with back pain, may require a further course if there is a prolonged relapse. Most practitioners would agree that pain relief can last for at least 5 years.

Prolotherapy research in sub-categories of low back pain

Sacroiliac dysfunction

A study in 2008 assessed 25 subjects with clinical symptoms and signs of sacroiliac dysfunction which had been refractory to conservative treatment for 6 months or more. The treatment consisted of 18% dextrose in three injections over 12 weeks, delivered to the interosseous ligaments under CT guidance. There was significant improvement in all pain and disability scores at 3, 12, and 24 months (Cusi et al. 2010).

Discogenic low back/leg pain

Miller et al. described a prospective series of subjects using disc space injections of 3 ml 25% dextrose with 0.25% bupivacaine for chronic degenerative discogenic leg pain, with or without low back pain (average duration 39 months). Seventy-six subjects with degenerative disc disease without herniation and with concordant pain reproduction with CT discography were included. All had failed physical therapies and epidural steroid injections. Patients underwent an average of 3.5 injections each. In the responders (33 of 76), the mean VAS scores were 8.9 at study entry, 2.5 at 2 months, and 2.6 at 18 months; 43 of 76 were considered non-responders (Miller et al. 2009).

Coccydinia

Khan studied 37 patients with chronic coccydynia which had been unresponsive to treatment: 25% dextrose/lidocaine solution was injected into the coccyx. Patients had up to three injections within 6 weeks. The mean VAS before prolotherapy was 8.5. It was 3.4 after the first and 2.5 after the second injection; 30 out of the 37 subjects reported good pain relief (Khan et al. 2008).

Non-spinal prolotherapy

First carpometacarpal (CMC) and inter-phalangeal joint osteoarthritis

A study by Reeves et al. in 2000 showed that improvement in pain with movement of fingers improved significantly with dextrose prolotherapy group (42%) versus a placebo control group (15%). Pain at rest and with grip improved more in the dextrose group, but not significantly. Flexion range of motion improved more in the dextrose group. Side-effects were minimal. The conclusion was that dextrose prolotherapy was clinically effective and safe in the treatment of pain on joint movement and range limitation in osteoarthritic finger joints (Reeves and Hassanein 2000).

Lateral epicondylosis

Prolotherapy has been shown in a systematic review to be more effective than placebo. Of several different treatments for lateral epicondylosis, the criteria for an effective treatment along with low risk of bias were only met by the prolotherapy trial included in the review (Krogh et al. 2012).

A randomized controlled trial (RCT) on prolotherapy for lateral epicondylosis, in 2008, reported significantly decreased pain scores for treatment with prolotherapy at 8 and 16 weeks. In addition, prolotherapy improved isometric strength significantly compared with controls, and grip strength compared with baseline. These improvements were sustained at 52 weeks (Scarpone et al. 2008).

Plantar fasciitis

A study published in 2009 reported on treatment of 20 patients with refractory plantar fasciitis of, on average, 21 months' duration; 25% dextrose was injected, under ultrasound guidance, on an average of three occasions. Pain scores significantly improved during activities of daily living by 49.7 points and during sport by 56.5 points; 16 out of 20 subjects reported a good or excellent effect of treatment (Ryan et al. 2009).

Patellar tendinopathy

A pilot study in 2011 evaluated ultrasound-guided hyperosmolar (25%) dextrose injection for patellar tendinopathy on 47 subjects after failed conservative treatment. A mean of four injections were carried out. At a mean of 45 weeks, there was a reduction in pain and an improvement in ultrasound appearance following the injections. Hypoechoic appearances improved as did neovascularity, in association with decreased pain scores. The results suggest that dextrose injections may modify tissue changes in patellar tendinopathy (Ryan et al. 2011). A case report in the *Archives of Physical Medicine and Rehabilitation* has demonstrated a similar effect on a series of MRI and ultrasound scans following prolotherapy in patellar tendinosis (Fullerton 2008).

Lateral ankle ligaments tears

A case report published in the *Archives of Physical Medicine and Rehabilitation* documented the repair of a chronic refractory anterior talofibular ligament (ATFL) tear following prolotherapy injections. The thickened, hypoechoic and anechoic areas improved in tissue echogenicity, uniformity of signal, and fibrillar pattern. The anechoic tear partially filled with new tissue and was no longer anechoic. The thickness of the main portion of the tendon returned to near normal thickness (Fullerton 2008). Similar case reports have shown tissue repair in the knee meniscus and Achilles and patellar tendons.

Achilles tendinopathy

In Achilles tendinosis, prolotherapy has been described using hypertonic injection around the Achilles tendon (Yelland et al 2007). Eccentric loading exercises, combined with prolotherapy, give more rapid improvements in symptoms than eccentric loading alone, but long-term Victorian institute of Sport Assessment - Achilles VISA-A scores were similar (Lind et al. 2006).

A case series in 2007 assessed prolotherapy in 36 subjects with Achilles tendinopathy; 25% dextrose was injected into hypoechoic areas in the Achilles tendon under ultrasound guidance. At 52 weeks, the VAS pain score had reduced by 78–88%. Also, tendon thickness had significantly decreased (Maxwell et al. 2007).

Lind et al. used the sclerosant, polidocanol, to obliterate neovascularization in persisting Achilles tendinosis. They concluded that

> . . . treatment with sclerosing polidocanol injections in patients with chronic painful mid-portion Achilles tendinosis showed remaining good clinical results at a 2-year follow-up. Decreased tendon thickness and improved structure after treatment might indicate a remodelling potential? (Lind et al. 2006)

Hip adductor groin pain/osteitis pubis

Topol et al. reported the use of 12.5% dextrose in 24 soccer and rugby players with an average of 15 months of groin pain, osteitis pubis, and/or adductor tendinopathy. Monthly injections were given into the entheses around the symphysis pubis. An average of 2.8 treatments were used. There was a 91.7% 'return to play' at a mean of 9 weeks. The mean improvement on VAS was from 6.3 to 1.0; 20 out of 24 had no pain and 22 out of 24 were unrestricted with sports at final data collection at 17 months (Topol et al. 2005).

Knee joint osteoarthritis

Reeves and Hassanein compared intra-articular knee injection of 10% dextrose against control injections. The authors concluded:

> Prolotherapy injection with 10% dextrose resulted in clinically and statistically significant improvements in knee osteoarthritis. Preliminary blinded radiographic readings (1-year films, with 3-year total follow-up period planned) demonstrated improvement in several measures of osteoarthritis severity. ACL laxity, when present in these osteoarthritic patients also improved. (Reeves and Hassanein 2000)

More recently, Rabago et al. (2013) showed that dextrose injections in and around the knee resulted in significant and sustained improvement of pain, function, and stiffness scores for knee osteoarthritis compared with blinded saline injections and home exercises.

Medial collateral ligament (MCL) injury

Grade 1 or 2 MCL tears are well known in sports medicine. The pain from these tears are amenable to treatment with prolotherapy and although the presence of robust controlled studies in the literature is limited, there is an abundance of anecdotal evidence that prolotherapy can help pain and instability in sufferers of this condition (Hauser 2001).

Neurogenic hamstring and recurrent injury

According to British football statistics, 'hamstring injuries account for 12% of the total injuries, with an average of five per club per season, resulting in 15 missed matches and 90 missed training days' (Woods et al. 2004) demonstrating just how much it affects the footballing population!

On the basis of the research by Vad et al. (2000), the majority of these hamstring injuries may be due to neurological problems arising from the central nervous system. Inflammation and irritation of the nerve roots exiting the vertebral foramen of the lumbar spine may, in fact, cause increased basal tone of the hamstring muscles, making them more susceptible to injury. A study by Kornberg and McCarthy (1992) found that there was a high incidence of positive slump tests in a group of injured football players compared with a control group. Research suggests that this abnormal neural tension or neural tethering may be responsible for the symptoms associated with 'neurogenic hamstrings'.

It has been proposed that these neural influences may predispose select groups of people to hamstring pain of a neurogenic origin, particularly those who engage in track and field sports such as sprinters and footballers. For this reason, amateur athletes and many elite athletes face ongoing problems with continued high-level training and competition.

In the author's opinion, it is conceivable that recurrent hamstring and calf tears, especially in football and athletics, may be associated with instability in the lumbar spine. This instability can result in degenerative discs and discogenic nerve root irritation resulting in central sensitization and changes in myotomal basal muscle tone. Thus, the susceptibility to muscle tearing is increased. Prolotherapy may indeed help reduce the frequency of these posterior chain injuries and is a potentially exciting topic for future research.

Neural prolotherapy

Neural prolotherapy is a more recently developed concept for the treatment of painful conditions along with joint, tendon, ligament, and muscle pain. The treatment involves a series of injections with a glucose solution, immediately under the skin, with a very fine needle, targeting the source of the pain. It can offer a success rate of greater than 75%.

Neural prolotherapy was developed by Dr John Lyftogt in New Zealand. His research focused on the treatment of Achilles tendon pain, with an apparent success rate of more than 90%. He has published two level 4 articles on Achilles tendon pain. The treatment of the Achilles tendon is different from the more usual prolotherapy in that the injections are given just under the skin (Lyftogt 2005).

A less invasive treatment than prolotherapy, neural prolotherapy, has been successfully used in the treatment of tennis elbow, painful knees, shoulders, neck, hips, ankles, muscle injuries, and low back pain. Two-year follow-up studies have shown promising success rates. An hypothesis was developed that glucose assists in the repair of connective tissue in nerve fibres under the skin similar to the way repair of connective tissue in ligaments and tendons is effected by the more usual type of prolotherapy. These nerves are now known to be involved in neuralgia and neuropathic pain pathways.

Teaching of prolotherapy techniques

The British Institute of Musculoskeletal Medicine and Blackberry Education are currently the only organizations teaching spinal prolotherapy techniques in the UK. The methods taught have evolved over many years, based on accumulated experience combined with the available evidence base. The advent of fluoroscopic guidance has further assisted in the accuracy and safety of the procedures.

Research into prolotherapy

Research into prolotherapy has always been hampered by the fact that the components of the commonly used proliferants are not open to pharmaceutical patent and, consequently, there is no pharmaceutical company likely to fund research into the usefulness of the technique. The first RCT appeared in 1987, systematic reviews were published in 2005 by Rabago and 2009 by the Cochrane Collaboration who concluded:

> Of the five studies we reviewed, three found that prolotherapy injections alone were not an effective treatment for chronic low-back pain and two found that a combination of prolotherapy injections, spinal manipulation, exercises, and other treatments can help chronic low-back pain and disability. (Dagenais et al. 2010)

Of the five published RCTs by Ongley, Klein, Dechow, Mathews, and Yelland on prolotherapy, two show a positive benefit when combined with an exercise programme and brief manipulative treatment (Klein et al. 1993; Ongley et al. 1987). The study by Yelland shows a sustained benefit of both prolotherapy and placebo groups over 2 years to rival that of any surgical intervention (Yelland et al. 2004).

Three studies that compared prolotherapy injections directly against control injections found no evidence that they are more effective (Dechow et al. 1999; Mathews et al. 1987; Yelland et al. 2004). However, these trials studied prolotherapy 'alone' in chronic LBP. All RCTs showed improvement in pain and disability in all chronic and moderate to severe LBP treatment groups. Yelland's study reported clinical improvement in excess of subjects' own perception of minimum improvement necessary for prolotherapy to be worthwhile (Yelland et al. 2000, 2004).

There is still a lack of consensus regarding the sub-groups of LBP which respond more readily to the treatment. In the UK, the injections tend to be carried out under fluoroscopic guidance to enhance accuracy and safety, but the debate on the best solution and treatment protocols continues. Recent research has focused on more specific groups of back pain patients to determine the most likely clinical features to correlate with the highest chance of success (Cusi et al. 2008).

It is the author's opinion that there is a variation in response to prolotherapy depending on the underlying LBP diagnosis, the extent of instability on videofluoroscopy, the adherence to a patient-centred exercise programme, and the motivation of the patient.

The literature indicates that the enthusiasm for the use of this technique has endured for over half a century. While it is by no means a panacea, prolotherapy offers a substantial chance for improvement. Many anecdotal cases with dramatic responses have greatly changed patients' quality of life. International rowers and footballers with career-threatening LBP have been able to continue in their chosen careers as a result of prolotherapy treatment. In many instances, prolotherapy may have led to the avoidance of spinal fusion or disc replacement.

An alternative to spinal fusion

In the NHS, surgical expenditure is the largest single component of expenditure for LBP, and the numbers of spinal fusions being performed was still rising when Gibson and Waddell published for the Cochrane database in 2005. Spinal fusion and disc replacement continue to generate controversy and, in any event, both of these interventions are far more costly, with a significantly higher number of reported complications than prolotherapy.

A recent study of over 725 workers' compensation cases that underwent spinal fusion discovered that 36% had surgical complications and 27% needed a second operation. After 2 years, only 26% had returned to work, compared to 67% of controls, 76% continued opiate use after surgery, and mean opiate use increased by 41% (Nguyen et al. 2011). Analgesic-related *mortality* after lumbar fusion in workers' compensation cases has been shown to be as much as 1% (Juratli 2009). It has been demonstrated that 2 years after surgery, in a study of workers' compensation cases, 63.9% of patients were disabled and the re-operation rate was 22% (Juratli et al. 2006).

The successful use of prolotherapy treatment may therefore well deter patients from seeking a surgical remedy for their LBP.

Side-effects of prolotherapy

A post-injection flare of pain is common but will last only one to three days. These flares usually respond to simple analgesia such as paracetamol or co-codamol. NSAID use is to be avoided if possible.

Adverse events following prolotherapy

Risk of allergic reaction, infection, and nerve damage is very low. Injections should only be performed by doctors trained in the technique and in a controlled environment while using sterile techniques. Although P2G is not licensed for use in the UK, this does not prohibit its use, and it has not been reported to cause significant side-effects or adverse reactions.

A survey in 2006 concluded that adverse reactions or events were no more common in spinal prolotherapy than in other spinal injections (Dagenais et al. 2006). There have been no significant adverse reactions from peripheral prolotherapy procedures.

Other forms of prolotherapy

- Autologous blood injection (ABI)
- Platelet-rich plasma (PRP)
- Autologous conditioned plasma (ACP)
- Dry needling
- Stem cell therapy

Rationale for proliferant treatments in tendinopathy

Tendinopathy is thought to be due to a combination of overuse microtrauma, genetic variants of matrix proteins, and metabolic disorders. It seems to be a failed healing response with fibrosis and neovascularization. The aberrant sensory nerves may explain excessive nociceptive afferent signalling. Also, release of neuronal mediators may contribute to the fibrotic changes seen in tendinopathy. Prolotherapy has been found in animal and human studies to stimulate inflammation, increase ligament size, produce hypertrophy of tendons and extracellular matrix, and cause fibroblastic proliferation.

Autologous blood injection, platelet-rich plasma, autologous conditioned plasma

Recent studies have demonstrated the effectiveness of ABI for lateral epicondylosis, plantar fasciitis, and patella tendinosis. It is assumed that ABI/PRP and ACP work via transforming growth factor beta (TGFβ) and basic fibroblast growth factor (BFGF) carried in the blood/plasma which act as mediators to induce the 'healing cascade'.

Neovascularization has been postulated as a cause for the symptom of pain in tendinosis but clearly the causes of the symptoms are more complex than can be attributed purely to the new vessel formation.

Using ultrasound scanning, it has been seen that following ABI there is a reduction in tendon thickness and inflammatory changes seen with the tendon. There is also a partial resolution of tendon tears following injection. One of the first studies on lateral epicondylosis by Edwards and Calandruccio (2003) showed that after an average follow up of 9.5 months, there was an improvement in pain and movement in 22 out of 28 patients. There have been several studies since showing similar success rates and over a longer duration of follow-up.

One injection is performed initially and there may occasionally be a requirement for a second injection 4 weeks later. Most pain relief occurs within the first 4–6 weeks. Patient selection and an accurate diagnosis are critical to the success of the procedure.

From recent studies, it would appear that autologous blood, PRP, and ACP injections have a more permanent effect on long-term benefit than that achieved with injection of corticosteroid. This is probably related to the healing benefits of ABI/PRP/ACP causing the tendon to return to its pre-injury state rather than simply relying on the anti-inflammatory action of corticosteroid injections (van Ark et al. 2011; Connell et al. 2001; Creaney et al. 2011; Edwards and Calandruccio 2003; Iwasaki et al. 1995; Khan and Cook 2001; Kraushaar and Nirschl 1999; Lian et al. 1996; Sheth et al. 2012).

Dry needling

The mechanism of short-term relief following dry needling is not fully understood but it may be that needle-induced trauma to the area of tendinosis or to a myofascial trigger point may initiate localized inflammation, triggering a wound-healing cascade, resulting in the deposition of new collagen. New collagen shrinks as it matures, enhancing strength of the new tissue. The effect can be optimized in the presence of injected autologous blood or from local bleeding.

Platelet-rich plasma and autologous conditioned plasma injections

PRP or ACP injection is yet another form of prolotherapy and is derived from a patient's whole blood. The blood is centrifuged, followed by an extraction method which separates out the plasma layer with the highest concentration of platelets and growth factors. The growth factors include transforming growth factor beta (TGF-β), platelet-derived growth factor (PDGF), insulin-like growth factor (IGF), vascular endothelial growth factor (VEGF), epidermal growth factor (EGF), and fibroblast growth factor-2 (FGF-2). These factors have been shown to stimulate bone and soft tissue healing, cell proliferation, collagen synthesis, and revascularization.

Laboratory studies have demonstrated that PRP can stimulate proliferation of stem cells and fibroblasts. In animal studies, it has been shown to promote osteochondral healing and enhance gene expression of key matrix molecules, suggesting a potential to heal damaged tendons, mainly in the early phase of healing.

Studies continue to appear in the literature regarding significant pain relief after treatment of tendinopathy with PRP versus control injections. Particular attention has focused on its use in lateral epicondylosis, plantar fasciitis, and patellar tendinopathy. It has also been used in the surgical treatment of osteochondritis dessicans to help re-attach the displaced chondral fragment.

A recent study from Italy has demonstrated its effect on pain relief in the degenerative knee. PRP injections showed more and longer efficacy than hyaluronic acid injections in reducing pain and other symptoms, along with recovering articular function. Better results were achieved in younger and more active patients with a low degree of cartilage degeneration (Kon et al. 2011).

PRP is a new technology that seems promising in respect of continuing publication on the subject and it may well prove to have numerous applications in the treatment of musculoskeletal injury (Mehta 2010).

Stem cell therapy

A number of different cell lines such as mesenchymal stem cells, tendon-derived cells, and dermal fibroblasts offer some promise in tendon engineering due to their 'proliferative' capacity and the potential of genetic modification to secrete tenogenic growth factors.

Even though cellular therapies offer some potential in treating tendon disorders, there have been few published trials to determine the ideal protocol for use.

There is much to be discovered in further research into cellular therapies and their role in treatment of tendon disorders. There is insufficient data to conclusively prove that these treatments are safe and effective. However, these therapies will probably become increasingly important in musculoskeletal and sports medicine (Young 2012).

Conclusion on prolotherapy in the UK

Prolotherapy has been used in its current form for almost a century, with hundreds of published articles, meta-analyses, and a handful of RCTs (Rabago et al. 2005). These studies stand out with their low 'risk of bias' in that proliferant solutions such as dextrose, P2G, and autologous blood have no pharmaceutical patent and, consequently, the studies do not attract corporate finance. The safety and efficacy of the treatments account for their advancing popularity in the western world.

In view of the scarcity of research establishments willing to promote high-quality research into the technique of prolotherapy, it may remain one of musculoskeletal medicine's best kept secrets for a few more years yet.

References

Alfredson H, Lorentzon R. Sclerosing polidocanol injections of small vessels to treat the chronic painful achilles tendon. *Cardiovasc Hematol Agents Med Chem (Netherlands)* 2007; 5(2):97–100.

Alfredson H, Ohberg L, Sclerosing injections to areas of neo-vascularisation reduce pain in chronic achilles tendinopathy: a double-blind randomized controlled trial. *Knee Surg Sports Traumatol Arthrosc* 2005; 13(4):338–44.

van Ark M, Zwerver J, van den Akker-Scheek I. Injection treatments for patellar tendinopathy. *Br J Sports Med* 2011; 45:1068–76.

Banks A. A rational for prolotherapy. *J Orthop Med* 1991; 13(3):54–9.

Cabraja M, Mohamed E, Koeppen D, Kroppenstedt S. The analysis of segmental mobility with different lumbar radiographs in symptomatic patients with a spondylolisthesis. *Eur Spine J* 2012; 21(2):256–61.

Cholewicki J, McGill S. Mechanical stability of the in vivo lumbar spine: implications for injury and chronic low back pain. *Clin Biomech* 1996; 11(1):1–15.

Connell D, Burke F, Coombes P, et al. Sonographic examination of lateral epicondylitis. *Am J Roent* 2001; 176:777–82.

Creaney L, Wallace A, Curtis M, Connell D. Growth factor-based therapies provide additional benefit beyond physical therapy in resistant elbow tendinopathy: a prospective, single-blind, randomised trial of autologous blood injections versus platelet-rich plasma injections. *Br J Sports Med* 2011;45:966–71.

Cusi M, Saunders J, Hungerford B, Wisbey-Roth B, Lucas P, Wilson S. The use of prolotherapy in the sacroiliac joint. *Br J Sports Med* 2010; 44(2):100–104.

Dagenais S, Ogunseitan O, Haldeman S, Wooley JR, Newcomb RL. Side effects and adverse events related to intra-ligamentous injection of sclerosing solutions (prolotherapy) for back and neck pain: a survey of practitioners. *Arch Phys Med Rehabil* 2006; 87:909–13.

Dagenais S, Yelland M, Del Mar C, Schoene M. Prolotherapy injections for chronic low-back pain. Cochrane collaboration. *Cochrane Database Syst Rev* (2) 2010.

Dechow E, Davies R, Carr A, Thompson P. A randomized, double-blind, placebo-controlled trial of sclerosing injections in patients with chronic low back pain. *Rheumatology*1999; 38:1255–9.

Dupuis P, Yong-Hing K, Cassidy J, et al. Radiologic diagnosis of degenerative lumbar spinal instability. *Spine* 1985; 10:262–76.

Dvorak J, Panjabi M, Chang D, et al. Functional radiographic diagnosis of the lumbar spine: flexion-extension and lateral bending. *Spine* 1991; 16:562–71.

Edwards SG, Calandruccio JH. Autologous blood injections for refractory lateral epicondylitis. *J Hand Surg* 2003; 28A:272–8.

Fullerton B. High-resolution ultrasound and magnetic resonance imaging to document tissue repair after prolotherapy: a report of 3 cases. *Arch Phys Med Rehab* 2008; 89(2):377–85.

Gibson J, Waddell G. Surgery for degenerative lumbar spondylosis. *Cochrane Database Syst Rev* 2005; (4):CD001352.

Hackett G, Hemwall G, Montgomery G. *Ligament and tendon relaxation treated by prolotherapy*. 5 Oak Park: Gustav A. Hemwall; 1993.

Hauser R, Hauser M. A retrospective study on dextrose prolotherapy for unresolved knee pain at an outpatient charity clinic in rural Illinois. *J Prolo* 2009; 1:11–21.

Hauser R, Hauser M. *Prolo your sports injuries away*. Beulah Land Press, 2001 USA.

Hayes M, Howard T, Gruel C, et al. Roentgenographic evaluation of lumbar spine flexion-extension in asymptomatic individuals. *Spine* 1989; 14:327–31.

Hicks G, Fritz J, Delitto A, et al. The reliability of clinical examination measures used for patients with suspected lumbar segmental instability. *Arch Phys Med Rehabil* 2003; 84:1858–64.

Hicks G, Fritz J, Delitto A, Mishock J. Interrater reliability of clinical examination measures for identification of lumbar segmental instability. *Arch Phys Med Rehabil* 2003; 84(12):1858–64.

Iwasaki M, Nakahara H, Nakata K, Nakase T, Kimura T, Ono K. Regulation of proliferation and osteochondrogenic differentiation of periosteum-derived cells by transforming growth factor-β and basic fibroblast growth factor. *J Bone Joint Surg* 1995; 77A:543–54.

Jensen K. *PhD dissertation: healing response of knee ligaments to prolotherapy in a rat model*. Madison: Biomedical Engineering, University of Wisconsin; 2006.

Juratli S, Franklin G, Mirza S, Wickizer T, Fulton-Kehoe D. Lumbar fusion outcomes in Washington State workers' compensation. *Spine* 2006; 31(23):2715–23.

Juratli SM, Mirza SK, Fulton-Kehoe D, Wickizer TM, Franklin GM. Mortality after lumbar fusion surgery. *Spine* 2009; 34(7):740–7.

Kanayama M, Abumi K, Kaneda K, Tadano S, Ukai T. Phase lag of the intersegmental motion in flexion-extension of the lumbar and lumbosacral spine. An in vivo study. *Spine* 1996; 21(12):1416–22.

Kasai Y, Morishita K, Kawakita E, Kondo T, Uchida A. A new evaluation method for lumbar spinal instability: passive lumbar extension test. *J Am Phys Ther Ass* 2006; 86(12):1661–7.

Khan KM, Cook, JK. Overuse tendon injuries. In: *Clinical sports medicine* (2nd edn). Sydney. McGraw-Hill; 2001.

Khan S, Kumar A, Varshney M, Trikha V, Yadav C. Dextrose prolotherapy for recalcitrant coccygodynia. *J Orthop Surg* 2008; 16:27–9.

Kim S, Stitik T, Foye P. Critical review of prolotherapy for osteoarthritis, low back pain, and other musculoskeletal conditions: a physiatric perspective. *J Phys Med Rehab* 2004; 83(5):379–89.

Klein G, Dorman T, Johnson C. Proliferant injections for low back pain; histological changes of injected ligaments and objective measurements of lumbar spine mobility before and after treatment. *J Neurol Orthop Med Surg* 1989; 10:123–6.

Klein RG, Eek BC, DeLong WB, Mooney V. A randomized double-blind trial of dextrose-glycerine-phenol injections for chronic, low back pain. *J Spinal Disord* 1993; 6(1):23–33.

Knutsson F. The instability associated with disc degeneration in the lumbar spine. *Acta Radiol* 1944; 25:593–609.

Kon E, Mandelbaum B, Buda R, et al. Platelet-rich plasma intra-articular injection versus hyaluronic acid viscosupplementation as treatments for cartilage pathology: from early degeneration to osteoarthritis. *Arthroscopy* 2011; 27(11):1490–501.

Kornberg C, McCarthy T. The effect of neural stretching technique on the sympathetic outflow to the lower limbs. *J Orth Sports Phys Ther* 1992; 16(6):269–72.

Kraushaar BS, Nirschl RP. Tendinosis of the elbow (tennis elbow). Clinical features and findings of histological, immunohistochemical and electron microscopy studies. *J Bone Joint Surg* 1999; 81–A:269–78.

Krogh T, et al. Comparative effectiveness of injection therapies in lateral epicondylitis. A systematic review and network meta-analysis of randomized controlled trials. *Am J Sports Med* 2012;41(6):1435–46.

Lian O, Holken KJ, Engebrestson L, Bahr R. Relationship between symptoms of jumper's knee and the ultrasound characteristics of the patellar tendon among high level male volleyball players. *Scand J Med Sci Sports* 1996; 6:291–6.

Lind B, Ohberg L, Alfredson H. Sclerosing polidocanol injections in mid-portion Achilles tendinosis: remaining good clinical results and decreased tendon thickness at 2-year follow-up. *Knee Surg Sports Traumatol Arthrosc* 2006; 14(12):1327–32.

Linetsky F, Rafael M, Saberski L. Pain management with regenerative injection therapy. In: Weiner R. (ed.) *Pain management*. Boca Raton: CRC Press; 2002; pp. 381–402.

Liu Y, Tipton C, Matthes R, Bedford T, Maynard J, Walmer H. An in-situ study of the influence of a sclerosing solution in rabbit medial collateral ligaments and its junction strength. *Connect Tiss Res* 1983; 11:95–102.

Lyftogt J. Prolotherapy and achilles tendinopathy: a prospective pilot study of an old treatment. *Austral Musculo Med* 2005; 10(1):16–9.

Manchikanti L, Singh V, Pampati V. Are diagnostic medial branch blocks valid? Results of a 2 year follow-up. *Pain Physician* 2003; 6(2):147–53.

Mathews J, Mills S, Jenkins V, et al. Back pain and sciatica: controlled trials of manipulation, traction, sclerosant and epidural injections. *Br J Rheumatol* 1987; 26(6):416–23.

Maxwell N, Ryan M, Taunton J, Gillies J, Wong A. Sonographically guided intra-tendinous injection of hyperosmolar dextrose to treat chronic tendinosis of the achilles tendon: a pilot study. *Am J Roent* 2007; 189(4):215–20.

Mehta V. Platelet-rich plasma: a review of the science and possible clinical applications. *Orthopedics* 2010; 33(2):111–15.

Miller M, Mathews R, Reeves K. Treatment of painful advanced internal lumbar disc derangement with intradiscal injection of hypertonic dextrose. *Pain Physician* 2006; 9:115–21.

Nachemson A. Lumbar spine instability: a critical update and symposium summary. *Spine* 1985; 10:290–1.

Nguyen, T, et al. Long-term outcomes of lumbar fusion among workers' compensation subjects. *Spine* 2011:36(4)320–31.

Oates J, Fitzgerald G, Branch R, Jackson E, Knapp H, Roberts LJ. Clinical implications of prostaglandin and thromboxane A2 formation. *New Engl J Med* 1988; 319(11):689–98.

Ongley M, Klein R, Dorman T, Eek B, Hubert L. A new approach to the treatment of chronic low back pain. *Lancet* 1987 18; 2:143–6.

Panjabi M. Clinical spinal instability and low back pain. *J Electromyogr Kinesiol* 2003; 13(4):371–9.

Panjabi M. The stabilizing system of the spine. Part II. Neutral zone and instability hypothesis. *J Spin Dis* 1992; 5(4):390–7.

Pitkänen M, Manninen H, Lindgren K, et al. Segmental lumbar spine instability at flexion-extension radiography can be predicted by conventional radiography. *Clin Radiol* 2002; 57:632–9.

Posner I, White A, Edwards W, et al. A biomechanical analysis of the clinical stability of the lumbar and lumbosacral spine. *Spine* 1982; 7:374–89.

Rabago D, Best T, Beamsly M, Patterson J. A systematic review of prolotherapy for chronic musculoskeletal pain. *Clin J Sports Med* 2005; 15(5): 376–80.

Rabago D, Best T, Zgierska A, Zeisig E, Ryan M, Crane D. A systematic review of four injection therapies for lateral epicondylosis: prolotherapy, polidocanol, whole blood and platelet rich plasma. *Br J Sports Med* 2009; 43(7):471–81.

Rabago D, Patterson J, Mundt M, et al. Dextrose prolotherapy for knee steoarthritis: a randomized controlled trial. *Ann Fam Med* 2013; 11(3):229–37.

Rabago M, Slattengren A, Zgierska A. Prolotherapy in primary care practice. *Primary Care* 2010; 37(1):65–80.

Reeves K, Hassanein K. Randomized prospective double-blind placebo-controlled study of dextrose prolotherapy for knee osteoarthritis with or without ACL laxity. *Altern Ther Health M* 2000; 6(2):68–80.

Reeves K, Hassanein K. Randomized, prospective, placebo-controlled double-blind study of dextrose prolotherapy for osteoarthritic thumb and finger (DIP, PIP, and trapeziometacarpal) joints: evidence of clinical efficacy. *J Altern Complem Med* 2000; 6(4):311–20.

Ryan M, Wong A, Gillies J, Wong J, Taunton J. Sonographically guided intra-tendinous injections of hyperosmolar dextrose/lidocaine: a pilot study for the treatment of chronic plantar fasciitis. *Br J Sports Med* 2009; 43:303–6.

Ryan M, Wong A, Rabago D, Lee K, Taunton J. Ultrasound-guided injections of hyperosmolar dextrose for overuse patellar tendinopathy: a pilot study. *Br J Sports Med* 2011; 45(12):972–7.

Scarpone M, Rabago D, Zgierska A, Arbogest J, Snell E. The efficacy of prolotherapy for lateral epicondylosis: a pilot study. *Clin J Sports Med* 2008; 18:248–54.

Shaffer W, Spratt K, Weinstein J, et al. The consistency and accuracy of roentgenograms for measuring sagittal translation in the lumbar vertebral motion segment: an experimental model. *Spine* 1990; 15:741–50.

Sheth U, Simunovic N, Klein G, et al. Efficacy of autologous platelet-rich plasma use for orthopaedic indications: a meta-analysis. *J Bone Joint Surg Am* 2012; 94:298–307.

Teyhen D, Flynn T, Childs J, et al. Fluoroscopic video to identify aberrant lumbar motion. *Spine* 2007; 32(7):220–9.

Topol G, Reeves K, Hassanein K. Efficacy of dextrose prolotherapy in elite male kicking-sport athletes with groin pain. *Arch Phys Rehabil* 2005; 86:697–702.

Vad V, et al. *An unusual cause for chronic pain in the proximal hamstring (buttock) area.*(Society for Tennis Medicine and Science; 2000. Available at: <http://www.stms.nl/april2000/artikel18.htm>

White A, Panjabi M. The problem of clinical instability in the human spine: a systematic approach.part4:The lumbar and lumbosacral spine. *Clin Biomech Spine* 1990; 2:342–61.

Wolfer L, Derby R, Lee J, Lee S. A systematic review of lumbar provocation discography in asymptomatic subjects with a meta-analysis of false-positive rates. *Pain Physician* 2008; 11:513–38.

Woods C, Hawkins RD, Maltby S, Hulse M, Thomas A, Hodson A. The Football Association Medical Research Programme: an audit of injuries in professional football—analysis of hamstring injuries. *Br J Sports Med* 2004; 38:36–41.

Yelland M, Glasziou P, Bogduk N, Schluter P, McKernon M. Prolotherapy injections, saline injections, and exercises for chronic low back pain: a randomized trial. *Spine* 2004; 29(1):9–16.

Yelland M, Sweeting K, Lyftogt, Ng S, Scuffman P, Evans K. Prolotherapy injections and eccentric loading exercises for painful Achilles tendinosis: a randomised trial. *Br J Sports Med* 2011; 45(5):421–8.

Yelland M, Yeo M, Schluter P. Prolotherapy injections for chronic low back pain: results of a pilot comparative study. *Austral Musculo Med* 2000; 5(2):20–30.

Yone K, Sakou T. Usefulness of Posner's definition of spinal instability for selection of surgical treatment for lumbar spinal stenosis. *J Spin Dis* 1999; 12:40–4.

Young M. Stem cell applications in tendon disorders: a clinical perspective. *Stem Cells Int* 2012; 637836.

Chapter 56

The use of neurodynamics in pain management

Toby Hall and Kim Robinson

Sub-classification of neural tissue pain disorders

In Chapter 15, we highlighted the relatively poor evidence supporting neural mobilization (Ellis and Hing 2008), which may be explained by poor patient selection, as well as by inappropriate treatment techniques for the nature and stage of the disorder being treated. To improve on this, we outlined a treatment-based classification system to identify sub-groups of neural pain disorders more suitable for management by neural mobilization (Schäfer et al. 2009a).

Evidence to support this approach is shown in a recent study of cervicobrachial pain. This study showed that when four sessions of neural mobilization were applied to patients with features of peripheral nerve sensitization (PNS), but without signs of compression neuropathy (CN), the outcome was positive when compared to advice to stay active (Nee et al. 2012). Numbers needed to treat favoured the neural mobilization for participant-reported improvement (2.7, 95% CI 1.7 to 6.5), neck pain (3.6, 95% CI 2.1 to 10), arm pain (3.6, 95% CI 2.1 to 10), Neck Disability Index (4.3, 95% CI 2.4 to 18.2), and the Patient Specific Functional Scale (3.0, 95% CI 19.9 to 6.7). Similarly, from the same research group, certain patient baseline characteristics were found to predict treatment outcome following neural mobilization (Nee et al. 2013). These characteristics included features of neuropathic pain identified by the Subjective Leeds Assessment of Neuropathic Symptoms and Signs (SLANSS) scale. In that study, 46% of the variance in outcome was explained by the absence of neuropathic pain determined, in part, by the SLANSS score. In addition, our research group investigated neural mobilization in patients with low back related leg pain and found similar findings (Schäfer et al. 2011). In that study, 77 patients received seven treatment sessions of neural mobilization, advice, and exercise. Subjects classified with PNS responded more favourably than those with CN, neuropathic pain with sensory hypersensitivity (NPSH), and musculoskeletal referred pain.

To better understand these issues, we can consider the classic example of carpal tunnel syndrome (CTS), purportedly involving entrapment of the median nerve in the distal forearm (Ibrahim et al. 2012). CTS is the most common peripheral neuropathy affecting 1.3 out of 1000 individuals, peaking in middle age (Bongers et al. 2007). There is a considerable body of knowledge regarding CTS; hence more is known about its pathophysiology than any other peripheral neuropathy. Unfortunately, a systematic review failed to find clear evidence of a benefit for neural gliding exercises in CTS (Medina McKeon and Yancosek 2008), which was also the finding of the latest Cochrane review (Page et al. 2012). One explanation for this is that neural mobilization is not effective for all patients with CTS. Indeed, CTS appears to be a constellation of different problems involving the median nerve including swelling (Hunderfund et al. 2011); mechanosensitivity (Fernandez-de-Las-Penas et al. 2010; Vanti et al. 2011); central sensitization (Fernandez-de-las-Penas et al. 2009); impaired longitudinal sliding (Nakamichi and Tachibana 1995); increased deformation from adjacent tendons (van Doesburg et al. 2012a); and increased transverse movement (van Doesburg et al. 2012b) among others. Hence clearly, neural mobilization is unlikely to benefit all of these problems. A protocol is required to guide the clinician to know when neural mobilization is likely to be of benefit.

Physical examination to assess for neural mobilization

In order to evaluate a client with a presenting disorder to identify when neural mobilization is likely to be effective, the clinician must carry out a comprehensive clinical examination. This will include a range of physical tests that do not presume the source of symptoms but that identify a sufficient number of signs correlating with and supporting each other in the formulation of a clinical diagnosis. It is important to state that physical treatment, in the form of manual therapy, cannot be prescribed from imagery or nerve conduction studies, although it may well be strongly influenced and guided by such studies, even to the degree that the results of either may contraindicate manual therapy.

As previously mentioned in Chapter 15, the classification of neural pain disorders is hierarchical. The first step is identifying NPSH using the LANSS scale. In the absence of this, the next criterion is significant neurological deficit determined through a comprehensive neurological examination. In the presence of normal conduction, the third step would be the identification of PNS. In this case, a number of very specific correlating signs must be present before confirmation of PNS can be made.

Peripheral nerve sensitization

The criteria to determine the presence of PNS are threefold and comprise hyperalgesic responses to active movement, neurodynamic tests, and nerve palpation. Reliability of this classification system has been demonstrated in both the upper and lower limb (Schäfer et al. 2009b; Tampin et al. 2012).

Peripheral nerve trunks are dynamic structures capable of movement independent of anatomical surrounding tissue and structures. Cadaveric evidence of independent nerve movement is substantial (Alshami et al. 2007; Breig 1978; Breig and Marions 1963; Coppieters et al. 2006a). Evidence is also seen *in vivo* through the wealth of ultrasonography literature showing sciatic nerve movement during various components of the straight leg raise (SLR) and slump tests (Ellis et al. 2012; Ridehalgh et al. 2012), and median nerve movement during various components of the median neurodynamic test (Dilley et al. 2003, 2007; van Doesburg et al. 2012a,b; Greening et al. 1999). This independence is to enable nerve trunks to adapt to body postural change and movement, enabling the clinician to physically examine nerve trunks in a selective manner.

Once nerve trunks become inflamed, they develop mechanosensitivity, showing non-compliance with movement due to pain. This non-compliance may present as limitation of movement due to increased muscle tone/activity in groups of muscles antagonistic to the painful direction of movement. Muscle contraction, as measured by electromyography, in response to provocation of neural tissue, has been demonstrated in both animal and *in vivo* human experiments (Balster and Jull 1997; Hall and Quintner 1996; Hall et al. 1998; Hu et al. 1995). In more severe cases of pain of neural tissue origin, the increased tone of muscles becomes widespread. The classic example of this is frozen shoulder, where movement is grossly limited in all directions. Clinically, we find up to one-third of patients with this condition present with PNS as the pain source driving the protective muscle response and limitation of movement.

Active screening

Using knowledge of applied anatomy, it becomes clearly evident that different positions of the limb joints and trunk will influence the peripheral trunks in different ways. In the upper limb, a landmark study has shown that a position of shoulder girdle depression, shoulder abduction/lateral rotation, elbow extension, and wrist/finger extension, with the cervical spine in contralateral lateral flexion, had the effect of placing the neural tissues of the brachial plexus and median nerve in a maximally lengthened position (Elvey 1979). While these movements were carried out passively on cadaveric specimens, it logical that active movements will influence the same neural tissues to the same degree and may be incorporated in physical examination tests. For example, during trunk flexion in standing, the sciatic nerve and its constituent roots will be elongated and neural structures are consequently stressed, and if sensitized, pain provoked. However, various musculoskeletal structures including intervertebral discs, sacroiliac joints, and muscles are also stressed and may induce pain.

To screen for the presence of PNS, the movement should be repeated with ankle dorsiflexion and cervical spine flexion (Figure 56.1). If the patient's concordant pain complaint is increased and range reduced, the potential for PNS as a contributing factor for pain is established. By itself, this screening test is insufficient evidence for diagnosis; many other confirmatory tests are required.

Similarly in the upper limb, various screening tests can be carried out to stress the median, radial, or ulnar nerve trunks and brachial plexus (Figures 56.2a,b,c). Obviously, in the presence of severe pain and movement limitation, such as in 'frozen shoulder', these tests would be greatly modified. For example, ipsilateral flexion of the neck may reduce the strain on the sensitized neural structures allowing increased range of shoulder abduction and flexion movement. This finding alone may increase the clinician's suspicion of PNS and indicate further PNS tests should be carried out.

This is a basic approach to active movement screening in the physical evaluation of PNS. With some thought to applied anatomy, the clinician can evaluate active movements in different directions and in various ways to support a clinical hypothesis formed at this early stage of evaluation. For example, a disorder of the C4/5 motion segment may sensitize the C5 nerve roots or spinal nerve. This may cause an observable dysfunction of shoulder abduction and movement of the hand behind the back because of the increased strain that these movements place on the suprascapular and axillary nerve trunks. Contralateral lateral flexion of the head and neck would increase the dysfunction.

Neurodynamic tests

Following on from an assessment of active movement, in the presence of positive PNS screening signs, the next step in the evaluation process of PNS are passive neurodynamic tests (Shacklock 2005).

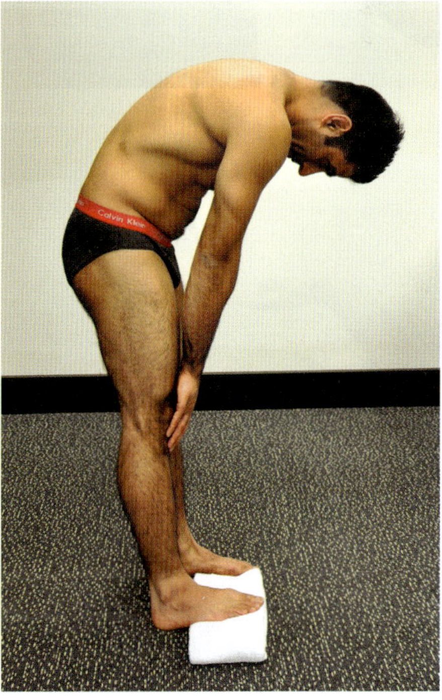

Figure 56.1 Active movement screening for peripheral nerve sensitization—lower limb.

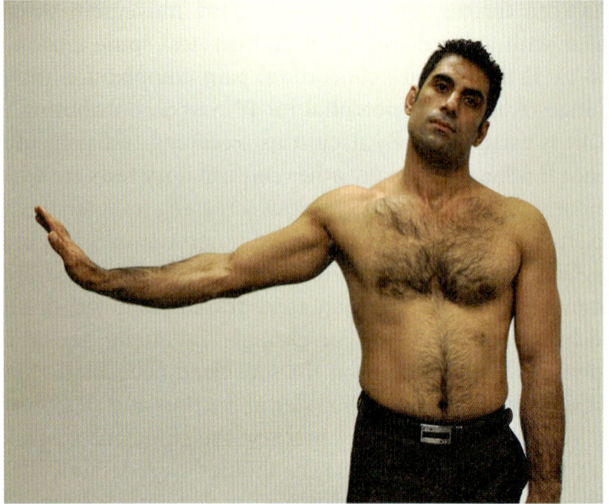

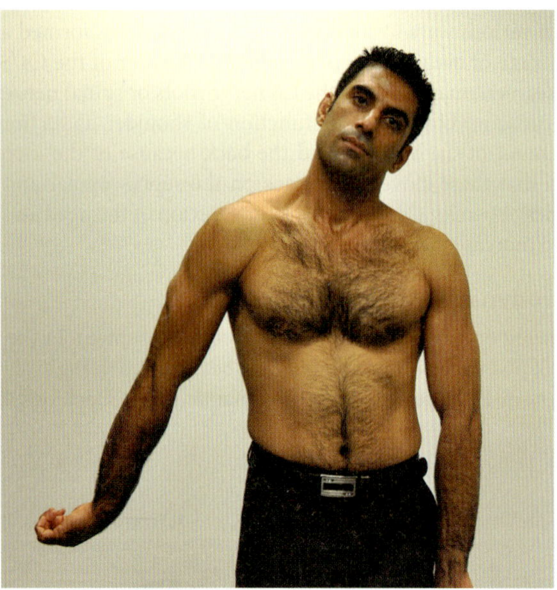

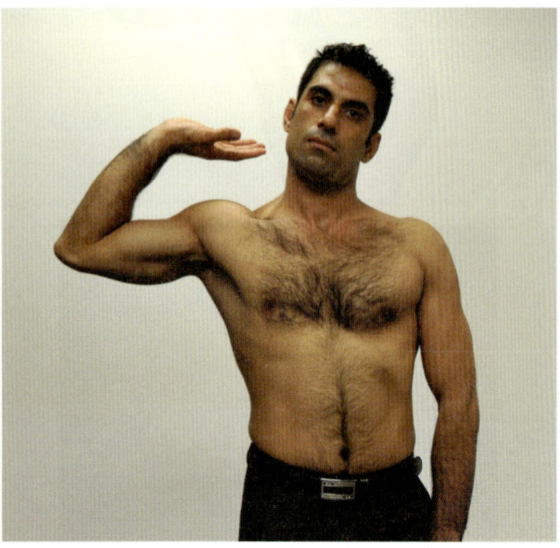

Figure 56.2 Active movement screening for peripheral nerve sensitization: (a) median nerve; (b) radial nerve; (c) ulnar nerve.

The purpose of these tests is to apply selective mechanical provocation to individual peripheral nerve trunks to identify pain and non-compliance to movement. A number of commonly used neurodynamic tests have been described to evaluate common problematic peripheral nerve trunks in the upper and lower quarter (Butler 1991; Hall and Elvey 2009, 2011; Shacklock 2005). However, with sound knowledge of nerve trunk anatomy, neurodynamic tests can be developed for any peripheral nerve in the body.

Commonly applied tests in the upper limb are the neurodynamic tests for the median, radial, and ulnar nerve (Figures 56.3a,b,c). The median nerve is elongated through a position of shoulder girdle depression, 90° shoulder abduction/lateral rotation, elbow extension, and wrist/finger extension, with the cervical spine in contralateral lateral flexion. Likewise, the radial nerve is in its most lengthened position with abduction/medial rotation of the shoulder, elbow extension, wrist/finger flexion in the position of the shoulder girdle depression, and cervical spine contralateral lateral flexion. The ulnar nerve is in its most lengthened position with abduction/lateral rotation of the shoulder, elbow flexion, wrist/finger extension, and again, with the same common position of the shoulder girdle and cervical spine.

Mechanical stress applied during neurodynamic tests undoubtedly influences musculoskeletal structures (Di Fabio 2001), including the fascia. Hence, to determine the presence of PNS requires structural differentiation (Butler 1991; Elvey 1997; Hall and Elvey 1999). This is a process whereby a distant body part is moved to increase or reduce the mechanical stress on the nerve during a neurodynamic test, and the associated responses noted. For example, during the median neurodynamic test, elbow extension in a position of wrist/finger extension, 90° external rotation, and 90° abduction (Figure 56.3a) may provoke concordant pain in the arm. If the neck is placed in contralateral lateral flexion and the test now provokes greater pain in the arm, this would be seen as positive for structural differentiation.

In the past, there has been criticism of neurodynamic tests, with questions raised as to whether these tests can selectively stress nerve trunks (Di Fabio 2001). Since then, a great deal of research has been undertaken investigating the validity of neurodynamic tests. For example, an experimental pain model was used to determine the specificity of a median nerve neurodynamic test in the differential diagnosis of hand symptoms (Coppieters et al. 2006b). Sensory responses to this test were unchanged by the presence of induced muscle pain in the hand, illustrating high specificity. Other studies have similarly demonstrated high sensitivity, but low specificity, for this test to identify patients with CTS (Wainner et al. 2005) and cervical radiculopathy (Wainner et al. 2005). For the interested reader, the validity of neurodynamic tests to detect peripheral neuropathic pain has been extensively reviewed (Nee et al. 2012).

A positive neurodynamic test indicating PNS is determined by three components. Most important is reproduction of concordant pain, followed by alteration in resistance determined by the therapist, and, finally, reduction in range of motion when compared with the contralateral side. Resistance is a measure of protective muscle activity associated with increased nerve trunk mechanosensitivity (Balster and Jull 1997; Hall et al. 1998; Jaberzadeh and Zoghi 2013; Jaberzadeh et al. 2005). Large side to side difference in range of motion has been reported during upper limb neurodynamic tests in asymptomatic people (Boyd 2012; Boyd and Villa 2012; Covill and Petersen 2011). One report for the median neurodynamic test

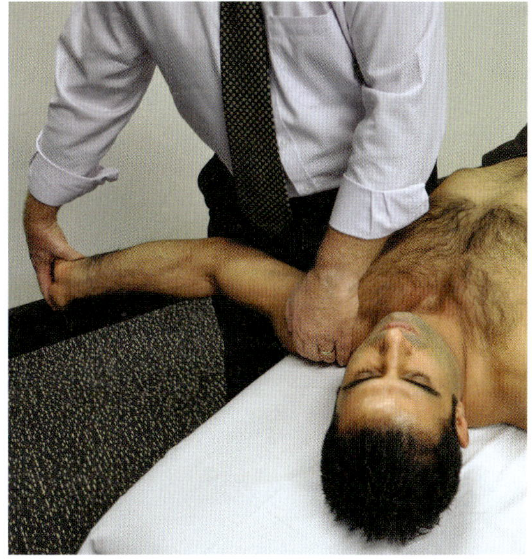

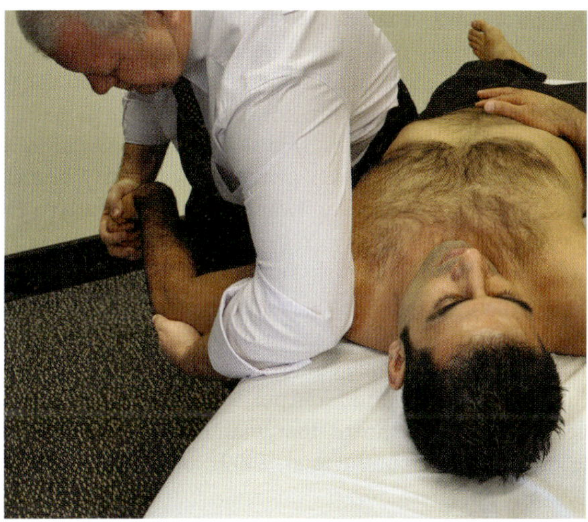

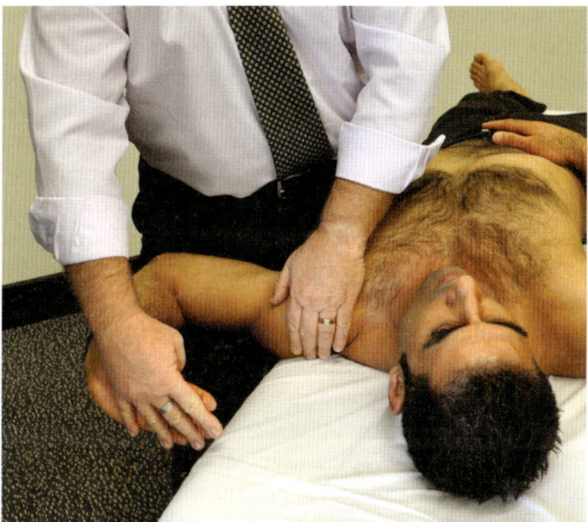

Figure 56.3 Neurodynamic tests: (a) median nerve; (b) radial nerve; (c) ulnar nerve.

indicated that range asymmetry of greater than 27° is required to be certain that the difference is not due to normal variation between sides (Covill and Petersen 2011). This was, however, for an incomplete median neurodynamic test sequence. Our research group found a smaller value of 15° was required to be certain that side to side difference in range of motion is greater than normal asymmetry (Stalioraitis et al. 2013).

Practitioners may be familiar with neurodynamic tests of the lower limb including the SLR, femoral nerve, and slump tests (Figures 56.4a,b,c). SLR and slump tests largely evaluate the same nerve tracts and may be used interchangeably (Walsh and Hall 2009a). Structural differentiation during the SLR test can be achieved by ankle dorsiflexion, lumbar lateral flexion, hip medial rotation or adduction, to identify PNS. As an example of the importance of structural differentiation, there is evidence of low levels of diagnostic accuracy for the SLR test in isolation. This was based on a report comparing the SLR test to a reference standard of magnetic resonance imaging (MRI) to determine lumbar disc herniation (Capra et al. 2011).

Neurodynamic tests can only be carried out within the available range of passive movement, which is governed by the severity of pain associated with the disorder. In more severe cases of PNS, the degree of limitation will be much greater, and standard neurodynamic tests may not be possible. Therefore, it is unrealistic to have a standard form of neurodynamic test for all presentations and the clinician is required to formulate test techniques for each individual patient. For example, a patient with severe neck and arm pain may present with gross limitation of shoulder movement. Standard neurodynamic tests may not be possible. In this case, the test order may be altered, so that cervical lateral flexion is performed in different positions of shoulder abduction/rotation with the elbow extended and wrist and fingers relaxed (Figure 56.5). In this way, even the most severely restricted patient may be evaluated for the presence of PNS.

It has been suggested that the sequence in which the various component movements are applied during neurodynamic tests are of importance as it provides information to the site of neural tissue pathology (Maitland 1985; Shacklock 2005). While this would be useful, it is unfortunately not supported by the literature (Boyd et al. 2013; Coppieters and Alshami 2007; Nee et al. 2010) and it may be that responses to neurodynamic sequencing may simply be due to the attention placed on the first of a combination of movements (Butler and Coppieters 2007). Again, the informed clinician will combine information from the whole examination, rather than that from one test in isolation. In the authors' opinion, nerve palpation is more likely to be able to localize origin of the PNS disorder.

Nerve palpation

Previous animal experiments confirm that, under normal circumstances, nerves are largely insensitive to gentle pressure, while when they are inflamed, there is a markedly increased response (Bove et al. 2003; Dilley et al. 2005). This has also been confirmed *in vivo* in people in the upper (Hall and Quintner 1996) and lower limb (Walsh and Hall 2009b). Validity of nerve palpation has been demonstrated in people with CTS and lateral epicondylalgia (Fernandez-de-Las-Penas et al. 2010). It makes sense that if inflamed neural tissues react to the mechanical stimulus of neurodynamic tests, then they should also react to the stimulus of gentle non-noxious digital pressure.

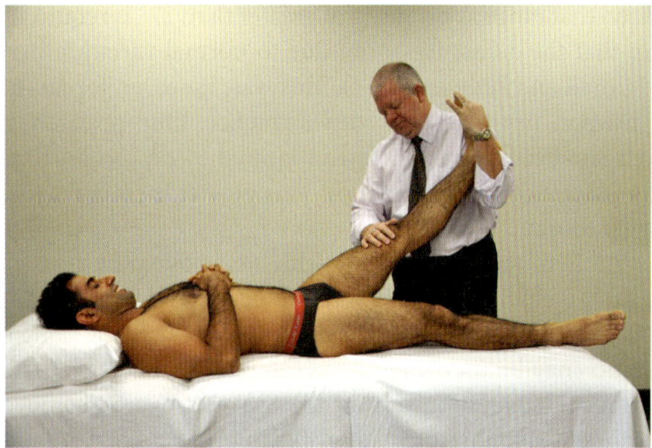

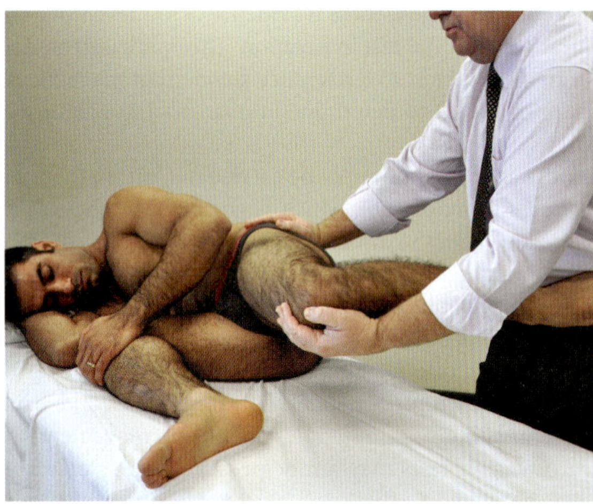

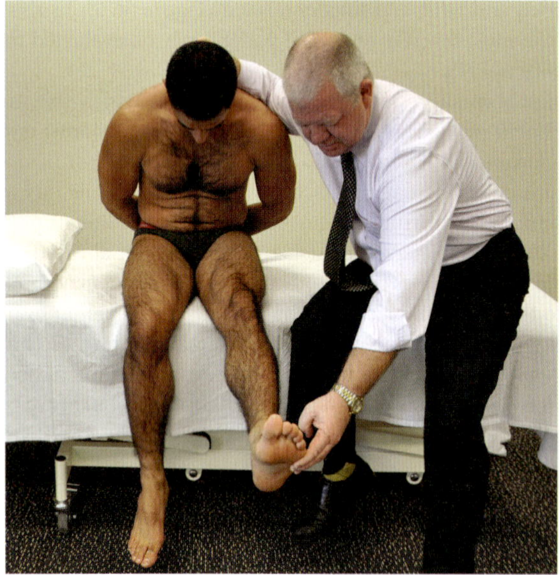

Figure 56.4 Neurodynamic tests: (a) SLR test: (b) femoral nerve test; (c) slump test.

With a good knowledge of applied anatomy, it is possible to selectively palpate various upper and lower limb nerve trunks. In many cases, it is possible to physically identify the nerve trunk and isolate it from its surrounding musculoskeletal structures. Good examples are the tibial nerve in the popliteal fossa, common peroneal nerve at the neck of the fibula, femoral nerve in the inguinal region, brachial plexus in the anterior neck, median nerve medial to biceps tendon, radial nerve in the mid humerus, and ulnar nerve at the medial epicondyle (Figures 56.6a–g). Many more locations accessible for nerve palpation are possible. Gentle thumb pressure should be used, enough to blanch the nail bed, and the non-involved side palpated first. Under normal circumstances, this should not cause pain. If the nerve is sensitized, then even gentle pressure may be painful. Stronger force may be used to 'twang' the nerve (Butler 1991) in less severe pain disorders.

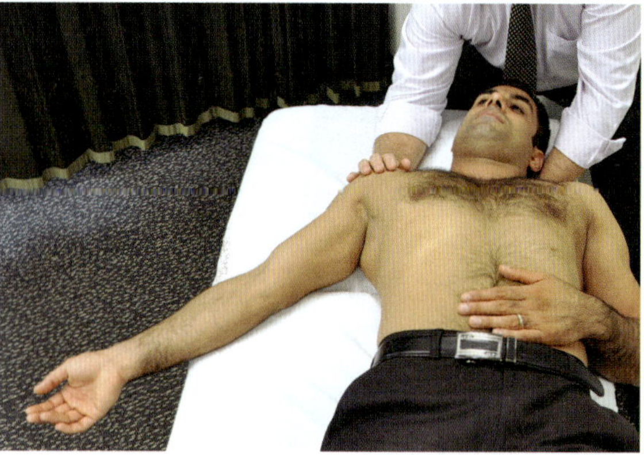

Figure 56.5 Neurodynamic tests using cervical lateral flexion for gross shoulder limitation.

It is important to distinguish Tinel's sign from nerve palpation. A positive Tinel's sign (shooting paraesthesia away from the site of nerve percussion) is indicative of a damaged regenerating nerve, which is a helpful sign when confirming the presence of CN.

Although nerve palpation has not been investigated to a great degree, studies have shown that manual palpation is reliable in the upper limb (Schmid et al. 2009) and lower limb (Walsh et al. 2012).

Evaluation for source of pathology

It is important to note that in disorders of nerve tissue, all of the aforementioned features of PNS may be found during a physical evaluation. However, this does not mean the condition is one suited to manual therapy management. It is quite possible that a painful neuropathy caused by a tumour infiltration or following damage from radiotherapy, for example, may cause all the features discussed thus far, including limitation of active movement and neurodynamic tests. An example is Pancoast tumour of the lung, which invades and sensitizes the brachial plexus causing pain and limitation of shoulder movement. The clinician must determine a cause for the neural sensitization to exclude such infrequent but clearly unsuitable conditions for manual therapy.

As an example, cervical intervertebral disk degeneration may result in radicular arm pain and specific cervical spine motion segment dysfunction. This would be manifested by lack of segmental movement and pain on spine segmental motions tests. For example, a C6 radiculopathy would present with abnormal responses to segmental movement tests at C5/C6. If the disorder were due to a Pancoast tumour of the lung, then no such spine dysfunction would be found.

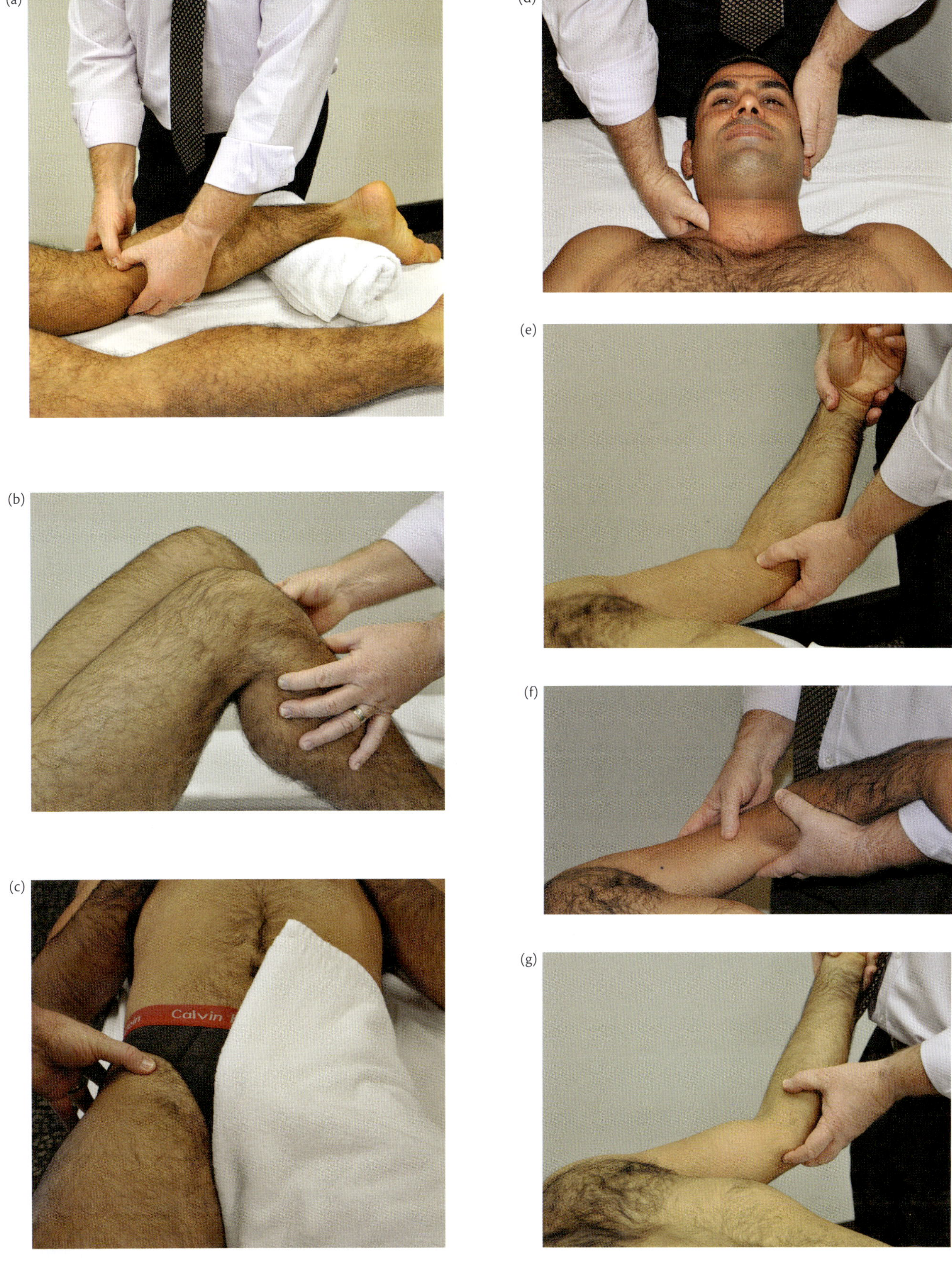

Figure 56.6 Nerve palpation sites in the upper and lower limb: (a) tibial nerve; (b) common peroneal nerve; (c) femoral nerve; (d) brachial plexus; (e) median nerve medial; (f) radial nerve; (g) ulnar nerve.

Neurological examination

An important aspect of the evaluation of neural tissue disorders is the assessment of neurological function. In the clinical setting, the neurological examination is the only means of determining the presence of axonal conduction loss. The neurological examination incorporates both subjective inquiry and physical tests of nerve function.

The clinician should not rely purely on dermatomal charts when determining the segmental origin of pain, as they are not the ideal diagnostic reference (Bove et al. 2005) due to significant overlap of innervation from adjacent nerve roots, in addition to much variability between individuals (Slipman et al. 1998; Wolff et al. 2001). In this respect, specific indicator sites for sensation loss may be more accurate (Nitta et al. 1993). Inter-observer reliability and agreement for the neurological examination is best achieved by incorporating the subjective history together with the combined neurological examination (Vroomen et al. 2000). Furthermore, diagnostic accuracy is increased when a cluster of physical examination tests are used (Wainner et al. 2003).

Management of neural pain disorders using neural mobilization

In this chapter and Chapter 15, a distinction has been made between different nerve disorders: NPSH, CN, and PNS. This distinction is important in regard to treatment selection, which conceptually should be different for each classification as each has different pathophysiology and underlying pain mechanisms.

NPSH is a disorder categorized by abnormal processing of sensory information. Patients thus classified do not respond to manual therapy techniques such as neural mobilization (Nee et al. 2013; Schäfer et al. 2011), as the problem is not amenable to physical treatment. Rather, a different treatment approach focused on reorganizing sensory input such as cognitive behavioural retraining (Butler and Moseley 2003), graded motor imagery (Butler et al. 2013), or mirror box therapy (Daly and Bialocerkowski 2009) would be more appropriate management. These approaches do not involve manual therapy. Ideally, a multidisciplinary team approach should be taken involving a pain specialist to advise on drug management, psychologists to advise on psychological approaches to pain management, as well as physiotherapy input.

For patients with evidence of CN, neural tissue mobilization, particularly that which attempts to lengthen or stretch the nerve, such as tensioners, would be contraindicated in all but the late stages of rehabilitation. This is particularly important in the acute to early chronic stage of the disorder, when the nerve trunk is physiologically vulnerable to hypoxia by lengthening (Topp and Boyd 2006). For patients fulfilling this category, treatment techniques aimed at decompressing the affected nerve are the priority, and later, gentle nerve sliding techniques can be included (Hall and Elvey 2009). For example, placing the lumbar spine in a position of flexion has been shown to reduce nerve root pressure when compared to extension (Morishita et al. 2009). Combining this position with manual techniques to enhance flexion can be helpful (Figure 56.7), as shown in a case series of people suffering from spinal stenosis (Murphy 2006).

A slider exercise for the median nerve is shown in Figure 56.8. Nerve slider exercises involve movement of the nerve bed along the course of the affected nerve, without increasing nerve tension. They would, therefore, be safer to use in the presence of neural hypoxia associated with vascular compromise from CN. Thus, conceptually, slider exercises improve circulation, nutrition, and axoplasmic flow, reduce oedema, and optimize repair (Coppieters and Butler 2007)—ideal attributes in the presence of nerve injury.

Treatment for patients fulfilling the third category, PNS, should consist of gentle manual therapy involving passive movement techniques, in which the tissues or structures surrounding the affected nerve or nerve root are gently mobilized. The cervical lateral glide is a very useful neural mobilization technique in this respect that has

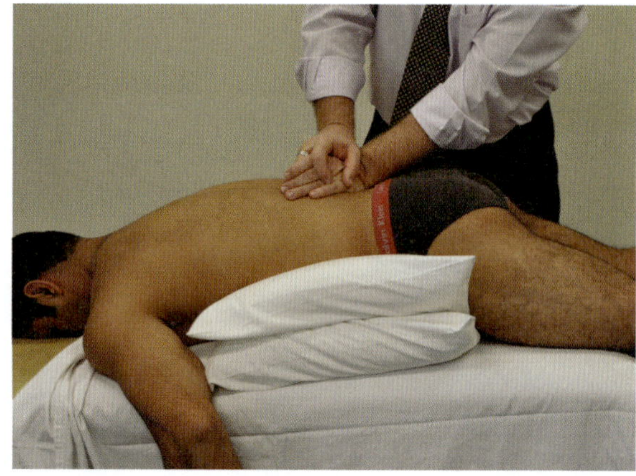

Figure 56.7 Flexion mobilization in lumbar spine flexion in prone position.

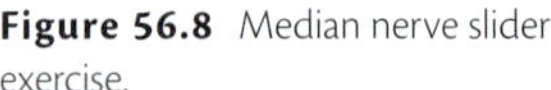

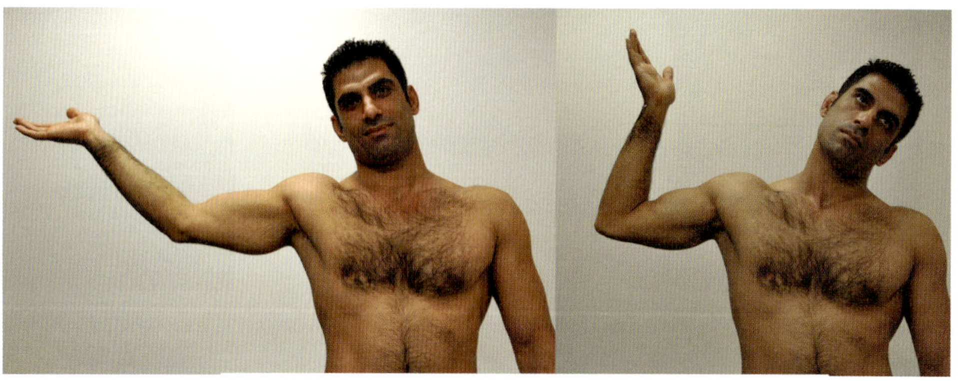

Figure 56.8 Median nerve slider exercise.

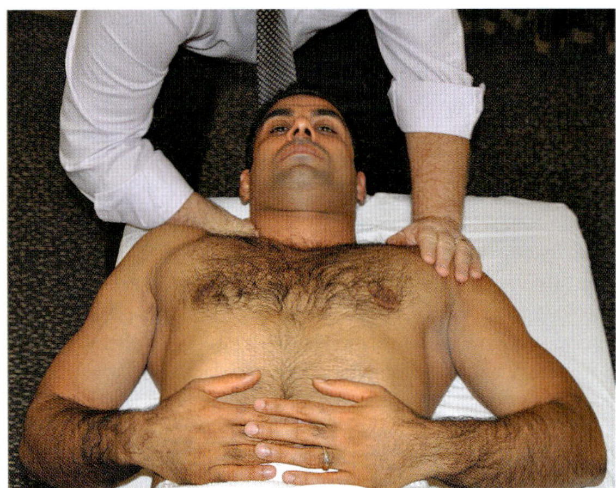

Figure 56.9 Cervical lateral glide technique.

been found to be effective in the management of upper limb PNS disorders (Allison et al. 2002; Nee et al. 2012, 2013).

Cervical lateral glide

With the patient lying supine, the clinician gently supports the shoulder girdle with one hand while supporting the patient's head and neck with the other (Figure 56.9). The affected motion segment is targeted and a lateral glide initiated. The patient's shoulder on the affected side should be slightly abducted and elbow flexed to about 90° such that the patient's hand rests on their abdomen. This position would be for a patient with more sensitized neural tissue and can be progressed into greater range of abduction and elbow extension as the condition improves and the sensitization allows.

Gentle controlled lateral glide to the contralateral side is performed in a slow oscillating manner up to a point in range where resistance is felt. Oscillation is performed for around 60 seconds and repeated up to five times. The most obvious indicator of successful treatment is an improvement in movement together with a reduction in the severity of pain. Evidence of the efficacy of the cervical lateral glide has been demonstrated in subjects with cervicobrachial pain (Allison et al. 2002; Coppieters et al. 2003; Cowell and Phillips 2002; Nee et al. 2012, 2013; Saranga et al. 2003; Sterling et al. 2010).

The cervical lateral glide technique mechanically influences neural tissue as far as the distal forearm and may be an effective treatment even if the source of the problem lies in the arm and not the cervical spine. For example, movement of the median nerve in the distal forearm was detected by ultrasonography during the cervical lateral glide technique (Brochwicz et al. 2013). In addition, evidence of the efficacy of the cervical lateral glide on distal pain disorders has been shown in lateral epicondylalgia (Vicenzino et al. 1996), a disorder involving PNS of the radial nerve (Yaxley and Jull 1993).

Self-treatment and management are most important. Slider exercises are an appropriate first exercise, as they are pain-free and promote desensitization (Coppieters and Butler 2007). Tensioning exercise should be avoided until the end stage of rehabilitation. Coppieters and Butler compared nerve strain during tensioning and sliding exercises (Coppieters and Butler 2007). They found an increase in nerve strain of 0.8% during a slider movement and 6.8% during a tensioner movement. Previously, 3% change in nerve length has been shown to initiate ectopic impulse generation in inflamed nerves (Dilley et al. 2005). Hence, tensioner movements are likely to provoke pain, while slider movements will not. Slider exercises may also disperse inflammatory products (Coppieters and Alshami 2007), hence reducing the original cause of mechanosensitization of the nerve trunk as well as reducing pain.

An example of an upper limb slider technique for the median nerve is shown in Figure 56.8 and shows the start and end point. The neck and elbow move simultaneously without raising significant nerve tension and should not cause pain or other symptoms. This movement is repeated 10 times and performed initially three times daily. This may appear unsubstantial, but it is essential to regard the movement as self-treatment. There are many other forms of slider exercises that can be developed for an individual patient, depending on which nerve is involved and at what point. Where possible, movement of the nerve should occur at the source of inflammation of the peripheral nerve trunk/plexus.

Conclusion to the use of neurodynamics in pain management

This chapter has described an evidence-based classification system for the identification and management of patients suitable for neural mobilization techniques. Neural mobilization techniques targeted at specific PNS disorders has been shown to be an effective treatment approach. However, clinicians should take care when prescribing neural mobilization to ensure that only appropriate patients receive this form of management.

References

Allison, G. T., Nagy, B. M., and Hall, T. (2002). A randomized clinical trial of manual therapy for cervico-brachial pain syndrome—a pilot study. *Man Ther* 7(2):95–102.

Alshami, A. M., Babri, A. S., Souvlis, T., and Coppieters, M. W. (2007). Biomechanical evaluation of two clinical tests for plantar heel pain: the dorsiflexion-eversion test for tarsal tunnel syndrome and the windlass test for plantar fasciitis. *Foot Ankle Int* 28(4):499–505.

Balster, S. and Jull, G. (1997). Upper trapezius muscle activity during the brachial plexus tension test in asymptomatic subjects. *Man Ther* 2(3): 144–9.

Bongers, F. J., Schellevis, F. G., van den Bosch, W. J., and van der Zee, J. (2007). Carpal tunnel syndrome in general practice (1987 and 2001): incidence and the role of occupational and non-occupational factors. *Br J Gen Pract* 57(534):36–9.

Bove, G. M., Ransil, B. J., Lin, H. C., and Leem, J. G. (2003). Inflammation induces ectopic mechanical sensitivity in axons of nociceptors innervating deep tissues. *J Neurophysiol* 90(3):1949–55.

Bove, G. M., Zaheen, A., and Bajwa, Z. H. (2005). Subjective nature of lower limb radicular pain. *J Manip Physiol Ther* 28(1):12–4.

Boyd, B. S. (2012). Common interlimb asymmetries and neurogenic responses during upper limb neurodynamic testing: implications for test interpretation. *J Hand Ther* 25(1):56–63; quiz 64.

Boyd, B. S. and Villa, P. S. (2012). Normal inter-limb differences during the straight leg raise neurodynamic test: a cross sectional study. *BMC Musculoskelet Disord* 13:245.

Boyd, B. S., Topp, K. S., and Coppieters, M. W. (2013). Impact of movement sequencing on sciatic and tibial nerve strain and excursion during the straight leg raise test in embalmed cadavers. *J Orthop Sports Phys Ther* 43(6):398–403.

Breig, A. (1978). *Adverse mechanical tension in the central nervous system: relief by functional neurosurgery*. Stockholm, Almquist and Wiksell.

Breig, A. and Marions, O. (1963). Biomechanics of the lumbosacral nerve roots. *Acta Radiologica* 1:1141–61.

Brochwicz, P., von Piekartz, H., and Zalpour, C. (2013). Sonography assessment of the median nerve during cervical lateral glide and lateral flexion. Is there a difference in neurodynamics of asymptomatic people? *Man Ther* 18(3):216–9.

Butler, D. S. (1991). *Mobilisation of the nervous system*. Melbourne, Churchill Livingstone.

Butler, D. S. and Coppieters, M. W. (2007). Neurodynamics in a broader perspective. *Man Ther* 12(1):e7–8.

Butler, D. and Moseley, G. (2003). *Explain pain*. Adelaide, Noigroup Publications.

Butler, D., Moseley, G., and Giles, T. (2013). *The graded motor imagery handbook*. Adelaide, Noigroup Publications.

Capra, F., Vanti, C., Donati, R., Tombetti, S., O'Reilly, C., and Pillastrini, P. (2011). Validity of the straight-leg raise test for patients with sciatic pain with or without lumbar pain using magnetic resonance imaging results as a reference standard. *J Manip Physiol Ther* 34(4):231–8.

Coppieters, M. W. and Alshami, A. M. (2007). Longitudinal excursion and strain in the median nerve during novel nerve gliding exercises for carpal tunnel syndrome. *J Orthop Res* 25(7):972–80.

Coppieters, M. W. and Butler, D. S. (2007). Do 'sliders' slide and 'tensioners' tension? An analysis of neurodynamic techniques and considerations regarding their application. *Man Ther* 13(3):213–21.

Coppieters, M. W., Alshami, A. M., Babri, A. S., Souvlis, T., Kippers, W., and Hodges, P. W. (2006a). Strain and excursion of the sciatic, tibial, and plantar nerves during a modified straight leg raising test. *J Orthop Res* 24(9):1883–9.

Coppieters, M. W., Alshami, A. M., and Hodges, P. W. (2006b). An experimental pain model to investigate the specificity of the neurodynamic test for the median nerve in the differential diagnosis of hand symptoms. *Arch Phys Med Rehabil* 87(10):1412–7.

Coppieters, M. W., Stappaerts, K. H., Wouters, L. L., and Janssens, K. (2003). The immediate effects of a cervical lateral glide treatment technique in patients with neurogenic cervicobrachial pain' *J Orthop Sports Phys Ther* 33(7):369–78.

Covill, L. G. and Petersen, S. M. (2012). Upper extremity neurodynamic tests: range of motion asymmetry may not indicate impairment. *Physio Theory Prac* 28(7):535–41

Cowell, I. M. and Phillips, D. R. (2002). Effectiveness of manipulative physiotherapy for the treatment of a neurogenic cervicobrachial pain syndrome: a single case study— experimental design. *Man Ther* 7(1):31–8.

Daly, A. E. and Bialocerkowski, A. E. (2009). Does evidence support physiotherapy management of adult complex regional pain syndrome type one? A systematic review. *Eur J Pain* 13(4):339–53.

Di Fabio, R. (2001). Neural mobilisation: the impossible. *J Orthop Sports Phys Ther* 31(5):224–5.

Dilley, A., Lynn, B., Greening, J., and DeLeon, N. (2003). Quantitative in vivo studies of median nerve sliding in response to wrist, elbow, shoulder and neck movements. *Clin Biomech (Bristol, Avon)* 18(10):899–907.

Dilley, A., Lynn, B., and Pang, S. J. (2005). Pressure and stretch mechanosensitivity of peripheral nerve fibres following local inflammation of the nerve trunk. *Pain* 117(3):462–72.

Dilley, A., Odeyinde, S., Greening, J., and Lynn, B. (2007). Longitudinal sliding of the median nerve in patients with non-specific arm pain. *Man Ther* 13(6):536–43.

van Doesburg, M. H., Henderson, J., Yoshii, Y., et al. (2012a). Median nerve deformation in differential finger motions: ultrasonographic comparison of carpal tunnel syndrome patients and healthy controls. *J Orthop Res* 30(4):643–8.

van Doesburg, M. H., Henderson, J., Mink van der Molen, A. B., An, K. N., and Amadio, P. C. (2012b).Transverse plane tendon and median nerve motion in the carpal tunnel: ultrasound comparison of carpal tunnel syndrome patients and healthy volunteers. *PLoS One* 7(5):e37081.

Ellis, R. F. and Hing, W. A. (2008). Neural mobilization: a systematic review of randomized controlled trials with an analysis of therapeutic efficacy. *J Man Manip Ther* 16(1):8–22.

Ellis, R. F., Hing, W. A., and McNair, P. J. (2012). Comparison of longitudinal sciatic nerve movement with different mobilization exercises: an in vivo study utilizing ultrasound imaging. *J Orthop Sports Phys Ther* 42(8):667–75.

Elvey, R. (1979). Brachial plexus tension tests and the pathoanatomical origin of arm pain. In: Idczak, R. (ed.) *Aspects of manipulative therapy*. Melbourne, Lincoln Institute of Health Sciences: pp. 105–10.

Elvey, R. L. (1997). Physical evaluation of the peripheral nervous system in disorders of pain and dysfunction. *J Hand Ther* 10(2):122–9.

Fernandez-de-Las-Penas, C., Ortega-Santiago, R., Ambite-Quesada, S., Jimenez-Garci, A. R., Arroyo-Morales, M., and Cleland, J. A. (2010). Specific mechanical pain hypersensitivity over peripheral nerve trunks in women with either unilateral epicondylalgia or carpal tunnel syndrome. *J Orthop Sports Phys Ther* 40(11):751–60.

Fernandez-de-las-Penas, C., de la Llave-Rincon, A. I., Fernandez-Carnero, J., Cuadrado, M. L., Arendt-Nielsen, L., and Pareja, J. A. (2009). Bilateral widespread mechanical pain sensitivity in carpal tunnel syndrome: evidence of central processing in unilateral neuropathy. *Brain* 132(6): 1472–9.

Greening, J., Smart, S., Leary, R., Hall-Craggs, M., O'Higgins, P., and Lynn, B. (1999). Reduced movement of median nerve in carpal tunnel during wrist flexion in patients with non-specific arm pain. *Lancet* 354(9174):217–8.

Hall, T. M. and Elvey, R. L. (1999). Nerve trunk pain: physical diagnosis and treatment. *Man Ther* 4(2):63–73.

Hall, T. and Elvey, R. L. (2009). Evaluation and treatment of neural tissue pain disorders. In: Donatelli, R. and Wooden, M. (eds) *Orthopaedic physical therapy*. New York, Churchill Livingstone.

Hall, T. and Elvey, R. L. (2011). *Neural tissue evaluation and treatment*. New York, Churchill Livingstone.

Hall, T. and Quintner, J. (1996). Responses to mechanical stimulation of the upper limb in painful cervical radiculopathy. *Austral J Physio* 42(4): 277–85.

M., Stalioraitis, V., Robinson, K. and Hall, T. (2014). Side-to-side range of movement variability in median and radial nerve neurodynamic test sequences in asymptomatic people. *Man Ther*, 19, 338–42.

Hall, T., Zusman, M., and Elvey, R. (1998). Adverse mechanical tension of the nervous system? Analysis of straight leg raise. *Man Ther* 3(3):140–6.

Hu, J. W., Vernon, H., and Tatourian, I. (1995). Changes in neck electromyography associated with meningeal noxious stimulation. *J Manip Physio Ther* 18(9):577–81.

Hunderfund, A. N., Boon, A. J., Mandrekar, J. N., and Sorenson, E. J. (2011). Sonography in carpal tunnel syndrome. *Muscle Nerve* 44(4):485–91.

Ibrahim, I., Khan, W. S., Goddard, N., and Smitham, P. (2012). Carpal tunnel syndrome: a review of the recent literature. *Open Orthop J* 6:69–76.

Jaberzadeh, S. and Zoghi, M. (2013). Mechanosensitivity of the median nerve in patients with chronic carpal tunnel syndrome. *J Bodyw Mov Ther* 17(2):157–64.

Jaberzadeh, S., Scutter, S., and Nazeran, H. (2005). Mechanosensitivity of the median nerve and mechanically produced motor responses during upper limb neurodynamic test 1. *Physiotherapy* 91:94–100.

Maitland, G. (1985). The slump test: examination and treatment. *Austral J Physio* 31(6):215–9.

Medina McKeon, J. M. and Yancosek, K. E. (2008). Neural gliding techniques for the treatment of carpal tunnel syndrome: a systematic review. *J Sport Rehabil* 17(3):324–41.

Morishita, Y., Hida, S., Naito, M., Arimizu, J., and Takamori, Y. (2009). Neurogenic intermittent claudication in lumbar spinal canal stenosis: the clinical relationship between the local pressure of the intervertebral foramen and the clinical findings in lumbar spinal canal stenosis. *J Spinal Disord Tech* 22(2):130–4.

Murphy, D. R., Hurwitz, E. L., Gregory, A. A. and Clary, R. 2006. A non-surgical approach to the management of lumbar spinal stenosis: a prospective observational cohort study. *BMC Musculoskelet Disord* 7: 16.

Nakamichi, K. and Tachibana, S. (1995). Restricted motion of the median nerve in carpal tunnel syndrome. *J Hand Surg Br* 20(4):460–4.

Nee, R. J., Jull, G. A., Vicenzino, B., and Coppieters, M. W. (2012). The validity of upper-limb neurodynamic tests for detecting peripheral neuropathic pain. *J Orthop Sports Phys Ther* 42(5):413–24.

Nee, R. J., Vicenzino, B., Jull, G. A., Cleland, J. A., and Coppieters, M. W. (2012). Neural tissue management provides immediate clinically relevant benefits without harmful effects for patients with nerve-related neck and arm pain: a randomised trial. *J Physiother* 58(1):23–31.

Nee, R. J., Vicenzino, B., Jull, G. A., Cleland, J. A., and Coppieters, M. W. (2013). Baseline characteristics of patients with nerve-related neck and arm pain predict the likely response to neural tissue management. *J Orthop Sports Phys Ther*. 43(6):379–91.

Nee, R. J., Yang, C. H., Liang, C. C., Tseng, G. F., and Coppieters, M. W. (2010). Impact of order of movement on nerve strain and longitudinal excursion: a biomechanical study with implications for neurodynamic test sequencing. *Man Ther* 15(4):376–81.

Nitta, H., Tajima, T., Sugiyama, H., and Moriyama, A. (1993). Study on dermatomes by means of selective lumbar spinal nerve block. *Spine* 18(13):1782–6.

Page, M. J., O'Connor, D., Pitt, V., and Massy-Westropp, N. (2012). Exercise and mobilisation interventions for carpal tunnel syndrome. *Cochrane Database Syst Rev* 6: CD009899.

Ridehalgh, C., Moore, A., and Hough, A. (2012). Repeatability of measuring sciatic nerve excursion during a modified passive straight leg raise test with ultrasound imaging. *Man Ther* 17(6):572–6.

Saranga, J., Green, A., Lewis, J., and Worsfold, C. (2003). Effects of a cervical lateral glide on the upper limb neurodynamic test 1: a blinded placebo-controlled investigation. *Physiotherapy* 89(11):678–84.

Schmid, A. B., Brunner, F., Luomajoki, H., et al. (2009). Reliability of clinical tests to evaluate nerve function and mechanosensitivity of the upper limb peripheral nervous system. *BMC Musculoskelet Disord* 10:11.

Schäfer, A., Hall, T., and Briffa, K. (2009a). Classification of low back-related leg pain—a proposed patho-mechanism-based approach. *Man Ther* 14(2):222–30.

Schäfer, A., Hall, T. M., Ludtke, K., Mallwitz, J., and Briffa, N. K. (2009b). Interrater reliability of a new classification system for patients with neural low back-related leg pain. *J Man Manip Ther* 17(2):109–17.

Schäfer, A., Hall, T., Muller, G., and Briffa, K. (2011). Outcomes differ between subgroups of patients with low back and leg pain following neural manual therapy: a prospective cohort study. *Eur Spine J* 20(3):482–90.

Shacklock, M. (2005). *Clinical neurodynamics*. Edinburgh, Elsevier.

Slipman, C. W., Plastaras, C. T., Palmitier, R. A., Huston, C. W., and Sterenfeld, E. B. (1998). Symptom provocation of fluoroscopically guided cervical nerve root stimulation. Are dynatomal maps identical to dermatomal maps? *Spine* 23(20):2235–42.

Sterling, M., Pedler, A., Chan, C., Puglisi, M., Vuvan, V., and Vicenzino, B. (2010). Cervical lateral glide increases nociceptive flexion reflex threshold but not pressure or thermal pain thresholds in chronic whiplash associated disorders: a pilot randomised controlled trial. *Man Ther* 15(2):149–53.

Tampin, B., Briffa, N. K., Hall, T., Lee, G., and Slater, H. (2012). Inter-therapist agreement in classifying patients with cervical radiculopathy and patients with non-specific neck-arm pain. *Man Ther* 17(5):445–50.

Topp, K. S. and Boyd, B. S. (2006). Structure and biomechanics of peripheral nerves: nerve responses to physical stresses and implications for physical therapist practice. *Phys Ther* 86(1):92–109.

Vanti, C., Bonfiglioli, R., Calabrese, M., et al. (2011). Upper limb neurodynamic test 1 and symptoms reproduction in carpal tunnel syndrome. A validity study. *Man Ther* 16(3):258–63.

Vicenzino, B., Collins, D., and Wright, A. (1996). The initial effects of a cervical spine manipulative physiotherapy treatment on the pain and dysfunction of lateral epicondylalgia. *Pain* 68(1):69–74.

Vroomen, P. C., de Krom, M. C., and Knottnerus, J. A. (2000). Consistency of history taking and physical examination in patients with suspected lumbar nerve root involvement. *Spine* 25(1):91–6; discussion 97.

Wainner, R. S., Fritz, J. M., Irrgang, J. J., Boninger, M. L., Delitto, A., and Allison, S. (2003). Reliability and diagnostic accuracy of the clinical examination and patient self-report measures for cervical radiculopathy. *Spine* 28(1):52–62.

Wainner, R. S., Fritz, J. M., Irrgang, J. J., Delitto, A., Allison, S., and Boninger, M. L. (2005). Development of a clinical prediction rule for the diagnosis of carpal tunnel syndrome. *Arch Phys Med Rehabil* 86(4):609–18.

Walsh, J. and Hall, T. (2009a). Agreement and correlation between the straight leg raise and slump tests in subjects with leg pain. *J Manip Physiol Ther* 32(3):184–92.

Walsh, J. and Hall, T. (2009b). Reliability, validity and diagnostic accuracy of palpation of the sciatic, tibial and common peroneal nerves in the examination of low back related leg pain. *Man Ther* 14(6):623–9.

Walsh, J., Raby, M., and Hall, T. (2012). Agreement and correlation between the self-report Leeds assessment of neuropathic symptoms and signs and Douleur Neuropathique 4 questions neuropathic pain screening tools in subjects with low back-related leg pain. *J Manip Physiol Ther* 35:196–202.

Wolff, A. P., Groen, G. J., and Crul, B. J. (2001). Diagnostic lumbosacral segmental nerve blocks with local anesthetics: a prospective double-blind study on the variability and interpretation of segmental effects. *Reg Anesth Pain Med* 26(2):147–55.

Yaxley, G. and Jull, G. (1993). Adverse tension in the neural system. A preliminary study in patients with tennis elbow. *Austral J Physio* 39(1):15–22.

Chapter 57

Trigger point injections

John Tanner

Aetiology and characteristics of trigger points

A trigger point is characterized by a focus of hyper-irritability in a muscle that is locally tender when compressed and, if sufficiently hypersensitive, gives rise to referred pain and tenderness (Travell and Simons 1983, 1998). A trigger point may produce autonomic phenomena. If the focus lies within a taut band of skeletal muscle and is active, it exhibits a local 'twitch' response when rolled under the palpating fingers. Each muscle tends to have characteristic locations of trigger points with typical patterns of referred pain (Figure 57.1).

Trigger points can be primary in the sense that they have become active as a result of direct influences on the muscle itself. This may follow a dynamic or a static postural strain. Indirectly, these points may be triggered as part of a referral pattern, from other parts of the musculoskeletal system or from visceral sources.

A final, and perhaps underestimated cause of trigger points with myofascial dysfunction is emotional distress, which may be mediated by increased sympathetic tone and circulating humoral factors.

Mechanical dysfunction of the spinal joints commonly causes referred pain with trigger point formation. When several trigger points can be found, the more peripheral ones tend to clear as range of motion improves with manipulative treatment (Fitzgerald 1991).

Microscopically, the histology of these irritable foci of muscle reveal little abnormality. However, it has been observed that trigger points commonly seem to be quite closely related to the motor points (the point at which the motor nerve enters the underlying muscle) and, in many instances, they are close to traditional acupuncture points (Melzack et al. 1977). Thermography may show areas of increased skin temperature or, in more chronic situations, reduced skin temperature. Hubbard and Berkoff (1993) showed that fine-needle electromyography (EMG) produces insertional activity when the hyper-irritable focus, which corresponds to an active muscle spindle, is directly penetrated.

Treatment of trigger points

Hubbard and Berkoff (1983) have also demonstrated the presence of direct sympathetic innervation of the muscle spindle. By using fine-needle EMG, the trigger points are located and a small dose of phenoxybenzamine (an alpha-adrenergic blocker) is delivered through a stylet to block the sympathetic efferent stimulation: this effectively stops activity of the trigger point. This procedure can give some significant soreness for up to 2 weeks. In therapeutic use, care must be taken not to inject too large a total dose in one session because of the risk of hypotension.

In recent years, botulinus toxin has become popular in the treatment of any, or all, refractory myofascial pain, particularly where neuropathic features of a chronic pain disorder are becoming manifest. However, a recent qualitative systematic review (Ho Ky 2007) of five controlled trials for myofascial trigger points found only one study with a positive effect compared to local anaesthetic, the rest showing no advantage. The negative studies received a higher validity score. For refractory trigger points this may prove to be a useful method.

Myofascial dysfunction can be treated in a variety of ways incorporating passive and active stretching techniques, improvement in posture, muscle balance, and attention to local joint or spinal dysfunction by appropriate mobilizing or manipulative techniques. If trigger points are persistent, then one may apply direct ultrasound, digital pressure-producing ischaemia and inhibition of the muscle, local anaesthetic injections with a small or large volume, and dry needling (intramuscular stimulation).

Different techniques of trigger point therapy for low back pain have been compared in two uncontrolled studies. Garvey et al. (1989) found stretching with a vapocoolant spray to be as effective as acupuncture or lidocaine (lignocaine) alone or with steroid, and Hong (1994) found that patients preferred lidocaine (lignocaine) trigger point therapy to dry needling, as it was less painful (though equally effective). In a controlled study, Kovacs et al. (1997) used a skin device for stimulating the trigger points and found it effective.

The technique recommended by Travell and Simons (1983, 1998) is careful palpation of the active trigger point between two palpating fingers and inserting a fine (23- or 25-gauge) needle to a point where intense aching or soreness is noted by the patient, and then injecting 0.5–1 ml of a low-concentration local anaesthetic, such as 0.5% procaine or lidocaine (lignocaine) (Figure 57.2). The patient

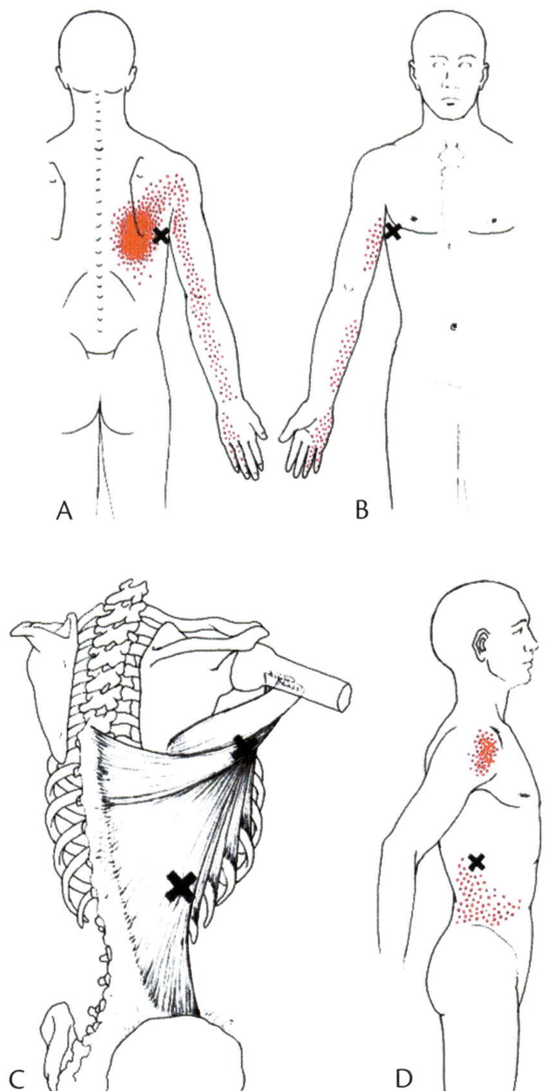

Figure 57.1 latissimus dorsi trigger points and zones of referral; A and B usual axillary location, C and D unusual lower location with referral zone;Travell and Simons.

is recommended to perform stretching exercises actively and regularly over the next few days.

Fischer (1981) proposes a larger-volume local anaesthetic injection (up to 10 ml 0.5% xylocaine) with multiple withdrawals and

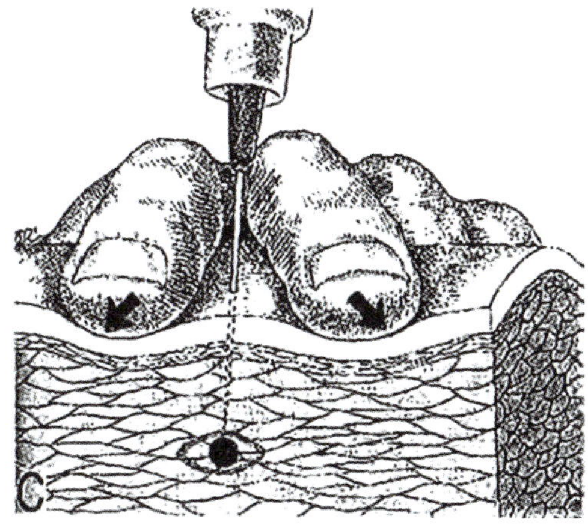

Figure 57.2 Injection of trigger point.

re-insertions in different directions to infiltrate larger bands of involved muscle.

References

Fischer, A. A. (1981) Thermography and pain. *Archives of Physical Medicine and Rehabilitation*, 62, 542.

Fitzgerald, R. T. D. (1991) Observations on trigger points, fibromyalgia, recurrent headache and the cervical syndrome. *Journal of Manual Medicine*, 6, 124–9.

Garvey, T. A., Marks, M. R., Wiesel, S. W. (1989) A prospective, randomised double-blind evaluation of trigger-point injection therapy for low-back pain. *Spine*, 14, 962–4.

Hong, C. Z. (1994) Lidocaine versus dry-needling to myofascial trigger points. The importance of the local twitch response. *American Journal of Physical Medicine and Rehabilitation*, 73, 256–63.

Hubbard, D. R., Berkoff, G. M. (1993) Myofascial trigger points show EMG activity. *Spine*, 18, 1803–7.

Kovacs, F. M., Abraira, V., Pozo, F., et al. (1997) Local and remote sustained trigger point therapy for exacerbations of chronic low back pain. *Spine*, 22, 786–97.

Ho Ky. (2007) Botulinus toxin A for myofascial trigger point injection: a qualitative systematic review. *European Journal of Pain*, 11(5), 519–27.

Melzack, R., Stillwell, D. M., Fox, E. J. (1977) Trigger points and acupuncture points for pain: correlations and implications. *Pain*, 3, 3–23.

Travell, J. G., Simons, D. G. (1983) *Myofascial pain and dysfunction. The trigger point manual.* Williams & Wilkins, Baltimore, USA.

Chapter 58

Soft tissue pain: treatment with stimulation-produced analgesia

C. Chan Gunn

The three phases of soft tissue pain

Wall (1978) saw pain as a reaction pattern of three sequential behavioural phases: immediate, acute, and chronic. Each phase may exist independently, or in any combination and proportion with the others. In the immediate nociceptive phase, primary afferent nerves (with mechanosensitive or mechanothermal-sensitive and C-polymodal fibres) transduce specific forms of energy (mechanical, thermal, or chemical) into electrochemical nerve impulses and transmit them to the central nervous system (CNS) via two main routes. One, the *spinoreticulothalamic tract*, has many synaptic relays and ends at the lower parts of the brain where it arouses the emotions and switches on the 'fight or flight' response. Its effects may, or may not, diffuse into the conscious brain; for example, nociceptive perception may not occur in the heat of battle (or the field of play) when there are other pressing distractions. The second tract, the *neospinothalamic*, evolved later and is more efficient, requiring only three relays to reach the sensory cortex that locates the pain. Thus, pain location occurs before its realization.

Nociception is usually transient, unless there is tissue injury and damaged cells result in the local release of algogenic substances (such as bradykinin, serotonin, histamine, hydrogen ions, potassium ions, prostaglandins, leukotrienes, nerve growth factors, and neuropeptides) to produce the inflammatory pain of Wall's acute phase. Anti-inflammatory drugs may have their application in this phase, but the abatement of inflammation with drugs can be counterproductive, because inflammation is the necessary prelude to healing.

After injury, most people heal rapidly and become pain-free, but in some, pain persists beyond the usual time for the healing process and becomes intractable. Chronic pain, or Wall's third phase, is likely to occur if there is:

- *on-going nociception*, e.g. an unhealed fracture, inflammation, rheumatoid arthritis
- *psychological factors* such as somatization disorders, depression, or adverse operant learning processes
- *abnormal function* in the nervous system.

The International Association for the Study of Pain defines injury, in its definition of pain, as 'an unpleasant sensory and emotional experience associated with actual or potential tissue damage, or described by the patient in terms of such damage'. However, pain need not be linked causally to injury. Injury does not always generate pain, nor does pain always signal injury. Pain perception can also arise from within the body when there is a functional disorder in the nervous system. The most common functional disorder, by far, is peripheral neuropathy stemming from spondylosis. This large and mundane category of pain was first referred to as 'pain following neuropathy' (Gunn 1978), but the term *neuropathic pain* has now been extended to include any acute or chronic pain syndrome in which the mechanism that sustains the pain is inferred to involve aberrant somatosensory processing in the CNS or peripheral nervous system. Spondylosis and segmental dysfunction are no longer implicit in the present definition. Instead, the term *radiculopathic pain* is now used to refer to spondylotic pain (Gunn 1997).

Clinical features of neuropathic pain

The identification of chronic pain caused by ongoing nociception or inflammation is usually straightforward, but the clinical features of neuropathic pain are less well known.

Peripheral neuropathy may be defined as a disease that causes disordered function in the peripheral nerve. Although sometimes associated with structural changes in the nerve, a neuropathic nerve can—deceptively—appear normal. It still conducts nerve impulses, synthesizes and releases transmitted substances, and evokes action potentials and muscle contraction. All fibres can be damaged: sensory, motor, and autonomic. Some features of neuropathic pain are listed in Box 58.1; in radiculopathy, these features appear in the distributions of both anterior and posterior primary rami (Bradley 1974; Fields 1987).

Myofascial pain syndromes

Myofascial pain syndromes affect muscles and their connective tissue attachments in any part of the body and are customarily named

Box 58.1 Features of neuropathic pain

Sensory

- Pain when there is no ongoing tissue-damaging process
- Delay in onset after precipitating injury; it takes about 5 days for supersensitivity to develop (Cannon and Rosenblueth 1949)
- Dysesthesia—unpleasant 'burning or searing' sensations
- Diffuse muscle tenderness and 'deep, aching' pain
- Pain felt in a region of sensory deficit
- Neuralgic pain—paroxysmal brief 'shooting or stabbing' pain
- Severe pain in response to a noxious stimulus (hyperalgesia)
- Severe pain in response to a stimulus that is not normally noxious (allodynia)
- Pronounced summation and after-reaction with repetitive stimuli

Motor

- Muscle shortening and pain caused by shortened muscle pulling on sensitive structures
- Loss of joint range

Autonomic

- Increased vasomotor, pilomotor, and sudomotor activity (hyperhidrosis)
- Trophedema
- Causalgic pain, reflex sympathetic dystrophy, or complex regional pain syndrome

Trophic

- Dermatomal hair loss
- Collagen degradation; weakness in tendons, offset by hypertrophy (enthesopathy)

Table 58.1 Myofascial pain syndromes

Syndrome	Shortened muscles
Achilles tendonitis	Gastrocnemii, soleus
Bicipital tendonitis	Biceps brachii
Bursitis: pre-patellar	Quadriceps femoris
trochanteric	Gluteus maximus, medius, gemelli, quadratus femoris
Capsulitis (frozen shoulder)	All muscles acting on the shoulder including trapezius, levator scapular, rhomboidei, pectoralis major/ minor, supra- and infraspinati, teres major/ minor, subscapularis, deltoid
Chrondromalacia patellae	Quadriceps femoris
De Quervain's tensynovitis	Abductor pollicis longus, extensor pollicis brevis
Facet syndrome	Muscles acting across the joint, e.g. rotatores, multifidi, semispinales
Fibromyalgia (diffuse myofascial syndrome)	Multisegmental, generally muscles supplied by cervical and lumbar nerve roots
Hallux vulgus	Extensores hallucis longus and brevis
Headaches: frontal	Upper trapezius, stenomastoid, occipitofrontalis
temporal	Temporalis, upper trapezius
vertex	Splenius capitis, cervicis
occipital	Suboccipital muscles
Intervertebral disc (early)	Muscles acting across the disc space, e.g. rotatores, multifidi semispinales
Low back sprain	Paraspinal muscles, e.g. iliocostalis lumborum and thoracis
Piriformis syndrome	Piniformis muscle
Rotator cuff syndrome	Supra- and infraspinatus, teres minor, subscapularis
Shin splints	Tibialis anterior
Temporomandibular joint	Masseter, temporalis, pterygoids
Tennis elbow	Brachioradialis, extensor muscles, anaconeus

according to the location of the painful part, e.g. 'tennis elbow', 'Achilles tendonitis', 'frozen shoulder', and even 'low back pain' (see Table 58.1). In neuropathy, muscles can shorten and mechanically stress their soft tissue attachments and joints. This can produce pain in many different parts of the body. Although musculoskeletal pain syndromes appear to have an astounding diversity, the common denominator is muscle shortening. Myofascial pain syndromes can be puzzling because they seem to arise and persist in the absence of detectable injury or inflammation. They are difficult to treat, because medications and physical therapies give only temporary relief. However, careful examination of myofascial pain conditions reveals them to be epiphenomena of neuropathy manifesting in the musculoskeletal system. Structural factors, such as muscle shortening and weakness of degraded collagen, also contribute to the pain.

The underlying problem is a functional disorder in the nervous system, and pain is a possible, but not inevitable, product of the neuropathy. The key to successful management of this important and widespread category of chronic pain is to understand neuropathy, how it can cause pain, and recognize it in its many disguises.

Electrophysiological features of neuropathy

Damaged primary afferent fibres demonstrate three electrophysiological features: spontaneous activity, exaggerated response to stimulus, and sensitivity to catecholamines. These features are explained by a fundamental physiological law: Cannon and Rosenblueth's (1949) law of denervation. This law points out that the normal physiology and integrity of all innervated structures are dependent upon the uninterrupted arrival of nerve impulses via the intact nerve to provide a regulatory or 'trophic' effect. When this flow—a combination of axoplasmic flow and electrical input—is obstructed, innervated structures are deprived of the vital factor that regulates cellular function. According to the law of denervation, atrophic structures become highly irritable and develop abnormal sensitivity. When a unit is destroyed in a series of efferent neurons, an increased irritability to chemical agents develops in the isolated structure or structures, the effect being maximal in the part directly denervated. All denervated structures—including skeletal muscle, smooth muscle, spinal neurones, sympathetic ganglia, adrenal glands, sweat glands, and brain cells—develop supersensitivity.

Cannon and Rosenblueth's original work was based on total denervation or decentralization for supersensitivity to develop: accordingly, they named the phenomenon *denervation supersensitivity*. It is now known that total physical interruption and denervation are not necessary. Any circumstance that impedes the flow of impulses for a duration of time can rob the effector organ of its excitatory input and disrupt normal physiology in that organ and in associated spinal reflexes (Sharpless 1975).

The importance of disuse supersensitivity cannot be overemphasized. Atrophic structures overreact to many forms of input, not only chemical but physical as well, including stretch and pressure. Supersensitive muscle cells can generate spontaneous electrical impulses that trigger false pain signals or provoke involuntary muscle activity (Culp and Ochoa 1982). Supersensitive nerve fibres become receptive to chemical transmitters at every point along their length instead of only at their terminals; sprouting may occur, and denervated nerves are prone to accept contacts from other types of nerves including autonomic and sensory nerve fibres. Short circuits are possible between sensory and autonomic (vasomotor) nerves and may contribute to 'reflex sympathetic dystrophy' or the 'complex regional pain syndrome'.

Disuse supersensitivity is basic and universal, yet not at all well known. Many pain syndromes of apparently unknown causation can be attributed to the development of supersensitivity in receptors and pain pathways.

Radiculopathy: its frequent relationship to spondylosis

It is not unusual for the flow of nerve impulses to be obstructed: peripheral neuropathy, often accompanied by partial denervation, is not exceptional. Of the numerous causes of nerve damage such as trauma, metabolic, and degenerative, spondylosis is easily the most prevalent.

Ordinarily, spondylosis follows a gradual, relapsing, and remitting course that is silent unless and until symptoms are precipitated by an incident often so minor that it usually passes unnoticed. The spinal nerve root is notably vulnerable to pressure, stretch, angulation, and friction, even from early prespondylosis (Gunn 1978). For pain to become a persistent symptom, affected fibres must have been previously irritated. After an acute injury to a healthy nerve, there is no prolonged discharge of pain signals, whereas injury to a neuropathic nerve can cause a sustained discharge (Howe et al. 1977). That is why some people develop severe pain after an apparently minor injury, and also why that pain can continue beyond a 'reasonable' period.

Physical irritation first entangles large-diameter nerve fibres—the axons of motor neurons and myelinated primary afferents from muscle proprioceptors. Muscle contracture with shortening is therefore an early feature of radiculopathy. Painless, tight knots can be felt in most individuals; not uncommonly, even in toddlers. Pain is not a feature until nociceptive pathways are involved. Many neuropathies are pain-free, such as hyperhidrosis and muscle weakness in ventral root disease.

Peripheral and central sensitization

Peripheral sensitization can follow tissue inflammation and peripheral neuropathy. There is increased transduction sensitivity of nociceptors caused by altered ionic conductances in the peripheral terminal. In inflammation, cells also produce growth factors and cytokines, which increase the sensitivity of nociceptors.

Central sensitization is a state of hyperexcitability in the dorsal horn. It can occur from damage to a peripheral nerve or from low-frequency, repetitive C-fibre input, as in arthritis. The spinal cord is not simply a passive conveyer of peripheral sensation to the brain: it can modify or amplify incoming signals. There is increased spontaneous activity of dorsal horn neurons, increased response to afferent input, expansion of receptive field size, reduction in threshold, and prolonged after discharges. Central sensitization leads to a cascade of molecular events, such as activation of the N-methyl-D-aspartate (NMDA) channel, increase in intracellular calcium, wind-up/wide dynamic range (WDR) neurone sensitization, and other phenomena (Munglani et al. 1996).

In central sensitization, low-intensity stimulation can be perceived as painful, i.e. severe pain can occur in response to a stimulus that is not normally noxious (allodynia); and high-intensity stimulation, which is normally painful, leads to hyperalgesia, i.e. there can be severe pain in response to a noxious stimulus. The receptive field size expands, and after discharges can occur. Pain often radiates several segments above and below the level of nociceptive input. This happens through propriospinal connections in adjacent layers of the dorsal horn where they make contact with WDR neurones. WDR neurones have immense fields compared to primary afferent neurones. Perceived pain can outlast the stimulus because a brief discharge from A-delta fibres or C-fibres can generate prolonged activity in WDR neurones.

Fibromyalgia has recently become a popular diagnosis, and many doctors now apply the American College of Rheumatology (ACR) 1990 criteria (Wolfe et al. 1990). Is fibromyalgia a distinctive syndrome (Gunn 1995) or does it merely describe the most extreme and extensive of the aches, pains, and tender muscles that we all have, in various degrees, at one time or other? Mildly tender points are not unusual in most individuals, and moderate to extremely tender points are not unusual in those who have a vulnerable back. Other features of fibromyalgia such as articular pain, coldness of extremities, irritable bowel, and trophedema also point to a functional disorder in the peripheral nervous system with downstream changes in the spinal cord. For example, large-diameter afferent neurones that normally transmit non-noxious stimuli now start to express substance P (which is normally associated with small-diameter C-fibres that transmit pain and temperature). The exact significance of this phenotypic switch by large-diameter fibres is not known, but it may explain how light touch and proprioceptive information (carried by A-beta fibres) may be misinterpreted as pain by the spinal cord (Munglani et al. 1996). In the spinal cord, there are changes in neuropeptide levels, such as an increase of substance P, glutamate, neurokinin A, and calcitonin gene-related peptide, and a decrease of serotonin level.

Diagnosis of neuropathic pain

Pain from ongoing nociception or inflammation is usually promptly recognized and appropriately dealt with. However, diagnosis of chronic neuropathic pain can be challenging, and depends almost entirely on the examiner's clinical experience and skill. The history gives little assistance. Pain frequently arises spontaneously with no history of trauma, and the degree of reported pain far exceeds that consistent with the injury.

Signs of neuropathy

The characteristic physical signs of neuropathy are different from the well-known ones of outright denervation, such as loss of sensation and reflexes (Gunn 1989). It is important to look for neuropathic signs because they indicate early neural irritation and dysfunction for which there is no satisfactory laboratory or imaging test. For example, thermography reveals decreased skin temperature, which is an indication of neuropathy, but does not by itself signify pain. Nerve conduction velocities usually remain within the wide range of normal values, and electromyography is not specific.

Diagnosis begins with a careful search for the signs of neuropathy—motor, sensory, and autonomic. Vasoconstriction differentiates neuropathic pain from inflammation pain: in neuropathic pain, the affected parts are perceptibly colder. There may be increased sudomotor activity, and the pilomotor reflex is often hyperactive and visible in affected dermatomes as 'goose bumps' (Figure 58.1). There can be interaction between pain and autonomic phenomena. A stimulus such as chilling, which excites the pilomotor response, can precipitate pain; vice versa, pressure on a tender motor point can trigger the pilomotor and sudomotor reflexes.

Increased capillary permeability can lead to local subcutaneous tissue oedema—neurogenic oedema or trophedema (Figure 58.2). This can be seen as *peau d'orange* skin (Figure 58.3) and can be confirmed by Gunn's 'matchstick' test. Trophedema is non-pitting to digital pressure, but when a blunt instrument such as the end of a matchstick is used, the indentation produced is clear-cut and persists for many minutes (Figure 58.4). This quick and simple test can demonstrate neuropathy earlier than electromyography. Trophic changes, including dermatomal hair loss, may also accompany neuropathy.

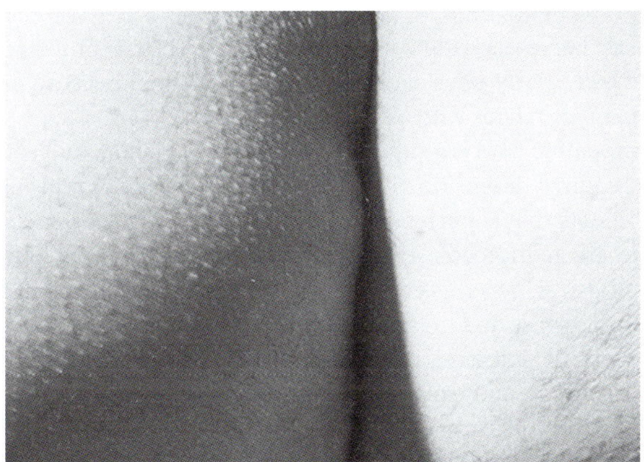

Figure 58.1 Goosebumps from a supersensitive pilomotor reflex on the left buttock, associated with muscle shortening in the gluteus maximus muscle.

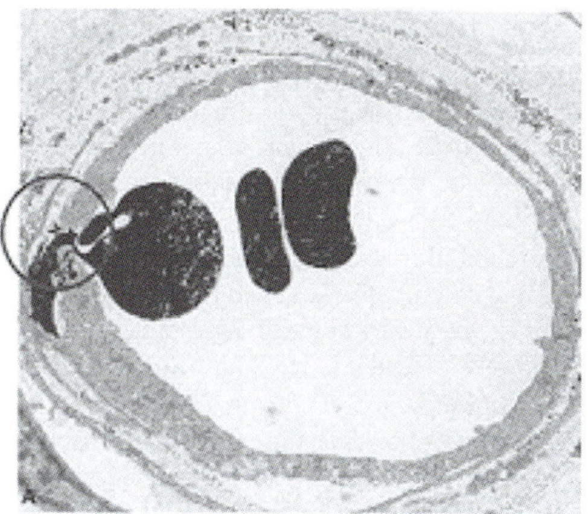

Figure 58.2 In neurogenic oedema, the permeability of small blood vessels is increased by transient gaps between endothelial cells, allowing fluid and plasma protein to escape into the extravascular space.
(Acute Respiratory Distress Syndrome (ARDS) successfully treated with low level laser therapy, *Journal of Complementary and Integrative Medicine*, Vol. 2, Issue 1, Art. 5)

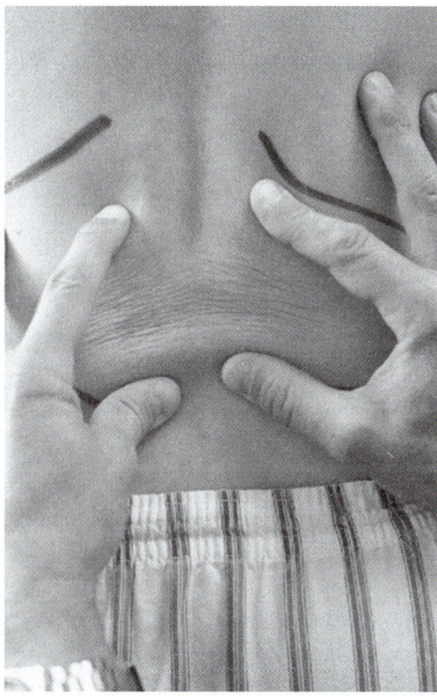

Figure 58.3 The 'peau d'orange' sign indicating neurogenic oedema or trophedema.
(Upper Lumbar Radiculopathy, seldom detected cause of BP, *JOM*, Vol. 29, No. 3, 2007, C. Chan Gunn, et al.)

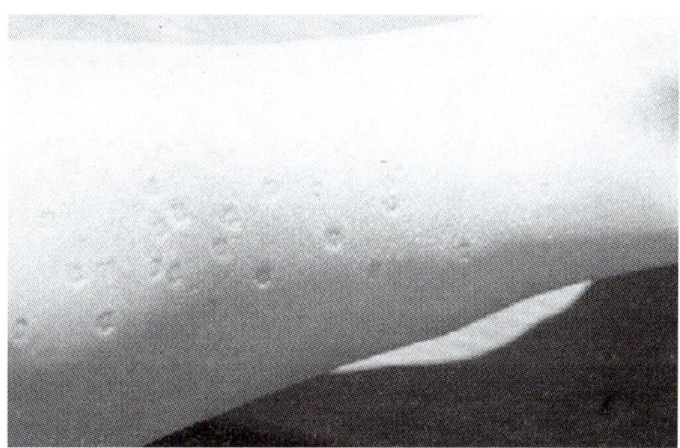

Figure 58.4 Gunn's matchstick test: trophedema is non-pitting to digital pressure but the end of a matchstick produces a clear-cut indentation that lasts for minutes.

Muscle signs

Neuropathic changes are most apparent and consistently found in muscle. Even when symptoms appear in joints or tendons, changes can be found in muscle. There is increased muscle tone; tenderness at motor points; taut, tender, and palpable contracture bands (trigger points); and restricted joint range.

Each constituent muscle can and must be palpated, and its condition noted. Palpation requires a good knowledge of anatomy, and palpatory skill comes with practice. Paraspinal muscles are often compound; for example, the longissimus muscle extends throughout the length of the vertebral column. Even when symptoms appear to be localized to one level, the entire spine must be examined. A knowledge of the segmental nerve supply to muscles points to the level(s) of segmental dysfunction.

Muscle shortening from contracture

Muscle contracture—the evoked shortening of a muscle fibre in the absence of action potentials—is a fundamental part of musculoskeletal pain (Figure 58.5). Muscle shortening can give rise to pain by its relentless pull on sensitive structures (Gunn 1996) (Figure 58.5). Muscle contracture occurs from:

- *Increased susceptibility*: Lessened stimuli, which do not have to exceed a threshold, can produce responses of normal amplitude.
- *Hyperexcitability*: The threshold of the stimulating agent is lower than normal.
- *Super-reactivity*: The capacity of the muscle to respond is augmented.
- *Superduration of response*: The amplitude of response is unchanged but its time course is prolonged.

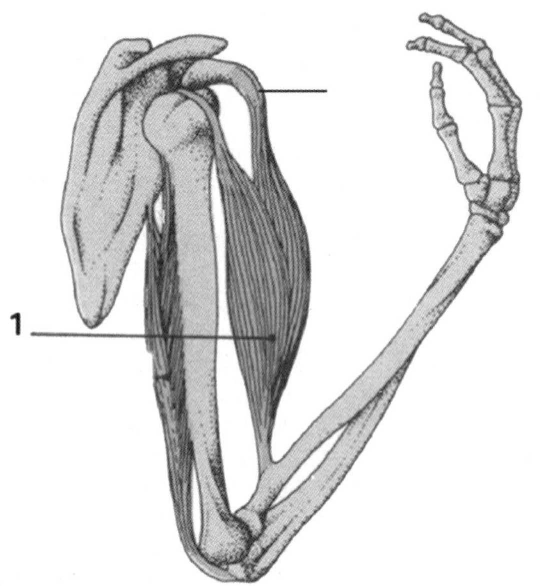

Figure 58.5 Muscle contracture can give rise to pain by its relentless pull on sensitive structures. Neuropathy degrades the quality of collagen, causing a tendon to thicken: enthesopathy. A shortened muscle pulling upon a tendon can produce 'tendonitis'. Increased tension in the synovial sheath causes tenosynovitis. Increased pressure of sesamoid bone on bone increases wear and tear, e.g. chondromalacia. Degraded collagen in a joint causes arthralgia and arthritis, eventually osteoarthritis.

Supersensitive skeletal muscle fibres overreact to a wide variety of chemical and physical inputs, including stretch and pressure. In normal muscle, acetylcholine acts only at receptors that are situated in the narrow zone of innervation, but in neuropathy, it acts at newly formed extrajunctional receptors or 'hot spots' that appear throughout the muscle. Additionally, their threshold to acetylcholine is lowered because of reduced levels of acetylcholinesterase. Acetylcholine slowly depolarizes supersensitive muscle membrane. It induces an electromechanical coupling in which tension develops slowly, and without generating action potentials.

The role of the needle: the Deqi response

The fine, flexible acupuncture needle is a unique tool for finding and releasing muscle contractures. Contracture is invisible to radiography, computed tomography (CT), or magnetic resonance imaging (MRI), and in deep muscles, it is beyond the finger's reach. The astonishing fact is that deep contracture can be discovered only by probing with a needle.

The needle transmits feedback information on the nature and consistency of the tissues it is penetrating. When penetrating normal muscle, it meets with little hindrance; when penetrating a contracture, there is firm resistance, and the needle is grasped by the muscle. This causes the patient to feel a peculiar, cramp-like, grabbing sensation which is referred to in acupuncture literature as the Deqi or Ch'i response (Gunn 1976). The intensity of the needle grasp parallels the degree of muscle shortening, and it gradually eases off during treatment as muscle shortening is released. Release can occur in seconds or minutes.

The Deqi response is associated with proprioceptors that sense muscle shortening: it is an important finding because it confirms the presence of neuropathy. The traditional acupuncturist painstakingly elicits the Deqi response to differentiate between pain that has the Deqi response (neuropathic), and pain that does not (nociceptive). This distinction is vital because of the different nature and treatment of the two pains.

Treatment of neuropathic pain

Clinical trials have shown that the pharmacological management of neuropathic pain is of limited effectiveness. Overall, there are no long-term studies of effectiveness to support the analgesic effectiveness of any drug beyond the short term (Kingery 1997).

Stimulation-induced analgesia

Physical therapy is widely used as a first-line treatment for neuropathic pain. Early physical treatment is advocated because earlier treatment correlates with better outcome.

Neuropathic pain is a supersensitivity phenomenon and its treatment requires desensitization. Lomo (1976) has shown in animal experiments that supersensitivity and other features of denervated muscle are reduced or reversed by electric stimulation. Physical therapy also achieves its effect by stimulation; for example, massage stimulates tactile and pressure receptors. Heat and cold act on thermal receptors. Exercise, manipulation, and dry needling stimulate muscle spindles and Golgi organs. These stimuli are sensed by their specific receptors, transduced into nerve impulses, and relayed to the dorsal horn. Stimulation then spreads out reflexively to the entire segment. All forms of physical therapy, including dry needling, are effective only when the nerve to the painful part is still intact.

When the nerve is not intact, neuropathic pain has been relieved by direct stimulation of the spinal cord (Howe et al. 1977).

All physical therapies have an inevitable limitation. They act as temporary substitutes for the body's own bioenergy, and their desensitization efforts do not persist: they last only as long as stimulation continues.

The current of injury

There is, serendipitously, an ideal source of energy—the body's own healing force—which can be tapped. Galvani, in a series of animal experiments that marked the beginning of electrophysiology, demonstrated in 1797 the existence of electricity in tissues. He was able to detect the electrical potential following tissue injury and called it the 'current of injury' (Galvani 1953). This intrinsic source of energy is the primary agent in promoting relief and healing. It is readily obtained, as in acupuncture and dry needling, by making minute injuries with a fine needle. Unlike extrinsic sources of energy, stimulation from the current of injury induced by the needle lasts for days until the miniature wounds heal. No injected medication is required.

The needle has another unique benefit offered by no other therapy: it promotes healing by releasing platelet-derived growth factor from blood. This substance induces cells to multiply and proliferate.

In chronic pain, fibrosis eventually becomes a major feature of the contracture. Response to dry needle treatment is then much less dramatic. The extent of fibrosis does not correlate with chronological age: scarring can occur after injury or surgery, and many older individuals have sustained less wear and tear than younger ones who have subjected their musculature to repeated physical stress. The treatment of extensive fibrotic contractures necessitates more frequent and extensive needling. To relieve pain in such a muscle, it is necessary to needle all tender bands. It is uncommon to encounter a muscle that is totally fibrotic and cannot be released by vigorous needling. Surgical release is usually unnecessary as the needle can reach deeply located shortened muscles.

Removing the cause of radiculopathy

For long-lasting pain relief and restoration of function, it is necessary to release muscle contracture in paraspinal muscle that is compressing a disc and entrapping the nerve root (Figure 58.6). Segmental dysfunction and pain are effectively resolved when pressure on the nerve root is relieved.

Treatment usually begins with simple measures such as heat and massage, escalating to more effective modalities such as transcutaneous electrical nerve stimulation (TENS), manipulation, and, ultimately, needling. The outcome of treatment depends not on the modality used but on the skill and experience of the therapist.

The Multidisciplinary Pain Center has, since 1985, successfully used a dry needling technique called intramuscular stimulation (IMS). In IMS, diagnosis, treatment, as well as progress during therapy are determined according to physical signs of neuropathy. Effective IMS requires a sound background in anatomy and physiology (Gunn 1996). The efficacy of IMS for chronic low back pain has been demonstrated by a randomized clinical trial involving a large group of Worker's Compensation Board patients. At their 7-month follow-up, the treated group was clearly and significantly better than the control group (Gunn and Milbrandt 1978).

It is a convincing experience to diagnose neuropathic pain by finding its unmistakable physical signs, then to treat the patient with IMS and witness the signs disappear, often within minutes. Objective evidence, directly witnessed, is the best form of evidence-based medicine.

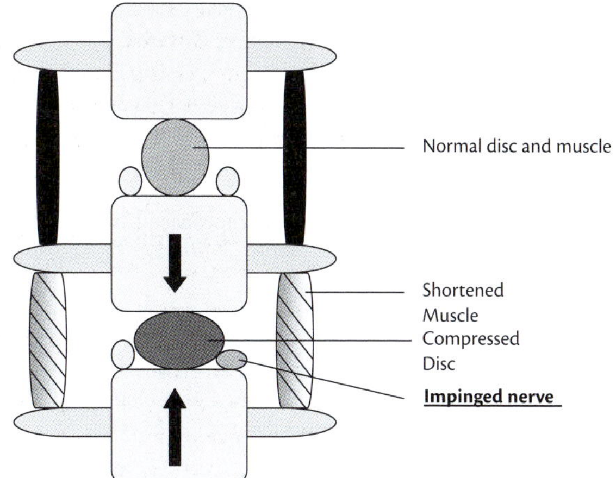

Figure 58.6 Muscle contracture across an intervertebral disc space can compress the disc which, in turn, can impinge on the spinal nerve.
(*The Gunn approach to the treatment of chronic pain: intramuscular stimulation for myofascial pain of radiculopathic origin*, printings 1989–2007, p. 31, http://www.istop.org/papers/neuropathicpain.htm)

Conclusions on neuropathic pain

The traditional definition of pain as a consequence of injury is often invalid. Chronic pain is commonly a manifestation of neuropathy and unrelated to nociception or inflammation. Neuropathic pain is now widely accepted, but its near-constant connection to spondylosis is not widely known. Signs of neuropathy are subtle and differ from those of outright denervation. Neuropathic pain has a proprioceptive component—pain cannot exist without muscle shortening. Shortened muscles are often the unsuspected cause of many conditions, such as tension headache and low back pain (see Table 58.1). Neuropathy degrades the quality of collagen and contributes to degeneration in weightbearing and activity-stressed parts of the body.

The underlying problem is neuropathy, and therapy should be directed to its cause. Drug treatment is unavailing; physical therapy is the best approach. The needle is a unique and effective tool for diagnosing and treating neuropathic pain. It is not by chance that acupuncture is based on the relief of neuropathy.

References

Bradley, W. G. (1974) *Disorders of peripheral nerves*. Blackwell Scientific Publications, Oxford, pp. 129–201; 253–67.

Cannon, W. B., Rosenblueth, A. (1949) *The supersensitivity of denervated structures*. Macmillan, New York, pp. 1–22, 185.

Culp, W. J., Ochoa, H. (1982) *Abnormal nerves and muscles as impulse generators*. Oxford University Press, New York, pp. 3–24.

Fields, H. L. (1987) *Pain*. McGraw-Hill, New York, pp. 133–64.

Galvani, A. (1953) *Commentary on electricity* (trans. Montraville Green, R.). Elizabeth Licht, Cambridge.

Gunn, C. C. (1976) Transcutaneous neural stimulation, needle acupuncture and 'Teh Ch'i' phenomenon. *American Journal of Acupuncture*, 4(4), 317–22.

Gunn, C. C. (1978) 'Prespondylosis' and some pain syndromes following denervation supersensitivity. *Spine*, 5(2),185–92.

Gunn, C. C. (1989) Neuropathic pain: a new theory for chronic pain of intrinsic origin. *Annals of the Royal College of Physicians and Surgeons of Canada*, 22(5), 327–30.

Gunn, C. C. (1995) Fibromyalgia: letter to the editor. *Pain*, 60, 349–52.

Gunn, C. C. (1996) *The Gunn approach to the treatment of chronic pain—intramuscular stimulation for myofascial pain of radiculopathic origin.* Churchill Livingstone, London.

Gunn, C. C. (1997) Radiculopathic pain: diagnosis and treatment of segmental irritation or sensitization. *Journal of Musculoskeletal Pain*, 5(4), 119–34.

Gunn, C. C., Milbrandt, W. E. (1978) Early and subtle signs in low back sprain. *Spine*, 3(3), 268–81.

Howe, J. F., Loeser, J. D., Calvin, W. H. (1977) Mechanosensitivity of dorsal root ganglia and chronically injured axons: a physiological basis for the radicular pain of nerve root compression. *Pain*, 3, 25–41.

Kingery, W. S. (1997) A critical review of controlled clinical trials for peripheral neuropathic pain and complex regional pain syndromes. *Pain*, 73, 123–39.

Lomo, T. (1976) The role of activity in the control of membrane and contractile properties of skeletal muscle. In: Thesleff, S. (ed.) *Motor innervation of muscle.* Academic Press, New York, pp. 289–315.

Munglani, R., Hunt, S. P., Jones, J. G. (1996) The spinal cord and chronic pain. In: Kaufman, L., Ginsburg, R. (eds) *Anaesthesia Review* 12, pp. 53–75.

Sharpless, S. K. (1975) Supersensitivity-like phenomena in the central nervous system. *Federation Proceedings*, 34(10), 1990–7.

Wall, P. D. (1978) The gate control theory of pain mechanisms—a re-examination and re-statement. *Brain*, 101, 1–18.

Wolfe, F., Smythe, H. A., Yunus, M. B., et al. (1990) American College of Rheumatology 1990 criteria for the classification of fibromyalgia: report of the Multicenter Criteria Committee. *Arthritis & Rheumatism*, 33, 160–72.

Chapter 59

Modern medical acupuncture

Anthony Campbell

There is no fully satisfactory way to refer to the modern version of acupuncture. Writers who wish to distinguish it from traditional acupuncture have coined terms such as 'dry needling' and 'intramuscular stimulation', but these are unfamiliar to many people—certainly to patients. 'Acupuncture' is itself a Western term and means simply the insertion of needles. In this chapter, 'acupuncture' will always refer to the modern version unless otherwise specified. In some cases, 'modern acupuncture' will be used to make the meaning completely clear.

The origins of modern acupuncture

Many people think of acupuncture as an esoteric and alien form of treatment that is based on ideas that have little if anything in common with those of modern science and medicine. Indeed, that difference is thought by some to be a positive merit; traditional Chinese medicine (TCM) is frequently praised for being more 'holistic' and 'natural' than mainstream medicine. That is probably largely a misunderstanding of TCM but, in any case, there is also a modern view of acupuncture which has little in common with the ancient ideas and instead treats it as a means of influencing the activity of the nervous system.

This is not an entirely new idea. Knowledge of acupuncture first reached the West at the end of the seventeenth century, and although it was considered a curiosity at first, acupuncture began to be used by doctors in Europe, mainly in France and Germany, in the nineteenth century. At that time, its Chinese roots were largely ignored and it was interpreted in the light of the medical knowledge of the day. However, in the first half of the twentieth century, Western doctors practicing acupuncture began to take on more traditional Chinese views, and that is still largely the case outside Britain and Sweden. In most European countries and in North and South America, acupuncture is mainly approached from a TCM standpoint, even by health professionals.

Events took a different course in Britain because, by the twentieth century, acupuncture was practically unknown here. It had flourished briefly in the early nineteenth century, when a young surgeon, James Morss Churchill, published a monograph on the subject in 1821. A number of doctors took it up, but interest soon faded away and, by the end of the century, it was practically unheard of. Its revival, beginning in the 1960s, was due largely to a young doctor, Felix Mann. He wanted to learn acupuncture but there was no one to teach him in the UK, so he went to Montpellier in France, to Munich, and to Vienna. The acupuncture he learned there was traditional because, as he said later, nothing else was then available. Returning to Britain in 1959, he set up an acupuncture practice in the West End of London—quite a bold undertaking at the time in view of the British public's unfamiliarity with the treatment. In the 1960s, he began teaching acupuncture to doctors, although at first, few came forward to learn. Then, however, his ideas about acupuncture began to change radically.

Central to the traditional system of acupuncture is the concept of acupuncture points: small areas of the body that produce distant or widespread effects when needled. Great precision is said to be necessary in locating them. It was this idea that Mann challenged. Although he initially practiced in the traditional way, because that was what he had been taught, he had a critical and inquiring mind and was always prepared to look at things in a different way. He began to experiment by putting needles in 'incorrect' places, and found that this worked just as well as putting them in the 'right' places. As time went by, he came to disbelieve the whole traditional theory of acupuncture, including the so-called meridians and the concept of *qi* or 'energy'. He now regarded it as a means of modifying the activity of the nervous system and as a treatment that could be explained in terms of the modern understanding of anatomy and physiology (Mann 2000).

According to his new view, neither acupuncture points nor the meridians exist as they are usually understood. Great precision in needle location is unnecessary, so instead of 'points', we should be thinking of areas. In many cases, these could be quite large: for example, Mann found a traditional site known as Liver 3, on the dorsum of the foot, to be particularly effective in many disorders, but needling anywhere below the knee seemed to have an equivalent effect for many patients. So, although he continued to use some of the traditional terminology, at least to begin with, this was simply for convenience, as a form of shorthand to record where the needles had been placed.

Mann introduced other departures from tradition as well. One was the use of periosteal needling, both to treat joint pain such as that due to arthritis and also to produce more generalized effects in a wide area. Another was his recognition of a subset of patients who responded particularly strongly to acupuncture, whom he called strong reactors. Disorders that usually do not respond to acupuncture might do so in a strong reactor. However, if a strong reactor were treated too vigorously, the results could be a worsening of their symptoms or a feeling of general malaise lasting for some hours or even days. Eventually, Mann came to believe that many traditionalists over-treated their patients, by putting in too many needles and leaving them in place for too long. Increasingly, he came to favour very gentle treatment, with few needles being inserted—sometimes only one—and the duration of needling being brief (seldom more than a minute or two and, quite often, just a few seconds).

Mann taught these ideas to the doctors who attended his courses in increasing numbers in the 1970s. He also went abroad to lecture, where his views, he reported, received a mixed reception. His former students constituted an informal medical acupuncture society. In 1980, matters were put on a more formal basis when the British Medical Acupuncture Society was founded, with Mann as its first President. The Society now has over 2000 members, all of whom are statutorily regulated health professionals such as doctors, physiotherapists, osteopaths, chiropractors, podiatrists, and nurses.

Changes in the scientific view of acupuncture

The new view of acupuncture that Mann was teaching in the 1970s arrived at a timely moment. In the 1960s, acupuncture was still thought of as a form of alternative or 'fringe' medicine, but attitudes began to change in the 1970s. There were several reasons for this. One was an event that occurred during President Nixon's visit to China in 1972. A journalist, James Reston, who was accompanying the mission, suffered acute appendicitis and was given acupuncture post-operatively to reduce his pain; he found this to be effective. Subsequently, Western surgeons visited Beijing and saw acupuncture being used instead of anaesthetics to prevent pain during surgery.

Two scientific developments at about this time appeared to provide the basis for a rational explanation of how acupuncture might work. A few years earlier, in 1965, Melzack and Wall had put forward the gate theory of pain. This was the signal for a new way of thinking about how the nervous system processes pain and how this could be modified by peripheral stimulation. Both these authors commented on the possible relevance to acupuncture. Then, in 1974, came the discovery of the endogenous opioids—'natural painkillers'. It quickly became apparent that these substances might have a role in acupuncture analgesia, and high levels of beta-endorphin were found in the cerebrospinal fluid of people receiving acupuncture (Clement-Jones and McLoughlin 1980). The pain-relieving effects of acupuncture were shown to be blocked by the morphine antagonist, naloxone (Mayer et al. 1977).

From this time on, acupuncture, at least in its modern form, began to attract increasing interest from Western researchers and clinicians. Today, *Acupuncture in Medicine,* the journal of the British Medical Acupuncture Society, is published by BMJ Journals.

Acupuncture today

Although most British health professionals who practice acupuncture would say they use the modern approach, they vary in how radical they are in disregarding TCM. Some seek to reinterpret at least some of the traditional ideas in terms of modern anatomy and physiology. This applies particularly to the acupuncture points, which many use as a guide to treatment, even without believing fully in their real existence. Others ignore them almost completely, preferring to base their practice on trigger points or other principles. Rather than a rigid division into two groups, therefore, there is a spectrum of opinion, with those who seek to preserve as much of the traditional ideas as possible at one extreme and complete modernists at the other.

Mechanisms of acupuncture

Currently, a number of different mechanisms are thought to be involved in acupuncture analgesia, operating in the local tissues, in the spinal cord, and in the brain (White et al. 2008).

Local effects

The insertion of a needle stimulates free nerve endings and the 'axon reflex', with the release of several kinds of neuropeptides, including calcitonin gene-related peptide (CGRP), nerve growth factor (NGF), vasointestinal peptide (VIP), and histamine. The effect, particularly of CGRP, is to promote vasodilatation and the formation of new vessels. These changes are likely to improve healing and may also influence structures nearby—for example, by increasing the flow of saliva from salivary glands.

Spinal cord effects

Acupuncture has been shown to produce changes in the spinal cord, both segmentally and extra-segmentally. The phenomenon of pain memory is important here. Long-term potentiation (LTP) is thought to be involved in chronic pain, by enhancing synaptic transmission between neurons in the pain pathways. The contrary phenomenon, long-term depression (LTD) will diminish this effect and this probably explains at least part of the effect of acupuncture in the relief of chronic pain (Sandkühler 2000, 2007).

Descending pathways in the spinal cord, originating mainly in the brain stem, are important in regulating pain perception. There is a constantly shifting balance in the central nervous system between excitation and inhibition. To diminish pain, one can either reduce excitation or increase inhibition. Acupuncture is likely to act by increasing inhibition.

The brain

In recent years, much attention has been directed to the role of central brain areas (limbic and paralimbic) in the modification of pain. The anterior cingulate cortex is particularly important in this respect: it is concerned with how unpleasant pain is felt to be. A number of studies have shown that acupuncture modifies (usually reduces) activity here, and this probably explains the common clinical observation that patients may feel less distressed by their pain after acupuncture, even if the pain is not completely eliminated (Hui et al. 2000).

More recently, new light has been thrown on the cortical representation of pain and its modification by sensory input. Acupuncture stimulates A-delta (small-diameter myelinated) nerve fibres preferentially and these project to a spatially-organized somatotopic map in the primary somatosensory cortex. This pain mapping is now known to be modified by sensory stimulation, not only of the skin and other tissues but also in other ways. This has been termed 'multisensory analgesia' (Haggard et al. 2013), which includes visual input—visual analgesia (Longo et al. 2009). Acupuncture supplies several different kinds of signal to the brain: touch in the preliminary examination for tender areas; needle stimulation, mainly of A-delta fibres; and sometimes, visual input from the patient's sight of the needle insertion. In the light of recent research, all these are likely to modulate pain (Campbell 2013).

Summary

This outline by no means exhausts all the information we currently have about acupuncture mechanisms, and new research is constantly shedding further light. For example, a recent study found that, in mice, acupuncture causes the release of adenosine (Goldman et al. 2010). This has anti-inflammatory properties and is an inhibitory neurotransmitter involved in promoting sleep and reducing arousal. Patients often feel relaxed by acupuncture and may find that their sleep quality is improved.

Myofascial trigger points and acupuncture

Most acupuncture modernists make use of the concept of myofascial trigger points (TPs). Practitioners who mainly rely on this approach often refer to it as dry needling (in contrast to 'wet needling', which refers to injection techniques).

Historically, the TP idea originated in work at University College Hospital in London in the 1930s, when a rheumatologist, J.H. Kellgren, was conducting experiments on volunteers (including himself) in whom he injected saline into muscles. He found that this gave rise to characteristic patterns of pain referral. He also found that injecting tender sites in patients suffering from musculoskeletal pain often alleviated their symptoms (Kellgren 1938).

In the 1940s, an American physician, Janet Travell, built on this work to develop the treatment of what she termed the myofascial pain syndrome (MPS). Later, she was joined by another physician, David Simons, and together they produced a large two-volume textbook on the subject (Simons et al. 1999; Travell and Simons 1992).

Although their approach was scientific, their work has not become well known to doctors, but practitioners of manual therapies (physiotherapists, osteopaths, chiropractors) generally are familiar with it and use it in treatment.

Some modern acupuncturists have interpreted modern acupuncture as consisting largely, if not wholly, in the treatment of TPs. It is often claimed, in the Western literature, that many of the traditional acupuncture points have a TP nearby, while conversely, nearly all the TPs described in the West have an acupuncture point nearby. Nevertheless, there is only limited evidence to show that needling TPs has a beneficial effect. A literature search by Tough and colleagues found that most published studies were of poor quality and only one supported this form of treatment (Tough et al. 2007). Their later review of the criteria used by 'experts' to diagnose TPs found considerable variations. Nearly all the studies cited Travell and Simons as the authoritative source, but most failed to apply their diagnostic criteria (Tough et al. 2009).

In spite of these reservations, the great majority of modernists do make considerable use of TPs. However, there are variations in the techniques they use to inactivate them. Some favour superficial (subcutaneous) acupuncture over the TP (Baldry 2002). Others prefer to use deep needling in an attempt to penetrate the actual TP and hope to get a muscle twitch as evidence of success (White et al. 2008). There is little objective evidence to show which, if either, of these methods gives better results. There are also different views about the number of TPs that should be treated in a session.

In summary, modern acupuncturists often needle TPs, but that is not the only method used. Needling non-tender areas can also work, and these cannot be termed TPs, since those are tender by definition. Another popular approach, based on neurophysiology, is to use the segmental innervation of the body as a guide. In this method, the needles are inserted in the dermatome, myotome, or sclerotome that contains the site of the problem to be treated. Additionally, a simpler idea is merely to insert the needles close to the site of pain. This was the main approach of acupuncturists in the nineteenth century.

As these remarks will indicate, there is no universally agreed way of deciding where to place the needles in modern acupuncture. In practice, many modernists take an eclectic approach and use a combination of TPs, body segments, and local tenderness, together with some classic TCM sites which they find to be effective (Campbell 1999). The following description summarizes these possibilities. Nearly all of modern acupuncture (and quite a lot of traditional acupuncture as well) fits into these categories, singly or in combination.

Placing of acupuncture needles

Needle the painful area itself

This is the simplest form of treatment and is often all that is required. For example, widespread back pain due to ankylosing spondylitis or osteoporosis often responds to needling in the paraspinal muscles of the affected region. Plantar fasciitis can often be relieved by needling the attachment of the plantar fascia to the medial calcaneal tubercle.

Needle a remote site that may relate to the site of pain

This depends on the phenomenon of referred pain. It therefore includes TP acupuncture and the use of spinal segments, although some treatments do not fall into either of these categories. An example would be needling the ulnar side of the hand for upper thoracic pain. (There is a traditional point here known as Small Intestine 3.) This presumably works because it is in the C8/T1 dermatome. Another example is needling the midpoint of the trapezius (which is a classic site called Gall Bladder 21). Radiation from this site can go up into the neck or down into the arm and is used to treat pain in those regions.

Needle the periosteum

This technique figures little, if at all, in the traditional system. It is most commonly used to treat intrinsic joint pain such as that due to osteoarthritis but it can also act on a wide area of the body. For example, needling the articular pillar in the neck can influence symptoms in the upper half of the body, and needling the pelvic periosteum in the region of the sacroiliac joint can do the same for the lower half.

Generalized (central) effects

Some patients, especially those classed as strong reactors, experience surprisingly profound generalized effects, presumably owing to central changes. Some degree of relaxation often occurs after the needles are inserted, and some patients become euphoric and feel as if they have had a few alcoholic drinks. They may report spontaneously that everything looks brighter. Others may laugh or cry, though they seldom know why this is happening. Effects of this kind can occur no matter where the needles are inserted but are particularly common when insertion is in the hands or feet. Sometimes such effects may come on later, perhaps an hour or more after treatment; it is therefore preferable for patients not to drive or operate machinery after acupuncture, especially on the first occasion. Patients often report that they sleep particularly soundly on the night after treatment. All these effects are suggestive of central changes.

Setting acupuncture in the modern context

Acupuncture can easily appear a strange and exotic form of treatment, but it is best considered as a form of manual therapy that overlaps with other manual therapies such as physiotherapy, osteopathy, and chiropractic (Figure 59.1). Indeed, it seems possible that all these treatments act in similar ways at the level of the nervous system. Practitioners who use these forms of treatment generally find that acupuncture fits well into what they are already doing.

Applications of acupuncture

The main application of acupuncture is for relief of pain. Its effectiveness depends, to a large extent, on the type of pain. It works well for musculoskeletal pain, both acute and chronic. Some forms of neurogenic pain, such as trigeminal neuralgia, also respond quite well. Chronic pain syndromes such as fibromyalgia respond less well; the effects are usually fairly short-lasting and partial. Acupuncture is used to treat miscellaneous disorders such as allergies, nausea and vomiting, and ulcerative colitis, but these are outside the scope of the present discussion. Pain due to malignancy will also not be discussed here.

It is important to understand that acupuncture is a technique, or set of techniques, and not a complete system of therapy. It is also best thought of as a means of relieving symptoms rather than producing 'cures'. This does not mean that it cannot produce permanent relief of symptoms in cases where spontaneous resolution may be expected to occur, as in acute disorders, but many patients with chronic disease may require occasional 'top-up' treatments over many months or years in order to maintain remission.

Because of its effect on symptoms, acupuncture may mask serious underlying disease for a time. For example, headache due to a space-occupying lesion may respond to acupuncture initially. Hence, patients receiving acupuncture should always have had an assessment to exclude red flag signs and symptoms.

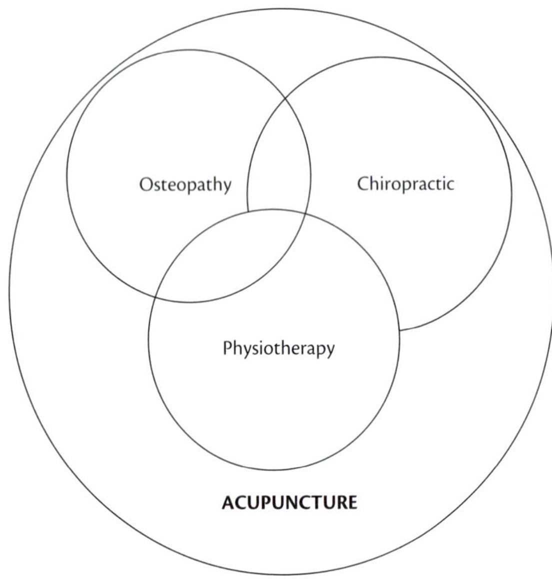

Figure 59.1 Types of acupuncture.

Different types of acupuncture

The original form of acupuncture consisted in the insertion of needles into the body. Other forms have developed from this over time. The different types of acupuncture alluded to in this section are included for information only, to give an idea of the range of acupuncture and allied treatments that exist (Figure 59.2), but will not be discussed further here.

Specialized forms of acupuncture

These are based on the idea that there are somatotopic maps of the body in particular areas. The best known of these is ear acupuncture (auriculotherapy), in which there is supposed to be a representation of the body in the auricle, with the feet at the top, the head at the bottom, and the spine at the outer margin. Other systems have maps in the scalp or in the hand, beside the first metacarpal. Whether such maps have any real existence is still contentious.

Electro-acupuncture

Electrical stimulation of the needles was tried in France in the nineteenth century, and more recently, the Chinese have used it to give prolonged stimulation for acupuncture analgesia during surgery. Electrical stimulation has often been used in research, probably because it gives a more precisely quantifiable intensity of stimulus than does manual stimulation. Some modern acupuncturists use electrical stimulation of the needles at least part of the time, but not everyone is convinced that it offers any advantage over manual stimulation and it is more time-consuming to perform. It is also not clear that manual and electrical stimulation are equivalent ways of modifying the activity of the nervous system.

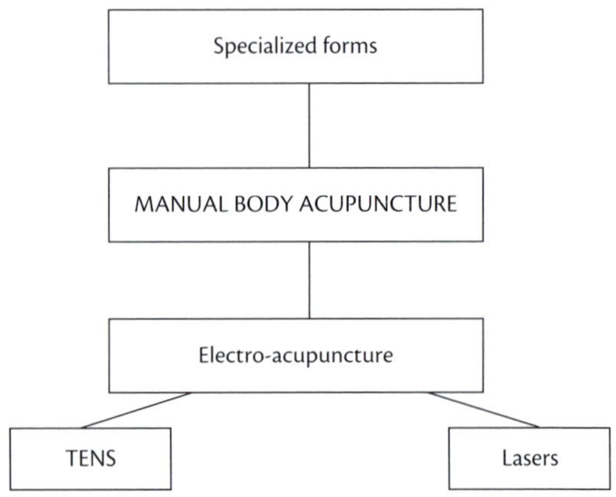

Figure 59.2 Acupuncture in relation to other manual therapies.

Electrical stimulation may be either slow (2–10 Hz) or fast (up to about 200 Hz). Slow and fast stimulation appear to have different biological effects. Machines offering various electrical wave forms and frequency patterns are available.

Allied treatments

Transcutaneous electrical nerve stimulation (TENS)

In this form of treatment, electricity is applied to the skin via conducting pads. Like electro-acupuncture it may be either slow or fast. TENS and acupuncture are used to treat pain and there is some overlapping between their effects, but some conditions respond differently to the two forms of treatment. As a rule, TENS gives pain relief only for as long as the current is flowing or for a short time afterwards, whereas acupuncture can give more prolonged or even permanent relief.

Lasers

These have been used in recent years as an alternative to needles. They have the advantage that they are painless and there is no risk of infection, but how useful they are clinically is still uncertain. Even if they do work, it is unclear how far their effect is similar to that of acupuncture.

Acupuncture treatment in practice

There are considerable variations in how acupuncture is performed. Most traditionalists use large numbers of needles (20 or more) and leave them in place for at least 20 minutes. During this time, the needles may be stimulated at intervals, either manually or electrically. Some modern acupuncturists also do this, while others use many fewer needles (sometimes only one) and leave them in for much shorter periods (seldom more than a minute or two and sometimes just a few seconds). There is little evidence to show that either of these methods is better than the other. All this means that it is practically impossible to describe a 'typical' acupuncture session, since what happens may vary so much according to the training and views of the acupuncturist.

Acupuncture 'dosage'

The concept of 'dosage' is often applied to acupuncture stimulation to refer to the amount of effect that is being produced on the patient. The following factors affect the strength of the treatment: number of needles inserted, thickness of needles, depth of insertion, and amount of manual or electrical stimulation applied. However, unlike what usually happens with drugs, there is not a simple relation between the intensity of acupuncture treatment and the occurrence of a therapeutic response. Paradoxically, some patients have a stronger response when minimal acupuncture is performed. How much stimulation to give in individual cases is very much a question of clinical judgement, and there are no firm rules.

Number of treatments

There is generally a build-up effect with repeated treatments until a 'plateau' is reached, after which no further improvement occurs. Usually, it takes up to about six treatments to produce the maximum response that the patient can expect, although this is a generalization and there are many variations. Some patients experience complete relief after one or two treatments, while others benefit from more than six.

Intervals between treatments

In chronic conditions, it is often convenient to start with weekly treatments. If there is improvement, the length between treatments can be increased. Once a 'plateau' (or complete relief of symptoms) has occurred, treatment is stopped, although occasional 'top-ups' may be needed, perhaps three or four times a year. Usually, only one treatment is required on these occasions to restore the remission.

Acute conditions are treated in much the same way but the intervals between treatments are shorter. So, perhaps two treatments might be given in the first week, and thereafter, the intervals between treatments are decided by the response, as for chronic disorders. It is seldom advisable to treat patients daily; enough time should be left between treatments for the effect to be observed.

Aggravations

Some patients experience a worsening of their existing symptoms after acupuncture. Such aggravations may mean that the patient was over-treated, although some will experience a mild aggravation after each treatment. Aggravations are generally short-lived and may be followed by an improvement.

Non-responders

Experience in the West indicates that approximately a fifth of patients do not respond to acupuncture. The reasons are unclear but it needs to be kept in mind when discussing the chances of improvement with a new patient.

Identifying non-responders

If acupuncture is going to work, there should usually be at least a little improvement after two or three treatments. If there is no response at all, it probably means that the patient is in the non-responder category.

Clinical evidence for acupuncture

Clinical research in acupuncture is bedevilled by the problem of finding a suitable control procedure with which to compare the treatment. A common method is to use so-called 'sham acupuncture'. There are two forms of this: inserting needles at non-acupuncture sites and using non-penetrating sham needles. Both of these are problematic (Lund and Lundeberg 2006) and, in any case, at best, they can be used in single-blind trials; double-blind trials are all but impossible.

In spite of the difficulties, a good deal of clinical research in acupuncture has been carried out in recent decades. In the broadest terms, this has tended to show that it is easy to demonstrate a significant difference between acupuncture and no treatment, but there is relatively little evidence for the specificity of 'acupuncture points' as understood in the traditional system. A good example is provided by the German insurance company studies (GERAC) which were carried out in the twenty-first century. They were the largest randomized controlled trials of acupuncture undertaken to date, with about 1000 patients in each. These were three-armed trials, comparing true acupuncture, sham acupuncture (needles inserted superficially at non-traditional sites), and conventional treatment. The acupuncture was performed by doctors who were trained in traditional acupuncture and believed in its efficacy.

For low back pain, both real and sham acupuncture were almost twice as effective as conventional treatment, but there was no significant difference between real and sham (Haake et al. 2007). The same was true of a trial of acupuncture for knee osteoarthritis (Scharf et al. 2006). In a trial of acupuncture for migraine prophyllaxis, too many patients withdrew to allow a comparison with conventional treatment, but once again, real and sham acupuncture were equally effective (Diener et al. 1996). Currently, the National Institute for Clinical Excellence (NICE) recommends acupuncture only for low back pain and migraine prophyllaxis.

In summary, acupuncture is used for a wide range of clinical conditions, especially musculoskeletal pain, but research evidence for efficacy in many of them is inconclusive. Elucidating the role of the needles themselves, in comparison with other elements of the treatment, is a challenging problem that is still a long way from being solved. Acupuncture is a complex procedure that cannot be validly reduced to the mere insertion of needles. There is often a preliminary manual examination for TPs and other clinical features that may be therapeutic in itself. These and other variables make the planning and interpretation of clinical trials in acupuncture difficult.

Safety of acupuncture

Acupuncture is an invasive procedure consisting in the insertion of needles into the tissues. Inevitably, this entails an element of risk, but the available evidence indicates that, if performed by a competent practitioner, it is remarkably safe (White 2004, 2006; White et al. 2001). To put this in context, the risk of having acupuncture is probably smaller than that of taking a non-steroidal anti-inflammatory drug.

The risks of acupuncture are of two main kinds: infection and anatomical damage.

Infection

Infection may be either bacterial or viral. Acupuncture should always be carried out with pre-sterilized disposable needles. This eliminates the danger that viral infections such as hepatitis B or human immunodeficiency virus (HIV) will be transmitted from patient to patient. Provided the acupuncturist uses standard precautions, the chance of causing bacterial infection is very low, but bacteria may be present on the patient's skin surface or in skin glands and hair follicles, and bacterial infections do occur, although rarely. There have been a few cases of septic arthritis, and diabetic or immunocompromised patients are at increased risk.

Some practitioners leave small stud needles in place for a week or more, usually in the ear. This entails the risk of causing bacterial endocarditis and should be avoided.

As in any procedure involving needles, the acupuncturist must take precautions to avoid needlestick injury. Immunization against hepatitis B is strongly advised but does not guarantee complete immunity.

Anatomical damage

Almost every organ in the body has been pierced by acupuncture needles at some time or other. Usually, this is due to insufficient anatomical knowledge on the part of the acupuncturist. In the West, the commonest serious anatomical injury is pneumothorax. Needling anywhere over the chest wall, including a well-known classic site at the midpoint of the trapezius (Gall Bladder 21), can cause pneumothorax. This is an emergency but will not be fatal provided it is treated immediately. However, delay can cause death if there is a tension pneumothorax or if the patient is severely emphysematous and cannot survive on the function of the remaining lung.

About 5–8% of the population has an ossification defect in the lower sternum. This site corresponds to a traditional acupuncture point known as Conception Vessel 17 (Ren 17). Needle insertion here has penetrated the pericardium and damaged coronary vessels, leading to a leak of blood into the pericardium and consequent cardiac tamponade; this may easily be fatal. The defect cannot be diagnosed with certainty by either palpation or X-ray, so periosteal acupuncture should never be performed at this site.

Apart from these structures, acupuncture should avoid internal organs, major blood vessels, and major nerves but, while the location of these is known, smaller vessels and nerves may be damaged and this cannot be totally guarded against. The acupuncturist must therefore know how to deal with bleeding, whether capillary, venous, or arterial. Certain patients are at increased risk of bleeding; they include those taking warfarin or the newer anticoagulants and aspirin, as well as those suffering from bleeding disorders such as haemophilia.

Damage to small nerves may give rise to altered sensation but this usually passes off quite quickly—within 24 hours or sooner. Just occasionally, however, pain due to nerve damage is longer-lasting—possibly even for many months. Of course, such undesirable effects are not confined to the use of acupuncture needles but may follow needle insertion for any reason, such as intramuscular injection.

Acupuncture in pregnancy

Acupuncture in pregnancy appears to be safe (Elden et al. 2005; Wedenberg et al. 2000; Park et al. 2014). In the traditional system, certain points are said to be 'forbidden' in pregnancy because they may cause abortion, but there is little evidence that the risk is real. All kinds of treatment are best avoided if possible in pregnancy, but the risks from acupuncture are probably smaller than those associated with drugs.

The future of acupuncture

Acupuncture is often described as a form of complementary/alternative medicine (CAM), and this is natural given its origins. It is associated with the mysterious East, and with ancient wisdom that is generally said to go back thousands of years. The alternative view, on which this chapter is based, is that acupuncture is best thought of as a treatment that can be explained in neurophysiological terms. Viewed in this way, it ceases to be CAM and becomes another therapeutic modality that can be fully incorporated into modern practice. This idea is unwelcome to traditionalists but it seems to be a logical development that will have benefits for patients by making the treatment more widely available.

Modern acupuncture can be thought of by analogy with astronomy and chemistry. Both of these have their roots in pre-scientific ways of thinking; astronomy arose from astrology, and chemistry from alchemy, but we do not approach them from those standpoints today. Acupuncture is beginning to follow a similar path.

No doubt the ancient Chinese made many correct clinical observations, but they interpreted them according to a pre-scientific philosophical system. It is better to see it today in the context of science.

This shift in outlook is already under way. The change will not occur overnight and it will be resisted by traditionalists, but there is no good evidence to show that acupuncture done according to TCM theory is any more effective than the modern version. If the trend towards modernization continues, acupuncture will become detached from its traditional roots, which will come to be seen as of historical interest only. An important consequence of understanding acupuncture in this way is that learning it need not be a lengthy or difficult process, and it could be built into the standard training of many health professionals.

References

Baldry P. Management of myofascial trigger point pain. *Acupunct Med* 2002; 20(1):2–10.

Campbell A. Acupuncture: where to place the needles and for how long. *Acupunct Med* 1999; 17(2):113–7.

Campbell A. Seeing the body: a new mechanism for acupuncture analgesia? *Acupunct Med* 2013; 31(3):315–8

Churchill JM. *A treatise on acupuncturation*. Simpkins & Marshall, London, 1821.

Clement-Jones V, McLoughlin L, Tomlin S, et al. Increased beta-endorphin but not met-enkephalin levels in human cerebrospinal fluid after acupuncture for recurrent pain. *Lancet* 1980; 316:948–57.

Diener H-C, Kronfeld K, et al. Efficacy of acupuncture for the prophylaxis of migraine: a multicentre randomised controlled clinical trial. *Lancet Neurol* 1996; 5(4):31–316.

Elden H, Lasfors K, Olsen MF, et al. Effects of acupuncture and stabilising exercises as adjunct to standard treatment in pregnant women with pelvic girdle pain: a randomised controlled trial. *BMJ* 2005; 220(7494):761–6.

Goldman N, Cen M, Fujita T, et al. Adenosine A1 receptors mediate antinociceptive effects of acupuncture. *Nat Neurosci* 2010; 13:883–8.

Haake M, Müller, H-H, et al. German acupuncture trials (GERAC) for chronic low back pain: randomized, multicenter, blinded, parallel-group trial with 3 groups. *Arch Intern Med* 2007; 167(17): 1892–8.

Haggard P, Ianetti GD, Longo MR. Spatial sensory organization and body representation in pain perception. *Curr Biol* 2013; 23:164–76.

Hui KS, Liu J, Makris N, et al. Acupuncture modulates the limbic system and subcortical gray structures of the human brain. Evidence from fMRI studies in normal subjects. *Hum Brain Map* 2000; 9(1):13–25.

Kellgren JH. Observations on referred pain arising from muscle. *Clin Sci* 1938; 3:175–80.

Longo MR, Betti V, Agliotti SM, et al. Visually induced analgesia: seeing the body reduces pain. *J Neurosci* 2009; 30:12125–30.

Lund I, Lundeberg T. Are minimal, superficial or sham acupuncture procedures acceptable as inert placebo controls? *Acupunct Med* 2006; 24(1):13–15.

Mann F. *Reinventing acupuncture: a new concept of ancient medicine* (2nd edn). Butterworth-Heinemann, Oxford, 2000.

Mayer DJ, Price DD, Rafii A. Antagonism of acupuncture analgesia in man by the narcotic antagonist naloxone. *Brain Research* 1977; 121:368–72.

Melzack R, Wall PD. Pain mechanisms: a new theory. *Science* 1965; 150:171–9.

Park J, Youngioo S et al. The safety of acupuncture in pregnancy: a systematic review. Acup med 2014; 21:257–266.

Sandkühler J. Learning and memory in pain pathways. *Pain* 2000; 28(2):113–8.

Sandkühler J. Understanding LTP in pain pathways. *Mol Pain* 2007; 3:9.

Scharf H-P, Mansmann U, et al. Acupuncture and knee osteoarthritis: a three-armed randomized trial. *Ann Intern Med* 2006; 145(1):12–20.

Simons DG, Travell JG, Simons LS. Myofascial pain *and dysfunction: the trigger point manual. Vol. 1: upper half of the body* (2nd edn). Lippincott, Williams & Wilkins, Philadelphia, 1999.

Tough EA, White AR, et al. Acupuncture and dry needling in the management of trigger point pain: a systematic review and meta-analysis of randomised controlled trials. *Eur J Pain* 2009; 13:3–10

Tough EA, White AR, et al. Variability of criteria used to diagnose myofascial trigger point pain syndrome—evidence from a review of the literature. *Clin J Pain* 2007; 23(3):278.

Travell JG, Simons DG. *Myofascial pain and dysfunction: the trigger point manual. Vol.2: the lower extremities*. Lippincott, Williams & Wilkins, Philadelphia 1992.

Wedenberg K, Moen B, Norling A. A prospective randomized study comparing acupuncture with physiotherapy for low back pain and pelvic pain in pregnancy. *Acta Obstet Gynaecol Scand* 2000; 79(5):331–5.

White A. A cumulative overview of the range and incidence of significant adverse events associated with acupuncture. *Acupunct Med* 2004; 22(3):122–33.

White A. The safety of acupuncture—evidence from the UK. *Acupunct Med* 2006; 24(Suppl):S53–S57.

White A, Cummings M, Filshie J. An introduction to Western medical acupuncture. Churchill Livingstone (Elsevier), 2008. Edinburgh, London, New York, Oxford, Philadelphia, St Louis, Sydney Toronto.

White AR, Hayhoe S, et al. Adverse events following acupuncture: prospective survey of 32,000 consultations with doctors and physiotherapists. *BMJ* 2001; 323:485.

Chapter 60

A pragmatic management strategy for low back pain—an integrated multimodal programme based on antidysfunctional medicine

Stefan Blomberg

Introduction to the STAYAC model of low back pain management

The *biopsychosocial model* (Waddell 1998) was an important move towards improved pain care. However, from the perspective of the extremely important somatically focused dysfunction theory,it is unfortunate that the 'bio-' prefix is so closely associated with the structural/pathomorphological paradigm. Patients with dysfunctional conditions certainly constitute the largest group of pain sufferers to which this paradigm should be applied. Moreover, possibly aside from purely psycho-existentially based conditions in which pain is not a feature, dysfunctional pain causes more suffering in the population than any other medical state and, from a societal perspective, it is also the most costly pain condition. This is especially true in primary healthcare settings, although it is a significant problem in many other disciplines too.

Furthermore, the existential dimension of pain suffering—an issue associated with obvious clinical consequences for the management of pain patients—is severely underestimated. It is unfortunate that the term 'bio-dysfunctio-psycho-socio-existential paradigm' is so cumbersome, as it accurately reflects the essence of the proposed STAYAC model for pain management.

The aim of this chapter is to interest the reader in the successful treatment results at the Stockholm Clinic—Stay Active (STAYAC). The therapeutic model includes manual therapy, steroid injections, muscle stretching, medical exercise therapy, traction modalities, and prolotherapy, closely incorporated in a cognitive behavioural and psychotherapeutic approach. The following constitute the key issues of the STAYAC method.

- *Profound pragmatism*. Since the real cause of (e.g. back) pain is rarely known, it is impossible to design high-precision target-based diagnostic measures as well as target-based treatment methods with an outcome that is satisfactorily predictable—all diagnostic measures have insufficient specificity, sensitivity, reliability, and validity. Consequently, it is impossible to satisfactorily identify in advance those patients who will respond to a specific single technique. This problem can only be resolved by pragmatic treatment/rehabilitation approaches, together with the recognition that pragmatism in this context is ultimately a recognition of the fact that diagnostic measures are insufficiently precise.
- A truly *eclectic* approach.
- *Metacognitive processes*, i.e. the therapists' continuous review of their own thought processes, attitudes, and beliefs.
- *Dysfunction theory*, including the concept of markers of dysfunction ('green flags') and *antidysfunctional therapy/medicine*. With regard to the nature of dysfunction, and the beneficial effects achieved by manual therapy, the underlying theoretical models are adapted to modern rationales, supported by recent neurophysiological research; mechanically oriented theories are rejected, and terms such as 'locking', 'blockage', 'subluxation', 'hypermobility', 'instability', and 'micro-instability' are abandoned.
- *Manual therapy* is a fundamental part of the algorithm, regardless of the duration of the symptoms, even after years of severe suffering. Manual techniques range from forceful thrust techniques, in which the 'traditional' Scandinavian concept of locking is aimed at directing the therapeutic forces exclusively to the dysfunctional segment (in which muscle energy therapeutic principles are integrated), to extremely gentle techniques in which 'pure' muscle energy principles are applied.
- Dysfunctional conditions are *treatable*, in spite of coexistent major pathomorphology such as clinically relevant herniated discs,

spinal stenosis, spondylolisthesis, and neighbouring acute compression fractures. Numerous 'classical' contraindications for manual therapy are abolished.

- *Evidence-based steroid injections* are included as one of the major treatment modalities in dysfunction-free states. Of these, the *parasacrococcygeal injection* is unique, extremely potent, and one of the most important items in the treatment arsenal.
- The concept of *hyper-reactivity*, with essential clinical implications, is introduced.
- Specified indications for *prolotherapy* are outlined, increasing the efficacy of the method.
- It is proposed that manual therapy/medicine relies largely on systemized *palpatory illusions*—a manageable, not a major problem, but one with important clinical implications.
- New pragmatic indications for the use of *antidepressants* are proposed. The benefits of high dosage are considered.
- *Antidysfunctional investigation* is undertaken over time.
- The *'ex juvantibus' diagnostic principle* (for explanation see 'Idiopathic pain—*ex juvantibus* diagnosis' in the section 'A macro-perspective of the algorithm') is consistently and systematically applied in virtually all patients.
- A new, structured *classification process* is utilized.
- Therapies are *combined* and a unique, *integrated approach* is shared by all members of the staff: receptionists, nurses, physiotherapists, behaviourists, psychologists/licensed psychotherapists, psychiatrists, physicians, etc. The ambition is to combine all evidence-based and empirically supported specific treatment modalities, and therefore potentially valuable therapeutic contributions, in a common concept, i.e. everything from psychoanalysis to fusion surgery, with manual therapy and steroid injections in between (the ultimate *'black box' concept*).
- *The stay-active concept is paramount.* There is a powerful synergy in applying the stay-active approach and antidysfunctional treatments in parallel, in a systematic, consistent, and integrated manner. The stay-active concept is not merely a matter of encouraging patients to increase activity simply by providing advice and prescribing physical exercise; another aspect, at least as important, is the effectiveness of the stay-active approach as a metacognitive method. Stay-active messages are conveyed while passive treatment, such as manipulation, is provided to the patients.
- The structured management protocol is aided by cost-effective routes of communication, with the aim of limiting the risk that patients remain at sub-optimal levels for long periods of time, and reducing the likelihood that treatment possibilities are missed.
- The *evidence-based integrated algorithm* for pain management encompasses both specific and non-specific categories of pain with confounding/contributing psycho-existential, social factors and other 'non-medical rehabilitation impediments'. Somatically focused treatment is utilized initially, usually as the first step in the 'antidysfunctional investigation', i.e. before psycho-existential and related moves are taken, thereby, through the '*Kierkegaard effect*', generating a therapeutic alliance between patient and clinician. The 'Kierkegaard effect' prepares the patient for psychosocial measures, which are applied later during the antidysfunctional investigation, only when indicated and when the patient is receptive for such procedures. This is true for more or less all pain patients regardless of genesis, duration, localization, and character of the symptoms. Consequently, the patients are offered a true 'somatic chance', i.e. the 'Kierkegaard effect'.
- Potent synergistic effects are achieved from the integrated approach of antidysfunctional medicine, with manual therapy as its core, and cognitive–behavioural therapy. The 'bone setter'/the manual therapist and the (cognitive) behavioural therapist are the same person, with the advantage that manual treatment may be replaced in appropriate patients by behavioural strategies, applied by the same therapist.
- '*Patient education*' is a new methodology within STAYAC, with the aim of minimizing the consequences of persisting symptoms; modifying beliefs, attitudes, fears, catastrophizing behaviour; and improving sense of coherence (Antonovsky 1987) and coping skills. It takes the form of interactive cognitive group therapy. The authority of the 'lecturing' physician (and also the behavioural therapist) is strengthened during the antidysfunctional investigation. Circumstances are created in which the patients are much less hesitant to discuss sensitive topics such as 'long-term sick leave illness', the stay-active concept, primary benefits, secondary benefits, basic crisis psychology, insufficient coping abilities, fear avoidance, catastrophizing, insufficient sense of coherence, pain behaviour, the pain-patient role, identity loss, development of pain identity, and life lies. One could say that patient education is a qualified and powerful mode of '*mental manipulation*'.
- *New psychological perspectives* with respect to the interaction between psycho-existential/social factors/other non-medical rehabilitation obstacles and the patients' pain and suffering are identified ('the third perspective'), with important clinical implications; three different basic perspectives are defined. In the STAYAC psychological paradigm, the denial of psycho-existential dimensions of pain suffering is considered to be the principal interfering psychological factor in pain syndromes. In the analyses of the patients' psycho-existential status, psychodynamic dimensions of their suffering are considered ('cognitive therapy with psychodynamic overtones').
- *The pain is virtually always regarded as nociceptive*, and only rarely of pure psychological origin. A model (the 'third perspective') is promoted, in which the pain is frequently 'used' by the patients to control and to facilitate repression of denied psycho-existential crises, which are externalized outside their own responsibility and control, as are the responsibility and control of their condition and their recovery. In the 'third perspective', unsatisfactory psycho-existential/social status of the patient at the onset of pain may induce inadequate consequences from the pain.
- The overriding objective of providing manual therapy initially, in advanced chronic perception-disturbed pain patients, is to create a *trusting doctor–patient relationship* and a satisfactory therapeutic basis for strategies based on psychodynamic theories, aiming at behavioural changes, improved coping strategies, and limited adverse consequences of the chronic pain. The initial manual therapy and steroid injections in the most severe cases is more or less a *ritual* ('The Kierkegaard effect' again)

to achieve these psychological effects, and to establish a long-standing therapeutic alliance—decreasing the patients' complaints by the treatment, from a physical perspective, is really not paramount. This way of utilizing manual therapy, with these premeditated intentions, has, as far as I know, not so far been described in the literature.

- Although patients with severe chronic pain frequently lack psychological awareness of important underlying factors such as their beliefs, attitudes, and behaviour, short-term psychotherapy is frequently very successful. The fundamental reason is that, from the patients' perspective, the primary problem, namely *their pain, is addressed throughout* (the 'Kierkegaard effect' again).
- *Patience* is necessary. We 'give up' extremely rarely. Within the described concept, there is virtually always another move to be taken when one measure has failed; even when pain is therapy-resistant, the patients' life situations are habitually brought under control. In advanced cases, several *parallel processes* may be undertaken (for example by the physician, psychiatrist, psychotherapist—one physiotherapist providing manual therapy; another, physical exercise; and a third, acupuncture). Intense communication between the therapists creates confidence and accelerates progress; and patient anxiety, by being referred to one therapist after another, in one clinic after another, is avoided.
- As a 'spin-off' effect, knowledge of the STAYAC model and its benefits improves professional confidence, thereby affecting the treatment results positively. In an optimal situation, all therapists in the team attend individual psychotherapy and receive tuition in psychotherapy.
- In conclusion, not only is a new somatically focused therapeutic paradigm presented, but a new psychological paradigm is introduced as well (or at least two new important Kuhnian, pre-paradigmatic phenomena; Kuhn 1962). The ultimate challenge is to manage unmotivated, psychologically unaware, and perception-disturbed chronic pain patients.

These key issues form the basis for the algorithm on which this chapter focuses (Figure 60.1).

Low back pain: background, evidence-based medicine, clinical trials, and literature reviews

Since the first edition of this textbook in 2005, the medical literature, including epidemiology, relevant to the contents of this chapter, has remained basically reliable. In developed countries, the incidence of acute low back pain requiring sick leave of 1 week or more is extremely high (80% according to Nachemson and Jonsson 2000). Although low back pain is usually self-limiting (most patients recover within weeks), it is a major diagnostic and therapeutic problem causing much suffering and large costs to the community (Nachemson and Jonsson 2000). Treatment has traditionally been conservative, consisting mainly of medication, prolonged bed rest, and the use of spinal supports. This passive regimen has been extensively criticized (Nachemson and Jonsson 2000), but scientific support for the use of virtually all alternative treatment modalities has been considered to be insufficient (Nachemson et al. 1991). Nachemson et al. concluded that, apart from surgery in a minority of patients with herniated discs, the treatment of non-specific low back pain was not a concern of medical care. The authors stated that the consequences of low back pain were exclusively related to lifestyle conditions, social factors, circumstances at work, smoking habits, and so forth, not to the access to treatment.

For centuries, physicians have been expected to work according to the Galenic principle or Hippocratic oath, i.e. empirical observations (experience) and sound scientific principles. However, over time, scientific society has realized that experience cannot always be trusted; many firmly established therapeutic traditions have been shown not to fulfil expectations of efficacy, when evaluated according to rigorous rules. Consequently, since the late 1980s, the era of 'evidence-based medicine' has emerged. The therapeutic society, especially when financed by the state, is expected to prioritize medical methods that are demonstrated to be effective in randomized controlled trials (RCTs). In addition, the governmentally supported methods have to be cost-effective (see also Chapter 3). A consequence of this is that the number of published RCTs increased exponentially during the 1990s and physicians have subsequently had to rely on literature reviews performed by 'evidence-based medicine institutes' such as the Cochrane Collaboration, the Rand Institute, and the SBU (Swedish Council on Technology Assessment in Health Care). These institutes have an extremely important assignment—their reports have to be accurate, trustworthy, and unbiased.

Approximately 55 RCTs on manual therapy have been published since 1956. In the studies, as well as in the literature reviews, conclusions with respect to efficacy of treatment are contradictory. The complexity of this area is reflected by the fact that there are more literature reviews published within this field than RCTs. Two of the reasons for this extreme inconsistency in conclusions are the lack of a consensus concerning reviewing methodology and the inappropriateness of both study designs and reviewing methods.

My thesis (Blomberg 1993a) includes a 44-page systematic review in which I concluded that manipulation was effective only in acute and subacute low back pain patients without radiating pain (Farrell and Twomey 1982; Fisk 1979; Hadler et al. 1987; Nwuga 1982; Rasmussen 1979; Wreje et al. 1992). In my opinion, with respect to evidence, the additional studies published since then have strengthened the position of manual therapy to a modest degree in acute neck pain and cervicogenic headache (Hoving 2002; Jull et al. 2002) and in chronic low back pain (Aure et al. 2003). Koes et al. (1992a,b,c) claim positive results achieved by manipulation in chronic patients, but the results should be considered to be inconclusive in view of flaws in reviewing methods and bias (Blomberg 1993a, pp. 28–9, 50–2). With respect to thoracic pain, low back pain with radiating pain, and chronic neck pain, there is still no evidence for the use of manual therapy. Bronfort et al. (2001) detected benefit from combined spinal manipulation and exercise for patients with chronic neck pain, but it was exercise that was evaluated by comparison with another group. This contradicts the published major literature reviews (see the following) but, in due course, results will be published by the group I am working with that support the long-term efficacy of manual therapy in conjunction with steroid injections in acute, subacute, and chronic low back pain patients, plus corresponding data in a short-term study (10 weeks) of acute/subacute low back pain with radiating pain (Blomberg et al. 2005a,b,c).

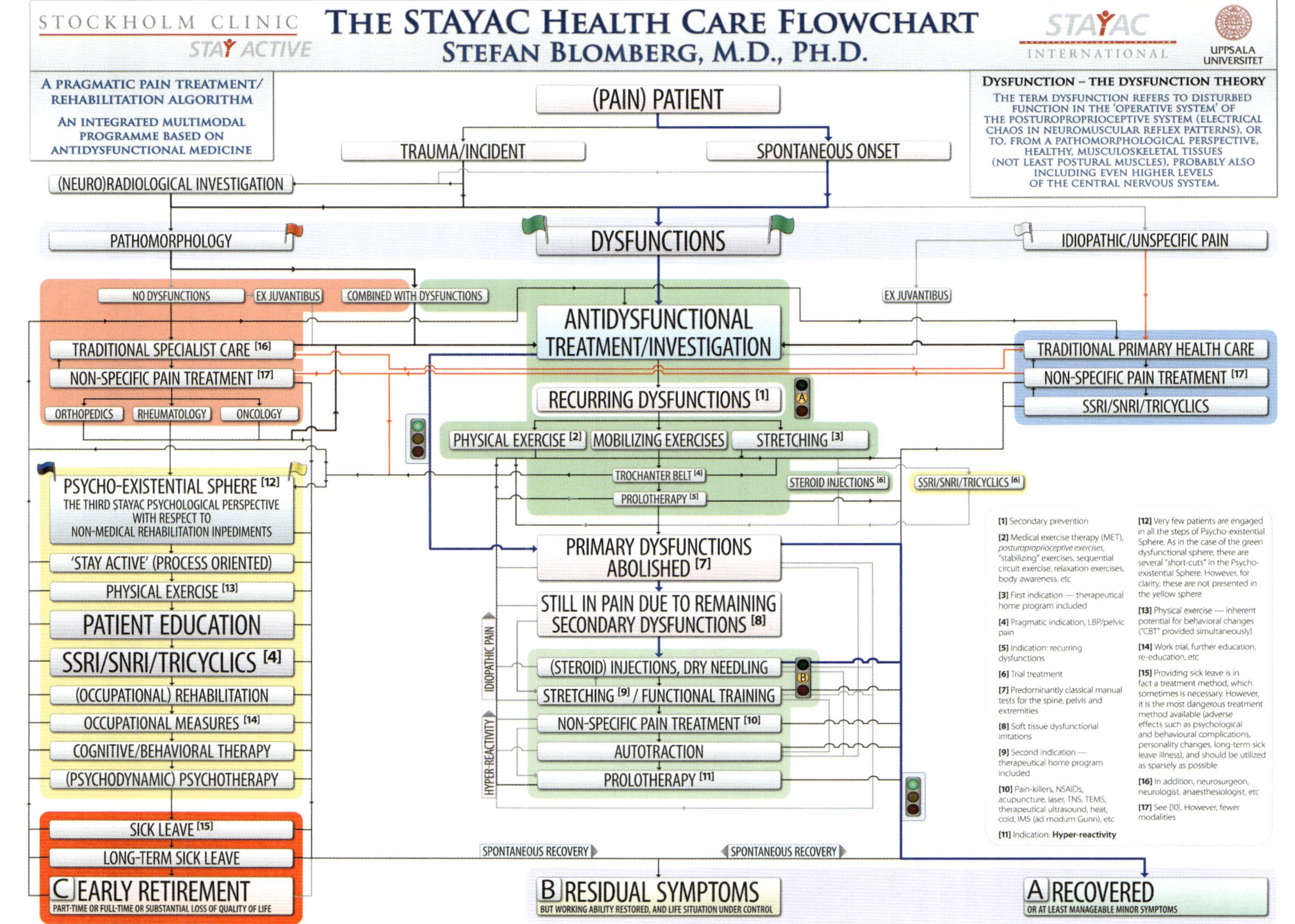

Figure 60.1 The STAYAC algorithm. (A larger coloured version of the algorithm is found on STAYAC's website, <http://www.stockholmclinic.se>. Printed and laminated copies are also available for those using the algorithm in clinical practice.) The patients 'start' at the top of the flowchart and there are three possible outcomes at the bottom of the scheme—no symptoms, or fully controllable minor symptoms, 'recovered'; residual symptoms reducing some aspect(s) of quality of life and/or some daily activities to some degree; long-term sick leave or early retirement or a substantial loss of quality of life. In between the top and the bottom, there are five different domains: • The 'specialist' sphere (upper left, red); • The 'general healthcare' area (upper right, blue); • The 'psycho-existential' sphere (left, yellow); • The 'antidysfunctional' domain: 'Yellow light A situation' (upper middle, darker green); • The 'antidysfunctional' domain: 'Yellow light B situation' (lower middle, lighter green). The flows between the different spheres and boxes are described in the text. Apart from the standard arrows, there are three different special arrows: • Grey lines: less usual flows; • Red lines: common, however unwelcome in a well-developed algorithm; • Thicker blue lines: most common flows. Thicker line = more common the flow; thinner line = less utilized flow. The flowchart is, in fact, designed as a 'street map': the arrows indicate the 'street'/line in question is a one-way 'street'; the 'streets' without arrows can be 'driven' in both directions. However, with respect to the latter, for simplicity, there are 'streets' without arrows that are actually one-way 'streets'—in these cases, it is obvious that only 'driving' in one direction is possible and logical.

It is apparent that several high-quality studies on the use of manual therapy/manipulation have commenced during recent years; hence, the evidence for manual therapy/manipulation may become stronger in future years.

In recent literature reviews, produced by different evidence-based medical institutes, there is a clear trend for an increasing number of manual therapies to be identified as effective (Bronfort et al. 2004; Harms-Ringdahl et al. 1999; Nachemson and Jonsson 2000; van Tulder et al. 1996). By contrast, in a meta-analysis of manipulation and low back pain, Assendelft et al. (2003) concluded that 'there is no evidence that spinal manipulative therapy is superior to other standard treatments for patients with acute or chronic low-back pain'. (The meta-analytical approach has deep flaws when attempting to compare a variety of therapeutic approaches.) The stay-active concept is generally acknowledged as the basic treatment approach of choice for non-specific low back pain. In addition, measures such as physical exercise, analgesics, non-steroidal anti-inflammatories (NSAIDs), manual therapy, behavioural therapy, and multidisciplinary treatment programmes are recommended, provided their respective indications and contraindications are considered.

A further consideration is that not all of these identified treatment strategies are shown to be effective in patients suffering from acute, subacute, and chronic neck or back pain. Nevertheless, it is obvious that the existence of a large variety of evidence-based and non-evidence-based treatment methods for back pain has not solved this enormous societal problem. Virtually all modes of treatment are available in Stockholm, for example, but nevertheless, the problem is expanding more rapidly than ever, not least from a cost perspective. Why is that? This chapter attempts to answer this question and offers an approach to management of spinal pain, and other localized or generalized pain, which is both evidence-based and pragmatic.

Gordon Waddell (1998) approached this problem in his thought-provoking and trail-blazing book *The back pain revolution*. He claims that (primarily) the physicians, but also their healthcare colleagues such as physiotherapists, chiropractors, and osteopaths, actually created the Western back pain problem: 'Back pain, the medical disaster of the 20th century'. Of course, he does not mean back pain *per se*; he is referring to the unreasonable consequences of back pain. He claims that epidemiological research demonstrates that the severity and prevalence of back pain is more or less the same in all countries in the world (Anderson 1984; Hoy et al. 2003; Wigley et al. 1994). Waddell blames the biomedical paradigm for far-reaching negative consequences in developed countries.

This paradigm has been extremely successful in numerous other medical fields, but it offers no solution to back pain patients except in a very few cases (see also Chapter 1). A simplistic and pathomorphologically based paradigm was foisted not only on everyone with an interest in back pain management, but also on society in general. Waddell formulates the problem brilliantly; unfortunately, he does not offer a genuine solution to it. In spite of being more complete than the biomedical paradigm, the biopsychosocial model does not, in my opinion, cover the entire problem complex either. I hope that this chapter will direct the reader, and in due course, also healthcare in general, towards a solution of the problem.

All hitherto published systematic literature reviews apply a dichotomized system in which diverse treatments are listed exclusively as 'effective' or 'not effective'. However, apart from the classification of patients suffering from neck pain or low back pain, and division into acute/subacute versus chronic complaints, there have been no attempts to evaluate which therapies are effective in which patients, and during which periods of their 'sickness career'. Furthermore, virtually nothing is known about the effectiveness of different therapies with respect to specified efficacy variables, or about the next cost-effective move through the chain of therapy when a certain therapeutic modality has failed. Moreover, the efficacy of certain therapies is not analysed hierarchically, despite the obvious fact that, although two different therapies may indeed be effective in a defined patient group, one therapy may be substantially more powerful than the other. In addition, questions have to be asked regarding which combinations of treatment methods are useful.

Although no algorithms are to be found in the evidence-based medicine literature, they have been published in different consensus reports, in which some components are evidence-based, while others are supported by 'best available evidence' or by experience, treatment traditions, and common sense (ACC 1997; AHCPR 1994; CSAG 1994; Kendall et al. 1997; RCGP 1996; Waddell 1998). However, all these algorithms are incomplete with respect to important aspects of (back) pain management, not least regarding manual therapy and other factors emanating from the dysfunction theory. Consequently, there is a need for a new, more comprehensive and inclusive algorithm.

Pragmatic treatment approach to low back pain

Why pragmatic treatment approaches?

One reason for the lack of more specific data in current literature reviews is obvious—the information extracted from the pool of RCTs is insufficient. The required research has hardly begun, and the research field that emerges when these perspectives are considered is huge.

The real cause of back pain is rarely known (Nachemson and Jonsson 2000). Consequently, in 'non-specific' (back) pain, it is impossible today to design high-precision target-based diagnostic measures as well as target-based treatment methods with an outcome that is satisfactorily predictable. This is why all diagnostic measures have insufficient specificity, sensitivity, reliability, and validity, especially at an individual level, but also at group level. Different diagnostic instruments, including those with behavioural or psychological orientation, diagnostic imaging, laboratory tests, and clinical tests, are indeed valuable at a group level in RCTs, and in clinical epidemiological research, but their precision for the purpose of predicting treatment outcome of a specific therapy, particularly for the individual patient, is unsatisfactory. When a patient is examined manually, something tangible is being palpated. However, something other than what is believed is being palpated. In addition, it is likely that benefits accrue during manual treatment for more complex reasons than are usually believed. Consequently, manual therapy/medicine may, to a large extent, rely on *systemized palpatory illusions*. However, this is academic as long as the treatment proves to be beneficial to the patients and cost-effective in conclusive RCTs, while we are waiting for the true explanations for the underlying mechanisms, achieved by experimental research;

evidence-based and cost-effective treatment models should be implemented in pain management even though they may be founded on incorrect theoretical models.

In conclusion, it is impossible to satisfactorily identify in advance those patients who will respond to a specific single technique. As long as we do not know the true cause of most low back pain, *this problem can only be addressed by pragmatic treatment approaches*. The essence of pragmatic treatment models is ultimately a recognition of the fact that diagnostic measures are insufficiently precise.

Why pragmatic trials?

In the context of RCTs, whatever measures are taken to select a patient group supposed to be susceptible to a specific treatment, the selected population will always contain a substantial subgroup of non-responders to the treatment in question. This may, in turn, seriously limit the power of the study, and may make it virtually impossible to detect the positive effects of a truly effective single treatment modality. Consequently, when conducting RCTs in this field, there is a need for pragmatic studies, in which there is a flexibility to change treatment modality when the treatment response is poor, as a result of the insufficient precision in predicting treatment response to a certain treatment modality in the individual patient. The choice of therapies and the number of visits is determined by the provisional/working diagnosis and the response to treatment at each visit.

Clinical trials using such approaches analyse the effect of a system of care, not the effect of single therapies or components of single therapies extracted from a complete treatment programme. In a pragmatic study, a multimodal therapeutic arsenal is utilized where the therapists are free to choose from the different treatment modalities according to need, after having assessed the patients at each consultation—the type, frequency, and duration of the treatment are at the discretion of the therapist, based on the patient's response. The treatment at each consultation is based on a functional diagnosis which, in turn, generates a treatment hypothesis. This hypothesis is either confirmed or rejected at the subsequent consultation, depending on the treatment response—the treatment hypothesis may have to be reconsidered and, consequently, the treatment strategy may be changed. The unravelling of structural (i.e. pathomorphological), social, psycho-existential, or dysfunctional factors associated with the patients' suffering is a process over time, i.e. a mapping procedure (see 'The antidysfunctional investigation' and 'Idiopathic pain—*ex juvantibus* diagnosis' in the section 'A macro-perspective of the algorithm').

In conclusion, a true pragmatic system for investigation and treatment is a process of consistent and systematic *ex juvantibus* diagnosis. Consequently, recurrences are treated throughout the course of a pragmatic study, thereby allowing as many treatment sessions as are considered necessary. Thus, the termination of the therapy is based on the patients' needs rather than on a rigid schematic study protocol, and the design of the intervention is aiming at emulating clinical reality. Considering the difficulty of predicting the treatment outcome of single 'fastidious' therapies, it is reasonable to postulate that the different items of a pragmatic treatment arsenal do not merely have additive effects but, rather, that they have 'synergistic' effects. This statement is substantiated by the results of our group's studies (see the following), and it is discussed more extensively in my thesis (Blomberg 1993a, pp. 122–7), and by Blomberg et al. (1994a).

Pragmatic trials are of the most immediate interest to the patients. However, this type of trial has a disadvantage: if one treatment is more successful than another, it may be difficult to identify which item in the therapeutic arsenal is responsible for the positive effects.

Fastidious trials—shortcomings and advantages

In rigorous 'fastidious' trials, all conditions are the same in both groups, except for one variable: a patient-blinded active treatment versus placebo. Optimally, a fastidious trial answers only one question. There are three major blinding possibilities: the patient, the physician, and the evaluator. Thus, in pharmacology, the term 'triple-blind design' would be more accurate than 'double-blind'. However, within the field of manual therapy, only two of these blinding possibilities are achievable: the evaluator and the patient. (A standardized therapeutic manoeuvre may be compared with a similar placebo treatment—with this design, the patient should not be able to distinguish whether or not they received active treatment.) Consequently, fastidious double-blind evaluations of specific components extracted from a complete (pragmatic) treatment programme are possible.

In pragmatic studies, only one blinding possibility is reasonable—the blinded evaluator. Consequently, these are open, observer-blinded studies. Fortunately, today, such designs are accepted, and are frequently found in the indexed journals. For many years, pragmatic studies were significantly more difficult to publish than fastidious trials; to a certain extent, this is still the case. In the literature, there are a couple of examples of trials (Bergquist-Ullman and Larsson 1977; Sloop et al. 1982) in which efforts have been undertaken to blind the patients. However, these study designs are very artificial.

In fastidious trials, the type, frequency, and duration of the treatment are strictly standardized in the study protocol, and equal in both groups—recurrences are not treated after the termination of the standardized treatment course. However, one of the important drawbacks is the obvious risk that fastidious trials of single therapies do not reveal detectable effects in controllable sample sizes. In addition, single treatments are of minor interest to the patients which, in turn, creates substantial risks of high drop-out rates, especially in long-term trials. Moreover, the results of single therapies may have only limited clinical applicability. Furthermore, using sham therapies as control intervention leads to methodological difficulties and ethical predicaments, and is far from clinical reality. Nevertheless, fastidious studies are necessary.

A pragmatic design is an advantageous first step in evaluating treatment programmes. If no differences in outcome between the groups in such a study are detected, the evaluation of the single items is of limited interest. Fastidious trials are needed to answer questions generated by pragmatic studies, such as the evaluation of separate treatment modalities extracted from a complete treatment programme. If a pragmatic management algorithm is shown to be effective, further similar, but less pragmatic research will evaluate the importance of additions or elimination of certain treatment modalities, changing of paths through the chain of therapy, alterations of indications within the scheme, measures to optimize cost effectiveness, and so forth. The subsequent studies may apply less pragmatic and more fastidious designs. However, in the subsequent research, it is important to consider the possible synergistic effects of a multimodal treatment programme—it may even be the case that long-term effects can only be detected in broad pragmatic treatment models (Blomberg 1993a, pp. 122–7), or possibly in treatment programmes that change the patients' beliefs and attitudes in a fundamental manner (Blomberg 1993a, p. 118). The longer the follow-up, the more valid is this statement. Moreover, it is reasonable to consider pragmatic studies more ethically acceptable for RCTs in the field of low back pain than fastidious studies.

If a pragmatic multimodal algorithm provides long-term efficacy in a pragmatic RCT, short-term effects achieved by the isolated items of the management in question in fastidious trials are sufficient; their possible contributions to the long-term effects in the evaluation of the entire concept have to rely on assumptions.

Scientific basis of the STAYAC management strategy for low back pain

There is evidence from two major studies of acute and subacute low back pain that a pragmatic approach incorporating a range of therapies is more effective than traditional care with respect to pain, disability, mobility, sick leave, general (psychosomatic) symptoms, quality of life, and costs.

The original study and the partial cross-over study

In my thesis (Blomberg 1993a, based on five papers: Blomberg et al. 1992, 1993a,b, 1994a, Blomberg et al. 1994b), it was demonstrated that a new pragmatic treatment of low back pain was superior to standardized and optimized conventional activity-based treatment by primary healthcare teams—the stay-active concept (Waddell 1998). The latter approach was the basic management in the experimental group also, but with the addition of a pragmatic multimodal treatment regime. The main items added were manipulation, specific mobilization, steroid injections, muscle stretching, and autotraction. After 1 month of follow-up, the proportion of patients on sick leave was six times larger in the conventionally treated group than in the experimental group. Furthermore, the 4-month follow-up showed considerable differences, again favouring the experimental group, in the two pain scores and the 15 disability rating scores. Moreover, measurements of mobility and movements causing pain, as well as the results of quality of life measurements and the presence of general symptoms of a psychosomatic character, favoured the experimental intervention. Pain drawings also showed substantial differences favouring the experimental group (Grunnesjö et al. 2005a,b).

The paper by Blomberg et al. (1992) provides the first indication in the literature of sick leave reduction (at 8 months) achieved by manual therapy. A 3-year follow-up showed that the reduction of sick leave in the experimental group remained (Bogefeldt et al. 2005a). In addition, the disability rating scores, followed for 2 years, indicated beneficial long-term effects as well. Such short- and long-term effects achieved by the pragmatic method in a population with chronic low back pain were also evident in a controlled partial cross-over study of 'failures' from the control group of the original study (Bogefeldt et al. 2005b).

The reproducibility study

Because of the pragmatic design of the first trial, it was not possible to draw firm conclusions about which items in the therapeutic arsenal were responsible for the positive effects. Consequently, a reproducibility study, with basically the same pragmatic design as the original study but with randomization to four groups, was undertaken to evaluate, separately, some of the components of the complete treatment arsenal. The results were consistent and basically similar to the results of the original study, so it was concluded that the second study was a successful replication of the original study (Blomberg et al. 2005a,b,c; Bogefeldt et al. 2004a,b; Grunnesjö et al. 2004a, 2005). Consequently, the pragmatic treatment programme can be communicated to other physicians and physiotherapists. In addition, the pragmatic concept, in combination with steroid injections, was shown to be superior to the corresponding treatment programme without steroid injections.

In our studies, not only do the differences favour the experimental treatment more substantially (even at 3 days) when compared with other RCT-evaluated treatment strategies, but the experimental intervention was also substantially less costly than standardized traditional management based on the stay-active concept within primary healthcare (the original study) and orthopaedic care (our reproducibility study). In addition, since it was shown that the population studied in the second trial was representative of the most severely affected acute/subacute low back pain patients (Bogefeldt et al. 2004b), the results should be valid in other acute/subacute low back pain populations too. Long-term effects were indicated by the fact that many differences in outcomes between the two groups in both studies increased over time (Blomberg et al. 1993a,b), and by the persisting differences in favour of the experimental treatment in the long-term follow-up in the original study and in the partial cross-over study. The treatment programme is one of the few to be reproduced in two subsequent trials according to a state of the art procedure.

In terms of cost effectiveness and long-term effects in an non-randomized group of patients with chronic low back pain, McGuirk et al. (2001) published their study of rural clinics. In this study, doctors who had post-graduate training in musculoskeletal medicine and who agreed to abide by evidence-based guidelines were compared with usual general healthcare with referral to physiotherapy or specialist if requested. There was less use of physiotherapy and opioid medication in the experimental group.

Behavioural aspects of manual therapy for low back pain

When undertaken sensibly, manual therapy is a suitable starting point and a good basis for a trustful patient–doctor relationship, a 'therapeutic alliance'. Unfortunately, excessive belief in manual therapy as a universal method, where the therapist holds (often subconsciously) that all pain problems can be solved by manual therapy, provided the therapist is skilful enough, is not uncommon. This attitude, often resulting in endless courses of passive treatment, may jeopardize the rehabilitation of the chronic 'perception-disturbed' patient by retaining or reinforcing their pain behaviour and the pain-patient role. It is crucial to prevent this, for example, by broadening and improving the education in manual therapy, and by explaining to patients the basis, purpose, and scope of manual therapy.

Nevertheless, it is important to emphasize that it is possible to *incorporate modern behavioural therapeutic thinking into manual therapy*: the two approaches are definitely compatible. Once pathomorphological changes relevant to the symptoms have been ruled out (such as herniated disc, fractures, tumours, inflammatory disorders—altogether less than 5% of the patients; Nachemson and Jonsson 2000), it is essential that all patients presenting with symptoms that may be associated with the locomotor system are subjected to examination with the aim of identifying dysfunctions treatable with manual therapy. This should be done before measures based on socio-psychological/psycho-existential considerations are undertaken. However, it is crucially important for the therapist to realize early when no further progress by manual therapy is possible. This is the point where psycho-existential factors must be taken into consideration.

I regularly meet chronic perception-disturbed pain patients whom I realize, during the first consultation, I will most probably not be able to help with manual therapy in a somatic sense. Despite this, I start by giving a short course (2–4 sessions) of manual treatment and/or steroid injections to give the patient a 'somatic chance', and to create a therapeutic alliance. In these patients, management from the beginning by physiotherapists trained in the stay-active concept parallels the investigation, over time, by the responsible physician, and a psychotherapist or psychiatrist may be included in the process early as well: the therapists communicate continuously and closely with each other. A small minority of these patients are treatable with antidysfunctional therapy alone, and since it is more or less impossible to predict these rare positive treatment responses, the only approach that avoids missing them is to perform the antidysfunctional investigation on all individuals in this patient category, regardless of severity and duration of pain.

Since the antidysfunctional treatment, once learned, is virtually free of additional costs, and since the associated risks are almost negligible (Nachemson and Jonsson 2000), this pragmatic approach is reasonable. However, the overriding objective of this process is to create a trusting doctor–patient therapeutic alliance and a satisfactory therapeutic basis for strategies aiming at behavioural changes, improved coping strategies, and limiting the consequences of the chronic pain. This is achieved through subliminal communication and through transference/counter-transference mechanisms according to psychodynamic theories, sometimes in explicit verbal terms. Furthermore, often subconsciously, the patients are also made aware that it is pointless to rely on a chiropractor or other therapist providing manual therapy or other somatically focused therapies.

Initial manual therapy and steroid injections are, in the most severe cases, more or less a ritual (the 'Kiekegaard effect', see the following) to achieve the desired psychological effects and to establish a long-standing therapeutic alliance—decreasing the patients' complaints by the treatment, from a physical perspective, is not paramount, even if it is extremely satisfying for the therapist in the few cases when it happens. This way of utilizing manual therapy, with these premeditated intentions, has, as far as I know, not hitherto been described in the literature, even if some therapists may do this to some degree, at least subconsciously.

The '*Kierkegaard effect*' (or, based on my understanding of him, I would suggest the '*postulate of Kierkegaard*') is highly applicable in and relevant for healthcare, not least in pain management. In my opinion, the following quotation from one of Kierkegaard's most famous texts (*The art of helping*) describes beautifully the roots of pain care failures, and identifies one of the most problematic system errors in healthcare today:

> If one is truly to succeed in guiding a person in a specific direction, one must first and foremost take care to find him where he is and begin there.
>
> This is the secret in the entire art of helping. Anyone who cannot do this is himself under a delusion if he thinks he is able to help someone else. In order truly to help someone else, I must understand more than he—but certainly first and foremost understand what he understands. If I do not do that, then my greatest understanding does not help him at all.

The pain experienced by patients is of course not experienced by the clinician whose traditional treatment or management of the symptoms is therefore based on manual investigation, manual treatment (carefully, through process-oriented, conscious, and thoroughly developed metacognitive abilities/skills, to avoid open or subliminal 'stay passive messages'), steroid injections, and so forth. These combined strategies represent the very core of antidysfunctional medicine, even if this field also includes all other reasonable pain management elements, not least psychological and behavioural dimensions, in a conceptualized unity. A premature attempted but inadequate psychological assessment of the pain patient's life situation, without a full understanding of his or her pain, is extremely common within traditional pain care. By breaking the 'postulate of Kierkegaard', dangerous nocebo factors are created, 'burying' the hurt, and placing the aggrieved and offended patient in a worse situation than he or she was in before the failed pain management.

Under the described circumstances, I radically revise my therapeutic attitude; the 'bonesetter' identity is left behind and cognitive–behavioural therapeutic principles are applied instead. Frequently, I never touch the patient again, and the continuing management focuses exclusively on behavioural strategies.

Although these behavioural potentials in manual therapy were not applied in this premeditated manner in our group's RCTs, the positive effects of the experimental treatment, not least the conspicuous long-term outcome, may partly be attributed to the inherent behavioural therapy effect of the treatment strategy we used. This may be deduced, for example, from the fact that the experimental patients not only had less pain but also stated, to a significantly greater extent than the conventionally managed group, that the treatment made it easier for them to cope with their residual pain both at work and during their leisure hours (Blomberg et al. 1993b). This effect may have been achieved by the inherent behavioural therapeutic potential of the treatment.

Many differences in outcomes between the two groups in our RCTs increased between the follow-ups at 2 and 4 months (Blomberg et al. 1993a). The behavioural aspects of management may also be partly responsible for this (Blomberg 1993a, p. 118). Differences between the groups persisted at the 2-year follow-up, and during the entire 3-year follow-up, the experimental management gave better results in terms of work absenteeism (Bogefeldt et al. 2005a). In the long term, the experimental management may change the sick leave behaviour of the patients (Blomberg 1993a, p. 118). The favourable long-term effects may also be explained by the perception of 'health', which was more positively influenced by the experimental management than the other 23 quality of life variables (Blomberg et al. 1993b). In another study (Eklund 1992), this measure was the most reliable predictor for an advantageous prognosis in occupational rehabilitation of low back pain patients on extended sick leave. Even lifestyle changes may occur, leading to a persistently increased level of physical activity or even participation in new activities: 80% of the patients in the experimental group stated that they had increased their level of physical activities after 2 years, compared with 40% in the control group (Bogefeldt et al. 2005a). This indicates that we succeeded in reducing the 'passivizing' risks of providing passive treatments. In addition, during the 2 years' follow-up, the experimental group consumed less healthcare resources than the control group. In another study (Cherkin et al. 1998), chiropractic care and management, according to McKenzie (1981), increased the utilization of healthcare. This difference could be explained by the potential for favourable behavioural changes inherent in the STAYAC algorithm.

A sensible manual therapeutic approach should include stay-active messages at an early stage: for example, informing the patients of the generally benign character of their condition and the adverse effects of inactivity and sick leave; making them understand that bed rest usually makes the situation worse and that it is generally not dangerous to work and take part in physical activities in spite of some pain.

Although manual therapy is a passive treatment modality, our therapeutic strategy seems to be an effective way to activate patients. This may seem paradoxical, but there are explanations:

- Pain creates anxiety and fear.
- Anxiety and fear create inactivity, leading to fear-avoidance behaviour and catastrophizing.
- This, in turn, generates increased sensitivity to loading of different soft tissues; decreased muscle strength; loss of fitness, postural control, and co-ordination.
- This process causes increased pain, and a vicious circle is established.

The evaluated treatment strategy might reduce and prevent the pain patient's anxiety, fear, and other phenomena such as personality changes. When patients notice that pain relief can be achieved by simple manual manoeuvres provided by a therapist, they may (subconsciously) realize that the symptoms cannot indicate dangerous tissue damage. Consequently, whether spontaneously or following encouragement from the physician and/or the physiotherapist, further moves towards more active behaviour are enhanced. To use behavioural therapeutic terminology, the physician and/or the physiotherapist become *reinforcers*.

Development of the STAYAC treatment algorithm for low back pain

Continuous development has been in progress for many years at the STAYAC clinic, where the evaluated treatment programme originated. Since the two trials were completed, the applied method has been broadened considerably. Although a behavioural approach has been an intrinsic part of the concept for a long time (Blomberg 1993a, pp. 128–9), behavioural and psychological measures have subsequently been integrated into the programme in a more focused manner. Our occupational rehabilitation, managed over a period of 6 years by a physician, a behavioural therapist, and a specialized physiotherapist, in a very special professional relationship, has had an important role in this process. One of the crucial characteristics of the STAYAC method is the close and integrated co-operation between all the staff members. A multidisciplinary team, in itself, is no guarantee of success. To achieve consistent results, a systematic algorithm, in which there is equal respect between the team members, has to apply.

Metacognition

The STAYAC model is largely a metacognitive approach. Metacognition (Flavell 1979; Jones and Rivett 2004) is a reflective process, and concerns the conscious (and, with time and experience, even pre- or subconscious) continuous scrutinizing and revising of the therapist's own thought processes, attitudes, and beliefs. Associated phenomena are *lateral thinking* (De Bono 1977) and *profound pragmatism*. In practice, this means that one has to be continually self-analytical, to reflect on whether one's actions and communication skills are optimal and of benefit for the patients. Although further discussion of this important aspect of management—in particular, the continuous scrutiny and revision of the therapist's own thought processes and beliefs—is outside the scope of this chapter, it should become apparent that the potential positive effects of metacognitive processes are identified in this chapter. In addition, there are numerous examples showing how inadequate metacognitive processes may affect the treatment results negatively. I believe that being aware of metacognition may optimize the treatment results more than any other factor. (An attempt to evaluate the impact on rehabilitation of physiotherapists' pain beliefs has been made by Daykin and Richardson (2004).) One could even state that the *STAYAC algorithm is a metacognitive method based on pragmatism with a core consisting of somatically focused therapies.*

Pragmatic approach

Considerable efforts have been made at the STAYAC clinic to eliminate the potentially negative aspects (i.e. passivity) of manual therapy within the multidisciplinary team. An inherent problem in traditionally passive treatment methods, such as manipulation, is the risk of subliminal 'stay passive' messages being transferred to the patients, usually non-verbally, at a subconscious level, but sometimes also by advice to limit activity. There are therapists whose 'treatment' strategies rely more or less exclusively on activity-limiting regimens, to avoiding pain at any price. One important reason for this is reliance on outdated, mechanistically oriented theoretical models.

Perhaps the integration of manual therapy into the stay-active concept is one of the main reasons for the success of our programme, when compared with other similar, also pragmatic and fairly recent studies in which the results of different kinds of manual therapy were indifferent (Cherkin et al. 1998; Rasmussen-Barr et al. 2003; Seferlis et al. 1998; Skargren et al. 1997).

The dysfunction paradigm (see later) becomes an excellent pedagogical model, which is fundamental in achieving this synergy between activity and 'passive' manual therapy. For many patients, it is impossible to live pain-free lives. For these patients, the only way forward is to challenge the pain, gradually increase their activity levels despite the pain, defeat it over time, and finally become able to live their lives normally as they once did. Preferably, during the entire process, a team of different therapists guides the patient, not infrequently, over long periods of time—a tremendous pedagogical challenge. A distinctive trait of the STAYAC model is patience. There is almost always another move to be taken when one measure has failed. Our greatest success has been the successful management of unmotivated, psychologically unaware, and perception-disturbed chronic pain patients who are no longer capable of managing the pressure of life or shouldering the responsibilities of their adult selves—the 'Peter Pan syndrome' (Kiley 1983).

We believe that our developmental project has led to the design of an *'ultrapragmatic' treatment programme*, with the ambition of combining all evidence-based and empirically supported specific treatment modalities ('best available evidence' according to Waddell 1998) and, therefore, potentially valuable therapeutic contributions in a common concept, i.e. everything from psychoanalysis to fusion surgery, with manual therapy and steroid injections in between (the ultimate *'black box' concept*). In fact, only a small minority of the treatment modalities are not evidence-based, and it is important to remember that the 'core package' (i.e. the 'antidysfunctional sphere') is evidence-based. We also believe that the pragmatic principle, both with regard to the study design and the experimental intervention, has been another important key to the successful outcome of our group's trials. (Many types of manual therapy, although at first glance seemingly closely related to the mode of manual therapy developed in our clinic, suffer from an obvious lack of pragmatism.)

Our group's results indicate that it is reasonable not only to include the complete evaluated pragmatic treatment programme in a new algorithm but that it should also play a major role from the beginning of the management of patients' back pain. Significant, clinically relevant differences in favour of our experimental intervention were demonstrated even after 3 days (Blomberg et al. 1994a). This constitutes a major difference between the STAYAC algorithm and all other previously published algorithms—manual therapies play minor roles, if any, in these other algorithms, with the exception of the UK guidelines (RCGP 1996) in which manipulation is recommended as one of the options during the first 6 weeks. (However, this algorithm is unclear about why and when manipulation should be provided and positioned in the scheme.) Moreover, current major literature reviews and algorithms recommend 'self-care' as the 'treatment' of choice during the early weeks, but STAYAC is opposed to this management philosophy. There are scientific and substantial observational data indicating that this strategy is not appropriate, so we suggest highly active management from the first day of pain. (Our studies indicate that this approach is cost-effective.) Manual therapy is a fundamental part of our algorithm, regardless of the duration of the symptoms.

In summary, the evidence-based integrated algorithm described in this chapter is used for all patients with locomotor system dysfunction, regardless of the genesis, duration, localization, and character of the complaints; regardless of whether or not the condition in question is complicated by psycho-existential or social factors; and regardless of whether the condition is specific or non-specific.

Evidence-based methods

What basically has been evaluated in our group's trials is the addition to the established stay-active concept of four treatment modes: manipulation/specific mobilization, steroid injections, muscle stretching, and autotraction. Individually, except for manipulation, these treatment modalities have a poor evidence base.

- According to the published systematic literature reviews, the overall results of manipulation are not very impressive, and its long-term effects remain to be demonstrated.
- There is only weak evidence for the benefit of epidural steroids for back pain (Nachemson and Jonsson 2000) (see also Chapter 52 for their use in sciatica). The use of steroid injections is a non-evidence-based treatment method in patients with low back pain. Additionally, this type of intervention has a mixed reputation, both among the majority of patients in developed countries, and among many physicians.
- Muscle stretching, as a clinical method for low back pain, is non-evidence-based; on the contrary, available studies imply moderately negative clinical effects (Bogefeldt et al. 2004a; Howell 1984). In one of the four groups of our reproducibility study, muscle stretching was incorporated as a single addition to the basic stay-active concept, and recovery was postponed in comparison to the group in which neither muscle stretching, manual therapy, or steroid injections were added to the basic management. Nevertheless, in the manual therapy group and the manual therapy/steroid injections combination group, stretching was in fact even more frequently applied than in the stay-active/stretching group. (However, the dysfunctions were treated before muscle stretching was applied— a core central principle in the STAYAC method.)
- Autotraction and other traction methods are not acknowledged as effective treatment modalities in any of the published systematic literature reviews (Harms-Ringdahl et al. 1999; Nachemson and Jonsson 2000).

How is it possible that a combination of four treatment modalities, with more or less doubtful efficiency, brought together in a common treatment programme, can be strikingly helpful in patients with low back pain? This paradox must be explained before our group's scientific results can be regarded as trustworthy. Accordingly, we must define a treatment algorithm based on a pragmatic approach, which will allow its application to everyday clinical practice. This chapter aims to define such an algorithm on the basis of the available evidence.

The lack of evidence-based algorithms for the management of back pain is a substantial problem. Consequently, an 'ultrapragmatic' RCT is currently being planned at STAYAC. This study will not evaluate effects achieved by specific treatment methods. Its starting point is the assumption that back pain is treatable and, furthermore, that resources for effective care are available, at least in an urban setting like Stockholm. The hypothesis of the study is that the main problem of back pain care is the lack of 'infrastructure' (the STAYAC flowchart constitutes such an infrastructure), i.e. an evidence-based multimodal algorithm for treatment/management of low back pain. All kinds of treatment modalities for back pain will be available in both groups (with no limitations in the control group), but care will be structured according to the STAYAC algorithm in the experimental group, whereas the control group will reflect the pathways according to poorly structured conventional care. Consequently, this infrastructure study will not evaluate the efficacy of any specific treatment modalities, but the possible effects of our treatment algorithm.

Dysfunction, markers of dysfunction, antidysfunctional treatment/medicine in relation to low back pain

The definitions used here are adapted to modern rationales, supported by recent neurophysiological research; (Johansson and Sojka 1991) on the nature of dysfunction and the underlying mechanisms of the beneficial effects achieved by manual therapy.

Dysfunction

The dysfunction theory

The term 'dysfunction' refers to disturbed function in musculoskeletal tissues (e.g. joints, muscles, ligaments, tendons), or in the neuromuscular reflex patterns within the 'operating system' of the postural muscles, probably also including higher levels of the central nervous system. *Dysfunctions occur in pathomorphologically damaged tissue, but also (and most frequently) in healthy tissues.* One of the many advantages of the dysfunction theory is that it is cause-neutral; the exact causes of pain are still unknown in most patients. Dysfunctions are diagnosed manually. Standard methods used within traditional healthcare for investigation of (back) pain including diagnostic imaging, scintigrams, sensory evoked potential, electromyography, electroneurography, and blood parameters (e.g. humoral markers of inflammation, hormones), aimed at identifying structural changes or abnormal biological processes, are of limited value. In the absence of a causal relationship between structural pathology and symptoms, the results of these investigations are frequently irrelevant: asymptomatic 'abnormalities' are common, particularly in diagnostic imaging (including magnetic resonance imaging (MRI) and computed tomography (CT)). The dysfunction model makes it possible to understand momentarily restored mobility, resolved compensatory scoliosis, and immediate pain relief after antidysfunctional treatment.

Our pain patients usually have no disease, according to the biomedical definition: it is only a question of their backs or necks not functioning optimally. With this attitude, from a behavioural and psychological perspective, inherent positive effects are evident. It is logical to stay active, to move, and not to rest unnecessarily. Fear avoidance and catastrophizing are counteracted, and the risk of subliminal stay-passive messages is reduced or even eliminated. The back is not 'worn out'; there is no real disease and patients are reassured. There are even patients in whom there is no further need for treatment if the condition recurs, once the pain has disappeared after antidysfunctional therapy. The comforting subliminal (or open) message is: 'If the pain disappears (even if it is only a temporary effect) with a simple treatment manoeuvre, it cannot be anything serious or dangerous.'

The concept of dysfunction is also applied within other medical disciplines. For instance, it is now accepted that 'gastritis' is an inappropriate diagnosis, since it is not an inflammatory condition: the mucosa of the stomach is dysfunctional, without pathomorphological/histological correlates, and the condition is now called 'dyspepsia'. Similarly, the dysfunctional 'irritable colon' (irritable bowel syndrome) was once thought to be an inflammatory disease. Dysfunctions are associated with many other relatively common symptoms including numbness, paresthesiae, vertigo, tinnitus, ear problems, micturition disturbances, blurred vision, voice changes, and even cardiac arrhythmias (see Chapter 10).

Many dysfunctional musculoskeletal conditions frequently mimic symptoms from other organ systems. For example, bowel pain may be referred from iliopsoas muscle and pelvic dysfunctions, and chest pain is commonly referred from dysfunctions in the thoracic column or rib joints. In addition, women with pelvic pain frequently interpret their condition as gynaecological, and undergo unsuccessful gynaecological investigations or even laparoscopy without positive findings. Urologists frequently see analogous cases in male patients. At STAYAC, there is an ongoing RCT evaluating the addition of antidysfunctional treatment to gynaecological management in women with pelvic pain who attend gynaecologists, either spontaneously (interpreting their pain as gynaecological) or by referral from physicians (who suspect gynaecological origin), and for whom there is no gynaecological explanation for the pain or gynaecological care fails. The preliminary results of this study indicate favourable and reliable results for antidysfunctional medicine in this female patient group. Clearly, to prevent unnecessary, expensive, and potentially stigmatizing investigations or even operations, education in antidysfunctional medicine should be made available not only to associated disciplines such as rheumatology, but also to other disciplines (for instance, cardiology, gynaecology, andrology/urology, genitourinary medicine) in which patients may suffer from dysfunctional conditions that give rise to symptoms that mimic symptoms from other organ systems. Unfortunately, there appears to be little systematic high-quality research in this field.

There is a problem with the term 'functional'. Paradoxically, this once had a similar meaning to 'dysfunctional', as defined in this chapter. However, the meaning of the word has changed over time. In Sweden, as in other countries, the term has become a coded deprecatory diagnosis for conditions with a primary psychogenic/psychosomatic background but no real 'sickness' (see discussion of the 'first perspective' in the section 'Pain-related syndromes—new psychological perspectives'), symptoms with an invented aspect, and even laziness. Consequently, I avoid the use of the term 'functional'. It should be appreciated that patients with dysfunctional conditions may present with symptoms that are as severe as, not infrequently worse than, those of patients suffering from pathomorphological conditions.

Dysfunction may sometimes be considered mechanical, insofar as it is caused by overuse, improper use, or strain, not least in dysfunctions of the extremities. However, it is my opinion that within manual therapy/medicine today, mechanical theories ('locking', 'blockage', 'subluxation', 'hypermobility', 'instability', etc.) are overemphasized and have to be balanced by more up-to-date rationales such as those suggested here. Many therapists get stuck in the 'biomechanical trap'. I believe that mechanical factors, as the primary cause of dysfunctions, are of minor importance, especially in the spine and pelvis. This belief is substantiated by the fact that symptomatic clinical features and signs in the extremities frequently disappear with manual treatment to the spine or pelvis, or with injections applied in areas distant from these symptoms. This is exemplified by many cases of apparent tendalgias at the shoulder, epicondalgias (see also Chapter 33), and plantar 'fasciitis'. Phenomena such as the momentary disappearance of paresthesiae, vertigo, blurred vision, and so forth can only be explained in a more general way, for instance as a reflex disturbance ('electrical chaos') localized in the 'operative system' of the posturo-proprioceptive system, rather than a mechanical dysfunction localized to a single vertebral segment (see the following).

To avoid confusion of terminology, particularly in those countries in which the meaning of 'dysfunction' is equivalent to '*general dysfunction*', indicating disturbance of activities of daily living (ADL) or impairment of functional capacity or disability, '*specific dysfunction*' indicates the type of dysfunction defined in this chapter.

The nature of the dysfunction

The 'dysfunction theory' is specific to antidysfunctional medicine. According to the best available evidence from modern neurophysiological research, the dysfunction is most probably a relatively generalized disturbance (and not specifically localized, as suggested by the dominating, mechanically oriented theories within manual therapy/medicine today). This generalized disturbance affects the intricate higher cerebral centres in addition to peripheral structures for postural control, with their complex, neuromuscular reflex patterns. The co-ordinating systems involved in postural control provide peripheral proprioceptive information to higher centres. The receptors situated in the vertebral segments and the sacroiliac joints may be the most important proprioceptive information centres. The small movements in the sacroiliac joints (Egund et al. 1978; Sturesson et al. 1989; Tullberg et al. 1998) are necessary for optimized proprioceptive input to the postural system. However, from a biomechanical perspective, these minor movements are not necessary for everyday mobility and movement.

According to Håkan Johansson's group's research in Umeå, Sweden, numerous proprioceptive receptors react to minor mechanical forces resulting in subtle, widespread, and complex modulation of muscle tension. Moreover, muscle spindles have virtually their own nervous system, the gamma system. The indications are that the ligaments function primarily as receptor organs, not as stabilizing structures; they are more or less an extension of the peripheral nervous system.

A dysfunction is a somatic cause of nociceptive pain in the locomotor system, most frequently not associated with simultaneous pathoneurophysiological or pathomorphological symptomatic manifestations in the back or its operative system. Of course, some type of abnormal electrical activity represents the dysfunction somewhere in the neuromuscular reflex systems. (This might be viewed as an 'electrical chaos' or an 'electrostorm', meaning that a certain number of molecules are out of place; for instance, on the 'wrong' side of cell membranes.) However, contrary to the situation in the wind-up phenomenon and/or neuropathic pain, the symptoms are reversible and are not represented by any permanent pathoneurophysiological process, biochemical correlates, or, of course, by anatomical, morphological, or histological changes; otherwise, the immediate effects achieved by manipulation, for instance, could not be understood (an excellent example of pragmatism, according to the dictionary definition).

Alternative mechanisms of back pain and effects achieved by manual therapy are discussed in my thesis (Blomberg 1993a, pp. 35–7, 125–6).

Antidysfunctional treatment

Dysfunctions are reversible conditions and are, by definition, treatable by different modes of manipulation, specific or non-specific mobilization, muscle stretching, autotraction, and steroid injections. Within the antidysfunctional paradigm, such treatment aims to normalize the function of the affected neuromusculoskeletal structure as a consequence of (sometimes quite forceful) reflex patterns, and to maintain the improved or normalized function by means of home-care programmes.

Self-maintained, disturbed pain-provoking reflex patterns in the postural system may be modified via gate-control mechanisms at the spinal level; additionally, as a consequence of (sometimes quite forceful) *proprioceptive* stimulation, 'reset' mechanisms may halt the electrical chaos triggered in the postural operative system. In the STAYAC model, the posturo-proprioceptive dysfunction theory is more vital and leads to a better, more comprehensive coverage and broadened understanding of many more pain conditions (and, thereby, substantially more treatment options in the locomotor system than the gate-control theory).

Dysfunctions may also disappear spontaneously or with activation (including physical exercise and other home exercises), or indirectly by behavioural, cognitive, or psychotherapeutically based approaches and other measures undertaken to modify the psycho-existential/social dimensions of the patient's suffering. Dysfunctions may also be positively and even causally influenced by drugs (for example, analgesics, NSAIDs, and antidepressants) and reflex therapy methods that inhibit vicious circles in neuromuscular reflex patterns (e.g. acupuncture, acupressure, massage).

In fact, notwithstanding the relevance of the gate-control theory, it may be the case that all therapeutic modalities with positive effects act through 'reset buttons' interfering with the systems previously described at different levels. This does not mean that they are equally effective; the efficacy of different modalities, or combinations of therapeutic modalities, has to be evaluated in RCTs. For back pain, particularly with radiating pain, it is my experience that the most effective 'reset button' is situated in the parasacrococcygeal structures, which are frequently injected with steroids at STAYAC.

Consequently, almost the entire treatment algorithm, even much of the specialist sphere, could be regarded as antidysfunctionally directed. There are many painful and dysfunctional conditions that are resistant to therapy before causal measures are undertaken for pathomorphological conditions, but treatable afterwards. An example is low back pain due to lumbar/pelvic dysfunction, obviously secondary to coxarthrosis. After surgery for the latter condition (and thereby cure of 'the disease component' of the patient's suffering), the dysfunctional component becomes treatable.

Antidysfunctional treatment may be passive (e.g. manipulation, steroid injections). However, it may also be active; most of the effects achieved by passive antidysfunctional treatments are also achievable by different kinds of home exercises. All physical exercises are antidysfunctional measures.

Markers of dysfunction

Dysfunctions are manifested by symptoms such as pain, stiffness, and disability. They are represented by *'markers of dysfunction'* (i.e. non-pathomorphological physical signs) on manual examination, such as localized tenderness, disturbance of segmental mobility and joint play, and positive functional, positional, and provocative tests for, for example, spinal and pelvic dysfunctions (see Chapter 10). Positive manual diagnostic tests are sometimes referred to as 'pathological' tests. However, the validity of many of these tests, for instance those that are supposed to evaluate the mobility of the sacroiliac joint and the position of the pelvic bones in relation to each other, has been disproved (Tullberg et al. 1998). Consequently, the term '*markers of dysfunction*' is cause-neutral and more appropriate.

Pathomorphological conditions cannot be treated by means of antidysfunctional therapy. However, at STAYAC, patients with pathomorphological conditions frequently improve or become symptom-free; this is explained by successful treatment of dysfunctional components of the patient's symptoms. This means that in patients with clear pathomorphological features who progress to full recovery, the structural findings are asymptomatic. The most frequent examples of this are herniated discs (30–65% of healthy and pain-free grown-up women and men have herniated discs without their knowledge), coxarthrosis (40% of healthy 60-year-old women and men have pain-free coxarthrosis), spinal stenosis (40% of a 60-year-old population have spinal stenosis without any symptoms—of course, substantially higher percentages in elderly), spondylosis (100% in elderly), and spondylolisthesis.

Subjects with structural pathology whose symptoms are not controlled after a reasonable number of steps through the algorithm are referred to relevant specialists, provided the symptomatology is sufficiently profound. Cases in whom there is an unsatisfactory margin in terms of cost–benefit analysis (i.e. expected improvement achieved by surgery weighed against the risks taken) are preferably managed within primary healthcare.

Hyper-reactivity

In the STAYAC model, the concept of *'hyper-reactivity'* supersedes concepts such as 'hypermobility', 'instability', and 'micro-instability', because it is more appropriate with regard to the pathogenesis of the 'classical hypermobility syndrome' than focusing on the mechanical properties of joints such as the degree of mobility and joint play. Experience of manual diagnosis suggests that the irritability of spinal segments is poorly related to mobility; the hyper-reactivity syndrome is more likely caused by seemingly 'permanent' distortion of proprioceptive afferents from the vertebral segment(s), which in turn, via misinformation ('computer viruses'), interfere with the operating system of the posturo-proprioceptive system. It is hypothesized that this operating system (including the cerebellum, the 'central computer') cannot interpret this misinformation and transforms it into adequate instructions to the postural muscles, so that agonists counteract antagonists, causing overload of different structures and a low-efficiency/energy 'crisis' of the entire system. Clinically, the hyper-reactivity syndrome has identical features to the 'hypermobility syndrome', including reliance on the history for diagnosis and clinical signs such as delayed and prolonged stretch pain on provocation tests.

A hyper-reactive segment may in fact be hyper, normo-, or even hypomobile. It could even be that *hypomobility* is more common than hypermobility in the severe cases, and that these are the ones most frequently and adequately subjected to surgical fusion. On the other hand, many markedly hypermobile subjects have no symptoms of hypermobility syndrome. The term hyper-reactivity is applicable to all joints of the body, including the sacroiliac joint, the hip joint, and peripheral joints.

Hyper-reactivity is a pathoneurophysiological disturbance that gives the appearance of permanency. It may have a post-traumatic and/or a degenerative background. Unlike dysfunctional conditions, hyper-reactivity is not easily causally treatable. However, it is hypothesized and also empirically supported, that symptoms associated with hyper-reactivity in all joints of the body are frequently alleviated by muscle stretching (not least the iliocrural muscles in low back pain, an important indication for this treatment modality within the STAYAC algorithm). Additionally, hyper-reactivity heals spontaneously over time and the associated symptoms subside. (Unfortunately, this may take years, even decades.) It is logical to believe that this healing process is attributable to the development of age-related spondylosis. This slowly decreases the mobility of the affected segment(s), resulting in less distortion of proprioceptive output, and finally, when there is little or no mobility, the postural control system is able to adapt to the abnormal situation, and the pain and other symptoms subside. This model could very well explain why virtually all back pain subsides with increasing age. I finish the 'patient education' (see subsequent section) by presenting this model. Its behavioural potential (e.g. reassurance) is obvious:

> I can see on the X-ray that the so-called 'degenerative changes' in your back are more pronounced today than they were 4 years ago. This is very good—your irritated back is definitely healing! What I see on the X-ray is not 'wear and tear', it's a healing process: the body's own capacity for fusion, which is much better than surgical fusion. Just live your life as usual and be active, while this healing process continues. Eventually, you will become pain-free.

We can also understand from this model why, although surgical fusion may seem successful initially, months or years later, patients may develop pain that is much worse than the condition that led to the operation. The fusion abolishes the distorted output (which is fine), but it also destroys other normal output that is needed for postural control. The mechanical rationales upon which fusion surgery is based are suspect, if one accepts the concept of hyper-reactivity. The same goes for the hypothesis that neighbouring segments become 'hypermobile' over time as a consequence of the stiff fused segment. In conclusion, rejecting mechanically oriented theories in favour of the 'posturo-proprioceptive model' is a good example of fruitful metacognition.

This *'posturo-proprioceptive model'* may even have a more important role in the syndrome than the local pain factor; furthermore, it allows the dissemination of nociceptive pain and other symptoms from the original focus to other distant parts of the body to be better understood. (This mechanism is not equivalent to 'referred pain', which is a central mechanism in the central nervous system (CNS) resulting from the inability of the pain-monitoring systems in the cortex to localize the pain to the proper part of the body—somatic 'pain' becomes 'pain' only at the point of time when nociceptive or neuropathic nervous input reaches the cortex. The posturo-proprioceptive model, although including central nervous mechanisms in the form of the operative system of postural control, is a matter of peripheral nociceptive pain mechanisms.)

Psycho-existential dimensions of pain suffering

The usual term for psychological factors in the context of pain is 'psychosocial'. However, from the psychological and social perspectives, the overall health, prosperity, and social status of people in developed countries are comparatively good. I therefore prefer the term *psycho-existential*. I believe that the existential dimension of pain suffering is severely underestimated; as I perceive the world of back pain, it is the dominating factor with respect to the consequences of pain conditions (see discussion of the 'third perspective' in the section 'Pain-related syndromes—new psychological perspectives'). This is not a matter of splitting hairs—the implementation of this paradigm in pain care, as an aspect of the metacognitive processes, is definitely associated with obvious clinical consequences.

A good example of the denial of the psycho-existential dimensions of the suffering, and denial of the role of the life situation in general, as a confounding factor with regard to the consequences of pain, is loss of work. In a society such as Sweden, largely driven by Lutheran ideals and morals, loss of work activates the existential crisis of not being needed, not being seen, not being heard, and, not infrequently, not feeling loved; and, finally, the utmost existential crisis of all, having no right to exist. Unemployment is for many an unfathomable situation for which pain and sick leave is 'convenient' in the short term but destructive and often disastrous for the individual patient in the long term. The mechanisms underlying 'long-term sick leave illness' (a condition/sickness caused by the long-term sick leave itself; a useful comprehensive term for all personality changes, behavioural changes, loss/distortion of identity, and loss of self-esteem and other psychological deviations that occur during long-term sick leave) are similar. Of course, unemployment and long-term sick leave could be perceived as purely social problems. However, in Western society, it is the profound existential dimensions of work loss and long-term sick leave, and their denial, that cause such destructive consequences.

Other relevant phenomena central to the STAYAC concept are poor quality of life, behavioural disturbances, insufficient coping strategies, and low sense of coherence (Antonovsky 1987).

Perception disturbances

The psychological phenomenon of perception disturbances develops in almost all patients with severe chronic pain, and frequently also in moderately affected subjects, during the destructive process of sick leave from the first day until the day of early retirement some years later. A stone becomes a mountain; it is as if numerous receptors in the perception system are turned to maximum volume, resulting in severe distortion. An illustrative situation arose during the early days of our occupational rehabilitation unit. When filling in questionnaires about their pain (after sitting quietly and apparently comfortably, listening to a 2-hour lecture), patients repeatedly indicated high visual analogue scale (VAS) scores for the item 'sitting for longer than a short period'. It was obvious that the instrument did not measure ability to sit (some patients even rated 110–120 on a 0–100 VAS scale!); it was much more likely that existential anxiety was recorded—a cry for help. This dimension of pain suffering is frequently the main obstacle to successful rehabilitation. If we, as therapists, are not aware of this phenomenon, we will have huge difficulties in managing these patients.

A macro-perspective of the STAYAC algorithm for management of low back pain

The following description of the STAYAC algorithm takes the form of a macro-perspective; providing the details is not within the scope of this chapter. However, this does not mean that other schools of pain treatment and manual therapy cannot integrate the STAYAC macro-perspective in their therapies. Our basic manual techniques are available in textbooks (Evjent and Hamberg 1985a,b; Kaltenborn and Evjent 1993), but their modifications and many details have to be learned on STAYAC courses. During recent years, the Mulligan manual techniques (Mulligan 2003; Reordan et al. 2012) have become a growing part of the STAYAC model. Other authors have influenced the Scandinavian manual therapy model and, thereby, also the STAYAC concept (Cyriax 1970; Janda 1976; Lewit 1991; Stoddard 1980). The reason for concentrating mainly on the wider perspective of the algorithm is that, to be able to improve pain care significantly, a better infrastructure in back pain care has to be developed and is paramount; the details are less important.

The STAYAC algorithm is genuinely pragmatic and eclectic, and aided by cost-effective routes of communication. The intention is to limit the risk that patients remain at sub-optimal levels (which might jeopardize their rehabilitation potential) for long periods of time, and to reduce the likelihood that treatment possibilities are missed. Central to the algorithm is a therapeutic philosophy emanating from the dysfunction theory, which applies to most pain patients, including those with neck and back pain. The therapeutic strategy directed by the dysfunction perspective is more scientifically based than other modes of treatment in an unselected patient group. In addition, the demonstrated effects appear more powerful in more important efficacy variables than other treatment approaches that have been evaluated in RCTs, not least with respect to sick leave. The protocol allows unsatisfactory progress to be detected early, which is important from the psychological perspective.

The core of the algorithm—the antidysfunctional domain—is evidence-based, and so are almost all of its other components. However, some aspects, as reflected by a series of statements and assumptions in this chapter and as stated in other algorithms (ACC 1997; AHCPR 1994; CSAG 1994; Kendall et al. 1997; RCGP 1996; Waddell 1998), are not supported by hard evidence, but based on best available evidence, observational data, and common sense. Patients' progress through the treatment protocol is based on the pooled experience of the clinic's staff members in mixing several management philosophies and methods over a 33-year period. Since the results of our algorithm are unique, it is important to publicize it to a broader circle of physicians, physiotherapists, and other people working with pain. The Swedish Social Insurance Agency (managed by the Swedish State) recorded that 80–85% of the patients in our year 2000 outcome cohort study who were on sick leave at the start of their rehabilitation (41 out of 125 patients), possibly even more (depending on analysing method), were working 8 years after the STAYAC rehabilitation. The self-reported duration of sick leave before rehabilitation was 2.6 years and the corresponding symptom duration was 8.2 years. An RCT evaluation of the entire algorithm is planned.

Possible outcomes

In terms of the diagram (Figure 60.1), all STAYAC patients enter the algorithm in the upper part of Figure 60.1 and progress downwards to one of three possible outcomes (at the bottom of Figure 60.1)—an ultimate 'black-box concept':

- *No symptoms or fully controllable minor symptoms*, without negative consequences. Neither quality of life nor work capability is disturbed. (The '*A box*' at the bottom of the flowchart in Figure 60.1.)
- *Residual symptoms reducing some aspects of quality of life and/or some daily activities to some degree*. However, the ability to perform the patient's usual work is retained. Retention of work capacity is not only the most important target in rehabilitation from a societal perspective, it is also the most important issue regarding long-term well-being in a general sense, not least in Lutheran Western societies, where a person's identity relies largely on the specific function they fulfil in society. Self-care will be appropriate as a short- and long-term strategy, and the chances of spontaneous recovery with time are excellent. The provision of relevant information, reassurance, and reinforcement and, when needed, patient education help the long-term situation. In other words, the general life situation is not fully optimal, but under control; there are no major psychiatric disorders such as depression, and the patient's psychological state is satisfactory. (The '*B box*' at the bottom of the flowchart in Figure 60.1.)

- *Long-term sick leave or early retirement (part- or full-time) or a substantial loss of quality of life*. The patient may regard sick leave as a reasonable solution for a life situation that is no longer manageable by other means. However, although the prescription of sick leave may occasionally be appropriate, it should be avoided whenever possible. It has to be remembered that the sick leave instrument is one of the most dangerous and potentially destructive treatments a physician can impose. This 'treatment' is associated with severe side-effects and complications. In Western societies, largely driven by Protestant morals and ideals, long-term sick leave—or worse, early retirement—is almost always a virtual disaster for the suffering patient. The lowest quality of life ever measured in a segment of the Swedish population is that of the early retired population. *From a strictly somatic pain perspective, long-term sick leave is rarely indicated*. (The '*C box*' at the bottom of the flowchart in Figure 60.1.)

The classification process

There are only three distinct factors that can explain and/or influence pain, the perception of pain, and the consequences of pain: the pathomorphological, the dysfunctional, and the psycho-existential spheres (Figure 60.2). In Figure 60.3, this is illustrated in another way and in more detail (see also Figure 60.4); the purpose is to illustrate the basis upon which the STAYAC concept relies.

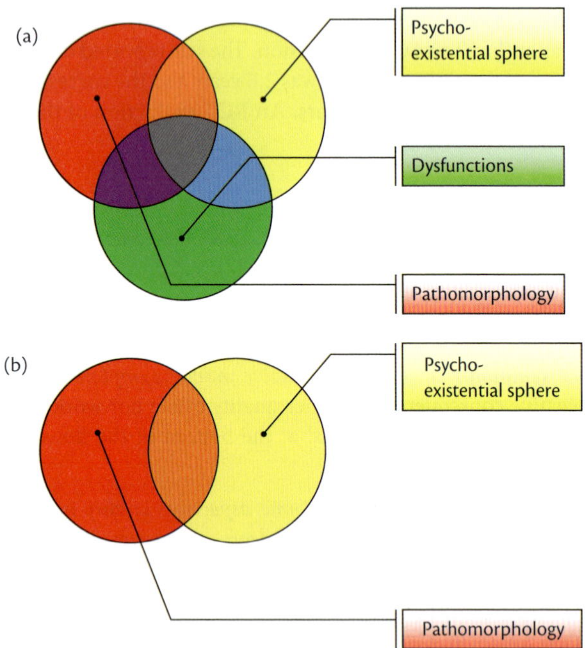

Figure 60.2 **(a)** Venn diagram shows the three basically different factors which can explain and/or influence pain, the perception of pain, and the consequences of pain. Any one factor may be the dominant (or single) factor, coexist in any combination, or all three may contribute simultaneously to the patient's condition (however, frequently with considerably different impact). Considering all three sectors is an essential requirement for optimal pain care. **(b)** Venn diagram shows the basic structure of today's pain care: managements based on the dysfunction theory are not systematically implemented in the 'cultural' pain care/currently dominating pain care paradigm (Kuhn 1962); with their 'subcultural'/pre-paradigmatic (Kuhn 1962) character, antidysfunctionally related treatment models are isolated from 'cultural'/'paradigmatic' medicine.

The large square in Figure 60.3a represents a population and the large circle corresponds to the proportion of the population that, according to numerous epidemiological studies, has experienced low back pain during the last 3 months (30–40%). The smaller circle represents the tiny group (at the most, 5% according to Nachemson and Jonsson 2000) of patients with low back pain in whom the pain has a causal relationship with pathomorphological changes in the structures of the spine and/or pelvis (i.e. disease as defined according to the biomedical paradigm). The somewhat larger dashed circle indicates that this figure may, by scientific progress, increase in size to a modest degree in the future. In Figure 60.3b, the larger proportion of psycho-existential factors is shown. Figure 60.3c illustrates patho-neurophysiological conditions (in which, for simplicity, hyper-reactivity is included). Examples of pathoneurophysiological conditions are central sensitization and the wind-up phenomenon; it may be that segmental hyper-reactivity is a type of wind-up phenomenon. The large dysfunction sphere is illustrated in Figure 60.3d. Everyone working within manual therapy/medicine knows that there are asymptomatic dysfunctions; opinions on whether or not they should be treated are usually represented by the extremes of 'never treat' or 'always treat'. In the STAYAC model, asymptomatic dysfunctions are treated in some situations, but not routinely.

In terms of the posturo-proprioceptive dysfunction theory, there is nothing strange in a patient promptly getting rid of headache after a lumbar/pelvic dysfunction has been treated (even when there is no low back pain); it is something that happens every now and then. There are many analogous examples, mostly associated with pelvic dysfunctions (such as groin pain interpreted as hip joint symptoms, knee problems, plantar 'fasciitis', and thoracic pain). Primary psychogenic pain is rare, and true simulators are even more infrequent (Figure 60.3e).

From Figure 60.3f, in which all the basic conditions are brought together within a common outline, it is obvious that the adoption of the dysfunction paradigm considerably decreases the proportion of pain patients whose pain cannot be understood or treated—idiopathic pain/unspecific neck and back pain are, according to the STAYAC paradigm, considered to be *specific* (dysfunctional) pain. However, also in the STAYAC Clinic are a smaller proportion of patients whose complaints, over time, during the antidysfunctional investigation, will come to be considered idiopathic. Nevertheless, this patient group is frequently helped in the end, guided at least to the 'B outcome', i.e. the 'almost healthy end result', after having passed through the flowchart, via many different pathways.

Initial stage. The first task of the physician (or the physiotherapist) is to consider the possibility of major 'red flag' conditions such as herniated discs, malignancies, fractures, and spondylolisthesis (see red box in upper left corner of the algorithm in Figure 60.1). The history (anamnesis) given by the patient is the most important tool in identifying these conditions; the classical aspects of the history, alerting the therapist to potential red flag conditions (Della-Giustina 1999), are described in several publications (Della-Giustina and Kilcline 2000; Deyo and Weinstein 2001). Laboratory or radiological investigations as a response to a suspicion of red flag conditions may be initiated at the first visit or at any point throughout the algorithm. However, they are unnecessary for the majority of acute low back pain patients after relevant screening questions for such conditions. (For discussion of features that suggest dysfunction(s), see Chapters 10 and 27.)

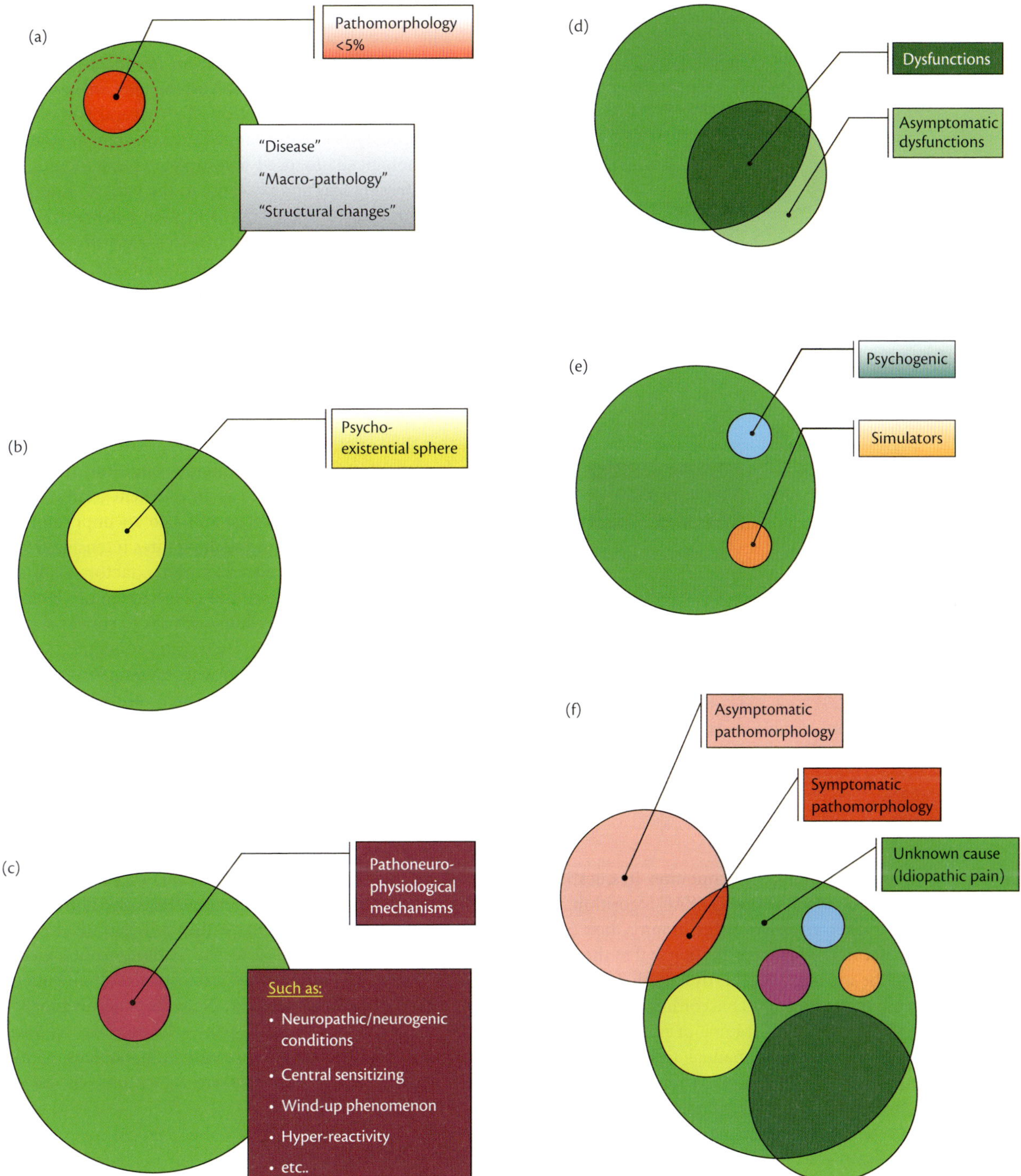

Figure 60.3 (a–f) The theoretical basis upon which the STAYAC concept relies. The squares represent a population and the circles, different underlying factors with respect to pain (a larger sphere represents a larger proportion of the population). See text for details.

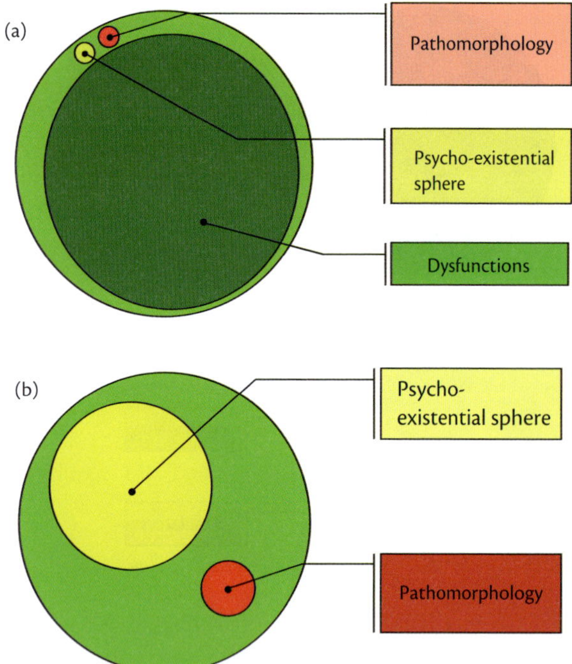

Figure 60.4 **(a)** In the acute phase, dysfunctions are the dominating cause of pain—pathomorphology and primary psycho-existentially based conditions are rare. Provided antidysfunctional treatment is carried out early, the vast majority of this patient category needs only a few steps in the antidysfunctional sphere. **(b)** Psycho-existential dimensions of the pain suffering dominate in patients with severe chronic disease. Such patients with purely dysfunctional conditions ('green flag' conditions) and therefore treatable with antidysfunctional therapy only, are rare, and consequently not represented here by a circle. With regard to chronic patients, the two figures represent the two extremes: there is an infinite variety of relationships between the three major spheres.

Another important issue is whether the condition in question is *traumatic or spontaneous in onset.* In the STAYAC algorithm, as illustrated by the short, thicker arrow from the 'trauma' box (see Figure 60.1), a consequence of the first consultation is that the majority of the patients will be managed (in the 'dysfunctional' green sphere; see centre green box in Figure 60.1) according to the same principles, whether there is a history of trauma or not. This is because there are virtually always gentle manual techniques (e.g. muscle energy techniques) for which trauma is no contraindication, when they are adjusted to the specific situation. Only a small minority of the patients (particularly after major trauma but also, for instance, when a herniated disc, fulfilling criteria for acute operation, is suspected) needs to undergo neuroradiological examination to confirm/reject red flags or exclude fractures before antidysfunctional treatment is begun. In most cases, after radiological examination, as illustrated by the thicker arrow from the '(neuro) radiological investigation' box (see Figure 60.1), the patients are allocated to the 'dysfunction' box (centre green box in Figure 60.1), and will thereafter follow the same path through the algorithm as other patients with dysfunctional conditions.

Investigations. In principle, with respect to radiography and neuroradiological imaging, we apply the criteria recommended in major evidence-based reports and consensus documents (Nachemson and Jonsson 2000; Waddell 1998). Neuroradiological imaging is regarded as a preoperative investigation. We use such investigations only if the clinical findings and history clearly indicate, for instance, a herniated disc, again fulfilling criteria for acute operation. Furthermore, the expected benefit from an operation should be weighed against the risk taken (the 'cost–benefit' analysis).

Not only does the demonstration of structural pathology such as disc prolapse by MRI *not* change the management strategy, but pathomorphologically focused investigations also incur a specific risk of transferring fear and passivity to the patient. Routinely refraining from diagnostic imaging is in itself behavioural therapy, and the result of a well-developed metacognitive process. On rare occasions, (neuro)radiological investigations are prescribed on psychological indications. However, such investigations should never be initiated just to satisfy the curiosity of the physician/physiotherapist or the patient. In this context, some patients bring huge piles of (neuro)radiological images (frequently on a CD) undertaken elsewhere. It is therapeutic if the clinician does not study them intensively or, even better, not at all, provided of course that this is not needed for the therapeutic/investigative process or for the assessment of the patient's condition. This also constitutes behavioural therapy and is an excellent example of well-developed metacognitive abilities, and also an important part of the reassuring process. Studying such pictures intensely, frowning, and looking troubled may indeed reinforce factors such as pain patient identity, fear avoidance, and catastrophizing. Doing so is also confusing for the patient when one tries to convey stay-active messages.

At STAYAC, the antidysfunctional investigation over time is virtually always completed before any additional investigations are undertaken, and such measures are not needed when patients recover satisfactorily. This approach restricts the need for MR/CT, radiography, and laboratory tests to a minimum—neuroradiological investigations may of course be carried out at any point in the flowchart, not only at the first visit. In the early phases only a few patients, whose complaints are not understandable or treatable from either a dysfunction or a pathomorphological perspective, i.e. their pain is unexplained, are allocated to the 'idiopathic pain' box. Since only a tiny minority of the trauma/incident subjects are allocated to the 'pathomorphological' box, after the initial triage has been undertaken, almost all patients are allocated to the 'dysfunction' box. Note that the diagnosis 'non-specific' (benign) (back or neck) pain—the dominating diagnosis within today's traditional pain care paradigm, not least within primary health care and in other current algorithms—is not used at all in the STAYAC algorithm.

The 'pathomorphology' box

Relevance of structural pathology. It is necessary to decide whether the pathomorphology is an isolated condition or if there are also markers of dysfunction. This step differentiates the STAYAC algorithm from other related methods and is important because, even in the presence of pathomorphology (sometimes major, such as acute vertebral compression fractures), the dysfunctions are treated within the STAYAC algorithm. In this context, suspected or confirmed herniated discs are the most frequent pathomorphology, but the same reasoning is also valid for spinal stenosis or spondylolisthesis.

By contrast, in other manual treatment programmes, important dysfunctions and injection sites are not only left undiagnosed, they are also untreated. In these situations, the possibility of referred pain from soft tissue irritations, mimicking true radicular pain, symptomatic spinal stenosis, or symptomatic spondylolisthesis is not considered. In traditional Swedish manual therapy, these patients are more or less exclusively treated by autotraction (Lind 1974; Natchew 1984) and/or by nerve mobilization techniques (see Chapter 56). At STAYAC, these techniques are rarely found to be effective if the dysfunctions and/or relevant sites of irritation are not treated/injected first. Consequently, in the STAYAC algorithm, there is an important flow from the 'combined pathomorphology/dysfunction(s)' box to the 'antidysfunctional' (re-functional) box (see Figure 60.1), where the patients are managed in a similar fashion to those with dysfunctional symptoms only. This approach is controversial, since it goes against conventional manual treatment algorithms, where several pathomorphological conditions, especially herniated discs, are considered strong contraindications for manipulation and specific mobilization.

Manual therapy. Our manual techniques range from relatively forceful thrust techniques to extremely gentle techniques. The 'traditional' Scandinavian concept of locking techniques (Evjent and Hamberg 1985a,b; Kaltenborn and Evjent 1993), aimed at optimizing the possibilities of directing the therapeutic forces exclusively to the dysfunctional segment, are applied and, in addition, muscle energy principles are integrated. As a consequence, these techniques may be applied to conditions such as herniated discs, spinal stenosis, spondylolisthesis, post-operative conditions, or even neighbouring acute compression fractures. Even patients with clinically relevant disc herniations, and in the presence of neurological signs from nerve root compression, and a classical positive Lasègue's sign of less than 30°, may be treated manually. When required, even rotational techniques in flexion and side-bending are applied in vertebral segments with MR-verified herniated discs. In these cases, gentle techniques are of course favoured but, when indicated, thrust techniques may also be applied. It should be emphasized that this statement does *not* concern treatment manoeuvres outside the STAYAC algorithm—we use non-locking techniques infrequently, and we have no experience of treating patients with coexistent pathomorphological conditions by means of non-specific techniques or therapeutic manoeuvres in which locking techniques are *not* applied. These manual techniques act only by treating dysfunctions and are not believed to influence pathomorphological conditions *per se*. This approach to combined dysfunctional/pathomorphological conditions may partly explain why our algorithm has been more successful than other related methods assessed in RCTs, not least those in which, as in our group's studies, unselected patient populations were recruited (Cherkin et al. 1998; Rasmussen-Barr et al. 2003; Seferlis et al. 1998; Skargren et al. 1997).

The locking techniques referred to in this chapter are of Norwegian origin and (to my knowledge) only published in Scandinavia (Evjent and Hamberg 1985a,b; Kaltenborn and Evjent 1993) and only taught by Scandinavians (e.g. outside Scandinavia, by Olav Evjent and by the Ola Grimsby Institute and its signatories). As these techniques may be important for our group's unique results, it is important to appreciate that the locking techniques used at STAYAC seem to be different from manipulation and mobilization techniques used elsewhere in the world.

Another important difference between the STAYAC algorithm and some other schools of manual therapy is that we almost always choose three-dimensional locking techniques in the most painful and movement-restricted direction (unlike some manual therapy philosophies, where treatment is preferably given in the pain-free direction). We state that treatment in the painful direction is more effective as well as time-saving. This is facilitated through the wide variety of different techniques including extremely gentle procedures with a combination of hold/relax, and muscle energy techniques, including coupled eye movements and synchronized breathing (Mitchel et al. 1979), in fact allowing patients to treat themselves with no application of external forces by the therapists whatsoever. Rarely, treatment in the painful direction is impossible; in those patients, according to the pragmatic principle, we simply try another direction first, and later, the (previously) painful direction, by which stage the dysfunction has resolved. Since the dysfunction has not infrequently already resolved after treatment in the 'wrong' direction, this subsequent treatment in the 'painful' direction is not always necessary.

Patient review. A common reason for therapeutic failures within manual therapy is over-emphasis on discogenic/true radicular symptoms. This is not only a problem in the lower back region, but also in patients with neck pain. In Sweden, this problem has paralleled the rapid dissemination of Butler's/Elvey's diagnostic and therapeutic principles among physiotherapists during recent decades. These principles have questionable validity with respect to reduced sliding of the nerves in their sheaths that they were, at one time, assumed to measure and treat. This statement is substantiated by the fact that during the patient's progress through the STAYAC algorithm, positive 'nerve stretch tests' are frequently normalized, even though no specific nerve 'mobilization' techniques have been applied. This normalization of the tests is frequently paralleled by disappearance of diffuse and complex peripheral, central, and general symptoms other than pain. Consequently, these observations suggest that positive 'nerve stretch tests' are not contraindications to manual treatment of symptomatic dysfunctions. Despite this (and the fact that there appears to be a limited evidence base for neural mobilization), neural tension tests/treatment may indeed be useful (for instance, in monitoring the progress of treatment, and sometimes as a therapeutic measure). However, therapists are often needlessly alarmed by positive 'nerve stretch tests', interpreting them as indicating true nerve impingement, as a consequence of which they refrain from treating symptomatic vertebral and pelvic dysfunctions.

Undue reliance on these tests in deciding which type of treatment should or should not be applied may have a negative effect on the overall treatment results. Dysfunctional aspects of the patient's suffering may not even be considered. I do not claim that Butler and Elvey necessarily caused this problem; it may very well be the case that some physiotherapists have misinterpreted their therapeutic approach. Indeed, the Butler–Elvey methodology is included in the STAYAC algorithm, rarely as a primary method, but late in the algorithm. The reason for this is that our experience suggests that in the antidysfunctional sphere, treatments such as manipulation, injections, and muscle stretching are considerably more effective. (For current thoughts on neurodynamics, see Chapters 15 and 56.)

In parallel with the popularity of neural mobilization in Sweden in recent years has been a heavy reliance on transversus abdominis exercises (Richardson, Hodges, Hides 2004). However, they should be used within the stay-active concept, and not replace effective antidysfunctional therapy. In conclusion, within the STAYAC concept, numerous 'contraindications' to manual therapy, of which only a few are mentioned here, have been abolished.

The 'antidysfunctional treatment' box—the antidysfunctional stack

The core, although not necessarily always the most important part, of the STAYAC algorithm is manual therapy. If there are markers of dysfunction, different kinds of manipulation and/or specific mobilization are applied as the first measure in virtually all patients. Of course there are exceptions. In some cases, it is obvious that manual therapy is not the appropriate primary treatment measure—physical exercises may be the preferable basic treatment, and specific manual therapy may be undertaken later.

Virtually all subjects referred to a clinic like STAYAC are in need of exercise. Even though the basic principle has to be the elimination of markers of dysfunction before initiation of physical exercise, this means that physical exercise is frequently initiated from the beginning of the antidysfunctional investigation, in parallel with the measures in the antidysfunctional domain. In other patients, the main problem is depression or psycho-existentially based conditions, requiring antidepressant medication and/or cognitive–behavioural measures respectively. Specific mobilizing exercises with the same intent as manipulation/specific mobilization, aimed at optimizing the treatment results and preserving increased mobility, are frequently taught to patients as an important part of the home-care programme. All the other boxes under the 'antidysfunctional box' belong to the antidysfunctional stack (situated centrally in the algorithm) (see Figure 60.1).

When the first edition of this book was published in 2005, the term 'green flags' was found neither in PubMed, Cochrane Library, nor in Embase. It is used here for markers of dysfunction and, consequently, implies dysfunctional conditions (see green-flagged 'dysfunctions' box near the top of the algorithm in Figure 60.1). In addition, this term also covers features in the patient's history indicating dysfunctional conditions (see also Chapters 10 and 27). Green flag conditions are therefore synonymous with dysfunctional conditions. One advantage of this term is avoidance of confusion in contexts where 'dysfunction' is equivalent to 'disability'.

The 'idiopathic/unspecific pain' box

The few patients whose pain cannot be understood (either from the 'pathomorphological' perspective or from the 'dysfunctional perspective') and cannot be easily explained by a 'psycho-existential perspective', will be regarded as *'idiopathic' pain patients with unspecific pain, e.g. in the neck or back region,* and allocated to this 'idiopathic/unspecific pain' box (see Figure 60.1).

The antidysfunctional investigation

A *trial treatment*, for instance a thrust manoeuvre, is provided according to an identified set of markers of dysfunction, all weighed together, fashioning a *'functional diagnosis'* (green flags); if an obvious positive treatment result is achieved, the provisional (functional) diagnosis is verified—this is called a *green light* (see the 'traffic light' symbol to the left of the 'antidysfunctional stack' in the flowchart in Figure 60.1). The diagnostic procedure is carried out over time, during which a series of provisional working hypotheses (i.e. functional diagnoses) are used, following the trial treatment, and either verified (shown in the algorithm by a green light, yellow light 'A', yellow light 'B'—the latter two symbols seen just to the right of the 'antidysfunctional stack' in the flowchart in Figure 60.1; see following text) or disproved (red light), depending on the response to treatment as assessed at the subsequent appointment with the physician or with the physiotherapist. *Red light* means no improvement, or even deterioration.

Provocation of *transient* symptoms after manual treatment is not uncommon; however, in most cases, the post-treatment pain subsides rapidly, and in others, the provoked pain disappears with steroid injections. The most frequent example in this context is (sometimes radiating) pain after lumbar/pelvic manipulation, which is nearly always a provocation of referred pain originating from the parasacrococcygeal structures and should not be misinterpreted as true radicular pain. Empirically, we are aware that focus on this anatomical region is even *the most important one* in the entire human body. This may be due to the fact that since the parasacrococcygeal structures contain masses of proprioceptive receptors, they are probably the end result of the evolutionary process during which human beings lost their tails, which are principal organs for the balance system for many animals. Although the parasacrococcygeal structures are a paramount and common source of pain, this is virtually unknown within the medical profession, internationally and in Sweden. In these cases, steroid injections in the appropriate area are extremely effective. Rarely, the provoked pain persists for up to a few weeks, and in 20 years, we have seen only a couple of long-term deteriorations, and neither of them had demonstrable true radicular pain.

The *yellow light 'A'* and *yellow light 'B'* outcomes indicate that treatment is on the right track, i.e. a substantial or temporary improvement, but the symptoms are not yet entirely under control. In the 'yellow light A' situation, the patient is improved or pain-free, but only for a limited period, for example a couple of days, and the markers of dysfunction (green flags) that disappeared immediately after the former treatment have recurred. The treatment may be repeated once or twice, but according to the STAYAC algorithm, not at subsequent visits without a reassessment of the functional diagnosis/treatment hypothesis. In 'the yellow light B' situation, the patient is persistently improved, the markers of dysfunction (green flags) at the previous visit are still absent, but there are residual symptoms still interfering with quality of life, everyday activities, or working capability. Again, the functional diagnosis and alternative strategies have to be reviewed.

Thus, the treatment hypotheses (on which the trial treatments are based) are continuously revised and changed when needed. In patients with complex pain, the dysfunctional, pathomorphological, and psycho-existential dimensions of the condition are comprehensively mapped—this process is called the antidysfunctional investigation. The procedure may, in complex conditions, take months. All available methods are tried in 'difficult' cases, as long as markers of dysfunction (green flags) persist. However, during this process (a mapping procedure), the passivizing risks have to be addressed and minimized by applying the stay-active concept from the first visit and, in addition, introducing physical exercises and the home-care programme at an early stage. By contrast, a simple dysfunctional case is 'mapped' after a single treatment and a final consultation at which no further treatment is required (green light situation).

Our ultra-pragmatic approach recognizes that our tests can only determine in which order we try the different items of a complete treatment arsenal. In theory, all treatment modalities in the algorithm should be tried before concluding that there is nothing more to offer the patient in question, who thereby is entirely therapy-resistant; this process is in fact, according to STAYAC 'philosophy', the only absolutely reliable manner to ensure that no treatment possibility is missed. In practice, this is not possible, but it is useful to keep in mind that the different items have to be tried systematically, in a specified order according to the algorithm.

Idiopathic pain—ex juvantibus diagnosis

Another important, although relatively rare, pathway in the algorithm is from idiopathic pain to the antidysfunctional investigation box. The principle of *ex juvantibus* diagnosis is applied when a diagnostic procedure/investigation does not lead to a clear diagnosis, but, despite this, a trial treatment is provided according to a hypothetical functional diagnosis; if an obvious positive treatment result is achieved, the provisional diagnosis is verified. In common with other antidysfunctional investigations, *ex juvantibus* diagnosis is a procedure that goes on over time, during which a series of provisional working hypotheses are either verified or disproved, depending on the response to treatment (i.e. the mapping procedure over time). Otherwise, there are no differences between the regular antidysfunctional investigation and the ultra-pragmatic *ex juvantibus* principle.

In the pragmatically based STAYAC algorithm, the *ex juvantibus* diagnostic principle is applied consistently and systematically in virtually all patients. An example is pain with a distribution consistent with sacroiliac joint pain in a subject free from markers of dysfunction (green flags), and also no provocation pain from the sacroiliac joint. In this situation, a diagnostic (and hopefully curative as well) injection of steroids and local anaesthetic may be given to the sacroiliac joint. A positive response, particularly if it persists, supports a diagnosis of sacroiliac joint 'irritation'. (A positive response to the injection does not indicate that a truly inflammatory condition has been treated.) Thus, an injection of 1.5 ml local anaesthetic and 1 ml steroid into the sacroiliac joint, even in the absence of green flag and positive provocation tests, may eliminate pain not only momentarily, but even permanently. This is true for pain localized to the region of the sacroiliac joint as well as for radiating pain (sometimes as far as the foot) in the presence of a positive straight leg raise (SLR) test. Consequently, where there has been a differential diagnosis of true radicular pain due to disc herniation, unnecessary (and therefore unsuccessful) surgery due to an asymptomatic disc herniation is avoided. In fact, *this pragmatic measure may be the only reliable method to detect whether or not a herniated disc is symptomatic.*

Another clinically important example of *ex juvantibus* diagnosis and treatment is the not unusual case of buttock pain, especially on sitting (particularly in a car), from the anatomical region of the ischial tuberosity. No remaining markers of dysfunction are present, there are no injection sites, range of movement in the hip joint is normal, there is no local tenderness, and so forth. According to our stretching philosophy (Evjent and Hamberg 1985a,b), there are four different stretching manoeuvres for the short and deep extensors of the hip joint (which are not palpable—consequently, an *ex juvantibus* diagnostic procedure); these are tested, and the most painful and perhaps most restricted one is chosen. The corresponding home exercise is taught. Although we do not know which structures are affected in these cases—it could be the hip joint, capsule, muscle(s), or nerves—this may be the only effective treatment, and, in addition, an excellent example of pragmatically based therapy.

Another example is the situation in which the diagnostic signs do not confirm L5 dysfunction. In some obese patients and in patients with well-developed musculature, a reliable segmental manual functional diagnosis is impossible, but despite this, a manipulation in the four different possible three-dimensional physiological directions is undertaken. If this is effective, it verifies an L5 dysfunction. In other situations, a trochanter belt (Figure 60.5) is sometimes successfully tried in cases without recurring markers of pelvic or lumbar dysfunction. Autotraction may be tried in *any* patient with low back pain, sometimes most effectively in spite of the absence of clinical signs of a herniated disc with or without radiating pain. According to conventional wisdom, autotraction is applied only in patients with radiating pain with a more or less clear nerve-root distribution and focal neurological signs; however, according to the STAYAC philosophy, autotraction is one of the antidysfunctional treatment modalities and not merely a treatment for herniated discs— another excellent and clinically important consequence of the pragmatic principle.

There are, of course, also patients with true idiopathic conditions in which the STAYAC concept cannot offer any specific treatment, because they do not respond positively to antidysfunctional investigation/treatment or to *ex juvantibus* treatment. They are represented by the small, vertically oriented 'idiopathic pain' pink box in the lower middle of the algorithm in Figure 60.1. These patients are managed within the yellow 'psycho-existential' stack to the left in the flowchart: non-specific adjuvant treatment, such as general physical exercise, the stay-active concept, behavioural strategies, patient education, and, sometimes, psychotherapeutic measures can be applied, with the intention of reducing the unwelcome consequences of the conditions. Applying the STAYAC algorithm in these patients consistently reduces, to a minimum, the risk of missing truly somatically oriented and treatable conditions, and thereby optimizes the number of patients whose symptoms cannot be brought under control.

In addition, there is a feedback flow from the yellow 'psycho-existential sphere' to the 'antidysfunctional treatment/investigation' box: in Figure 60.1, all the arrows from the 'psycho-existential sphere' coalesce in a common long feedback loop far to the left, which continues all the way back to the 'antidysfunctional treatment/investigation' box (see the smaller descending arrow close to the left of the thick arrow going from the 'dysfunctions' box to the 'antidysfunctional' domain). This feedback loop takes account of patients in the 'psycho-existential sphere' in (renewed) need of antidysfunctional treatment, not least those who were subjected to physical exercise as the initial main management early in the antidysfunctional investigation.

Yellow light B situations

Steroid injections

Frequently, antidysfunctional treatment, such as manipulation, soon leads to 'primary dysfunctions abolished' (the upper pale pink box in the middle of the 'green flags' sphere), followed by freedom from pain and other associated complaints (i.e. the thick blue arrow exiting right from this box, going further down to the 'A' or 'B' boxes). However, despite the apparent resolution of dysfunction, pain will persist in a group of patients at 'primary dysfunctions abolished'; these patients continue down to the next pale pink box in the middle of the 'green flags' sphere—'Still in pain due to remaining secondary dysfunctions' (i.e. soft tissue dysfunctional irritations). This is when a steroid injection should be considered, not earlier. Steroid injections undertaken in patients with ongoing

(a)

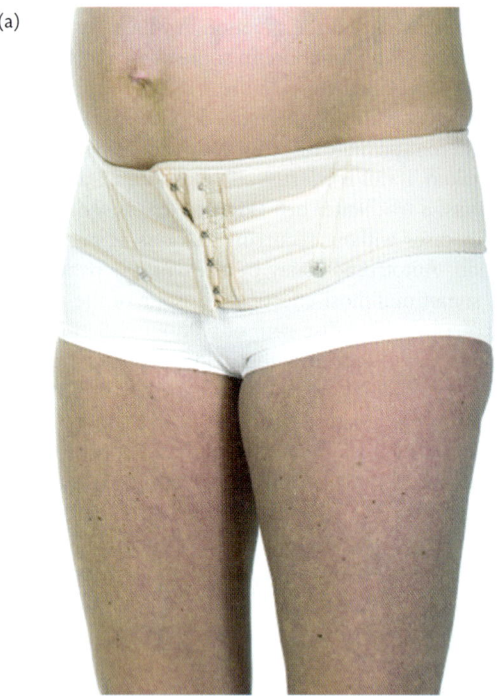

(b)

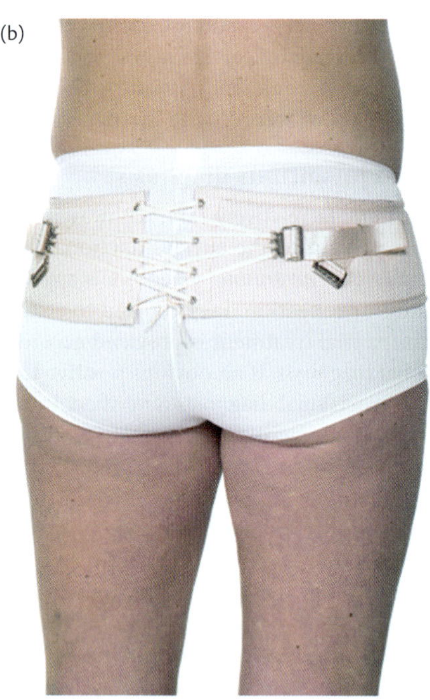

Figure 60.5 (a,b) A trochanter belt is used following manipulation in both male and female patients with recurring markers of pelvic dysfunction. It is non-stretchable, strapped on with permanent fasteners, and has groin straps to prevent the belt from sliding upwards (Camp, 'Tro-Camp').

dysfunctions are considerably less effective and, in addition, long-term effects seem to be limited or non-existent. As indicated by the 'steroid injections' box (between the symbols for yellow light A and for yellow light B, close to the 'green flags' stack in Figure 60.1), there is one rare exception: steroid injections are sometimes tried as a secondary prevention measure when other such moves have failed to achieve a 'primary dysfunctions abolished' state. Occasionally, the phenomenon of recurring dysfunctions is brought to an end in this way.

Not all patients need steroid injections: approximately 40–50% of the most severely affected patients with acute/subacute low back pain are treated by steroid injections (Blomberg et al. 1994b; Grunnesjö et al. 2004a&b). Consequently, there is an important 'short cut' from 'still in pain due to remaining secondary dysfunctions' to 'stretching/ functional training'. Moreover, as represented in the algorithm by the arrow in the reverse direction, some patients who have primarily been managed by physiotherapists are referred for steroid injections when treatment has not been sufficiently effective. The flow of patients between doctors and physiotherapists works best when both disciplines have been trained in the indications, possibilities, limitations, and effectiveness of each other's treatment methods. This is achieved by training doctors and physiotherapists together in shared courses, covering the needs of both professional groups—an important approach within the STAYAC concept.

Since, in spite of its complex structure, the STAYAC algorithm is still a simplification of the clinical reality in which therapists are educated in the pragmatic treatment programme, there are many more 'short cuts' that are exceptions to the main flows, and which for simplicity are not included in the algorithm. Paler lines to the right of the green 'antidysfunctional sphere' indicate some of the less frequent shortcuts. The most important of these is the one on the far right: the small subgroup of patients who, at an early stage during the antidysfunctional investigation, have been diagnosed as suffering from significant idiopathic pain, enter the antidysfunctional sphere, follow the paler arrow directly to the 'primary dysfunctions abolished' and 'still in pain due to remaining secondary dysfunctions' boxes and, as indicated by the vertically arranged 'idiopathic pain' box in the middle of the algorithm, proceed to the 'psycho-existential sphere', via the long grey ascending line that connects with all the different levels of the green antidysfunctional sphere.

A second fairly important short cut is the one from 'still in pain due to remaining secondary dysfunctions' directly to 'autotraction'. This refers to the tiny minority of patients with verified herniated discs, but without any treatable dysfunctions; they are directed from the 'no dysfunctions' box (in the upper left corner of the algorithm) to 'antidysfunctional treatment', via 'combined with dysfunctions'. Thereafter, the flow follows the main route to 'still in pain due to remaining secondary dysfunctions' and hence to autotraction. The patients are either non-surgical cases or candidates for operation, but, with the aim of avoiding surgery, autotraction and/or nerve mobilization are tried first. The *ex juvantibus* principle may be applied in cases with suspected symptomatic herniated discs.

When steroid injections are applied in a 'primary dysfunctions abolished' state, they are usually effective, and the effect is dependent on the uniquely integrated co-operation between the doctors and the physiotherapists at STAYAC, together keeping the patients persistently in a 'primary dysfunctions abolished' state. In the few cases that are refractory to steroid injections, or in whom the steroid effect is only temporary (some weeks), wet needling (i.e. with local anaesthetics, 5 or 6 times, 5–10 days in between, and with a steroid on the first occasion) to the structure(s) in question is provided. The most common sites for a series of wet needling are the piriformis and the teres minor muscles, lateral epicondalgia ('epicondylitis'), and the origin of the patellar tendon in the condition of apex patellae ('apicitis', 'distal patellalgia'). Although some authorities claim that this is incorrect, the periosteum should, in my opinion, be intensively needled—a procedure that definitely reinforces the treatment results. Dry needling without local anaesthetic (Lewit 1991) is infrequently applied by the doctors at STAYAC, since it is less effective than wet needling. However, nowadays, dry needling is, to an increasing extent, undertaken by our specially educated physiotherapists. For optimized therapeutic effects of extra-articular injections (with the exception of parasacrococcygeal injections), wet needling should always combine local anaesthetic with steroid. In addition, the muscle in question is always stretched after injection with local anaesthesia. Combined treatments are a STAYAC trademark.

According to the literature (Zulian et al. 2003), triamcinolone hexacetonide is the drug of choice, often in combination with needling and local anaesthetics (lidocaine is normally used at STAYAC). The injections are given according to manual diagnostic findings, i.e. pain by palpation, isometric contraction, and/or stretching. However, according to the ultra-pragmatic approach, to avoid over-reliance on the predictive value of clinical findings, only one of these diagnostic requirements needs to be fulfilled, and sometimes not even that. Sometimes the *ex juvantibus* principle is applied, i.e. the treatment is given although none of these signs is present.

Several types of injections are undertaken at STAYAC. Some examples of important injection sites in the lower back region are listed in Box 60.1. All these 'irritations' are rarely seen without a co-existent lumbar/pelvic/thoracic/cervical dysfunction. The same is more or less true for injections in the extremities. According to the pragmatic STAYAC principle, in which dysfunctions are considered to represent disturbances of the posturo-proprioceptive system/postural control organization, 'electrical chaos' or an 'electrostorm' occurs. These disturbances are normally halted by antidysfunctional treatment (comparable to the electrical shock conversion of cardiac, atrial, or ventricular fibrillation or cardiac arrest), home exercises, physical exercises, the 'stay-active concept', and so on, or subside spontaneously. The disturbances are, in turn, generated by one or more of an unknown amount of postulated *'sinus nodes'* involved in the process of the posturo-proprioceptive system losing control. It is not possible to distinguish between lumbar and pelvic dysfunctions; they always come together.

The most important and most frequent injection, which is probably unique to the STAYAC concept, is described here. This injection—to painful and sometimes spastic parasacrococcygeal structures—is responsible for a good deal of our treatment results. 'Parasacrococcygeal' is preferred to the more common term 'paracoccygeal', as the injection site is most frequently located more cranially in the area of the apex of the sacrum and near the cranial part of the coccyx, not only adjacent to the latter.

Cyriax (1970) stated that the sacrotuberous and sacrospinal ligaments were common foci for pain, but it is obvious that contractile tissues also are involved. This anatomical region does indeed incorporate the origins of the sacrotuberous and sacrospinal ligaments, but also the musculus coccygeus and musculus levator ani pars iliaca, and maybe also the origin of the piriformis muscle. To my knowledge, this area was first described as a site for (bimanual) injection by the late Sven-Otto Myrin (Myrin 1972), and the bi-manual injection technique seems to have been developed by him in the 1960s (teaching me the technique in 1985).

Originally, the patient lay on one side, but prone positioning seems more functional. The needle is usually introduced through the skin about 2 cm below the crena ani and 1 cm lateral to the midline. To simplify the manoeuvre, the medial/upper part of the buttock is pushed away from the midline with the thumb of the hand palpating the rectum. In this way, the distance from the surface of the skin to the bone is rarely more than 1 cm and a 0.7-mm × 50-mm needle is almost always sufficient. (On rare occasions, a 0.8-mm × 80-mm needle is needed.) After bone contact with the

Box 60.1 Some examples of injection sites in the lower back region

Dorsal aspect of the lower back and pelvis, in order of frequency

- Parasacrococcygeal structures
- Painful insertions on the greater trochanter of the piriformis muscle (also, less frequently, the origin/insertion of the gluteus medius/minimus and the submedius bursa)
- Sacroiliac joint (provocation-positive but dysfunction-free)
- Muscle insertions and other structures on the ischial tuberosity
- 'Kissing spines' (i.e. interspinal tenderness, considered by some authors to be a bursitis)
- Origin of the tensor fascia lata (lateral aspect)
- Transverse processes
- Iliolumbar ligaments*
- Posterior sacroiliac ligaments
- Epidural steroid injections**

Anterior aspect of the lower back and pelvis, in order of frequency

- Hip joint
- Bursa iliopectinea
- All adductors (most frequently, the adductor longus)
- Lateral femoral cutaneous nerve (in meralgia paresthetica)
- Ilioinguinal nerve

* The iliolumbar ligaments attach to the anterior aspect of os ilia and are reachable with an 80-mm needle. Injections into tender soft tissues in this anatomical area are frequently to muscular structures. Nevertheless, they may sometimes prove beneficial. However, cases of significant hyper-reactivity in the lower lumbar spine usually manifest considerable tenderness here, resulting in only temporary effects from steroid injections. Despite this, injection may be tried, although not repetitively.

** Epidural steroid injections (through the hiatus sacralis) are an important contribution to the STAYAC algorithm. However, this measure is introduced later than other steroid injections, after autotraction, and never as a primary measure. Epidural injections are needed in only a tiny minority of patients as a late move in the antidysfunctional investigation. The approach is pragmatic, i.e. it may, at an appropriate point of time, be applied in any patient with low back pain, not only when radicular pain or dural irritation is suspected.

apex of the sacrum is made, the needle penetrates further laterally/caudally in the tissues. During this process, the tip of the needle is palpated by the gloved index finger of the other hand, which is inserted in the patient's rectum. The distance between the index finger and the tip of the needle is probably a few millimetres. A quick oscillation of the syringe and the needle, with minimal amplitude, makes it easier to palpate the tip of the needle *per rectum*. One ml of steroid and 5–10 ml of local anaesthetic is injected on the affected side. (Bilateral irritation is considerably more common than unilateral pain.) The injected fluid should be spread in the area while successively re-penetrating the needle in a fan-shaped pattern. Note that the skin is penetrated only once on each side.

The most painful parts of the area are injected, which frequently means (a) the entire area as previously described but, not uncommonly, only (b) the tissue adjacent to the inferior lateral angle of the apex sacri (ILA, the Michigan osteopaths) or (c) the lateral and somewhat more distant parts. The bi-manual injection technique seems necessary in order to enable the steroid to be injected deeply enough to affect the symptomatic tissue. In STAYAC, where approximately 20 different physicians altogether have provided at least 15,000 parasacrococcygeal injections since 1985, no complications, except for one infection treated successfully in a hospital, have ever been observed.

After the injection, the parasacrococcygeal structures are also stretched *per rectum* (Midttun et al. 1983), a method that can be used as a primary alternative to the injection just described. However, parasacrococcygeal stretching seems to be less effective and frequently, in our experience, has to be repeated four or five times; in addition, applied as a primary measure, the stretching is considerably more painful than the injection. (Stretching the structures after local anaesthetic has been injected is not painful.) Nevertheless, our specially trained physiotherapists sometimes apply *per rectum* stretching—they perform diagnostic manoeuvres *per rectum* frequently though—with excellent results in cases where it is not too painful (see following text). Sometimes, *deep frictions* from outside work sufficiently.

Tissue irritation in this region (the posterior part of the pelvic floor) is a common cause of pseudoradicular pain in the leg, frequently extending all the way down to the foot. Referred pain frequently emanates from irritable foci at the insertion of the piriformis muscle and from sacroiliac joints, in addition to the parasacrococcygeal structures. In some patients, particularly those who have not received appropriate treatment for a long time (frequently for many years), all three irritable foci have to be injected. The clinical picture seems repeatedly to be misinterpreted as true radicular pain (see previous text), and there is an obvious risk of operation for an asymptomatic herniated disc. In fact, this pragmatic measure may be the only reliable method of detecting whether or not a herniated disc is symptomatic.

In patients in whom the steroids achieve merely temporary effects, the parasacrococcygeal structures may be re-injected once or twice, not more. If the tenderness persists, the situation is usually resolved after a series of five or six parasacrococcygeal *per rectum* stretching sessions (habitually performed by our specially trained physiotherapists). Occasionally, this procedure (stretching without local anaesthetics) is extremely painful, and under these circumstances a physician takes care of the stretching series, each time after local anaesthesia (no steroid), administered in the same manner as the usual parasacrococcygeal injections. Sometimes *botulinum toxin* is used instead of steroids, especially in the few cases where steroids do not supply a persistent pain relief in the parasacrococcygeal structures, or no pain relief at all; at times, botulinum toxin provides better results than steroids.

From the general principles listed in Table 60.1, it should be possible to estimate reasonable procedures when injecting other locations. According to our latest outcome study, the average number of injections per patient, including the most severely troubled patient category, is 1.9 (0.29 injections per visit), a moderate number in comparison to what is provided in some pain clinics.

How do steroids exert their effects?

Only a tiny minority of extra-articular irritations are true inflammations, deserving an '-itis' suffix. Consequently, leading rheumatologists suggest the abolition of terms such as 'epicondylitis' and suggest 'epicondalgia' and 'tendalgia'. From a behavioural perspective, this is important. Using words stronger than necessary in communication with patients, implying that patients are more sick than they actually are, may influence them negatively, i.e. in a stay-passive direction. Furthermore, if the physician/therapist thinks in terms of inflammation, the risk of subconscious transferring of stay-passive messages increases (insufficient metacognition and lateral thinking). Regrettably, limiting regimens due to this phenomenon are also frequently conveyed consciously. In communication with the patient, the word 'irritation' (of a muscle insertion, for instance) should be used. If a steroid injection is curative, it does not necessarily mean that a true inflammatory condition was eliminated; there are other, largely unknown, mechanisms suggesting that only a minor part of the entire inflammatory complex (e.g. antiprostaglandin effects) is involved. For the time being, as long as we have not identified a true inflammatory condition for sure, the soft tissue irritations are regarded as dysfunctions. Again, this illustrates the metacognitive aspects of the STAYAC approach.

Alternatives to steroid injections

There are numerous alternative treatment modalities that may be used instead of steroid injections at this stage, although in general they are less effective: function massage, deep frictions, acupuncture, laser (today, evidence-based), intramuscular stimulation (IMS) (Gunn 1996; see Chapter 58), dry needling (see Chapter 59), wet needling (with local anaesthetics), transcutaneous nerve stimulation, transcutaneous electrical muscular stimulation, therapeutic ultrasound, etc. Physiotherapists with appropriate training may undertake these treatment modalities. These methods are not infrequently used within the STAYAC concept, but never as primary methods; in the presence of ongoing dysfunctions, these treatment modalities will certainly offer poor treatment results and are not cost-effective.

Which method is used is, to a large extent, a matter of personal preference. However, one has to be prepared to repeat the treatment, and in many patients, a steroid injection will be necessary in the end anyway. Consequently, administering steroids from the beginning of this phase in the antidysfunctional investigation (still in pain due to remaining secondary dysfunctions) is obviously more cost-effective. Steroid injections may, however, be viewed as aggressive (not least by some patients). This is irrational; in reality, depot steroids have negligible side-effects and complications (not least in comparison with the NSAIDs and opioids frequently used outside the STAYAC approach). Every physician has to develop an

Table 60.1 Needle sizes, volumes of steroid, and local anaesthetic for some of the most common injections

Structure	Triamcinolone (ml)	Prilocaine (ml)	Needle size (mm)
Lig. iliolumbale	1 (20 mg)	4–10 (unilateral injection)	0.8 × 80 (0.7 × 50)
Parasacrococcygeal inj.	1 per side	5–10 per side	0.7 × 50 (0.8 × 80)
Sacroiliac joint	1	1	0.8 × 80
Piriformis	1	4–6	0.7 × 50 (0.8 × 80)
Tensor fascia latae	1	4–6	0.7 × 50
Hip joint	2	3–4	0.8 × 80
Bursa iliopectinea	1	4–6	0.7 × 50
Adductor longus origin	1	2–6	0.7 × 50
Lev. scapulae, insertion	1	3–4	0.7 × 50
Teres minor, insertion	1	2–4	0.7 × 50
Supraspinatus, insertion	1	2–4	0.7 × 50
Subacromial bursa	1	3–4	0.7 × 50
Acromioclavicular joint	0.5–0.7	0[a]	Intracutanous needle
Lat. epicondalgia	1	2–4	0.7 × 30
Med. epicondalgia	1	2–3	0.7 × 30
Kissing spines	1	1–2	0.7 × 50

[a]There is no room for local anaesthetics in this small joint. Preferably, anaesthetize the skin and deeper structures such as the periosteum with 2–3 ml lidocaine before injecting the joint (particularly if you are not fully trained in injection techniques). Other small joints in which the same method may be applied are the finger joints, the toe joints, and the sacrococcygeal joint. In many joints, injection is facilitated by letting an assistant (physiotherapist or nurse) apply traction simultaneously with the injection procedure (not only in small joints, but also in the hip joint, shoulder joint and subacromial bursa, ankle joint, etc.).

educational model to handle patients' scepticism. Preferably, this is done in the patient education groups (see the subsection 'The 'stay active' and the 'patient education' boxes').

Few physicians are adequately trained for these procedures: in order not to overload them, it is valuable for physiotherapists to have access to alternative treatments, which they may try before asking their cooperating physician to administer steroid injections.

Muscle stretching: second indication

Muscle stretching, according to the 'second indication' (see the corresponding box in the 'green flags' stack of the algorithm in Figure 60.1), is shown as an alternative or complementary treatment to the injections. The theoretical rationales for muscle stretching are that dysfunctionally shortened muscles may be an important source of pain (at their origin, belly, and/or insertion) and that they may secondarily cause joint, joint capsule, or ligament pain (or disseminated diffuse pain in a system of joints) by altering the biomechanics, even in the absence of diagnosable primary dysfunctions. Examples are pain from the thoracolumbar junction due to shortened iliopsoas muscle(s), and knee pain due to shortened muscles involved in knee function.

The stretching approach applied within the STAYAC concept, which seems to be the most advanced one available, has been developed by Evjent and Hamberg (1985a,b). Stretching is an important treatment in all regions of the body, including the hands and feet. An essential difference between this model and some other stretching philosophies is that even *considerable pain in the muscle in question is allowed*, as long as the patient can tolerate it, and in spite of the pain is able to relax the muscle during the stretching phase. This procedure is time-saving and more effective, particularly in patients with considerable shortening of muscles in whom it is impossible to make progress with pain-free stretching, whether therapeutic or as home exercises. Only dysfunctionally shortened muscles are stretchable. Contrary to what some authorities claim, it is virtually impossible to damage muscles or any other anatomical structures during muscle stretching. In contractures (i.e. pathomorphology with permanently changed plasticity), only further shortening may be counteracted, and in spastic muscles, e.g. due to disturbed (dysfunctional) complex neuromuscular reflex patterns in the posturo-proprioceptive control system, muscle stretching may, as shown in our research, provoke pain, and the treatment results are poor.

One important issue is whether or not we really stretch muscles. Analogous reasoning has to be applied as in the case of neurodynamics according to Elvey and Butler: numerous structures may be stretched other than muscles—nerves, fasciae, veins, arteries, skin, fat, other subcutaneous tissues, and so forth. A further possible mechanism for the beneficial effects of muscle stretching is the posturo-proprioceptive model (described in 'Antidysfunctional treatment' in the section 'Dysfunction, markers of dysfunction, antidysfunctional treatment/medicine') in which it is logical to stretch muscles that may not even be shortened: 'electrical chaos'/'electrostorm' may be halted by 'control/alt/delete' and 'reset' mechanisms (see previous text); the stretching home programme may likewise (like physical exercise and the specific mobilizing exercises for the entire spine—see following text) contribute to the process of keeping the patients in a 'primary dysfunctions abolished' state. If and when 'muscle stretching' becomes evidence-based, further fundamental research may be able to map out the underlying mechanisms.

Home exercises aiming at optimizing the treatment results and preserving the increased muscle lengths are almost always taught to the patients as an important part of the home-care programme. This is true also with respect to muscle stretching according to the 'first indication' (see the corresponding box in the 'green flags' stack of the algorithm in Figure 60.1). The Evjent/Hamberg 'autostretching' book (Evjent and Hamberg 1990) covers advanced stretching techniques for iliocrural muscles and all muscles of the extremities, as well as specific mobilizing exercises for the entire spine, including locking techniques. In addition, some other home exercises are included in our home programmes (Lewit 1991).

Non-specific pain treatment

The constituents of 'non-specific pain treatment' are primarily those associated with medical disciplines outside manual medicine/manual therapy. Since all these methods, as demonstrated in our research, are considerably less effective than other items in the antidysfunctional sphere, especially if applied as primary measures, they have a comparably minor role in the STAYAC algorithm.

Medication (for example, diazepam as a muscle relaxant, or opioids) is used only occasionally as a primary measure, usually to facilitate specific antidysfunctional treatment in extremely acute cases of neck or back pain with significant regional muscle spasm. Other methods of handling such situations are strictly applied muscle energy principles (sometimes this works better than thrust techniques) and locking techniques, or using the autotraction couch as a primary measure, i.e. as a 'mobilization device'. This is a rather non-specific mobilization; however, despite significant muscle spasm, it is possible to move the dysfunctional segment(s) in the desired direction three-dimensionally during significant traction, simultaneously utilizing mechanical traction, gravitational traction, and traction applied by the patient himself/herself (the latter constituting the 'auto'-component of the autotraction method). Otherwise, non-specific pain treatment modalities are usually not applied until after manipulation, muscle stretching, and steroid injections have been tried with insufficient results.

Examples of non-specific pain treatments are analgesics, muscle relaxants, NSAIDs, acupuncture, evidence-based laser, transcutaneous nerve stimulation (TENS), transcutaneous electrical muscular stimulation (TEMS), therapeutic ultrasound, intramuscular stimulation (IMS) (see Chapter 58), heat, cold, cryostretching (Travell 1983–1992), and so forth. With respect to NSAIDs (an evidence-based treatment modality in acute low back pain), there is a tiny subgroup of pain patients, without confirmed inflammatory conditions, in whom NSAIDs are the only therapeutic measure that works, at least in combination with antidysfunctional treatment modalities. These patients are preferably identified during the selection process of the algorithm, and NSAIDs in these cases should of course be prescribed for continuous use, over years if necessary, with relevant annual tests of blood parameters. Over-enthusiasm for manual therapy may cause clinicians to overlook this small but important patient group.

Non-specific pain treatment—acupuncture

Acupuncture plays an essential role in 'non-specific pain treatment', having become a frequently used treatment modality. At this stage in the algorithm flowchart, acupuncture sometimes appears to be the only effective treatment, especially in cases of widespread regional muscle/soft tissue tenderness (of course, again, in a 'primary dysfunctions abolished' state—otherwise, acupuncture has seemingly modest effects), provided the acupuncturist is adequately trained and has satisfactory experience in this technique. Having scrutinized the results of different acupuncturists in the clinic for many years, I am now convinced that the original Chinese/Eastern mode of acupuncture is superior to acupuncture adapted to the Western biomedical paradigm/thinking, despite the lack of hard evidence indicating this.

The muscle tenderness previously referred to is frequently described as '*myofascial pain*'. Unfortunately, at least in Sweden, this perspective has become overused and, according to our experience, too much focus on acupuncture (or IMS) as a single 'silver bullet' therapy yields poor and cost-ineffective treatment results. As usual within the STAYAC concept, '*primary dysfunctions*' and, not least, soft tissue '*secondary dysfunctions*' have to be treated initially with other modalities, and the appropriate steroid injections have to be provided first. This may sound a bit harsh; however, anyone working within the STAYAC paradigm may sometimes try different needles primarily (without steroids and local anaesthetics), but not endless ineffective series. Another important reason for this approach is that, empirically, in many patients, virtually all trigger points (for example, in the back muscles, from the lower back up to the neck) quickly disappear, seconds after manual treatment of, for example, lower lumbar and pelvic dysfunctions. Consequently, within the STAYAC concept, *trigger and tender points are considered a secondary manifestation* of the more or less generalized '*electrical chaos*' in the posturo-proprioceptive system, and not viewed as primary conditions.

Consistently disappointed by poor treatment results from dry needling of trigger points (the same is true for steroids directed to trigger points), I now only rarely inject trigger points with steroids and local anaesthetics (since triamcinolone hexacetonide is not to be administered intramuscularly, methylprednisolone is used), especially if the physiotherapists have problems with one or two symptomatic and therapy-resistant trigger points and, after having tried everything else without benefit, ask me to do so. In summary, in a fairly small subgroup of our patients, Chinese/Eastern acupuncture is an essential treatment method at STAYAC. IMS is probably a useful alternative to acupuncture at this stage of the flowchart.

Most important, acupuncture is *never* to be allowed to become an alternative to physical exercise or any other item of the flowchart—definitely, too much primary, passive, single-tool 'silver-bullet' acupuncture is applied to patients all over the world.

Traction modalities, including autotraction

Autotraction (Knutsson et al. 1988; Lind 1974; Ljunggren et al. 1984; Natchew 1984) and other traction methods are usually applied only in patients who are free from primary and secondary dysfunctions and after soft tissue foci of irritation have been injected with steroids. The elimination of 'pseudo-neurological' signs achieved by autotraction (which is an antidysfunctional treatment) is most probably not a question of reduction of nerve root pressure. Neuropathology caused by a herniated disc cannot be treated by autotraction or any other antidysfunctional therapy. In addition, the original theory that the herniation was 'sucked back into the disc' during autotraction, has been disproved (Gillström et al. 1985). This retraction was attributed to a negative pressure during traction: on the contrary, it has been shown that the intradiscal pressure increases during autotraction (Andersson et al. 1984).

The warning about the dangerous and passivizing regimen applied by some clinicians after prolotherapy goes for autotraction too. Unfortunately, the originator of this therapeutic modality (Lind 1974), and many autotraction therapists, believed in mechanistically oriented models, and many therapists are still stuck in this 'biomechanical trap'. Patients were not allowed to leave their bed for weeks or even longer, and were transported by ambulance to and from the treatment sessions. The risk of the patients perceiving this as a dramatic procedure, with potentially negative consequences, is evident. Adherence to these outmoded theories has contributed to the fact that this very useful treatment method, which flourished in the 1970s in Sweden and elsewhere, has today more or less disappeared outside manual therapy circles. Patients treated by autotraction should be encouraged to be active and disabused of the previously applied passivizing regimens. Autotraction is perceived at STAYAC as an antidysfunctional treatment, with effects similar to manipulation (a 'reset' manoeuvre), and combined with maintenance of activities of daily living.

Autotraction seems to be considerably less effective in patients with untreated dysfunctions, and with uninjected irritable soft tissue foci, not least in the presence of referred radiating pain mimicking true radicular pain (e.g. from parasacrococcygeal structures, from the sacroiliac joint, from the musculus piriformis and gluteus medius/minimus). Since only a few patients need prolotherapy, there is of course an important short-cut from the 'non-specific pain treatment' box to the 'autotraction' box (shown as a paler line in the algorithm in Figure 60.1).

Prolotherapy: first indication

In the few patients in whom the pain is not controlled at this stage, prolotherapy (see corresponding box in the 'green flags' stack of the algorithm in Figure 60.1) may be provided in relevant cases. The indication is *segmental hyper-reactivity*. The originator of prolotherapy (Hackett 1958) believed that it brought about proliferation of connective tissue in the spinal column, which, in turn, leads to 'stabilization' of 'hypermobile' vertebral segments or sacroiliac joints.

Although I have experienced good treatment results from prolotherapy, when applied according to specific indications, my impression is that the spinal mobility of the patients *increases*, as supported by a dynamic radiography report (Tilscher 1995, 1996). I am convinced that the underlying mechanism is not mechanical: rather, I believe that this treatment, as is the case with other antidysfunctional treatment modalities, addresses the electrical chaos caused in central elements of the posturo-proprioceptive control system by disturbed proprioception from a damaged and hyperreactive vertebral segment. In other words, prolotherapy is equivalent to a *forceful and aggressive reset manoeuvre*.

It is important to avoid the 'hypermobility' model, in which rest is perceived as advantageous after prolotherapy. By contrast, most of our patients work as usual after treatment sessions, except for some that have to stay at home for a day or two because of temporary post-treatment pain. They walk, exercise, ride on horseback, and so forth, and I am entirely convinced that the treatment results have improved considerably since the introduction of this activity modification of prolotherapy. Being a fairly aggressive and expensive treatment method (lumbar/pelvic prolotherapy in STAYAC's protocol takes 10 treatment sessions), it is not appropriate for use as a primary approach, especially in patients with ongoing dysfunctions. In fact, my use of prolotherapy has diminished considerably since the 1980s, paralleled by a corresponding enforcement of behavioural/psychodynamic thinking (nowadays permeating the entire concept), metacognition, the development of patient education since 1988, and so forth. (For a further discussion of prolotherapy, see Chapters 54 and 55.)

Nerve mobilization

Nerve mobilization is included in the STAYAC concept. It is appropriate to introduce this treatment approach in the cases when autotraction is not applicable or successful, and of course in other parts of the body (e.g. extremities) when the patients have not responded to other antidysfunctional therapy, or in the few cases in which true dysfunctional nerve pain is suspected. (True neuropathic pain cannot be treated by means of nerve mobilization.) For simplicity, and since these techniques rarely provide additional positive treatment effects when the earlier measures in the antidysfunctional domain have been undertaken, this approach is not represented by a box of its own in the algorithm—it may be introduced as a trial treatment in many stages of the flowchart.

Yellow light A situations

Recurring dysfunctions

Patients whose dysfunctions recur despite 2–4 antidysfunctional treatments fall into the *'recurring dysfunctions'* or *'yellow light A category'*. The positive effect(s) of manipulations or specific mobilizations may be substantial, but short-lived, and more than 3 or 4 repetitions of similar specific treatment manoeuvres is inappropriate. The three, often parallel, procedures that should be applied early in this instance are physical exercise (including functional training), mobilizing home exercises, and muscle stretching. This last measure is applied according to its first indication in the algorithm, namely 'recurring dysfunctions' (the second indication being primary, e.g. see previous discussion of muscle pain treatment). In the lower back/pelvic region, the most common muscles subjected to stretching are the hamstrings, rectus femoris, adductors, iliopsoas, tensores fasciae latae, and piriformis, but all muscles in the region are frequently stretched. A common name for this muscle group is the *'iliocrural muscles'*, even though a couple of them have an origin other than the os ilium.

The aim of the home exercise protocol is not only to maintain restored or improved function, achieved by the specific therapy; a proportion of the patients are even able to treat recurring dysfunctions themselves by stretching. Consequently, physical exercises, mobilizing home exercises, muscle stretching, the use of a trochanter belt, and prolotherapy for recurring dysfunctions are classified as *secondary prevention measures* for recurring dysfunctions. Two additional measures for secondary prevention are antidepressants (see later discussion) and steroid injections (see previous text).

Trochanter belt

In patients with recurring lumbar pain with recurring markers of pelvic dysfunctions, in spite of regular physical exercises and normalized muscle lengths, a trochanter belt (see Figure 60.5) is applied. The indication for this measure is simple and pragmatic. In recurring pelvic/lumbar dysfunctions, the application of the belt is *post-manipulative,* and has nothing to do with 'sacroiliac joint instability', post-partum low back pain, and so forth (i.e. the 'classical' indications for a trochanter belt in manual medicine). This means that the belt, originally developed for women with pelvic pain during or after pregnancy, is applied in male patients almost as frequently as in female patients. Thus, if the condition is not controlled at this stage, the belt should be applied following manipulation, and should be worn 24 hours a day for 6 weeks, and during the day only, for another 6 weeks. Stretchable trochanter belts with self-adhesive straps are not firm enough to prevent recurrence of pelvic dysfunctions: the belt should be non-stretchable and strapped on with permanent fasteners. In most patients, groin straps are needed to prevent the belt from sliding upwards.

The 'classical' mechanistic rationale for the use of this belt ('keeping the pelvic bones together in the correct position') is probably not valid—a proprioceptive effect (a slow but more or less continuous) 'reset' process is more likely. In most cases, the dysfunctions resolve within 12 weeks, after which most patients remain free of primary dysfunctions for extended periods without the belt.

There are no corresponding measures for patients with neck or thoracic pain, although epicondalgia bandages and knee orthoses may have similar effects.

Prolotherapy: second indication

Prolotherapy is indicated in the few cases in which dysfunctions continue to recur despite the measures taken so far in the algorithm. This is the second indication for prolotherapy (the first indication being a primary treatment for hyper-reactivity, as previously described).

For treatment success with prolotherapy, strict indications are needed. At this stage, through the selection process within the algorithm, the patients frequently have been suffering for a long time, and psycho-existential/social dimensions/complications are common. This is also true for prolotherapy according to the first indication. An essential criterion that has to be fulfilled before prolotherapy is considered is that major psycho-existential dimensions to patients' symptoms are ruled out by means of a suitable psychological instrument, that can be done in many different ways. The patients should also have been undertaking continuous physical exercise for at least 6 months, and have pursued this in a well-motivated manner. Prolotherapy should never be carried through as an alternative to physical exercise—these two managements should always go hand in hand. Disappointing results for prolotherapy may be obtained if strict criteria are not used (Dechow et al. 1999; Yelland et al. 2004). Otherwise, it is an excellent method.

Although it is not yet considered sufficiently evidence-based (Nachemson and Jonsson 2000), very few patients fail to benefit from it if provided at an appropriate stage. Substantive support for the use of prolotherapy is provided by Ongley et al. (1987) who treated patients with chronic pain. Klein et al. (1989) demonstrated increased lumbar spinal mobility after prolotherapy, and Klein et al. (1993) also showed borderline differences in favour of prolotherapy in a double-blind RCT.

Note that in the algorithm (Figure 60.1) there are short cuts to the 'no dysfunctions' box from all the 'secondary prevention' boxes in the upper half (darker green) of the antidysfunctional stack, indicating that only a minority of patients are in need of trochanter belt and prolotherapy respectively.

'Primary dysfunctions abolished' state

The 'primary dysfunctions abolished' state is defined as follows: there are no remaining markers of 'primary dysfunctions' (predominantly classical manual tests for the spine, pelvis, and extremities), *ex juvantibus* treatment has not shed light on the situation, and/or there are no reasonable indications that *ex juvantibus* diagnosis would be meaningful. When the algorithm has been followed so far, a 'primary dysfunctions abolished' state is almost always established. However, some patients are still in pain at this stage. These patients will follow the same pathways as those who achieved a 'primary dysfunctions abolished' state already, during the early treatment steps of the algorithm, without the described measures of secondary prevention.

In conclusion, there is, due to persisting 'green flag' conditions, still pain; 'secondary dysfunctions' (i.e. soft tissue irritations) are still to be found.

Successful outcomes: 'recovered' (alternative A) or 'residual symptoms' (alternative B)

From the 'stack' of antidysfunctional measures, there are pathways to the right at all levels, representing the recovered cases or instances with minor symptoms, without the need for further treatment, and without significant consequences for patients' quality of life and ability to work (outcome alternative A). In the acute phase, dysfunctions are the dominating cause of pain—see Figure 60.4a (pathomorphology and primary psycho-existentially based conditions are rare).

- Consequently, according to our clinical trials (Blomberg 1993a,b), in acute and subacute patients, after one or two treatments, the pathway (thick blue line—a short cut on the *left* side of the antidysfunctional green stack in the algorithm in Figure 60.1) leading to the 'primary dysfunctions abolished' state is the most common scenario (an important short cut in the algorithm). After this, they progress (again, via a thick but longer blue line—a short cut on the *right* side of the green stack) to 'recovered' (outcome alternative A) or to a status of 'residual symptoms' (outcome alternative B).
- Another substantive group of patients make the same progress, after steroid injections (a somewhat shorter thick blue line—again, a short cut on the *right* side of the green stack), to outcome A or B.
- A group of patients, still in some pain, reaches this state (the A outcome) over time, via the same route, through 'spontaneous recovery'/improvement.
- In addition, another group of patients, with partly therapy-resistant pain, reaches outcome B (see the *right* broad, light-blue arrow at the bottom and centre of the flowchart).

- Later, these and other outcome B patients, again via 'spontaneous recovery', reach outcome A in the reverse direction (again, see *right* broad, light-blue arrow at the bottom and centre of the flowchart).
- A fifth group of patients are still in some pain, after having been guided through the 'psycho-existential sphere' (see the *left* broad, light-blue arrow at the bottom and centre of the flowchart).

As illustrated in Figure 60.4b, psycho-existential dimensions of pain suffering are dominant in severe chronic patients. Severe and chronic patients with purely dysfunctional conditions (green flag conditions), consequently treatable with antidysfunctional therapy only, are rare; thus, these patients are not represented by a circle in Figure 60.4b. There is an infinite variety of relationships between the three major circles: Figures 60.4a and 60.4b represent two extremes. Generally, chronic patients, in whom the dysfunctions and the relevant sites for injections have been untreated, sometimes for years, require on average more treatment steps than acute and subacute patients. Very few pain patients need to proceed through the entire antidysfunctional sphere or, of course, the entire algorithm. If antidysfunctional treatment is given early enough, most patients in this category need only a few treatment steps.

Outcome alternative B is somewhat less successful than alternative A, but still satisfactory. The ability to work is restored and circumstances are under control, although residual complaints still disturb everyday function and/or quality of life to some degree. In these patients, the process of self-recovery (see *both* broad, light-blue arrows at the bottom and centre of the flowchart in Figure 60.1), facilitated by long-term and tailor-made self-care programmes, and occasional manipulation provided by the physiotherapist, will finally lead to recovery.

The psycho-existential sphere (yellow flags)

The second important major 'stack' of therapeutic measures deals with the psycho-existential sphere ('yellow flags'). We know that the correlation between impairment (organ level) and perceived (dis)ability (individual level) is very weak (Waddell 1998). Consequently, we all meet patients who cope well with severe conditions and function well in most aspects including working ability, whereas others, whose impairment is minor (on objective assessment), perceive themselves as more or less completely disabled (see also 'Perception disturbances' in the section 'Dysfunction, markers of dysfunction, antidysfunctional treatment/medicine').

Nevertheless, patients with minor dysfunctional conditions, but who perceive themselves as disabled for instance with respect to working capability, should, according to the STAYAC method, virtually always be treated in the first instance with somatically oriented antidysfunctional therapy before steps are taken to deal with the psycho-existential dimensions of their suffering, although it is unlikely, alone, to solve the patient's life situation; it is all a matter of the 'Kierkegaard effect' and of founding a trustful therapeutic alliance. (See the section 'Behavioural aspects of manual therapy for low back pain' for a discussion of antidysfunctional therapy for established chronic patents and of the 'Kierkegaard effect'.) Unfortunately, this rarely happens in today's healthcare; a premature psychological approach may even reduce a patient's chances of moving forward (see discussion of the 'first perspective' in the section 'Pain-related syndromes—new psychological perspectives'). The patient's pain must be addressed, but the risk of passivizing the patients with pointless courses of antidysfunctional treatment has, according to metacognitive notions, to be continually kept in mind. Regrettably, as illustrated in Figure 60.6a, there is a widespread lack of awareness in manual therapy of psycho-existential factors, and endless series of passive treatments are too frequently provided. This leads to the reinforcement of pain behaviour and the development of pain identity, with adverse consequences.

Focusing on dysfunctional factors without attention to psycho-existential factors is not optimal, but the converse also applies (Figure 60.6b). As reflected by the two rudimentary algorithms in Figure 60.6, I believe that today's pain care in general is simultaneously over-somatized and over-psychologized (see also the discussion of the 'first' and 'second' perspectives in the section 'Pain-related syndromes—new psychological perspectives').

Figures 60.7a–d constitute a further series of rudimentary algorithms, also reflecting today's clinical reality. These are coexisting, but not connected or integrated, and in my opinion, this total lack of infrastructure is the main reason for the complete failure of healthcare with respect to the management of pain. The schemes illustrated in Figures 60.7a–d are discussed in later sections.

Consequently, in all stages of the antidysfunctional exploration, it is important to be constantly aware of psycho-existential factors that may jeopardize the rehabilitation process. In the algorithm (Figure 60.1), this awareness is represented by a series of lines on the left side of the 'green flag' domain, each directed from the different steps of the antidysfunctional domain to the yellow psycho-existential area (yellow flags). The lowest line from the autotraction box represents the point where the constituents of the psycho-existential sphere, in a deeply pragmatic manner (see following), should be considered at the absolute latest. The need for such measures may be assessed by means of predictive questionnaires (Linton and Halldén 1998) and/or an algorithm specially designed for the identification of yellow flags (Kendall *et al.* 1997), but is not necessary in the vast majority of cases. However, these philosophies suggest applying questionnaires which are not sufficiently reliable with respect to predictability on an individual level; they are useful in the process of assessing groups within research. The only solution to this problem is the truly pragmatic approach to the individual patient.

However, failure to heed the psycho-existential factors early in the programme is even worse and increases the risk of chronicity and progression to an unfavourable outcome such as early retirement. Theoretically, there is a possibility of spontaneous recovery, as represented by a flow from the C box to the A and B boxes in Figure 60.6a (see corresponding grey line between these boxes in the algorithm in Figure 60.1). However, probably as a result of the stigmatizing effect of long-term absence from work and 'long-term sick leave illness', this is rare. As illustrated in Figures 60.6a and 60.6b and Figures 60.7a–d, the reason for this is the lack of co-ordination of the different therapeutic resources—slow and extended management at inappropriate levels of care, during incorrect periods of patients' 'pain careers', and with barriers hindering patients from entering appropriate levels. Their rehabilitation potential is eventually destroyed. In the more difficult cases, close co-operation between all the healthcare professionals involved, the family, workplace representatives, and social services, combined with well-defined behavioural attitudes and capable metacognition skills, is paramount to avoid this slide into early retirement, its associated unhappiness, and even the 'living dead state'.

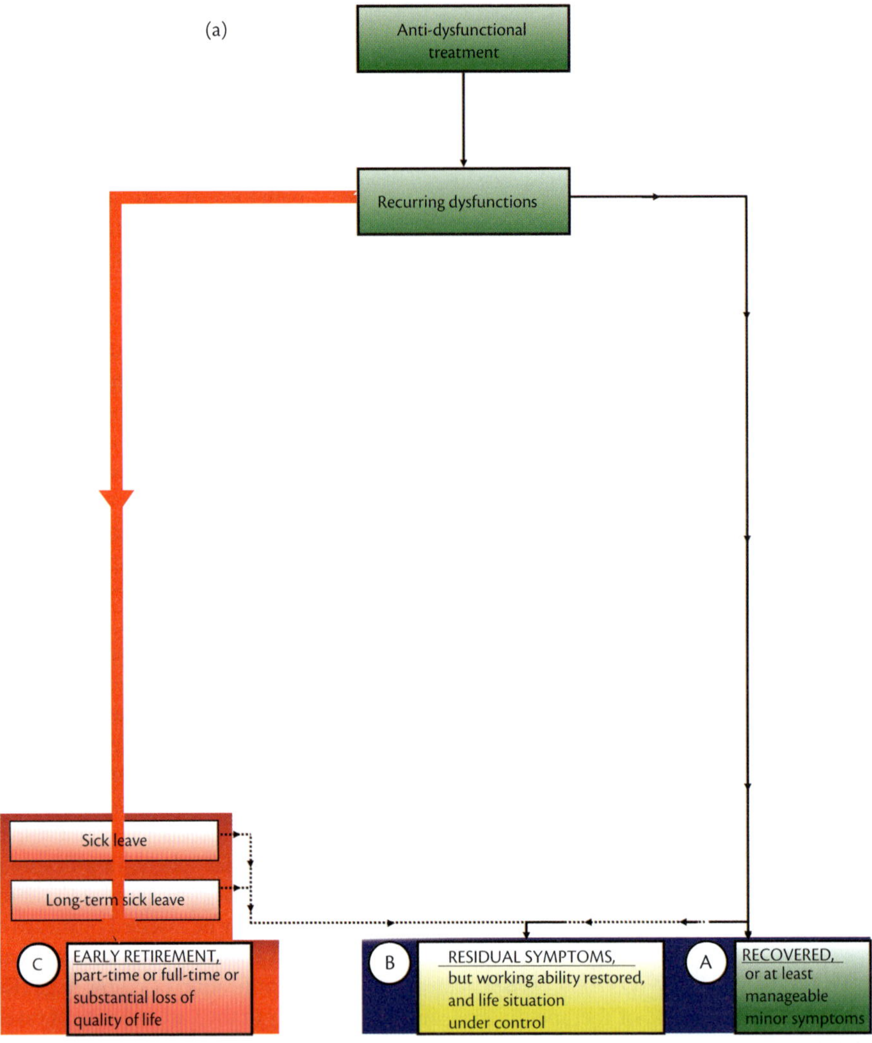

Figure 60.6 (a) Lack of awareness of psycho-existential factors and over-reliance on antidysfunctional/manual therapy, too frequently resulting in an endless series of passive treatments.

The 'stay active' box

The stay-active concept (see corresponding box in Figure 60.1) is not merely a matter of encouraging patients to increase their levels of activity just by providing advice and reassurance, and prescribing physical exercise. Another aspect, which is at least as important, is the stay-active approach as a metacognitive method. Without metacognitive processes, the activating strategies of the patients will never be optimal. In the STAYAC model, the metacognitive aspect means that every word communicated to the patient should contain (not infrequently subliminal) stay-active messages, not least while providing passive treatment such as manipulation.

Most pain management programmes focus on the stay-active approach, and it is now considered the most solidly evidence-based method of back pain care (Koes et al. 2001; Nachemson and Jonsson 2000; Waddell 1998). Nevertheless, the stay-active concept is insufficiently implemented in healthcare generally. All too often, management consists mainly of the passive prescription of medication and sick leave.

There is a synergy in a systematic and consistent parallel application of the stay-active approach and antidysfunctional treatments: a therapeutic combination, which is all too infrequent today. The stay-active concept (evaluated by Indahl et al. 1995; Malmivaara et al. 1995; and Torstensen et al. 1998) includes encouraging patients to take part in physical and other activities. Providing information about the benign character of the condition, and the adverse effects of inactivity and sick leave, encourages the patient to be more active.

'Staying active' is not only a matter of increasing physical activity. Relatively 'passive' activities such as going to the movies for the first time in 10 years (if the fear-avoidance thinking of the patient has hindered them from doing so), or going away on holiday for the first time in years, can be the key to rehabilitation success. Regrettably, these crucial but simple and frequently effective 'treatment' possibilities are often overlooked. The stay-active concept is a basic therapeutic principle, which is adopted from the first visit onwards. However, before the stay-active philosophy is applied in a goal-oriented manner—according to the considerations within the 'postulate of Kierkegaard' that states that the patient has to be met where he/she is, namely in his/hers pain, and nowhere else—the possibility of dysfunctional factors must be considered. This is an important difference between the STAYAC approach and the widespread recommendation that only (unspecified) 'self care' should be applied during the first weeks of acute low back pain. From our results, it is evident that active antidysfunctional treatment should be applied from the first visit, not least from a societal perspective; at this early stage, a decrease of only 2 days of sick leave on average

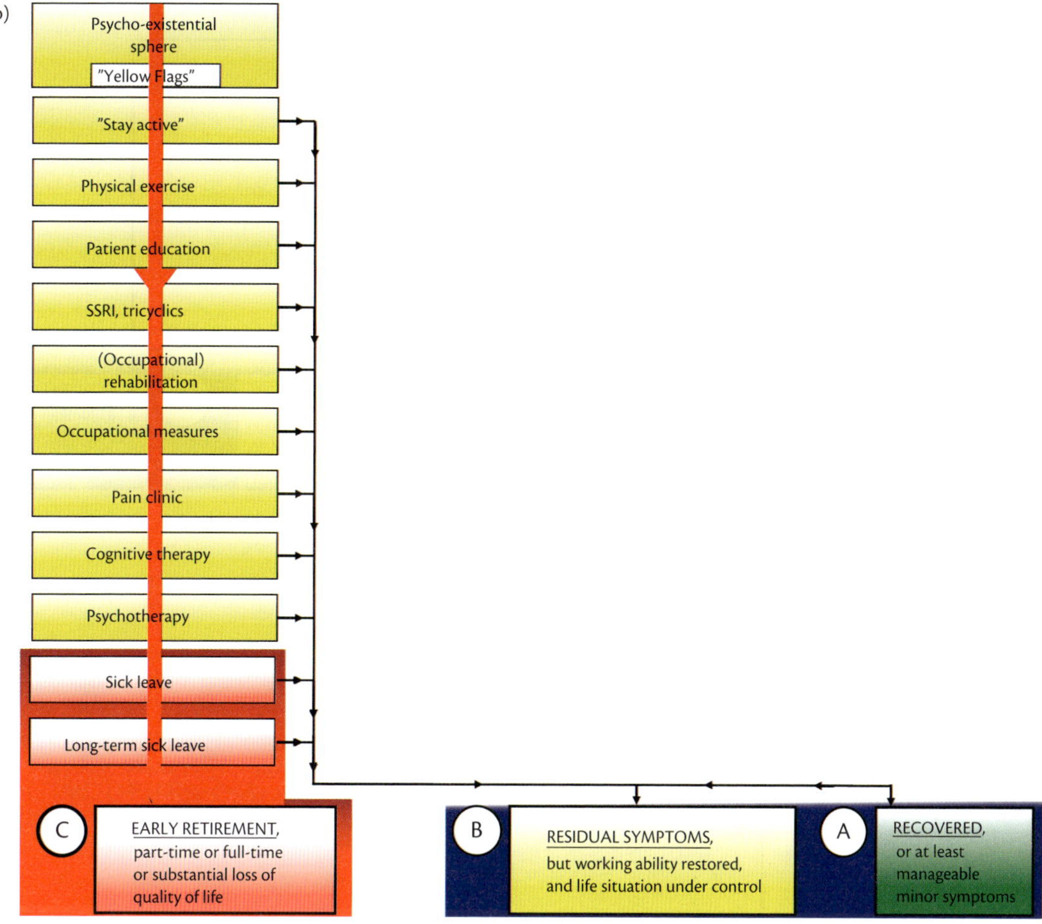

Figure 60.6 (b)The converse situation to that shown in Figure 60.6(a): a unidimensional focus on psycho-existential factors.

per patient would be extremely cost-effective (Hadler et al. 1987; Hadler et al. 1987).

Physical exercise—another 'self care' box

The STAYAC algorithm is basically an activity approach, which includes physical exercises, enhanced by manipulation and steroid injections. The '*Physical exercise*' box, in the yellow psycho-existential area (see Figure 60.1), not only includes exercises under the supervision of physiotherapists, but also constitutes a 'self care' box. It includes non-specific exercise, such as athletics or horse-riding, and stimulation to increase enjoyable, physically demanding leisure-time activities such as walking (Indahl et al. 1995) or any physical activity that the patient may have given up, frequently because of the pain (fear avoidance being a frequent underlying factor).

During recent years, the most frequently applied exercise philosophy has become functional exercise/training by means of the 'muscle action quality' concept (MAQ). This exercise methodology seems to be even better than medical exercise therapy (MET) (see following text) with regards to the optimizing of the function of the posturo-proprioceptive system. The idea of this model is to provide a minimum of restrictions, thereby creating a maximum of possibilities. Training/exercise is executed systematically and effectively to develop mobility, control, balance, and strength. It is about movement quality, doing the right things in the right order. MAQ is based on knowledge and experience gained from two decades of sports exercise and rehabilitation. The method begins with understanding and the exercise: it becomes a tool in combination with other treatment modalities to achieve certain goals. Integrated within the STAYAC algorithm, we use the MAQ concept to build up a good base, a good function, an optimal technique, and capacity to help the individual to get the function that is required to achieve and retain a pain-free status (Johansson and Larsson 2007).

Other exercise philosophies such as MET (Holten and Torstensen 1991; Torstensen 1997; Torstensen et al. 1998) sequential exercises are also employed and integrated in the STAYAC exercise model. Physical exercise is an evidence-based method (Harms-Ringdahl et al. 1999; Nachemson and Jonsson 2000; van Tulder et al. 2000; Waddell 1998). In a literature review, it was concluded that 'the reviewed trials provided strong evidence that exercise significantly reduces sick days during the first follow-up year' (Kool et al. 2004). Relaxation exercises, body awareness exercises, African dance, yoga, hathayoga (hatha means 'powerful'), 'grounding', Qi Gong, breathing exercises, 'liberating dance', 'dance of the senses', and Feldenkrais and Nordic walking are provided in the STAYAC rehabilitation today; all the items are available in different combinations by a specially trained physiotherapist. These modalities have, for simplicity, been allocated to this 'physical exercise' box, but are never used as primary measures and not applied in the (other) 'physical exercise' box in the green antidysfunctional sphere. Rosen therapy and Alexander therapy are other useful methods. The following are two important and different dimensions.

(a)

Pain clinic
Sick leave
Long-term sick leave
C
EARLY RETIREMENT, part-time or full-time or substantial loss of quality of life
B
RESIDUAL SYMPTOMS, but working ability restored, and life situation under control
A
RECOVERED, or at least manageable minor symptoms

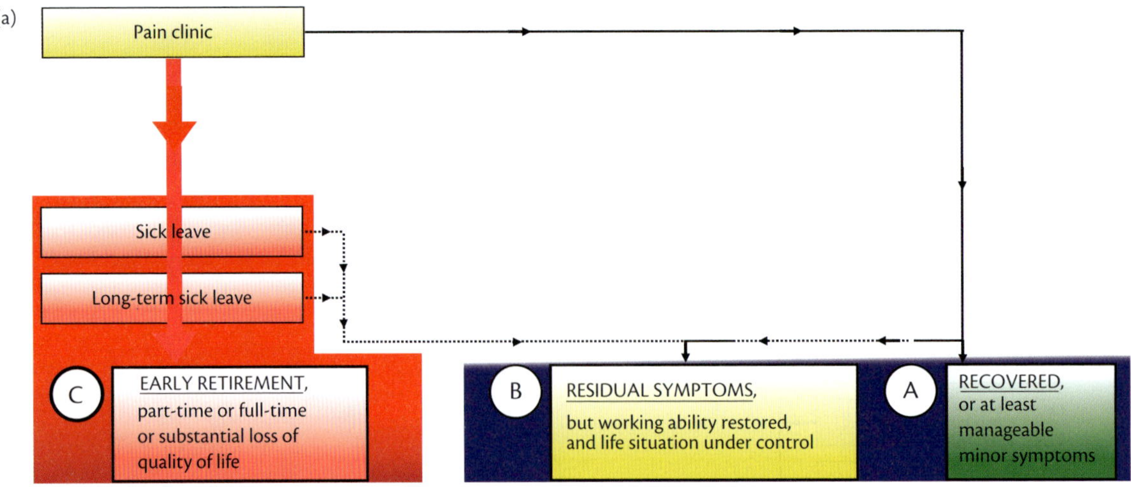

(b)

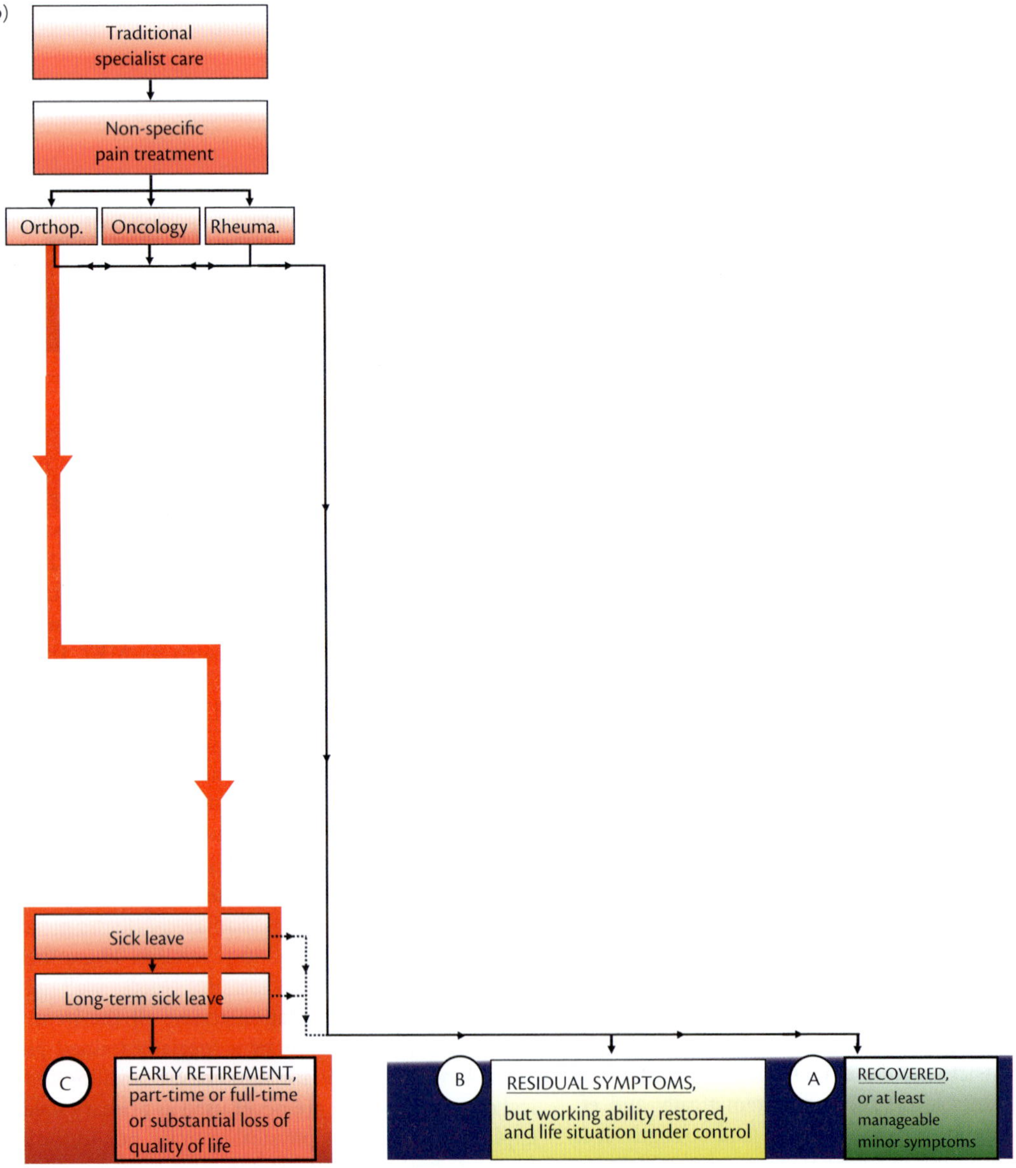

Traditional specialist care
Non-specific pain treatment
Orthop.
Oncology
Rheuma.
Sick leave
Long-term sick leave
C
EARLY RETIREMENT, part-time or full-time or substantial loss of quality of life
B
RESIDUAL SYMPTOMS, but working ability restored, and life situation under control
A
RECOVERED, or at least manageable minor symptoms

Figure 60.7 (a–d) A series of rudimentary algorithms, reflecting today's clinical reality. See text for details.

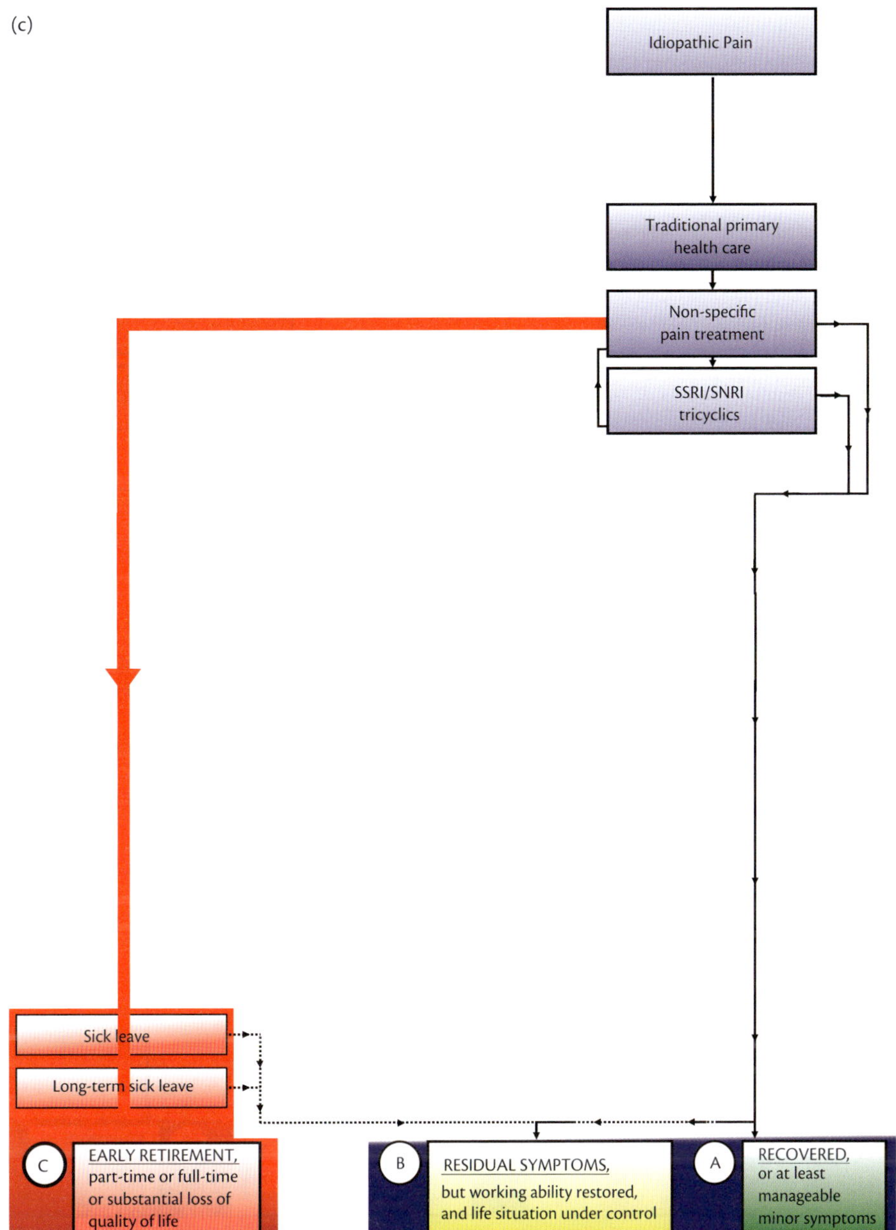

Figure 60.7(a–d) *(continued)*

According to the dominant, mechanically oriented theories among physiotherapists, the apparent advantageous effects are achieved by, for example, 'stabilization' of 'unstable' vertebral segments. There is a huge variety of 'stabilization exercises' through which extreme positions of 'unstable' joints are supposed to be avoided in everyday life, and certain protective movement patterns are taught. There is an obvious risk of transferring subliminal and subconscious stay-passive messages to the patients. The net effect of the stay-passive messages weighed against the positive effects achieved by the exercises may even be negative. On the other hand, it is possible to convey stay-active messages while providing passive treatment, such as manipulation. An increased awareness of subliminal stay-passive messages is extremely important. This could be achieved, as in the STAYAC algorithm, by updating the rationales behind hyper-reactivity and improving the terminology. Mechanically oriented terms such as 'hypermobility', 'instability', and 'micro-instability' should be avoided. The exercises could instead be described as helping postural control and co-ordination, optimizing the function of the posturo-proprioceptive system control and the operative system of the muscle spindles, improving peripheral proprioceptive functions, and compensating disturbed proprioceptive functions by improving the function of higher centres in the central nervous system (CNS).

Within this paradigm of the 'operative system' of the posturo-proprioceptive control organization, it becomes logical to stay active, move, and so forth. This is metacognition: fear avoidance and catastrophizing are counteracted, and the risk of subliminal stay-passive messages is reduced or even eliminated. In conclusion, the

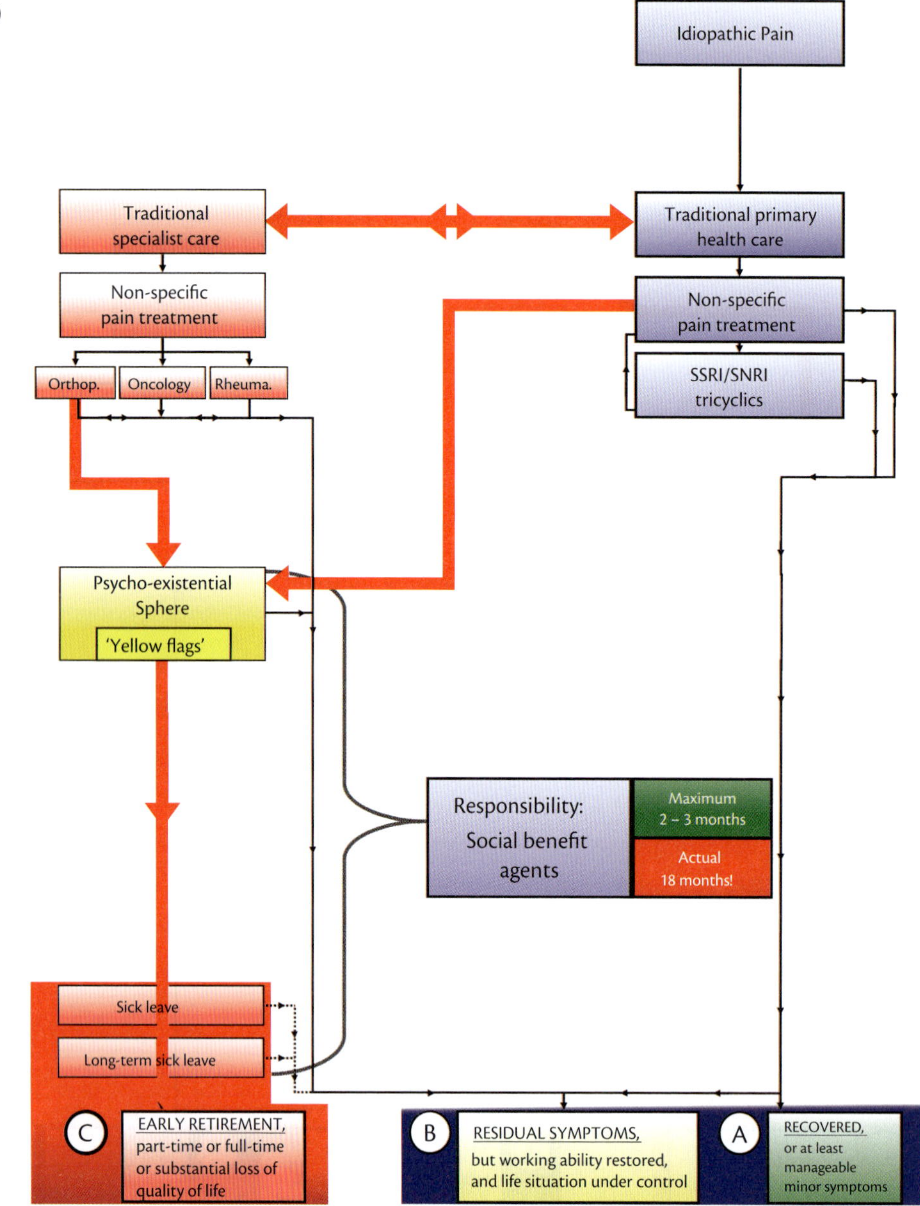

Figure 60.7(a–d) (*continued*)

beneficial effects of physical exercises in hyper-reactivity may be achieved by optimizing the function of the 'software' in order to compensate for minor weaknesses in the 'hardware'. Thus, the contents of this section illustrate a metacognitive aspect of the STAYAC algorithm.

In addition, beneficial non-specific somatic effects may be achieved from increased strength, endurance, improved co-ordination, and fitness. (For alternative views on stabilization, see Chapter 63.)

Of course, there are patients with more severe hyper-reactivity syndromes that cannot be controlled or cured solely by individualized exercise (or prolotherapy). As indicated by the vertically aligned 'hyper-reactivity box (bottom left of green dysfunctional area in Figure 60.1), by following the subsequent grey paths in the psycho-existential sphere (the stay-active concept, reassurance, behavioural measures, and so forth), patients' coping strategies will become strengthened, while their conditions heal spontaneously over time and the consequences of their suffering are reduced in various ways. At this point in the algorithm, these principles have to be applied in a more process-oriented manner.

Fortunately, progression to chronic low back pain is rare; only a tiny minority needs prolotherapy, and an even smaller number of patients are referred to specialized orthopaedic surgeons for fusion surgery (see the corresponding grey line from the left of the 'physical exercise' box in Figure 60.1). Except in clearly demonstrated pathomorphological cases (e.g. unstable and significant spondylolisthesis) in which the symptoms of the patients, with high probability, are truly correlated to the findings in MRI/CT, fusion surgery is controversial. One study (Fritzell et al. 2001) provides only weak scientific support for surgery. In spite of this, I believe that surgery is appropriate for a tiny proportion of patients with chronic low back pain.

Unfortunately, moderate or even severe psycho-existential dimensions frequently seem to be overlooked by surgeons, leading to poor operation results. This is of course also true for all those dysfunctional conditions without any symptomatology, not at all correlated to findings at diagnostic imaging; this may even be a larger problem than forgetfulness with respect to psycho-existential dimensions of patients' sufferings. I believe that if patients for surgical treatment were pre-selected by careful and systematic application of the STAYAC algorithm, the results would improve considerably.

Physical exercise—the inherent potential for behavioural change

An underestimated aspect of physical exercise is its behaviour-modifying potential. Exercises carry positive subliminal messages. During the process of antidysfunctional analysis, the physician/therapist has built an alliance of trust and mutual respect ('I respect and understand your pain, which has a physical component'; 'I have the competence to treat your pain'). By prescribing exercises, the therapist conveys to the patient their belief that the patient's condition is not dangerous. The patient's back is not 'worn out'—if it was, physical activities would aggravate the condition, and the therapist would not prescribe exercises. Tendencies to fear avoidance and catastrophizing are thereby prevented. This inherent effect of physical exercise may be one of the reasons why no differences between the large numbers of different exercise modes have been demonstrated at group level in RCTs (Harms-Ringdahl et al. 1999; Nachemson and Jonsson 2000; van Tulder et al. 2000; Waddell 1998).

Experienced physiotherapists may communicate this message to the patients more or less subconsciously, without the specific goal-oriented intention of altering patients' behaviour. However, if a physiotherapist who is specially trained in both behavioural and manual therapy can invoke this dimension of physical exercise by a process-oriented (metacognitive) and premeditated application of exercises as a behavioural therapy, the ability of the method to stabilize the patient's life situation will probably be enhanced further. (A physiotherapist and a psychologist/licensed psychotherapist may also work together in group settings.) The patient's fear of pain associated with exercise, everyday life, and treatment is minimized or even eliminated. In many instances, the behavioural dimension of physical exercise may be more important than improvement of strength, endurance, fitness, and even co-ordination and posturo-proprioceptive control.

The 'patient education' box

The education of patients—with the aim of modifying their beliefs, attitudes, fear, and behaviour—begins at the first visit and permeates the entire flowchart. However, in the absence of sufficient therapeutic response at this stage of the algorithm, this approach has to be carried out using a new 'patient education' methodology that has been developed at STAYAC. A more focused and goal-oriented approach to influence various behavioural disturbances, long-term sick leave illness, coping skills, sense of coherence, learned helplessness (Miller and Seligman 1975; Miller et al. 1975), and poor self-efficacy (Bandura 1977) are needed in a substantive subgroup of patients at this stage. The patients are usually in chronic pain and on extended sick leave; the diagnoses are idiopathic pain including somatoform syndromes, hyper-reactivity, fibromyalgia, whiplash-associated disorders (WAS), and so forth.

The patient education takes the form of cognitive behavioural group therapy, aiming to minimize the consequences of persisting symptoms (see the 'third perspective' in the section 'Pain-related syndromes—new psychological perspectives'). This therapeutic method involves interactive sessions (of 4 hours' duration on five occasions) by the responsible physician and physiotherapist, with whom the patients have become familiar during their antidysfunctional management. The basic idea is that the 'bone setter'/manual therapist and the (cognitive) behavioural therapist are the same person.

This approach increases the patient's confidence not only that the responsible clinician has the competence to take care of, or to initiate, all measures necessary to reduce the pain by means of somatically oriented treatment methods, but also that all such measures really have been carried through thoroughly or at least considered. In the analyses of patients' psycho-existential status, psychodynamic dimensions of their suffering are considered, so this is cognitive therapy with psychodynamic overtones, but traditional psychotherapy is not provided at this level of the algorithm.

Cognitive behavioural therapy, as a stand-alone therapy, is considered solidly evidence-based (Nachemson and Jonsson 2000), and this cognitive behavioural group therapy seems highly successful with regard to the enhancement of the patient's sense of coherence (Antonovsky 1987) and coping skills. Sometimes it is not even paramount for the preceding management to alleviate the somatic component of the patient's suffering. The patient's 'escape routes' are closed by the conveyance of the subliminal messages previously mentioned, and circumstances are created in which patients are much less hesitant to discuss relevant matters. The 'teacher' can make a gradual shift from standard topics, such as pain mechanisms, anatomy, and the dysfunction perspective, to potentially controversial subjects such as long-term sick leave, the stay-active concept, primary and secondary benefits, the 'Peter Pan' syndrome (Kiley 1983), the 'Humpty Dumpty' syndrome, and basic crisis psychology. Other sensitive topics include insufficient coping abilities, insufficient sense of coherence, pain behaviour, the pain patient role, identity loss, development of pain identity, and life lies.

Much of the content of the sessions is too abstract for many patients. However, this does not matter, and it is not necessary for them to remember much—basically, patient education is a matter of repeating five or six basic stay-active messages, largely without the patients noticing. However, it is obvious to the clinician that, after these sessions, there are frequently dramatic changes in patients' attitudes to work and sick leave, improved coping strategies, and so forth, even in those who evidently disliked the sessions. Some of the most successful cases have been in patients who were clearly irritated and annoyed by patient education. Irritating the patients is not a goal in itself, although the method may be experienced by some as partly provocative. In conclusion, one could even say that the core of patient education is a qualified and powerful mode of 'mental manipulation'. (For another view on patient education, see Chapter 49.)

Optimally, all therapists in the team should attend sessions of individual long-term psychotherapy, and/or individual guidance, by an experienced psychotherapist. This is at least as important as guidance for psychotherapists, where such supervision is considered a matter of course. At STAYAC, we have not yet reached this goal; however, we regularly have a Balint-type group conducted by our psychiatrist/psychoanalyst and our psychologist/licensed psychotherapist and in which even secretaries, receptionists, and nurses take part.

Antidepressants

The next therapeutic modality, the use of antidepressants (see corresponding box in the yellow psycho-existential area in the algorithm in Figure 60.1), is well established. Low dosages of tricyclic antidepressants, such as clomipramine and amitriptyline, are a well-documented treatment method for chronic pain. We have had experience of the use of higher antidepressive doses of tricyclic antidepressants for chronic pain since the mid 1980s. The dose–response curve seems linear, i.e. the higher the dose, the higher the therapeutic response. Supported by these observational data, I applied the same therapeutic principle, i.e. dosages towards the top end of the permitted range, when the selective serotonin/noradrenaline reuptake inhibitors (SSRIs/SNRIs) arrived in Sweden around 1990. After experience of this approach over many years, it seems obvious that the linear dose–response curve in the treatment of chronic pain is valid for SSRIs/SNRIs as well. Today, there is reliable evidence of efficacy for the use of SSRIs/SNRIs in chronic pain problems, especially with respect to fibromyalgia, and it is also evidence-based that low dosages of SSRIs/SNRIs for pain have lesser positive effects than maximum allowed doses (as recently evaluated in RCTs).

Potential adverse effects. There are compliance problems with tricyclic antidepressants, because of relatively frequent adverse events. The SSRI/SNRIs have fewer side-effects, and after a slow and gradual increase to maximum dosages, they may be as effective as tricyclics in chronic pain patients, and even more useful. The apparent linear dose–response graph is similar to the treatment strategies in patients with obsessive-compulsive disorders (OCD), social phobia, and panic anxiety syndromes, in which the linear dose–response relationship is well established. By contrast, the dose–adverse effect curve is apparently non-linear. Consequently, increasing the dosage of SSRI/SNRIs (after any initial side-effects have subsided) rarely causes any further problems. In some patients, the adverse effects do not subside, and I have seen a handful of cases demonstrating moderate signs of too high levels of serotonin in the postsynaptic space, such as early wakening (early 'serotonergic syndrome'). However, these situations have been rapidly solved by reduction of the dosage or by a change to another SSRI/SNRI drug.

Benefits. Generally, in the context of pain management, *the therapeutic potential of antidepressants is underestimated* and, consequently, this type of treatment is under-used. Aside from pain reduction/elimination, modulation of pain perception appears to be an important effect of SSRI/SNRI treatment in pain patients. Instead of focusing primarily on their pain, they may constructively plan their future return to a worthwhile life; the pain no longer rules their lives to the same extent. This frequently happens despite undiminished pain—a phenomenon which is exciting to observe. There is also a growing consensus that antidepressants neutralize central sensitization, probably the main factor behind fibromyalgia and a part of the symptomatology in the vast majority of other chronic pain patients. Thus, according to our experience, this treatment approach is useful not only in advanced idiopathic somatoform pain syndromes, but also in other chronic conditions.

In the STAYAC algorithm (Figure 60.1), when management at this stage has failed to provide sufficient pain control and in accordance with the pragmatic approach (as previously mentioned), antidepressants are tried in *all* pain patients whose quality of life, everyday functioning, and/or working capacity are reduced. Whether or not there is a coexistent depression is not essential; the patient will report this after some weeks of medication (see also 'Idiopathic pain—*ex juvantibus* diagnosis' in the section 'A macro-perspective of the algorithm'). Additionally, there are no reliable instruments with sufficient precision to predict accurately whether the pain will respond to this therapy. This is an excellent example of truly pragmatic management. Consequently, in the pragmatic approach, the method, when needed, is simply tried at a relevant stage, at full dosage, regardless of the patient's apparent psychiatric status. This seems to be a very fruitful approach, supported by one of the leading Swedish specialists in antidepressive medication, Lars von Knorring (personal communication). He considers SSRIs/SNRIs not to be antidepressants, but rather, a general restorative of the serotonergic/noradrenergic systems; these medications modulate numerous other aspects of perception, and depression is becoming merely one indication among many others. Certainly, antidepressants may be introduced at any level in the algorithm, and if the patient is obviously depressed, or has a chronic and severe pain condition, they may be recommended them at the first visit.

Evidence. Since 1990, I have acquired experience of virtually all SSRIs/SNRIs available. In this context, I would like to share some empirical knowledge concerning some of them. (There are an insufficient number of RCTs available to support my experience, but I believe that, since 1985, I have been one of the doctors in Sweden to treat most pain patients with antidepressants.). *Citalopram* was the first SSRI to arrive in Sweden and my experience from that substance was definitely encouraging from the beginning, provided the patients received maximum allowed doses. The arrival of *escitalopram* (also SSRI) constituted a definite increase of the treatment results and became my treatment of choice for many years, also with less adverse effects, especially with respect to sexual dysfunction compared with citalopram. The first combined SSRIs/SNRIs coming after escitalopram were, in spite of my high expectations, a disappointment. Probably owing to a weak noradrenaline effect, my impression was that, in spite of trying them all, the effects were less positive than for escitalopram. Due to insufficient effects in some patients, at this point of time, I still used tricyclics in some cases. (Basically, with regards to tricyclics, I have experience only of *clomipramine* and *amitriptyline*, both preferably in high doses of 150 mg, although I have had patients on 300 mg. In spite of what has previously been said, a high dose frequently works after the 'Kierkegaard effect' (previously discussed), paralleled with some pedagogic work.)

Results. The greatest step towards considerably better treatment results was the arrival of duloxetine (combined SSRI/SNRI), which is my absolute treatment of choice today, despite somewhat more problems with adverse effects than those of the earlier SSRIs and SSRIs/SNRIs (although however, sexual dysfunction is definitely though). Today I use tricyclics infrequently, *not* because of better effects achieved by duloxetine but, in fact, because there are a handful of patients who tolerate the tricyclics better than duloxetine.

Duloxetine is the first modern and selective antidepressant with an effect that equals that of the tricyclics, not only in the serotonin system, but also in relation to adrenaline, and with considerably less adverse effects than the tricyclics.

The results achieved by duloxetine in dysfunction-free patients, after having passed the entire green antidysfunctional area in the middle of the flowchart (see Figure 60.1), and after patient education, is amazing, and has dramatically increased the treatment results in this STAYAC patient group. For some considerable time, our strong impression is that patient education effectively decreases the 'placebo/expectation adverse effects'. Again, high doses are definitely more effective, which is evidence-based for fibromyalgia: you start with 30 mg once a day, with a gradual escalation by 30 mg per approximately one week, up to 120 mg per 24 hours. Some patients receive 180 mg. A considerable advantage with duloxetine is that the dose–adverse effects graph is obviously *not* linear—most of the side-effects are transient (subside within 2–3 weeks), and when the body's systems have adapted to the substance, you can usually escalate to maximum doses without any problems whatsoever. A handful of patients, especially those with strong central sensitization (who need duloxetine more than any other patient group), cannot start with 30 mg; the capsule can be divided and the initial dose may be 15 mg, 7.5 mg, or, sometimes, even less. The substance is preferably dissolved in apple juice. (Just to reassure the reader, I am not paid by Lilly!)

Conclusion. According to the STAYAC algorithm, antidepressants are used frequently, and this type of therapy commonly resolves the patient's adverse life situation, not always by alleviating depressive symptoms, but often by relieving pain, and/or by modulating the perception of pain to a manageable level. However, patients' resistance to a trial of antidepressants is widespread. This seems to be especially valid for pain patients, but less of an issue in patients who spontaneously identify themselves as suffering from depression. To deal with the patient's concerns about antidepressant medication, it is desirable to have a refined pedagogical model to provide an understandable explanation of potential benefits, rationales, and adverse effects of antidepressants used for pain. This motivational process may be provided in individual consultations if necessary, but it is time-consuming, and is preferably carried out in groups as part of the standard patient education procedure.

In some studies, positive effects have been demonstrated with the use of SSRIs in non-depressive patients (Harmer *et al.* 2003; Knutson et al. 1997, 1998; Loubinoux et al. 2002; Shores et al. 2001; Tse and Bond 2002). For instance, there was improvement in coping with everyday situations, stress thresholds, and the ability to cooperate in groups, and a 'smoothing' of the less favourable aspects of their personalities. *This suggests that our SSRI strategy may in fact bring about its positive effects by 'super-normal' levels of serotonin in the CNS, leading to biochemically induced, artificially strengthened coping strategies.* Consequently, it seems that this strategy is not necessarily a matter of treating 'masked depressions' (see discussion of the 'first perspective' in the section 'Pain-related syndromes—new psychological perspectives'), even though that diagnosis is indeed relevant in some of the chronic pain patients. This hypothesis needs to be tested in experimental and clinical studies such as RCTs.

We have, according to the pragmatic principle, noticed another phenomenon that is not easily understood. (Hypothetically, it may be explained by serotonin and noradrenaline being involved in the function of the posturo-proprioceptive system). In a subgroup of patients with recurring dysfunctions that are difficult to bring under control, after some weeks on antidepressants, the situation is suddenly stabilized, and the markers of dysfunction do not recur. This phenomenon should be regarded as a measure of secondary prevention (see the yellow 'SSRI/SNRI/tricyclics' trial treatment box to the right of the darker green 'yellow light A situation' in Figure 60.1).

Occupational rehabilitation

The next step in the algorithm is occupational rehabilitation. There is evidence that this approach is effective in the management of back pain (Bendix et al. 1998a,b, 2000). The fundamental difference between our approach and other multidisciplinary rehabilitation concepts is that all the previously discussed measures are undertaken before our patients are subjected to our occupational rehabilitation, and that the method itself is predicated upon the same fundamental principles as the rest of the algorithm, i.e. the inherent behavioural potential of the antidysfunctional approach, exploited (with respect to the content) in a process-oriented manner. A related approach, aside from the antidysfunctional management, is the pragmatic approach to low back pain used at Volvo, Gothenburg (Lindström et al. 1992) in which a graded activity programme, including a back school and graded individualized exercise programmes, is the core, and the operant conditioning behavioural concept is essential too. This concept was found to decrease sick leave and to increase mobility, strength, and fitness in comparison to unspecified, uncontrolled 'traditional care'.

It has been demonstrated that the elimination of dysfunctional factors from patients' suffering considerably enhances their ability to take part in physical activities (Blomberg et al. 1993a,b) and, thereby, of course, rehabilitation programmes as well. This is substantiated by data from the reproducibility study: muscle stretching was the treatment most frequently considered painful by patients, which was expected. However, the second most painful treatment modality was the physical exercises in the two groups in which manual therapy (and steroid injections) were not provided. In these groups, the physical exercises were experienced as painful more frequently than manipulation and injections in the experimental groups. The physical exercises were only rarely experienced as painful in the two groups in which manual therapy (and steroid injections) were allowed (Blomberg et al. 2005a). Accordingly, as much as possible of the antidysfunctional treatment/investigation is completed before occupational rehabilitation.

These major differences from other rehabilitation programmes are probably the main reasons behind the extraordinarily successful results achieved by our 6-week/half-time rehabilitation programme with follow-ups after 1 and 3 months (and, in some subjects, continuous follow-up for longer periods of time), as evaluated in a hitherto unpublished outcome study. The population of this study suffered from advanced persistent pain syndromes refractory to earlier managements. The mean duration of pain in the first 76 patients was 4 years, and the pain debut averaged 10 years; 10% of the patients had suffered from pain for more than 20 years. The mean period of sick leave was 18 months, and only 10% of the patients had suffered periods of work absenteeism for less than 1 year. The quality of life score was extremely low, and the rating of symptoms, mainly of a psychosomatic character, was complex. The final assessment was performed between 6 months and 2 years after the rehabilitation period: from a societal perspective (with respect to reduction of sick leave), the rehabilitation was successful in 81% of cases. Consequently, the proportion of patients at definite risk

of early retirement was only 19%, as compared with the realistic expected risk of early retirement of close to 100%. Most of the successfully rehabilitated subjects (81%) returned to their normal work, and the remainder returned to modified work tasks, or reduced their proportion of sick leave (in Sweden, 25%, 50%, 75%, or 100% sick leave can be prescribed), or were able to carry out different procedures with a realistic aim of
returning to some type of work task that they could not do before the rehabilitation.

Occupational measures (blue and black flags)

The next suggested step, occupational measures (see corresponding box in Figure 60.1) could be applied at any point in the algorithm. These measures include a graded return to work, light duties, retraining, re-education, further education, and referral to special establishments for people with permanently reduced working ability. It is not uncommon to discover during the first visit that this measure has been neglected. If the patient has been offered poor advice and lacks guidance and direction, this measure should be initiated promptly. At the other extreme, in Sweden, occupational measures are unfortunately far too often initiated at early stages in individuals for whom a variety of treatment possibilities have not been taken into consideration, not least the STAYAC model. This is not a cost-effective strategy. For simplicity, there are no boxes in the algorithm in Figure 60.1 representing 'blue flags' and 'black flags'. *Blue flags* include fear of being laid off, lack of job satisfaction, poor relationship with work colleagues, a claim against an employer, and organizational climate (Waddell 1998). *Black flags* comprise factors beyond individual influence such as governmental policies and work regulations, and also workplace conditions associated with the onset of low back pain and the development of disability (Bartys et al. 2002). These factors are often considered at this stage not infrequently, parallel to occupational measures.

Cognitive behavioural therapy

The 'cognitive behavioural therapy' box refers to extended therapy over a longer period of time, individually or in closed or open groups. At this stage, a few patients are in obvious need of such management, which indeed is available in some pain clinics, some psychiatric clinics, and within medical or occupational rehabilitation. The STAYAC concept underpins cognitive behavioural therapeutic principles at all stages of the algorithm. Obviously, there are extremely potent synergistic effects in the integration of antidysfunctional medicine, with manual therapy as its core, and cognitive behavioural therapy. Unfortunately, there is a widespread misconception that these two therapeutic principles are incompatible. Long-term behavioural therapy may be perfectly well executed by general practitioners (GPs) or physiotherapists with appropriate insight and training: referral to a specialist is not always necessary.

Psychotherapy

The principal underlying psychological factor in pain syndromes is, I believe, denial of the psycho-existential dimensions of the suffering and denial of the role of the life situation in general as a non-medical factor with regard to the consequences of the pain. The pain is virtually always nociceptive (see the following section on the 'third perspective'). However, the pain is 'used' by the patient to control and to facilitate repression of denied psycho-existential crises, which are *externalized* (the STAYAC model generally enhances the process of *internalizing* these psycho-existential conflicts) outside their own responsibility and control, as are the responsibility and control of their conditions and their recoveries; thus, this is the 'function' of the pain. However, the pain only rarely has a primary psychological origin.

The 'psychotherapy' box (lower left corner of the algorithm in Figure 60.1, in the yellow sphere) is controversial. As a consequence of their lack of psychological awareness with respect to important underlying factors such as their beliefs, attitudes, and behaviour, most patients with severe pain are usually considered unsuitable for psychotherapy. Some degree of awareness of one's own situation is a requirement for successful psychotherapy of any kind. There is a definite risk that a patient whose pain is uncontrolled, and who primarily considers him/herself innocently stricken by pain outside his/her own control, may take offence and be further distressed by a therapeutic strategy that is too psychodynamically focused and/or introduced prematurely. This may also reinforce feelings of guilt and shame in some patients; being driven by these feelings is a common aspect of the pain patient personality.

However, even powerful and profound psychotherapy, when indicated, is frequently very successful if undertaken at an appropriate stage of the algorithm. Even short-term therapies are commonly effective. At this point in the algorithm, most patients are 'mature' (i.e. well-motivated) for psychotherapeutic processes, and have no resistance to them. The fundamental reason for this is that the primary problem, as perceived by the patient (namely their pain), is addressed all the way through the algorithm—the 'Kierkegaard effect'. This, in turn, facilitates the patient's understanding of psycho-existential, emotional, social psychodynamic, behavioural, and cognitive dimensions—the psycho-therapeutic process is shortened and thereby cost-optimized.

Another facilitating factor is that, at this stage, the patient's life crises have frequently been controlled through cognitive behavioural measures, resulting in improved coping strategies, and at least some degree of reduction of pain is virtually always achieved by the antidysfunctional management. Moreover, an increased awareness of how ability to cope with everyday difficulties is connected to the patient's behaviour pattern is achieved. *A feeling of hope is generated,* and the patients develop confidence and self-respect. The importance of a complete picture when providing individuals with information has been stressed (Magnusson and Mahoney 2001). The multidimensional treatment of the patient, with touching and psychotherapy, creates parasympathetic reactions, thereby increasing motivation and trustfulness, facilitating the endurance of pain, and engendering a more positive attitude to life situations (Arn 1999).

Several psychotherapeutic methods, both reality/cognitive and emotionally oriented, are used; these include traditional psychotherapy, identity therapy, psychodrama, hypnotherapy, family therapy, and self-supporting therapy. The psychotherapy is both individual and group-based, sometimes combined with antidysfunctional physical therapy on the same occasion.

Pain-related syndromes—new psychological perspectives

According to a recent and so far unpublished outcome study, we achieve excellent outcomes in a high percentage of patients with extremely complex problems, for whom numerous different approaches to pain management have failed.

Psychotherapy has an important role in the therapeutic process, in exploring the interaction between psycho-existential/social factors and the patient's pain and suffering. In the STAYAC concept, we have identified and defined three different basic perspectives with respect to the psychological approach:

- **The first perspective:** The first group comprises patients who present physical problems, with an underlying psychological traumatic experience or a psychodynamic process resulting in pain instead of, for instance, open anxiety, which is thereby avoided (a primary benefit). This perspective could be exemplified by different kinds of *somatization syndromes*. Numerous models for pain are to be found in the psychosomatic/psychological/psychotherapeutic/psychiatric literature, all apparently relating to the first perspective.
- **The second perspective:** The second group contains patients who have somatically based problems generating psychological disorders such as depression. This perspective is frequently adopted within different schools of manual therapy and musculoskeletal/manual medicine: 'If you have had pain long enough, you will of course be depressed and feel bad. Let me treat your (somatic) pain, and everything will become as it was before you were stricken by pain.' Manual therapists advocating this perspective as the fundamental approach frequently talk in terms of 'somatopsychic' conditions.
- **The third perspective:** The third group comprises patients in whom neither physical nor psychological problems are the dominating cause of the pain—both basic factors interact in a complex way. The pain is 'real', physical, nociceptive, and of somatic origin. However, an unsatisfactory psycho-existential/social status of the patient at the debut of pain may induce inadequate consequences from the pain. Thus, '*consequences*' is the key word in this paradigm; it is an essential concept for the success of treatment. The pain is frequently 'used' by the patients to control and to facilitate repression of denied psycho-existential crises, and for enhancing their abilities to bury their life lies.

The aforementioned reasoning is basically a 'hen and egg' discussion.

A conscious or subconscious over-reliance on, or incorrect application of, the first two perspectives is extremely common. For instance, mistrustful patient–therapist relationships are created by over-reliance on, unfortunately dominating, the *first perspective* (Figure 60.6b). On the other hand, by over-reliance on the *second perspective* (Figure 60.6a) and regression according to psychodynamic theories (making it easier for the patient to 'hand over' to the therapist, the responsibility for control of their conditions and their recoveries, enhancing destructive repression of denied psycho-existential crises and enhancing externalization), there is unhelpful reinforcement of behavioural disturbances such as identity loss and development of a pain identity. Reinforcement in this context of the 'injury' or the 'lesion', and a reliance on continuing manual treatment, can be extremely disadvantageous to the patient, leading to chronicity of symptoms (see also Chapter 20).

In the STAYAC model, all three perspectives are relevant. However, *the third perspective should be applied for most patients* as true 'psychogenic' pain (hysteria, conversion neuroses, pure somatization syndromes, etc.) is rare, and the second perspective is overemphasized, especially within manual medicine/therapy. The third perspective permeates the entire algorithm, as it does this entire chapter: attitudes, patient communication, metacognitive processes (the therapist's continuous review of their own thought processes), and so forth. Unfortunately, in clinical reality, to the disadvantage of pain patients, the third perspective is rarely applied today—in general, pain care is extremely polarized between advocates of the first perspective and the second perspective.

I am convinced that the consequent appliance of the 'third perspective' thinking, to an essential part, contributes to the unique treatment results of STAYAC.

Sick leave, long-term sick leave, and early retirement

The next phase is sick leave, long-term sick leave, and early retirement; see corresponding boxes in the darker red area, bottom left in the algorithm (Figure 60.1). Sick leave is in fact a treatment method, but its dangers are not universally understood. It has a high risk of adverse effects and complications such as 'long-term sick leave illness' and alcoholism. Work absenteeism is the most powerful risk factor for the development of alcoholism. A further predicament in this context is that it is largely the patients themselves, and not the physicians, who decide whether or not sick leave is necessary and/or adequate (Englund 2000).

Sick leave may of course be prescribed at any point of the algorithm, but should be used with the greatest caution and to the most limited extent possible. Not only may inappropriate sick leave be disastrous for individual patients, the danger of its widespread use is the legitimization of socio-cultural ills and problems. I am convinced that pain as a general societal predicament could be reduced to a minimum provided an appropriate infrastructure within pain care could be developed, departmentalization of the 'pain market' could be abolished, and the lack of knowledge with respect to possibilities as well as limitations within 'competing' and related disciplines could be taken care of.

Nevertheless, sick leave, including long-term sick leave and even early retirement, is sometimes therapeutic and is indicated for a tiny minority of pain patients.

Pain clinic

STAYAC nowadays is a full-grown pain clinic (I am also a licensed pain specialist myself), with very few exceptions where an anaesthesiologist are needed. As a consequence, pain clinics are excluded from the flowchart in this second edition. Instead, the anaesthesiologists are included in the red specialist sphere (bottom left corner of algorithm), and the neurologists and neurosurgeons have been managed in the same manner (also, bottom left corner of algorithm). For the small minority of pain patients in which their input is needed, these patients are referred to anaesthesiologists (at very late stages in antidysfunctional investigation); they are usually located in traditional pain clinics. Some examples of indications for referral to anaesthesiologists are for radio frequency (heat for destruction of the dorsal rami, empirically very useful in a handful of patients, e.g. some whiplash-associated disorder (WAD) patients), stimulation of the dorsal horns, epidural infusions, rhizolysis, phenol, and alcohol blockades.

In Sweden, during the last years, the number of pain clinics has diminished, probably due to the poor treatment results that have been generally observed, not least by their patients and the healthcare stakeholders. The medical management profile in traditional pain clinics varies considerably from unit to unit. There is no supporting evidence for the effectiveness of the (often extensive) series of blockades/injections that are provided, more or less, as a single-tool therapy, with the exception of medication, in some pain clinics. In addition, such treatment strategies are expensive. The indications for injections within the STAYAC concept are very different from the indications within those pain management clinics in which series of blockades are not supported by specific functional diagnoses. Consequently, within the STAYAC concept, with the exception of the few patients that are subjected to lumbar prolotherapy (10 treatments), costly series of injections are *never* provided. In addition, the injections in the STAYAC concept are evidence-based (Blomberg et al. 2005a).

Cryostretching and IMS are two other methods that are frequently applied by Swedish pain specialists, but they have the same problems: the high cost, the lack of evidence, and their frequent appliance as single-tool 'silver bullet' therapy. In spite of this, these methods are used within the STAYAC concept, but *never* primarily and only at late stages in a tiny minority of the patients, because they are seldom needed. (For a contrasting view with respect to IMS, see Chapter 58.)

However, the essential problem in traditional pain medicine is the lack of the dysfunction perspective. Although the underlying principles within this discipline are focused on (neuro-)physiological/biochemical peripheral and central pain mechanisms, rather than on structural factors, these are still, in principle, exclusively pathomorphologically oriented and an application of the biomedical paradigm. With respect to the diagnosis of '(pseudo) neuropathic pain', many patients with chronic pain have features of dysfunctional conditions ('green flag' conditions) that are treatable with antidysfunctional treatment.

A number of clinical features that are regarded within traditional pain medicine as more or less pathognomonic for true neuropathic/neurogenic pain are frequently present in dysfunctional conditions, both axially (chest, lower back, and abdomen) and in the extremities. In addition, when of dysfunctional origin, symptoms such as hypoesthesia, hyperesthesia, dysesthesia, analgesia, paresthesia, and even reflex disturbances are reversible, resolving rapidly after antidysfunctional therapy, sometimes within seconds. In these situations that occur frequently during antidysfunctional management, it is obvious to the clinician that pathomorphological states or neuropathic diagnoses are of no relevance. Consequently, the lack of the dysfunction perspective within traditional pain medicine creates a substantial risk of overdiagnosing of neuropathic/neurogenic pain and a corresponding overuse of medication such as antiepileptics. This is unfortunate, considering the adverse effects, and the frequently unsatisfactory treatment results, especially in patients with symptoms of a dysfunctional origin. Furthermore, for the same reason, an over-reliance on psychological factors as the primary cause of pain is common ('psychogenic pain') (see the 'first perspective' in the previous subsection 'Pain-related syndromes—new psychological perspectives'). Another regrettable but frequent consequence is an insufficient application of the stay-active concept. Figure 60.7a illustrates the rudimentary algorithm of suboptimal pain clinics as described here.

Thus, according to extensive observational data, in many cases antidysfunctional investigation, over time, is the most reliable method of differentiating true neuropathic/neurogenic pain from 'pseudoneurological' features.

Of course, antiepileptics are used also in the STAYAC model; however, for a minority of the patients and at late stages during the antidysfunctional investigation. Similarly, this reasoning is applied in the context of differentiation between true radicular pain and referred pain by antidysfunctional management (see previous text), and in numerous other situations in which there is a differential diagnosis of pain syndromes, both with respect to the locomotor apparatus and within other medical disciplines (e.g. gynaecological issues are discussed in 'The nature of dysfunction' subsection). The mechanisms behind 'pseudo-neurological' signs may be related to the theories concerning the nature of the dysfunction that are postulated in this chapter (see previous text): there may be dispersal effects between posturo-proprioceptive, sensory systems and the autonomous nerve system ('cross-talking', as in the case of referred pain). Patients with true neuropathic/neurogenic pain are frequently treatable with SSRI/SNRIs and/or antiepileptics such as pregabalin, gabapentin, or carbamazepine.

Some pain specialists advocate double-blind injections of morphine, local anaesthetics, and placebo to differentiate neuropathic, peripheral nociceptive, central, and psychogenic pain, whereas others doubt the validity of this diagnostic method.

There are indeed pain clinics that provide adequate occupational rehabilitation and cognitive behavioural therapies of different types. However, these rehabilitation strategies are still problematic, due to the lack of implementation of the *dysfunction theory* and its paramount consequences. Premature and routine referral to traditional pain clinics should be avoided.

Figure 60.7 shows some further examples of malfunctioning, rudimentary, coexistent, but isolated, algorithms: over-reliance on pain medicine, specialist care, and primary healthcare respectively. Clinical reality today is no better than the one presented in Figure 60.7d.

Traditional specialist care domain: red flag 'no dysfunctions' box

Close to the upper left corner of the algorithm (see Figure 60.1), in the red sphere, is the 'no dysfunctions' box (5% or less of patients with low back pain) (Nachemson and Jonsson 2000); see Figure 60.3a. This area represents the 'specialist sphere'. In this context, the discussion within the earlier 'Classification process' section has a clear relevance.

In our concept, the management of this patient group is consistent with other published guidelines for (back) pain. Consequently, there is no need here for an in-depth discussion of the management of symptoms of pathomorphological origin (i.e. 'red flags'). The algorithms and guidelines, currently available elsewhere, are mainly focused on management of such conditions, and therefore aimed at not overlooking them (ACC 1997; AHCPR 1994; CSAG 1994; Kendall et al. 1997; RCGP 1996; Waddell 1998). Consequently, they are indeed helpful in the management of the small subgroup of 'pure' red flag patients but of limited usefulness in the management of most patients who have benign, 'non-specific' (dysfunctional/ 'green flag') pain. Nevertheless, it is essential not to miss treatable, potentially disabling, dangerous, or life-threatening red flag conditions (e.g. symptomatic herniated discs fulfilling the indications for operation, tumours, symptomatic spinal stenosis again fulfilling the indications for operation, true inflammatory conditions, infections), and there should be a continual awareness of these possibilities regardless of where the patient is in the algorithm at any moment in time, not least during the antidysfunctional investigation and in the yellow psycho-existential sphere. In Figure 60.1, grey lines from the different levels of the green anti-dysfunctional and the yellow psycho-existential spheres represent this awareness—all these lines coalesce in a common feedback loop to the different modes of pathomorphologically oriented management. The lines from the antidysfunctional stack in the middle bypass the 'stay active' box in the psycho-existential section.

The 'non-specific pain treatment' box

With the exception of the respective different specialists' specific measures within this red sphere such as operations, advanced anti-inflammatory treatment, and antineoplastic agents, the dominant therapeutic treatments are the different items in the 'non-specific pain treatment' box. This box is of course present in all five major domains of the algorithm (see previous text).

Basically, these are similar items to those applied in the antidysfunctional stack, but at a considerably earlier stage (frequently the only stage) as basic core treatment modalities, and utilized to a far greater extent than in the STAYAC concept, where they are usually used only as adjuvant treatment, infrequently as a primary measure (see previous text). However, the contents of this box are definitely more limited than the corresponding box in the STAYAC model, in which a larger variety of non-specific measures against pain is found. In STAYAC, they are also applied on more specific indications—as shown in my thesis (Blomberg 1993a), 100% of the patients in the experimental group experienced medication as effective, compared with the 60% of the control group.

Traditional measures are NSAIDs, painkillers, and traditional physical therapy such as therapeutic ultrasound, heat, cold, TNS, and TEMS. With the exception of NSAIDs, none of these measures is evidence-based. (It is claimed in the back/neck pain SBU report (Nachemson and Jonsson 2000), however, that painkillers are evidence-based; unfortunately, this conclusion is incorrect.)

The domain of 'traditional specialist care' includes referral to pathomorphologically focused specialists such as orthopaedic surgeons, rheumatologists, and oncologists. In addition, the sector covers neurologists, neurosurgeons, and anaesthesiologists, although they are not represented by boxes of their own in the scheme.

Antidysfunctional filtering of the patients in this sector will substantively reduce unnecessary overloading of the specialists with patients to whom they cannot offer any relevant treatment other than what GPs are able to execute. Their treatment results should then be improved by reducing excessive focus on pathomorphologically oriented rationales (which, in turn, frequently lead to nihilistic treatment attitudes and, paradoxically enough, also to overuse of sometimes aggressive therapeutic measures like unnecessary operations).

If dysfunctional and psycho-existential factors have been taken care of before referral to the specialist sphere, the pathomorphological conditions will be more 'refined' at the start of the pathomorphologically oriented investigation, and the symptoms less 'diluted' by dysfunctional factors. This is true not only in the context of back surgery, neurology, and so forth. New, easily treatable, 'green flag' conditions in patients with known inflammatory diseases are frequently, indeed automatically, interpreted as manifestations of their basic inflammatory disease. These patients may be subjected unnecessarily to (sometimes) aggressive pharmacological treatments (e.g. gold salts or even anti-neoplastic agents). A suboptimal specialist algorithm is presented in Figure 60.7b.

From the sphere of traditional specialist care, there are two lines pointing to the right (see Figure 60.1), representing successful treatment outcomes.

Primary healthcare

The upper blue section on the right at the top of the algorithm (Figure 60.1) represents the GPs, conventional physiotherapists, occupational therapists, and sometimes psychologists within primary healthcare. Regrettably, pain management and corresponding referral strategies from within primary care are extremely variable, dependent to a large degree on a practitioner's post-graduate education in manual/musculoskeletal medicine and awareness of psycho-existential factors.

The thicker black lines from the blue primary health care zone, and from the red specialist sphere respectively, both leading to the green antidysfunctional zone, represent the importance of *not* holding patients back from antidysfunctional investigation. This works poorly in today's healthcare, and it is to be hoped that orthopaedic surgeons, rheumatologists, GPs, and others will make increased referrals for antidysfunctional treatment (see following text). The thicker red arrows leading back and forth between the blue and the red zones, in an infinite manner, are extremely destructive paths for patients, representing how their rehabilitation potential is consumed month by month, year by year.

There are patients who are referred back to primary healthcare after treatment in the antidysfunctional sector, for final management when control of pain and the patient's life situation is established, or when no further specialized management is required or possible. (See the ascending long black arrow on the far left of the algorithm in Figure 60.1, collecting all the feedback loops from the psycho-existential and antidysfunctional spheres to the specialist domain, which continues all the way back to the 'antidysfunctional treatment' box and further, to the primary healthcare zone as well.)

Thus, patients are usually referred directly to the specialist sphere (thicker red arrow). Consequently, many patients are denied antidysfunctional management by unnecessary referral to the specialist sphere from the blue primary healthcare zone. In addition, a substantial group of these patients, after referral from GPs, are referred back to their GPs and physiotherapists (according to the corresponding thicker red arrow). These patients too often therefore remain somewhere in these two sectors until often unnecessary early retirement. This is definitively not a cost-effective procedure, and is why the flows between these spheres are marked with thicker red arrows: until education in antidysfunctional medicine within the specialist and primary healthcare sectors is sufficient, these flows should be avoided. In an optimized algorithm, the only reliable way in which to rule out dysfunctional and psycho-existential factors before referral to the specialist sphere (and vice versa) is by antidysfunctional investigation and, when indicated, psycho-existentially focused management in a unit like STAYAC.

In primary care, most patients are classified as idiopathic (very few patients in STAYAC) or as having psychogenic conditions (see 'the first perspective' in the earlier subsection 'Pain-related syndromes—new psychological perspectives'). This is almost exclusively a group of patients with 'green flag' symptoms and, therefore, treatable conditions, provided they are referred for appropriate antidysfunctional management in time. Non-specific pain treatment, with limitations as discussed previously, constitutes the core treatment, but antidepressant medication is sometimes utilized (although too rarely and, most frequently, in too low dosages). Despite the obvious overall poor treatment results within the primary healthcare zone, and the lack of cost effectiveness, passive modalities such as therapeutic ultrasound, TENS, and TEMS are frequently applied in pain patients as primary measures. Nevertheless, in a dysfunction-free state, these methods appear to be helpful in a minority of patients.

The suboptimal management of pain patients within primary healthcare is illustrated in Figure 60.7c. Figures 60.6a and b and Figures 60.7a–d may, of course, be perceived as unfair, not least considering the thick red arrows to the 'early retirement' boxes. This does not indicate that most patients are pensioned off early. However, it indicates that some may take early retirement unnecessarily, and that a large majority of those who do not—and are not subjected to causal-specific therapy in the different specialist spheres—heal spontaneously, instead of having an accelerated recovery achieved by relevant antidysfunctional therapy or measures within the psycho-existential sphere. Nevertheless, clinical reality today is no better than the view presented in Figure 60.7d.

As demonstrated in the algorithm (thicker red arrow, Figure 60.1), there is also a flow of patients from the Traditional (GP) primary health care sphere to the psycho-existential sphere, together with a corresponding flow from the 'non-specific treatment' box in the specialist sphere (again a thicker red arrow). Generally, these routes do not function well today, and many patients 'get stuck' at inappropriate levels of the algorithm, managed passively with the prescription of medication and longer and longer periods of passive sick leave, without a plan for rehabilitation. Disappointingly, in many cases, numerous adequate measures are never taken. Consequently, these flows are marked with thicker red arrows, as are those between the primary healthcare sector and the specialist sphere (see previous text), the reason again being to assure the exclusion or confirmation of dysfunctional dimensions before premature referral to a psychologist, for instance. In a fully developed STAYAC model, there will virtually be no patient flows along the thicker red arrows in the algorithm.

In conclusion, there is a huge amount of developmental, educational, and scientific work to be done before healthcare will be able to offer an effective service for patients with pain from neuromusculoskeletal disorders—a service that reduces the suffering and the costs to society of this patient group, costs that at the moment run riot.

Additional therapeutic measures in the management of low back pain

For simplicity, some constituents of the algorithm demonstrated in Figure 60.1 have been omitted. It should be noted, however, that in practice some of them, such as the following examples, are fairly frequently used.

Sleep disorders and the linked lack of daily routines

A well-established essential factor and frequent problem in pain patients is sleep disorders and the linked lack of daily routines. There is no need for this to take room in the flowchart in Figure 60.1 and also no need to describe this predicament in depth in this chapter: this factor is so classical and we deal with this problem within the STAYAC model in the same way as do other units. In this context, the importance of improved sleep and strict daily routines cannot be overemphasized.

A *'sleep school'* is included in the STAYAC concept. Sometimes sleeping pills are necessary—the shorter this treatment, the better. Sleep is also frequently normalized by *SSRIs/SNRIs/tricyclics*, which is the preferable long-term solution.

Cork wedges

The compensation of anatomical true leg-length differences (5–15 mm) by means of cork wedges (a secondary prevention measure) seemingly decreases the frequency of recurrence of pelvic/lumbar dysfunctions, or even eliminates recurrences. Differences larger than 15 mm have to be compensated by a combination of a cork wedge inside the shoe and the building up of the heel of the shoe, or preferably, the entire sole. It is important to appreciate that, since patients with ongoing dysfunction(s) in the pelvic/lumbar region always manifest false (dysfunctional) leg-length differences, measuring leg length by means of a tape measure or by conventional radiography is meaningless. The final decision to compensate for leg-length differences should be undertaken in a stable and definite dysfunction-free state and, even better, when the patient is pain-free. The purpose of the cork wedge is to achieve a horizontal pelvis, and this can only be undertaken by means of relatively sophisticated manual techniques in the standing and the lying position. The difficulty of this procedure is severely underestimated and, consequently, even more incorrectly prescribed cork wedges have to be discarded than new cork wedges prescribed.

Posture exercises and posture correction

To change posture permanently is rarely necessary, and it is also time-consuming, costly, and extremely difficult for the patient. Consequently, such measures have a minor role in the STAYAC concept. They are never undertaken as primary measures, but are occasionally appropriate for secondary prevention, usually late in the antidysfunctional sphere. These cases may be referred to specialized physiotherapists who work with this measure exclusively.

Ergonomic advice

As secondary prevention, this is also a late and fairly rare move in the algorithm, the reason simply being that it is rarely necessary when some steps in the antidysfunctional investigation have been undertaken. Adjusting the environment of the patient who has ongoing and treatable dysfunctions does not make sense. Indeed, when possible, which it almost always is, enabling the patient to work in any workplace by means of optimizing their function is a preferable approach. However, sometimes a stable situation for the patient is achievable only in this way. Some of our physiotherapists visit workplaces for this purpose, but external specialists are sometimes engaged instead. The purpose of visiting workplaces, often in cooperation with the company's occupational care unit, is more often to analyse the workplace milieu from a social/psycho-existential perspective, involving colleagues, managers, and so forth.

Spinal supports, orthoses, special chairs, special, beds, etc.

Such measures are occasionally necessary, but only as one of the final measures that are undertaken within STAYAC; although in some other paradigms, they constitute the core 'management'. We are especially disappointed with the use of spinal supports, which are virtually never used at STAYAC. In this context, of course, trochanter belt constitutes an important exception.

Oestrogen withdrawal

Although this is controversial, there is some support in the literature for the hypothesis that oestrogen therapy in women, for treatment of postmenopausal syndromes (Brynhildsen et al. 1998) as well as for contraception (Wreje et al. 1995, 1997), increases the risk of lower back and pelvic troubles. Seemingly, in some therapy-resistant women with recurring lower lumbar/pelvic dysfunctions, withdrawal of such medications is the only correct move, at the right point of time and carefully weighed against the medication's significance for the quality of life. This measure is considered extremely late in the antidysfunctional investigation, when it is absolutely necessary for the condition in question. Nevertheless, as it is frequently possible to withdraw the oestrogen after some years of medication without recurrence of any postmenopausal symptoms, this seems to be the solution for some women. The indication for this move is recurring dysfunctions in the lower back and the pelvis. However, in both young and elderly women, it may take 6–12 months before the situation is stabilized after this measure.

Omissions from the STAYAC algorithm for management of low back pain

Dietary measures

With respect to pain management, very few therapeutic possibilities are not included in the STAYAC algorithm. As evident elsewhere in this chapter, some modalities have a minor role, and one or two are not included at all. In addition, we have not yet adopted dietary measures, omega-3, or antioxidants systematically, a strategy that is advocated by a growing number of physicians and physiotherapists, not least within manual therapy/medicine. To gather experience from this field may be one of the future steps in the further development of the STAYAC algorithm, or we may wait for conclusive studies to support the inclusion of dietary measures in the management of pain patients. In this context, vitamin D constitutes an exception; there is a growing consensus, partly evidence-based, that the role of vitamin D depletion in pain cannot be unnoticed, especially not in fibromyalgia, and, during the last 2–3 years, our impression is that vitamin D substitution is helpful in some patients. Regrettably, the vitamin D test is costly.

Activity-limiting regimens

In the STAYAC concept, regardless of the condition (dysfunctional, WAD, herniated discs, coxarthrosis, and so forth), *no activity-limiting regimens at all are inflicted on the patients*. This essential part of the STAYAC algorithm will certainly be perceived as controversial within numerous medical fields, including manual therapy/medicine. Nevertheless, we have approximately at least 20 years of experience of this approach. We probably practice the stay-active concept more extensively than within any other pain management paradigm. More or less all patients have already limited themselves unnecessarily, but extensively, when they first attend. Patients are encouraged to return gradually to their accustomed levels of activity. If an activity-limiting regimen is inflicted, the subliminal message will be that I, 'the expert', believe that structures in your body are (pathomorphologically) 'injured', that doing this or that may be dangerous, jeopardize your long-term prognosis, and so forth. This is a powerfully negative and unwanted message.

The expected benefit of inflicting activity-limiting advice is improvement of the short-term and long-term prognosis of the patient. Firstly, there is no evidence that this is possible. Secondly, the cost aspect of the measure is easily forgotten. All active medical measures are associated with calculated risks; if a physician prescribes penicillin for a sore throat, he takes a minimal risk that the patient dies from the medicine. Even seemingly innocent measures may be associated with considerable risks for the patients. Imagine that a patient has waited 20 years for his recent retirement, enabling him to play golf full-time. The quality of life of this patient is entirely dependent on his ability to play golf. If you advise him *not* to play golf (to avoid rotational movements in the back), you may more or less have destroyed his life, because you have overlooked the cost–benefit analysis. If a 35-year-old man who loves mogul skiing has a herniated disc, attempt to stimulate him to try! If he cannot do it, he will not do it. What could happen? In the worst case, surgery has to be undertaken, but there is no evidence that it is possible to heal a herniated disc by inactivity. In this patient, activities of daily living, such as lifting his child, are just as likely to precipitate surgery within a few weeks. In point of fact, I am still, after 20 years, waiting for the first patient to come back to me, saying 'You told me that I could do anything in spite of my pain; see what happened!'

Conclusion on the STAYAC management strategy for low back pain

The STAYAC concept is definitely not finally developed, once and for all; in clinical practice, we continually and systematically try to evaluate new treatment and exercise modalities, change the paths through the algorithm, and reconsider the indications within the scheme. A lot of research has to be performed to support such potential modifications; the first step will be the infrastructure study. Ten years have passed since I wrote the first edition of this chapter; numerous, sometimes seemingly small changes have been executed since then, presented in this second edition. In another 10 years, the algorithm will be different from the one presented here, but I am sure that *the core of the algorithm will continue to be the antidysfunctional sphere including manual therapy*.

The STAYAC algorithm is usable in clinical management of all kinds of pain associated with the locomotor system. If a patient has not responded positively to any provided treatment, and you feel insecure about the next step, you can follow their path through the algorithm. This makes it easy to realize whether some box has been forgotten, or what should be the next reasonable cost-effective step in the antidysfunctional investigation when the current measure has failed.

As some of the examples given in this chapter demonstrate, *numerous other medical disciplines would benefit from the application of the 'dysfunction/green flag' paradigm* and its consequences. With appropriate and, in some instances, minor alterations, the algorithm could also be used in other medical fields outside pain management. The basic principle would be the same: with the exception of the few patients fulfilling indications for acute pathomorphologically focused specialist care, dysfunctional explanations for patients' symptoms should be considered before pathomorphologically or psychologically focused investigations are initiated.

References

ACC (1997) *New Zealand acute back pain guide.* Accident Rehabilitation & Compensation Insurance Corporation of New Zealand and the National Health Committee, Wellington, New Zealand.

AHCPR (1994) *Management guidelines for acute low back pain.* Agency for Health Care Policy and Research, U.S. Department of Health and Human Services, Rockville, MD.

Anderson, R. T. (1984) An orthopedic ethnography in rural Nepal. *Med Anthropol*, 8, 46–58.

Andersson, G. B. J., Schultz, A. B., et al. (1984) Intervertebral disc pressures during traction. *Scand J Rehab*, 16, 88–91.

Antonovsky, A. (1987) *Unravelling the mystery of health; hoe people manage stress and stay well.* Jossey-Bass, San Francisco.

Arn, I. (1999) *A biopsychological analysis of functional gastrointestinal disorders and a clinical trial of its treatment with psychodrama.* Dissertation, Division of Psychosocial Factors and Health, Department of Public Health Sciences, and the National Institute for Psychosocial Factors and Health, Karolinska Institute, Stockholm, Sweden.

Assendelft, W. J. J., Morton, S. C., Yu, E. I., et al. (2003) Spinal manipulative therapy for low back pain. A meta-analysis of effectiveness relative to other therapies. *Ann Intern Med*, 138, 871–81.

Aure, O. F., Nilsen, J. H., et al. (2003) Manual therapy and exercise therapy in patients with chronic low back pain. A randomized, controlled trial with 1-year follow-up. *Spine*, 28, 525–32.

Bandura, A. (1977) Self-efficacy: toward a unifying theory of behavioural change. *Psychol Rev*, 84, 191–215.

Bartys, S., Burton, K., Watson, P. J., et al. (2002) *Organisational obstacles to recovery—the role of 'black flags' in the implementation of an early psychosocial intervention for back pain.* Paper presented at BritSpine, Birmingham.

Bendix, A. E., Bendix, T., et al. (1998a) A prospective, randomized 5-year follow-up study of functional restoration in chronic low back pain patients. *Eur Spine J*, 7(2), 111–9.

Bendix, A. F., Bendix, T., et al. (1998b) Functional restoration for chronic low back pain. Two-year follow-up of two randomized clinical trials. *Spine*, 23(6), 717–25.

Bendix, T., Bendix, A., et al. (2000) Functional restoration versus outpatient physical training in chronic low back pain: a randomized comparative study. *Spine*, 25(19), 2494–500.

Bergquist-Ullman, M., Larsson, U. (1977) Acute low back pain in industry. A controlled prospective study with special reference to therapy and confounding factors. *Acta Orthop Scand Supp* 170, 1–117.

Blomberg, S. (1993a) *A pragmatic approach to low-back pain including manual therapy and steroid injections. A multicentre study in primary health care.* Thesis, Uppsala University.

Blomberg, S. (1993b) Resultaten giltiga om de kan reproduceras. *Sjukgymnasten*, 8, 43–5.

Blomberg, S. A retrospective outcome study (with respect to an eight years, follow-up of sick leave, a prospective outcome study) evaluating the efficacy of the STAYAC method—a pragmatic approach to patients with low back pain and other pain-related diagnoses. Outcome study no 2.

Blomberg, S. E. I., Bogefeldt, J. P., Grunnesjö, M. I., et al. (2005a) A randomized clinical trial comparing four different treatment regimens: manual therapy including steroid injections, manual therapy, muscle stretching and orthopaedic care. Pain scores and functional variables. Submitted for publication.

Blomberg, S. E. I., Bogefeldt, J. P., Grunnesjö, M. I., et al. (2005b) A randomized controlled trial of stay-active care versus manual therapy combined with steroid injections in addition to stay-active care in low-back pain radiating to the leg(s), and below the knee(s) respectively. Functional variables and pain. In manuscript.

Blomberg, S. E. I., Bogefeldt, J. P., Grunnesjö, M. I., et al. (2005c) A randomized controlled trial of stay-active care versus manual therapy combined with steroid injections in addition to stay-active care in low-back pain. Quality-of-life score and a general psychosomatic symptom profile. In manuscript.

Blomberg, S., Hallin, G., et al. (1994b) Manual therapy with steroid injections—a new approach to treatment of low back pain. A controlled multicenter trial with an evaluation by orthopedic surgeons. *Spine*, 19(5), 569–77.

Blomberg, S., Svärdsudd, K., et al. (1992) A controlled, multicentre trial of manual therapy in low-back pain, Initial status, sick-leave and pain score during follow-up. *Scand J Prim Health Care*, 10, 170–8.

Blomberg, S., Svärdsudd, K., et al. (1993a) A controlled, multicentre trial of manual therapy with steroid injections in low-back pain, functional variables, side-effects and complications during four months' follow-up. *Clin Rehab*, 7, 49–62.

Blomberg, S., Svärdsudd, K., et al. (1993b) Manual therapy with steroid injections in low-back pain. Improvement of quality of life in a controlled trial with four months' follow-up. *Scand J Prim Health Care*, 11(2), 83–90.

Blomberg, S., Svärdsudd, K., et al. (1994a) A randomized study of manual therapy with steroid injections in low-back pain. Telephone interview follow-up of pain, disability, recovery and drug consumption. *Eur Spine J*, 3(5), 246–54.

Bogefeldt, J. P., Grunnesjö, M. I., Svärdsudd, K. F., et al. (2004b) Diagnostic differences between general practitioners and orthopaedic surgeons in a randomised controlled trial of manual therapy in low back pain. Submitted for publication.

Bogefeldt, J. P., Grunnesjö, M. I., Svärdsudd, K. F., et al. (2005a) A randomised clinical trial of manual therapy combined with steroid injections—the Säter low-back pain study. Results from the three-year follow-up. In manuscript.

Bogefeldt, J. P., Grunnesjö, M. I., Svärdsudd, K. F., et al. (2005b) A randomized clinical trial of manual therapy combined with steroid injections in chronic patients—a partial crossover study. In manuscript.

Bogefeldt, J. P., Grunnesjö, M. I., Wedel, H., et al. (2004a) Sick-leave measures as outcome in a randomised controlled clinical trial of manual therapy combined with steroid injections for low-back pain. The Gotland low-back pain study. Submitted for publication.

Bronfort, G., Evans, R., Nelson, B., et al. (2001) A randomized clinical trial of exercise and spinal manipulation for patients with chronic neck pain. *Spine*, 26, 788–99.

Bronfort, G., Haas, M., Evans, D. C., et al. (2004) Efficacy of spinal manipulation and mobilization for low back pain and neck pain: a systematic review and best evidence synthesis. *Spine*, 4, 335–56.

Brynhildsen, J. O., Bjors, E., et al. (1998) Is hormone replacement therapy a risk factor for low back pain among postmenopausal women? *Spine*, 23, 809–13.

CSAG (1994) Report on back pain. Clinical Standards Advisory Group, HMSO, London.

Carroll, L. (undated) *Alice in wonderland* and *Through the looking glass.* Collins Clear Type Press, London.

Cherkin, D. C., Deyo, R. A., et al. (1998) A comparison of physical therapy, chiropractic manipulation, and provision of an educational booklet for the treatment of patients with low back pain. *New Engl J Med*, 339(15), 1021–9.

Cyriax, J. (1970) *Textbook of orthopaedic medicine.* Baillière Tindall, London.

Daykin, A. R., Richardson, B. (2004) Physiotherapists' pain beliefs and their influence on the management of patients with chronic low back pain. *Spine*, 29, 783–95.

De Bono, E. (1977) *Lateral thinking.* Penguin, London.

Dechow, E., Davies, R. K., Carr, A. J., et al. (1999) A randomized, double-blind, placebo-controlled trial of sclerosing injections in patients with chronic low back pain. *Rheumatology*, 38, 1255–9.

Della-Giustina, D. A. (1999) Emergency department evaluation and treatment of back pain. *Emerg Med Clin N Am*, 17(4), 877–93, vi–vii.

Della-Giustina, D., Kilcline, B. A. (2000) Acute low back pain: a comprehensive review. *Comp Ther*, 26(3), 153–9.

Deyo, R. A., Weinstein J. N. (2001) Low back pain. *New Engl J Med*, 344(5), 363–70.

Egund, N., Olsson, T. H., et al. (1978) Movements in the sacroiliac joints demonstrated with roentgen stereophotogrammetry. *Acta Radiol Diag*, 19, 833–45.

Eklund, M. (1992) Chronic pain and vocational rehabilitation: a multifactorial analysis of symptoms, signs, and psycho-socio-demographics. *J Occup Rehab*, 2(2), 53–66.

Ellis, R. M., Remvig, L., Airaksinen, O., et al. (2006) The rationale for invasive treatment in manual/muscular medicine. *J Orthoped Med*, 28, 545–50.

Englund, L. (2000) *Sick-listing—attitudes and doctors' practice with special emphasis on sick-listing practice in primary health care.* Acta Universitatis Upsaliens. Digital comprehensive summaries of dissertations from the Faculty of Medicine, University of Uppsala, no. 956.

Evjent, O., Hamberg, J. (1985a) *Muscle stretching in manual therapy, a clinical manual, the extremities.* Alfta Rehab Förslag, Alfta.

Evjent, O., Hamberg, J. (1985b) *Muscle stretching in manual therapy, a clinical manual, the spinal column and the temporomandibular joint.* Alfta Rehab Förlag, Alfta.

Evjent, O., Hamberg J. (1990) *Autostretching. The complete manual of specific stretching.* Alfta Rehab Förlag, Alfta.

Farrell, J. P., Twomey L. T. (1982) Acute low back pain. Comparison of two conservative treatment approaches. *Med J Austral*, 1, 160–4.

Fisk, J. W. (1979) A controlled trial of manipulation in a selected group of patients with low back pain favouring one side. *New Z Med J*, 10, 288–91.

Flavell, J. H. (1979) Metacognition and cognitive monitoring: a new area of cognitive-developmental inquiry. *Am Psychol*, 34, 906–11.

Fritzell, P., Hägg, O., Wessberg, P., et al. (2001) Volvo award winner in clinical studies: lumbar fusion versus nonsurgical treatment for chronic low back pain: a multicenter randomized controlled trial from the Swedish lumbar spine study group. *Spine*, 26, 2521–32.

Gillström, P., Ericson, K., et al. (1985) Computed tomography examination of the influence of autotraction on herniation of the lumbar disc. *Arch Orthop Trauma Surg*, 104, 289–93.

Grunnesjö, M. (2011) *Low-back Pain. With special reference to manual therapy, outcome and its prognosis.* Acta Universitatis Upsaliensis. Digital comprehensive summaries of Uppsala dissertations from the Faculty of Medicine, Uppsala University, no. 691.

Grunnesjö, M., Bogefeldt, J., Blomberg, S., Delaney, H., Svärdsudd, K. (2006) The course of pain drawings during a ten week treatment period in patients with acute and sub-acute low back pain. *BMC Musculo Dis*, 7, 65.

Grunnesjö, M. I., Bogefeldt, J. P., Blomberg, S. E. I., Strender, L-E., Svärdsudd, K. F. The contribution of pain drawings in the prediction of return to work in patients with acute or subacute low-back pain.

Grunnesjö, M. I., Bogefeldt, J. P., Svärdsudd, K. F., et al. (2004a) A randomised controlled clinical trial of stay-active care versus manual therapy in addition to stay-active care; functional variables and pain. *J Manip Physiol Ther*, 27, 431–41.

Grunnesjö, M. I., Bogefeldt, J. P., Svärdsudd, K. F. et al. (2004b) The course of pain drawings relative to time and treatment in acute and subacute low back pain.

Grunnesjö, M. I., Bogefeldt, J. P., Svärdsudd, K. F., et al. (2005a) A randomised clinical trial of manual therapy combined with steroid injections—the Gotland low-back pain study. Pain drawings.

Grunnesjö, M. I., Bogefeldt, J. P., Svärdsudd, K. F., et al. (2005b) A randomised clinical trial of manual therapy combined with steroid injections—the Säter low-back pain study. Pain drawings.

Gunn, C. C. (1996) *The Gunn approach to the treatment of chronic pain—intramuscular stimulation for myofascial pain of radiculopathic origin.* Churchill Livingstone, London.

Hackett, G. S. (1958) *Ligament and tendon relaxation treated by prolotherapy* (3rd edn). Charles C. Thomas, Springfield, IL.

Hadler, N. M., Curtis, P., et al. (1987) A benefit of spinal manipulation as adjunctive therapy for acute low-back pain: a stratified controlled trial. *Spine*, 12(7), 703–6.

Harmer, C. J., Bhagwagar, Z., et al. (2003) Acute SSRI administration affects the processing of social cues in healthy volunteers. *Neuropsychopharmacology*, 28(1), 148–52.

Harms-Ringdahl, K., Holmström, E., et al. (1999) *Evidensbaserad sjukgymnastisk behandling. Patienter med ländryggsbesvär.* Rapport 102:99. SBU (Swedish Council on Technology Assessment in Health Care), Stockholm, Sweden.

Holten, O., Torstensen, T. A. (1991) Medical exercise therapy—the basic principles. WCPT Congress, London, 1991. Special issue of *Fysioterapeuten*, 58, 27–32.

Hoving, L. J. (2002) *Neck pain in primary care—the effects of commonly applied interventions.* Thesis. VU University Medical Centre, Amsterdam.

Howell, D. W. (1984) Musculoskeletal profile and incidence of musculoskeletal injuries in lightweight women rowers. *Am J Sports Med*, 12, 278–82.

Hoy, D., Toole, M. J., Morgan, D., et al. (2003). Low back pain in rural Tibet. *Lancet*, 361, 225–6.

Indahl, A., Velund, L., et al. (1995) Good prognosis for low back pain when left untampered: a randomized clinical trial. *Spine*, 20, 473–7.

Janda, V. (1976) *Muskelfunktionsdiagnostik.* Steinkopff, Dresden.

Johansson, P., Larsson, L. (2007) *Muscle action quality* (2nd edn). Bulls Graphics AB, Halmstad.

Johansson, H., Sojka P. (1991) Pathophysiological mechanisms involved in genesis and spread of muscular tension in occupational muscle pain and in chronic musculoskeletal pain syndromes: a hypothesis. *Med Hypoth*, 35, 196–203.

Jones, M. A., Rivett, D. A. (2004) Chronic low back and coccygeal pain. In:Hodges, P. (ed.) *Clinical reasoning for manual therapists.* Butterworth-Heinemann, London, Chapter 7.

Jull, G., et al. (2002) A randomized controlled trial of exercise and manipulative therapy for cervicogenic headache. *Spine*, 27(17), 1835–43.

Kaltenborn, F. M., Evjent O. (1993) *The spine, basic evaluation and mobilization techniques.* Olaf Norlis Bokhandel, Oslo.

Kendall, N. A. S., Linton, S. J., Main, C. J. (1997) *Guide to assessing psychosocial yellow flags in acute low back pain: risk factors for long term disability and work loss.* Accident Rehabilitation & Compensation Insurance Corporation of New Zealand and the National Health Committee, Wellington, New Zealand, pp. 1–22.

Kiley, D. (1983) *Peter Pan syndrome: men who have never grown up.* Dodd Mead, USA.

Klein, R. G. Dorman, T. A., Johnson, C. E. (1989) Proliferant injections for low back pain: histologic changes of injected ligaments and objective measurements of lumbar spine mobility before and after treatment. *J Neurol Orthop Med Surg*, 10, 123–6.

Klein, R. G., Eek, B. C., DeLong, W. B., et al. (1993) A randomized double-blind trial of dextrose-glycerine-phenol injections for chronic, low back pain. *J Spinal Disord*, 6, 23–33.

Knutson, B., Cole, S., et al. (1997) Serotonergic intervention increases affiliative behavior in humans. *Ann New York Acad Sci*, 807, 492–3.

Knutson, B., Wolkowitz, O. M., et al. (1998) Selective alteration of personality and social behavior by serotonergic intervention. *Am J Psychiat*, 155(3), 373–9.

Knutsson, E., Skoglund, C. R., et al. (1988) Changes in voluntary muscle strength, somatosensory transmission and skin temperature concomitant with pain relief during autotraction in patients with lumbar and sacral root lesions. *Pain*, 33, 173–9.

Koes, B. W., Bouter, L. M., van Mameren, H., et al. (1992a) The effectiveness of manual therapy, physiotherapy, and treatment by general practitioner for chronic non-specific back and neck complaints: a randomized clinical trial. *Spine*, 17, 28–35.

Koes, B. W., Bouter, L. M., van Mameren, H., et al. (1992b) A blinded randomized clinical trial of manual therapy and physiotherapy for chronic back and neck complaints: physical outcome measures. *J Manip Physiol Ther*, 15, 16–23.

Koes, B. W., Bouter, L. M., van Mameren, H., et al. (1992c) Randomised clinical trial of manipulative therapy and physiotherapy for persistent back and neck complaints: results of one year follow-up. *BMJ*, 304, 601–5.

Koes, B. W., van Tulder, M. W., et al. (2001) Clinical guidelines for the management of low back pain in primary care. An international comparison. *Spine*, 26(22), 2504–14.

Kool, J., de Bie, R., Oesch, P., et al. (2004) Exercise reduces sick leave in patients with non-acute non-specific low back pain: a meta-analysis. *J Rehab Med*, 36, 49–69.

Kuhn, T. S. (1962) *The structure of scientific revolutions*. University of Chicago Press, Chicago.

Lewit, K. (1991) *Manipulative therapy in rehabilitation of the locomotor system*. Butterworth-Heinemann, London.

Lind, G. A. M. (1974) *Auto-traction. Treatment of low back pain and sciatica. An electromyeographic, radiographic and clinical study*. Linköping, Sweden.

Lindström, I., Öhlund, C., et al. (1992) Mobility, strength, and fitness after a graded activity program for patients with subacute low back pain. A randomized prospective clinical study with a behavioral therapy approach. *Spine*, 17(6), 641–52.

Linton, S. J., Halldén, K. (1998) Can we screen for problematic back pain? A screening questionnaire for predicting outcome in acute and subacute back pain. *Clin J Pain*, 14, 209–15.

Ljunggren, A. E., Weber, H., et al. (1984) Autotraction versus manual traction in patients with prolapsed lumbar intervertebral discs. *Scand J Rehab Med*, 16, 117–24.

Loubinoux, I., Pariente, J., et al. (2002) A single dose of the serotonin neurotransmission agonist paroxetine enhances motor output: double-blind, placebo-controlled, fMRI study in healthy subjects. *Neuroimage*, 15(1), 26–36.

Magnusson, D., Mahoney, L. (2001) *A holistic person approach for research on positive development*. Report 76, Research Program on Individual Development and Adaption, Department of Psychology, Stockholm University.

Malmivaara, A., Hakkinen, U., et al. (1995) The treatment of acute low back pain—bed rest, exercises, or ordinary activity? *New Engl J Med*, 332(6), 351–5.

McGuirk, B., King, W., Govind, J., et al. (2001) Safety, efficacy and cost-effectiveness of evidence-based guidelines for the management of acute low back pain in primary care. *Spine*, 26, 2615–22.

McKenzie, R. (1981) *The lumbar spine. Mechanical diagnosis and therapy*. Spinal Publications, Waikanae, New Zealand.

Midttun, A., Bojsen-Traeden, J., et al. (1983) *Syndroma ligamenti sacrotuberalis—a case for manual therapy*. Scandinavian Association for the Study of Pain, Annual Meeting 5.

Miller, W. R., Seligman, M. E. (1975) Depression and learned helplessness in man. *J Abnorm Psychol*, 84, 228–38.

Miller, W. R., Seligman, M. E., et al. (1975) Learned helplessness, depression, and anxiety. *J Nervous Ment Dis*, 161, 347–57.

Mitchel, F., Moran, P., et al. (1979) *An evaluation and treatment manual for osteopathic muscle energy procedures*. Mitchel, Moran and Protozoa, Valley Park.

Mulligan, B. R. (2003) *Self treatments for back, neck and limbs*. Plane View Services Ltd., New Zealand.

Myrin, S-O. (1972) *Varo add on rigged*. Bokförlaget Robert Larsson, Täby, Sweden.

Nachemson, A., Jonsson, E., et al. (1991) *Ont i ryggen—orsaker, diagnostik och behandling*. SBU (Swedish Council on Technology Assessment in Health Care), Stockholm, Sweden.

Nachemson, A. L, Jonsson, E. (eds). (2000) *Neck and back pain: the scientific evidence of causes, diagnosis, and treatment*. Lippincott, Williams & Wilkins, Philadelphia.

Natchew, E. (1984) *A manual on auto-traction treatment for low back pain*. Folksam Scientific Council, Stockholm.

Nwuga, V. C. B. (1982) Relative therapeutic efficacy of vertebral manipulation and conventional treatment in back pain management. *Am J Phys Med*, 61(6), 273–8.

Ongley, M. J., Dorman, T. A., et al. (1987) A new approach to the treatment of chronic low back pain. *Lancet* (18 July), 2(8551), 143–6.

RCGP (1996) *Clinical guidelines for the management of acute low back pain*. Royal College of General Practitioners, London.

Rasmussen, G. G. (1979) Manipulation in treatment of low back pain: a randomized clinical trial. *Man Med*, 1, 8–10.

Rasmussen-Barr, E., Nilsson-Wikmar, L., et al. (2003) Stabilizing training compared with manual treatment in sub-acute and chronic low-back pain. *Man Ther*, 8, 233–41.

Reordan, D., Chevan, J., Clapis, C. (2012) *The Mulligan concept. Physical therapy management of low back pain: a case-based approach*. Jones & Bartlett Publishers.

Richardson, C, Hodges, PW, Hides, J (2004). Therapeutic exercise for lumbsopelvic stabilisation, 2nd ed. Churchill Livingstone.

Seferlis, T., Németh, G., et al. (1998) Conservative treatment in patients sick-listed for acute low-back pain: a prospective randomised study with 12 months' follow-up. *Eur Spine J*, 7, 461–70.

Shores, M. M., Pascualy, M., et al. (2001) Short-term sertraline treatment suppresses sympathetic nervous system activity in healthy human subjects. *Psychoneuroendocrinology*, 26(4), 433–9.

Skargren, E. I., Öberg, B. E., et al. (1997) Cost-effectiveness of chiropractic and physiotherapy treatment for low back pain and neck pain. Six-month follow-up. *Spine*, 22(18), 2167–77.

Sloop, P. R., Smith, D. S., et al. (1982) Manipulation for chronic neck pain. A double-blind controlled study. *Spine*, 7(6), 532–5.

Stoddard, A. (1980) *Manual of osteopathic technique*. Hutchinson, London.

Sturesson, B., Selvik, G., et al. (1989) Movements of the sacroiliac joints. A roentgen stereophotogrammetric analysis. *Spine*, 14(2), 162–5.

Tilscher (1995 and 1996) A dynamic radiography report of spinal mobility before and after prolotherapy: the mobility of the lumbar spine is increased by prolotherapy. Personal communication (to be published).

Torstensen, T. A. (1997) The physical therapy approach. In: Whitecloud III, T. (ed.) *The adult spine: principles and practice*. Lippincott-Raven, Philadelphia, pp. 1797–805.

Torstensen, T. A., Ljunggren, A. E., et al. (1998) Efficiency and costs of medical exercise therapy, conventional physiotherapy, and self-exercise in patients with chronic low back pain. A pragmatic, randomized, single-blinded, controlled trial with 1-year follow-up. *Spine*, 23, 2616–24.

Travell, J. S. D. (1983–92) *Myofascial pain and dysfunction—the trigger point manual*. Williams & Wilkins, Baltimore, MD.

Tse, W. S., Bond, A. J. (2002) Serotonergic intervention affects both social dominance and affiliative behaviour. *Psychopharmacology (Berlin)*, 161(3), 324–30.

Tullberg, T., Blomberg, S., et al. (1998) Manipulation does not alter the position of the sacroiliac joint. A Roentgen stereophotogrammetric analysis. *Spine*, 23(10), 1124–9.

van Tulder, M., Malmivaara, A., et al. (2000) Exercise therapy for low back pain: a systematic review within the framework of the Cochrane collaboration back review group. *Spine*, 25(21), 2784–96.

van Tulder, M. W., Ostelo, R., Vlaeyen, J. W. S., et al. (1996) Behavioral treatment for chronic low back pain. A systematic review within the framework of the Cochrane back review group. *Spine*, 26, 270–81.

Waddell, G. (1998) *The back pain revolution*. Churchill Livingstone, Edinburgh.

Wigley, R. D., Zhang, N. C., Zeng, Q. Y., et al. (1994). ILAR-China study comparing the prevalence of rheumatic symptoms in northern and southern rural populations. *J Rheumatol*, 21, 1484–90.

Wreje, U., Isacsson, D., et al. (1997) Oral contraceptives and back pain in women in Swedish community. *Int J Epidem*, 26(1), 71–4.

Wreje, U., Kristiansson, P., et al. (1995) Serum levels of relaxin during the menstrual cycle and oral contraceptive use. *Gynecol Obstet Invest*, 39, 197–200.

Wreje, U., Nordgren, B., et al. (1992) Treatment of pelvic joint dysfunction in primary care—a controlled study. *Scand J Prim Health Care*, 10, 310–5.

Yelland, M. J., Glasziou, P. P., Bogduk, N., et al. (2004) Prolotherapy injections, saline injections, and exercises for chronic low-back pain: a randomized trial. *Spine*, 29, 9–16.

Zulian, F., Martini, G., Gobber, D., et al. (2003) Comparison of intra-articular triamcinolone hexacetonide and triamcinolone acetonide in oligoarticular juvenile idiopathic arthritis. *Rheumatology*, 42, 1254–9.

Chapter 61

Dynamic neuromuscular stabilization: exercise in developmental positions to achieve spinal stability and functional joint centration

Alena Kobesova, Marcela Safarova, and Pavel Kolar

Introduction to dynamic neuromuscular stabilization

Kolar's approach to dynamic neuromuscular stabilization (DNS) is a complex approach that encompasses principles of developmental kinesiology during the first year of human life (Kolar et al. 2010). Further, it includes defining posture, breathing pattern, and functional joint centration from a 'neurodevelopmental' perspective. DNS assessment is based upon the comparison of the patient's stabilizing pattern to the one of a healthy infant. The treatment approach is based on ontogenetic postural locomotor patterns. Optimizing the distribution of internal forces of muscles that act on each segment of the spine and/or any other joint is the primary goal of this treatment approach.

When assessing a patient with pain in the locomotor system and searching for its primary cause, the morphological aspects and external biomechanical impacts affecting the spine and the joint as well as the internal, stereotypically repeating forces developed by the patient's own musculature need to be considered. Current research literature addresses the importance of the deep spinal stabilizing muscle system (Bouche et al. 2011; Kim et al. 2010; Watanabe et al. 2010). However, not only 'deep muscles' provide spinal and extremity joint stability. Through postural-locomotion kinematic chains, nearly every muscle is involved in stabilization function. Muscle co-ordination is directly controlled by the central nervous system (CNS). Therefore, the quality of postural stabilization depends on the quality of sensorimotor control. Any phasic or purposeful movement is preceded by the automatic activation of the stabilizers (Borghuis et al. 2008; Hodges 2004; McGill et al. 2009). Therefore, body posture influences quality of purposeful movements and vice versa.

Postural stabilization is an automatic, subconscious function that is frequently compromised in patients with musculoskeletal pain and with various neurological diagnoses. Postural function is interdependent with respiratory function, which is an important aspect for consideration. Postural misalignment may result in an abnormal breathing pattern and vice versa. Since this coupled, automatic postural-respiratory function is not completely under voluntary control, it may be difficult to train and improve it with traditional rehabilitation approaches.

Assessment of sensorimotor central control and postural-locomotion function should be an integral part of clinical assessment in rehabilitation practice. Based on functional assessment, a 'key link' (or clinically most relevant dysfunction) should be identified and addressed by treatment. The goal of DNS is to improve or normalize quality of postural, respiratory, and locomotion patterns as defined by developmental kinesiology (early ontogenesis) and integrate the proper postural-locomotion and respiratory function within activities of daily living and sport performance.

Definition of an ideal body posture from a developmental perspective

Normal early progress during the first year of life usually leads to the development of an optimal stabilization pattern, meaning ideal co-ordination between the cervical and thoracic spinal flexors (longus colli, longus capitis, rectus capitis anterior, and lateralis muscles) and the extensors (semispinalis cervicis and capitis, splenius

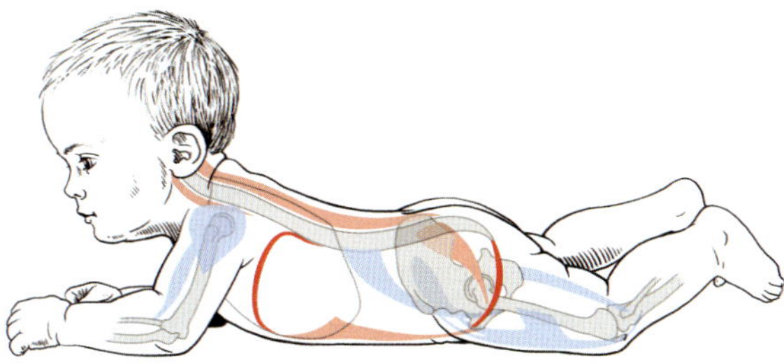

Figure 61.1 (a) A 3-month-old infant in prone position can hold its head against gravity, utilizing bilateral elbows and the pubic symphysis for support. To maintain this posture, the core must be stabilized via muscle synergy (muscles pictured in red). The cervical and upper thoracic spine are stabilized by balanced co-contraction between the deep neck flexors and extensors. The lower thoracic and lumbar spine are stabilized anteriorly by intra-abdominal pressure arising from co-ordinated activity of the diaphragm, pelvic floor, and abdominal wall musculature. This muscle synergy must be in balance with spinal extensors. Cervical extension, or uprighting, is initiated at the mid-thoracic spine (at the origin of the deep neck flexors).

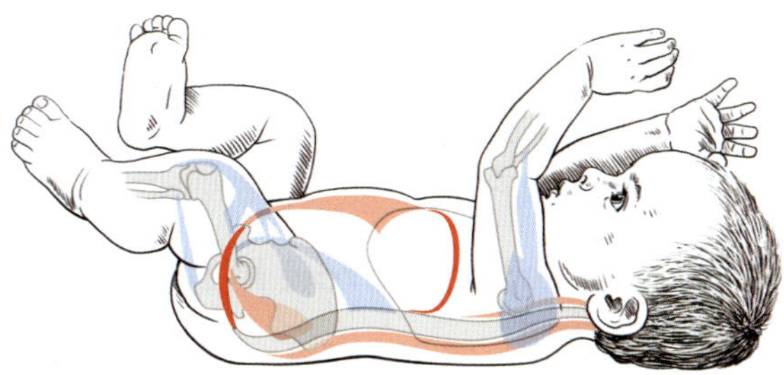

Figure 61.1 (b) A 3-month-old infant in supine position can hold its legs above the floor against gravity, utilizing the upper sections of the gluteal muscles, nuchal line, and back for support. The spine is stabilized using the same muscle synergy as described for prone position in Figure 61.1(a).

cervicis and capitis muscles). The lower thoracic and lumbar spine are stabilized via co-ordinated activity between the diaphragm, pelvic floor, and abdominal wall (i.e. muscles that regulate intra-abdominal pressure) (Figure 61.1a,b). Such muscle balance and optimal co-ordination can already be observed in a 3-month-old baby. At this age, the development of the stabilization function is completed in both prone (Figure 61.1a) and supine positions (Figure 61.1b), and is later utilized in more mature developmental postural positions such as side-lying, quadruped, tripod, bear position, squat, standing, and gait (see Chapter 8).

Aetiology of atypical posture

This optimal muscle synergy can be compromised by several mechanisms. Congenital skeletal dysplasia may prevent optimal stabilization. For example, pectus excavatum or carinatum, or congenitally fused vertebral bodies (Klippel-Feil syndrome) do not necessarily stand for atypical postural function, but may be inconvenient for ideal postural-locomotion muscle function. Such innate skeletal abnormalities usually do not respond well to any conservative treatment and may need to be corrected surgically.

Abnormal postural development during the first year of life is the second cause of atypical stabilization function (see Chapter 8) Depending on the type of developmental screening tests, developmental scales, and motor assessment instruments used during the evaluation of motor development of newborns and toddlers, various incidence of abnormal motor development is reported in literature (Zafeiriou 2004). Delayed or abnormal postural development classified as cerebral co-ordination disturbance (CCD) by Vojta (Imamura et al. 1983) is found in about 30% of infants and may result in a fixation of less than ideal co-ordination among stabilizers and may persist for the rest of life. Such abnormal postural muscle synergy may be even fostered by inadequate sports training or workload and potentially lead to pain syndromes.

The third common reason for faulty stabilization includes a habitual cause. For example, women, in order to look slim, constantly perform abdominal wall hollowing. In the end, a so- called 'hourglass syndrome' (Figure 61.2) becomes fixated as an abnormal stabilization pattern. Such abdominal wall imbalance keeps the diaphragm elevated, preventing it from maintaining a more neutral position and descending caudally during postural tasks. Lack of diaphragmatic postural function is then usually compensated for by paraspinal muscles, which become overloaded, develop trigger points, physiologically shorten, cause spinal joint dysfunction, and, finally, lead to degenerative spinal changes in an attempt to adjust for the permanent imbalance of stabilizing musculature. Similar consequences may occur as a result of incorrect weight training or

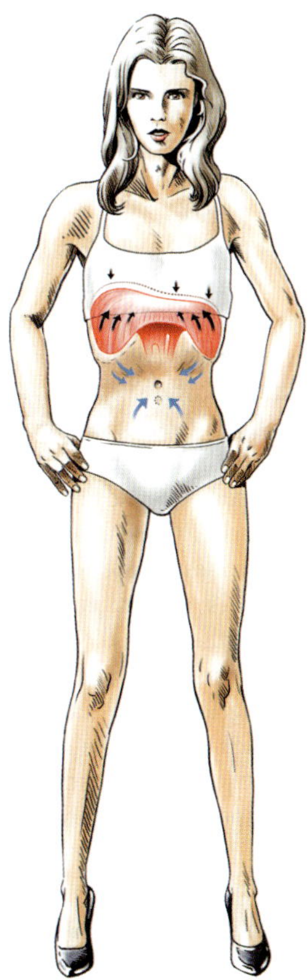

Figure 61.2 'Hourglass syndrome': intentional hollowing, i.e. constant concentric activation of the abdominal wall muscles (blue arrows pointing towards the umbilicus, which moves upwards and inwards) pushes the diaphragm cranially, leading to limited excursions of the diaphragm during postural tasks (the difference between dotted and continuous red line indicating the upper contour of the diaphragm). During postural tasks, an 'inverse' diaphragm activation occurs (indicated by black arrows on the diaphragm, pointing towards the centrum tendineum).

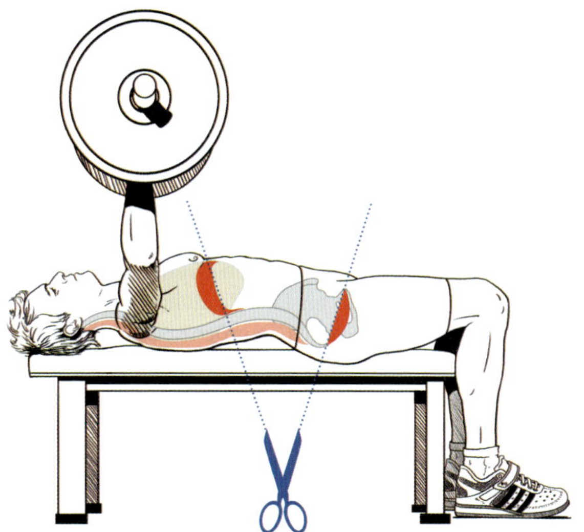

Figure 61.3 'Open scissors syndrome': oblique alignment of the diaphragm and the pelvic floor during weightlifting does not allow for sufficient intra-abdominal pressure increase and it is compensated for by hypertrophic paraspinal muscles. Neck stabilization may also be compromised by this poor training strategy—note the position of the shoulders, neck extension, and atypical head support (should be nuchal line optimally).

erroneous methodology in sports training. For example, excessive strengthening of upper chest stabilizers (pectorales, upper trapezius) and paraspinal muscles may change the alignment between the chest and the pelvis, leading to an 'open scissors syndrome' and inefficient stabilization (Figure 61.3).

The fourth cause of abnormal stabilization is a protective postural pattern. Janda (1980) already described, several decades ago, characteristic patterns of muscle hyper- and hypo-activity leading to predictable postural and gait disturbances and the stereotypical types of an 'antalgic posture' (Page et al. 2010). Also, Lewit describes 'chain reactions' that lead to abnormal postural patterns, such as 'forward drawn posture' and 'pelvic shear dysfunction syndrome', often originating from a pelvic girdle or a foot dysfunction (Lewit 2010). In other words, in case of any pathology (functional or structural, e.g., kidney stones, disc lesion, meniscus tear, respiratory disease), an individual's posture automatically and subconsciously changes to protect the injured or affected body part. This protective postural pattern becomes consistent, sometimes clinically obvious, even in scenarios where the individual is still pain-free. Musculoskeletal pain is a protective signal leading to changes in movement patterns that serve to unload the painful tissue (Henriksen et al. 2011). This aspect is very important not only in a primary locomotor system dysfunction, but also in viscero-somatic patterns (Bitnar 2012). It is important for a clinician to remember that recurring muscle trigger points, joint restrictions, soft tissue dysfunction with a hyperalgic zone, and stereotypical changes in postural or stabilizing pattern may primarily originate from a visceral pathology that must be diagnosed and treated first.

Functional joint centration from a developmental perspective

When the CNS develops and functions optimally, in any postural situation, the joints are in the most suitable position for weightbearing (greatest possible stability at any angle) and are in the most favourable condition for further movement. During childhood, bone growth is linked to muscle activity. An optimal muscle pull will lead to a normal joint development. Furthermore, optimal joint position will be essential for both muscle pull and ligament orientation.

Traditionally, clinicians determine joint centration or decentration ('subluxation') by X-rays. Functional joint centration, however, is a broader term. It is not just the one position depicted on an X-ray. Functional joint centration is a dynamic neuromuscular strategy allowing for maximum interosseous contact and best biomechanical advantage in any joint position. Perfect muscular co-ordination, stabilizing the joint, is considered essential for therapeutic procedures. In a functionally centrated position, static loads are best tolerated based on the anatomical structures that can be found only in humans and, thus, making human locomotion unique and different from any animal (Lee at al. 2012; Ogihara et al. 2012; Sylvester and Pfisterer 2012; Zeinigner et al. 2011). During development, the principles controlling posture determine the formation of anatomical structures and are the expression of a centrally controlled programme. In DNS, clinical assessment is based on evaluation of muscle co-ordination related to a joint position (centration), with a therapeutic goal to restore such muscle co-ordination and joint centration as defined by developmental kinesiology.

Zones of support: their role in stabilization and locomotion

Zones of support form the basis for erect posture and any locomotion is initiated from these zones. They are stable points at which a muscle pull is anchored. Zones of support (i.e. supporting segments) play an important role in proprioception and exteroception and facilitate stabilization and locomotion functions (stepping and supporting function of extremities). In DNS, proper positioning, such as the functional centration of supporting segments, is critical. The CNS determines the zones of support based on the intended movement. Based on the developmental models, DNS describes functional joint centration for each exercise position in order to allow for ideal biomechanical loading with maximal congruence of articular surfaces. Starting an exercise by using functional centration in the supporting segment helps achieve centration in other joints as well. By contrast, incorrect position in the supporting segments may prevent ideal muscle co-ordination and joint centration elsewhere.

Functional assessment of dynamic neuromuscular stabilization

In addition to traditional musculoskeletal assessment, such as assessment of joint range of motion, soft tissue mobility, trigger points, or movement patterns (Janda 1980), DNS emphasizes functional assessment of core stabilization. DNS assessment is based on the comparison of the patient's stabilizing pattern to the developmental stabilization pattern of a healthy infant.

Functional stabilization is a global pattern. If one muscle (or even a part of it, such as the muscle section containing trigger points) is dysfunctional, then the entire stabilizing function is disturbed and the quality of purposeful movement is compromised. Compensatory mechanisms are developed in an attempt to provide some degree of segmental stability. These compensations typically involve certain muscle groups causing overload of joint and spinal discs, muscle overuse, and repetitive strain. Perpetuation of imbalance in the locomotor system and decreased spinal stability eventually result in painful conditions. The functional diagnostic system of DNS presents a set of functional tests to analyse the quality of functional stability and to define a 'key link' of dysfunction that should be primarily addressed by functional treatment.

1. Diaphragm test

Under normal conditions, the diaphragm fulfils combined respiratory, postural, and sphincter functions. Its function is challenging and often compromised. Disorders of breathing and continence have a stronger link to back pain than obesity and physical activity (Smith et al. 2006). Breathing and continence mechanisms may interfere with the physiology of spinal control and may provide a link to back pain. This relationship may be explained by physiological limitations in co-ordination of postural, respiratory, and continence functions of trunk muscles (Smith et al. 2006). Therefore, the diaphragm test is considered to be a key functional test in the DNS approach. It assesses the diaphragm's respiratory and postural functions as well as its co-ordination with other trunk stabilizers, i.e. the pelvic floor and all the muscles of the abdominal wall. These muscles regulate, or more precisely, increase the intra-abdominal pressure during postural tasks helping to stabilize the lower thoracic and lumbar spine.

During clinical assessment, the patient sits on the table, legs unsupported, arms relaxed on the table. First, the patient's breathing pattern is observed. The examiner places his/her fingers between and under the patient's lower ribs and asks the patient to take a deep breath in (Figure 61.4a). Optimally, the lower intercostal spaces widen as a result of external intercostal muscle activation. At the same time, as the diaphragm descends caudally with inspiration, the abdominal wall below the lower ribs expands proportionately in all directions (eccentric activity). Many individuals prefer to engage accessory respiratory muscles in their breathing, especially the sternocleidomastoid, scalenes, pectoralis major and minor, and the upper trapezius. In such case, the activation under the clinician's fingers is minimal and the patient's clavicles and shoulders are observed to elevate with each inhalation. This still does not indicate any real functional pathology or, at least, such a stereotype does not necessarily result in musculoskeletal pain conditions as long as the patient can modify it. To learn the patient's ability to modify their respiratory stereotype, the patient is instructed to relax their shoulders and take a deep breath under the examiner's palpating fingers (Figure 61.4a). Now, a significant and symmetrical expansion of the lower thoracic cavity in a lateral direction should be palpated and observed while the abdominal wall below the lower ribs should also expand in dorsolateral and anterior directions. Optimally, when observing the respiratory breathing from the front and palpating the lower abdominal wall, the inspiratory wave should go as far as the groin and the activation should also be felt under the examiner's fingers just above the hip joints (Figure 61.4b).

To assess postural diaphragmatic function, the patient is instructed to exhale (diaphragm is in a cranial position) and then to expand actively the abdominal wall below the lower ribs in all the directions (the diaphragm descends caudally as a result of purely postural function, the person does not breathe). The amount of expansion correlates with postural function of the diaphragm (Kolar et al. 2010). In order to expand the abdominal wall, the eccentric activation of external and internal obliques along with the transversus and rectus abdominis are necessary. In addition, the concentric activation of the diaphragm (descends caudally during postural tasks) is needed to exert pressure on abdominal content from above and work in harmony with the pelvic floor muscles, which contract concentrically at the same time and provide pelvic support. Abdominal wall activation follows diaphragm and pelvic floor activation, modifying the amount of eccentric activation (expansion) to the activity of the diaphragm and the pelvic floor. From the front, the examiner can check if a person can actively expand the lower abdominal wall above the groin. Once again, this is possible only if the diaphragm properly fulfils its postural function, along with pelvic floor and subsequent abdominal wall activation (Figure 61.4b).

In reality, the diaphragm must fulfil respiratory and postural functions at the same time. In clinical assessment, however, it appears to be convenient to assess the respiratory and postural functions separately, as just described. It is more indicative of a person's ability to control the function of the diaphragm.

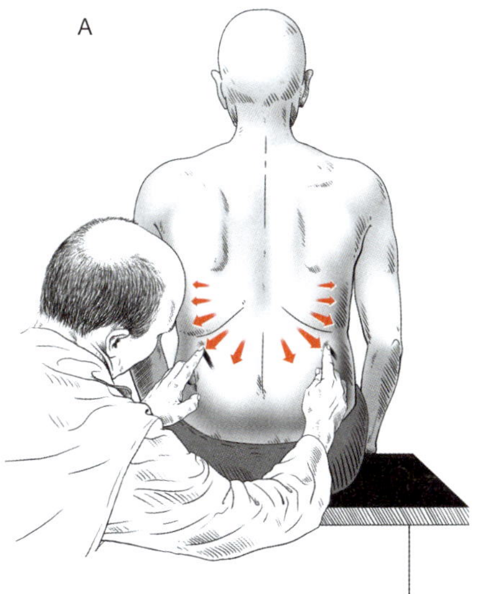

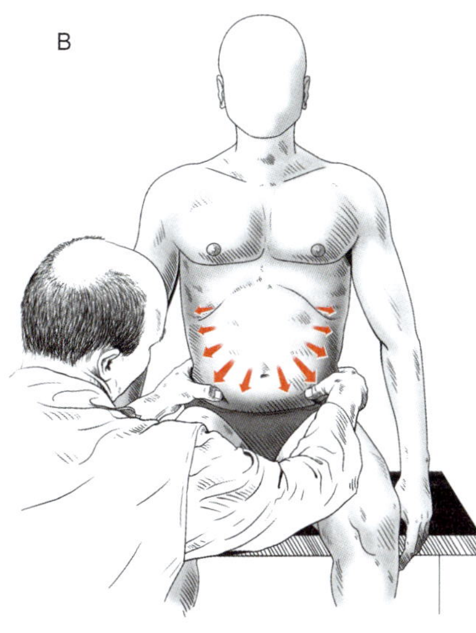

Figure 61.4 Diaphragm test: (**a**) optimal activation, assessment from behind; (**b**) optimal activation, assessment from the front.

2. Intra-abdominal pressure test

The patient lies supine, with legs lifted above the table and flexed to 90° at the hips and knees. Knees are pelvic width apart. Initially, the examiner supports the patient's legs and then slowly removes the support. The patient's stabilizing pattern is observed during this postural task. Under normal conditions, posturally increased intra-abdominal pressure forces the patient's lower back towards the table and the chest remains aligned with the pelvis in such a way that the chest and pelvic axes remain parallel. Frequently, a descent of the diaphragm becomes evident, observed by a caudal movement of the umbilicus towards the pubic symphysis. Shoulders are relaxed. The entire abdominal wall activates eccentrically and proportionately in all directions. Co-ordinated activation between hip abductors and adductors and external and internal rotators keeps the hips in a neutral position (Figure 61.5a).

The following errors can be observed if postural function is compromised (Figure 61.5b):

(1) Insufficient intra-abdominal pressure increase is compensated for by excessive activation of paraspinal superficial muscles, leading to an open scissors syndrome.

(2) Patient's lumbar lordosis increases and the lower back does not adhere to the table; lack of intra-abdominal and intra-pelvic pressure causes hollowing above the groin.

(3) Diastasis recti can be observed and palpated.

(4) Patient elevates and protracts their shoulders (excessive activation of the upper trapezius and pectoralis).

(5) Poor trunk stabilization does not anchor hip flexors properly and the patient cannot maintain neutral hip position as a result; lower extremities become 'too heavy' and fall back on the table; hip abduction increases.

3. Trunk and neck flexion test

The trunk flexion test is performed in supine position with arms positioned along the trunk. The patient slowly performs trunk flexion until the lower scapular angles come off the table. Ideally, the proportional eccentric activation of abdominal wall musculature in all directions is observed and palpated. Diastasis recti should not be observed. The thoracolumbar junction and lumbar spine adhere to the table as a result of an increased intra-abdominal pressure. Lower ribs are well stabilized via the oblique abdominal muscle slings (external and internal obliques, transversus abdominis) and do not flare out. The movement is smooth and effortless; the patient can maintain the end positions for at least 20 seconds (only lower scapular angles are in contact with the table). Lower extremities remain on the table during the testing (Figure 61.6a).

Common signs of insufficiency (Figure 61.6b) include:

(1) Diastasis recti;

(2) Disproportional activation of abdominal wall with the upper section of the rectus abdominis predominant and the dorsolateral sections insufficient (bulging);

(3) Lower rib flaring;

(4) Hollowing above the groin;

(5) Trunk shaking (muscle weakness).

The neck flexion test is also performed in supine position. Ideally, the deep cervical flexors (longus capitis, longus colli, and rectus capitis anterior) are the primary muscles activated while the sternocleidomastoids and the scalenes assist. In a normal scenario, smooth, arc-shaped cervical flexion is observed, with the chin reaching as far as the jugular fossa at the end of the movement. This end position should be maintained for at least 20 seconds (Figure 61.7a).

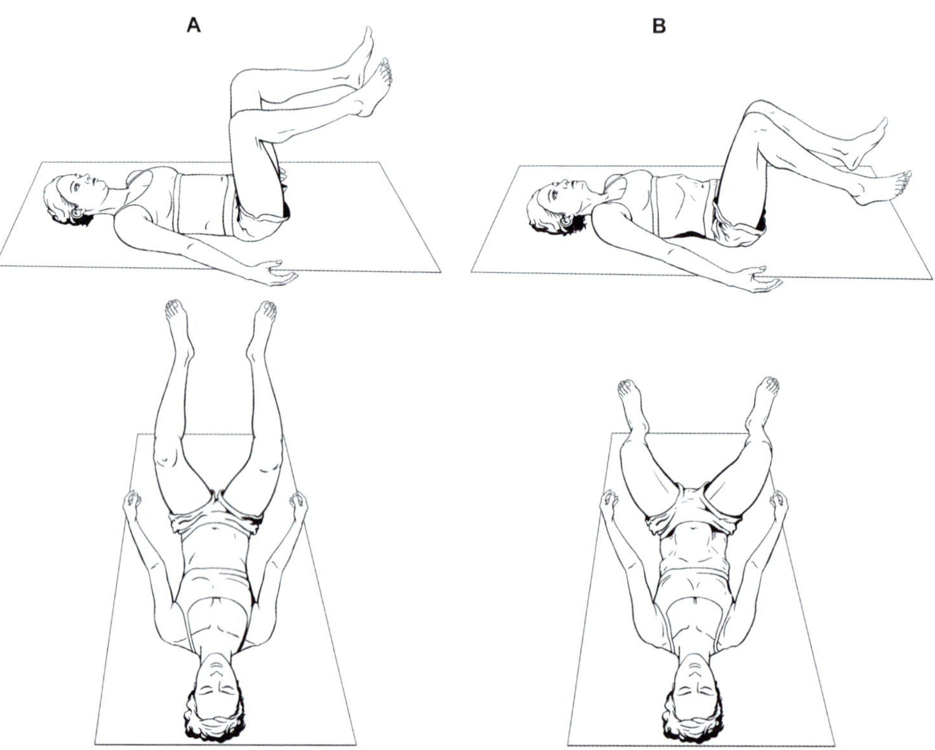

Figure 61.5 Intra-abdominal pressure test: (**a**) optimal activation; (**b**) abnormal activation.

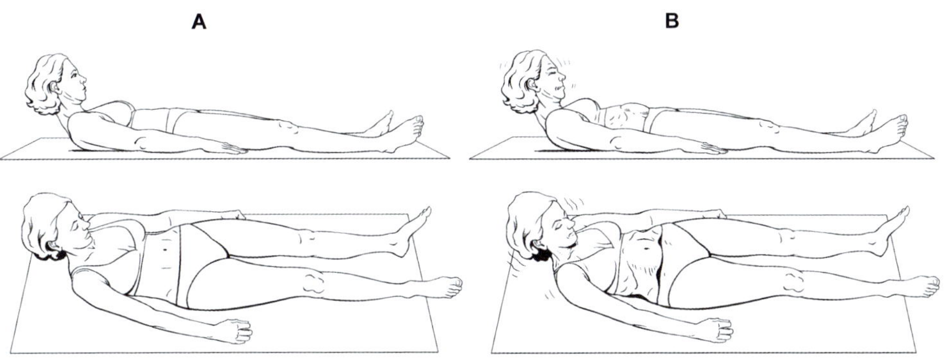

Figure 61.6 Trunk flexion test: (**a**) optimal activation; (**b**) abnormal activation.

The deep neck flexors are often weak and substituted for by superficial muscles, mainly the sternocleidomastoid muscles. In such a case, the arc-shaped, proportionally segmental, cervical flexion pattern is altered and flexion takes place mainly in the lower cervical and upper thoracic segments while extension occurs in the upper cervical segments. At initiation of the movement, the chin juts forward. The movement is often shaky as a result of muscle weakness (Figure. 61.7b).

The test can also be enhanced by a slight resistance against the patient's forehead to confirm inadequate stabilization by the deep cervical flexors.

4. Trunk and neck extension test

The patient performs trunk extension in prone position with arms relaxed along the trunk. Ideally, gradual extension is observed in the cervical and thoracic segments. Shoulder blades remain in a neutral position with medial scapular borders being almost parallel to the spine. Eccentric activation of the dorsolateral sections of the abdominal wall occurs, counterbalancing the paraspinal muscle activity. The pelvis maintains its neutral position with the pubic symphysis and bilateral anterior superior ilias spine (ASIS) becoming zones of support. Lower extremities remain on the table with the gluteal muscles relaxed (Figure 61.8a).

Common signs of insufficiency (Figure 61.8b) include:

(1) Thoracic spine maintains a rigid kyphosis and gradual cervicothoracic segmental extension is replaced by extension at the cervicothoracic and thoracolumbar junctions only.

(2) Shoulder blades are elevated and externally rotated with protruding medial borders.

(3) Hyperactive superficial paraspinal muscles compensate for weak and bulging dorsolateral abdominal wall sections.

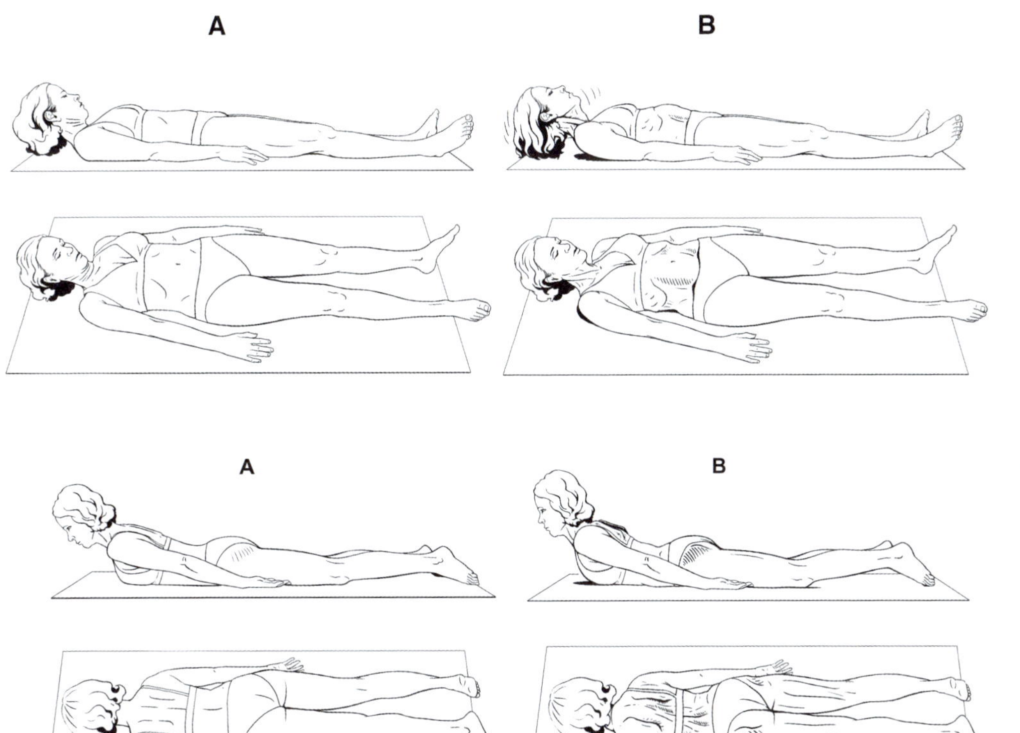

Figure 61.7 Neck flexion test: (**a**) optimal activation; (**b**) abnormal activation.

Figure 61.8 Trunk and neck extension test: (**a**) optimal activation; (**b**) abnormal activation.

(4) Anterior pelvic tilt occurs as a result of insufficient frontal lumbar stability, which is often compensated for by superficial paraspinal muscles and hamstrings; patient may lift their legs off the table.

(5) Concentric activation of the gluteal muscles may also occur as a compensatory pattern assisting in pelvic stabilization with the patient squeezing their buttocks together.

5. Quadruped rock forward test

The patient is in a quadruped position using hands and knees for support. Then, slowly, the patient shifts their head and trunk forward and stays in this position for approximately 30 seconds. The hand position (supporting function) and the trunk stabilization pattern are observed.

Ideally, both hands provide support while maintaining functionally centrated position; i.e. the thenar and hypothenar areas are equally loaded, fingers are 'freely' extended rather than hyperextended or flexed, both hands are 'grasping' the floor providing support. Shoulder blades are in a neutral position, adhering to the rib cage, medial borders nearly parallel to the spine. The spine elongates, the thoracolumbar junction is firm and stable, proportionate activation of the muscles of the abdominal wall occurs (Figure 61.9a).

Under pathological conditions, a decentration of the hands occurs. Usually, the hypothenar area is weightbearing more while the thenar section loses contact with the table. As a result, flexion at the elbow occurs. Often, the scapula on the ipsilateral slide loses its neutral position; it is pulled cranially, its lower angle rotating externally and the medial border protruding. A collapse at the thoracolumbar junction is often related to an anterior pelvic tilt (Figure 61.9b).

6. Squat test

The patient performs a squat. The pattern of trunk stabilization, head position, and the support function of the feet are evaluated. Ideally, the cervical spine is elongated, proportional co-ordination between the neck flexors and extensors keeps the head in a neutral position. During the squat, shoulders and knees are aligned, the chest is not pulled forward in front of the knees, and the knees are not moving over the big toes. Proportional eccentric activation of all the sections of the abdominal wall can be palpated. The chest axis is parallel to the pelvic axis. Gluteal muscles are activated eccentrically demonstrating a hemispheric shape. Knees are pelvic width apart. Feet are functionally centrated, the longitudinal arch does not collapse, the first and fifth metatarsophalangeal regions and the heel form a supporting tripod. The toes are 'grasping' the floor and assisting in stabilization (Figure 61.10a).

Signs of insufficiency (Figure 61.10b) include the following:

(1) Hyperextension at the cervicocranial junction (deep neck flexor insufficiency);

(2) Hyperactivity of paraspinal muscles;

(3) Chest moves forward and the chest axis is not properly aligned with the pelvic axis;

(4) Pelvis tilts anteriorly leading to open scissors syndrome;

(5) Insufficient activation of lower abdominal wall;

(6) Disproportional or insufficient activation of the gluteal muscles is manifested by flattening of the gluteal region, hip internal rotation, and knees collapsing inward;

(4) Decentrated supporting foot function manifests itself by longitudinal arch collapse; insufficient supporting function of the first toe is common; the patient lifts the first toe or all the toes from the ground or, on the contrary, grasps the floor with the toes too forcefully.

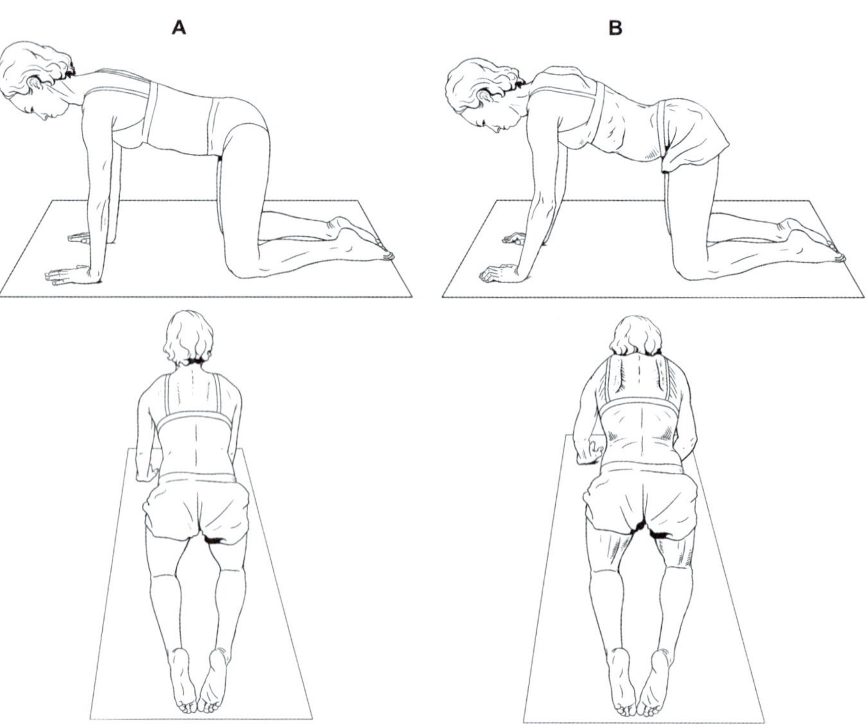

Figure 61.9 Quadruped rock forward test: (**a**) optimal activation; (**b**) abnormal activation.

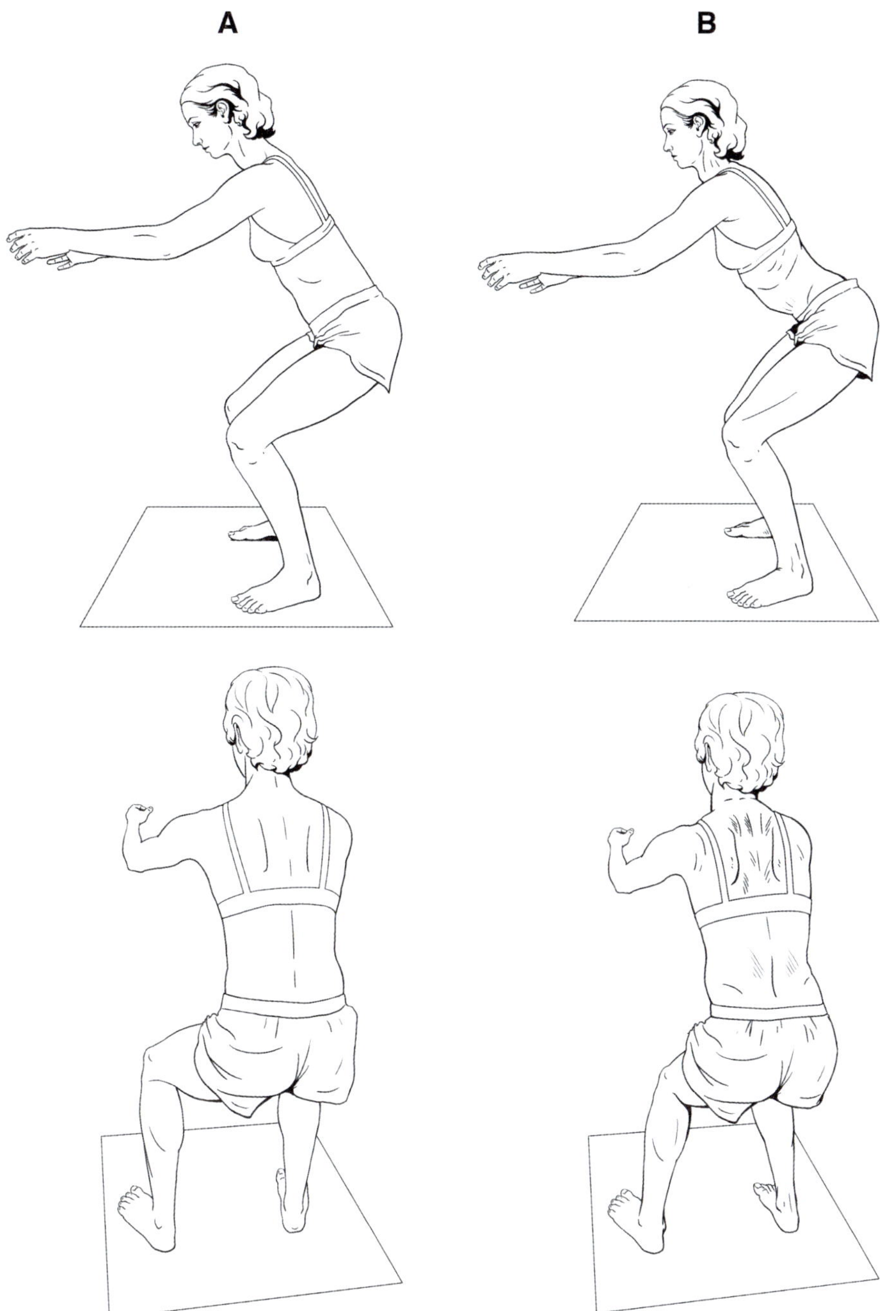

Figure 61.10 Squat test: (**a**) optimal activation; (**b**) abnormal activation.

The functional tests described here are just examples. In DNS, any positions can be used for both functional assessment and exercise positions. Each position is a snapshot of a partial pattern of the entire locomotor pattern. Ideally, muscle co-ordination has to be balanced at each snapshot, stabilizing the core properly and allowing for the most efficient pattern of stepping, grasping, and supporting extremity function as well as head movement.

Dynamic neuromuscular stabilization training based on developmental positions

In addition to traditional manual techniques, such as joint mobilization, soft tissue mobilization, and muscle stretching, patient's education in exercise and self-treatment procedures form a critical component of the DNS concept. Active exercise needs to address CNS control to alter and correct motor patterns. Hence, patient participation and compliance are important. A patient is expected to exercise on a daily basis. 'Brain education' is the ultimate goal to achieve ideal muscle balance and functional joint centration in an attempt to avoid overloading and to control movement patterns in a more efficient way. Patient's exercise needs to be fully 'conscious': the patient must be aware of movement quality, which is much more important than quantity. The patient must feel both the correct and incorrect movement pattern and be able to differentiate them. This depends on adequate body awareness. Only then can the patient exercise independently at home.

Movement should be slow and the patient should pay full attention to it, always looking for functional joint centration. Supporting segments form the basis for posture, and locomotion is initiated from these segments. If the supporting segment is decentrated, the decentration will reflect throughout the entire system, and the exercise may promote further pathology instead of correcting the problem.

Every patient is unique and DNS training must always be modified for each individual. The progression is from simple and basic to more advanced or challenging positions and exercises. Finally, the patient should be able to activate correct movement patterns not only during DNS exercise but also during activities of daily living and sports performance. The greater the number of modifications of the movement pattern the patient can execute with good control, the better the prognosis and success of the programme, i.e. the greater the variety of motor programmes available to the patient.

In DNS, any developmental position (physiological) can be used in self-treatment. More mature positions (i.e. ontogenetically younger) are always based on the less mature ones (i.e. ontogenetically older). Usually, ontogenetically younger positions are more difficult than the older ones, but this is not a rule. Since DNS is mostly an educational programme focusing on the improvement of the stabilizing system, its therapeutic effect can usually be observed after 6 or more weeks. It requires discipline and patience from both the clinician and the patient. However, the final effect can be quite remarkable and long-lasting.

Since stabilization function is inseparable from respiratory function, training of a proper breathing pattern is an essential part of DNS. Often, the first step is to release soft tissues of the trunk and the fasciae of the back, mobilize the thoracic spine and vertebrocostal joints to achieve neutral position of the chest. The neutral position consists of balance between the upper chest stabilizers (pectorales, upper trapezius, sternocleidomastoid muscle (SCM), scalenes), which are often short and overloaded, and the lower chest stabilizers (abdominal muscles, diaphragm), which may be posturally insufficient in some sections. Chest and pelvic axes need to be in parallel alignment in such a way that the lower thoracic cavity is positioned just above the pelvis.

The following positions described can be used in stabilization training, but the entire DNS system offers much more. If one videos a healthy infant, older than 3 months, in any position, any snapshot from the video can be used as an exercise position. If the baby is developing normally, any position demonstrates ideal core stabilization, joint centration, and an ideal locomotion pattern as a result of a genetically determined CNS programme. In DNS, the patient's position and movement are compared to the physiological developmental positions and movements.

Initially, just holding the position and focusing on proper breathing can be quite challenging and serve as a sufficient exercise for a patient. Once the patient masters the position easily, it can be progressed by moving extremities against resistance bands (resistance against stepping, reaching, or supporting extremity function; see Chapter 8). When exercising against resistance, the resistance must be adequate; in other words, the amount of resistance must correlate to the strength of the weakest part of the stabilizing system. Resistance training should not be performed before correct stabilization and breathing are mastered. Also, the transitions from one position to another can be trained (e.g. supine to side-lying, side-lying to side-sitting or prone). The exercise can be performed on unstable surfaces or with weights (barbells, dumb-bells). Any modification and progression can be used as long as the patient maintains ideal stabilization co-ordination and breathing pattern. Only as many repetitions should be performed as for which the patient can demonstrate perfect stabilization and a high-quality locomotion pattern.

1. Supine position equivalent to 3 months of age (Figure 61.11)

Initial position: Supine, legs above the table, approximately 90°Flexion at hips and knees, slight hip external rotation. Initially, the legs may be supported.
Zones of support: Nuchal line, thoracolumbar junction, upper gluteal muscles.
Instructions: Relax the shoulders, maintain neutral (caudal) position of the chest throughout the entire respiratory cycle, breathe into your groin, and breathe into the dorsolateral sections of your abdominal wall.
Modification and progression: Legs unsupported; exercise against resistance band; holding a heavy ball in both hands, moving it few centimetres to each side and/or up and down; the clinician gives unexpected perturbations as the patient resists while maintaining proper trunk position and abdominal wall co-ordination; exercise cervical flexion (deep neck flexor activation).

2. Prone position equivalent to 3 months of age (Figure 61.12)

Initial position: Prone, elbow support, approximately 125–135° angle between the trunk and the arm.
Zones of support: Medial epicondyles of bilateral elbows, bilateral ASIS, and pubic symphysis.
Instructions: Focus on elbow support, spine elongation, pulling down the shoulder blades, chin tuck, breathing into the groin, and breathing into dorsolateral sections of the abdominal wall.

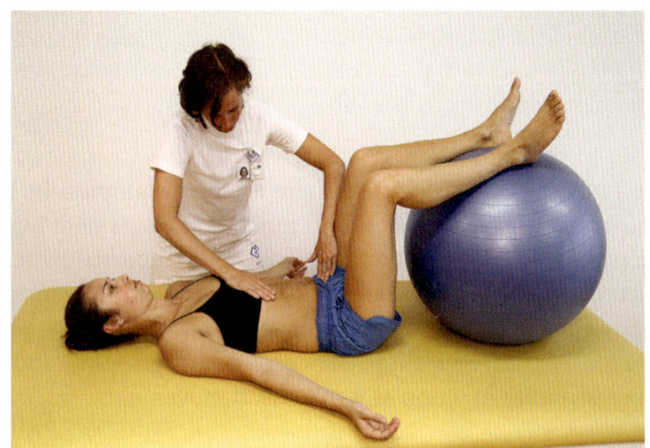

Figure 61.11 Exercise in supine position equivalent to 3 months of age. The clinician helps the patient maintain neutral (caudal) position of the chest by slightly pushing the chest caudally (while avoiding pressing it towards the table); the other hand, placed on the lower abdominal wall, cues the patient to activate the lower abdominal wall with inhalation and/or a postural task.

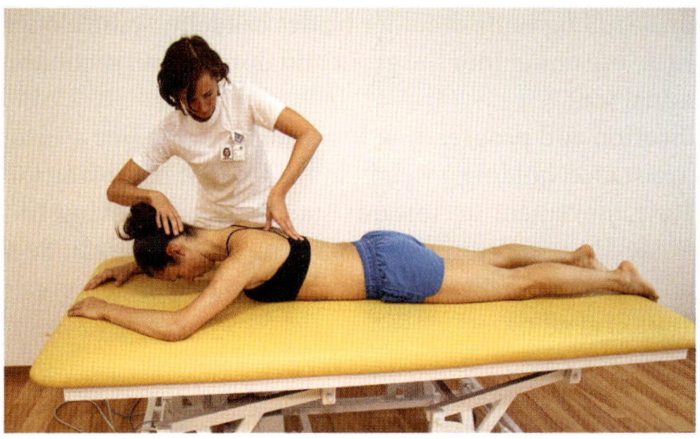

Figure 61.12 Exercise in prone position equivalent to 3 months of age. The clinician helps elongate the spine and align the neck in a neutral position by placing one hand on the nuchal line and the other hand on the mid-thoracic spine. The clinician guides the patient to initiate cervical extension from this specific area.

Modification and progression: Exercise segmental extension in the mid-thoracic spine, initiating the movement at T4–5 and then extending the spine in a cranial direction, segment by segment at a time; exercise rotation of the cervical and upper thoracic spine, imagine that neck rotation initiates at the mid-thoracic segments.

3. Side-lying position equivalent to 5 months of age (Figure 61.13)

Initial position: Side-lying, head may be supported, pillow height correlating with the distance between the patient's bottom shoulder and the neck, 90°Flexion at shoulder and elbow of the bottom arm, top leg placed in front of the bottom leg.
Zones of support: Deltoid and greater trochanter areas (mastoid, lateral nuchal line if head supported).
Instructions: Spine elongation, weightbearing through the deltoid and greater trochanter area, pulling the bottom shoulder blade caudally (Figure 61.13a), breathing into the groin and dorsolateral sections of the abdominal wall.
Modification and progression: Exercise against resistance band—top arm is reaching against resistance, bottom forearm is pronating against resistance (Figure 61.13b); holding barbell or dumb-bell in each hand, focusing on a breathing pattern and spinal elongation; initiating rolling by shifting the support from the deltoid area towards the elbow of the bottom arm; clinician gives unexpected perturbations rolling the patient forwards and backwards, the patient resists while maintaining proper core stabilization.

4. Supine position equivalent to 6 months of age (Figure 61.14)

Initial position: Supine, legs lifted, hands grasping the feet. If uncomfortable, patient's buttocks are supported with a towel.
Zones of support: Nuchal line, upper sections of the gluteal muscles, and thoracolumbar junction.
Instructions: Spine elongation, pulling shoulder blades caudally, breathing into the groin and dorsolateral sections of the abdominal wall.
Modification and progression: Shifting support from the gluteal region towards the thoracolumbar junction; trying to lift the pelvis and low back as one unit towards the ceiling; rolling the entire body from one side to the other side; bracing the entire core; exercising cervical flexion (deep neck flexor activation).

5. Side-sitting position equivalent to 8 months of age (Figure 61.15)

Initial position: Side-sitting, supporting hand is in line with the bottom greater trochanter, top leg in front of or behind the bottom leg, slight hip and knee flexion of the bottom leg.
Zones of support: bottom palm with weightbearing throughout the entire palm, bottom greater trochanter.
Instructions: Focusing on proportional support of the hand and weightbearing throughout the trochanter area, pulling the bottom shoulder blade caudally, elongating the spine, tucking in the chin, breathing into the groin and dorsolateral sections of the abdominal wall.
Modification and progression: Reaching with the top arm against band resistance; holding a weight in the top hand; moving forward towards quadruped position and back; resisting the clinician's unexpected perturbations.

6. Tripod position equivalent to 9 months of age (Figure 61.16)

Initial position: Modified kneeling.
Zones of support: Knee, ipsilateral hand, and contralateral foot.
Instructions: Focusing on proportional foot support, distributing the weight between the first and fifth metatarsophalangeal joints and the heel, focusing on proportional support through

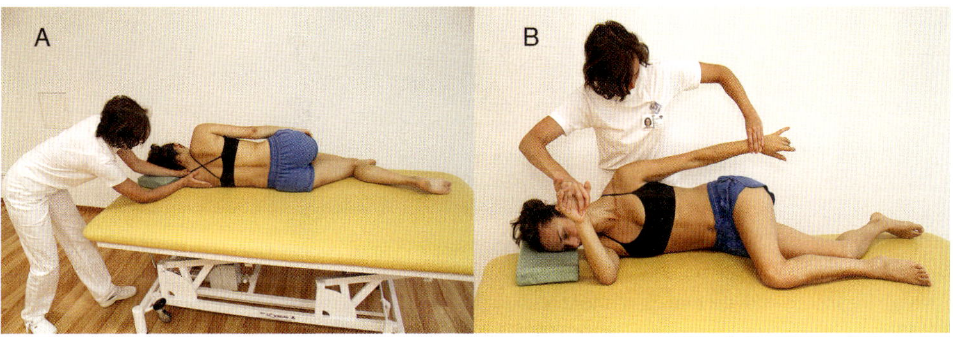

Figure 61.13 Exercise in side-lying position equivalent to 5 months of age: (**a**) the clinician facilitates a neutral position of the bottom supporting shoulder blade, which the patient then attempts to maintain by him/herself throughout the exercise; (**b**) the clinician resists reaching movement of the patient's top arm (forearm supination) and the supporting movement of the bottom arm (forearm pronation).

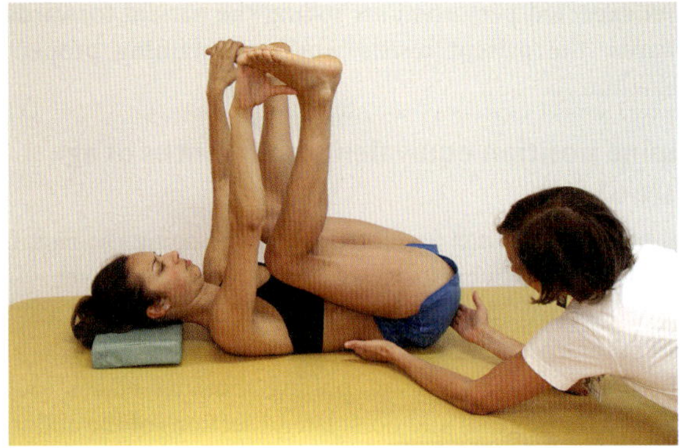

Figure 61.14 Exercise in supine position equivalent to 6 months of age. The clinician instructs the patient to lift the buttocks and lumbar spine, shifting support from the upper gluteal sections towards the thoracolumbar junction, while guiding the patient's breathing into the dorsolateral sections of the abdominal wall.

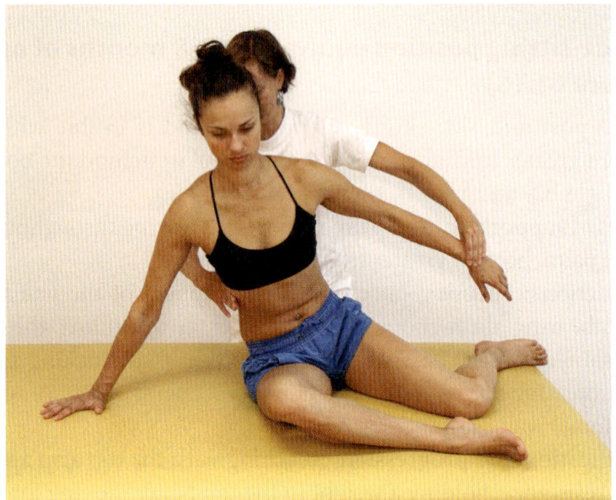

Figure 61.15 Exercise in side-sitting position equivalent to 8 months of age. The clinician's one hand assists the patient in maintaining a neutral chest position and guides proper breathing pattern, while the other hand resists the patient's reaching movement with the top arm.

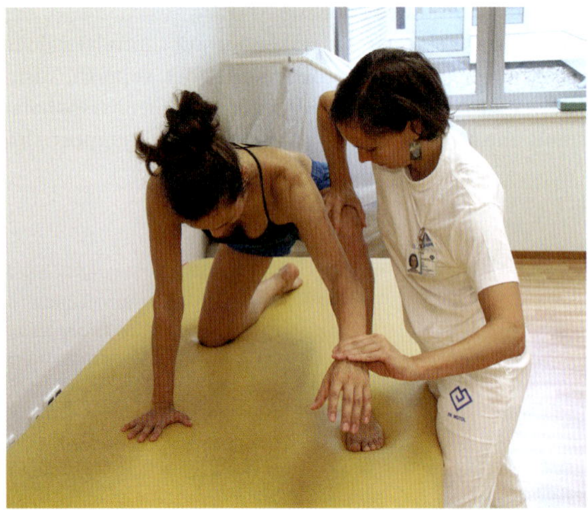

Figure 61.16 Exercise in tripod position equivalent to 9 months of age. The clinician helps to centrate the knee, pushing through the knee towards the supporting foot and resisting the patient's reaching arm.

the hand, pulling both shoulder blades caudally, spine elongation, chin tuck, breathing into the groin and dorsolateral sections of the abdominal wall.

Modification and progression: Reaching with the free arm against band resistance; holding a weight in the free hand; moving forward (initiating movement up towards standing) and moving back towards side-sitting position. The range of movement can be small, only initiating the change in the position, but maintain proper core stabilization at all times.

7. Squat position equivalent to 10 months of age (Figure 61.17)

Initial position: Unsupported squat or, initially, buttock support (upper gluteal sections leaning on the edge of a table), arms in front of trunk.

Zones of support: Centrated feet (and upper gluteal muscles).

Instructions: Focusing on centration of both feet, maintaining longitudinal arch on bilateral feet, weightbearing through the first and fifth metatarsophalangeal joints and the heel, keeping knees above the forefeet, spine elongation, pulling the shoulder blades caudally, breathing into the groin and dorsolateral sections of the abdominal wall.

Modification and progression: Arm movement against band resistance; holding heavy ball, moving the ball up and down and/or sideways; moving the body up and down several centimetres (moving between deeper and higher squat) while maintaining proper foot centration, knee position, and core bracing; squatting on a soft or unstable surface.

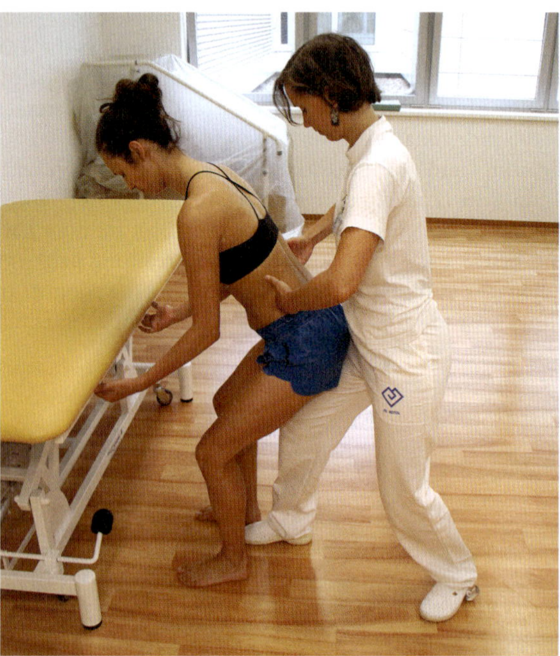

Figure 61.17 Exercise in squat position equivalent to 10 months of age. The clinician provides support and helps stabilize the patient's posture while guiding their breathing pattern. Gradually, the support may be removed and the patient may move lower to a deeper squat.

Acknowledgements

The authors thank Eliska Gerzova, MPT and Lucie Doubkova, MPT for their assistance with the photographs.

References

Bitnar P. Viscero-somatic relationships and its influence on spinal stabilization. *Int Musculo Med* 2012; 34(2):51–3.

Borghuis, J., Hof, A.L., Lemmink, K.A. The importance of sensory-motor control in providing core stability: implications for measurement and training. *Sports Med* 2008; 38(11):893–916.

Bouche, K.G., Vanovermeire, O., Stevens, V.K., et al. Computed tomographic analysis of the quality of trunk muscles in asymptomatic and symptomatic lumbar discectomy patients. *BMC Musculo Disord* 2011; 12:65. DOI: 10.1186/1471-2474-12-65.

Henriksen, M., Rosager, S., Aaboe, J., Bliddal, H. Adaptations in the gait pattern with experimental hamstring pain. *J Electromyogr Kinesiol* 2011; 21(5):746–53. DOI: 10.1016/j.jelekin.2011.07.005.

Hodges, P. Lumbopelvic stability: a functional model of biomechanics and motor control. In: Richardson, C. (ed.) *Therapeutic exercise for lumbopelvic stabilization*. Churchill Livingstone, Edinburgh, 2004, pp. 13–28.

Imamura, S., Sakuma, K., Takahashi, T. Follow-up study of children with cerebral coordination disturbance (CCD, Vojta). *Brain Dev* 1983; 5(3):311–4.

Janda, V. Muscles as a pathogenic factor in back pain. In: OPTP (eds) *Janda compendium, volume I*. OPTP, Minneapolis, 1980, p. 43–70.

Kim, K., Lee, S.K., Kim, Y.H. The biomechanical effects of variation in the maximum forces exerted by trunk muscles on the joint forces and moments in the lumbar spine: a finite element analysis. *Proc Inst Mech Eng H* 2010; 224(10):1165–74.

Kolar, P., Sulc, J., Kyncl, M., et al. Stabilizing function of the diaphragm: dynamic MRI and synchronized spirometric assessment. *J Appl Physiol* 2010; 109(4):1064–71. DOI: 10.1152/japplphysiol.01216.2009.

Lee, L.F., O'Neill, M.C., Demes, B., et al. *Joint kinematics in chimpanzee and human bipedal walking*. 2012. Available at: <http://www.asbweb.org/conferences/2012/abstracts/335.pdf>

Lewit, K. Clinical aspects of locomotor system dysfunction (vertebrogenic disorders). In: Lewit, K. (ed.) *Manipulative therapy. Musculoskeletal medicine*. Churchill Livingstone/Elsevier, Edinburgh, 2010, p. 302–61.

McGill, S.M., McDermott, A., Fenwick, C.M. Comparison of different strongman events: trunk muscle activation and lumbar spine motion, load, and stiffness. *J Strength Cond Res* 2009; 23:1148–61.

Ogihara, N., Kikuchi, T., Ishiguro, Y., Makishima, H., Nakatsukasa, M. Planar covariation of limb elevation angles during bipedal walking in the Japanese macaque. *J R Soc Interface* 2012; 9(74):2181–90. DOI: 10.1098/rsif.2012.0026.

Page, P., Frank, C.C., Lardner, R. Pathomechanics of musculoskeletal pain and muscle imbalance. In: Page, P. (ed.) *Assessment and treatment of muscle imbalance*. Human Kinetics, Champaign, 2010, p. 43–55.

Smith, M.D., Russell, A., Hodges, P.W. Disorders of breathing and continence have a stronger association with back pain than obesity and physical activity. *Austral J Physio* 2006; 52:11–16.

Sylvester, A.D., Pfisterer, T. Quantifying lateral femoral condyle ellipticalness in chimpanzees, gorillas, and humans. *Am J Phys Anthropol* 2012; 149(3):458–67. DOI: 10.1002/ajpa.22144.

Watanabe, S., Kobara, K., Ishida, H., Eguchi, A. Influence of trunk muscle co-contraction on spinal curvature during sitting cross-legged. *Electromyogr Clin Neurophysiol* 2010; 50(3–4):187–92.

Zafeiriou, D.I. Primitive reflexes and postural reactions in the neurodevelopmental examination. *Pediatr Neurol* 2004; 31(1):1–8.

Zeininger, A., Richmond, B.G., Hartman, G. Metacarpal head biomechanics: a comparative backscattered electron image analysis of trabecular bone mineral density in Pan troglodytes, Pongo pygmaeus, and Homo sapiens. *J Hum Evol* 2011; 60(6):703–10. DOI: 10.1016/j.jhevol.2011.01.002.

Chapter 62

Exercise therapy: limbs

Bryan English, Diego Rizzo, and Stefano Della Villa

Introduction to the rehabilitation process

Rehabilitation is easy to do badly and difficult to do well. A technically excellent operative procedure can be undermined by poor rehabilitation and an average procedure can be complimented by expert rehabilitation.

Rehabilitation is carried out by a variety of specialists and the closer that they work as a team, then the more successful is the end result. Rehabilitation is not the focus of one practitioner. It may be mainly carried out by one practitioner but the construction, judgement, and case management of the process needs to have input from several professionals with differing areas of training and expertise. However, someone needs to take responsibility for the whole process and the most appropriate person within a large medical team would be the physician with training and expertise within this field.

There are many ways to rehabilitate a medical problem. In relation to orthopaedics, such functional rehabilitation can fall into five phases:

1 Decrease pain and swelling.

2 Achieve full range of movement and flexibility.

3 Achieve full power and endurance.

4 Restore top levels of proprioception and co-ordination.

5 Restore sport-specific activities and achieve a safe return to play, with future problems prevented.

It is important to follow some form of structure in rehabilitation. Structure that is preferably, but not essentially, backed with some form of science/evidence gives the patient, as well as the rehabilitation team, confidence and reassurance that all is going to be well. Education of the staff and the patient throughout the process is important as each patient brings their own challenges. Previous history, expectations, operative success, and time availability for rehabilitation (prior to necessity of return to work) will lead to a case by case personal rehabilitation plan rather than a heavy protocol-based prescription. Constant review of the success/failure of the rehabilitation process is healthy to avoid following a path that may lead to failure. For this reason, measurements such as range of movement of a joint, heart response to exercise, maximal speed, ability to decelerate, and many others can demonstrate to the rehabilitation team and the patient that progress is being made. Return to full training can be set as a target to provide both a focus for patient motivation and also criteria for those carrying out the assessments and treatments.

Assessment of the rehabilitation phases can encompass state of the art scientific evaluation such as high-speed video analysis, accelerometers, and global positioning system (GPS) satellite data. However, it can also be done by using a stopwatch and some sticks in the ground! In other words, the process should be creative and imaginative for the practitioner, while being enjoyable, possible, and affordable for the patient.

The five phases of functional rehabilitation

Phase 1: Decrease pain and swelling

After an injury or an operation, the main focus is to keep swelling to a minimum and, with this, one would hope that the pain will also be minimized. Pain and swelling will prevent progress towards phase 2.

There are many methods to alleviate swelling; however, compression, cooling, and elevation appear to be the mainstays of treatment (van den Bekerom et al. 2012; Waterman et al. 2012) (Figure 62.1). One should also include 'decreased function', as an early lack of swelling and pain can lead to complacency and attempts by the patient to 'try it out'. The importance of rest and recovery, even if just for 48 hours (depending on the case), can be very productive. The patient should be educated as to why this is important. If the surgery has been elective, then hopefully, steps will have been made by the patient to create a support network to assist in this phase when at home (as returning home as soon as possible is beneficial to all).

Gentle, resisted muscle activation is possible at this stage, and indeed this can be electrically induced to avoid the muscle-damaging effect of pain and swelling.

Aquatic therapy is an excellent modality to ease swelling and pain, due to the compressive effect of water and the beneficial effect of minimal movement in deep water (Bushman et al. 1997; DeMaere and Ruby 1997; Eyestone et al. 1993; Killgore 2012; Killgore et al. 2006; Masumoto et al. 2009; Mercer and Jensen 1997; Wilcox et al. 2007) (Figure 62.2). Naturally, there may be anxiety with regards to wound protection; however, such anxiety should be countered by expertise in wound protection and management. Aquatic

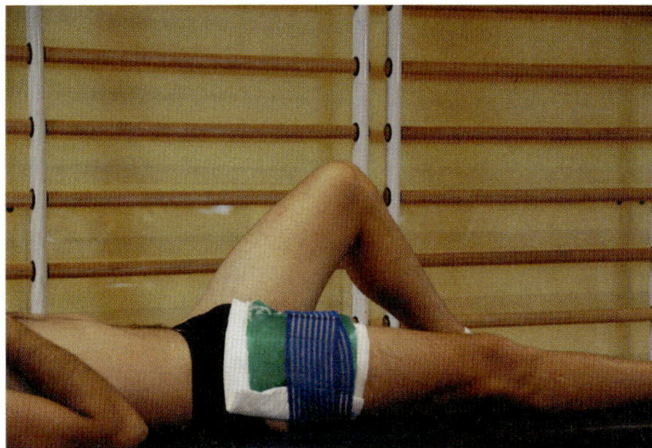

Figure 62.1 Compression and cryotherapy.

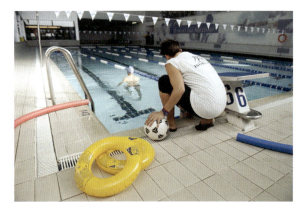

Figure 62.2 Rehabilitation in the pool.

therapy in these circumstances should not be contraindicated as there is no evidence that the chemicals in a well-maintained pool should cause a problem (especially when the wound can be covered with waterproof dressing) (Pool Water Treatment Advisory Group 2009; Villalta and Peiris 2012).

Analgesia has its place at this stage to decrease inflammation and allow the patient to become more mobile and, importantly, to adopt as normal a gait as possible, as early as possible.

Manual therapy/effleurage is a useful way to make the patient feel that he or she is being looked after (do not underestimate the power of this) and gentle passive mobilization will start to produce less fear in the patient that movement will cause pain. The manual therapist will get a feeling of the degree of swelling, warmth, and range of the injured area and the reactivity of the contractile tissues. This hands-on knowledge is valuable in determining progression or regression in this initial crucial phase. Wound breakdown, bleeding, and infection are issues that can be easily avoided with care and diligence from experienced professionals. An over-zealous rehabilitation team or over-ambitious, impatient patient can disturb the healing phase at this stage and send the plan completely off course. Leadership and guidance at this stage is a priority to support those responsible for the success or failure of rehabilitation. Good communication between all parties will hopefully see the patient through phase 1 as soon as is possible, without fear and with a positive expectation of phase 2 (which naturally overlaps with phase 1, on a case by case basis).

Can progress in phase 1 be measured? Yes: swelling can be measured daily, by limb girth; pain can be measured by many methods, such as the visual analogue scale (VAS).

Phase 2: Achieve full range of movement and flexibility

The range of movement of the joints and contractile tissues involved (proximal and distal to the injury) should be mobilized as soon as possible. Fear and pain should not stand in the way unless there is a specific reason to restrict movement. Increased range can be encouraged by passive and active movements of the joints and soft tissues, and these movements should be observed, documented, and, where possible, measured with reproducibility. Methods for measuring should be standardized and discussed by the rehabilitation team to encourage good inter-measurer reliability, while recognizing that intra-tester testing may be ideal.

Knowledge of the pre-injury range of movement is helpful, which is why annual musculoskeletal screening/profiling is beneficial in sport. However, the contralateral limb offers a good comparison, with obvious assumptions being made about pre-injury symmetry.

The patient is often anxious in this phase and needs to be educated that increasing movement range is not often a pain-free process. Warming up the joint (applied heat or exercise) prior to end of range movement can help. Cradling of the joint with experienced hands can provide reassurance during the passive movement phase. Active movements can be encouraged with the use of aquatic therapy, along with many other tools such as static cycling.

Daily measurement can provide a visual for the medical team and the patient, with goal-setting providing a target. Such measurements also act as a guide as to whether mobilization is excessive (resulting in increased swelling and decreased range of movements, especially first thing in the morning).

Can range of movement be measured in phase 2? Yes: goniometers are still a useful tool to measure range of movement of a joint while recognizing that the range may be restricted due to swelling, tight soft tissues, pain, bone, etc.

Flexibility is less easy to measure as such measurements tend to be more global than local. Ability to touch one's toes with extended knees (for fear of using a rather clumsy example) covers movements of the spine, sacroiliac joints, hip, knee, and ankle along with associated ligament, tendon, muscle, fascia, and neurovascular structures. However, this should not deter the medical team from addressing all these structures in order to obtain full range of movement. The use of passive and active stretches, manual therapy, active resisted techniques (hold, contract, stretch), and techniques to decrease hypertonic tissue (heat, electrical therapy) can all be considered as part of the arsenal to create as much range as possible (van der Wees et al. 2006) (Figure 62.3).

Can flexibility be measured in phase 2? Yes: the knee to wall test, for example, can demonstrate flexibility of the calf muscle and/or deep flexors of the foot and ankle as well as range of movement of the ankle. It would be up to the practitioner to determine whether this restriction is due to lack of range or lack of flexibility. Such tests can be arranged for any joint and they can be combined with 'range' assessment.

The importance of experience in this phase cannot be underestimated. It is paramount to achieve good range early (extension, post anterior cruciate surgery, for example) with sympathy for the restriction and information provided from the tissues during the treatment process. Careful mobilization may indicate that the joint

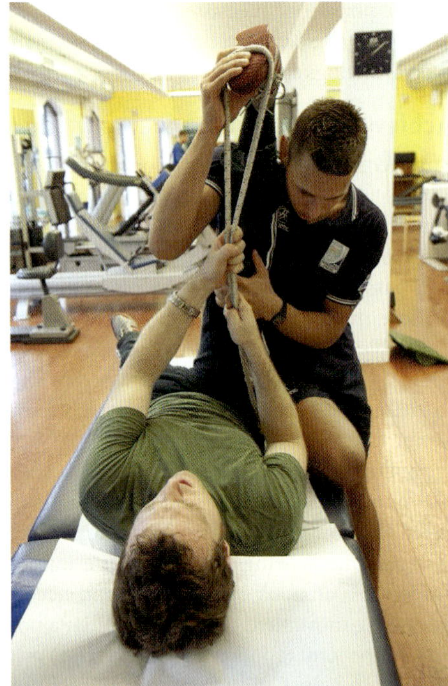

Figure 62.3 Flexibility exercises.

is just not ready for the range, with too much swelling, too much pain, or indeed a defective surgical procedure. When dealing with living human tissue one can 'listen' to the structure rather than just mobilizing and forcing the restriction.

This phase, like many of the others, can be very individual. Some joints will respond well and one can accelerate through the process; others will react and will need more patience. Therefore, progression should be the target and goal-setting should not be hastened by unrealistic time schedules. Occasionally, 'rest' for 48 hours can allow the joint to settle and follow a much more productive phase.

Phase 3: Achieve full power and endurance

The overlap between phase 1 and 2 is marked. However, there is little overlap between phase 2 and 3 because progress in phase 3 is limited and even switched off. For example, the vastus medialis switches off with a knee effusion and, in the author's opinion, the tibialis posterior switches off with an ankle effusion (Kulig et al. 2011; Palmieri et al. 2004). One cannot get the power back in these areas and exercise them fully until one has got past phases 1 and 2 completely. In contrast, the early stages of phase 4 can be introduced in the mid stages of phase 3.

Power is an expression from the muscle of full physiological function and it is one of the most easily measured of the modalities (using weights, scales, dynanometers, isokinetic machines, to name but a few). The progress can easily be recorded, showing maximal effort or exercise to fatigue (can you do 10 lunges, for example), with both scientific, laboratory-based assessment or field testing of functional movement patterns.

Can power be measured in phase 3? Yes: exercise is the key in this phase. Isometric and isotonic exercises are cheap and easy to do as a self-management process and can be done with the joint isolated (for example, knee extension while sitting) or, as one may prefer, using the whole kinetic chain (the standing jump, for example). These movements can be measured and are repeatable and reliable (Crow et al. 2009; Engebretsen et al. 2010; Holmich et al. 1999, 2004; Verrall et al. 2005).

Can endurance be measured in phase 3? Yes: repeated calf raises to fatigue can be measured; however, quality of movement needs to be supervised. Repeated concentric loading at a certain speed can be accurately measured with an isokinetic machine (Figure 62.4). These tests can measure isolated endurance.

Whole body endurance is also important at this stage and this can be measured with lactate testing on treadmill running, for example (or devising another exercise for a multidirectional athlete). Lactate testing involves using sequential blood samples to measure the increase in body lactate as a response to increasing exercise. The less fit an individual, then the sooner their body lactate rises. A less invasive way to measure fitness can be field testing and by judging heat rate response to a sub-maximal exercise (such as the 'Yo-Yo' test) (Bendiksen et al. 2012).

Whole body endurance work can be wrongfully ignored in phase 3, due more to practitioner's fear than anything else. After passing phase 2, the patient should not be viewed as a fragile being who is going to break down. The injured area can be respected while the body performs heavy cardiovascular work. The heart can be worked hard in the water, for example. There are numerous ways to exercise in deep water to produce a significant cardiorespiratory challenge. The big muscle groups can be challenged with power repetitions to produce/reinforce range, power, flexibility. The exercises can be entertaining to aid compliance and the practitioner should, ideally, be of a physical state to join in and demonstrate such work to the patient (with intermittent breaks, with such as 'head tennis' in the water, for recovery).

A higher state of monitoring can involve the wearing of a heart rate monitor throughout the working day to produce an estimate of cardiovascular 'work done'.

Phase 4: Restore top levels of proprioception and co-ordination

This is arguably the most important rehabilitation phase. The authors' opinion is that phase 4 is easy to dismiss by the improving athlete eager to get to phase 5 and beyond. Phase 4 requires concentration and discipline from the practitioner and the patient. However, understanding human nature, the practitioner may wish to drop in aspects of phase 5 to provide a taste of things to come when phase 4 has been successfully mastered.

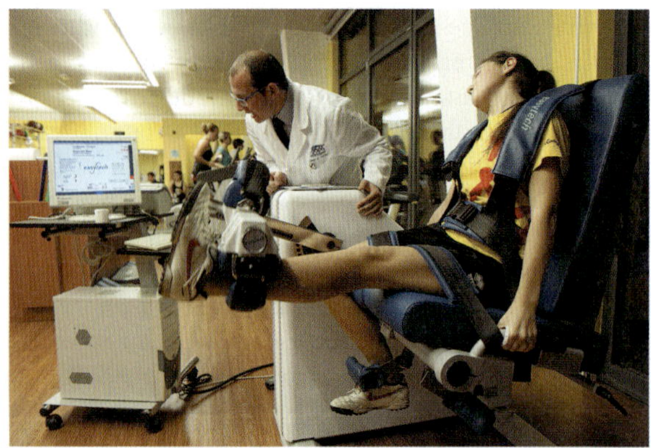

Figure 62.4 Isokinetic Training.

This phase also allows for the artistry and imagination of the practitioner to flourish. In the discipline of balance, proprioception, and co-ordination, it can be rewarding to find a variety of ways to enable the patient to master body control (Figure 62.5). Movements that test and train proprioception and co-ordination need to be diverse, challenging, entertaining, and relevant to the person's future activity (as this helps with compliance).

There are a plethora of examples on how to do this work (Figure 62.6). Taking one simple example, the 'hop and hold' test highlights deficiencies to the patient who may notice the asymmetry with this basic movement (and therefore understand that phase 5 is not possible without being able to control function in phase 4). This test can be progressed onto different surfaces such as sand or a trampoline. The complexity of the test can be heightened by asking the patient to catch a ball after landing (i.e. the 'hold' phase) (Garrison et al. 2012; Narducci et al. 2011; Postle et al. 2012; Thomeé et al. 2011, 2012).

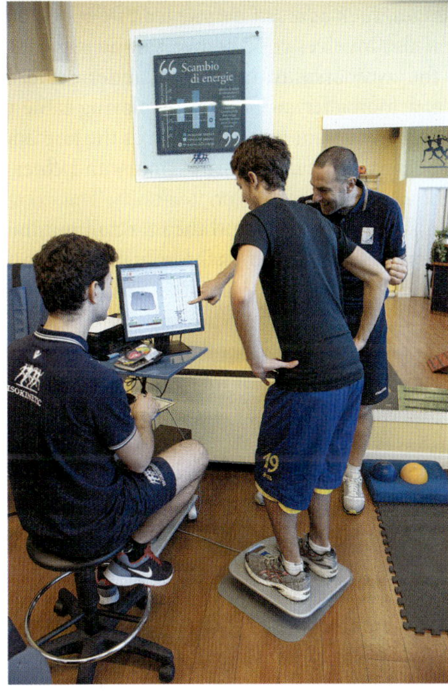

Figure 62.5 Proprioception evaluation.

The aim here is to safely increase the complexity of the work that is being done by the body, time and time again. The execution of the work has to be good otherwise the patient may be learning abnormal movement patterns that will be difficult to undo at a later stage. If the body learns highly complex tasks and performs these well, then the introduction of phase 5 will take place safely.

Can proprioception and co-ordination be measured in phase 4? Yes: balancing and hop and hold tests can be visualized and videoed. The amount of sway can be measured on force platforms, as can the quality of foot strike and propulsive force (if one wishes, such measurements can be taken in the biomechanics laboratory).

Re-visiting phase 4 with the new challenge of different surfaces such as sand and the trampoline can lead to a higher level of function and increase the challenge for the patient and player (Aragão et al. 2011; Binnie et al. 2012; Hugh et al. 2005; Kidgell et al. 2007; Kvist 2006).

Phase 5: Restore sport-specific activities and achieve a safe return to play, with future problems prevented

This phase of the rehabilitation programme takes place mainly on the field (Figure 62.7). Phase 5 is the exciting phase as the patient starts to feel as though they are 'nearly there'. So it is a very positive phase, but also a long and dangerous one. There are some important skills left to learn. The patient and the player may now be under pressure to return to full activity as they are seen to be functioning at a high level. For example, following an injury to the ankle syndesmosis, the player now has:

- no ankle swelling or pain and good range of movement
- good power of the calf, deep flexors, peroneals, and thigh/buttock musculature
- good cardiovascular endurance compared to previous testing (as shown by the Yo-Yo test)
- symmetry, as shown by basic proprioception and co-ordination in water and on sand, trampoline, and grass.

So what does the player do now?

- Perform tasks relating to his/her sport such as kicking, jumping, twisting, sprinting, tackling.

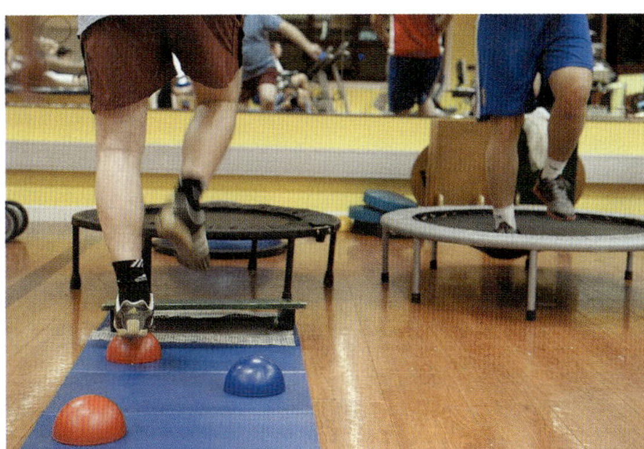

Figure 62.6 Proprioception and coordination.

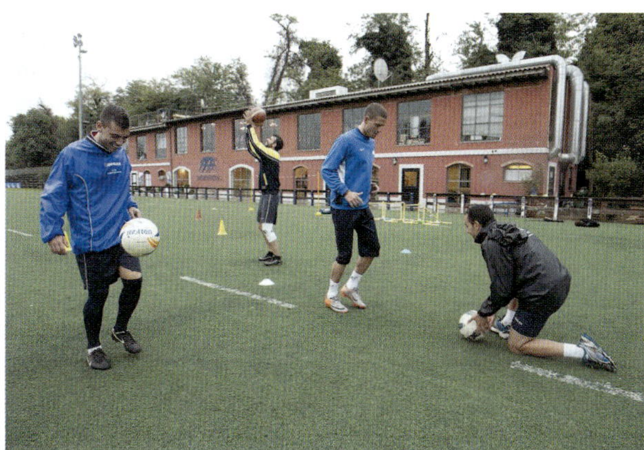

Figure 62.7 Rehabilitation on the field.

- Perform these tasks with increasing load such as a heavier ball, greater speed of movement, tighter angle of movement, involving contact from other players or trainers.
- Repeat these tasks hundreds of times with precise execution and quality of movement, to start to match the demands of full training.

Return to training criteria can be set in the initial stages of rehabilitation and may take several forms. For example, in a 75-year-old bowls player recovering from an ankle arthroscopy, the criteria might be:

- Maximal ankle range as compared to 'normal side' or acceptable range
- No swelling or pain
- Ability to walk up and down stairs pain-free
- Ability to get out of a chair using both legs (separately)
- Ability to perform crown green bowling for an hour
- An understanding of self-management strategies

However, for a professional football player recovering from the same operation, the criteria might be:

- Maximal joint range as compared to the other side/pre-injury range
- No pain or swelling
- Maximal isotonic/isokinetic power of lower leg musculature
- Maximal jump test as compared to previous measures (compare left to right)
- Ability to perform hop and hold test with maximal proprioception/agility
- Reach pre-injury levels of number and quality of maximal accelerations and decelerations, comparing right to left side
- Ability to cope with striking a ball and endurance work on the grass for up to time spent in normal training session
- An understanding that self-management work is accepted and will be complied with

These are just two examples of return to training criteria that may go into the thought process of judging when a patient is ready to return to their sport, without support, but with the knowledge that compliance of self-management strategies will be high. Unrealistic/unreasonable demands are counter-productive and may lead to frustration and disappointment. Realistic goal setting is the aim. A visual display/chart can be used (similar to VAS) to show how towards the target the patient has progressed over the previous days or weeks.

Can phase 5 be measured? Yes: there is continuous measurement of a player's skills. One can measure the speed and movement of the individual. The quality of movement and agility can be seen on video or measured with accelerometers in the field. The accuracy of kicking a moving ball can be seen and felt by the rehabilitator. Although some of the skills-related work may be difficult to measure, there is a type of VAS for this form of work. The rehabilitator/trainer may mention that the quality of short-ball striking is 10 out of 10; however, the long-ball striking is 8 out of 10 for power and 6 out of 10 for accuracy.

Technology offers a multitude of support to assess function of human movement. Scales, cameras, dynanometers, accelerometers, GPS systems, heart rate monitors, and stopwatches are pieces of equipment that can measure the most basic of human movements up to the most dynamic. These measurements are reproducible and can be collected and digitized to create a library of functional analysis. The processing of the data and its application is dependent upon the interest and education of the clinician. Reams of meaningless and difficult to apply data can cause a great loss of time and money. Data that is easy to apply can prevent a 'nearly healed' injury from being over- or under-exposed in the rehabilitation process.

The final goal of the rehabilitation programme is to return to play, safely. Prevention is the great challenge when leaving this last phase. Compliance requires an education in and understanding of the need for prevention. For example, an arthritic ankle in a tennis player may require assessment, on occasions, to check the range of movement of the joint and to ensure that work complies with an increase to that range (if it is found to be quietly decreasing). So, although asymptomatic, the work on range of movement may prevent other issues, such as a calf muscle tear, from occurring.

Prevention also involves good recovery strategies (nutrition, rest, sleep) and the avoidance of over- and under-exercising. Cross-training (e.g. a footballer swimming or playing table tennis) and executing good movement patterns (such as the hop and hold test) should also be part of the discipline of injury and illness avoidance (Figure 62.8).

Prevention is hard to measure within a small number of people and over a short period of time, as the only measure is the percentage of injury recurrence (which is multifactorial). Although difficult to assess, the value of education to the individual will hopefully lead to that person taking on the responsibility for self-managing their future (in a similar way to which we advise people on how to manage their dental health with daily self-care and regular check-ups).

Return to play is multifactorial, seen not only from the individual patient's perspective but also from that of the decision makers. In team sports, the people involved in the decision to return to play can be the doctor (clinical evaluation shows the patient is continuing to improve with increased load and demands of training), the scientist (satisfied with the performance-related data), the fitness coach (satisfied that the player has completed enough skill- and agility-related activity), and the coach (satisfied that the player has had enough time training in order to meet the requirements of the next game). Other stakeholders, such a player's agent or the directors

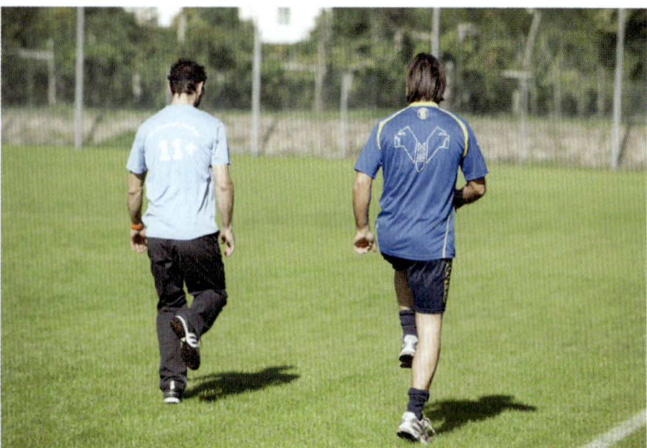

Figure 62.8 Prevention.

of a club, are involved with professional sport. However, the most important stakeholder is the player, who needs to feel ready—and this can cover a plethora of psychological as well as physical issues.

From a medical point of view, a successful return to play means that there will be no recurrence of the injury, as well as a secondary desire that the performance of the player is as good, and possibly better, than it was before the injury (with the exception of certain aspects of the game that can only be achieved by performance in the competitive environment). Return to play can involve reassurance from the support/rehabilitation staff that 'everything will be okay', with reminders of the success of progress to date. Psychological reassurance throughout all stages of the rehabilitation process should not be undervalued.

There may be occasions when a player's load can be managed to enable him to play. For example, a player suffering from recurrent Achillodynia may be managed by removal from the training group the day after a game. The player's first recovery day may be spent in the water and for the second day of recovery, the loading (that can be measured as stated before using heart rate and GPS) can be restricted to whatever percentage the prevention team view as appropriate. The use of these modalities is in its infancy and their reliability depends on the positioning of satellites around the world. In areas of reliable coverage, current devices are thought to be up to 15% inaccurate. Such loading data should be viewed with an artistic mind at this stage, but it will possibly become more defined in the future so that 'true loading' can be matched alongside cause and effect (Nielsen et al. 2012; Scott et al. 2012).

Summary of exercise therapy for limbs

Rehabilitation is easy to do badly and difficult to do well. Many people are involved in the process and they need to act as a team to support the patient, with good communication and good team play (supporting the process). There should be a nominated head of the rehabilitation team and the case manager, in these circumstances, is the physician. The case manager needs to evaluate the patient on a regular basis and be involved in the decision making throughout the rehabilitation. The case manager shares information within the team and makes the decision as to when to progress or when to arrest treatment.

The whole process can be satisfying to all concerned when dealing with motivated and enthusiastic patients. Measuring the process is achievable and gives credibility and backup to the initial hypothesis of the individual's rehabilitation programme.

Rehabilitation involves creativity, combining science and art, with the end result being the ultimate achievement of the patient to return to a normal life or to return to play (depending on the nature of the individual and the injury).

References

Aragão FA, Karamanidis K, Vaz MA, Arampatzis A. Mini-trampoline exercise related to mechanisms of dynamic stability improves the ability to regain balance in elderly. *Journal of Electromyography and Kinesiology* 2011; 21(3):512–8.

van den Bekerom MP, Struijs PA, Blankevoort L, Welling L, Van Dijk CN, Kerkhoffs GM. What is the evidence for rest, ice, compression, and elevation therapy in the treatment of ankle sprains in adults? *Journal of Athletic Training* 2012; 47(4):435–43.

Bendiksen M, Ahler T, Clausen H, Wedderkopp N, Krustrup P. The use of Yo-Yo IR1 and Andersen testing for fitness and maximal heart rate assessments of 6–10 year old school children. *Journal of Strength Conditioning Research* 2013; 27(6):1583–90.

Binnie MJ, Peeling P, Pinnington H, Landers G, Dawson B. Effect of training surface on acute physiological responses following interval training. *Journal of Strength Conditioning Research* 2013; 27(4):1047–56.

Bushman BA, Flynn MG, Andrea FF, Lambert CP, Taylor MS, Braun WA. Effect of 4 weeks of deep water run training on running performance. *Medicine & Science in Sports & Exercise* 1997; 29(5):694–9.

Crow J, Pearce A, Veale J, et al. Hip adductor muscle strength is reduced proceeding and during the onset of groin pain in elite junior Australian football players. *Journal of Science and Medicine in Sport* 2009; 13(2):202–4

DeMaere JM, Ruby BC. Effects of deep water and treadmill running on oxygen uptake and energy expenditure in seasonally trained cross country runners. *Journal of Sports Medicine and Physical Fitness* 1997; 37(3):175–81.

Engebretsen A, Myklebust G, Holme I, et al. Intrinsic risk factors for groin injuries among male soccer players: a prospective cohort study. *American Journal of Sports Medicine* 2010; 38(10):2051–7.

Eyestone ED, Fellingham G, George J, Fisher AG. Effect of water running and cycling on maximum oxygen consumption and 2-mile run performance. *American Journal of Sports Medicine* 1993; 21(1):41–44.

Garrison JC, Shanley E, Thigpen C, Geary R, Osler M, Delgiorno J. The reliability of the Vail Sports Test as a measure of physical performance following anterior cruciate ligament reconstruction. *International Journal of Sports Physical Therapy* 2012; 7(1): 20–30.

Hölmich P, Hölmich LR, Bjerg AM. Clinical examination of athletes with groin pain: an intraobserver and interobserver reliability study. *British Journal of Sports Medicine* 2004; 38:446–51.

Hölmich P, Uhrskov P, Ulniths L, et al. Effectiveness of active physical training as a treatment for long-standing adductor-related groin pain in athletes: randomised trial. *The Lancet* 1999; 353:439–43.

Kidgell DJ, Horvath DM, Jackson BM, Seymour PJ. Effect of six weeks of dura disc and mini-trampoline balance training on postural sway in athletes with functional ankle instability. *Journal of Strength Conditioning Research* 2007; 21(2):466–9.

Killgore GL. Deep water running: a practical review of the literature with an emphasis on biomechanics. *The Physician and Sports Medicine* 2012; 40(1):116–26. 40(1).

Killgore GL, Wilcox AR, Caster BL, Wood TM. A lower-extremities kinematic comparison of deep-water running styles and treadmill running. *Journal of Strength & Conditioning Research* 2006; 20(4):919–27.

Kulig K, Popovich JM, Noceti-Dewit LM, Reischl SF, Kim D. Women with posterior tibial tendon dysfunction have diminished ankle and hip muscle performance. *Journal of Orthopaedic and Sports Physical Therapy* 2011; 41(9):687–94.

Kvist J. Sagittal plane knee motion in the ACL-deficient knee during body weight shift exercises on different support surfaces. *Journal of Orthopaedic Sports Physical Therapy* 2006; 36(12): 954–62.

Masumoto K, Delion D, Mercer JA. Insight into muscle activity during deep water running. *Medicine & Science in Sports & Exercise* 2009; 41(10):1958–64.

Mercer JA, Jensen RL. Reliability and validity of a deep water running graded exercise test. *Measurement in Physical Education and Exercise Science* 1997; 1:213–222.

Narducci E, Waltz A, Gorski K, Leppia L, Donaldson M. The clinical utility of functional performance tests within one year of post ACL reconstruction: a systematic review. *International Journal of Sports Physical Therapy* 2011; 6(4):333–42.

Nielsen RO, Cederholm P, Buist I, Sørensen H, Lind M, Rasmussen S. Can GPS be used to detect deleterious progression in training volume among runners? *Journal of Strength Conditioning Research* 2013; 27(6):1471–8.

Palmieri RM, Ingersoll CD, Hoffman MA, et al. Arthrogenic muscle response to a simulated ankle joint effusion. *British Journal of Sports Medicine* 2004; 38(1):26–33.

Pinnington HC, Lloyd DG, Besier TF, Dawson B. Kinematic and electromyography analysis of submaximal differences running on a firm surface compared with soft, dry sand. *European Journal of Applied Physiology* 2005; 94:242–53.

Pool Water Treatment Advisory Group. *Swimming pool water. Treatment and quality standards for pools and spas* (2nd edn). 2009. Gosling H

Postle K, Pak D, Smith TO. Effectiveness of proprioceptive exercises for ankle ligament injury in adults: a systematic literature and meta-analysis. *Manual Therapy* 2012; 17(4):285–91.

Scott BR, Lockie RG, Knight TJ, Clark AC, Janse de Jonge X AK. A comparison of methods to quantify the in-season training load of professional soccer players. *International Journal of Sports Physiology and Performance* 2013; 8(2):195–202.2.

Thomeé R, Kaplan Y, Kvist J, et al. Muscle strength and hop performance criteria prior to return to sports after ACL reconstruction. *Journal of Knee Surgery, Sports Traumatology and Arthroscopy* 2011; 19(11):1798–805.

Thomeé R, Neeter C, Gustavsson A, et al. Variability in leg muscle power and hop performance after anterior cruciate ligament reconstruction. *Journal of Knee Surgery, Sports Traumatology and Arthroscopy* 2012; 20(6):1143–51.

Verrall G, Slavotinek J, Barnes P, et al. Description of pain provocation tests used for the diagnosis of sports-related chronic groin pain: relationship of tests to defined clinical (pain and tenderness) and MRI (pubic bone marrow oedema) criteria. *Scandinavian Journal of Medicine and Science in Sports* 2005; 15(1):36–42.

Villalta EM, Peiris CL. Early aquatic physical therapy improves function and does not increase risk of wound-related adverse events for adults post orthopedic surgery: a systematic review and meta-analysis. *Archives of Physical Medicine and Rehabilitation* 2013; 94(1):138–48.

Waterman B, Walker JJ, Swaims C, et al. The efficacy of combined cryotherapy and compression compared with cryotherapy alone following anterior cruciate ligament reconstruction. *Journal of Knee Surgery* 2012; 25(2):155–60.

van der Wees PJ, Lenssen AF, Hendriks EJ, Stomp DJ, Dekker J, de Bie RA. Effectiveness of exercise therapy and manual mobilisation in ankle sprain and functional instability: a systematic review. *Australian Journal of Physiotherapy* 2006; 52(1):27–37.

Wilcox KC, Woodall WR, Stubbs PL. Development of a multifaceted aquatic exercise program for rehabilitation of athletes with patellar tendinopathy. *Journal of Aquatic Physical Therapy* 2007; 15(2):1–9.

Chapter 63

Exercise therapy: spine

Mark Comerford

Introduction: movement control impairments

For many years, clinicians have been convinced that impairments of movement control play an important role in the development and recurrence of painful conditions of the neuromusculoskeletal system (Comerford and Mottram 2001a, 2012, 2014; Janda 1985, 1995; Richardson et al. 1999; Sahrmann 2002, 2011). There is an evolving understanding of the importance of movement control, dynamic and static joint stability, and the co-ordination of muscle synergies in the management of neuromusculoskeletal impairments (Comerford and Mottram 2001a, 2012, 2014; Hides et al. 1996; Hodges and Richardson 1996; Jull 1997,1998; Lee 1996; Mottram 1997; Mottram and Comerford 1999; O'Sullivan 2000; Richardson and Jull 1995; Richardson et al. 1999, 2004; Sahrmann 2002, 2011). Recent research has demonstrated the need to consider how movement is co-ordinated and controlled in the treatment of low back pain (LBP) (Hides et al. 1996; Hodges and Richardson 1996; O'Sullivan et al. 1997a; Richardson et al. 2004), cervical pain, and headaches (Jull et al. 1999).

The correction of movement control impairments or uncontrolled movement (UCM) should be based on a sound clinical assessment and clinical reasoning. The approach in the clinic should include three points: the best skills from current therapies, the best information from science, and the best therapeutic relationship with a particular patient (Butler 1998). This chapter highlights an approach to managing symptoms, impairments and disability, or activity limitations through assessing movement control impairments (uncontrolled movement) in the spine.

Concepts of muscle function and movement control

It is useful to consider the classification of muscles in relation to function when considering movement control and dynamic stability. The concept of classifying muscles by function gained general acceptance with Rood's concept of stabilizer and mobilizer muscles (Goff 1972). Rood's concept of differentiating stabilizer and mobilizer muscles has been further developed by Janda (1985) and Sahrmann (1993, 2002, 2011). Stabilizer muscles are described as having the characteristics of being mono-articular or segmental, deep, working eccentrically to control movement, and having static holding capacities. Mobility muscles on the other hand are described as bi-articular or multi-segmental, superficial, working concentrically with the acceleration of movement, and producing power. No other clinically accepted classification system was described until Bergmark presented the concept of local and global muscle systems when describing mechanical modelling of the spinal system (Bergmark 1989). In the local system, all muscles have their origin or insertion at the vertebrae and this system is used to control the curvature of the spine and provide stiffness to maintain mechanical stability of the lumbar spine. In the global system, the muscles are more superficial and link the thorax and pelvis. These muscles produce large torque/force.

Based on these concepts a new model of functional classification has been proposed (Comerford 1997; Comerford and Mottram 2001a, 2012, 2014) (Table 63.1). This model provides a subgrouping of muscles according to three distinct functional roles—a local stability muscle role, a global stability muscle role, and a global mobility muscle role (Comerford and Mottram 2001a, 2012, 2014; Mottram and Comerford 1999). The characteristics and function of the local stabilizer, global stabilizer, and global mobilizer muscles are described in Table 63.2. Examples are illustrated in Table 63.3.

Muscle characterization: categorization according to role

Although these three different functional roles for muscles now appear to be well accepted, it has not been possible to characterize every muscle in the locomotor system according to one single subgroup or another. Understanding a muscle's primary role is not always simple. Some muscles can easily be categorized into a subgroup, having only one specific functional role; however, other muscles appear to be capable of performing more than one of these functional roles (Comerford and Mottram 2012, 2014) Some muscles clearly exhibit all the characteristics of one subgroup and minimal characteristics of the others. They appear to have a single, very specific role and therefore their primary role can be defined as a local stabilizer or global stabilizer or global mobilizer. These muscles are single-task specific muscles. However, some muscles exhibit characteristics of more than one subgroup which cannot be explained by poor research methodology or misinterpretation of

Table 63.1 Model of reclassification of muscle function (by combining the strengths of the two previous models)

Stabilizer		Mobilizer
Local	Global	
Local stabilizer function	Global stabilizer function	Global mobilizer function

transversus abdominis, vastus medialis obliquus) or a global stabilizer role (e.g. external obliquus abdominis) or a global mobilizer role (e.g. rectus abdominis, hamstrings, iliocostalis lumborum). In the presence of pathology and/or pain, very specific impairments develop which are associated with the recognized specific primary functional role. The specific impairments are highly predictable and almost always present if they are assessed for. Very research results. They appear to be less specific and seem to be able to participate in a variety of different functional muscle roles without demonstrating impairment or dysfunction. These muscles are multi-taskcapable muscles (Comerford and Mottram 2012).

Single-task specific muscles

These muscles have a specific task-orientated role associated with being characterized as having *only* a local stabilizer role (e.g. specific retraining or correction strategies have been advocated in the treatment of the recovery of these predictable impairments (Hodges and Richardson 1996, 1997, 1999; Jull 2000; O'Sullivan 2000). This very specific training or corrective intervention is usually non-functional and as such is designed to correct very specific elements of impairment and dysfunction (Comerford and Mottram 2012). This specific retraining or correction may or may not integrate into normal functional activity. There is no way at

Table 63.2 The function and characteristics of the three different muscle functional roles

Local Stabilizer Role	**Global Stabilizer Role**	**Global Mobilizer Role**
Function & characteristics ◆ ↑ Muscle stiffness to control segmental motion ◆ Controls the *neutral* joint position ◆ Contraction = no/min; length change therefore does not produce range of motion ◆ Activity is often anticipatory to functional load or movement to provide protective muscle stiffness prior to motion stress (feed-forward recruitment) ◆ Activity is independent of direction of movement ◆ Continuous activity throughout movement ◆ Proprioceptive input re: joint position, range, and rate of movement	Function & characteristics ◆ Generates force to *control range* of motion ◆ Contraction = *eccentric* length change; therefore control throughout range, especially inner range ('muscle active' = 'joint passive') and hyper-mobile outer range ◆ Functional ability to: (i) shorten through the full inner range of joint motion; (ii) isometrically hold position; (iii) eccentrically control the return against gravity and control hyper-mobile outer range of joint motion if present ◆ Low load deceleration of momentum (especially axial plane: rotation) ◆ Non-continuous activity ◆ Activity is direction- dependent	Function & characteristics ◆ Generates torque to *produce range* of movement ◆ Contraction = *concentric* length change; therefore concentric production of movement (rather than eccentric control) ◆ Concentric acceleration of movement (especially sagittal plane: flexion/ extension) ◆ Shock absorption of load ◆ Activity is direction- dependent (predominately in the sagittal plane) ◆ Non-continuous activity (on:off phasic pattern)

Table 63.3 Examples of classification of muscle functional roles

Local Stabilizer Role	**Global Stabilizer Role**	**Global Mobilizer Role**
For example: ◆ Transversus abdominis ◆ Segmental lumbar multifidus ◆ Psoas (posterior fascicles) ◆ Diaphragm ◆ Pubococcygeus ◆ Deep sacral gluteus maximus ◆ Longus colli (longitudinal) ◆ Sub-occipital cuff ◆ Clavicular fibres of upper trapezius	For example: ◆ Oblique abdominals ◆ Superficial multifidus ◆ Spinalis ◆ Deep gluteus maximus ◆ Deep gluteus medius ◆ Psoas (anterior fascicles) ◆ Levator ani ◆ Longus colli (oblique fibres) ◆ Semi-spinalis cervicus	For example: ◆ Rectus abdominis ◆ Iliocostalis ◆ Longissimus ◆ Latissimus dorsi ◆ Quadratus lumborum (lateral fibres) ◆ Rectus femoris ◆ Tensor fascia latae (+ anterior iliotibial band) ◆ Hamstrings ◆ Superficial gluteus maximus (+ posterior iliotibial band) ◆ Piriformis ◆ Levator scapulae ◆ Scalenae ◆ Sternocleidomastoid

the moment to predict or clinically measure automatic integration into normal function. In many subjects, this integration may need to be facilitated.

Multi-task capable muscles

These muscles appear to have a multi-tasking function associated with being characterized as having the potential to perform more than one role. That is, there is good evidence to support both a local role and a global role, or the evidence may support the muscle having a contribution to both stability and mobility roles (e.g. gluteus maximus, infraspinatus, and pelvic floor). They appear to contribute to combinations of local stabilizer, global stabilizer, and global mobilizer roles when required in normal function. In the presence of pathology and/or pain, a variety of different impairments and dysfunctions may present. These impairments can be identified as being associated with either one or several of the multi-tasking roles and appear to be related to recruitment deficiencies in an individual's integrated stability system (Comerford and Mottram 2012). Treatment and retraining has to address the particular impairment or dysfunction that presents, usually needs to be multi-factorial, and should emphasize integration into 'normal' function.

Muscle physiology, pain, and recruitment

All human muscles have both fast and slow motor units and the function of the muscle is dependent on the recruitment of the motor units (Table 63.4). Dynamic postural control and normal low load functional movement is primarily a function of low threshold slow motor unit (tonic) recruitment. Low load (not high load or overload) exercise tends to optimize slow motor unit recruitment training. High load activity or strength training (endurance or power overload training) is a function of both slow (tonic) and fast (phasic) motor unit recruitment.

There is consistent evidence of altered recruitment in the presence of pain. Pain affects slow motor unit recruitment more significantly than fast motor unit recruitment. Pain does not appear to significantly limit an athlete's ability to generate power and speed so long as they can mentally 'put the pain aside'. Research (Hodges and Moseley 2003) indicates that in the pain-free state, the brain and the central nervous system (CNS) are able to utilize a variety of motor control strategies to perform functional tasks and maintain control of movement, equilibrium, and joint stability. However, in the pain state, the options available to the CNS appear to become limited.

Recent research on musculoskeletal pain has focused on motor control changes associated with the pain state. This research has provided important new information regarding chronic or recurrent musculoskeletal pain. A large number of independent research groups are all reporting a common finding in their studies. They have consistently observed and measured that in the presence of chronic or recurrent pain, subjects change the patterns or strategies of synergistic recruitment that are normally used to perform low load functional movements or postures. They demonstrate that these subjects employ strategies or patterns of muscle recruitment that are normally reserved for high load function (e.g. lifting, pushing, pulling, throwing, jumping, running), for normal postural control, and low threshold functional activities. These altered (or limited) motor control strategies present as consistent co-contraction patterns, usually with exaggerated recruitment of the multi-joint muscles over the deeper segmental muscles, or as uncontrolled movement with impairments of movement control strategies (Comerford and Mottram 2012).

These altered strategies or patterns have been described in the research and clinical literature as 'substitution strategies', 'compensatory movements', 'muscle imbalance' between inhibited/lengthened stabilizers and shortened/overactive mobilizers, 'faulty movements', 'abnormal dominance of the mobilizer synergists', 'co-contraction rigidity', and 'control impairments'.

Table 63.4 Key features of slow and fast motor unit recruitment

Function	Slow Motor Units (low threshold or tonic recruitment)	Fast Motor Units (high threshold or phasic recruitment)
Load threshold	Low (easily activated)	High (requires greater stimulus)
Recruitment	Primarily recruited at low% of maximum voluntary contraction (<25%)	Increasingly recruited at higher% of maximum voluntary contraction (>40%)
Speed of contraction	Slow	Fast
Contraction force	Low	High
Fatiguability	Fatigue-resistant	Fast-fatiguing
Role	Fine control of postural activity and non-fatiguing low load 'normal' functional movements	Rapid or accelerated movement and fatiguing high load activity

Concept of restrictions and compensations to maintain functional movements

Movement control impairments may present as a disorder of articular translational movements at a single motion segment, e.g. abnormal articular translational motion. They may also present as a myofascial disorder in the functional movements across one or more motion segments, e.g. abnormal myofascial length and recruitment or as a response to neural mechanosensitivity. These two components of the movement system are inter-related and consequently articular translational and myofascial impairments often occur concurrently.

The inability to dynamically control movement at a joint segment or region may present as uncontrolled movement (UCM) or as an impairment of movement control. UCM is defined as a lack of active (or cognitive) low-threshold control of the local or global muscle's ability to control motion at a particular site (joint or region of the body) in a particular direction or specific plane of motion (Comerford and Mottram 2012, 2014). UCM can present as a lack of control of normal functional motion or hypermobile range. It may be identified in the physiological or functional movements of joint range, or in the accessory translational gliding movements of a joint (Table 63.5). UCM is commonly (but not always) associated with a loss of motion or 'restriction' (Comerford and Mottram 2012, 2014).

Table 63.5 Key elements of restriction and uncontrolled compensation

Restriction	Compensation (uncontrolled movement)
Articular restriction	*Uncontrolled translation*
Intra-articular and inter-articular joint hypomobility	Uncontrolled intra-articular and inter-articular joint hypermobility
Myofascial restriction	*Uncontrolled range*
Lack of myofascial extensibility restricting range of motion	Myofascial inability to control range of motion

The restriction may be associated with limitation of articular translation and a lack of extensibility of the connective tissue (intra-articular or peri-articular) at a motion segment. This presents with a loss of translational motion at a joint and is confirmed with manual palpation (e.g. Maitland et al. 2005). The restriction may be associated with a lack of extensibility of contractile myofascial tissue or neural tissue. The muscles may lose extensibility because of:

i) increased low threshold recruitment or 'over activity' (Janda 1985; Sahrmann 2002, 2011)

ii) a lack of range because of length-associated changes (Goldspink and Williams 1992; Gossman et al. 1982)

iii) a lack of normal neural compliance and a protective response associated with abnormal neural mechanosensitivity (Balster and Jull 1997; Edgar et al. 1994; Hall and Elvey 1999; Hall et al. 1998).

These restrictions are confirmed with myofascial extensibility tests.

Movement control impairments can result in abnormal movement about several motion segments. When a muscle contracts it generates tension across motion segments at both ends, and if there is inadequate stability or control at any segment, then inappropriate motion may develop at this site. There is frequently, but not always, a restriction of normal motion (loss of physiological or accessory movement) at one or more motion segments, which contributes to compensatory excessive movement at adjacent segments in order to maintain function.

UCM often results from uncontrolled compensation for restriction. These movement control impairments may present as uncontrolled translation or uncontrolled range. When the UCM presents as uncontrolled translation, it is associated with laxity of articular connective tissue. Panjabi (1992) defined spinal instability in terms of laxity around the neutral position of a spinal segment called the neutral zone. Maitland et al. (2005) have described joint hypermobility. The end result of this process is abnormal development of uncontrolled movement and a loss of functional or dynamic stability. Articular translational UCM can compensate for:

i) articular restriction in the same joint (restriction and compensation at an intra-articular level),

ii) articular restriction in an adjacent joint (restriction and compensation at an inter-articular level),

iii) myofascial restriction (restriction and compensation at a regional level).

When the UCM presents as uncontrolled range, it is associated with excessive length or poor control of myofascial tissue. This is the usual compensation for:

i) myofascial restriction at an adjacent region (restriction and compensation at a regional level),

ii) abnormal mechanosensitivity at an adjacent region (restriction and compensation at a regional level),

iii) segmental articular translational restriction at an adjacent joint (restriction and compensation at an inter-articular level).

Uncontrolled translation and uncontrolled range can present in isolation without restriction. Common examples of this type of presentation are:

i) a traumatic incident (capsular/ligamentous laxity or instability),

ii) inhibition associated with pain and pathology,

iii) sustained postural strain positioning.

The UCM may be due to muscle inhibition associated with abnormal neural mechanosensitivity.

In the functional movement system, the site of UCM is the site of the movement control impairment (Comerford and Mottram 2012, 2014). The uncontrolled segment or region is the most likely source of pathology and symptoms of mechanical origin. The direction of UCM relates to the direction of tissue stress or strain and pain-producing movements (Comerford and Mottram 2012; Sahrmann 2002, 2011). It is important, in the assessment of movement control impairments, to identify the region and the direction of UCM and relate it to the symptoms and pathology.

The clinical testing for movement control impairments identifies the *segment* and the *direction* of uncontrolled movement that are related to the direction of symptom- producing movement. The identification of UCM into excessive uncontrolled lumbar flexion, under flexion load, may place abnormal stress or strain on various tissues and result in flexion-related symptoms. Likewise, the identification of UCM into uncontrolled lumbar extension, under extension load, produces extension-related symptoms; while uncontrolled lumbo-pelvic rotation or side-bend/side-shift, under unilateral load, may produce unilateral symptoms. Stiff or restricted segments are not usually the source of pain during normal functional movement or loading, although pain may be elicited under abnormal movement or load. *Generally, the stiff or restricted segment may be a cause of compensatory UCM at an adjacent joint.*

Restriction → Compensation → Uncontrolled Movement (UCM)→ Pathology → Pain

Although it is commonly observed that restrictions are compensated for by increasing movement elsewhere in the body, it is incorrect to assume that all compensation is uncontrolled. A compensation that demonstrates efficient active or cognitive control during testing for movement control impairments is a normal compensation strategy and does not constitute UCM and usually does not contribute to symptoms. However, compensation that fails to demonstrate this is an aberrant compensation strategy (Comerford and Mottram 2012, 2014).

It is important to relate the site and direction of UCM to symptoms and pathology and to the mechanisms of provocation of symptoms. Management of the movement control impairment that relates to the symptoms and pathology becomes the clinical

Table 63.6 Lumbar spine movement control impairments

Lumbar spine movement control impairment	Direction of UCM (uncontrolled compensation)	Common symptom presentation
Lumbar flexion UCM	Lumbar flexion under flexion load	Pain in lumbar spine (+/− referred)—aggravated or provoked by flexion load, movements, or flexed postures
Lumbar flexion rotation UCM	Lumbar rotation and flexion under unilateral load	Unilateral pain in lumbar spine (+/− referred)—aggravated or provoked by unilateral load or flexion load, movements, or flexed postures
Lumbar extension UCM	Lumbar extension under extension load	Pain in lumbar spine (+/− referred)—aggravated or provoked by extension load, movements, or extended postures
Lumbar extension rotation UCM	Lumbar rotation and extension under unilateral load	Unilateral pain in lumbar spine (+/− referred)—aggravated or provoked by unilateral load or extension load, movements, or extended postures
Lumbar global (multi-directional) UCM	Lumbar flexion and extension and rotation under related load tests	Pain in lumbar spine (central or unilateral) (+/− referred); flexion symptoms provoked by flexion load or movements (especially prolonged sitting); extension symptoms provoked by extension load or movements (especially prolonged standing); unilateral symptoms provoked by unilateral load or movements (especially static asymmetrical postures)

Table 63.7 Cervical spine movement control impairments

Cervical spine movement control impairments	Direction of UCM (uncontrolled compensation)	Common symptom presentation
Upper cervical extension UCM	Upper cervical extension under extension load	Upper cervical pain (+/−headaches or referral)—aggravated or provoked by extension load, movements, or postures
+/− rotation/sidebend	Cervical extension or lateral flexion during rotation	Unilateral pain in upper cervical spine—aggravated or provoked by unilateral load or movements
Low cervical flexion UCM	Low cervical flexion under flexion load	Low cervical pain (+/− referred)—aggravated or provoked by flexion load, movements, or postures
+/− rotation/sidebend	Cervical lateral flexion during rotation	Unilateral pain in upper cervical spine—aggravated or provoked by unilateral load or movements
Mid cervical translation UCM	Mid cervical (usually translational shear C3-4 or C4-5) under extension load	Mid cervical pain (+/−referred)—aggravated or provoked by extension load, movements, or postures
+/− rotation/sidebend	Cervical extension or lateral flexion during rotation	Unilateral pain in upper cervical spine—aggravated or provoked by unilateral load or movements
Upper cervical flexion UCM	Upper cervical flexion under flexion load	Upper cervical pain (+/− headaches or referral)—aggravated or provoked by flexion load, movements, or postures (often traumatic involving upper cervical ligamentous laxity, e.g. forced flexion injury)
+/− rotation/sidebend	Upper lateral flexion during rotation	Unilateral pain in upper cervical spine—aggravated or provoked by unilateral load or movements

priority. UCMs that may be evident, but do not relate to symptoms, are not a priority of pathology management. However, it may indicate a potential risk for the future. The movement control impairment can be labelled (or diagnosed) by the side and direction of UCM. Common patterns seen in the clinic are described in Tables 63.6 and 63.7.

Evidence of movement control impairment

Movement control impairments can be identified in the local and global muscle systems (Table 63.8). They can occur as aberrant recruitment and motor control of the deep local muscle stability system, resulting in poor control of the neutral joint position (Hides et al. 1996; Hodges and Richardson 1996; Jull et al. 1999; O'Sullivan et al. 1997b; Richardson et al. 1999, 2004). This literature demonstrates a motor control deficit associated with delayed timing or inefficient low threshold recruitment in the local stability system. These changes may decrease the efficiency of muscle action around a motion segment and potentially result in poor segmental control and instability (Cholewicki and McGill 1996).

Hodges and Richardson (1996) investigated the contribution of the transversus abdominis to spinal stabilization in subjects with and without LBP. The delayed onset of contraction of the transversus abdominis in subjects with LBP indicates a deficit of motor control and, as a result of this, the authors hypothesize that there would be inefficient muscular stabilization of the spine. From the evidence to date, it would appear that in all back pain subjects, the transversus abdominis has a recruitment impairment that is independent of the type or nature of pathology, while subjects who have never had significant back pain do not have this impairment (Hodges and

Table 63.8 Recruitment impairment in the three muscle functional roles

Local Stabilizer Role	Global Stabilizer Role	Global Mobilizer Role
Impairment: ◆ ↑ Motor control deficit associated with delayed timing or recruitment deficiency ◆ Reacts to pain and pathology with inhibition ◆ ↑ Muscle stiffness and poor segmental control ◆ Loss of control of joint neutral position	*Impairment:* ◆ Muscle lacks the ability to (i) shorten through the full inner range of joint motion; (ii) isometrically hold position; (iii) eccentrically control the return ◆ Muscle active shortening = joint passive (loss of inner range control) ◆ If hyper-mobile—poor control of excessive range ◆ Poor low threshold tonic recruitment ◆ Poor eccentric control ◆ Poor rotation dissociation	*Impairment:* ◆ Loss of myofascial extensibility—limits physiological and/or accessory motion (which must be compensated for elsewhere) ◆ Over-active low threshold, low load recruitment ◆ Reacts to pain and pathology with spasm
Result: **Local inhibition**	**Global imbalance** ⟷ (inefficient, centrally down-regulated global stabilizer)	**Global imbalance** (overactive/short, centrally up-regulated global mobilizer)

Richardson 1996; Richardson et al. 2004). The recruitment impairment is related to motor control deficits, not strength.

There is evidence of lumbar multifidus muscle reduction in a cross-sectional area ipsilateral to symptoms in patients with acute/subacute LBP (Hides et al. 1994). This decrease in size of the multifidus was seen on the side of the symptoms with the reduced cross-sectional area observed at a single vertebral level, suggesting segmental pain inhibition. This evidence suggests that pain and impairment are related (Stokes and Young 1984). In acute onset back pain, this immediate inhibition of the lumbar multifidus does not automatically return when symptoms settle. It has been observed that recovery of symmetry was more rapid and more complete in patients who received specific, cognitive, localized multifidus and transversus abdominis muscle recruitment retraining (Hides et al. 1996).

Dangaria and Naesh (1998) assessed the cross-sectional area of the psoas major in unilateral sciatica caused by disc herniation. There was significant reduction in the cross-sectional area of the psoas at the level and site of disc herniation on the ipsilateral side. Segmental inhibition due to pathology and pain may be responsible for the psoas reduction in the cross-sectional area.

Inhibition of the local stability system has also been demonstrated in subjects with headaches (Jull et al. 1999). Deep neck flexor muscle contraction was significantly inferior in the cervical headache group.

There is a common model of stability in the lumbar spine relating it to a cylinder. Richardson et al. (1999, 2004) use a cylinder concept to describe the local stability system for the lumbo-pelvic region. They suggest the transversus abdominis and the spinal column make up the wall of the cylinder, with the diaphragm and pelvic floor muscles making up the top and bottom respectively. In the light of recent research, perhaps the stability cylinder model can be updated (Figure 63.1). Consider the spine as a flexible segmented structure embedded in the wall of the cylinder. The role of the cylinder is to support and stabilize this flexible structure while it moves. The cylinder can be portrayed as having an inner (local) core and an outer (global) shell (Comerford and Mottram 2012). The wall of the inner local core of the cylinder is made up of the transversus abdominis providing lateral control and resistance to segmental displacement laterally. The spine is stabilized posteriorly by segmental attachments of the lumbar multifidus and stabilized anteriorly by segmental attachments of the psoas (posterior fascicles). These two muscles provide sagittal and axial control and resistance to antero-posterior and rotatory segmental displacement. Their longitudinal fibre placement contributes to axial compression to enhance stability throughout the spinal range of motion. Tension generated by these muscles also contributes to increasing fascial tension to improve the load-bearing ability of the spine.

The cylinder requires a top and bottom if it is to increase internal pressure, known as intra-abdominal pressure (IAP), to enhance spinal stability. If IAP is to assist in spinal stabilization, it must be able to generate pressure independently from respiratory and continence functions. It has been demonstrated that the costal part of the diaphragm has a stability role independent from respiration, although it also contributes to respiratory function (Hodges and Gandevia 2000). It is theorized that the pubo-visceral muscles (e.g. pubococcygeus) have the stability role within the pelvic floor (Sapsford et al. 1997).

If the model of a local core is valid, then these muscles must have efficient recruitment and have sophisticated co-ordination and integration processes. It seems logical that if any one of these muscles is dysfunctional, then the stability of the cylinder will be compromised unless the other muscles (or some other process) can adequately compensate.

The outer global shell of the cylinder consists of the global stabilizer muscles and the global mobilizer muscles acting around the trunk (Comerford and Mottram 2012). The global stabilizer muscles, such as the oblique abdominals, anterior fasiculus of psoas, superficial multifidus, and spinalis, act to eccentrically control range of motion and decelerate rotational forces across the trunk. The global mobilizer muscles, such as the rectus abdominis, iliocostalis, longissimus, and quadratus lumborum, act to produce fast, large-range, and forceful movement. When the integrated local cylinder function can be achieved, then the local core and the global shell should be retrained to ensure co-ordinated normal function.

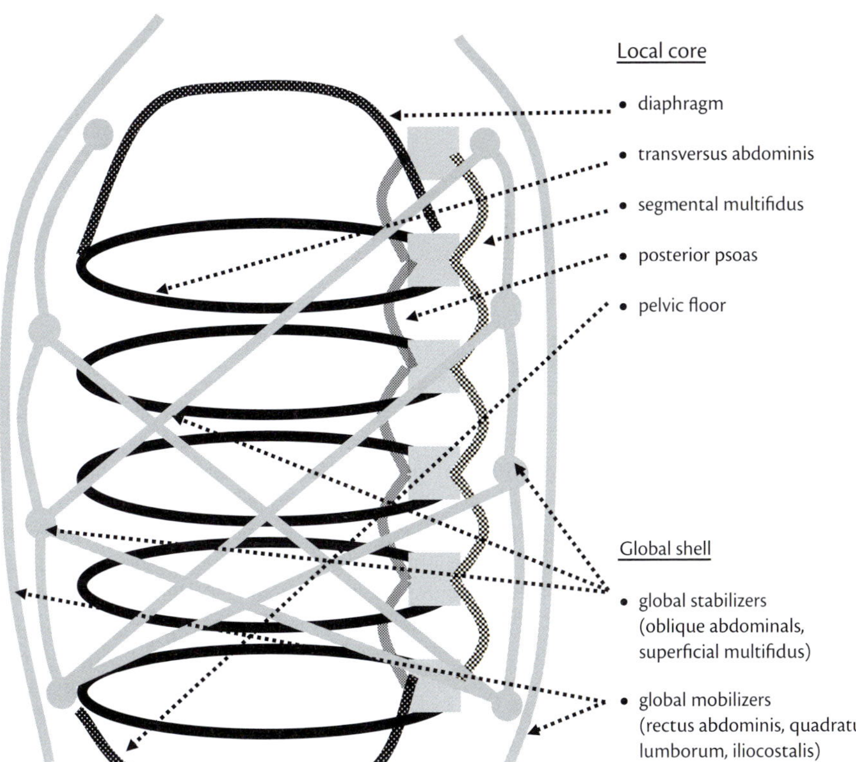

Figure 63.1 Functional stability cylinder for the trunk (reprinted with permission from Movement Performance Solutions).

The global stability of the trunk is essential for proximal control of the spine and girdles during limb motion and functional loading. If the local cylinder has re-established normal efficient function, then under low load normal functional demands, it should recruit automatically whenever the global system is required to work.

Movement control impairments can occur globally as imbalance between the mono-articular stabilizers and the bi-articular mobilizers or movement-producing muscles (Rood, as reported by Goff 1972; Janda 1985; Kankaanpaa et al. 1998; Sahrmann 1993, 2002). This imbalance presents in terms of alteration in functional length tests and recruitment patterns of these muscles.

Clinically, it can be seen that the global stability muscles lack the ability to shorten through the full range of joint motion. They also demonstrate poor low load or low threshold recruitment (Janda 1995; Sahrmann 2002, 2011) and poor low load eccentric control of rotation (Comerford and Mottram 2002a,b,c,d; Sahrmann 2002, 2011). For example, gluteal dysfunction has been associated with lumbo-pelvic pain (Janda 1985; Kankaanpaa et al. 1998). With over-activity in the global mobility muscles, clinical examination demonstrates myofascial shortening which limits motion (Sahrmann 2002, 2011). For example, the over-activity of the rectus abdominis, rectus femoris, tensor fascia latae, and the hamstrings can have a significant influence on the compensatory movement of the pelvis and lumbar spine. A similar influence can be observed in the cervical spine with over-activity and/or shortness of, for example, the levator scapulae and scalanae.

Recruitment impairment in the global muscle system may result in abnormal centrally mediated up-regulation and 'over-activity' of muscles with a global mobilizer role, along with concurrent centrally mediated down-regulation and inefficiency of muscles with a global stabilizer role. This 'imbalance' in the control and co-ordination of recruitment between joint stabilizer muscles and their joint mobilizer synergists results in altered forces acting around a motion segment. The loss of ideal or normal local or global control may result in abnormal stress or strain being imposed on the joint, its supporting soft tissue structures, and related myofascial tissue and neural tissue. As a result of these movement control impairments, tissue stress and microtrauma may exceed the tissues' tolerance and ability to recover, with pathology and pain developing over time.

The assessment for movement control impairments must identify changes in the recruitment of muscles in the local stability system and recruitment, length, and force efficiency changes in the global stability system (Comerford and Mottram 2012).

Clinical examination for movement control impairment

The clinical examination aims to identify movement control impairments and relate these impairments to pain in the movement system. The movement system is made up of articular, myofascial, neural, and connective tissue systems of the body. Good function requires the integrated and co-ordinated interaction of these systems. Each system needs to be examined and the influence of one system on the other needs to be considered. For example, pain, pathology, disuse, and abnormal proprioceptive input can inhibit muscle recruitment (Brumagne et al. 1999; Hurley and Newham 1993; Stokes and Young 1984; Taimela et al. 1999). This inhibition can be noted in muscles with a local stability role and a global stability role. Noxious input, for example pain, may produce muscle

Table 63.9 Differentiation between low threshold recruitment impairment and high threshold strength/speed performance

Movement and performance dysfunction	Low threshold movement control impairments	High threshold strength/ speed impairments
Assessment	Identified by the failure to control movement under non-fatiguing low-load testing	Identified by the failure to perform movement under fatiguing high-load testing
Result	Results in the development of uncontrolled movement, pathology, and pain	Results in weakness and loss of performance

'spasm' (Schaible and Grubb 1993). Clinically, this 'spasm' is primarily observed in the global mobility muscles. This is seen as a typical pattern in patients with LBP, i.e. over-activity and centrally mediated up-regulation in the large superficial erector spinae, while at the same time, inhibition is observed in the segmental fibres of the lumbar multifidus.

Proprioception can influence muscle function at peripheral joints (Hurley 1997) and may have an influence on spinal muscle function (Brumagne et al. 1999; Taimela et al. 1999). Pain, pathology, sensitized neural tissue, and altered proprioceptive input can all influence recruitment of muscles that perform a local or global stability role, thus affecting functional stability and movement control. Therefore, it is important to assess function and impairment in all components of the movement system.

Sahrmann (1993, 2002, 2011) emphasizes the importance of considering the factor of cumulative microtrauma as a cause of musculoskeletal pain and states, 'faulty movement can induce pathology, not just be a result of it'. This cumulative microtrauma can result from repetitive activities or from complex changes in patterns of multi-joint movements. For this reason, movement patterns need to be examined in detail, and a history of activities and functional activities analysed. In view of the changes in muscle function in the local and global systems, the physical examination must include an assessment of muscle function: local stability muscles, global stability muscles, and global mobility muscles. Specific tests need to be considered (Table 63.9).

The diagnosis of uncontrolled movement (UCM): direction control

In pain-free function, all muscles work and co-activate in integrated patterns to produce and control movement during all normal functional activities. All functional activities impose stress and strain forces on the movement system in varying loads and in all three planes or directions of motion, and normal functional movements rarely eliminate motion from one joint system while others move through range. Functional movement rarely occurs in only one plane.

However, everybody has the ability to perform patterns of movement that are not habitually used in 'normal function' (e.g. pat the head and rub the stomach). Performance of some of these unfamiliar movements is a test of motor control (skill and co-ordination). The ability to activate muscles to isometrically hold position or to control/prevent motion at one joint system, while concurrently actively producing a movement at another joint system in a specific direction, is a test of movement control efficiency (Comerford and Mottram 2012).

The process of dissociating movement at one joint from movement at another joint has potential benefits for retraining the stability muscles to enhance their recruitment efficiency to control direction-specific stress and strain. The global and the local stability muscle systems can be trained to recruit in co-activation patterns to prevent movement in a specific direction at a vulnerable, painful, or unstable joint, while an adjacent joint is loaded in that direction. In this way, the movement control system can be trained to control a specific site and direction of UCM (Comerford and Mottram 2012).

The global muscles react to pain and pathology with functional length and recruitment impairments. The assessment of global muscle function considers the ability to dissociate direction and control of through-range motion. The global stability muscles are required to control directional strain, i.e. cognitively or actively control the excessive UCM into flexion/extension or rotation to certain benchmark standards. The assessment for the ability of the global stability muscles to control direction- related stress and strain involves actively controlling and preventing movements of the spine into flexion, extension, rotation, or sidebending, while moving the limbs independently into flexion, extension, rotation, and other directions. These movement control tests are not natural or 'normal' functional movements, but rather, are movement patterns that everybody should have the ability to perform given the instruction to do so and a short period of teaching and familiarization (Comerford and Mottram 2012; Hamilton 1998; Sahrmann 2002, 2011). Some examples of movement control tests that are used to identify the site and direction of UCM are highlighted here.

In the cervical spine, a symmetrical range of cervical rotation should be achieved. Symmetry is important but range is variable. The common directions of UCM are *upper cervical—extension UCM* (chin poke associated with poor recruitment efficiency of the deep neck flexor stabilizer muscles) and *cervical—lateral flexion UCM* during rotation (associated with a coupling dysfunction in the articular system and/or poor recruitment efficiency of the deep neck flexors) (Figure 63.2). A significant asymmetry of rotation or an obvious decrease in range of motion is seen when the UCM is actively or passively controlled. Restriction may occur from articular translational dysfunction or myofascial dysfunction or related neural sensitivity.

Two useful tests for lumbar flexion UCM are the *standing forward lean test* and the *sitting forward lean test.*

- *Standing forward lean test* (Comerford and Mottram 2012; Sahrmann 2002) (Figure 63.3): the subject is instructed to stand tall and to bend or 'bow' forwards from the hips, keeping the back straight (neutral spine), and prevent or control any lumbar flexion or posterior tilt increasing at the lumbar pelvic area. Ideally,

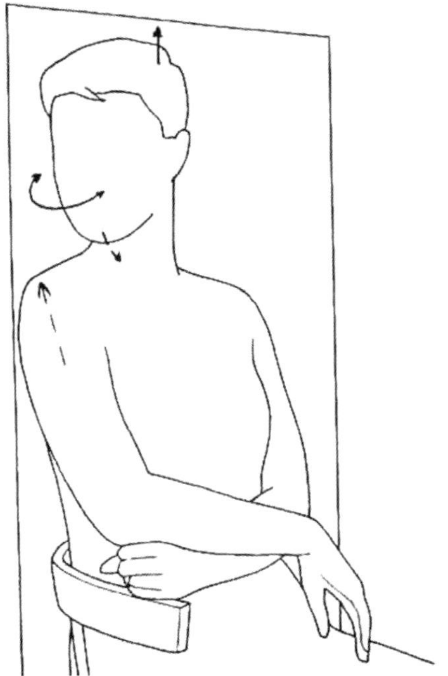

Figure 63.2 Cervical rotation control (reprinted with permission from Physiotools).

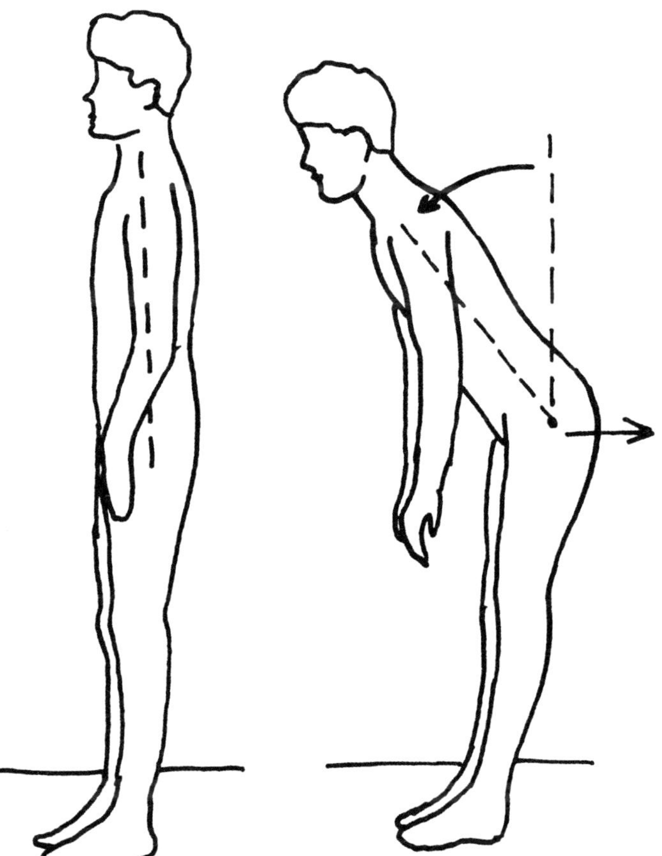

Figure 63.3 Lumbar flexion control—standing forward lean (reprinted with permission from Physiotools).

the subject should have the ability to dissociate the lumbar spine from hip flexion as evidenced by 50° forwards lean while preventing or controlling lumbar flexion and maintaining the lumbar spine neutral position. A positive test for *lumbar flexion UCM* will demonstrate a lack of ability to control or prevent lumbar flexion throughout the benchmark range of direction control to 50° forwards leaning.

- *Sitting forward lean test* (Comerford and Mottram 2012; Hamilton 1998; Sahrmann 2002) (Figure 63.4): the subject is instructed to sit tall and to lean forwards from the hips, keeping the back straight (neutral spine). Ideally, the subject should have the ability to dissociate the lumbar spine from hip flexion as evidenced by 30° of forwards lean with maintenance of the lumbar spine neutral position. A positive test for *lumbar flexion UCM* will demonstrate an inability to control or prevent lumbo-sacral flexion and posterior tilt occurring before the benchmark of 30° forwards leaning. A positive test for *lumbar extension UCM* will demonstrate an inability to control or prevent lumbar extension and anterior tilt occurring before the benchmark of 30° forwards leaning.

Supine bent knee fallout (Comerford and Mottram 2012; Sahrmann 2002) is a useful test to identify a *lumbo-pelvic rotation UCM* (Figure 63.5). With the subject lying supine and with legs extended and the feet together, both anterior superior iliac spines (ASISs) are checked for symmetry in the antero-posterior plane. The subject is instructed to slide one heel up beside the other knee. Ideally, the pelvis should not rotate and the ASIS remains level. If the pelvis stays stable and does not rotate, the subject is instructed to slowly lower the bent leg out to the side, keeping the foot supported beside the straight leg. There is usually some slight rotation of the pelvis at this stage. The subject is then instructed to repeat the 'bent leg fallout' but not to allow the pelvis to rotate at all. Ideally, the bent leg should be able to be lowered through the available range of hip abduction and lateral rotation (at least 50°) and returned, without

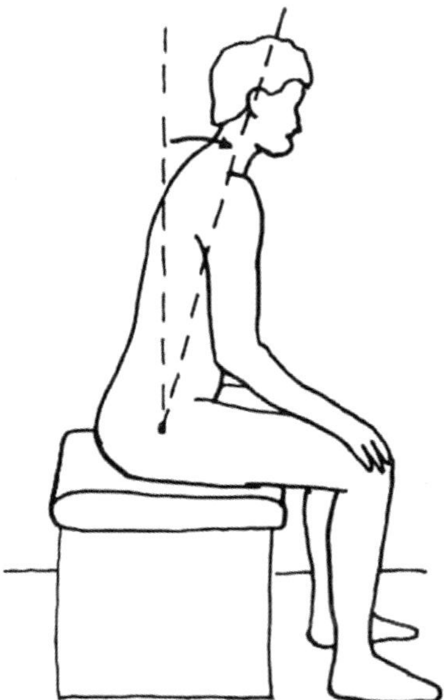

Figure 63.4 Lumbar flexion control—sitting forward lean (reprinted with permission from Physiotools).

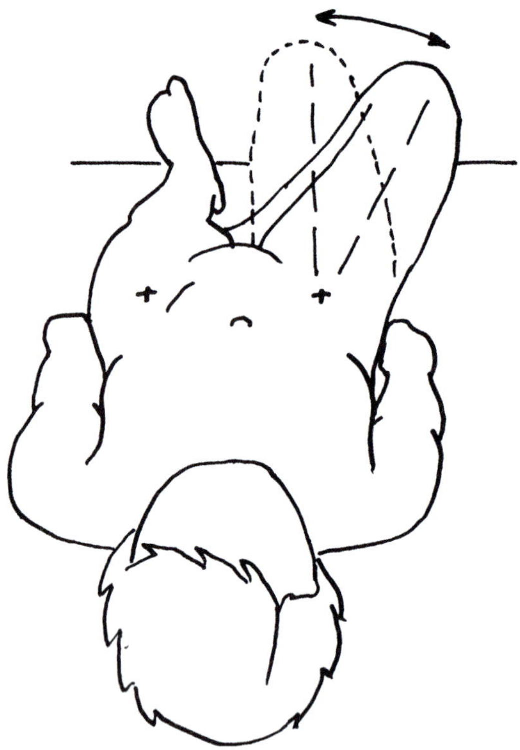

Figure 63.5 Lumbar rotation control—bent knee fallout (reprinted with permission from Physiotools).

associated pelvic rotation. A positive test for *lumbo-pelvic rotation UCM* will demonstrate an inability to control or prevent pelvic rotation occurring before the benchmark of 50° leg abduction and lateral rotation out to the side.

Local stability muscle role: control of intersegmental displacement in neutral joint position

In the presence of regional pathology or pain, the local stability muscles demonstrate recruitment impairments, and specific tests have been designed to assess these impairments (Hides et al. 1996; Hodges and Richardson 1996; Jull 1998; Jull et al. 1999; Richardson and Jull 1995; Richardson et al. 1999, 2004). These tests must identify and exclude substitution strategies from the global muscles, e.g. during a low abdominal hollowing recruitment strategy for the transversus abdominis, observe and palpate for excessive activity of the external obliques and rectus abdominis.

To test for the stability function of the deep neck flexors (longus colli), the subject is positioned in supine position with the spine, temporomandibular joint (TMJ), and scapula in a neutral position (head supported on towel). The subject is instructed to perform a very slight upper cervical flexion action (cranio-cervical flexion), which causes a slight cervical flexion and flattening of the cervical curve. A pressure biofeedback unit ('Stabilizer', manufactured by the Chattanooga Group, Australia) can be used to measure function (Jull 1998, 2000, 2001) (Figure 63.6). There should be no substitution (for example, from the scalenae or sternocleidomastoid) or fatigue. A flattening pressure (6–8 mmHg in 2-mmHg increments)

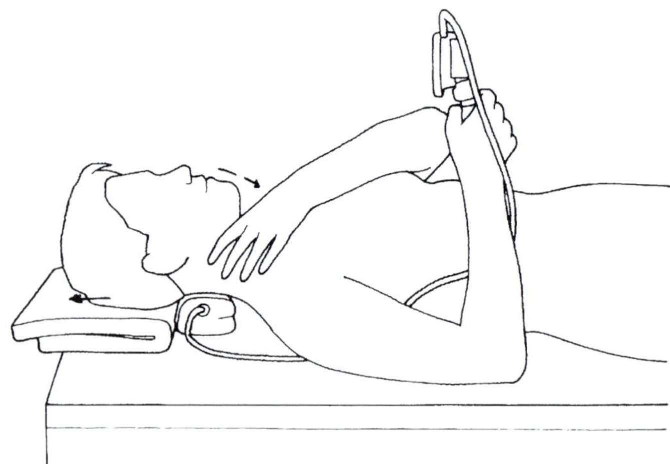

Figure 63.6 Deep neck flexor control of neutral position (reprinted with permission from Physiotools).

should be sustained for 10 seconds with 10 repetitions (Jull 1998). There should be minimal range of movement.

The transversus abdominis will tension the low abdominal fascia and hollow the low abdominal wall. This 'drawing in' or 'low abdominal hollowing' action should be specifically localized to the lower abdominal region and there should be minimal spinal or pelvic tilt or rib cage movement. It should not cause lateral flaring of the waist. A pressure biofeedback unit ('Stabilizer', manufactured by the Chattanooga Group, Australia) can be used to measure a function of transversus abdominis recruitment in prone lying (Figure 63.7) (Cairns et al. 2000; Hodges et al. 1996; Richardson et al. 1999, 2004). For good motor control patterns, the patient needs to be able to specifically activate a dominant transversus contraction using the lower abdominal hollowing strategy, and maintain this contraction consistently during relaxed breathing. The activation strategy should be repeated several times in a variety of different functional postures such as lying, supported sitting, and supported standing. A useful guide is a 10-second hold with 10 repetitions (Richardson and Jull 1995; Richardson et al. 2004).

To test for lumbar multifidus function, the multifidus is consciously activated against the facilitating pressure of a thumb/finger (Hides et al. 1996; Richardson et al. 1999) (Figure 63.8). This contraction ideally should be maintained for 10 seconds and consistently repeated 10 times. Substitution strategies, for example, excessive substitution of the erector spinae or lumbar extension/pelvic tilt, should be avoided.

To test for recruitment of a local stability role for the psoas major (posted fascicles), the patient lies on one side with both legs bent. The top femur is supported horizontally with the spine, pelvis, and

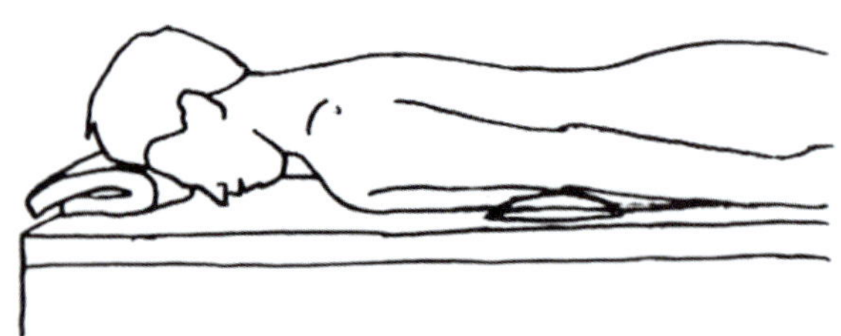

Figure 63.7 Transversus abdominus activation in neutral position (reprinted with permission from Physiotools).

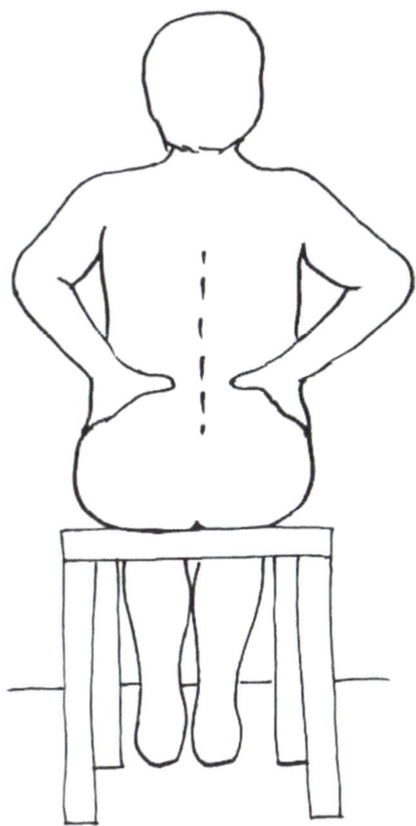

Figure 63.8 Lumbar bifidus activation in neutral position (reprinted with permission from Physiotools).

upper trunk all in neutral alignment. The local stabilizer role of the psoas major is evaluated with a longitudinal activation strategy. The psoas is facilitated by gently distracting the top leg longitudinally and the patient is instructed to 'gently pull the hip back into the socket' without moving the spine or pelvis (Comerford and Mottram 2014). Facilitation may be localized segmentally. The therapist manually palpates the relative stiffness at that level, attempting to translate the spinous process side to side. The psoas activation is facilitated and resistance to manual translation (stiffness) is reassessed (Comerford and Emerson 1999). Ideally, a significant increase in resistance to manual displacement should be noted when the psoas is activated. The contraction (and increased stiffness) should be maintained for 10 seconds and consistently repeated 10 times. This response should be noted at all lumbar segmental levels.

Segmental psoas recruitment impairment is identified by identifying the level that does not increase resistance to manual translation when compared to adjacent levels (which do increase resistance to translation when the psoas is activated with the longitudinal activation strategy). A lack of increased resistance to manual displacement during psoas activation indicates a probable loss of segmental control of the local stability role of the psoas (Comerford and Mottram 2014).

Global muscle imbalance—recruitment synergies: global stabilizer down-regulation

In normal pain-free function, the one-joint global stability muscles are designed to have the ability to move body segments against gravity through the full available range of joint motion. The global stabilizers are normally dominant to their multi-joint global mobilizer synergists during non-fatiguing submaximal normal function. The global mobilizer synergists are designed to be dominant to the global stabilizers for high load fatiguing function. When global stability muscles demonstrate recruitment impairment, for example during episodes of musculoskeletal pain, they present with centrally mediated down-regulation or inhibition. They respond less efficiently to non-fatiguing loads and low threshold stimuli and demonstrate an inability to move the body segments throughout the full inner range of joint motion. For example, through range control of the cervico-thoracic stabilizing extensors (semi-spinalis) is required to control segmental cervico-thoracic extension and eccentric cervico-thoracic flexion. Clinically, it is frequently observed that the gluteus maximus loses the ability to control hip extension to the inner range. The global stability muscles must have the ability to move the joint through the full available range in normal non-fatiguing function. These examples are illustrated here.

- *Semi-spinalis inner-range control* (Comerford and Mottram 2014)—through-range control of the cervico-thoracic stabilizing extensors (Figure 63.9): The subject starts by resting prone on elbows, with the scapulae and thoracic spine neutral and the head hanging in flexion. The subject is instructed to maintain the upper cervical spine in flexion or neutral and lift their head with independent extension of the low cervical spine through the full range and lower the head to return to the starting position. Ideally, the subject should have the ability to independently extend the lower cervical spine through the full range of extension and hold in the shortened range position for 10 seconds without fatigue or substitution; then return, with eccentric control, to the starting position in the outer range without substitution. Activation of the mobility muscles under load is normal. When the movement is performed correctly (without substitution or fatigue), the range that can be controlled actively equals the available passive range of cervical flexion.
- *Gluteus maximus inner-range control* (Comerford and Mottram 2014)—hip extension with knee flexed, prone position (Figure 63.10): With the subject lying prone and one knee flexed to past 90°, the lumbo-pelvic region is manually stabilized and the hip passively lifted into extension to check the available range of hip extension. The subject is instructed to lift the knee (hip

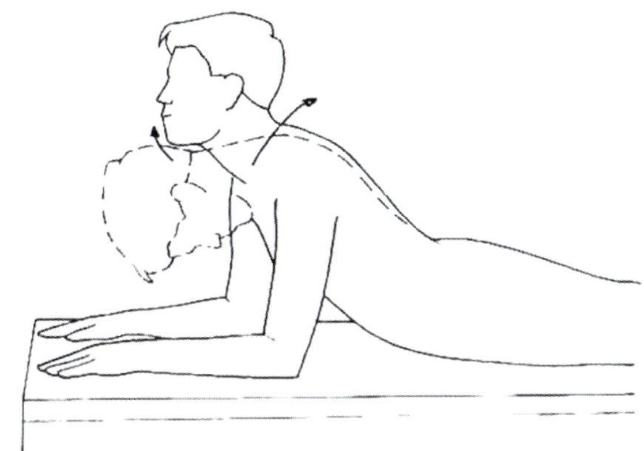

Figure 63.9 Cervico-thoracic extensor stabilizers—through-range control (reprinted with permission from Physiotools).

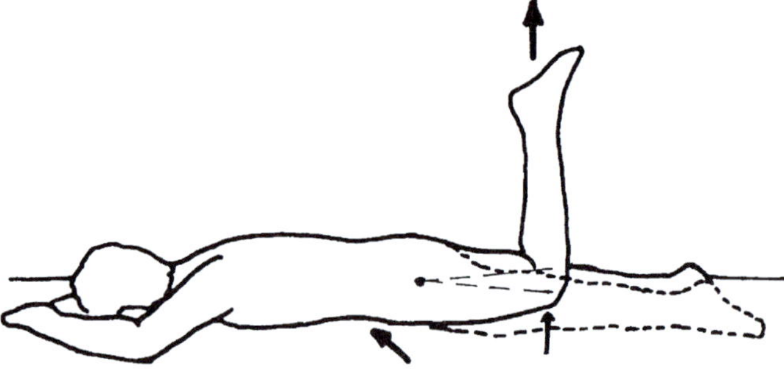

Figure 63.10 Gluteus maximus—inner-range control (reprinted with permission from Physiotools).

extension) approximately 3 to 5 cm (1 to 2 inches). Note any lack of gluteal participation, cramping of the hamstrings, or excessive lumbar extension or rotation under hip extension load. Ideally, the lumbo-pelvic region should maintain a neutral position as the hip actively extends (approximately 10–15°). Hip extension should be initiated and maintained by the gluteus maximus. The muscle should have the ability to shorten sufficiently and hold the limb load in the joint inner-range position for 10 seconds, and repeat the movement 10 times (without the inner-range hold) and without substitution or fatigue. The hamstrings will participate in the movement but should not dominate. There will be paraspinal muscle activation (asymmetrically biased) but there should be no gross hyperextension, segmental shear (pivot), or rotation in the lumbar spine.

Global muscle imbalance—recruitment synergies: global mobilizer up-regulation

In the presence of chronic or recurrent musculoskeletal pain, one-joint global stabilizer synergists become inhibited and less efficient. In this situation, the global mobilizer synergists appear to become up-regulated and demonstrate increased recruitment of slow motor units, 'taking over' from the global stabilizers to become the dominant synergists to perform postural control tasks and non-fatiguing functional movements. Over time, as the global mobilizers participate excessively with increased tonic, slow motor unit recruitment in postural control tasks, the global mobilizer muscles lose extensibility. This loss of extensibility usually requires that some other motion segment increases movement as a compensation to maintain function. When the global mobility muscles lose extensibility, there may be changes in the contractile or connective tissue elements of the muscle. Recruitment issues or mechanical issues may influence these elements. The global mobility muscles need to be examined for length and recruitment changes.

- *Assessment for hamstring extensibility* (Comerford and Mottram 2014) (Figure 63.11): The subject sits with the spine and pelvis in neutral alignment, the acromion vertically positioned over the ischium, the hips flexed at 90° and the feet unsupported. The operator monitors the lumbo-pelvic position and passively extends the knee until either resistance to extension is felt (stretch in the posterior thigh) or there is a loss of lumbo-pelvic neutral position. Ideally, with maintenance of lumbo-pelvic neutral position and the hip flexed to 90°, the knee should be able to extend to within 10° of full extension. The lumbar spine should not flex and the pelvis should not posteriorly tilt or rotate. The shoulders should stay vertically aligned over the ischium and not lean back into hip extension.
- *Assessment for levator scapula extensibility* (Comerford and Mottram 2014) (Figure 63.12): Position the subject with cervical spine and scapula in neutral position (lying). The cervical spine

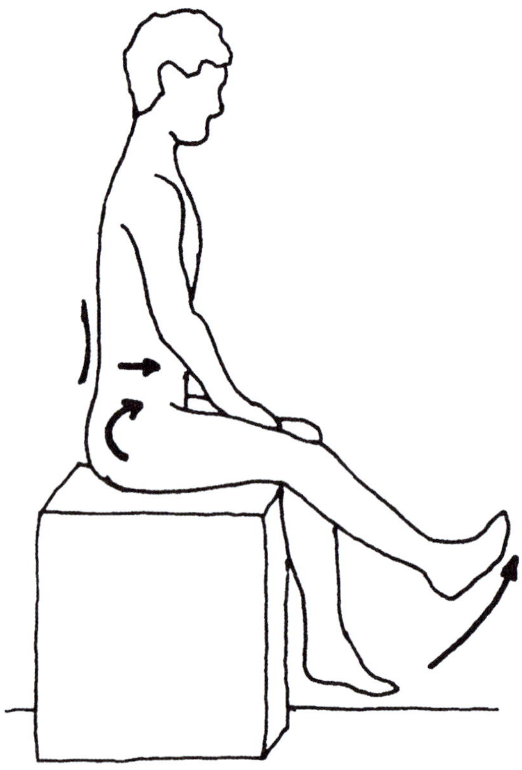

Figure 63.11 Hamstrings extensibility (reprinted with permission from Physiotools).

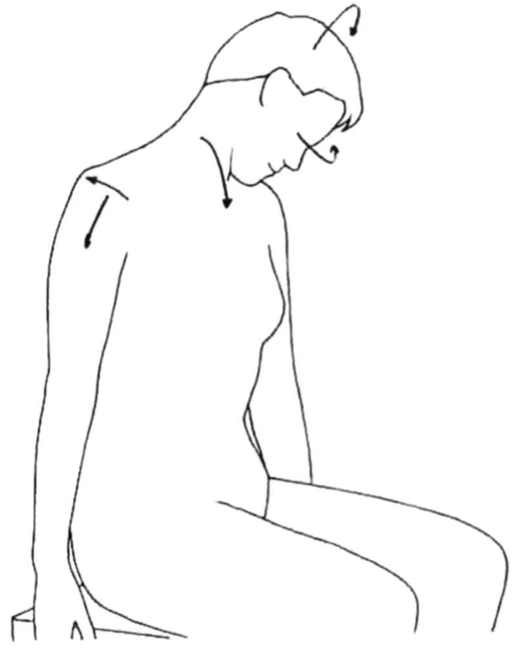

Figure 63.12 Levator scapulae extensibility (reprinted with permission from Physiotools).

is flexed, the head rotated and laterally flexed away from the side to be assessed. The head is moved until the extensibility limit of the levator scapula is reached or the scapula elevates to follow the muscle. Maintain this position and take tension off the muscle by passively elevating the shoulder. Then attempt to move the head into more range of lateral flexion. If there is no further available range, the cervical spine is at the limit of motion and the levator scapula muscle is not short. If there is more range available, then the levator scapula is short and limiting function.

Rehabilitation strategies for regaining control of uncontrolled movement

The retraining of movement control impairments will depend on the pattern of the impairment and the site and direction of the UCM. From the assessment of articular translational and myofascial restriction and for uncontrolled translation and range, retraining priorities can be identified. Making a diagnosis of the site and direction of UCM using movement control impairment tests, and then using this diagnosis to begin direction control retraining is a good first step in managing mechanical musculoskeletal pain. Correcting movement control impairments and recruitment patterns is the priority in the rehabilitation of the local stability system. Correcting length and impairments in the patterns of synergist recruitment between global stabilizers and global mobilizers is the priority of the global system. Addressing the restriction on uncontrolled compensation is the key to rehabilitation (Table 63.10) (Comerford and Mottram 2001b, 2012).

As well as dealing with mechanical components of movement dysfunction, the pathology must be addressed and non-mechanical issues identified and managed (Figure 63.13) (Comerford and Mottram 2001b, 2012). Fitness and exercise programmes have been shown to be an effective treatment approach for chronic LBP (Frost et al. 1998; Torstensen et al. 1998). Consideration of psychosocial factors is essential in the management of LBP (Kendall and Watson 2000; Main and Watson 1999; Watson 2000; Watson and Kendall 2000). Cognitive behavioural approaches have a significant role in the management of chronic LBP (Klaber Moffet et al. 1999; Waddell 1998; Watson 2000).

A useful guide for rehabilitation has been described using four principles of low load movement and stability rehabilitation (low threshold stability training) (Comerford and Mottram 2001b, 2012) (Table 63.11).

Principle I: Control of the site and direction of UCM

Principle II: Local control of translation in neutral position

Principle III: Global stabilizer control through range

Principle IV: Global mobilizer extensibility

Once these four principles have been achieved, an additional three principles of high threshold ('core') stability training can be integrated into high load function (Comerford and Mottram 2014).

Principle V: Control during overload training

Principle VI: Control during slow spinal and girdle movements

Principle VII: Control during high-speed movements

This chapter will not detail these last three principles of high threshold 'core' stability.

Principle I: Control of the site and direction of UCM

The key goal to effective retraining is to re-establish control of the UCM and regain normal mobility of motion restrictions. The direction control tests that diagnose the site and direction of UCM can also become the retraining strategies. The aim is to change the recruitment pattern and actively control movement at the site and in the direction of stability dysfunction (Comerford and Mottram 2001b, 2012, 2014).

This is a process of sensory motor re-programming. For example, if the movement control impairment is diagnosed as *lumbar flexion UCM*, the therapist would instruct the subject actively to control or prevent lumbar flexion (while using visual and palpation feedback) while bending forwards independently at the hips (hip flexion) (e.g. Figure 63.3) or while lowering the thoracic spine into flexion independently of any lumbar movement. The movement control retraining focuses on the joint region where the movement is actively being controlled or limited (lumbar flexion), not the joint that is producing the movement (hip flexion or thoracic flexion) that is challenging the ability to control the UCM. This involves active cognitive recruitment of the lumbar extensor stabilizer muscles to isometrically control lumbar flexion during slow repetitions of the exercise. The flexion movement at the hip or the thoracic spine creates a flexion loading challenge that the lumbar extensor stabilizer muscles have to continually work against.

Worsley et al. (2013) have demonstrated the clinical effectiveness of using this process in patients with shoulder impingement pathologies. They measured significant shoulder pain and disability, failure of a scapula movement control test, aberrant scapula muscle recruitment

Table 63.10 Rehabilitation strategy for restrictions and uncontrolled compensation

	Translation	Range
Uncontrolled movement (UCM)	The UCM may be uncontrolled translation, i.e. it is associated with laxity of joint connective tissues and aberrant recruitment of local stabilizer muscles, resulting in an abnormal control of translation and displacement of the PICM at an articular segment.	The UCM may be uncontrolled range, i.e. it is associated with excessive length or inefficient recruitment of global stabilizer muscles, resulting in increased relative flexibility.
	Articular	**Myofascial**
Restriction	The restriction may be articular, i.e. it is associated with a lack of mobility of the joint and its connective tissues (e.g. capsule), resulting in an abnormal decreased translation and displacement of the PICM at an articular segment.	The restriction may be myofascial, i.e. it is associated with a lack of extensibility of contractile myofascial tissue (especially global mobilizer muscle) or neural tissue, resulting in increased relative stiffness.

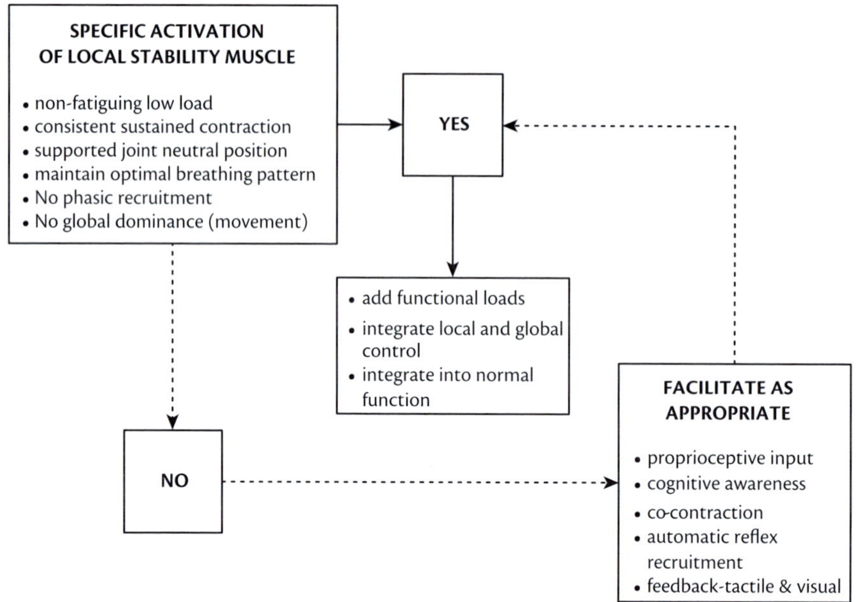

Figure 63.13 Model of rehabilitation (reprinted with permission from Movement Performance Solutions).

Table 63.11 Principles of movement control retraining

Principle I: Control of site and direction of UCM		Retrain control of the movement control impairments in the direction of symptom producing movements. Use the low threshold recruitment to control and limit motion at the segment or region of UCM and then actively move the adjacent restriction. Only move through as much range as the restriction allows or as far as the UCM is cognitively and efficiently controlled.
Principle II: Local control of translation in neutral position		Retrain low threshold activation of the local stabilizer muscle roles to increase muscle stiffness and control intersegmental displacement in the neutral training region.
Control of recruitment synergy imbalance	**Principle III: Global stabilizer control through range**	Retrain the global stabilizer muscle roles to actively control the full available range of joint motion. These muscles are required to be able to actively shorten and control limb load through to the full passive inner range of joint motion against gravity. They must also be able to control any hyper-mobile outer range. The ability to control rotational forces is an especially important role of global stabilizers. This is optimized by low-effort, sustained holds in the muscle's shortened position with controlled eccentric lowering.
	Principle IV: Global mobilizer extensibility	When the two-joint global mobilizer muscles demonstrate a lack of extensibility due to up-regulation or adaptive shortening, compensatory overstrain or UCM occurs elsewhere in the movement system in an attempt to maintain function. It becomes necessary to lengthen or inhibit over-activity in the global mobilizer muscles to eliminate the need for compensation to keep function.

(both delayed onset of activation and early termination of recruitment of the serratus anterior lower trapezius muscles) during arm movements, and altered scapula kinematics (reduced upward rotation and backward tilt) during arm movements. They showed that a 10-week movement control retraining programme, using scapular direction control retraining, achieved significant improvements in pain and disability, correction of movement control impairment, recovery of scapula muscle recruitment (onset of activation in termination of recruitment) to match normal controls, and recovery of normal scapula kinematics (increased upward rotation and backward tilt).

Another example of direction control retraining is for *cervical rotation UCM* where the subject needs to regain control of pain provocative cervical rotation (Figure 63.2). Position the cervical spine and scapula neutral, and rotate the head through the available range without substitution strategies (lateral flexion and chin poke). It may be useful to passively unload the ipsilateral scapula (taping, passive support). As range improves and symptoms decrease, the patient should begin to actively control the scapula position. This exercise can be started in a sitting position with support but should be progressed into function.

The sitting and standing bow tests can be used to retrain lumbar spine flexion stability dysfunction (Figures 63.3 and 63.4). The bent knee fallout test (Figure 63.5) can be used to retrain lumbo-pelvic rotation UCM.

Key points for rehabilitation

Retrain control of the site and direction of UCM:

- Specific recruitment and control exercise programmes need to be practised to restore normal muscle function (Comerford and Mottram 2001b, 2012; Sahrmann 2000).

- Control the UCM and move the restriction.
- Use conscious activation of the stability muscles to control or prevent the provocative movement and move the adjacent joint or motion segment.
- Movement at the adjacent joint should be independent of the region of poor movement control.
- Movement must be controlled eccentrically as well as concentrically.
- Move at adjacent joint only as far as:
  - control of the UCM can be maintained
  - the restriction at the adjacent joint allows.
- Try to use low to moderate effort to facilitate tonic recruitment. Maximum effort (co-contraction rigidity) is to be discouraged.
- The movement control impairment is direction-dependent and relates to the type and nature of pathology.
- Direction control movements are not stretches or strengthening exercises: Low force! No stretch! No strain! No substitution! No fatigue! No pain!

Principle II: Local control of translation in neutral position

Retraining the local stabilizer muscles to recover their low threshold recruitment and timing deficiencies in order to regain control of inter-segmental displacement or translation requires specific activation of the local stabilizer muscles, without substitution strategies. There is evidence that the transversus abdominis is controlled independently of other abdominal muscles (Hodges and Richardson 1999). The contraction needs to be sustained with the joint in neutral position and under low physiological load, independently of normal related reading and without movement (substitution with the global muscle system). The emphasis here is on motor control and recruitment and not strength and flexibility. The goal is to regain the normal automatic recruitment and timing of the local stabilizer muscle roles for the lumbar and cervical spines.

Teaching the specific activation of the local stability muscle role requires good clinical observation and instruction skills from the therapist. Local muscle retraining often requires specific facilitation techniques as appropriate (Figure 63.14) (Comerford and Mottram 2012, 2014). Facilitation techniques will help to improve proprioceptive awareness and cognitive activation, thus assisting in recovery of low threshold, slow motor unit recruitment.

Re-education of the local stabilizer role of the deep neck flexors requires the patient to learn a pure head nodding action (cranio-cervical flexion), which the clinician must carefully teach (Jull 1998; Jull et al. 2000). The gentleness and precision of the action needs to be reinforced. The aim is to train 10-second holds, with 10 repetitions, with the appropriate pressure change (Jull 1998) (Figure 63.6). As control and recruitment improves, the ability to sustain the optimal pressure change without substitution 'feels easy'.

The specific activation of the transversus abdominis is taught by asking the patient to gently draw in (hollow) the low abdominal wall (Hodges et al. 1996; Richardson and Hodges 1996; Richardson and Jull 1995; Richardson et al. 1999, 2004) (Figure 63.7). Facilitation and learning techniques can be employed to assist the patient.

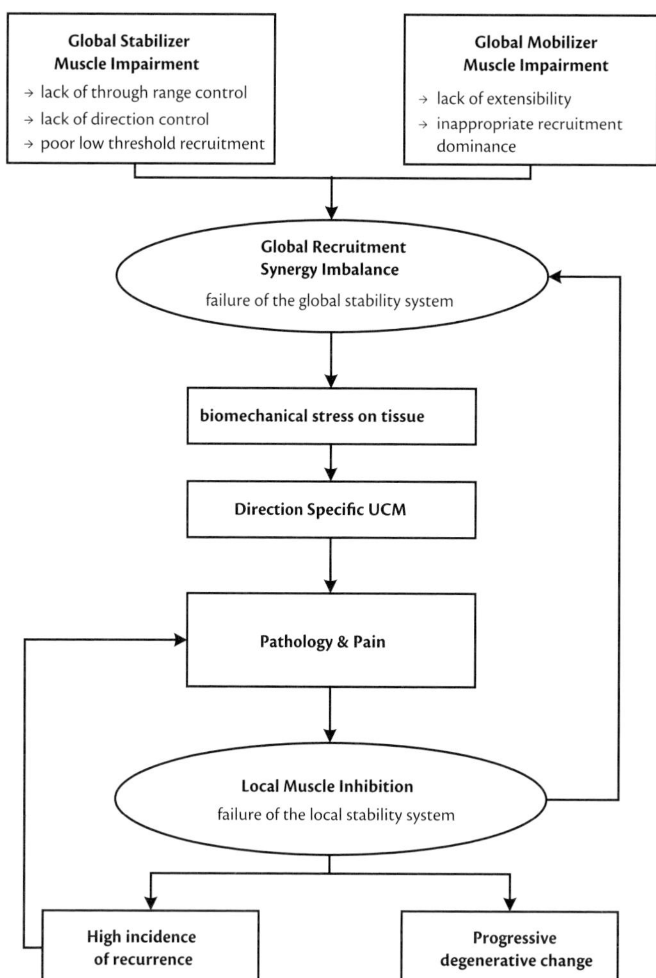

Figure 63.14 Specific recruitment of the local stability system (reprinted with permission from Movement Performance Solutions).

These include visualization and instructional cues (e.g. 'draw your lower abdomen up and in' to encourage conscious activation), tactile feedback, breathing control, and facilitation through a pelvic floor contraction or multifidus co-activation. Any facilitation through co-activation of other muscles should ideally be a short-term option, with specific cognitive activation using visual and palpation feedback being a preferable strategy.

Recruiting a sustained and repeatable multifidus contraction needs specific instruction (Hides et al. 1996) (Figure 63.8). Again, visualization and cues are useful facilitators, as is achieving a joint neutral spinal position (Hamilton 1998; Richardson et al. 1999).

The re-education of the local stabilizer role of the psoas major involves the action of longitudinal compression; for example, 'shortening the leg' or attempting 'to pull the hip into the socket'. Psoas contraction should increase stiffness segmentally in the lumbar spine and should resist motion segmentally rather than produce it. Optimal facilitation and retraining requires providing an appropriate low load facilitation and feedback. This training is best started in supine, side-lying, or inclined sitting position before progressing into function. Useful facilitation techniques are co-activation with the pelvic floor, breathing control, and low effort lateral rotation of the femur (Comerford and

Mottram 2012, 2014). During active retraining of the psoas, it is also essential to identify and eliminate various substitution strategies and faults.

The patient must at all times be able to maintain consistent specific recruitment of the local stabilizer muscle from their breathing pattern. Subjects with back pain have demonstrated difficulty dissociating respiration from recruitment of the lumbar stability muscles (Cairns et al. 2000; Richardson et al. 2004).Once activation has been achieved in the clinic, the patient needs to practise so that the motor control pattern becomes integrated into all functional positions (see Box 63.1) (Comerford and Mottram 2012, 2014).

O'Sullivan et al. (1997a) have demonstrated the clinical effectiveness and importance of the integration of the deep stability muscle system into functional movements, activities of daily living, and even to high loads and provocative positions.

Key points for rehabilitation

Activation of local and global stability muscles to control the neutral joint position:

- Specific activation of the deep local stability muscles in the neutral joint position.
- The contraction is biased for the local stability muscles.
- The contraction is isometric.
- The contraction should be biased for slow motor unit recruitment (low force).
- It is a conscious activation requiring motor planning and proprioceptive feedback.
- The ability to sustain a consistent low force hold is paramount for rehabilitation of motor control deficits.
- Optimal facilitation is dependent on identification and elimination of substitution strategies and overload or fatigue.

Box 63.1 Integration of local stability muscle recruitment into normal function

1. Activation in neutral alignment with a variety of different postures or positions (progression: supported → unsupported)
2. Activation in neutral alignment without co-contraction rigidity (for the trunk: activation with normal relaxed breathing; for the limbs: activation without resistance to passive rotation)
3. Activation in neutral alignment on an unstable base (add a proprioceptive challenge)
4. Activation during directional control exercises (dissociation or recruitment reversals)
5. Activation during normal physiological movements (the trunk and girdles actively move away from neutral position)
6. Activation during functional activities (normal movements of the unloaded limbs and trunk—'red dot' exercise)
7. Activation during stressful or provocative movements and positions (pathology- and symptom-specific)
8. Activation during occupational, recreational, or sport-specific skills

Reprinted with permission Movement Performance Solutions

- A high sensation of effort is permissible initially, but as control and functional integration return, a low sensation of effort activation should dominate.
- There should be no fatigue or substitution.
- Recruitment of the stability muscles to control the joint neutral position must be non-provocative and pain-free.
- Low threshold motor control retraining is the intention—not strength training.

Principle III: Global stabilizer through range control

When spinal stability can be maintained during movements of the limbs into flexion, extension, rotation, or abduction, then the global stability muscles can be retrained to achieve through-range control. Global stabilizer muscles are designed to be the dominant synergist producing and controlling motion during non-fatiguing functional movements and postural control tasks. Muscles with a global stabilizer role are therefore required to have the ability to:

- Concentrically shorten to synergistically contribute to joint motion in the full physiological inner-range position with no greater resistance than limb load against gravity, without substitution of the global mobilizer synergists.
- Isometrically hold this (or any other) position to sustain postural alignment or support functional trunk or limb load.
- Eccentrically control the return through range (limb lowering against gravity). The muscles are required to eccentrically control or decelerate rotational strain at all joints, especially the trunk and girdles. They should contribute significantly to rotation control in all functional movements.
- Control whatever functional range is available. Therefore, the global stabilizers should demonstrate efficient control of both normal and hypermobile ranges of motion.

There are five key elements to retraining the global stabilizer muscles to produce and control non-fatiguing range of motion (Comerford and Mottram 2012, 2014):

1. Retrain low threshold recruitment (low force/low load exercise). The stabilization force must be low actual effort—in the range of less than 30% of maximum voluntary contraction (MVC) to ensure efficient recruitment of low threshold slow motor units for non-fatiguing function.
2. Retrain holding time. Increasing the holding time of muscle activation aims to facilitate low threshold slow motor unit recruitment. The ability to sustain this contraction seems to be important for prevention of recurrence and for return of function (Hides et al. 1996; Hodges and Richardson 1996; Richardson and Jull 1995; Richardson et al. 2004). Optimal holding times may vary but the general clinical guide is of a 10-second, consistently sustained contraction, repeated 10 times.
3. Retrain the muscle's shortened position (inner-range hold) to increase force efficiency in ranges of postural control. The low-force, sustained contractions ideally should be performed in the muscle's shortened range, and at the point that can be comfortably held for 10 seconds, to facilitate muscle inner-range control and recovery of low threshold recruitment.
4. Retrain eccentric control muscle lengthening, especially during limb lowering against gravity. The eccentric control of the active

movement from the muscle's shortened position is important to retrain as part of the low-force, sustained hold. Poor eccentric control is commonly observed clinically. Eccentric control of the outer range of movement is especially important for movement control. If hypermobile range of motion is evident, eccentric control of that range has high priority.

Through-range control of the cervico-thoracic stabilizing extensors (semi-spinalis) is required to produce controlled low survival extension and rotation into shortened range and to eccentrically control the low cervical flexion through range (Figure 63.9). When movement is performed correctly (without substitution or fatigue), the range that can be controlled actively equals the available passive range of cervical extension.

5 Retrain the global stabilizer muscle's holding time to the point that through range can be controlled without substitution (ideally, 10-second hold for 10 repetitions).

Through-range control of the hip stabilizing extensors (gluteals) is required to produce controlled hip extension into shortened range and eccentrically control hip flexion through range. The patient supports their trunk on the edge of a bench, table, or bed with both feet supported on the floor and the knees slightly flexed. The lumbar spine is positioned in neutral alignment. The abdominal and gluteal muscles are co-activated to control the neutral spine and to prevent excessive lumbar extension. The patient is instructed to bend one knee to 90° and then lift that bent leg into hip extension. The hip extension must be independent of any lumbo-pelvic motion. The leg is extended only as far as the neutral lumbo-pelvic position can be maintained without cramping or over-activation of the hamstrings. At this point, the leg is slowly lowered back towards the floor. Initially, the patient may only be able to dissociate the lumbar spine (neutral) from hip extension to within 40°Flexion from horizontal.

As the ability to control lumbo-pelvic extension gets easier and the pattern of dissociation feels less unnatural, the exercise can be progressed to hip extension level with the horizontal (0°) and, eventually, to 10–15° of extension above the horizontal. When the patient can lift the leg horizontal (to 0° hip extension), and control lumbo-pelvic neutral position, the exercise can be progressed in prone position (Figure 63.10). The patient is positioned prone with a pillow under the pelvis (hips flexed to approximately 10–15°) to allow the gluteals to work from an efficient length. The subject is instructed to bend one knee past 90° (to relax the hamstrings) and then lift that knee (hip extension) approximately 3 to 5 cm (1 to 2 inches). The leg may lift into extension only as far as the neutral lumbo pelvic position can be maintained without cramping or over-activation of the hamstrings. At this point, the leg is slowly lowered back towards the floor while also maintaining the lumbo-pelvic neutral position.

Key points for rehabilitation

Low threshold recruitment, through-range control of the global stability muscles:

- Low force to encourage slow motor unit recruitment.
- Increasing the holding time of muscles that have a stability function has priority over strengthening. This is to facilitate recruitment of tonic fibres and train specificity of anti-gravity holding function.
- Shortened muscle position—a basic requirement of stability function is that the global stabilizer muscles have the ability to move the limbs (functional load) through their available range; or at least move the limbs through the same range that the synergistic global mobilizers can.
- Eccentric control is important to control the joint through range.
- The rotatory component of global stabilizer muscle action must be controlled during the low-force, sustained hold. Therefore, it is important to have reasonable rotation direction control ability prior to retraining the global stabilizer function.
- Exercise in a closed kinetic chain environment (distal fixation or weightbearing) allows better low threshold recruitment and also provides additional proprioceptive afferent information.
- No phasic recruitment or dominance of global muscles should be allowed.

Principle IV: global mobilizer extensibility

The global mobility muscles with centrally mediated up-regulation and over-activity have also frequently lost extensibility. There is a need to inhibit or down-regulate their excessive tonic, slow motor unit recruitment and to regain their ideal physiological length and extensibility. There are many appropriate techniques that can be employed to achieve this goal, e.g. inhibitory muscle lengthening, soft tissue techniques, and myofascial release. Rehabilitation should ensure that these multi-joint global mobilizers are not the dominant synergists for non-fatiguing functional movements and postural control tasks (Comerford and Mottram 2012, 2014). Their primary role is for high-load/high-speed activity.

Key points for rehabilitation

Regain extensibility and inhibit the short or over-active global mobility muscles:

- The aim here is to target the tight tissue, and techniques can be used to address the tight contractile or connective tissue. Techniques for regaining length and inhibition of over-active muscles include myofascial release, proprioceptive neuromuscular facilitation, muscle energy techniques, and active inhibitory restabilizations.
- An inhibitory lengthening technique, 'active inhibitory restabilization', is a useful technique for regaining length. It involves the operator gently and slowly lengthening the muscle until the resistance causes a slight loss of proximal girdle or trunk stability (into the stability dysfunction). The operator then maintains the muscle or limb in this position. The subject is then instructed to actively restabilize the proximal segment that has lost stability and sustain the correction for 20–30 seconds, repeat this 3–5 times. This encourages reciprocal inhibition of the over-active muscle and bonus proximal stability (Figures 63.11 and 63.12).

None of the corrective exercises to directly improve dynamic stability (Principles I, II, and III) should produce or provoke any symptoms at all. If any symptoms are aggravated or provoked by corrective exercises, first check that the exercise is being performed correctly, with appropriate low load and control. Overload is the most common cause of provocation. If an appropriate exercise is performed correctly but is still provocative, then other issues must be considered—acute inflammatory pathology, gross segmental instability, neurogenic or neuropathic pain, visceral pain, or serious medical pathology.

Conclusion: movement control impairments

There is a growing volume of evidence which suggests that improving muscle recruitment strategies and thresholds to restore ideal function, by assessing and correcting movement control impairments, is an integral part of the management of patients presenting with spinal pain of neuromusculoskeletal origin. Research evidence shows that patients with LBP may demonstrate movement control impairments in both the local and global stability systems, resulting in uncontrolled movement which can be diagnosed in terms of the site and direction of cognitive movement control deficiencies. Local muscle role impairments present as a change in the recruitment of the deep local stability muscles that have a role in maintaining dynamic stability at the spinal motion segments. Global movement control impairments present as a lack of global muscle control of direction, especially rotation, but also flexion, extension, and other directions. Global stabilizer muscle impairments also present as an imbalance in the recruitment thresholds and strategies between the one-joint global stabilizer and multi-joint global mobilizer synergists. The global stabilizer synergists demonstrate central down-regulation and inhibition, contributing to a lack of efficiency of through-range control of joint motion and poor low threshold postural recruitment. The global mobilizer synergists demonstrate central up-regulation and a loss of myofascial extensibility, together with inappropriate dominance of low threshold postural function. These changes are associated with the presentation of spinal pain, disability, and movement control impairments (Figure 63.15).

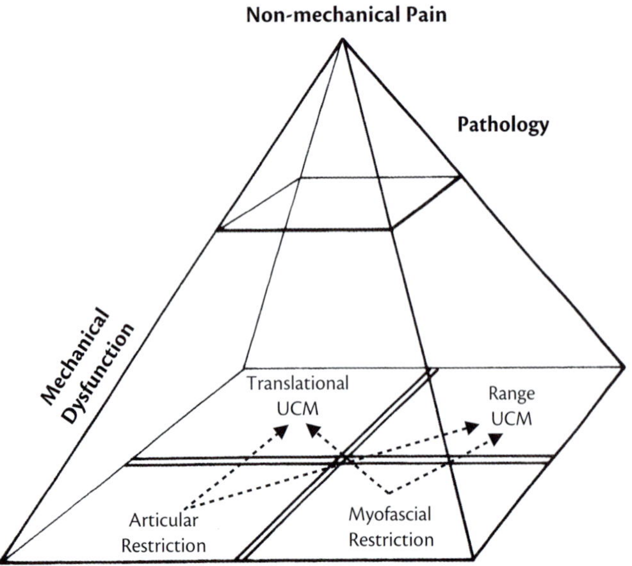

Figure 63.15 Movement dysfunction model (reprinted with permission from Movement Performance Solutions).

Assessment procedures and rehabilitation strategies for retraining movement control impairments in regaining control of the site and direction of UCM have been described (Comerford and Mottram 2001a,b, 2012; Richardson et al. 1999, 2004) and there is evidence of effectiveness for movement control retraining programmes (Beeton and Jull 1994; Grant et al. 1997; Hides 1998; O'Sullivan et al. 1997a, 1998).

The ability to assess movement function and correct movement control impairments is a key clinical skill required when managing neuromusculoskeletal pain and dysfunction. Evidence suggests that therapists would benefit from having the skills to assess for UCM and rehabilitate movement control impairments in patients attending the clinic with spinal pain, both acute and chronic.

References

Balster SM, Jull GA (1977) Upper trapezius muscle activity during the brachial plexus tension test in asymptomatic subjects. *Manual Therapy* 2(3):144–9.

Bergmark A (1989) Stability of the lumbar spine: a study in mechanical engineering. *Acta Orthopaedica Scandinavica* 230(60):20–4.

Brumagne S, Lysens R, Swinnen S, Verschueren S (1999) Effect of paraspinal muscle vibration on position of lumbosacral spine. *Spine* 24(13): 1328–31.

Butler D (1998) Integrating pain awareness into physiotherapy—wise action for the future. In: Gifford L (ed.) *Topical ssues in pain*. CNS Press, Falmouth, pp. 1–23.

Cairns MC, Harrison K, Wright C (2000) Pressure biofeedback: a useful tool in quantification of abdominal muscular dysfunction? *Physiotherapy* 86(3):127–38.

Cholewicki J, McGill SM (1996) Mechanical stability of the in vivo lumbar spine: implications for injury and chronic low back pain. *Clinical Biomechanics* 11(1):1–15.

Comerford M (1997) *Dynamic stabilisation—evidence of muscle dysfunction*. Conference Proceedings, British Institute of Musculoskeletal Medicine, London

Comerford MJ, Emerson (1999) Personal communication.

Comerford MJ, Mottram SL (2001a) Functional stability retraining: principles and strategies for managing mechanical dysfunction. *Manual Therapy* 6(1):3–14.

Comerford MJ, Mottram SL (2001b) Movement and stability dysfunction—contemporary developments. *Manual Therapy* 6(1):15–26.

Comerford MJ, Mottram SL (2012) *Kinetic control: the management of uncontrolled movement*. Elsevier, Australia.

Comerford MJ, Mottram SL (2014) *The movement solution: assessment and retraining of uncontrolled movement*. (Course manual). Movement Performance Solutions, Chichester, UK.

Dangaria TR, Naesh O (1998) Changes in cross-sectional area of psoas major muscle in unilateral sciatica caused by disc herniation. *Spine* 23(8): 928–31.

Edgar D, Jull G, Sutton S (1994) The relationship between upper trapezius muscle length and upper quadrant neural tissue extensibility. *Australian Journal of Physiotherapy* 4:99–103.

Frost H, Lamb S E, Klaber Moffet JA, Fairbank JC, Moser JJ (1998) A fitness programme for patients with chronic low back pain: 2 year follow up after a randomized controlled trial. *Pain* 75:273–9.

Goff B (1972) The application of recent advances in neurophysiology to Miss Rood's concept of neuromuscular facilitation. *Physiotherapy* 58(2): 409–15.

Goldspink G, Williams P (1992) Muscle fibre and connective tissue changes associated with use and disuse. In: Ada L, Canning C (eds). *Physiotherapy: foundations for practice. Key issues in neurological physiotherapy*. pp. 197–217.

Gossman MR, Sahrmann SA, Rose SJ (1982) Review of length-associated changes in muscle. *Physical Therapy* 62(12):1799–808.

Grant R, Jull G, Spencer T (1997) Active stabilisation training for screen based keyboard operators—a single case study. *Australian Journal of Physiotherapy* 43(4):235–42.

Hall TM, Elvey RL (1999) Nerve trunk pain: physical diagnosis and treatment. *Manual Therapy* 4(2):63–73.

Hall T, Zusman M, Elvey R (1998) Adverse mechanical tension in the nervous system? Analysis of straight leg raise. *Manual Therapy* 3(3):140–6.

Hamilton C (1998) *Active control of the neutral lumbopelvic posture; a comparison between back pain and non-back pain subjects*. Proceedings of 3rd Interdisciplinary World Congress on Low Back and Pelvic Pain, Vienna.

Hides JA (1998) *The lumbar multifidus: evidence of a link to low back pain*. Proceedings of 3rd Interdisciplinary World Congress on Low Back and Pelvic Pain, Vienna.

Hides JA, Richardson CA, Jull GA (1996) Multifidus recovery is not automatic after resolution of acute, first-episode low back pain. *Spine* 21(23):2763–9.

Hides JA, Stokes MJ, Saide M, Jull GA, Cooper DH (1994) Evidence of multifidus wasting ipsilateral to symptoms in patients with acute/subacute low back pain. *Spine* 19(2):165–77.

Hodges PW, Richardson CA (1996) Inefficient muscular stabilisation of the lumbar spine associated with low back pain: a motor control evaluation of transversus abdominis. *Spine* 21(22):2640–50.

Hodges PW, Richardson CA (1999) Transversus abdominis and the superficial abdominal muscles are controlled independently in a postural task. *Neuroscience Letters* 265(2):91–4.

Hodges PW, Moseley GL (2003) Pain and motor control of the lumbopelvic region: effect and possible mechanisms. *J. Electromyogr. Kinesiol.* 13(4):361–70.

Hodges PW, Richardson CA, Jull GA (1996) Evaluation of the relationship between laboratory and clinical tests of transversus abdominis function. *Physiotherapy Research International* 1:30–40.

Hodges PW, Gandeva SC (2000) Activation of the human diaphragm during a repetitive postural task. *J. Physiol.* 5222(Pt 1):165–175.

Hurley MV (1997) The effects of joint damage on muscle function, proprioception and rehabilitation. *Manual Therapy* 1(5):11–17.

Hurley MV, Newham DJ (1993) The influence of arthrogenous muscle inhibition on quadriceps rehabilitation of patients with early, unilateral osteoarthritic knees. *British Journal of Rheumatology* 32:127–31.

Janda VL (1985) Pain in the locomotor system—a broad approach. In: Glasgow, et al. (eds) *Aspects of manipulative therapy*. Churchill Livingstone, pp. 148–51.

Janda VL (1994) Muscles and motor control in cervicogenic disorders: assessment and management. In: Grant R (ed.) *Physical therapy of the cervical and thoracic spine*. Churchill Livingstone, pp. 195–216.

Jull G (1997) Management of cervical headache. *Manual Therapy* 2(4):182–90.

Jull G (1998) Physiotherapy management of neck pain of mechanical origin. In: Giles LGF, Singer KP (eds) *Clinical anatomy and management of cervical spine pain*. Butterworth-Heinemann, Oxford, pp. 168–91.

Jull GA, Richardson CA (2000) Motor control problems in patients with spinal pain: a new direction for therapeutic exercise. *J. Manipulative Physiol.* 23(2):115–7.

Jull G, Barrett C, Magee R, Ho P (1999) Further clinical clarification of the muscle dysfunction in cervical headache. *Cephalalgia* 19(3):179–85.

Kankaanpaa M, Taimela S, Laaksonen D, Hanninen O, Airaksinen O (1998) Back and hip extensor fatigability in chronic low back pain patients. *Archives in Physical Medicine and Rehabilitation* 79:412–7.

Kendall N, Watson P (2000) Identifying psychosocial yellow flags and modifying management. In: Gifford L (ed.) *Topical issues in pain 2—biopsychosocial assessment and management*. CNS Press, Falmouth, pp. 131–9.

Klaber Moffet JA, Torgerson D, Bell-Syer (1999) Randomized controlled trail of exercise for low back pain: Clinical outcomes, costs, and preferences. *British Medical Journal* 319:279–83.

Lee DG (1996) Rotational instability of the mid-thoracic spine: assessment and treatment. *Manual Therapy* 1(5):234–41.

Main CJ, Watson PJ (1999) Psychological aspects of pain. *Manual Therapy* 4(4):203–15.

Maitland G, Hengeveld E, Banks K, English K (2005) *Maitland's vertebral manipulation* (7th edn). Elsevier.

Mottram SL (1997) Dynamic stability of the scapula. *Manual Therapy* 2(3):123–31.

Mottram SL, Comerford M (1999) Stability dysfunction and low back pain. *Journal of Orthopaedic Medicine* 20(2):13–18.

O'Sullivan PB (2000) Lumbar segmental 'instability': clinical presentation and specific stabilizing exercise management. *Manual Therapy* 5(1):2–12.

O'Sullivan PB, Twomey L, Allison G, Sinclair J, Miller K, Knox J (1997a) Altered patterns of abdominal muscle activation in patients with chronic low back pain. *Australian Journal of Physiotherapy* 43(2):91–8.

O'Sullivan PB, Twomey L, Allison G (1997b) Evaluation of specific stabilising exercises in the treatment of chronic low back pain with radiological diagnosis of spondylosis or spondylolisthesis. *Spine* 22(24):2959–67.

O'Sullivan P, Twomey L, Allison G (1998) Altered abdominal muscle recruitment in back pain patients following specific exercise intervention. *Journal of Orthopaedic Sports Physical Therapy* 27(2):114–24.

Panjabi MM (1992) The stabilising system of the spine. Part 1: Function, dysfunction, adaptation, and enhancement. *Journal of Spinal Disorders* 5(4):383–9.

Richardson CA, Jull GA (1995) Muscle control—pain control. What exercises would you prescribe? *Manual Therapy* 1:1–9.

Richardson C, Hodges P, Hides J (2004) *Therapeutic exercise for lumbopelvic stabilization: motor control approach for the treatment and prevention of low back pain* (2nd edn). Churchill Livingstone.

Richardson C, Jull G, Hodges P, Hides J (1999) *Therapeutic exercise for spinal segmental stabilization in low back pain: scientific basis and clinical approach*. Churchill Livingstone.

Sahrmann SA (1993) *Movement as a cause of musculoskeletal pain*. Proceedings of the 8th Biennial Conference of the Manipulative Physiotherapists' Association of Australia, Perth.

Sahrmann SA (2002) *Diagnosis and treatment of management impairment syndromes*. Mosby, USA.

Sahrmann SA (2011) *Movement system impairment syndromes of the extremities, cervical and thoracic spines*. Elsevier, USA.

Sapsford RR, Hodges PW, Richardson CA (1997) Activation of pubococcygeus during a variety of isometric abdominal exercise, Abstract, International Continence Conference, Japan.

Schaible H, Grubb BD (1993) Afferent and spinal mechanisms of joint pain. *Pain* 55:5–55.

Stokes M, Young A (1984) The contribution of reflex inhibition to arthrogenous muscle weakness. *Clinical Science* 67:7–14.

Taimela S, Kankaanpaa M, Luoto S (1999) The effects of lumbar fatigue on the ability to sense a change in lumbar position. *Spine* 24(13):1322–7.

Torstensen TA, Ljunggren AE, Meen HD, et al. (1998) Efficiency and costs of medical exercise therapy, conventional physiotherapy, and self-exercise in patients with chronic low back pain. *Spine* 23(23):2616–24.

Waddell G (1998) *The back pain revolution*. Churchill Livingstone, Edinburgh.

Watson P (2000) Psychosocial predictors of outcomes from low back pain. In: Gifford L (ed.) *Topical issues in pain 2—biopsychosocial assessment and management*. CNS Press, Falmouth, pp. 5–109.

Watson P, Kendall N (2000) Assessing psychosocial yellow flags. In: Gifford L (ed.) *Topical issues in pain 2—biopsychosocial assessment and management*. CNS Press, Falmouth, pp. 111–29.

Worsley P, Warner M, Mottram S, et al (2013) Motor control retraining exercise for shoulder impingement: effects on function, muscle activation, and biomechanics in young adults. *Journal of Shoulder and Elbow Surgery* 22:e11–e19.

Chapter 64

Chronic pain management

Grahame Brown

Introduction to chronic pain management

In order to manage pain, its function and basic physiology needs to be understood. Despite the huge advances in our scientific understanding of pain as the result of research over the past few decades, today, most people and many health professionals still do not understand pain.

The nature of pain has puzzled humanity for centuries. Many different models of pain have been put forward over the years and our thinking is always constrained by prevailing conceptual models.

The Cartesian model of pain was developed in the seventeenth century after French philosopher, Rene Descartes, and based on a fundamental dualistic view of mind and body. The legacy of this model is still very prevalent in clinical practice and society, in that pain is still viewed as either organic (i.e. in the tissues—think of the language many clinicians continue to use as they search for 'pain generating tissues') or psychological. Logical to this concept is that clinicians will do many and repeated investigations and treatments aimed at the tissues when a patient presents with pain, and only when this fails to relieve pain, as it often does, will any thought be given to the psychological and social determinants of pain and a referral to the 'pain clinic' be made, by which time the patient will often be in a state of despair, feeling helpless and hopeless. In many healthcare systems, the concept of rehabilitation is viewed in a similar way: something that is done only when all possible biomedical interventions have been exhausted (Waddell and Burton 2004).

The biopsychosocial model allows us to understand a person's experience of their pain in the context of their life, culture, hopes and aspirations, past experiences, thoughts, feelings, and relationships, influenced by information gained both consciously and subconsciously from family, friends, media, and healthcare professionals. Despite the overwhelming evidence for the effectiveness of this approach to someone in pain, especially chronic pain, it is depressingly common to see evidence of the damage done to patients by what has been said to them by healthcare professionals, especially after magnetic resonance imaging (MRI) scanning of the spine.

The concepts of pain management discussed here are intended to be integrated into every contact with a patient who consults with a pain problem, wherever they might be on the spectrum from acute, chronic (from here on, meaning persistent over time), or acute flare-up of a chronic problem. Identifying, and modifying where possible, risk factors that predict chronicity (Linton 2000), at every clinical encounter, is vital to help reduce the risk of a slide into disability and chronicity. There is an excellent and well-validated tool available to help determine those persons with back pain at increased risk of chronicity when they first present in a primary care setting (Hill et al. 2008).

As soon as a clinician hears that a pain persists, is spreading, is worsening, and is unpredictable, and that lots of movements (even small ones) hurt, then the pain is more related to central nervous system processes than tissue processes (clearly assuming that, in some patients, tests will need to be done if possible serious or destructive pathology is suspected). Patients with this type of pain will often collect a number of different diagnostic labels depending on who they have seen; for example, myofascial pain syndrome, somatic dysfunction, non-specific back pain, neuropathic pain, fibromyalgia, psychosomatic pain, degenerative disc disease. The signs and symptoms of these 'diagnoses' can readily be explained at a biological level by sensitization of all or part of the central nervous system.

Important concepts of pain

All pain experiences are real and normal: *pain is a response from the brain when it computes that there is a threatening situation.* Many parts of the central nervous system (CNS) are involved in the pain response. Even when pain is chronic, it hurts because the brain has concluded, for one reason or another, often completely subconsciously, that there is a threat. Even if there are no problems whatsoever in the tissues or immune system, it will still hurt if the brain computes that there is danger. *The key is finding out why the brain has come to this conclusion* (Butler and Moseley 2003).

No one wants pain. Once a person has it, they naturally want to get rid of it. Pain demands attention: this is the very thing that makes it so effective and a given of life. Pain protects; it makes a person behave, move, and think differently to facilitate healing. It can be so effective that it suspends thinking, feeling, or the ability to focus on anything else (Butler and Moseley 2003).

Occasionally, the pain system acts in odd ways (Melzack and Wall 1996): tissue injury but no pain (for example, advanced osteoarthritis of a hip joint on X-ray when a patient presents with loss of hip mobility but no pain), pain persisting way beyond tissue healing time (for example, chronic low back pain), or pain in the absence of tissues (phantom limb). Sometimes, the pain system fails (for example, it fails to give early warning of many cancers). Sometimes, the peripheral nerves are damaged as a result of disease and fail to alert to danger (for example, leprosy and diabetic neuropathy).

The threat value of pain contributes directly to the pain experience. By helping people to understand what is happening inside their bodies, clinicians can reduce the threat. This must be done at every clinical encounter and alongside whatever tissue treatment that may be provided. By doing so, intervention treatments will be more effective.

There are many and varied cues that relate to the pain experience; for example, movements, thoughts, anticipation, emotions, attention, memories, sounds, visual experiences, the environment. However, it is the brain that decides whether something hurts or not: there are no exceptions. If there is no pain, it means that changes in the tissues are not perceived by the brain to be threatening (Butler and Moseley 2003).

Pain relates to context. It is going to hurt much more if the threat is perceived as affecting at least one important *need* met in life (Box 64.1); for example, the need for status, which might be met at work or in sport. It is also going to hurt more if a grievance is being carried together with a believe that someone else should be blamed for pain and if there is a desire to right a perceived wrong through the civil tort system, or if there is compensation available.

The language that is used, especially amongst healthcare professionals, directly affects the pain experience. For example, pain that persists is often described as *neuropathic*, implying that there is an organic pathological process at work. This might be the case in some conditions such as diabetic neuropathy. It sounds very scary, especially if the patient is in a state of high anxiety. The vast majority of people with chronic pain have disordered functioning within the CNS, i.e. neurogenic pain. Musculoskeletal clinicians will be acquainted with the harm caused to people with back pain by repeated reference to terms like 'degenerative disc disease', 'arthritis of the spine', 'discs out', and so on: all potentially very disempowering for a person in pain, and likely to increase fear and avoidant response.

Nociception (literally 'noxious reception' or 'danger reception') in the tissues is *neither sufficient nor necessary for pain* (remember phantom limb pain) (Butler and Moseley 2003).

Danger-alert nerve pathways multiply with use in the dorsal horn of the spinal cord—a process known as sensitization (Doubell et al. 1999). This process is also known to occur in the brain (Flor et al. 1997). Consequently, over time, the area that hurts seems to hurt more and with less provocation and the pain gradually spreads. The increased traffic down the *facilitating* pathway from the brain to the spinal cord dorsal horn causes these circuits to increase in number, thus increasing the sensitization, or, put another way, turning up the gain control. Activity down the facilitating pathway from the brain to the dorsal horn can be thought of as an amplification system, and traffic down this pathway is stimulated by focused attention on the hurting area (i.e. introspection), also a key feature of depression, anxiety, fear, and anger. These strong emotional responses also keep the chemical and hormonal 'fight or flight' system primed, which increases the sensitization. The immune system is also impaired, over time, under these chronic stress influences.

Absolutely critical to understand is that the descending *inhibitory* pathway from the brain to the dorsal horn of the spinal cord is *the most powerful analgesic*. It can be thought of as a muting system. Activity down this pathway is stimulated by distraction, deep relaxation (meaning stimulation of the parasympathetic nervous system by breathing training), satisfying activity that absorbs our attention, at least one satisfying close relationship, fun and laughter, pleasurable physical activity, and a feeling of being in control. Pain management programmes must aim to help a person focus on meeting these needs for themselves and thus, at a biological level, stimulate and reactivate the descending inhibitory pathway from the brain to the dorsal horn of the spinal cord.

Box 64.1 Emotional *needs* and *resources* to allow fulfilment of potential

When these needs, which are genetically programmed into humans, are not being met, or if the resources are misused are damaged through development or organic brain disease, then poor emotional health is experienced (Griffin and Tyrrell 2013).

Emotional needs include:

- Security—safe territory and environment
- Attention—to give and receive
- Sense of autonomy and control
- Being emotionally connected to others
- Being part of a wider community
- Friendship, fun, love, intimacy
- Sense of status within social groupings
- Sense of competence and achievement
- Meaning and purpose—which come from being stretched in what a person does and thinks
- Time for quietness and reflection

The resources nature has given to help in meeting these needs include:

- The ability to develop complex long-term memory, which enables adding to innate knowledge and learning
- The ability to build rapport, empathize, and connect with others
- Imagination, which enables focus of attention away from the emotions and to problem solve more creatively and effectively
- A conscious, rational mind that can check emotions, question, analyse, and plan (left hemisphere)
- The ability to 'know'—understand the world unconsciously through metaphorical pattern matching (right hemisphere)
- An observing self—that part of the mind which can step back, be more objective, and recognize itself as a unique centre of awareness, apart from intellect, emotion, and conditioning (frontal lobes)
- A dreaming brain that preserves the integrity of the genetic inheritance every night by metaphorical defusing of emotionally arousing introspections not acted out the previous day.

These are known as the 'human givens'.

The APET model

The APET model, out of which effective counselling and psychotherapy happen, offers the most psychologically sophisticated and physiologically accurate view of mind–body functioning available for psycho-behavioural interventions for depression, anxiety disorders, anger problems, chronic pain, etc. (Griffin and Tyrrell 2013).

The 'A' in APET stands for activating agent—a stimulus from the environment—that is taken in through the senses and processed in the pattern ('P') matching part of the brain (subconscious). This, in turn, gives rise to an emotion ('E') which may or may not initiate certain thoughts ('T'). Most pattern matching is unconscious and does not necessarily result in a thought.

An important advantage of this holistic, scientific model is that the practitioners who operate from it can more easily see how to make interventions, as appropriate, at any stage in therapy. They can work to change the stimulus in the environment that is causing the problem or they can put in bigger, more useful patterns, using reframes and metaphors (P), lower emotional arousal (E), and work on thinking style (T).

The RIGAAR method

A recommended framework for a solution-focused approach to a consultation with a patient in chronic pain is the RIGAAR model, in which 'R' stands for rapport building, 'I' for information gathering, 'G' for goal setting, 'A' for accessing resources, 'A' for agreeing a strategy for change, and 'R' for rehearsing the strategy for change. This framework is also a basis for motivational interviewing.

Rapport building

Before a clinician can have a beneficial effect for a patient, a relationship has to be built with them, both at the verbal and non-verbal level. Non-verbally, rapport is created through matching the behaviour and the characteristics of the patient. This is an instinctive process; for example, whenever possible, walk into the consulting room with the patient. At the verbal level, it is very helpful, initially, to use truisms and 'yes sets'. Walking into the room with the patient provides an early opportunity; for example:

PRACTITIONER: 'Well done, you found our office then?'
PATIENT: 'Yes.'
PRACTITIONER: 'And your name is John?'
PATIENT: 'Yes.'
PRACTITIONER: 'It's a lovely day out there isn't it?'
PATIENT: 'Yes.'

'Yes sets', used sparingly like this, help to bypass resistance and prepare the client for change. Develop empathy (which is not the same as liking) by matching tonality of voice and body language. Aim to enter the client's mode of reality through a process of *reflective* listening.

Information gathering

What is needed is high-quality information from a patient, and not an exhaustive diary of the treatment investigation process (the patient often thinks that clinicians want to know all this as a priority). Important to know, for example, is what else was going on in the patient's life at or shortly before the time they started to experience their pain or during flare-ups. It is very common to uncover major negative life events that occurred in the weeks or months before the onset of the pain, which the client had never thought relevant to the pain problem.

Listen to the description of the symptoms from the patient using their own words. Generally, the terms used will fall into one of three main categories: *sensory, cognitive-evaluative*, or *emotional* (Melzack 1975). Pay attention not just to *what is said* but, crucially, *how it is said,* as a strong affect may be present and, if identified, needs to be reflected back to the patient as part of the reflective listening process. In this way, the patient will feel understood and will more likely confide useful information; for example, 'As I understand it John, you have been experiencing this intense and often burning pain in the back, buttock, and thigh for over 6 months, and the way it has started to dominate your life has left you feeling quite angry.'

Also important is the need to know how the client has tried to deal with their pain and what, through their own efforts, they have found helpful for providing relief and enabling them to cope. Aim to have a good idea of the patient's attitudes and beliefs surrounding their pain, as well as their anxieties about it. How do they behave in response to their pain, especially flare-ups? What is the patient expecting from the consultation? It is easy for a health professional to assume what the patient wants, but when this question is asked, the response can often be surprising.

The physical examination is so important, especially in this age of high-tech medicine and scanning: it provides a unique opportunity for rapport building, as well as for assessing the tissues, and, in chronic pain problems, the skill of palpation provides an invaluable window on the sensitized CNS (Gunn 1997). Be curious to find out what the patient thinks is the cause of their problem and what their preferences for treatments are.

Throughout this process, look out for any instances where the client is not getting their essential emotional needs (Box 64.1) met; with practice, this becomes an instinctive process.

> Fear generates anxiety and anxiety focuses the attention. The more attention is locked, the worse the pain.
>
> Dr Patrick Wall (1925–2001)

Goal setting

Establish where the patient wants to go. All too commonly, the patient wants 'to be out of pain'; aiming for the absence of something so abstract is very hard and often unachievable. It is also a focus on the negative. Encourage the client, and persist if necessary, to identify positive goals which are *specific, **m**easurable, **a**chievable, **r**elevant* to the client, and ***t**ime-oriented* (SMART). For example: 'What would you like to be *doing* [next week, in six months, in a year] that you cannot do at present because of your pain?' Notice how this powerful question forces the patient to look forward, to use their imagination, and to focus away from feelings into action and doing. It also identifies motivation for change.

Then, identify for the patient any *obstacles* to achieving that goal, for example, fear of pain, depressed mood, sleep disturbance, difficulty relaxing, physical deconditioning, work factors, and so on. Remember that there may be social, financial, and occupational/vocational barriers to progressing towards some goals, which are beyond the influence of clinical intervention or even the patient's efforts. Help the client to identify these if necessary, as it will ultimately reduce anxiety and help with problem solving.

All of this process places the patient in problem-solving mode. Move towards helping the client gain control over their pain and life, and to meeting their unmet *needs* rather than *wants.*

Access resources

Having agreed an outcome together, aim to motivate the patient to feel able to take on the large task of making the necessary changes in their life. In chronic conditions, the patient is likely to have low self-esteem and feel incapable of making changes. It is from a state of self-empowerment that people believe it is possible to make changes happen, so do something straight away to increase the client's confidence. Often a quick way of doing this is to get the client to recount successes and achievements they have already had in their lives. This raises their sense of self-sufficiency and can also be a source of metaphors to use. Find out what they like doing that gives pleasure and use these resources in metaphor.

> It is much more important to know what sort of a patient has a disease than what sort of a disease a patient has.
>
> Sir William Osler (1849–1919)

Agreeing a strategy for change/management

This is the place for providing information that might include the biology of pain and the major differences between acute and chronic pain, the dysfunction in the musculoskeletal system and nervous system, or interpretation of scans. This cognitive approach is very helpful of course, *but only if* the patient is relaxed enough to have an open and therefore problem-solving state of mind. A highly aroused person (through fear, anxiety, depression, or anger) will experience an 'emotional hijack' of their cognitive functions and will be thinking, as the emotional brain does, in only two dimensions: black or white, right or wrong, total pain or no pain. If by this stage of the consultation, it has been difficult to lower emotional arousal, then work at a cognitive level is a waste of time and effort. It might be prudent to invite the patient to return for another appointment.

A behavioural approach might be agreed, such as becoming more physically active (always important in patients with depression or chronic pain). Eliciting such behavioural change will always be more effective when working with the resources of the patient. For example, it might occur to the clinician that exercise in a gym or swimming pool is likely to be most helpful, and it may be *if* the patient does it! However, if the patient prefers gardening or dancing or country walks with their dog, then adherence to, and sustaining of, a more active lifestyle is likely to be more effective by encouraging these activities. While obvious, it is surprising how many healthcare professionals fail to recognize this.

Where the patient resists making changes to a dysfunctional view, then metaphor and stories are very powerful at bypassing cognitive resistance. If the clinician has the skills and it is appropriate in the context of the clinical encounter, guided imagery, after relaxing the client, is immensely powerful in these situations. Very few people will resist the offer, well intended, to be able to relax a little more.

Sometimes it can become apparent that the single biggest obstacle to progress in a chronic pain patient is post-traumatic stress. Look out for this if the onset of pain occurred following trauma of any kind. It might be at a level below which a diagnosis of post-traumatic stress disorder (PTSD) would be made; what psychotherapists call 'sub-threshold trauma'. The author believes this to be common in musculoskeletal medicine practice: simply ask a patient who tends to catastrophize flare-ups of acute to chronic pain to rewind for a few moments and recall what thoughts and feelings they experienced when they had their very first episode of pain in that part of their body. The APET model already described allows for an understanding of this process in the subconcious brain. Also, a large number of patients who experience chronic whole-body pain, fatigue, unrefreshing sleep, and other somatic symptoms (commonly described as fibromyalgia) have a history of an unhappy childhood. In such people who have persistent post-traumatic stress in the context of chronic pain, trauma-focused cognitive behavioural therapy (NICE 2005) and other brief solution-focused therapies such as 'Human Givens' (Griffin and Tyrrell 2013) and EMDR (eye movement desensitization reprocessing) (NICE 2005), within the context of a multidisciplinary clinic setting, can have hugely beneficial effects for the patient's rehabilitation, provided always, of course, that the patient is ready to engage with such treatment.

Rehearsing the strategy for change

This is achieved through the brain's reality simulator—in other words, getting the patients to use their imagination. This is a tool that nature has given to enable rehearsal of changes before they are made. Quite simply, it entails asking the patient to imagine themselves carrying out the changes that they want to make. This creates a template for success in their minds and links what has been discussed with the outside world. They are visualizing the actual events and reactions they are going to encounter, and their own desired reactions to them. Going through the reality simulator provides the patient with an opportunity to check out how realistic their therapeutic strategies are. Patients in pain are frequently reassured to know that most elite sportspeople use these same techniques to maximize performance. If the client needs any resources or additional help, or if the goals need to be divided into smaller ones, it can be done at this stage. These techniques can also be very useful in assisting a player to return to sport participation after trauma.

This exercise can be done in different ways. Particularly useful for the musculoskeletal practitioner is to demonstrate one or two simple exercises for the patient to do and project them into the context of the patient's life: this might be a forward rolling of the spine in the standing position (from yoga) that can be done in the office or kitchen, or a diaphragm breathing exercise to relieve tension in the neck that can be done as mini-break exercise in 3–5 minutes while sitting or standing almost anywhere.

Valuable communication skills when dealing with patients in chronic pain

There are additional communication skills, not already referred to, that are useful when dealing with patients in chronic pain.

Reframing statements

This helps the patient to see their problems in a different and wider context. For example, used with a man who is excessively introspecting about why he should have developed backache (with no serious pathology) at the age of 50, one could say: 'Well done for reaching 50 without being troubled by this complaint before. It most commonly starts much earlier. You must have a stronger back than most.' Similarly, used with a patient who believes his spinal nerves are damaged: 'Well, they are at present certainly over-active and firing excessively and, sometimes, inappropriately.' For someone with sciatica who believes her nerve is trapped: 'The nerve sleeve is very sensitive and likely to be swollen due to inflammation.'

Challenge a client's belief systems

Unhelpful and illogical thoughts and beliefs offered to explain problems are very common in pain patients, and obstacles to progress. Gently challenge these and begin to break them down early (but not too soon) in the consultation process. Many are examples of black and white thinking, fuelled by emotional arousal. For example: 'I am always going to be in pain' (permanentalizing); 'Anybody who has pain all the time must have something seriously wrong. If only "they" could find it, I'd be cured' (pathologizing); 'I've got this terrible pain. My life will never be the same again' (catastrophizing). Separate opinions from facts.

Separate the clinical problem from the person: 'you are not your pain'

For example: 'Jenny is concerned about a persistent pain that affects her buttock and right leg' sounds altogether different from 'Jenny has chronic pain which she complains about all of the time'. This is very powerful therapeutically and helps the person into their 'observing self' (Box 64.1) and consequently into problem-solving mode.

Watch out for and challenge nominalizations

These are abstract nouns derived from verbs and, as such, mean different things to different people. For example: the verb *to depress* is turned into the noun *depression;* the verb *to fear* is turned into the noun *fear.* The process of nominalization is vitally important for all healthcare practitioners to observe and understand since it always means that essential information is being deleted—namely, precisely who is doing precisely what to precisely who. To fill in the missing gaps in the information when a nominalization is heard, the subconscious brain seeks to identify a matching experience from the past to give meaning to these words when someone says them. They are word snares that can trap the receiver if allowed to do so. Listen to the orations of politicians and salespeople and there will be many nominalizations used as a method of influence.

The clinician needs to be on guard for the patient's nominalizations as they can make the clinician dysfunctional. This is likely to be the mechanism if the clinician is feeling somewhat gloomy and depressed after meeting with a patient. Just think of the language people use to describe their situation: 'I feel so *gloomy* and *depressed*. My life is full of *pain*. I'm *useless* and *hopeless*. I just want to be *happy* again.' It is folly for a clinician to attempt to reassure an anxious patient when it is not known *precisely* what they are anxious about. For example, *fear* is often present in patients with pain. However, what specifically are they fearful of? It might be (and there are others that can be added):

- Pain
- Not being believed
- The seriousness of the cause of the pain
- Re-injury
- Making things worse with activity
- Not being able to work
- Not being able to play with the kids
- Not being able to have kids
- Having sex
- Not playing sport
- Getting old
- Ending up in a wheelchair
- Drug addiction
- Not being compensated
- Failing again
- Relapse

Wherever possible, scale problems

A useful score for pain is on a scale of 1–10 verbally, or 0–10 on a visual analogue scale, where 10 represents the client's worst imaginable pain. Ability to function can also be scored in patients with pain and, in clinical practice, it is strongly recommended. The most useful scales for back pain sufferers are the Oswestry Disability Index and the Roland and Morris Disability Questionnaire. These scales all provide some degree of objectivity to the assessment, and response to interventions can be demonstrated. They provide very useful feedback for the client, which helps to break down black and white thinking and forces the client to be objective about their situation.

Metaphors

As already described, the subconscious brain is a pattern-matching organ. Humans naturally communicate by metaphor and storytelling; it is instinctive and a given of human nature. In the information gathering from a patient, listen out for the metaphors they use; they may give valuable clues as to what might be underlying and driving their pain state when usual treatments are not working. Remember that the patient will often have no insight whatsoever about these mind–body connections until they are gently and sensitively discussed. Once this happens, the patient will usually feel unshackled and can then begin to let go of pain and rehabilitate. The clinician does not have to solve these problems for the patient; simply bringing them into the open and acknowledging strong associated feelings is often therapeutic in itself. Here are some examples (remembering it is not simply *what* is said but *how* it is said):

- 'The pain feels like a heavy weight across my shoulders': Who or what is perceived as a burden for them?
- 'My shoulder is so stiff and painful all of the time': Is there a broken relationship (given 'the cold shoulder')?
- 'It feels like a knife is stabbing me between my shoulder blades': The term 'backstabber' is often used to describe difficult behaviour in a person who says one thing directly then does something else that undermines a person's integrity. Is the patient in this type of relationship with someone?
- 'The pain is all around my chest' (non-cardiac): Is the patient heartbroken or suffering loss or grief?
- 'It feels like my back is splitting in two': Possibly, the patient is struggling to cope with expectations and responsibilities and feeling unsupported.
- 'The pain is always in one half of my body or the other': There could be an unresolved conflict that might be contradicting a person's core values (a common psychological phenomenon called cognitive dissonance).

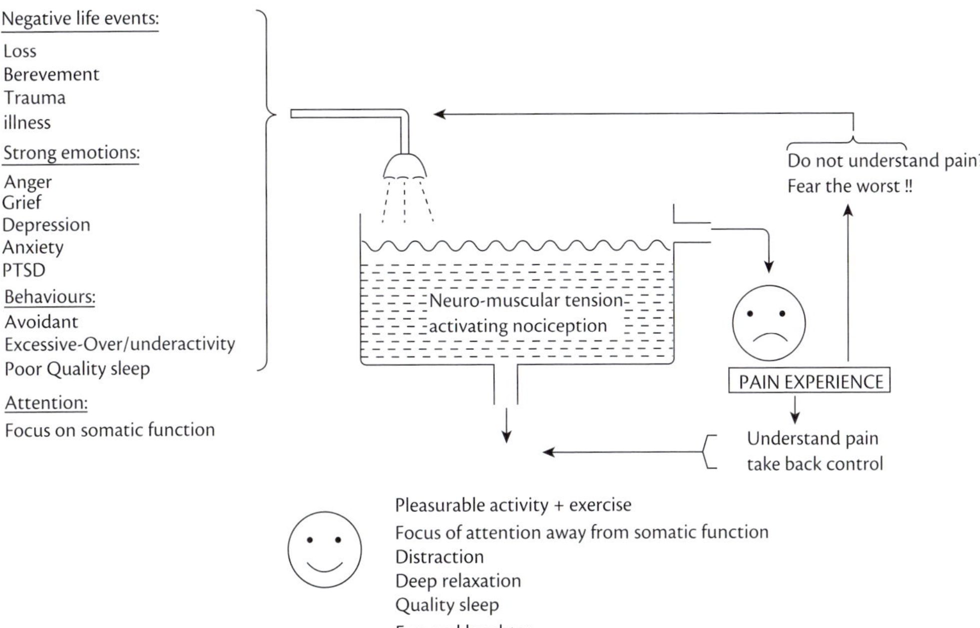

Figure 64.1 The overflowing bath-tub.

- 'It feels like my hips do not support me' (outer hip pain): On the brain's body map, the hip is the part of the body that is involved in supporting the upright posture. Could this patient be feeling very unsupported in an important part of his/her life?

Metaphors are invaluable when communicating concepts to patients that can be difficult to understand. Some examples:

- At examination, hyperalgesia or allodynia is elicited, indicating a sensitized nervous system: 'This part of your body is set to danger, red alert.'
- An episode of severe pain occurs with seemingly very little provocation: 'The water in a bath-tub (i.e. the level of neuromuscular tension in the body) has spilled over into the overflow pipe' (Figure 64.1) which brings the danger alert system to the attention of the brain. This is a very powerful visual metaphor that works well at an individual level and in groups. A useful and therapeutic discussion can develop when, with the help of the patient, the clinician lists those things that fill up the bath-tub; for example, negative life events, poor sleep, unresolved conflict or a difficult relationship with important other people, anger, fear, lack of exercise, work–life imbalance. List what helps with distraction: fun and laughter, a good night's rest, some treatments, etc. By this means, the patient can be helped to see their pain problem in the context of their life events.

Is the patient ready to engage with a process of rehabilitation and pain management?

If, on clinical evaluation, there is no objective evidence of organic pathology consistent with the presenting symptoms, then dysfunction in the tissues and sensory neural and motor system will be present to some extent or other. In the clinical encounter and for recovery to take place, a therapeutic relationship with the clinician is a prerequisite. A shared understanding of what is wrong and a treatment plan evolves, which in all cases will involve the patient making changes and contributing to their own recovery. This might be a reframing of their perception of what is wrong and behavioural changes such as exercise, returning to work, or facing up to, and problem solving, conflicts; in other words, accepting some personal responsibility for getting better. This concept is called, by psychologists, 'locus of control' (Bennett et al. 1999; Kendell et al. 2001).

It is normal for humans to be on a spectrum from external locus(someone else's responsibility) to internal locus (total personal responsibility), for different aspects of life at different times. Remember that many patients with chronic pain will have become heavily conditioned to be passive recipients of treatment based on the medical model of healthcare. It needs courage to face up to one's personal problems, especially those buried away in the subconscious and perhaps *too painful* (a metaphor the patient might use) to acknowledge, and to make lifestyle changes. Any person can feel helpless and hopeless when subjected to repeated treatments, no doubt well-intended, that do not work for the pain. While patently no person can be responsible for, nor control, everything that happens to them, believing that most things are beyond individual control is disadvantageous for health. Belief in one's own ability to influence recovery is always advantageous. *How ready is the patient to shift to taking back some responsibility for their own recovery?*

Using a guiding rather than a directing style of consultation, and with motivational interviewing skills, most people will engage. However, there can be many reasons why a patient is not ready to engage, and will rarely explicitly disclose what these are. It is up to the clinician to assess readiness, which may not become noticeable until more rapport is developed with the patient. The clinician may encounter what is called 'resistance', either consciously or subconsciously, from the patient, and this usually reflects their ambivalence about change. It is vital to identify ambivalence and reflect this back to the patient since if the clinician pushes on with action talk (with the best of intentions of course), more conscious or subconscious resistance from the patient is usually encountered.

Here are some of the more common reasons for not being ready to engage:

- The patient may have firmly held beliefs in a missed diagnosis or that some biomedical intervention will 'fix' their pain problem once and for all. They might wish to be put to sleep and wake up with everything fixed; very understandable for someone who tends to be a 'passive coper' and who has an external locus of control.
- The patient may be seeking a patho-anatomical disease diagnosis, for whatever reason, and an explanation based on dysfunction of the neuromuscular system with a focus on rehabilitation is unacceptable. The underlying reason for this conflict can sometimes be that the patient (or on occasions, the patient's partner) needs a disease-based label to self-justify a health belief or to support a claim, or intended claim, for benefits or compensation. These obstacles can be very difficult to overcome and can act as barriers to rehabilitation.
- There may be role reversals within the family unit subsequent to the pain problem. Others within the family unit will need to change too.

With excellent rapport and communication skills, the clinician may be able to elicit these conflicts and reflect back to the patient the ambivalent state that they are in.

Gauging readiness to change is a key skill when assessing persons suitable to join a functional restoration programme, and in this respect, the *readiness to change model* is useful (Figure 64.2). This model states that a person moves through each stage at a time, and can move back again. Some people move very quickly; others can be stuck at one stage, especially ambivalence, for a very long time. Remember that there are often factors outside of clinical influence (the 'black flags') that may be acting to keep a person stuck in ambivalence.

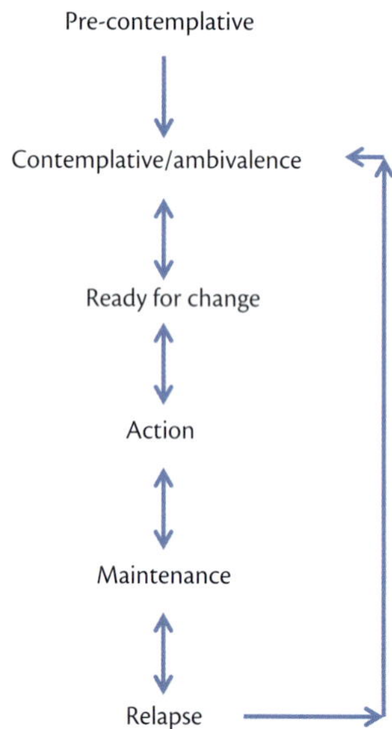

Figure 64.2 The readiness to change model.

In the experience of the author, the length of time a person has been experiencing pain problems is a relatively minor obstacle to functional restoration and managing pain. Far more significant barriers to rehabilitation are very firmly held and nurtured negative health beliefs and established social and economic constructs in the patient's life that reinforce pain-related disability (the 'black flags').

'Black flags' are socioeconomic and occupational obstacles to recovery outside of clinical influence. Some examples include:

- Settlement of a claim that depends on how much pain and pain-related disability a person is experiencing
- Application or appeals for, and the ongoing maintenance of, awards or benefits that depend on pain-related disability
- Very generous sick leave 'entitlement' when a person is feeling disaffected and unhappy at work (unhappiness at work is an individual's *perception*, hence known as a 'blue flag').

When identified, these issues need to be discussed in a solution-focused and non-judgemental manner before rehabilitation based on achieving functional goals can proceed. Sometimes, time is needed to resolve these issues before rehabilitation. Nortin Hadler (1999) summed up this whole dilemma as 'the vortex of disability determination' and 'how can a person get better when they are having to prove they are ill'.

Functional restoration and pain management programmes

For a clinician specializing in musculoskeletal medicine, brief psychotherapy and counselling skills are essential items in their toolkit of skills. The patient will be rewarded with more satisfactory outcomes using fewer interventions. For the clinician, there will be enhanced job satisfaction with reduced risk of 'burn-out'. A practitioner of musculoskeletal medicine can integrate all of the aforementioned methods as part of a treatment plan, on a one to one basis, with most patients. As with all skills, practice and an attitude of continual improvement is necessary.

There are, however, situations when a person's recovery will be better served within a small-group setting, usually called a 'functional restoration programme' (FRP). There is good evidence for their effectiveness and they are recommended in the NICE guidelines for the treatment of common low back pain in the UK (where they are called 'combined psychological and physical treatment') (NICE 2009). Time commitments vary considerably: generally, 12 hours, spread over the course of 4 weeks, and a follow-up a month later, is a minimum (Rogers et al. 2014). Others concentrate everything in 10 full days, over 2 weeks, and a follow-up day. Some centres offer FRPs and pain management programmes full-time, over 6 or more weeks.

As with all treatments, careful patient selection is key for a successful outcome. There can never be a 'one treatment fits all' approach to patients presenting with health problems as complex and multifactorial in origin as chronic pain. There are three general groups of patients who can benefit from such treatments. All will have at least one important functional goal they want to achieve and be ready to engage:

1. One group comprises those with regional pain problems who have 'failed' at least one course of one-on-one treatment and have

a strong locus of control, low fear-avoidant beliefs and behaviours, and a low tendency to boom–bust behaviour. In general, these patients will be able to get on with their lives despite their discomfort. These groups can be led by a physiotherapist or fitness instructor in a hospital gymnasium or community setting. Circuit training exercise will be the key element, with coaching to maintain motivation for a more active lifestyle beyond the programme.

2 Another group comprises those who have regional pain problems and at least one 'failed' one-on-one treatment course, fear-avoidant beliefs and behaviours, and/or boom–bust activity patterns. Disability attributable to the pain should not have been established for much more than a year or two. In general, pain will now be dominating these patients' lives. There should be an interdisciplinary team to lead these programmes, the elements of which must consist of therapeutic education on the biology of the human pain system, pacing activity, dealing with flare-ups, medication use and misuse, and maintaining progress. Relaxation skills should ideally be coached, and group sessions lend themselves favourably for this. As resources allow, an introduction to mindfulness (Burch 2008) and visualization skills are very worthwhile. The exercise regime will be based on functional exercises for activities of daily living, with an emphasis on movement rehabilitation. Individuals are coached to find their own baseline for each activity and to progress in a step by step way, working below the level that fires off their pain alarm system. These types of programmes are also ideally suited for those who are running into short- term or long-term sickness absence problems but, crucially, still have a job to return to (occupational rehabilitation).

3 A final group comprises those who have well-established pain disability and usually substantial social and vocational difficulties, who will often have been unemployed for some time because of pain problems. These persons, in addition to the aforementioned elements of the FRP, will require more input for family members, occupational therapy, and vocational rehabilitation. These programmes usually run over the course of at least 4 consecutive weeks and will require participants to be resident on site or in the vicinity. There are very few centres offering this level of service in the UK for the obvious reason of financing the treatment, the accommodation, the time commitment for the patient and family members, and the professional human resources required.

Patient's functional relationship with pain and dealing with flare-ups

It is very important for a musculoskeletal clinician to have a working knowledge of whatever point on the spectrum a patient with a pain problem is, when examined. This is just as important in the sports injury clinic and the primary care musculoskeletal clinic as in secondary care and the FRPs.

Activity relationships with pain

There are generally two activity relationships with pain:

- *The gradual decline pattern* (Figure 64.3): Pain kicks in at a certain amount of activity and the response, naturally, is to stop the activity when the pain starts. Over time, the amount of activity at which the pain is experienced slowly reduces, eventually leading to disuse, deconditioning, and, very probably, depression. This pattern is more common in people who are afraid of pain and re-injury and for people who tend to have a strong external locus of control.
- *The 'boom–bust' pattern* (Figure 64.4): Pain comes on but the person perseveres, tolerating as much as they can ('no pain no gain' might have been drummed into them long ago). They try to ignore the pain and keep going, using distraction, until, often suddenly, it is unbearable and they crash down ('bust'), usually in a crisis, flooding their system with stress chemicals. Such people will often fear the worst during these events. They struggle for several days, weeks, or even months, gradually picking themselves up in order, unwittingly of course, to start the process all over again. Such persons are often perfectionists, will often be high achievers tending to over-strive, and be (or used to be) very energetic. They are frequently encountered in the sports injury clinics. They can be very hard on themselves when they perceive that they are failing to meet their targets, and such negative self-talk floods more stress arousal chemicals into the system, thus increasing an already sensitized nervous system.

The net effect of both of these patterns is a decline into pain-related disability and loss of control.

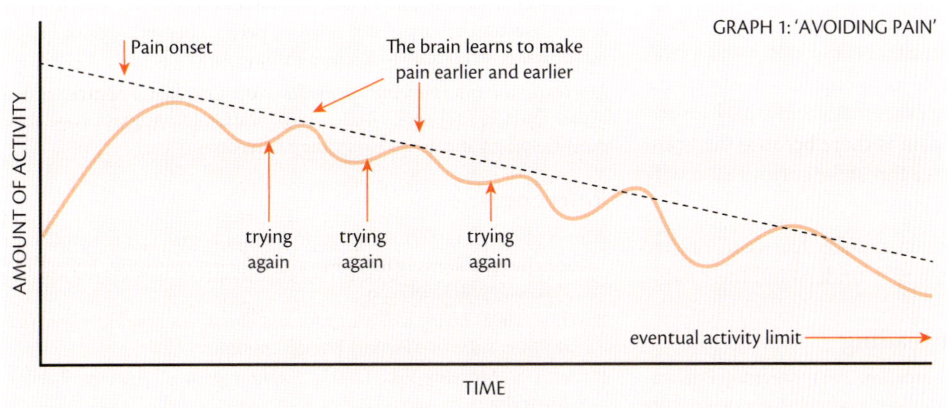

Figure 64.3 The gradual decline pattern. Pain kicks in at a certain amount of activity and the response to the pain is to stop the activity. Over time, the amount of activity at which the pain is experienced slowly reduces.
Source: Adapted from *Explain Pain* by Butler, Moseley and Sunyata.

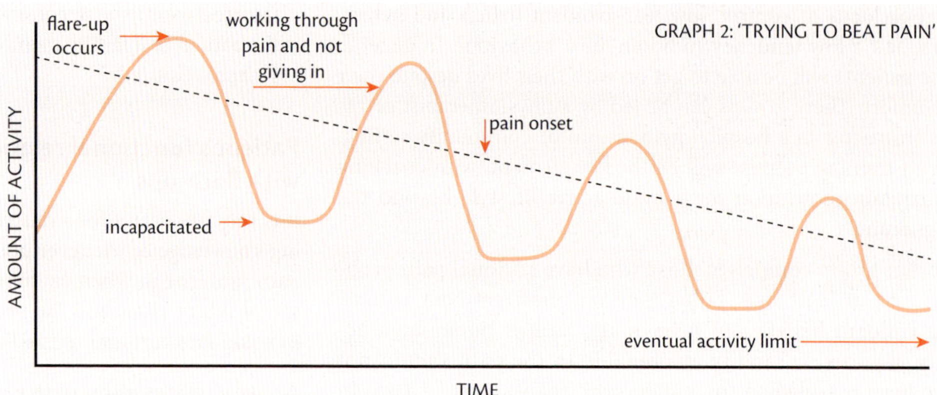

Figure 64.4 The 'boom–bust' pattern. Pain comes on but the person perseveres, trying to ignore it, until suddenly, the pain is unbearable and they crash down ('bust'), usually in a crisis, flooding their system with stress chemicals.
Source: Adapted from Explain Pain by Butler, Moseley and Sunyata

Dealing with flare-ups

Flare-ups are inevitable and to be planned for when pain has become chronic. The pain alarm system is sensitive and changes its threshold over time. Even many persons who recover from a first episode of low back pain can expect another one within a year. Clinicians must help patients to deal with these flare-ups and a five-point plan is recommended:

1 Calm down, because the pain locks attention and drives up emotional arousal making the pain experience much worse. Bring in breathing training skills at this point: 7/11 breathing (Box 64.2) is easy to teach and learn and highly effective in any situation. Practise these relaxation skills before they are needed in an emergency.

2 When calmed down, think things through by doing a body scan. Is this the usual pain (even though the intensity may of course vary)? If there are symptoms that are very unfamiliar or about which you are unsure, seek medical advice.

3 Watch the self-talk and *stop* self-defeating negative statements. Practise phrases such as 'This will come to pass' and 'I have the resources to get through this'.

4 Practise, as soon as possible (before needing them as an emergency), one or two tried and tested gentle stretching exercises to release muscle tension and joint tightness. Remember to breath out while moving into the stretch. Take analgesics if they have been helpful in the past. Modify activities but do not stop doing them completely.

5 Reflect on the event: congratulate yourself on coming through it. Learn from it: spot any triggers? These triggers can include a thought or a cue from the environment and not just a physical event (for example, the thought of going into a workplace associated with unhappiness or the exacerbation of a pain on approaching a clinical setting). The pain is there because the brain is responding to what it perceives as a threat: be curious as to why the brain is doing this.

By repeating this sequence, a person quickly learns to master their pain. They can only do this when they understand their pain.

Box 64.2 7/11 relaxation breathing technique

Count to 7 on the in breath and count to 11 on the out breath, doing this for 3–10 minutes. Focus all of the attention on the breathing. If 7/11 is too long, count 5/8. The parasympathetic nervous system is stimulated. When put into practice, diaphragm breathing usually follows naturally. 7/11 is easier to learn and remember and easier to use in an emergency than deep breathing or diaphragm breathing alone. In an emergency situation, many people who have been told to do 'deep breathing' actually make matters worse for themselves (until this is pointed out to them) by speeding up their breathing and, in effect, hyperventilating. This floods their already sensitized nervous system with stress chemicals and hormones.

Recommendations for further reading

Explain pain (David Butler and Lorimer Moseley, 2003, Noigroup Publications, Adelaide) An outstanding book written in plain English and beautifully illustrated. A must read for clinicians: it will change how you work with patients in pain.

The science of suffering (Patrick Wall, 1999. Weidenfield & Nicholson, London) Dated now, but this book remains a classic.

How to liberate yourself from pain: a practical help for sufferers (Grahame Brown and Denise Winn, 2009, HG Publishing, London) One of a series of practical guides based on the 'Human Givens' organizing ideas. Very useful to recommend to patients who you are working with.

Coping successfully with pain (Neville Shone, 1995, Sheldon Press, London) One man's guide to confronting and overcoming chronic pain.

Hypnotise yourself out of pain now! (Bruce N. Elmer, 2nd edition, 2008, Crown House Publishing, Carmarthen) An excellent self-help guide to a cognitive behavioural and self-hypnosis method to control pain.

Living well with pain and illness: the mindful way to free yourself from suffering (Vidyamala Burch, 2008, Piatkus Books, London) A guide to the use of mindfulness techniques to manage chronic pain.

Motivational interviewing in health care (Stephen Rollnick, William R. Miller, and Christopher C. Butler, 2008, The Guildford Press, New York/London) Helping patients to change their behaviour.

References

Bennett P, et al. (1999) Affective and social-cognitive predictors of behavior change following first myocardial infarction. *British Journal of Health Psychology*, 4(3):247–56.

Burch V. (2008) *Living well with pain and illness. The mindful way to free yourself from suffering*. Piatkus Books: London.

Butler DS, Moseley GL. (2003) *Explain pain*. Noigroup Publications: Australia.

Doubell TP, Mannion RJ, Woolf CJ. (1999) The dorsal horn: state dependent sensory processing, plasticity and the generation of pain. In: Melzack R, Wall PD (eds). *Textbook of pain*. Churchill Livingstone: Edinburgh.

Flor H, et al. (1997) Extensive reorganisation of somatosensory cortex in chronic back pain patients. *Neuroscience Letters* 244:5–8.

Griffin J, Tyrrell I. (2013) Human givens: the new approach to emotional health and clear thinking (2nd edn). HG Publishing: London.

Gunn CC. (1997) Radiculopathic pain: diagnosis and treatment of segmental irritation or sensitization. *Journal of Musculoskeletal Pain*, 5(4):119–34.

Hadler NM. (1999) Occupational musculoskeletal disorders (2nd edn). Lippincott, Williams & Wilkins: Philadelphia.

Hill JC, Dunn KM, Lewis M, et al. (2008) A primary care screening tool identifying patient subgroups for initial treatment. *Arthritis & Rheumatism* 59:1–10.

Kendell K, et al. (2001) Psychological factors associated with short term recovery from total knee replacement. *British Journal of Health Psychology*, 6(1):41–52.

Linton SJ. (2000) A review of psychological risk factors in back and neck pain. *Spine* 25:1148–56.

Melzack R. (1975) The McGill Pain Questionnaire: major properties and methods. *Pain*, 1:277–99.

Melzack R, Wall PD. (1996) *The challenge of pain* (2nd edn). Penguin: London.

NICE (2005) *NICE guideline CG26 (post-traumatic stress disorder)*. NICE: London. Available at: <https://www.nice.org.uk/guidance/cg26/chapter/guidance>.

NICE (2009) *NICE guideline CG88 (low back pain)*. NICE: London. Available at: <https://www.nice.org.uk/guidance/cg88>.

Rogers D, Gardner A, MacLean S, Brown G, Darling A. (2014) *A retrospective analysis of a functional restoration programme for patients with persistent low back pain*. Available in the Wiley Online Library (<http://www.wileyonlinelibrary.com>). DOI: 10.1002/msc.1078.

Waddell G, Burton AK. (2004) Concepts of rehabilitation for common health problems. The Stationery Office: Norwich.

Chapter 65

An integrated approach to musculoskeletal medicine

Adam Ward and Michael Hutson

Introduction: an integrated approach to musculoskeletal medicine

Those readers of this textbook who have diligently studied a substantive number of chapters will understand that the intention of the editors is to have produced an eclectic mix of opinion. The intention throughout has been to allow experienced practitioners to impart their views with the guarantee that although authors of chapters may hold challenging beliefs, this constitutes a healthy situation for our medical specialty. We take the view that we have promoted an integrated approach to medical practice. However, what is meant by an integrated approach?

> 'When *I* use a word,' Humpty Dumpty said, in rather a scornful tone, 'it means just what I choose it to mean— neither more nor less.'
>
> Chapter VI, *Through the looking glass* (Lewis Carroll, 1872)

Words are important not only as a function of description but also as an indicator of the evolutionary and contextual development of ideas. They even affect the way that both we and our patients think.

The words 'integrated' and 'integrative' go back, like so many English words, to the Latin: (*integer*—untouched or undiminished, a whole). Etymology dates the first English use of the word to around 1450, to describe something intact and unblemished. Over 600 years later, in the 1990s, it was used in a medical context by physicians in the USA interested in integrating complementary and alternative approaches such as acupuncture, hypnotherapy, and massage into general medical practice. Out of that came the now commonly used acronym CAM (complementary and alternative medicine).

Since then, however, the use of the words 'integrative' or 'integrated' has cascaded into all areas of healthcare, involving not just the choice of therapies but also 'whole patient' care and health service structures. This is certainly not merely a recent concept. Hippocrates (460—377BC) embraced a holistic approach towards sick patients ('treatment of the whole person'), in which lifestyle and personal characteristics were deemed important, whereas modern medicine has tended to concentrate more on the characteristics of illness itself. Have the beliefs of compassionate doctors and therapists changed so much since then?

The views of H.R.H. the Prince of Wales (2012), in which he extols the virtues of an approach that incorporates 'the best of' technological advances, current understanding of the nature of ill health, and 'ancient wisdom' (perhaps 'empiricism' and 'acquired wisdom' would be more appropriate concepts), have identified and highlighted the humanistic aspect of musculoskeletal medicine, as advanced in many of the chapters of this textbook.

These underpinning concepts and associated management strategies are not only of direct relevance to musculoskeletal medicine; it has been argued in this textbook that a post-modern approach, in which patients' views are respected and incorporated into healthcare approaches, is at the heart of this medical specialty.

Integrated care can be usefully grouped into three broad categories: firstly, the provision of healthcare service structures; secondly, the integration of different therapies and medical disciplines; and thirdly, patient-centred 'whole person' care.

Integration of healthcare services in musculoskeletal medicine

A leading article in the *British Medical Journal* (2014), discussing the recently published 'Independent Commission on Whole Person Care', which was commissioned by the UK Labour Party, draws attention to the fact that fewer than 4% of people who live with long-term conditions currently have a care plan. It goes on to state that an understanding of how diverse organizations can be successfully integrated is only just emerging.

According to the Arthritis and Musculoskeletal Alliance, expenditure in the UK on musculoskeletal conditions accounts for the fourth highest area of National Health Service (NHS) programme budget spend and, in 2009–10, amounted to £4.76 billion. In the relatively affluent countries internationally, it is recognized that musculoskeletal disorders, particularly back pain, are the commonest cause of disability, creating an enormous financial burden on healthcare systems. Accordingly, it would be reasonable to assume that a policy of systematic integration of available healthcare, to include services that have a known impact on musculoskeletal health (for instance, the provision of tailored exercise and weight-loss plans, when appropriate), would prevail. However, it is doubtful if scientific advice regarding fitness has been implemented to an effective level in the European communities or elsewhere.

When 'integration' is viewed as an overarching concept, musculoskeletal medicine has, by dint of necessity, traditionally linked a range of different services in order to provide diagnosis, treatment, rehabilitation, and lifestyle management. These include hospital- and community-based treatments, combining different professional input from physicians, surgeons, nurse therapists, physiotherapists, occupational therapists, nutritionists, exercise and motivational therapists, and psychologists. All are linked in with community and social service support networks. The specific, and vastly important, responsibility of the general practitioner (family doctor), who continues to exercise the medical gatekeeper role on behalf of patients with musculoskeletal (and allied complaints) in the UK, is described by numerous authors in this textbook (see Chapters 4, 5, and 6). There is little argument that this role provides not only a triaging capability but also an opportunity for a fully integrated approach to diagnosis and treatment of somatic symptoms, based on the knowledge of psycho-socio-cultural factors specific to the patient. The benefit of early referral for physiotherapy triage is identified in Chapter 48.

An integrated approach to treatment/ management in musculoskeletal medicine

Integration of therapies

The current level of knowledge of musculoskeletal conditions is identified by many authors in this book. While acknowledging that 'truths' (including scientific truths) are contemporary, contextual, and often ethno-cultural, the importance of meaningful inter-observer understanding of the reproducibility of diagnostic techniques (see Chapter 3) and the profound difficulties associated with bias in the search for evidence through randomized controlled trials is stressed in the text where appropriate. Integration of therapies is generally understood within the context of chronic pain, though the benefits of a multidisciplinary approach are not always appreciated outside of primary care.

Clinical musculoskeletal practice demands significant degrees of tactile feedback for both diagnosis and treatment, in addition to empathy (comprising structured compassion) and holism. There should always be a place for discussion with the patient about complementary and alternative treatments when circumstances suggest its relevance.

Concerns surrounding mechanistic approaches

The technological revolution within the developed world has been an extraordinary feature of recent decades. The developments within musculoskeletal medicine—diagnostic, therapeutic, and pedagogical—have escalated in recent years and have led to significant benefits in specific situations. However, too much reliance on technology can cause concern. The introduction of guided injections, for example, should be reviewed on the basis of its advantages, when they exist, with respect to outcome and safety. The use of interventional medical techniques and how they are delivered remains an area of continuing debate (see, for example, Chapters 25, 51, 52, 53, and 57).

There are multiple research papers in the medical literature concerning evidence to support the use of guided invasive procedures. There are also numerous studies that conclude that reliance on guided injections is not always necessary. Longitudinal studies need to clearly demonstrate patient benefit from concurrent imaging over the long term and not just evidence that, for example, the placement of injections is more precise. A key question is whether guided injections, irrespective of their greater potential for accuracy, produce significantly different outcomes, both in terms of safety and efficacy (Hutson 2013). This is in addition to the continuing debate about the safety and efficacy of the injections themselves. The classic study of accurate (ultrasound-guided) steroid injections for shoulder pain, which showed no difference in long-term benefit compared to landmark-guided placement and also simple intra-muscular injection (Bloom et al. 2012), should lead to reflection. Jones et al. (1993) demonstrated that in a group of rheumatologists of mixed seniority (consultant, senior registrars, and research registrars), intra-articular injections were often inaccurate. Hany Elmadbouh (Chapter 25) writes: 'Until we have good evidence that image-guided injections in routine therapeutic practice are both more clinically effective and cost-effective, it seems reasonable to conclude that most peripheral injections can be given using an anatomical landmark approach.'

Advice against the unnecessary use of surgery is contained in an analysis of the most recent, high-quality systematic reviews comparing surgery with conservative treatments for the treatment of patients with chronic low back disorders. In a list of key points, it states that spinal surgery should not be offered as a first-line treatment for non-specific low back pain, as insufficient evidence exists for greater effectiveness of surgical interventions over conservative treatment (Peul et al. 2014).

However, making a diagnosis of non-specific low back pain is not always straightforward and symptoms may mask causes which require specific interventions. 'Red flags' are a well-established aid to identifying the possibility of more serious causes of back pain, some of which, such as cauda equina syndrome, may require urgent surgery. An editorial in the *British Medical Journal* on the use of red flags for back pain carried the subheading 'A popular idea that didn't work and should be removed from guidelines' (Underwood and Buchbinder 2013). In the same edition of the journal, a survey of 14 studies which evaluated a total of 53 red flags revealed significant disparities and poor levels of predictability (Downie et al. 2013). Nevertheless, red flags continue to be used throughout the world and referral of patients is often still based upon the presence or absence of red flags.

This further confirms the importance of integrating all aspects of back pain management. It is important to identify those cases that will benefit from specific invasive treatments but it is also essential to protect the majority of back pain sufferers, who do not require such interventions, from unnecessary and possibly harmful investigations and procedures. It can be difficult always to do this with accuracy and more work is needed to refine our processes.

Manual diagnostic and palpatory techniques and skills underpin musculoskeletal practice and should not be replaced, but used in conjunction with other diagnostic aids. At an international conference some years ago, Professor Karel Lewit, founder of the Prague School of Manual Medicine and Rehabilitation, stated:

> The examination and assessment of dysfunction of the motor system, by far the most frequent cause of so-called non-specific pain, cannot yet be done by apparatus, but only those most sophisticated instruments, the human hands and eyes and a little thought.

This sentiment is expressed in many of the chapters in this textbook by authors from diverse backgrounds and disciplines.

Placebo effect

Musculoskeletal medical practice is predominantly concerned with pain and dysfunction and with patients who are in pain and worried about their mobility and ability to lead a normal life. In such cases, knowledge of the possibility of the effects of a placebo is particularly important both for good and ill (nocebo). A placebo (or 'contextual') effect, which is common in clinical practice, can be described as a clinical interaction between the clinician and patient but not due to the intrinsic powers of a substance administered or specifically to the therapeutic procedure.

Cohen (Chapter 21) eloquently describes the interaction or 'integration' of non-placebo and placebo effects within the healing process and the need for recognition by clinicians of contextual factors in their management strategies. A direct quote from Cohen is relevant here:

> Every interaction with medical or other therapeutic professionals plays a role in determining the contextual (placebo) component of a person's future response to treatment. Factors include aspects of a doctor or therapist's behaviour such as friendliness; consideration of a patient's concerns; provision of time; clear explanations of diagnosis, prognosis, and treatment; enthusiasm for treatment; and the choice of words, gestures, or other non-verbal forms of communication.

Reference is made, in a number of chapters in this textbook, to the needle effect as exemplified in acupuncture and dry needling, where no physical agent is injected. The possible modes of action have stimulated much debate. A thoughtful review by Campbell (Chapter 59) provides a balanced assessment of the background to the use of acupuncture/dry needling, the reading of which is highly recommended in view of its extensive use for musculoskeletal pain.

Recent advances

While recognizing the importance of manual diagnostics, modern diagnostic aids can lead to potentially important advances in musculoskeletal practice; a pertinent example being MAST (Modic antibiotic spinal treatment) which offers a new approach in the treatment of a subgroup of patients with chronic low back pain and degenerative disc disease. The idea that an infection of the intervertebral disc might be a factor in the degenerative change seen in back pain is not new. However, with the introduction of magnetic resonance imaging (MRI), it became possible to categorize spinal changes seen on MRI scans based upon an interpretation of vertebral end-plate changes. These were first described by Dr Michael Modic and colleagues in 1988 (Modic et al. 1988a,b) and are generally referred to as Modic changes.

Over the following years, the clinical relevance of Modic changes seen on MRI have been a subject of much debate. The Research Department of the Spine Centre of Southern Denmark, University of Southern Denmark, Odense, led by Hanne B. Albert, has pursued the hypothesis that Modic MRI changes might be used in the identification of patients with chronic back pain who have possible chronic infection affecting the intervertebral discs and their adjacent vertebrae (Albert and Manniche 2007; Albert et al. 2008).

Papers published by Albert and her research group (Albert et al. 2013a,b) suggest that long-term oral antibiotics over a course of 100 days could lead to significant improvement. Nevertheless, diagnosis still requires a thorough clinical history and examination by an experienced practitioner, and the treatment is not without hazard. A thoughtful editorial by Max Aebi in the same edition of the *European Spine Journal* stresses the need for further research.

In an attempt to create a balance here with respect to prevailing views within the musculoskeletal community on back pain, it is worth recollecting the statement of Professor A.L. Cochrane, 35 years ago: 'The most fundamental problem is uncertainty about the nature of back pain, of how the complaint arises, and of the significance of various attributes that may be associated with it' (Cochrane, AL, 1979).

Multidisciplinary integration

Care programmes in which educationalists, psychologists, physiotherapists, exercise therapists, nutritionists, social and community workers, and others work together with medical specialists are the aim.

Integrative personal care in musculoskeletal medicine

The notion of integrated care also applies to 'holistic' or 'whole person' care, with emphasis upon the 'biopsychosocial'. Interestingly, the constitution of the World Health Organization, which came into force on 7 April 1948, presaged these ideas in its definition of health as being a state of 'complete physical, mental and social well-being and not merely the absence of disease or infirmity'. We are very aware of the implications to health of social deprivation, and suggest that Chapter 5 on the social determinants of pain is essential reading.

The concept of 'whole person' health benefits, with particular reference to the interaction between a relevant amount of physical exercise and the musculoskeletal system in patients from all backgrounds, is stressed by a number of authors.

An integrated approach to musculoskeletal medicine: summary

Musculoskeletal medicine is one of the most exciting of the developing medical specialties. Not only does it take in the technological medical advances of twenty-first-century medicine but it also recognizes the importance of the overall health of autonomous, individual patients through its integrative approaches to care which have always been at the heart of its development. Musculoskeletal patients form the largest single group of all those presenting with chronic pain in both primary and secondary care, and musculoskeletal dysfunction increasingly affects the mobility and quality of life of a population blessed with increasing longevity. We are entrusted with the healthcare of patients with musculoskeletal problems at a time when the need for the full integration of musculoskeletal medicine has never been more necessary.

References

Albert HB,Manniche C. (2007) Modic changes following lumbar disc herniation. *Eur Spine J*; 16(7):977–82.

Albert HB, Kjaer P, Jensen TS, Sorensen JS, Bendix T,Manniche C. (2008) Modic changes, possible causes and relation to low back pain. *Med Hypotheses*; 70(2):361–8.

Albert HB, Lambert P, Rollason J, et al. (2013a) Does nuclear tissue infected with bacteria following disc herniations lead to Modic changes in the adjacent vertebrae? *Eur Spine J*; 22(4):690–6. (See more at: <http://www.arthritisresearchuk.org/health-professionals-and-students/reports/synovium/synovium-summer-2013/antibiotics-low-back-pain.aspx#sthash.JJ0wur2t.dpuf>.)

Albert HB, Sorenson JS, Christensen BS, Manniche C. (2013b) Antibiotic treatment in patients with chronic low back pain and vertebral bone edema (Modic type 1 changes): a double-blind randomized clinical controlled trial of efficacy. *Eur Spine J*; 22(4):697–707. (See more at: <http://www.arthritisresearchuk.org/health-professionals-and-students/reports/synovium/synovium-summer-2013/antibiotics-low-back-pain.aspx#sthash.JJ0wur2t.dpuf>.)

Arthritis and Musculoskeletal Alliance (ARMA) (2010) Liberating the NHS: transparency in outcomes-a framework for the NHS, ARMA consultation response, London, www.arma.uk.net/pdfs

Cochrane AL (1979) Report to the Secretary of State for Social Services of a working group on back pain, London, HMSO

Downie A, Williams CM, Henschke N, Hancock MJ, et al. (2013) Red flags to screen for malignancy and fracture in patients with low back pain: systematic review. *BMJ*; 347:f7095.

H.R.H. the Prince of Wales (2012) Integrated health and postmodern medicine. *J R Soc Med*; 105:496–8.

Bloom, JE, Rischin A, Johnston RV, Buchbinder R. (2012) *Cochrane Rev*; 8. Available at: <http://www.thecochranelibrary.com>.

Jones A, Regan M, Ledingham J, Pattrick M, et al. (1993) Importance of placement of intra-articular steroid injections. *BMJ*; 307:1329–30.

Hutson MA. (2013) Ultrasound-guided soft tissue injections: safety and effectiveness. *Int Musc Med*; 35 (2):49–51.

Independent Commission on Whole Person Care for the Labour Party (2014) BMJ, 348:g2136

Modic MT, Steinberg PM, Ross JS, et al. (1988a) Degenerative disk disease: assessment of changes in vertebral body marrow with MR imaging. *Radiology*; 166(1):193–9.

Modic MT, Masaryk TJ, Ross JS, Carter JR. (1988b) Imaging of degenerative disk disease. *Radiology*; 168:177–86.

Underwood M, Buchbinder R. (2013) Red flags for back pain—a popular idea that didn't work and should be removed from guidelines. *BMJ*; 347:f7432.

Peul WC, Bredenoord AL, Jacobs WCH. (2014) Avoid surgery as first-line treatment for non-specific low back pain. *BMJ*; 349:g4214.

Index